Medical Microbiology

An Introduction to
Infectious Diseases

Second Edition

Editor

John C. Sherris, MD, FRCPath
Professor Emeritus, Department of Microbiology
School of Medicine
University of Washington
Seattle, Washington

James J. Champoux, PhD
Professor, Department of Microbiology
School of Medicine
University of Washington
Seattle, Washington

Lawrence Corey, MD
Professor and Head, Clinical Virology Division
Departments of Laboratory Medicine and Microbiology
School of Medicine
University of Washington
Seattle, Washington

Frederick C. Neidhardt, PhD
Frederick G. Novy Distinguished
University Professor
Department of Microbiology and Immunology
University of Michigan
Ann Arbor, Michigan

James J. Plorde, MD
Professor, Departments of Laboratory Medicine and Medicine
School of Medicine
University of Washington
Chief, Microbiology Section, Laboratory Services
Veterans Administration Medical Center
Seattle, Washington

C. George Ray, MD
Professor, Departments of Pathology and Pediatrics
Chief, Virology and Immunoserology Sections
College of Medicine
University of Arizona
Tucson, Arizona

Kenneth J. Ryan, MD
Professor, Departments of Pathology and Microbiology
Chief, Clinical Microbiology Section
College of Medicine
University of Arizona
Tucson, Arizona

Chapter 62.
Dental and Periodontal Infections, contributed by
Murray R. Robinovitch, DDS, PhD
Professor and Chairman, Department of Oral Biology
School of Dentistry
University of Washington
Seattle, Washington

Medical Microbiology

An Introduction to Infectious Diseases

Second Edition

Editor

John C. Sherris

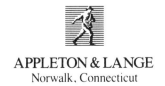

APPLETON & LANGE
Norwalk, Connecticut

Copyright © 1990 by Appleton & Lange
Simon & Schuster Business and Professional Group

93 94 95 96 97 / 10 9 8 7 6 5 4 3 2 1

Prentice Hall International (UK) Limited, *London*
Prentice Hall of Australia Pty. Limited, *Sydney*
Prentice Hall Canada, Inc., *Toronto*
Prentice Hall Hispanoamericana, S.A., *Mexico*
Prentice Hall of India Private Limited, *New Delhi*
Prentice Hall of Japan, Inc., *Tokyo*
Simon & Schuster Asia Pte. Ltd., *Singapore*
Editora Prentice Hall do Brasil Ltda., *Rio de Janeiro*
Prentice Hall, *Englewood Cliffs, New Jersey*

ISBN 0-8385-6210-8

Library of Congress Catalog Card Number: 92-055058

PRINTED IN THE UNITED STATES OF AMERICA

To our families, colleagues, and students,
for their support,
and to the late John D. Lawrence
whose encouragement led to
the first edition of the book

Contents

Preface

This second edition of *Medical Microbiology: An Introduction to Infectious Diseases* has been modified considerably in the light of new developments in the field and feedback from students and instructors who used the first edition. The major changes have included a substantial increase in the depth of coverage of basic microbiology in a manner that we believe will facilitate understanding of the more applied aspects of the discipline and which reflects recent advances in knowledge. We have added a chapter giving an introduction to the specific immune response, because we found that a number of students using the book had not been exposed to immunology and had difficulty in understanding discussions of immune mechanisms in other parts of the book: This chapter in no sense replaces the need for more detailed study of immunology. We have also included new chapters on retroviruses, DNA tumor viruses, and the acquired immunodeficiency syndrome because of the increasing importance and significance of these topics.

We have retained the general format of the book and have kept the number of contributors small to help achieve continuity and balance. The marginal notes have been modified and expanded to highlight key points and facilitate review of the material, and we have also substantially increased the Glossary. Tables and appendices have again been used to illustrate the greater depth of the subject rather than material to be learned. We have added two appendices at the end of the book. One summarizes the characteristics of some organisms and diseases that are rarely seen in Western countries and are not included in the text. The second is an historical table that notes many of those who have made major contributions to the field of medical microbiology. We have retained both the overview chapter (Chapter 1) to help the student see how the different sections of the book interrelate and the syndromic chapters (Chapters 59–73) so that information on specific organisms and diseases may be reviewed in the context in which they may be encountered. Selected monographs, reviews, and papers that we consider to be especially helpful have been cited at the end of most of the microbiological chapters for students who wish to pursue the topics in more depth. Comprehensive bibliographies are beyond the scope of the book, and we consider that further readings to illustrate the processes of scientific thought and advance are best selected by course instructors who will also be indicating the degree of emphasis to be placed on the different topics covered.

We are very cognizant of the difficulties faced by students of medicine and the other health sciences as a result of the explosion in knowledge and the conflicting academic demands on their time and attention. We have thus tried to develop the subject in a form that is easy to read, to which it is easy to refer, and that clearly stresses the major principles and facts on which future studies of infectious diseases will be based. We will have succeeded if we have helped catch the student's interest and enthusiasm for the study of microbiology and its application to infectious diseases.

John C. Sherris
Editor

Acknowledgments

The authors wish to thank Drs. Bruce Gilliland, Neal Groman, William Kirby, Stephen Lory, Sheila Lukehart, Raymond Nagle, and Peter Rabinovitch for reviewing some individual chapters of this edition and for their helpful suggestions. The final results are, of course, the sole responsibility of the authors. We also wish to thank the many friends and colleagues who reviewed chapters for the first edition.

The mycology and parasitology drawings and marginal illustrations for the first edition were the work of Sam C. Eng, Clinical Technologist of the Clinical Laboratories of the University Hospital, University of Washington. The great majority of the other illustrations were prepared by Marilyn Pollack-Senuta. Their expertise and friendly cooperation are gratefully acknowledged.

We also wish to indicate our appreciation of the staff members of Elsevier who took over a complicated assignment in bringing the book to publication and did so with skill, patience, and good humor.

Finally, we wish to acknowledge with gratitude and affection the work of Elizabeth Sherris. She typed most of the new chapters, transposed the innumerable modifications for this edition, and was an unfailing source of help and encouragement to the editor.

Medical Microbiology

An Introduction to Infectious Diseases

Second Edition

1
Overview

John C. Sherris

The science of microbiology as it applies to medicine dates back to the pioneering studies of Pasteur and Koch and is, thus, only a little over a century old. The period between about 1875 and 1910 can be regarded as the first golden age of medical microbiology and was one of extraordinary advance. Many bacterial diseases were defined, and the organisms responsible for them were seen microscopically. Techniques, some still of great importance today, were developed for growing bacteria and studying their phenotypic characteristics. The existence of antibodies and complement as mediators of immune responses to infection were recognized, and the first steps taken to extend the principles of vaccination for smallpox described by Jenner in 1796 to other infectious diseases. Some diseases were shown to be caused by more complex organisms and others by filterable agents (viruses) that could not be grown in culture but that caused disease in experimental animals and elicited immune responses. As a result of these developments, the aura of mysticism and helplessness that surrounded infectious diseases was dispelled, their epidemiology was clarified, and avenues for control were opened. The period from 1910 to 1944 can be regarded as one of extension and consolidation of the earlier discoveries. Many new pathogenic organisms were described, and there were great advances in public health and the epidemiological control of infectious diseases. The discoveries of penicillin by Fleming in 1929 and sulfonamides by Domagk in 1935 opened the way to the great developments in chemotherapy that were to come. Contemporaneously, there were great advances in the fields of general, environmental, and industrial microbiology.

During the past 40 years or so, there has been a quantum leap in understanding of the biology and genetics of microbes, the processes by which pathogens cause disease, and the elegant complexities of the defense mechanisms of the host. Electron microscopy clarified the ultrastructure of bacteria, fungi, and protozoa and has demonstrated the shape and structure of viral particles. The science of molecular biology, which developed from studies on bacteria, has led to an understanding of microbial genetics and of the processes by which bacteria control protein synthesis, maintain their identity, and adapt to different environments. The chemical nature of some viruses has been almost completely defined, and the complex interactions between them and their host cell have been elucidated. Details of the precise mechanisms by which microorganisms cause disease are being increasingly uncovered. Numerous antimicrobial agents, some tailored to particular needs and targets, have been developed and provide the clinician with powerful weapons to control infections.

A major effect of the knowledge and understanding gained during this second golden age of microbiology (which is continuing) is that phenomena that were learned simply as facts in the past can now be explained. Much of the material in the first chapters of this book are devoted to these concepts and fundamental processes because they have application to the topics considered subsequently. All the advances in the past century have derived from basic and applied research, and the end result has been control of many of the infectious scourges that have afflicted our species, and a level of understanding that opens the way to controlling those that remain. Some of the most significant discoveries and those who made them are listed in the historical appendix at the end of the book.

Entry into microbial world

At birth, the normal infant, previously protected from the environment by the mother's placenta and immune system, enters an enormously complex microbial world that has evolved over the past 3.5 billion years. Some inhabitants of this ecosystem have adapted to colonize the external, alimentary, upper respiratory, and vaginal surfaces of humans (and other creatures) in vast numbers—generally to their mutual benefit. A few have the capacity to cause disease by invading the tissues, producing toxic substances, or both. Most, however, are free living and nonparasitic to other organisms, and many play a central part in shaping the environment of our planet. Without these microbes other life forms as we know them could not exist.

Roles of microorganisms in nature

Microorganisms, which are by definition invisible to the unaided eye, are responsible for much of the breakdown and natural recycling of organic material in the environment. Some can fix atmospheric nitrogen and synthesize nitrogen-containing inorganic and organic compounds that contribute to the nutrition of living things that lack this ability. Some can use atmospheric carbon dioxide as a source of carbon for organic compounds; others (the oceanic algae) produce oxygen through their use of atmospheric CO_2 for photosynthesis. Thus, microorganisms play central roles in the nitrogen and carbon cycles and contribute to maintaining the atmospheric oxygen level.

Microbial diversity

Very few areas on the surface of the planet do not support microbial life, because microorganisms have an astounding range of metabolic and energy-yielding abilities, and many can exist under conditions that are lethal to other life forms. For example, some bacteria can oxidize inorganic compounds such as sulfur or ammonium ions to generate energy, and some can survive and multiply in hot springs at temperatures over 75°C. Many microorganisms can only metabolize fermentatively, using substances other than oxygen as terminal electron acceptors and can thus multiply under highly reduced conditions. Some of these are cellulolytic and can multiply rapidly in masses of decaying vegetation in the absence of oxygen. To many, oxygen is rapidly lethal.

Symbiosis

Some microbial species have adapted to a symbiotic relationship with higher forms of life. For example, bacteria that can fix atmospheric nitrogen colonize root systems of legumes and of a few trees such as alders and provide the plant with its nitrogen requirements. When the plant dies or is plowed under, the fertility of the soil is enhanced by nitrogenous compounds originally derived from the metabolism of the bacteria. Ruminants can use grasses as their prime source of nutrition, because the abundant flora of anaerobic bacteria in the rumen breaks down cellulose and other plant-compounds to usable carbohydrates and amino acids and synthesizes essential nutrients including some amino acids and vitamins. These few examples illustrate the protean nature of microbial life and their essential place in our ecosystem.

Human exploitation of the microbial world

The metabolic heterogeneity and diverse synthetic abilities of microorganisms have led to their application to human purposes. These uses include alcoholic fermentation in the production of wines, beers, and spirits; composting techniques; and the mass production of complex organic compounds such as vitamin B_{12} and various antibiotics or their precursors. In many cases, because microorganisms multiply rapidly and have a relatively simple genome, mutants that improve quality and yield have been readily selected in the laboratory. More recently, through the use of recombinant DNA techniques, genes encoding the synthesis of complex biologically active substances, such as human growth hormone and some immunologic mediators have been added to the genetic makeup of bacteria or yeasts, which then synthesize the desired product in culture. Because of this relatively simple and manipulable genetic structure, molecular biological studies on bacteria continue to help illuminate the complexities of cellular regulation and differentiation in higher life forms.

Classes of microorganisms that interact with humans

It is because these organisms are essential to the existence of life on our planet that the study of general microbiology and of the role of microorganisms in nature is of such great interest and importance. This book, however, has a narrower anthropocentric focus and is concerned with those microorganisms directly involved in the maintenance of health or causation of disease in humans. Within this context, we will consider the four broad classes of microorganisms that interact with humans: bacteria, fungi, viruses, and protozoa. We have extended the definition of microbiology to include some disease-producing multicellular parasites—the helminths and flukes—that are macroscopic at some stages of their life cycles; indeed, intestinal tapeworms can measure many feet in length and become discomfortingly obvious.

Fungi and protozoa

Among the microorganisms that infect or coexist with humans, the fungi and protozoa have many of the cellular characteristics found in mammalian or plant cells: nuclear membranes, several chromosomes, mitotic apparatus, mitochondria, sterol-containing cell membranes, and, in many cases, the ability to reproduce sexually. These microorganisms are termed *eukaryotes* because of their "true" nuclear structure. Their size is quite variable; although width or diameter rarely exceeds 10 μm (0.01 mm), length may be much greater. Most fungi and some protozoa can be grown in culture on artificial media.

Bacteria

The bacteria are generally smaller, simpler, and probably more primitive than the fungi and protozoa. Their nuclear material comprises a single, double-stranded, but very large DNA molecule without a structural nuclear membrane. They are thus described as *prokaryotic;* they are haploid with no true sexual mode of reproduction. Many possess autonomous self-replicating smaller circular DNA molecules, termed *plasmids,* which are transmissible between bacteria and often encode properties that facilitate

Table 1.1 Distinctive Features of Prokaryotic and Eukaryotic Cells

Cell Component	Prokaryotes	Eukaryotes
Nucleus	No membrane, single circular chromosome	Membrane bounded, a number of individual chromosomes
Extrachromosomal DNA	Often present in form of plasmid(s)	In organelles
Organelles in cytoplasm	None	Mitochondria (and chloroplasts in photosynthetic organisms)
Cytoplasmic membrane	Contains enzymes of respiration. Active secretion of enzymes. Site of phospholipid and DNA synthesis	Semipermeable layer not possessing functions of prokaryotic membrane
Cell wall	Rigid layer of peptidoglycan (absent in *Mycoplasma*)	No peptidoglycan (in some cases cellulose present)
Sterols	Absent (except in *Mycoplasma*)	Usually present
Ribosomes	70S in cytoplasm	80S in cytoplasmic reticulum

their survival under adverse conditions. Bacteria have no mitochondria, their cytoplasmic membranes generally contain no sterols, and they have a unique and usually very rigid cell wall structure. Most divide by binary fission and can be grown in artificial culture, often with extraordinary rapidity. For example, many bacteria have a doubling time under ideal conditions of about 20 min; thus, under optimal growth conditions, a single organism can yield a population of more than 10^9 after only 8 hr. Such growth rates are rarely, if ever, achieved in the human body; severe bacterial disease, nevertheless, can develop very rapidly. The major differences between prokaryotic and eukaryotic cells are listed in Table 1.1.

Viruses

The viruses, a totally distinct group of infecting agents, are strict intracellular parasites of other living cells—not only of mammalian and plant cells but also of simple unicellular organisms, including bacteria (the bacteriophages). The viruses are simple forms of replicating, biologically active particles that carry genetic information in either DNA or RNA molecules, but never both. Most mature viruses have a protein coat over their nucleic acid and sometimes a lipid surface membrane derived from the cell that they infect. They lack the protein-synthesizing enzymes and structural apparatus for their own replication; they bear essentially no resemblance to a true eukaryotic or prokaryotic cell.

The origin of viruses is obscure; they share characteristics with genes, plasmids, and certain simple obligately intracellular bacteria. Indeed, different groups of viruses show such disparate characteristics that some could conceivably have originated from each of these sources. Viruses replicate by using their genetically active nucleic acids to subvert the metabolic activities of the cell that they infect to bring about the synthesis and reassembly of their component parts. A cell infected with a single viral particle may thus yield many thousands of viral particles, which can be assembled almost simultaneously under the direction of the viral nucleic acid. With many viruses, cell death and infection of other cells by the newly formed viruses result. Sometimes, viral and cell reproduction proceed simultaneously without cell death, although cell physiology may be affected. The close association of the virus with the cell sometimes results in the integration of viral nucleic acid into the functional nucleic acid of the cell, producing a latent infection that can be transmitted intact to the progeny of the cell.

Viral integration and latent viral infections

Integration may be an inherent property of the virus or be facilitated by mutational changes in the host or viral nucleic acid. The integrated viral genome can be silent, producing no metabolic effect; can alter the expression of the genome of the host cell; or may encode the production of a biologically active protein. For example, diphtheria toxin is encoded by a bacteriophage integrated into the chromosome of the diphtheria bacillus.

Carriage of viral nucleic acid may be passed not only to the progeny of cells within the host, but also longitudinally through each successive generation of inbred animals. Some latent viral infections are associated with a high incidence of specific tumors in animals, and there is increasing evidence that some human tumors are associated with certain viral infections. The integrated viral nucleic genome can sometimes be activated by mutational or other stimuli, leading to production of complete viral particles and death of the host cell. Other types of viral latency occur: for example, latency between clinical attacks of herpes simplex infection may not be consequent to viral integration but probably to a balance between the ability of the virus to replicate and some immunologic response of the host: when host immunity declines, relapse occurs.

Normal bacterial flora

Although certain viruses can coexist with humans without causing disease, most of the known normal microbial inhabitants of humans are bacteria and yeasts. The skin and the alimentary, upper respiratory, and vaginal tracts all play host to numerous bacteria that are amazingly well adapted to survive under the physiologic and nutritional conditions found in these sites. These organisms often maintain themselves by adhering specifically to epithelial cells and multiplying on their surfaces without damaging them. In some cases, organisms of the normal flora are directly beneficial to the host: they prime the immune system or synthesize nutritionally useful products, such as vitamin K. The normal flora also benefits the host indirectly by providing formidable competition to colonization and infection by pathogenic bacteria. Elimination of this competition by removal of normal floral organisms with antibiotic treatment increases susceptibility to many bacterial and yeast infections.

Endogenous infections

Many members of the normal flora have pathogenic potential: if sufficient numbers reach normally sterile areas of the body (for example, tissues, peritoneal cavity, bladder, or lower respiratory tract), they may cause severe or even fatal infections. These infections can result from mechanical causes, such as a ruptured intestine, or from a congenital or acquired failure of some critical component of the immune system that normally helps to prevent organisms from transgressing body surfaces or removes them when the day-to-day minor accidents of life deposit them in the tissues. This process is largely effected by the phagocytic cell system and enhanced by the early inflammatory response.

Exogenous infections

The initial stages of infection by extraneous organisms (those not part of the body's indigenous flora) may be secondary to structural or functional damage to surface structures that normally exclude them (for example, a third-degree burn of the skin, the bite of an insect vector, or damage to the bronchial ciliated epithelium from smoking). Other organisms can infect healthy individuals with intact epithelia, and these are particularly associated with epidemic spread. A major attribute of these pathogens is the ability to adhere to target epithelial cells and establish a primary site of infection. Viruses and a few other organisms pass into the target cell and replicate there; others pass through or between the cells, and some produce toxins that destroy the cells and thus gain access to the tissues. In some diseases toxins alter the physiology of the epithelial target cells without destroying them and produce disease in this way. An example is the massive outpouring of fluid in cholera.

Organisms that invade and multiply in the tissue of individuals with intact cellular and humoral immune mechanisms have specific determinants of virulence that allow them to avoid eradication by the body's first line of defense, including ingestion by phagocytic cells. Such organisms usually possess several characteristics needed for virulence, and these vary with different pathogens. Some organisms are resistant to phagocytosis, some produce substances that kill phagocytes or inhibit their migration, and some are resistant to destruction after phagocytosis. Intracellular existence and multiplication protect viruses and some bacteria, fungi, and protozoa from phagocytic and humoral immune mechanisms as long as they remain within the cell. Some bacteria produce enzymes that destroy surface-secreted antibody, (immunoglobulin A). In most cases, the ability to circumvent the body's defenses is relative, and organisms must be numerous to initiate an infection that may then progress with simultaneous destruction and multiplication of the infecting agent.

Determinants of virulence

The mere presence of microorganisms multiplying in the tissues does not necessarily produce disease. Many produce toxic substances. Some of these are highly potent and pharmacologically specific and facilitate spread of infection or damage local and remote organs. Viral diseases often result from direct or immunological destruction of infected cells or from alterations in cellular function. Damage also results from the body's response to infection through inflammation, through immediate or delayed hypersensitivity to microbial antigens, or through local or remote tissue responses to immune complexes. Some organisms can cause disease without penetrating mucous membranes through the effects of their highly potent toxins. Such toxins are often produced in the intestinal tract or, in some cases, in food before ingestion.

Mechanisms of damage to host

During the course of an infection, the body's adaptive immune mechanisms, both specific and nonspecific, come into play. The local inflammatory reaction mobilizes phagocytes and serum antimicrobial factors. Polymorphonuclear leukocytosis often develops in bacterial infections and increases the number of phagocytic cells; fever may slow multiplication of some infecting agents and increase the effectiveness of specific antimicrobial processes in the body. Antigen, often processed by macrophages, primes and leads to multiplication of specific immunologically active lymphoid cells of both the T and B series. Antibody with specific attachment sites for the infecting agent and for phagocytic cells increases the efficiency of phagocytosis or abrogates the effectiveness of antiphagocytic surface components of some bacteria, a process in which the normal serum complement system collaborates. In some cases, direct killing of the pathogen results from the action of complement on antibody-coated cells; in others, antibody blocks attachment sites on the surface of strict intracellular parasites such as viruses, thus halting the cycle of spread from cell to cell. Cell-mediated immune mechanisms serve to increase the activity of macrophages and of other mechanisms directed against intracel-

Immune responses of host

lular pathogens. Interferon production, which plays a major role in blocking the intracellular replication of viruses, also appears to interact with natural killer cells to increase their efficiency in destroying virus-infected cells. These processes are but a few of the diverse and often interacting defense mechanisms that the body mounts against infecting agents.

Outcome of infection

The outcome of an infection is determined by the size of the infecting dose, the site of infection, the virulence of the organism, and the speed and effectiveness of the immune response. Most infections transmitted between humans are ultimately controlled by the body's defenses, even without therapeutic intervention, because selective pressures over the course of human history have been toward a balanced state of parasitism that ensures survival of both host and parasite. This does not apply to infections with pathogens that have a primary reservoir in nonhuman hosts (eg, rabies) or to organisms that have not been previously or recently experienced by our species. These are frequently of unusual virulence. Examples are the 1918–1919 influenza pandemic that took more lives than World War I and the present pandemic of acquired immunodeficiency syndrome (AIDS). The origin of such "new" highly virulent organisms is uncertain, but may have arisen by mutation in pathogens of other species or by recombinational events within or between human and animal pathogens.

Epidemic spread

Many infections, other than those caused by members of the normal flora, may spread epidemically. Epidemics range from those in small, closed communities or hospitals to those with massive, worldwide spread. The factors determining the occurrence, spread, and resolution of epidemics are complex, but can often be influenced by medical and public health intervention. To produce a transmissible epidemic, an organism must have a sufficient degree of infectivity and virulence, and conditions must exist that permit spread. These conditions may include direct contact (impetigo), aerial transmission (influenza), blood and body fluid transmission (AIDS), contaminated food or water (typhoid), or the presence of essential insect vectors (malaria). The degree of innate and acquired immunity in the population must be sufficiently low for the rate of infection to be amplified as the disease spreads. Epidemic spread and disease are facilitated by malnutrition, poor socioeconomic conditions, natural disasters, and hygienic inadequacy. In previous centuries, epidemics, sometimes caused by the introduction of new organisms of unusual virulence, often resulted in high morbidity and mortality and massive dislocation of society because of the pervasive fear and helplessness that they produced. The possibility of recurrence of old pandemic infections, especially of influenza, remains, and we are currently witnessing a pandemic of a new, if more chronic, infection in the case of AIDS. Fortunately our understanding of the etiology, epidemiology, and immunology of individual disease points the way to their control. As the focus of medicine moves increasingly toward prevention, it becomes even more important for all health care workers to understand the principles and control of epidemic spread.

Chemotherapy

Over the past 40 years, therapeutic tools of remarkable potency and specificity have become available for the treatment of bacterial infections. These include all the antibiotics and an array of synthetic chemicals that kill or inhibit the infecting organism, but have minimal or acceptable toxicity for the host. These antibacterials exploit the structural and metabolic differences between bacterial and eukaryotic cells to provide the selectivity necessary for good antimicrobial therapy. Penicillin, for example, interferes with the synthesis of the bacterial cell wall, a structure that has no analog in human cells. After Fleming's discovery of penicillin, the earlier effective antibiotics were discovered by screening many fungi and bacteria for their possible production of antimicrobial agents. This approach yielded a rich harvest that included, among many others, such agents as streptomycin, chloramphenicol, the tetracyclines, and erythromycin. More recently, research and development have focused on molecular modification of naturally occurring agents to improve their ranges of activity, to enhance their pharmacologic characteristics, or to make them insusceptible to the resistance mechanisms that some bacteria have developed to their earlier congeners. There are fewer antifungal and antiprotozoal agents, because of closer metabolic and structural similarities between the eukaryotic cells of the host and those of the parasite. Nevertheless, there are a series of significant differences, and effective therapeutic agents have been discovered or developed to exploit them.

Specific therapeutic attack on viral disease has posed more complex problems, because of the intimate involvement of viral replication with the metabolic and replicative activities of the cell. Thus, most substances that inhibit viral replication have unacceptable toxicity to host cells. In recent years, however, advances in molecular virology have identified specific viral targets that can be attacked. Some successful antiviral agents have resulted, including agents that interfere with the liberation of viral nucleic acid from its protective protein coat or with the processes of viral nucleic acid synthesis and replication. Some experimental antiviral agents act indirectly by stimulating production of interferons, a group of antiviral proteins usually produced by virally infected host cells.

With increased understanding of the molecular biology of viral replication, it seems certain that new synthetic compounds targeted to interfere with essential viral processes such as attachment, replication, or assembly will be developed and that similar approaches will increase the number of chemotherapeutic agents available for use against eukaryotic parasites.

Microbial resistance to chemotherapy

The response of bacteria, and to a lesser extent of protozoa and fungi, to the widespread use of specific antimicrobial agents in therapy and prophylaxis reflects their extraordinary genetic plasticity. Resistant strains have appeared among many species that were previously fully susceptible to a particular agent. This resistance has resulted from mutation in the microbial genome and, in the case of bacteria, from the acquisition of genetic determinants of resistance on extrachromosomal, self-replicating portions of DNA (plasmids). Some individual genetic sequences can move from plasmid to plasmid or from plasmid to chromosome or vice versa (transposons). Some plasmids carry multiple resistance determinants against several antibiotics and can be transferred within or between bacterial species. Thus, the selective pressure of a single antimicrobial agent can lead to the predominance of multiple resistance in a previously fully susceptible strain. These developments have had major implications for successful prevention and treatment of many bacterial infections, and the selective factors that have contributed to the spread of resistance must be understood and acted on if some of the benefits of the antibiotic revolution are not to be lost through excessive or inappropriate use. Mutational resistance to antivirals is also encountered and may, for example, pose problems in the treatment of AIDS.

Prevention by immunization

As indicated previously, new developments and understanding in medicine are increasing the emphasis on prevention of disease, and nowhere is this more important than in infectious diseases. Specific immunization by parenteral injection of nonliving purified or complex antigens has long been shown effective in preventing diphtheria, tetanus, pertussis, poliomyelitis, and influenza infections if immunization schedules are rigorously applied and maintained with appropriate boosters. More recently, vaccines of purified capsular antigens have been used for preventing pneumococcal, some meningococcal, and some *Haemophilus* infections in populations at particularly high risk of serious disease with these organisms. Inactivated vaccines have also been developed to help protect burn victims and other highly susceptible patients from certain opportunistic organisms that can produce dangerous infections.

Live vaccines, using organisms of reduced virulence (attenuated) that undergo limited multiplication in the body, have also been used for many decades in the prevention of smallpox, rabies, poliomyelitis, and tuberculosis. This approach has been extended more recently to measles, rubella, and mumps and has effected dramatic changes in the overall occurrence of childhood infections with their toll of poor health, school absences, serious complications, and even death. Live vaccines provide prolonged immunologic stimuli and thus obviate the need for repeated boosters.

Many infectious diseases have not yet been controlled by vaccines, either because effective immunization antigens have not been discovered or because the parenteral routes of immunization are ineffective. Particular attention is being paid to the development of vaccines that stimulate local (IgA) immunity at the initial site of infection. Some are mutants that have lost certain determinants of virulence but continue to produce the immunizing antigen and thus resemble the oral poliomyelitis vaccine. Another promising avenue is the production of hybrid organisms by genetic engineering in which genes encoding immunizing antigens of the pathogen are introduced into nonpathogenic organisms capable of colonizing the susceptible area of the body. These approaches are being applied particularly to intestinal diseases such as bacillary dysentery.

Other prophylactic approaches

Other methods of prevention are being exploited. Chemoprophylaxis with specific antibiotics for brief periods has extended the range of surgical procedures that can be performed safely; for example, patients with implanted heart valves or artificial hips can be protected from infection by organisms that gain access during surgery and may then lead to loss of the prosthesis. Identification of the chemical nature of specific receptors for bacterial toxins or viruses may allow them to be used therapeutically. For example, attachment of receptor material to non-absorbable particles could bind enteric toxins before they could attack living cells. Perhaps most importantly, there is increasing emphasis on stimulation of the body's nonspecific phagocytic and cytotoxic immune system and on the physiologic and nutritional factors that influence resistance to infection. For example, it has been shown that a key factor in preventing the severely burned patient from succumbing to infection is the maintenance of general nutritional balance by parenteral feeding with essential nutrients. Those who have read George Bernard Shaw's *The Doctor's Dilemma* will deduce that we are coming full circle and that "stimulation of the phagocytes," a major focus of research in the 1920s, is highly relevant today.

Diagnostic microbiology

Detection and identification of microorganisms or their products in clinical material are undertaken in clinical or public health microbiology laboratories. Most bacteria and fungi can be grown in artificial culture, studied for a variety of key taxonomic characteristics, and speciated within a day or two. Once grown, they can be tested for their susceptibility to antimicrobial agents in the test tube, and the results used in the rational selection of therapy. Most viruses can be grown in cultures of eukaryotic cells derived from human or mammalian tissues, then speciated by appropriate techniques, such as reactivity with specific antibodies. These processes take several days, and much more rapid diagnostic procedures are now being used increasingly. In some cases, specific products of infecting organisms can be detected in clinical specimens using highly sensitive and specific chemical or immunological techniques. In others, nucleic acid probes have been developed by gene cloning that can detect specific portions of a microbial genome in infected cells or in clinical exudates. Procedures have also been developed that amplify even rare integrated viral nucleic acid sequences to detectable levels. These approaches have already proved their value in the rapid diagnosis of a number of diseases, establishing the etiology of an infection when other methods fail, detecting genes encoding specific determinants of virulence, and tracing the interspecies spread of antibiotic resistance genes.

Sometimes, diagnosis of an infection is only practicable by detecting antibodies produced by the patient in response to the infecting organism (serodiagnosis). Procedures for accomplishing this have been in use for some diseases since the turn of the century but have now increased greatly in sensitivity and specificity. This approach is of particular value in the diagnosis of chronic infection such as syphilis and AIDS in which the causative organism can either not be recovered or only isolated with great difficulty and expense. Serodiagnosis has limited value in the diagnosis of acute life-threatening infections because of the inherent delay in mounting an immune response. It is, however, of great value epidemiologically in detecting and tracing the occurrence of epidemic diseases, especially those caused by viruses.

The isolation or detection of a potentially pathogenic organism, particularly in material from a site with a normal flora, often does not provide sufficient evidence of etiology. Knowledge of potential sources of contamination, the constituents of the normal flora, and the probability of a particular pathogen's association with the clinical manifestation must all be considered in arriving at a probable or confirmed diagnosis. Likewise, interpretation of the significance of antibodies to an organism in a patient's serum involves recognition that they could result from a previous infection or sometimes from cross-reaction with another organism. A single test, which cannot detect an increasing immunological response, is usually of value only in diseases that are chronic or for epidemiological studies. Informed judgment thus plays a critical role in presumptive laboratory diagnosis of many specific infectious diseases and in the interpretation of all laboratory results. It is essential that the student grasp the principles, methods, and pitfalls of these approaches if the potentialities of the laboratory are to be applied correctly and errors and misinterpretations avoided.

It is hoped that this overview will help the reader to understand how the different topics in this book relate to one another and the reasons why the authors believe that a student who will practice in any branch of medicine should understand the material presented. There is much specific information in the book, some of which illustrates principles that must be understood and some of which must be learned. We offer no apologies for the fact that some rote memorization is essential. For example, one cannot deduce the major characteristics of a staphylococcus or the manifestation of a staphylococcal infection from first principles. They must be learned, and memory continually reinforced and extended. Memorization without understanding, however, is no basis for the application of a discipline to the care of patients and to the diagnosis and treatment of disease: it is essential that the underlying principles be firmly grasped.

Interpretation of diagnostic tests

2

The Bacterial Cell:
Structures for Growth, Survival, and Colonization

Frederick C. Neidhardt

General Morphology, Body Plan, and Composition

The bacterial cell that is seen today is closer in form to the primordial cells of our planet than is any animal or plant cell. Despite this similarity, bacteria are the product of close to 3 billion years of natural selection and have emerged as immensely diverse and successful organisms colonizing almost all parts of the world and its inhabitants. Because they have remained microscopic, it can be concluded that very small size per se is not a disadvantage in nature and may very well provide unique opportunities for survival and reproduction. Thus, the first major principle to help us understand bacteria is their small size.

Bacteria are by far the smallest living cells, and some are considered to have the minimum possible size for an independently reproducing organism. Individuals of different bacterial species range from 0.1 to 10 μm ($1 \mu m = 10^{-6}$ m) in their largest dimension. Most spherical bacteria have diameters of from 0.5 to 2 μm, and rod-shaped cells are generally from 0.2 to 2 μm in width and 1 to 10 μm in length. At the lower end of the scale, bacteria (rickettsias, chlamydia, and mycoplasmas) overlap with the largest viruses (the poxviruses), and at the upper end there are some rod-shaped bacteria with a length equal to the diameter of some eukaryotic cells (Figure 2.1). As a shorthand approximation, bacteria are sole possessors of the 1 μm size.

> Most bacteria are in the range of 1–8 μm

A wealth of structural detail cannot be discerned in bacteria even with the best of light microscopes because of their small size and because they are nearly colorless and transparent and have a refractive index similar to that of the surrounding liquid. Shape, however, can easily be discerned with appropriate microscopic techniques, and distinctive shapes are characteristic of broad groupings of bacteria (Figure 2.2). The major forms that can be recognized are: spheres, rods, bent rods, and spirals. Spherical or oval bacteria are called *cocci* (singular: *coccus*). Rods are called *bacilli*

11

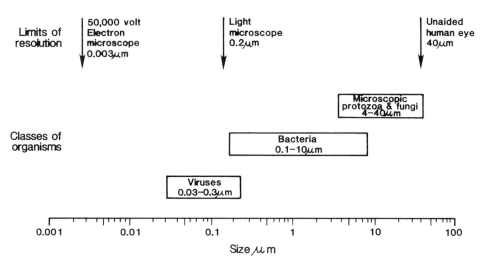

2.1 Relative sizes of microorganisms.

Variety of shape and cell arrangements

(singular: *bacillus*). Very short rods that can sometimes almost be mistaken for cocci are called *coccobacilli.* Some rod-shaped bacteria have tapered ends and are therefore termed *fusiform,* whereas others are characteristically club shaped at one end. Short rods that are curved or bent are sometimes referred to as *vibrios.* Spiral-shaped bacteria are called *spirilla* if the cells are rigid and *spirochetes* if they are more flexible and undulating.

In addition to shape, distinctive arrangements of groups of cells can readily be observed for some bacterial genera (Figure 2.3). The reason one can speak of arrangements of unicellular organisms is that there is a tendency, varying with different genera, for newly divided cells to stick together. The nature of the aggregates formed depends on the degree of stickiness (which can vary with growth conditions) and on the plane of successive cell divisions. Among the cocci, pairs (*diplococci*), chains (*streptococci*), cubical arrays (*sarcinae*), and irregular clusters (*staphylococci*) are found. A few genera of bacteria were named for their distinctive shape or cell arrangement. There are many thousands of species of bacteria, however, so it should be clear that the shape and arrangement of cells cannot be taken far in identifying the particular organism in a given sample or culture. A further caution for medical microbiologists is the tendency

Some antimicrobics affect cell morphology

of some bacteria to take on altered shapes and arrangements when in contact with various antimicrobics.

Whatever the overall shape of the cell, the 1-μm size could not accommodate the familiar eukaryotic cell plan. There is insufficient room for mitochondria, nucleus, Golgi apparatus, lysosomes, endoplasmic reticulum, and the like in a cell that is itself only as large as an average mito-

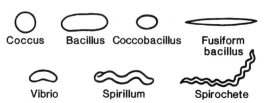

2.2 Shapes of some different bacteria.

2.3 Arrangement of spherical bacterial cells.

Diplococcus Tetrad Streptococcus Staphylococcus

chondrion. The design of the bacterial cell must thus differ fundamentally from that of other cells. As we have seen in Chapter 1, this is precisely the case, and the unique design is designated *prokaryotic*.

A generalized bacterial cell is shown in Figure 2.4. The major structures of the cell belong either to the multilayered *envelope* and its *appendages* or to the interior core consisting of the *nucleoid* (or nuclear body) and the *cytosol*. In contrast to the alien nature of this body plan, the general chemical nature of the bacterial cell is more familiar to a eukaryotic cell biologist. Greater than 90% of its dry mass consists of five macromolecularlike substances similar to those found in eukaryotes: proteins (about 55% of the dry mass); RNA, consisting of the familiar mRNA, tRNA, and rRNA (about 20%); DNA (about 3%); carbohydrate (about 5%); and phospholipid (about 6%). In addition there are a few macromolecules unique to prokaryotes: a peptidoglycan called *murein* is found in all walled bacteria, and a few other unique molecules (lipopolysaccharide and teichoic acids) are found in specific groups of bacteria.

As we shall see, it is small size and extraordinarily simple design that help explain the success of bacteria in nature. Small size facilitates rapid exchange of nutrients and metabolic by-products with the environment, whereas simplicity of design facilitates the assembly of cell structures and the formation of new cells by division. Both features contribute to a distinctive functional property of bacteria—their ability to grow at least an order of magnitude faster than eukaryotic cells. At the molecular level,

Prokaryotic cell design is unique

Chemical similarities to eukaryotic cells

Small size and simple design facilitates rapid growth

2.4 Schematic of structures of a dividing bacterium.

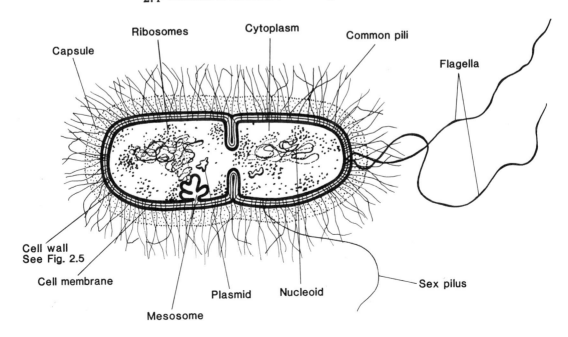

Capsule Ribosomes Cytoplasm Common pili Flagella

Cell wall
See Fig. 2.5

Cell membrane

Mesosome Plasmid Nucleoid Sex pilus

however, bacteria are far from simple, and it is necessary to learn something of their complexity at this level to understand the ability of some of them to colonize humans or to cause disease.

The Envelope and Appendages

As a first approximation, bacteria can be said to have a plain interior and a fancy exterior. The cell core, consisting solely of nucleoid and cytosol, is incredibly simple and almost structureless compared to the interior of a eukaryotic cell. It fits our notion that simplicity facilitates rapid growth. The envelope, on the other hand, is an exceedingly baroque part of the cell, consisting of structures of great complexity that vary in detail among the different major groups of bacteria. This can be readily understood by appreciating three important principles of bacterial functional anatomy: 1) the envelope is responsible for many cellular processes that are the province of the internal organelles of eukaryotic cells; 2) the envelope is the primary site of functions that protect the bacterial cell against chemical and biological threats in its environment; and 3) the envelope and certain appendages make possible the colonization of surfaces by bacteria.

Complexity of prokaryote structure and function of cell envelope

Differences in envelope structure and composition (Table 2.1) are the basis of the assignment, described below, of all eubacterial species to one of three major groups: Gram-negative bacteria, Gram-positive bacteria,

Table 2.1 Components of Bacterial Cells

Structure	Composition	Distribution[a]		
		Gram-Negative Cell	Gram-Positive Cell	Mollicutes (Mycoplasma)
ENVELOPE				
Layers				
Capsule (slime layer)	Polysaccharide or polypeptide	+ or −	+ or −	−
Wall		+	+	−
Outer membrane	Proteins, phospholipids, and lipopolysaccharide	+	−	−
Peptidoglycan layer	Murein (+ teichoate in G +)	+	+	−
Periplasm	Proteins and oligosaccharides in solution	+	−	−
Cell membrane	Proteins, phospholipids	+	+	+
Appendages				
Pili (fimbriae)	Protein (pilin)	+ or −	+ or −	−
Flagella	Proteins (flagellin plus others)	+ or −	+ or −	−
CORE				
Cytosol	Polyribosomes, proteins, carbohydrates (glycogen)	+	+	+
Nucleoid	DNA with associated RNA and proteins	+	+	+
Plasmids	DNA	+ or −	+ or −	+ or −
ENDOSPORE				
	All cell components plus dipicolinate and special envelope components	−	+ or −	−

[a] "+" indicates the structure is invariably present; "−" indicates it is invariably absent; "+ or −" indicates that the structure is present in some species or strains and absent in others.

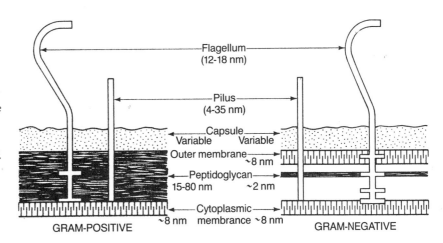

2.5 Schematic representation comparing the envelopes of Gram-positive and Gram-negative bacteria. *(Reproduced with permission from Ingraham, J., Maaløe, O., and Neidhardt, F.C., 1983. Growth of the Bacterial Cell. Fig. 14, p. 26. Sinauer Associates, Sunderland, Mass.)*

and the mollicutes (mycoplasma). Figure 2.5 shows schematically the major differences between the envelopes and appendages of Gram-positive and Gram-negative bacteria.

Capsule

Many bacterial cells surround themselves with one or another kind of hydrophilic gel. This layer is often quite thick; commonly it is thicker than the diameter of the cell. Because it is transparent and not readily stained, this layer is usually not appreciated unless made visible by its ability to exclude particulate material, such as India ink (Chapter 14). If the material forms a reasonably discrete layer, it is called a *capsule;* if it is amorphous in appearance, it is referred to as a *slime layer.* Almost all bacterial species can make such material to some degree. Most capsules or slime layers are polysaccharides made of single or multiple types of sugar residues; some are simple (though unusual) polypeptides, such as the polymer of D-glutamic acid, which forms the capsule of *Bacillus anthracis,* the causative agent of anthrax (Chapter 17); a few are proteins. Encapsulated bacteria give rise to smooth, often mucouslike colonies, but unencapsulated variants are common, particularly with long-term laboratory cultivation. Their colonies are nonmucoid and described as "rough."

Capsules can protect bacteria. Within animal and human hosts capsules impede ingestion by leukocytes. *Streptococcus pneumoniae,* the causative agent of pneumococcal pneumonia, in large measure owes its virulence to the ability of its copious polysaccharide capsule to interfere with phagocytosis (Chapter 16). The pneumococcal polysaccharide, as is the case with most capsular material, is antigenic (elicits the production of specific antibodies, see Chapter 8), and when specific antibody attaches to it, phagocytosis can occur. A mouse–pneumococcus experimental model is instructive. Unencapsulated pneumococci are tolerated by mice, but a single encapsulated cell injected intraperitoneally will kill a mouse—unless the mouse has been immunized with capsular material of the specific antigenic type of the infecting pneumococcus, in which case it is protected. More than 80 capsular serotypes of this organism are known, reflecting a diverse genetic capacity of the species to produce capsular polysaccharides of differing chemical structure.

Protection against phagocytosis is only part of the much broader function of bacterial capsules in nature, which is to aid colonization, primarily

Capsule is a hydrophilic gel; not readily stained

Most capsules are polysaccharide; a few are polypeptide or protein

Antiphagocytic effect of some capsules is major virulence determinant

Role of some capsules in adherence and colonization

by assisting the cell to attach to surfaces. For example, the ability of *Streptococcus mutans* and *Streptococcus salivarius* cells to adhere to the surface of teeth is in large measure a function of the polysaccharide capsules of these oral bacteria (Chapter 62).

Capsule synthesis depends on growth conditions

Capsules do not contribute to growth and multiplication and are not essential for cell survival in artificial culture. Capsule synthesis is greatly dependent on growth conditions. For example, the capsule made by the caries-producing *S. mutans* consists of a dextran carbohydrate polymer made only in the presence of sucrose.

The Cell Wall

Rigid structure unique to prokaryotes

Internal to the capsule (if one exists), but still outside the cell proper, a rigid *cell wall* surrounds all eubacterial cells except mollicutes (mycoplasma). The structure and function of the bacterial wall is so distinctive as to constitute a hallmark of the prokaryotes; nothing like it is to be found elsewhere.

Prevents osmotic lysis, determines shape, and protects against toxins

Unlike the capsule, which is dispensable for survival outside the body of the host, the wall has vital functions. It protects the cell from mechanical disruption and from being burst by the turgor pressure resulting from the hypertonicity of the cell interior relative to the environment. The wall also provides a barrier against certain toxic chemical and biological agents. Being rigid, its form is responsible for the shape of the cell.

Bacterial evolution has led to two major solutions to the challenge of constructing a wall that can protect a minute, fragile cell from chemical and physical assault, while still permitting the rapid exchange of nutrients and metabolic by-products required by rapid growth. Long before these solutions were understood in ultrastructural terms, it was recognized that bacteria could be divided into two groups depending on their reaction to a particular staining procedure devised a century ago by the Danish microbiologist, Hans Christian Gram. This procedure, the Gram stain, is described in detail in Chapter 14. It depends on the differential ability of ethanol or ethanol–acetone mixtures to extract iodine–crystal violet complexes from bacterial cells. These complexes are readily extracted from one group of bacteria, termed *Gram negative,* which can be subsequently stained red with an appropriate counterstain. They are retained by the other, termed *Gram positive,* which are thus stained violet by the retained crystal violet. The Gram stain response of a cell reflects which of the two types of wall it possesses.

Significance of Gram stain reactions

Virtually all of the eubacteria with walls can be assigned a Gram response. The few exceptions, however, include some medically important organisms. For example, the mycobacteria (such as *Mycobacterium tuberculosis,* the causative agent of tuberculosis) are Gram positive on the basis of their wall structure, but fail to stain because of interference by special lipids present in their walls. The spirochetes, including *Treponema pallidum* (the causative agent of syphilis), although Gram negative by structure, are too small to be resolved in the light microscope when stained by simple stains.

The Gram-Positive Cell Wall. The Gram-positive cell wall contains two major components, peptidoglycan and teichoic acids, plus additional carbohydrates and proteins depending on the species. A generalized scheme showing the arrangement of these components is shown in Figure 2.6.

Gram-positive walls contain peptidoglycan and teichoic acid

The chief component is *murein,* a peptidoglycan, which is found nowhere except in prokaryotes. Murein consists of a linear glycan chain of

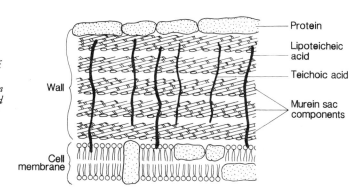

2.6 Schematic representation of the wall of Gram-positive bacteria. *(Redrawn with permission from Ingraham, J., Maaløe, O., and Neidhardt, F.C. 1983. Growth of the Bacterial Cell. Fig. 10, p. 66. Sinauer Associates, Sunderland, Mass.)*

Murein comprises linear glycan chains of alternating NAG and NAM cross-linked in three dimensions by peptide chains

Scaffoldlike murein sac surrounds cell

two alternating sugars, *N*-acetylglucosamine (NAG) and *N*-acetylmuramic acid (NAM), in 1:4 linkages (Figure 2.7). Each muramic acid residue bears a tetrapeptide of alternating L- and D-amino acids. Adjacent glycan chains are cross-linked into sheets by peptide bonds between the third amino acid of one tetrapeptide and the terminal D-alanine of another. The same cross-links between other tetrapeptides connect the sheets to form a three-dimensional, rigid matrix. The cross-links involve perhaps a third of the tetrapeptides and may be direct or may include a peptide bridge, as, for example, a pentaglycine bridge in *Staphylococcus aureus*. The cross-linking extends around the cell, producing a scaffoldlike giant molecule, termed

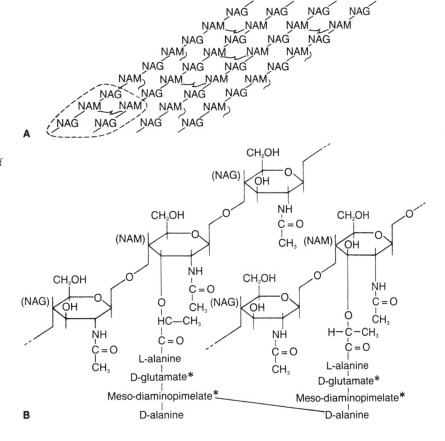

2.7 Schematic representation of the peptidoglycan, murein. NAG = *N*-acetylglucosamine; NAM = *N*-acetylmuramic acid. *(Reproduced with permission from Ingraham, J., Maaløe, O., and Neidhardt, F.C. 1983. Growth of the Bacterial Cell. Fig. 10, p. 17. Sinauer Associates, Sunderland, Mass.)*

the *murein sac,* or *sacculus.* Murein is much the same in all bacteria, except that there is diversity in the nature and frequency of the cross-linking bridge and in the nature of the amino acids at positions 2 and 3 of the tetrapeptide.

The murein sac derives its great mechanical strength from the fact that it is a single, covalently bonded structure; other features contributing strength are the β-1,4 bonds of the polysaccharide backbone, the alternation of D- and L-amino acids in the tetrapeptide, and extensive internal hydrogen bonding.

Rare or unique components of murein provide resistance to most mammalian enzymes

Biological stability is contributed by components of murein that are not widely distributed in the biological world or in fact are unique to murein: these include muramic acid, D-amino acids, and diaminopimelic acid (an amino acid found in the tetrapeptide of some species). Most enzymes found in mammalian hosts and other biological systems do not degrade peptidoglycan; one important exception is lysozyme, the hydrolase present in tears and other secretions, which cleaves the β-1,4 glycosidic bond between muramic acid and glucosamine residues (Figure 2.7). On the other hand, bacteria themselves are rich in hydrolases that degrade peptidoglycan, because the murein sac must be constantly expanded by insertion of new chains as the cell grows and forms a cross wall preparatory to cell division. As we shall learn, disruption of the fine control that bacteria exert over the activity of these potentially lethal enzymes is the means by which a large number of antibiotics and other chemotherapeutic compounds work (Chapter 13).

Bacterial enzymes insert new murein chains during growth and provide targets for antimicrobics

The role of the murein component of the cell wall in conferring osmotic resistance and shape on the cell is easily demonstrated by removing or destroying it. Treatment of a Gram-positive cell with penicillin (which blocks formation of the tetrapeptide cross-links and activates the cell's own murein hydrolases) or with lysozyme (which directly hydrolyzes the glycan chains) destroys the murein sac, and the wall is lost. Prompt lysis of the cell ensues. If the cell is protected from lysis by suspension in a medium approximately isotonic with the cell interior, such as 20% sucrose, the cell rounds up and forms a sphere called a *protoplast.* Some protoplasts can grow, and their formation within patients treated with penicillin-type antibiotics has been postulated to account for some persistent infections. Superficially, protoplasts resemble the mollicutes (mycoplasmas) that are naturally wall-less bacteria.

Loss of cell wall leads to lysis in hypotonic media or protoplasts in isotonic media

A second component of the Gram-positive cell wall is a *teichoic acid.* These compounds are polymers of either glycerol phosphate or ribitol phosphate, with various sugars, amino sugars, and amino acids as substituents (Figure 2.8). The lengths of the chain and the nature and location of the substituents vary from species to species and sometimes between strains within a species. Up to 50% of the wall may be teichoic acid, some of which is covalently linked to occasional NAM residues of the murein. Of the teichoic acids made of polyglycerol phosphate, much is linked not to the wall, but to a glycolipid in the underlying cell membrane. This type of teichoic acid is called *lipoteichoic acid* and seems to play a role in anchoring the wall to the cell membrane.

Teichoic and lipoteichoic acids are components of Gram-positive cell wall

Teichoic acids are found only in Gram-positive cells and constitute major antigenic determinants of their cell surface individuality. For example, *S. aureus* polysaccharide A is a teichoic acid and *Streptococcus faecalis* group D carbohydrate is a lipoteichoic acid.

Different teichoic acids occur in different Gram-positive genera

Beside the major wall components—murein and teichoic acids—Gram-positive walls usually have lesser amounts of other molecules. Some are polysaccharides, such as the group-specific antigens of streptococci; others

A

D-alanine

          OH   H   O   H   OH
          | | ‖ | |
     — O — P — O — C — C — C — O — P — O —
          ‖ | | | ‖
          O   H   H   H   O

          └────── Repeating subunit ──────┘

2.8 Schematic reproduction of teichoic acids. (**A**) Glycerol teichoic acid. (**B**) A ribitol teichoic acid in which R may be glucose or succinate in different species.

B

                    R   D-alanine
                    | |
          OH   H O OH O   H   OH
          | | | | | | |
     — O — P — O — C — C — C — C — C — O — P — O —
          ‖ | | | | | ‖
          O   H H H   H   H   O

          └────────── Repeating subunit ──────────┘

are proteins, such as the M protein of Group A streptococci. The detailed arrangement of the various antigens in some of the more complex Gram-positive walls is still being worked out, but minor components are thought to protect the peptidoglycan layer from the action of such agents as lysozyme and sometimes to promote colonization by sticking the bacteria to the surfaces of host cells.

Other cell wall components may offer protection and promote colonization

Gram-Negative Cell Wall.   The second kind of cell wall found in bacteria, the Gram-negative cell wall, is depicted in Figure 2.9. Except for the presence of murein, there is little chemical resemblance to cell walls of Gram-positive bacteria, and the architecture is fundamentally different. In Gram-negative cells, the amount of murein has been greatly reduced, with some of it forming a single-layered sheet around the cell and the rest forming a gel-like substance, the *periplasmic gel,* with little cross-linking. External to this *periplasm* is an elaborate *outer membrane.*

Thin murein sac is imbedded in periplasmic murein gel

2.9 Schematic representation of wall of Gram-negative bacteria. LPS = lipopolysaccharide with endotoxic properties. (*Redrawn with permission from Ingraham, J., Maaløe, O., and Neidhardt, F.C. 1983. Growth of the Bacterial Cell. Fig. 12, p. 67. Sinauer Associates, Sunderland, Mass.)*

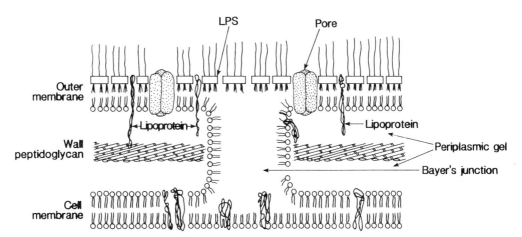

The concept of a "periplasmic gel" is relatively new. Earlier electron micrographs had suggested that the small amount of murein in Gram-negative cells, such as *Escherichia coli,* formed a single sheet around the cell, and that this murein sac was floating in a space, the *periplasmic space,* containing a fairly concentrated solution of proteins and oligosaccharides. Recent evidence modifies this picture and indicates that the "space" is a gel formed by murein peptidoglycan chains with little or no cross-linking.

Whatever its precise nature, the *periplasm* contains a murein sac, with a unit peptidoglycan structure quite similar to what we have seen in Gram-positives. Despite its reduced extent in the Gram-negative wall, the murein sac still is responsible for the shape of the cell and is vital for its integrity. As in the case of Gram-positive cells, removing or damaging the peptidoglycan layer leads to cell lysis. If the cells are protected from osmotic lysis during lysozyme or penicillin treatment, they assume a spherical shape. Because such spheres cannot be totally stripped of wall material, they are called *spheroplasts,* in contrast to the *protoplasts* formed from Gram-positive cells. Spheroplasts of some species can multiply.

The proteins in solution in the periplasm consist of enzymes with hydrolytic functions (such as alkaline phosphatase), sometimes antibiotic inactivating enzymes, and various binding proteins with roles in chemotaxis and in the active transport of solutes into the cell (Chapter 3). Oligosaccharides secreted into the periplasm in response to external conditions serve to create an osmotic pressure buffer for the cell.

The periplasm is an intermembrane structure, lying between the cell membrane (discussed below) and a special membrane unique to Gram-negative cells, the *outer membrane.* This has an overall structure similar to most biological membranes with two opposing phospholipid–protein leaflets. In composition, however, it is unique in all biology. Its inner leaflet consists of ordinary phospholipids, but these are replaced in the outer leaflet by a special molecule called *lipopolysaccharide* (LPS). LPS is extremely toxic to humans and other animals and is called *endotoxin;* even in minute amounts, such as the amount released by antibiotic therapy of a patient with a Gram-negative infection, this substance can sometimes produce fever and shock (*Gram-negative shock* or *endotoxic shock*).

LPS consists of a toxic *lipid A* (a phospholipid containing glucosamine rather than glycerol), a *core polysaccharide* (containing some unusual carbohydrate residues and fairly constant in structure among related species of bacteria), and *O-antigen polysaccharide side chains* (Figure 2.10). The last component constitutes the major surface antigen of Gram-negative cells (which, it will be recalled, lack teichoic acids).

The presence of LPS in the outer leaflet of the outer membrane results in the covering of Gram-negative cells by a wall that should block the passage of virtually every organic molecule into the cell. Hydrophobic molecules (such as some antibiotics) would be blocked by the hydrophilic layer of O-antigen; hydrophilic solutes, including most nutrients, such as sugars and amino acids, would face the barrier created by the lipid portion of the outer membrane. Clearly this is a trade-off that cannot be made, the Gram-negative cell, for whatever benefit is afforded by possessing a wall with an outer membrane, must make provision for the rapid entry of nutrients. Active transport (described in Chapter 3) is part of the solution, and another part is contributed by a particular structural feature of the outer membrane. Special proteins, called *porins* or *matrix proteins,* form pores through the outer membrane that make it possible for hydrophilic solute molecules of molecular weight less than about 800 to diffuse through it and into the periplasm.

Structural significance of murein sac; removal results in spheroplasts

Periplasmic proteins have transport, chemotactic, and hydrolytic roles

Gram-negative outer membrane is phospholipoprotein bilayer

Outer layer is LPS endotoxin

Lipid A is toxic moiety of LPS; polysaccharides are antigenic determinants

Impermeability of outer membrane is overcome by active transport and porins

2.10 Schematic representation of lipopolysaccharide. The O-specific side chain is highly variable among species and sub-species and is a major determinant of antigenic specificity. *(Redrawn with permission from Ingraham, J., Maaløe, O., and Neidhardt, F.C. 1983. Growth of the Bacterial Cell. Fig. 9, p. 16. Sinauer Associates, Sunderland, Mass.)*

Murein lipoprotein is an abundant component

The outer membrane does not contain the variety of proteins present in the cell membrane, but those that are present are quite abundant. In addition to the porins, there is a protein called *Braun's lipoprotein* or *murein lipoprotein,* which is probably the most abundant protein in Gram-negative cells, such as *E. coli.* This protein is covalently attached at its carboxyl end to the third amino acid in the murein tetrapeptide, and at its amino end it is attached to a lipid imbedded in the outer membrane. It is believed that this forms the major attachment of the murein layer to the outer membrane of the wall in *E. coli* (Figure 2.9).

The LPS is exclusively in the outer leaflet, so the outer membrane is distinctly asymmetric. The innermost leaflet is contiguous in regions (called *Bayer's junctions*) with the outermost leaflet of the cell membrane (Figure 2.9).

Outer membrane has many functions

In evolving a cell wall containing an outer membrane, Gram-negative bacteria have succeeded in 1) creating the periplasm, which holds digestive and protective enzymes and proteins important in transport and chemotaxis; 2) presenting an outer surface with strong negative charge, which is important in evading phagocytosis and the action of complement (Chapter 8); and 3) providing a permeability barrier against such dangerous molecules as host lysozyme, β-lysin, bile salts, digestive enzymes, and many antibiotics.

The Cell Membrane

Basic structure is phospholipid–protein bilayer membrane
Sterols are absent

Generally the cell membrane of bacteria is similar to the familiar bileaflet membrane, containing phospholipids and proteins, that is found throughout the living world. However, there are important differences. The bacterial cell membrane is exceptionally rich in proteins (up to 70% of its weight) and does not (except in the case of mycoplasmas) contain sterols. It possesses convoluted infoldings called *mesosomes.* The bacterial chromosome is attached to the cell membrane, which plays a role in segregation

Role in synthetic, homeostatic, and electron transport processes and cell division

of daughter chromosomes at cell division, analogous to the role of the mitotic apparatus of eukaryotes. The membrane is the site of synthesis of DNA, cell wall polymers, and membrane lipids. It contains the entire electron transport system of the cell (and, hence, is functionally analogous to the mitochondria of eukaryotes). It contains receptor proteins that function in chemotaxis. Like cell membranes of eukaryotes, it is a permeability barrier and contains proteins involved in selective and active transport of solutes. It is also involved in secretion of proteins to the exterior (exoproteins), including exotoxins and hydrolytic enzymes involved in the pathogenesis of disease.

Cell membrane is functional equivalent of many eukaryotic organelles

The bacterial cell membrane, therefore, is the functional equivalent of most of the organelles of the eukaryotic cell and is vital to the growth and maintenance of the cell.

The cell membranes of Gram-positive and Gram-negative cells are similar in composition, structure, and function except for the modification, already described, in Gram-negative cells that places the outer membrane of the wall and the cell membrane in intimate contact (Bayer's junctions).

The Flagella

Flagella are molecular organelles of motility found in many species of bacteria, both Gram positive and Gram negative. They may be distributed around the cell (an arrangement called *peritrichous:* Greek, trichos = hair), at one pole (*polar* or *monotrichous*), or at both ends of the cell (*lophotrichous*). In all cases, they are individually helical in shape and propel the cell by rotating at the point of insertion in the cell envelope. The presence or absence of flagella and their position are important taxonomic characteristics.

Flagella are rotating helical organs of locomotion

The flagellar apparatus is complex, but consists entirely of proteins,

2.11 Schematic representation of the flagellar apparatus. *(Reproduced with permission from De Pamphilis, M.L., and Adler, J. 1971. Fine structure and isolation of hook-basal body complex of flagella from Escherichia coli and Bacillus subtilis. J. Bacteriol. 105:384–359, Fig. 25.)*

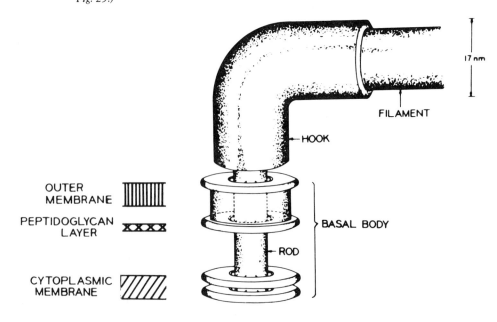

encoded in genes called *fla* (for *fla*gella). They are attached to the cell by a *basal body* consisting of several proteins organized as rings on a central rod (Figure 2.5). In Gram-negative cells, there are four rings, an outer pair that serve as bushings through the outer membrane and an inner pair located in the peptidoglycan gel and the cell membrane. In Gram-positive cells, only the inner pair is present. The *hook* consists of other proteins organized as a bent structure that may function as a universal joint. Finally, the long *filament* consists of polymerized molecules of a single protein species called *flagellin* (Figure 2.11).

Flagella have bushing rings in cell envelope

Flagellar filament is composed of flagellin protein

Motility and chemotaxis, both important properties contributing to colonization, are discussed in Chapter 3.

The Pili

Pili are proteinaceous hairlike projections

Pili are molecular hairlike projections, composed of protein, which are found on the surface of cells of many Gram-positive and Gram-negative species. There are two general classes, common pili and sex pili (Figure 2.12). *Common pili* cover the surface of the cell. They are, in many cases, *adhesins,* which are responsible for the ability of bacteria to colonize surfaces and cells. To cite only one example, the pili of *Neisseria gonorrhoeae* are necessary for the attachment to the urethral epithelial cells prior to penetration: without pili, the bacterium cannot cause gonorrheae. Thus, common pili are often important virulence factors. Some bacteriologists use the name *fimbriae* to refer to surface proteins forming more of a fuzz than a hairlike growth, but the distinction is not easily made. The *sex pilus* is diagnostic of a male bacterium and is involved in exchange of genetic material between some Gram-negative bacteria. There is only one per cell. It is composed of molecules of a protein called *pilin* arranged to form a tube with a minute, hollow core. The function of the sex pilus will be discussed in Chapter 4.

Common pili have adherence roles

Male Gram-negative cells of some species have single tubular sex pili

Some pili are encoded not by chromosomal, but by plasmid genes (see

2.12 On the left-hand side is a "male" *E. coli* cell exhibiting many common (somatic) pili and a sex pilus by which it has attached itself to a "female" cell that lacks the plasmid encoding the sex pilus. As discussed in Chapter 4, the sex pilus facilitates exchange of genetic material between the male and female *E. coli*. In this preparation, the sex pilus has been labeled with a bacterial virus that attaches to it specifically. *(This electron micrograph was kindly provided by Charles C. Brinton and Judith Carnahan.)*

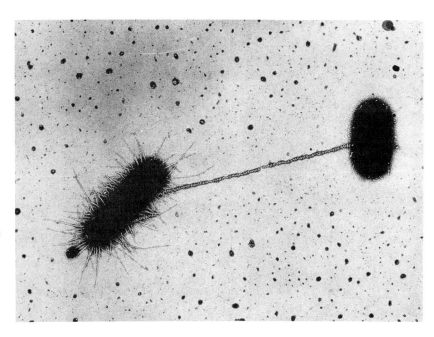

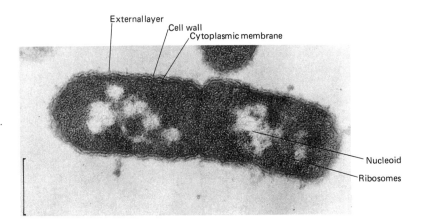

External layer
Cell wall
Cytoplasmic membrane

2.13 Electron micrograph of a Gram-negative bacterium. *(Kindly provided by the late Dr E.S. Boatman.)*

Nucleoid
Ribosomes

Some pili are plasmid encoded

Chapter 4). This fact means that both sex and virulence are properties conferred on many bacteria by a foreign genome.

The Core

In contrast to the structural richness of the layers and appendages of the cell envelope, the interior seems relatively simple in transmission electron micrographs of thin sections of bacteria (Figure 2.13). There are two clearly visible regions, one granular (the cytosol) and one fibrous (the nucleoid). In addition, many bacteria possess plasmids that are circular double-stranded DNA bodies in the cytosol separate from the larger nucleoid.

The Cytosol

The dense *cytosol* is bounded by the cell membrane. It appears granular because it is densely packed with ribosomes, which are much more abundant than in the cytoplasm of eukaryotic cells. This is a reflection of the higher growth rate of bacteria. Each ribosome is a ribonucleoprotein particle consisting of three species of rRNA (5S, 16S, and 23S) and about 56 proteins. The overall subunit structure (one 50S plus one 30S particle) of the 70S bacterial ribosome resembles that of eukaryotic ribosomes (which are 80S, composed of one 60S and one 40S particle), but it is smaller and differs sufficiently in function that a very large number of antimicrobics have the prokaryotic ribosome as their target. The number of ribosomes varies directly with the growth rate of the cell (Chapter 3). At all but the slowest growth rates about 70% of the ribosomes at any one time exist as polysomes and are engaged in translating mRNA.

Abundant 70S ribosomes with 50S and 30S subunits; that are targets for some antimicrobics

Except for the functions associated with the cell membrane, all of the metabolic reactions of the cell take place in the cytosol. Accordingly it is found to be the major location of a great fraction of the 2000–3000 different enzymes of the cell.

The cytosol of some bacterial species also contains nutritional storage granules, *reserve granules*. The most prevalent kinds consist of glycogen or polymetaphosphate. They have some diagnostic value, although, as might be expected, their presence and abundance depends on the nutritional state of the cell.

The Nucleoid

Large circular chromosome of supercoiled double-stranded DNA

The bacterial genome resides on a single chromosome and consists of about 4000 genes encoded in one, large, circular molecule of double-stranded DNA containing about 5 million nucleotide base pairs. This molecule is over 1 mm long, and it therefore exceeds the length of the cell by some 1000 times. Needless to say, tight packing is necessary, and it is this packing that displaces all ribosomes and other cytosol components from the regions that appear clear or fibrous in electron micrographs of thin sections of bacterial cells (Figure 2.13). These regions can also be visualized in specially stained cells with the light microscope or even in living bacteria by phase-contrast microscopy.

Bacteria have no nuclear membranes

Each region thus contains a chromosome, coated perhaps by polyamines and some specialized DNA-binding proteins, but not with the structural organization of a eukaryotic chromosome. Because it is not surrounded by a membrane, it is not correctly called a nucleus, but rather a *nucleoid* or *nuclear body*. The manner in which the DNA molecule is packed to form a nucleoid is not yet totally known. It is known that the DNA is attached to the cell membrane, and that the double-helical DNA chain is twisted into supercoils. Evidence indicates that the entire chromosome is attached to some central structure, perhaps RNA, at a large number of points (12–80), creating folds of DNA, each of which is independently coiled into a tight bundle. Gentle methods of lysing cells permit nucleoids to be isolated as compact particles from which DNA loops can be sprung out.

Nucleoid is attached to cell membrane and central structures

Cell may contain 2–4 nucleoids during growth

Each nuclear body visible in a stained cell corresponds to a DNA molecule. The number of nuclear bodies varies as a function of growth rate; resting cells have only one, rapidly growing cells may have as many as four. As will be described in Chapter 4, bacteria are genetically *haploid*, because all the chromosomes are identical and are segregated at random into daughter cells.

The absence of a nuclear membrane confers on the prokaryotic cell a great advantage for rapid growth in changing environments. As described in Chapter 3, ribosomes can be translating mRNA molecules even as the latter are being made; no transport of mRNA from where it is made to where it functions is needed.

Plasmids

Plasmids are nonchromosomal, small, circular, double-stranded DNA molecules

Many bacteria contain small, circular, covalently closed, double-stranded DNA molecules separate from the chromosome. More than one type of plasmid may be present in the cell, or several copies of a single plasmid. Many plasmids carry genes coding for the production of enzymes that protect the cell from toxic substances. For example, antibiotic resistance is often plasmid determined. Many attributes of virulence, such as production of some pili and of some exotoxins, are also determined by plasmid genes. Some plasmids code for production of the male sex pilus and are transmissible to other bacteria. They are thus "infectious," are nonhomologous to the bacterial chromosome, and provide a rapid method for acquisition of valuable genetic traits. This topic is considered in more detail in Chapter 4.

Many encode protective enzymes, virulence determinants, and transmissibility

Spores

Endospores are resistant, quiescent forms of some Gram-positive bacteria

Endospores are small, dehydrated, metabolically quiescent forms that are produced by some bacteria upon nutrient limitation or a related sign that tough times are coming. Very few species produce spores (the term is loosely used as equivalent to endospores), but they are particularly prevalent in the environment and some sporing bacteria are of great importance in medicine, causing such diseases as anthrax, gas gangrene, tetanus, and botulism. All spore-formers are Gram-positive rods. Some grow only in the absence of oxygen (eg, *Clostridium tetani*), some only in its presence (eg, *Bacillus subtilis*).

Spore allows survival of cell under adverse conditions

The bacterial endospore is not a reproductive structure. One cell forms one spore under adverse conditions (the process is called *sporulation*). The spore may persist for a long time (centuries) and then upon appropriate stimulation rise to a single bacterial cell (*germination*). Spores, therefore, are survival rather than reproductive devices.

Resistance due to dehydrated state, calcium dipicolinate, and specialized spore coats

Spores of some species can withstand extremes of pH and temperature, including boiling water, for surprising periods of time. The thermal resistance is brought about by the low water content and the presence of a large amount of a substance found only in spores, calcium dipicolinate. Resistance to chemicals and, to some extent, to radiation is aided by extremely tough, special coats surrounding the spore. These include a *spore membrane* (equivalent to the former cell membrane), a thick *cortex* composed of a special form of peptidoglycan, a *coat* consisting of a cysteinrich, keratinlike, insoluble structural protein, and finally an external lipoprotein and carbohydrate layer called an *exosporium*.

Germination reproduces cell identical to that which sporulated

The metabolic signal for sporulation is not fully understood. A nucleoid and its surrounding cytosol becomes walled off initially by invagination of the cell membrane, and later the special spore layers are added. Germination begins with activation (by heat, acid, and reducing conditions). Initiation of germination leads eventually to outgrowth of a new vegetative cell of the same genotype as the cell that produced the spore.

Additional Reading

Davis, B.D., Dulbecco, R., Eisen, H.N., and Ginsburg, H.S. 1980. *Microbiology.* 3rd ed. Hagerstown, Md.: Harper & Row. Chapters 2 and 6 (the former chapter written by B.D. Davis, the latter by L.L. Leive and B.D. Davis) of this classic text in medical microbiology are scholarly presentations of bacterial structure, with excellent electron micrographs.

Ingraham, J.L., Maaløe, O., and Neidhardt, F.C. 1983. *Growth of the Bacterial Cell.* Sunderland, Mass.: Sinauer Associates, Inc. A very readable description of the composition, organization and structure of the bacterial cell is presented in Chapter 1. The focus on structure geared to growth is particularly appropriate for the enteric cell the authors use as their paradigm of a bacterial cell. A good list of references for further reading is included.

Stanier, R.Y., Ingraham, J.L., Wheelis, M.L., and Painter, P.R. 1986. *The Microbial World.* 5th ed. Englewood Cliffs, N.J.: Prentice-Hall. Many parts of this excellent, general text are of interest to medical microbiologists. Chapter 6 is a superb account of the relationship between structure and function in the prokaryotic cell.

3

The Bacterial Cell:
Processes Involved in Growth, Survival, and Colonization

Frederick C. Neidhardt

In this chapter we will examine how the structural and chemical components of bacteria function in the growth and survival of these cells and in their colonization of the human host.

Cell Growth

Growth of single-celled organisms is accomplished by an orderly progress of metabolic processes followed by cell division by binary fission. The subject of growth has three areas for study: metabolism, which produces cell material from the nutrient substances present in the environment; regulation, which coordinates the progress of the hundreds of independent biochemical processes of metabolism to result in an orderly and efficient synthesis of cell components and structures in the right proportions; and cell division, which results in the formation of two independent living systems from one.

Bacterial growth requires metabolism, regulation, and division by binary fission

Bacterial Metabolism

We shall not review in depth the many aspects of (mostly mammalian) metabolism customarily learned in biochemistry courses. Many of the principles, and even some of the details of metabolism, are universal. Indeed, the principle known as the *unity of biochemistry* is underscored by the fact that much of what we know of metabolic pathways is derived from work with *Escherichia coli*. We shall focus, rather, on the unique aspects of bacterial metabolism that are important in medicine.

The broad differences between bacteria and human eukaryotic cells can be summarized as follows:

Metabolic distinctions between prokaryotic and eukaryotic cells

1. The metabolism of bacteria is geared to rapid growth and proceeds 10–100 times faster than in cells of our bodies.

2. Bacteria are much more versatile than human cells in their ability to use various compounds as energy sources and in their ability to use oxidants other than molecular O_2 in their metabolism of food stuffs.

3. Bacteria are much more diverse than human cells in their nutritional requirements, because they are more diverse with respect to the completeness of their biosynthetic pathways.

4. The simpler prokaryotic body plan makes it possible for bacteria to synthesize macromolecules by far more streamlined means than our cells employ.

5. Some biosynthetic processes, such as those producing murein, lipopolysaccharide (LPS), and teichoic acid, are unique to bacteria.

Each of these differences contributes to the special nature of the human/microbe encounter, and each provides a potential means for designing therapeutic agents to modify the outcome of this interaction.

Bacterial metabolism is highly complex. The bacterial cell synthesizes itself and generates energy for active transport, motility (in some species), and other activities by as many as 2000 chemical reactions. These reactions can be helpfully classified according to their function in the metabolic processes of *fueling, biosynthesis, polymerization,* and *assembly.*

Fueling Reactions

Fueling reactions provide the cell with energy and with the 12 precursor metabolites used in biosynthetic reactions (Figure 3.1).

Nutrient entry despite envelope permeability barriers

The first step is the capture of nutrients from the environment. Both Gram-positive and Gram-negative cells have surrounded themselves with envelopes designed in part to exclude potentially harmful substances and, therefore, have had to evolve a number of ways to assure rapid transport of selected solute molecules through the envelope. Methods used by Gram-negative cells are summarized in Figure 3.2.

Almost no important nutrients enter the cell by *simple diffusion,* because the cell membrane is too effective a barrier to most molecules (the exceptions are CO_2, O_2, and H_2O). Some transport is by *facilitated diffusion* in which a protein carrier in the cell membrane, specific for a given compound, participates in the shuttling of molecules of that substance from one side of the membrane to the other. Glycerol enters *E. coli* cells in this manner, and in bacteria that grow in the absence of oxygen (anaerobic bacteria; see below) it is reasonably common for some nutrients to enter the cell and for fermentation by-products to leave the cell by facilitated diffusion. Because no energy is involved, this process can work only with, never against, a concentration gradient of the given solute.

Facilitated diffusion across cell membrane requires shuttling by carrier protein

Active transport, like facilitated diffusion involves specific protein molecules as carriers of particular solutes, but the process is energy linked and can therefore establish a concentration gradient (active transport can pump "uphill"). Active transport is the most common mechanism in aerobic bacteria. Gram-negative bacteria have two kinds of active transport systems. In one, called *shock-sensitive* because the components are released from the cell by osmotic shock treatments, solute molecules cross the outer membrane either by diffusion through the pores of the outer membrane (as in the case of galactose) or by a special protein carrier (as in the case of maltose). In the periplasm the solute molecules bind to specific *binding proteins,* which interact with carrier proteins in the cell membrane.

Active transport can move nutrients against concentration gradient

Shock-sensitive transport involves periplasmic binding proteins and ATP-derived energy

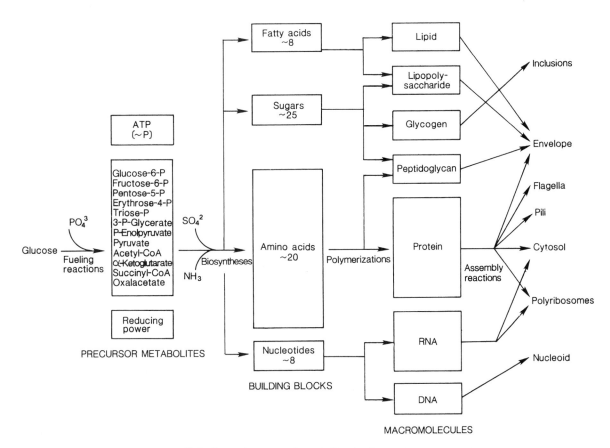

3.1 General pattern of metabolism leading to the synthesis of a bacterial cell from glucose. Boxes indicating building blocks and macromolecules are proportional to their need in making an *E. coli* cell. *(Adapted from Ingraham, J.L., Maaløe, O., and Neidhardt, F.C. 1983. Growth of the Bacterial Cell, Fig. 1, p. 51. Sinauer Associates. Sunderland, Mass.)*

Shock-sensitive systems couple the transport across the cell membrane with the hydrolysis of ATP.

Shock-insensitive transport at cell membrane requires proton gradient energy

The other type of active transport involves only cell membrane components (hence is *shock insensitive*) and is distinctive in that solute transport is coupled to the simultaneous passage of protons (H^+) through the membrane. The energy for this type of active transport is therefore derived not from ATP hydrolysis, but from the proton gradient set up by electron transport within the energized cell membrane.

Group translocation involves chemical conversion of transported molecule

Finally, *group translocation* is an extremely common means of transport in the absence of oxygen. It involves the chemical conversion of the solute into another molecule as it is transported. The phosphotransferase system for sugar transport, which involves the phosphorylation of sugars such as glucose by specific enzymes, is a good example.

Iron is an essential nutrient, but is sequestered by host Fe-binding proteins

The transport of iron and other metal ions needed in small amounts for growth is special and of particular importance in virulence. There is little free Fe^{3+} in human blood or other body fluids, because it is sequestered by iron-binding proteins (eg, *transferrin* in blood and *lactoferrin* in milk). Bacteria must have iron to grow, and their colonization of the

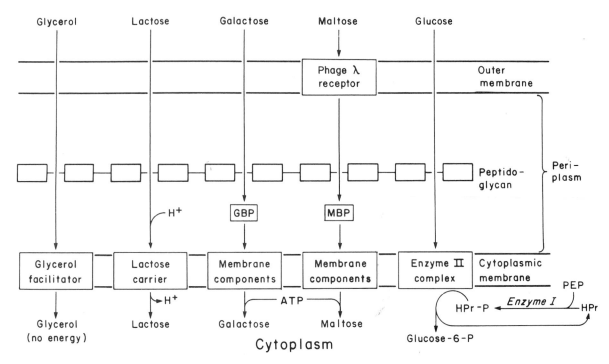

3.2 Schematic representation of the various modes of carbohydrate transport by *E. coli*. *Facilitated diffusion* is demonstrated by glycerol transport; *proton gradient energized transport,* by lactose uptake; *shock sensitive ATP-dependent transport,* by galactose and maltose uptake; and *group translocation,* by glucose uptake. *(Reprinted with permission from Lin, E.C.C., Goldstein, R., and Sylvanen, M. 1984. Bacteria, Plasmids, and Phages. Harvard University Press. Cambridge, Mass., p. 40.)*

Bacterial siderophores chelate the iron and are actively transported into cell

human host requires capture of iron. Bacteria secrete *siderophores* (Fe-specific chelators) to trap Fe^{3+}; the Fe-containing chelator is then transported into the bacterium by specific active transport. One example of a siderophore is *aerobactin* (a citrate-type of hydoxamate), another is *enterobactin* (a catechol). Some siderophores are produced as a result of enzymes encoded not in the bacterial genome, but in that of a plasmid, providing another example of the many ways in which plasmids are involved in virulence.

Once inside the cell, sugar molecules or other sources of carbon and energy are metabolized by the Embden–Meyerhof glycolytic pathway, the pentose phosphate pathway, and the Krebs cycle to yield the carbon compounds needed for biosynthesis. Some bacteria have central fueling pathways (eg, the Entner–Doudoroff pathway) other than those familiar in mammalian metabolism.

Unidirectional central fueling pathways produce biosynthetic precursors

The central fueling pathways function unidirectionally to produce the 12 precursor metabolites, but connections to *fermentation* and *respiration* pathways allow the reoxidation of reduced coenzyme NADH to NAD^+ and the generation of ATP. Bacteria make ATP by substrate phosphorylation in fermentation, or by a combination of substrate phosphorylation and oxidative phosphorylation in respiration (photosynthetic bacteria are not important in medicine).

Fermentation and respiration pathways regenerate ATP and NAD^+

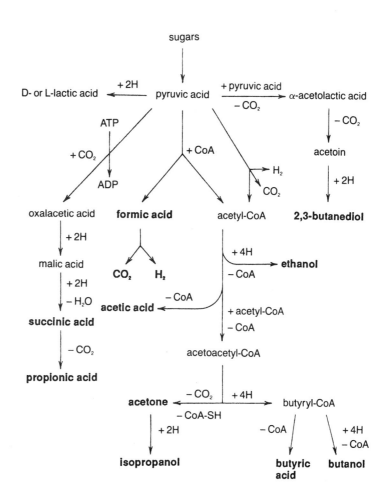

3.3 Principle pathways of fermentation of sugars through pyruvate in bacteria. The end products are shown in boldface type. Individual species of fermentative bacteria have one or more of the pathways shown. *(From Stanier, R.Y., Ingraham, J.L., Wheelis, M.L., and Painter, P.R., 1986. The Microbial World. 5th ed. Fig. 4.24, p. 95. Reproduced by permission of Prentice-Hall Inc., Englewood Cliffs, N.J.)*

Fermentation uses direct electron and proton transfer to final organic receptor

Fermentation produces organic acids and alcohols; low ATP-generating efficiency

Respiratory chain of electron carriers; oxygen usually the terminal acceptor

Respiration is efficient energy producer

Fermentation is the transfer of electrons and protons directly to an organic acceptor. Pyruvate occupies a pivotal role in fermentation (Figure 3.3). Fermentation is an inefficient way to generate ATP, and consequently huge amounts of sugar must be fermented to satisfy the growth requirements of bacteria anaerobically. Large amounts of organic acids and alcohols are produced in fermentation. Which compounds are produced depends on the particular pathway of fermentation employed by a given species, and therefore the profile of fermentation products is a diagnostic aid in the clinical laboratory.

Respiration involves fueling pathways in which substrate oxidation is coupled to the transport of electrons through a chain of carriers to some ultimate acceptor, frequently, but not always, molecular oxygen. These are efficient generators of ATP. Respiration in prokaryotes as in eukaryotes occurs by membrane-bound enzymes (quinones, cytochromes, and terminal oxidases), but in prokaryotes the cell membrane rather than mitochondrial membranes serve this function. The passage of electrons through the carriers is accompanied by the secretion from the cell of protons, generating an H^+ differential between the external surface of the cell and the cell interior. This differential, called the *protonmotive force,* can then be used to 1) drive transport of solutes by the shock-insensitive systems of active transport (see above); 2) power the flagellar motors that rotate the filaments and result in cell motility in the case of motile species; and 3) generate ATP by coupling the phosphorylation of ADP to the passage of protons inward through special channels in the cell membrane. The latter, anachronistically called *membrane ATPase,* can in fact function in either direction, coupling ADP phosphorylation to the inward passage of protons down the gradient or hydrolyzing ATP to accomplish the secretion of protons to establish a protonmotive force. The latter process explains how cells can generate a protonmotive force anaerobically (in the absence of electron transport).

In evolving to colonize every conceivable nook and cranny on this planet, bacteria have developed distinctive responses to oxygen. They are conveniently classified according to their fermentative and respiratory activities, but much more generally by their overall response to the presence of oxygen. The response depends on their genetic ability to ferment or respire, but also on their ability to protect themselves from the deleterious effects of oxygen.

Oxygen, though itself only mildly toxic, gives rise to at least two extremely reactive and toxic substances, *hydrogen peroxide* (H_2O_2) and the *superoxide anion* (O_2^-). Peroxide is produced by reactions (catalyzed by flavoprotein oxidases) in which electrons and protons are transferred to O_2 as final acceptor; the superoxide radical is produced as an intermediate in most reactions that reduce molecular O_2. Superoxide is partially detoxified by an enzyme, *superoxide dismutase,* found in all organisms (prokaryotes and eukaryotes) that survive the presence of oxygen. Superoxide dismutase catalyzes the reaction: $2O_2^- + 2H^+ \rightarrow H_2O_2 + O_2$. Hydrogen peroxide is degraded by *peroxidases* by the reaction: $H_2O_2 + H_2A \rightarrow 2H_2O + A$, where A is any of a number of chemical groups (in the case in which H_2A is another molecule of H_2O_2, the reaction yields $2H_2O + O_2$, and the peroxidase is called *catalase*). Bacteria that lack the ability to make superoxide dismutase and catalase are exquisitely sensitive to the presence of molecular O_2 and, in general, must grow anaerobically using fermentation. Bacteria that possess these protective enzymes can grow in the presence of oxygen, but whether they utilize the O_2 in metabolism or not depends on their ability to respire. Whether these oxygen-resistant bacteria can grow anaerobically depends on their ability to ferment.

Various combinations of these two characteristics (oxidation resistance and the ability to use molecular oxygen as a final acceptor) are represented in different species of bacteria, resulting in the five general classes shown in Table 3.1. There are important pathogens within each class. Both the nature of the diseases they cause and the methods for cultivating and identifying them in the laboratory are dictated to a large extent by their response to O_2.

Biosynthesis

Biosynthetic reactions form a network of pathways that lead from 12 precursor metabolites (provided by the fueling reactions) to the many amino acids, nucleotides, sugars, aminosugars, fatty acids, and other building blocks needed for macromolecules (Figure 3.1). In addition to the carbon precursors, large quantities of NADPH, ATP, amino nitrogen, and some source of sulfur are needed for biosynthesis of these building blocks. These pathways are similar in all species of living things, but bacterial species differ greatly as to which pathways they possess. Because all cells require the same building blocks, those that cannot be produced by a

---

Marginal notes:

Varying responses to oxygen

Production of peroxide and toxic oxygen radicals; detoxifying enzymes

Superoxide dismutase and peroxidase allow growth in air; absence requires strict anaerobiosis

Organisms growing in air may or may not have respiratory pathway

Aerobes, anaerobes, facultatives, indifferents, and microaerophils

Biosyntheses require 12 precursor metabolites, energy, amino nitrogen, and sulfur

Table 3.1 Classification of Bacteria by Response to Oxygen

Type of Bacteria	Growth Response		Possession of Catalase and Superoxide Dismutase	Comment	Example
	Aerobic	Anaerobic			
Aerobe (strict aerobe)	+	−	+	Requires oxygen; cannot ferment	*Mycobacterium tuberculosis* *Pseudomonas aeruginosa* *Bacillus subtilis*
Anaerobe (strict anaerobe)	−	+	−	Killed by oxygen; ferments in absence of O_2	*Clostridium botulinum* *Bacteroides melaninogenicus*
Facultative	+	+	+	Respires with O_2; ferments in absence of O_2	*Escherichia coli* *Shigella dysenteriae* *Staphylococcus aureus*
Indifferent (aerotolerant anaerobe)	+	+	+	Ferments in presence or absence of O_2	*Streptococcus pneumoniae* *Streptococcus pyogenes*
Microaerophilic	(+)[a]	+	(+)[a]	Grows best at low O_2 concentration; can grow without O_2	*Campylobacter jejuni*

[a] (+) = small amounts of growth or catalase and superoxide dismutase.

Differing nutritional requirements

given cell must be obtained preformed from the environment. Nutritional requirements of bacteria, therefore, differ from species to species and serve as an important practical basis for laboratory identification.

There are relatively few unique reactions in the domain of biosynthesis that form the basis for specific therapeutic attack on the microorganism rather than the host. The effectiveness of sulfonamides is one of these exceptions; it relates to the requirement of many bacteria to synthesize folic acid rather than being able to use it preformed from their environment as human cells do.

Polymerization Reactions

DNA polymerization is called *replication*. In bacteria it involves 12 or more proteins acting at a small number of sites (replication forks) where DNA is synthesized from activated building blocks (dATP, dGTP, dCTP, and dTTP). Replication always begins at special sites on the chromosome called *oriC* (for *origin* of replication) and then proceeds bidirectionally around the circular chromosome (Figure 3.4). Synthesis of DNA at each repli-

Bidirectional semiconservative DNA replication occurs at replication forks

cation fork is termed *semiconservative* because each of the DNA chains serves as the template for the synthesis of its complement, and, therefore, one of the two chains of the new double-stranded molecule is conserved from the original chromosome. One of the two new strands must be synthesized in chemically the opposite direction of the other; this is accomplished by having each new strand made in short segments, 5' to 3', which are then ligated by one of the DNA synthesizing enzymes (Figure 3.4). Interestingly, an RNA primer is involved in getting each of these segments

3.4 Schematic representation of DNA replication in bacteria. **(A)** A portion of a replicating chromosome shortly after replication has begun at the origin is shown. The newly polymerized strands of DNA (wavy lines) are synthesized in the 5′ to 3′ direction (indicated by the arrows) using preexisting DNA strands (solid lines) as templates. The process creates two replication forks that travel in opposite directions until they meet on the opposite side of the chromosome. **(B)** A more detailed view of one replicating fork showing the process by which short lengths of DNA are synthesized and eventually joined to produce a continuous new strand is shown. For purposes of illustration, four segments are shown at various stages. In the first (1) primer RNA (thickened area) is being synthesized by RNA polymerase (R Pol). In the second (2), DNA is being added to it by DNA polymerase 111 (pol 111). In the third (3), a preceding RNA primer is being hydrolyzed and DNA is being polymerased in its place by DNA polymerase 1 (Pol 1). Finally, the completed short segment of DNA (4) is joined to the continuous strand (5) by the action of DNA ligase (ligase). *(From Stanier, R.Y., Ingraham, J.L., Wheelis, M.L., and Painter, P.R. 1986. The Microbial World. 5th ed. Fig. 5.41, p. 133. Reprinted by permission of Prentice-Hall, Inc., Englewood Cliffs, N.J.)*

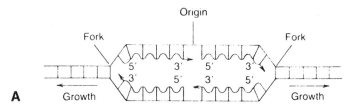

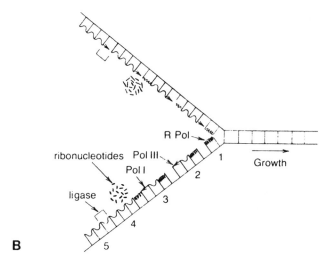

DNA gyrase inhibitors

One RNA polymerase synthesizes all forms of bacterial RNA

Bacterial mRNA needs no special means of transport to ribosomes

initiated. The two replication forks meet at the opposite side of the circle. The frequency of initiation of chromosome replication (and therefore the number of growing points) varies with cell growth rate; the chain elongation rate is rather constant.

Some chemotherapeutic agents derive their selective toxicity for bacteria from the unique features of prokaryotic DNA replication. The antibiotic, *novobiocin,* and the synthetic compound, *nalidixic acid,* inhibit DNA gyrase, one of the many enzymes participating in DNA replication.

Transcription is the synthesis of RNA. Transcription in bacteria differs from that in eukaryotic cells in several ways. One way is that all forms of bacterial RNA—mRNA, tRNA, and rRNA—are synthesized by the same enzyme, RNA polymerase. Like the several eukaryotic enzymes, the single bacterial RNA polymerase utilizes activated building blocks (ATP, GTP, CTP, and UTP) and synthesizes an RNA strand complementary to whichever strand of DNA is serving as template.

A second major difference is that bacterial mRNA need not be transported to the cytoplasm through a nuclear membrane, and hence no poly(A) cap is needed and no special means of transport exists. In fact, because each mRNA strand is directly accessible to ribosomes, binding of the latter to mRNA to form polysomes begins at an early stage in the synthesis of each mRNA molecule (Figure 3.5).

As in eukaryotic cells, all stable RNA molecules are made from giant precursor molecules that must be processed by nucleases and then ex-

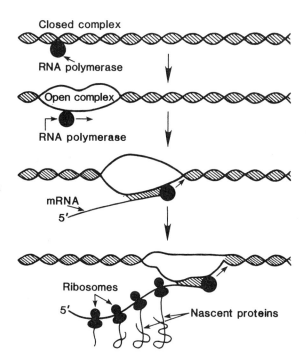

3.5 Schematic representation of the coupling of transcription and translation in bacteria.

tensively modified to produce the mature product (the tRNAs and rRNAs).

Bacterial RNA polymerase is the target of the *rifamycin* series of antimicrobics (including the semisynthetic compound *rifampin*). They block initiation of transcription. Other substances of biological origin block extension of RNA chains or inhibit transcription by binding to DNA. They have been of great value in molecular biological studies, but are toxic also to human cells and thus are not used in human therapy.

Rifampin inhibits RNA polymerase

Translation is the name given to protein synthesis. Bacteria activate the 20 amino acid building blocks of protein in the course of attaching them to specific transfer RNA molecules. The aminoacyl-tRNAs are brought to the ribosomes by soluble protein factors, and there the amino acids are polymerized into polypeptide chains according to the sequence of codons in the particular mRNA that is being translated. Having donated its amino acid, the tRNA is released from the ribosome to return for another aminoacylation cycle.

Proteins made by polymerizing amino acid residues from specific tRNAs

This description fits translation in eukaryotic as well as prokaryotic cells, but major differences do exist. The initiation of translation of a new polypeptide chain requires fewer proteins in bacteria. The ribosomes of bacteria are smaller and simpler in structure. Bacterial mRNA is largely polycistronic, that is, each mRNA molecule is the transcript of more than one gene (cistron) and, therefore, directs the synthesis of more than one polypeptide. No processing or transport of the mRNA is necessary. RNA polymerase makes mRNA at about 55 nucleotides per second (at 37°C) and ribosomes make polypeptide chains at about 18 amino acids per second. Therefore, not only does translation of each mRNA molecule occur simultaneously with transcription, but it occurs at the same linear rate (55

Bacterial mRNA is polycistronic; requires no processing or transport

mRNA translation and
transcription occur
simultaneously

nucleotides per second / 3 nucleotides per codon = 18 amino acids per second). This means that ribosomes are traveling along each mRNA molecule as fast as RNA polymerase makes it. This coupling plays a role in several aspects of regulation of gene expression unique to bacteria.

These special features of translation in bacteria contribute to the streamlined efficiency of the process. The bacterial cytosol is packed with polyribosomes. Each ribosome functions near its maximal rate, and therefore, the faster the growth rate of the cell, the more ribosomes are needed for protein production. It can be estimated that during growth in rich media, over half the mass of the *E. coli* cell consists of ribosomes and other parts of the translation machinery.

Many antimicrobics act on
translation mechanisms

Many antimicrobics derive their selective toxicity for bacteria from the unique features of the prokaryotic translation apparatus. In fact, protein synthesis is the target of a greater variety of antimicrobics than is any other metabolic process (Chapter 13). Some inhibit the ribosomal large subunit (eg, *chloramphenicol, lincomycin,* and *erythromycin*), some the small subunit (eg, *tetracyclines, streptomycin,* and *spectinomycin*), some the soluble protein factors involved in initiation or elongation steps of peptide synthesis (eg, *fusidic acid*).

Other polymerization reactions involve synthesis of peptidoglycan, phospholipid, LPS, and capsular polysaccharide. All of these reactions involve activated building blocks that are polymerized or assembled within, or on the exterior surface of, the cytoplasmic membrane.

Peptidoglycan (murein) synthesis occurs in three compartments of the cell (Figure 3.6).

N-Acetyl muramic acid and
attached peptide synthesized
in cytosol; attached to carrier
bactoprenol

1. In the cytosol a series of reactions leads to the synthesis, on a nucleotide carrier (UDP), of an *N*-acetylmuramic acid residue bearing a pentapeptide (the tetrapeptide found in mature murein plus an additional terminal D-alanine).

N-Acetyl glucosamine and
bridge amino acids added in
cell membrane

2. This precursor is then attached, with the release of UMP, to a special, lipidlike carrier in the cell membrane called *bactoprenol* (or *undecaprenol*). Within the cell membrane *N*-acetyl glucosamine is added to the precursor, along with any amino acids that in this particular species will form the bridge between adjacent tetrapeptides.

Glycan polymer and peptide
cross-links formed in
periplasm or wall

PBPs are involved in murein
assembly, expansion, and
shaping

3. Outside the cell membrane (in the periplasm of Gram-negative cells and the wall of Gram-positive cells), this disaccharide subunit is attached to the end of a growing glycan chain and then cross-links between chains are formed by a transpeptidization using the energy transduced by the release of the terminal D-alanine—the extra amino acid on the tetrapeptide. Eventually, release from the carrier occurs. Many enzymes, called *penicillin-binding proteins* (PBPs) from their property of combining with this antibiotic, are involved in forging, breaking, and reforging the peptide cross-links between glycan chains. This dynamic process is necessary to permit expansion of the murein sac during cellular growth, to shape the envelope, and to prepare for cell division. It is this process that goes awry in the presence of penicillin and related antimicrobics, the action of which can be broadly stated as preventing formation of stabilizing peptide cross-links.

Uniqueness of wall offers
target for several
antimicrobics

The whole process of synthesizing peptidoglycan (murein), which is completely absent from eukaryotic cells, offers many vulnerable attack points for antibiotics and other chemotherapeutic agents. Some of these are shown in Figure 3.6; others are described more fully in Chapter 13.

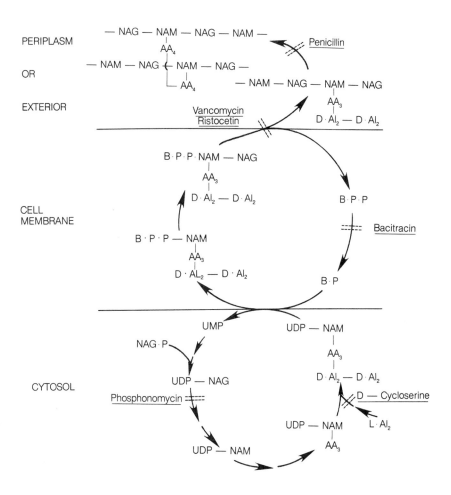

3.6 Schematic representation of murein synthesis with sites of action of some antibiotics. NAG = N-acetylglucosamine; NAM = N-acetylmuramic acid; BP and BBP = bactoprenol phosphate and bactoprenol pyrophosphate, respectively; AA_3 = tripeptide residue that in *E. coli* is L-alanyl-D-glutamyl-*m*-diaminopimelic acid; $D-AL_2$ and $L-AL_2$ = D-alanine and L-alanine, respectively; UMP and UDP = uridine mono- and diphosphate, respectively. Some of the arrows represent more than one chemical reaction. See the text for a description of this process.

Assembly Reactions

Assembly of cell structures occurs both by spontaneous aggregation (*self-assembly*) and by special, specific mechanisms (*guided assembly*). Some macromolecules are made at the sites of assembly (such as LPS in the outer membrane), and others must be transported to them (porin is made in the cytosol, but ends up in the outer membrane). Self-assembly is illustrated by two cell structures that will spontaneously assemble in a test tube from their component macromolecules: flagella and ribosomes. Guided assembly is illustrated by the formation of the envelope. A problem is posed by the difficulty of getting macromolecules out of the cell and into their proper place in the wall, outer membrane, and capsule. This process is only beginning to become understood. Important parts of envelope assembly include special mechanisms for the secretion of proteins, the use of Bayer's zones of adhesion (Chapter 2, Fig. 2.9) to form the phospholipid/protein leaflets of the membranes, and the use of carrier molecules (eg, bactoprenol) to transport hydophilic compounds within the lipid portions of the membrane.

Bacitracin and *vancomycin* interfere with the function of bactoprenol as a carrier in polymerization and assembly reactions. The *polymyxins* partially disassemble the cell membrane, leading to an interference in envelope assembly, but, probably more importantly, causing leakage of essential compounds from the cell.

Self-assembly (eg, of ribosomes) can occur in vitro

Guided assembly requires transport of components within cell

Cell Division

Many genes involved

Bacteria multiply by binary fission. More than 30 genes in *E. coli* are known to be involved in the process that involves the polar separation of the daughter chromosomes, the formation of the cross-wall and envelope at the point of cell division, and ultimately the separation of the two newly formed cells. In rich medium at 37°C the entire process in *E. coli* and many pathogenic species is completed in 20 min. The most astounding aspect of this feat is that the replication of the chromosome in these cells takes approximately 40 min, largely independently of the nature of the medium. The trick of dividing faster than the chromosome can replicate is accomplished by a mechanism that triggers the start of a new round of replication before an earlier one has been completed. In other words, during rapid growth there are multiple pairs of replication forks at work on a given chromosome, and a newborn cell inherits chromosomes that have already been partially replicated. Bacteria maintain a constant ratio of cell mass:DNA, and because rapidly growing cells have extra DNA (due to the multiple replication forks), cell size obviously is related to growth rate; the faster bacteria grow, the larger is their average size.

Multiple replication forks allows faster cell division than chromosome replication

Cell division must be precisely coordinated with the completion of a round of DNA replication, or nonviable offspring will be produced. This coordination does not just happen; it requires a special regulatory system. Mutants are known that are defective in this regulation. Under some growth conditions, such mutants fail to synchronize cell division with DNA replication, and one of the daughter cells, called a *minicell*, is born without a chromosome. Minicells are useful research tools to study metabolic processes in the absence of instruction from endogenous chromosomal DNA or to study the specific functions of plasmids (including recombinant plasmids) introduced into them.

Uncoordinated division and DNA replication yields anucleate minicells

The complexity of cell division would lead one to expect that it might be easily disrupted by chemotherapeutic agents. This is the case. Nonlethal concentrations of antimicrobics that act, even indirectly, on the polymerization or assembly reactions of the cell wall cause the formation of bizarre and distorted cells. Long filaments can result from incomplete cell division in the case of rod-shaped bacteria such as *E. coli*. Such forms are frequently encountered in direct examination of specimens from patients treated with antibiotics.

Distortion of division and morphology by some antimicrobics

Growth of Bacterial Cultures

Definitions

Solutions of nutrients that will support the growth of bacteria are called *media* (singular, *medium*). These can be solidified by the incorporation of agar (see Chapter 14). The introduction of live cells into liquid sterile media or onto the surface of solidified media is called *inoculation*. A population of bacterial cells is referred to as a *culture*. If the population is genetically homogeneous (ie, if all cells belong to the same strain of the same species), it is called a *pure culture*. Identification of bacteria from clinical specimens usually requires study of pure cultures. These can be obtained in several ways (Chapter 14). The most common is to spread a very dilute suspension of a mixed culture on the surface of media solidified with agar. Growth of individual cells deposited across the surface of solidified media leads to visible mounds of bacterial mass called *colonies*. The cells in a colony are usually descended from a single original cell and, in this case, constitute a *clone*. There is little difference between a pure culture and a clone, except that a pure culture may have been produced by the

Growth as colonies on solid media

Difference in colonial morphologies and consistency

original inoculation of several identical cells. Colonies of different species and strains show marked differences in size, form, and consistency resulting from differences in growth rates, surface properties of the organisms, and their response to the gradients of nutrients and metabolites that develop within the colony as it enlarges. This facilitates subculturing to pure cultures.

Monitoring growth in liquid media by colony counts

Growth of a liquid bacterial culture can be monitored by removing samples at timed intervals and placing suitable dilutions in or on solidified medium order to obtain a count of the number of colonies that develop. The count can be directly extrapolated to the number of *viable units** in the original sample. Growth can also be measured by determining the number of *total cells* in each sample. Direct count with a microscope is simple but tedious; more sensitive and accurate counts can be made with the aid of an electronic particle counter. More often, the turbidity of the culture is measured, because bacterial cultures above approximately 10^6 cells/ml are visibly turbid, and turbidity is proportional to the total mass of bacterial protoplasm present per milliliter. Turbidity is quickly and easily measured by means of a spectrophotometer.

Monitoring growth turbidimetrically

The growth rate of a bacterial culture depends on three factors: the species of bacterium, the chemical composition of the medium, and the temperature. The time needed for a culture to double its mass or cell number is in the neighborhood of 30–60 min for most pathogenic bacteria in rich media. Some species can double in 20 min (*E. coli* and related organisms), and some (eg, some mycobacteria) take almost as long as mammalian cells—20 hr. In general, the greater the variety of nutrients provided in the medium, the faster growth occurs. This superficially simple fact actually depends on the operation of metabolic regulatory devices of considerable sophistication, which, as we shall see in the next section, assure that building blocks provided in the environment not be wastefully synthesized by the cells. For each bacterial species, there is a characteristic optimum temperature for growth, and a range, sometimes as broad as 40°, within which growth is possible. Most pathogens of warm-blooded creatures have a temperature optimum for growth near normal body temperature, 37°C; growth will often occur at room temperature, but slowly; therefore, incubators set at 35–37°C are employed for culture of most clinical specimens. Exceptions to this rule include some organisms causing superficial infections for which 30°C is more suitable. As a group, bacteria have the widest span of possible growth temperatures, extending virtually over the entire range of liquid water, 0°C to 100°C. Bacteria that grow best at refrigerator temperatures are called *psychrophiles*, those that grow above 50°C are called *thermophiles*; between are the *mesophiles*, including all pathogens.

Some species can divide every 20 min, others much more slowly

Growth rate dependent on nutrient availability, pH, and temperature

Wide ranges of growth temperatures

Phases of growth; metabolic activity in lag phase

When first inoculated, liquid cultures of bacteria characteristically exhibit a *lag period* during which growth is not detectable. This is the first phase of what is called the *culture growth cycle* (Figure 3.7). During this lag, the cells are actually quite active in adjusting the levels of vital cellular constituents necessary for growth in the new medium. Eventually net growth can be detected, and after a brief period of *accelerating growth*, the culture enters a phase of constant, maximal growth rate, called the *exponential* or *logarithmic phase* of growth, during which the generation time is constant. During this phase, cell numbers and total cell mass and the

---

* A viable unit may be a small clump or chain of certain bacteria. It may not, therefore, represent the number of bacterial cells.

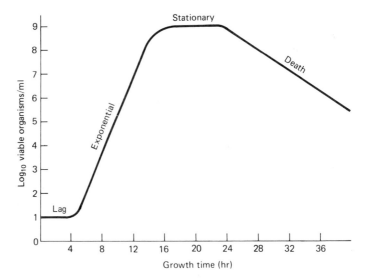

3.7 Phases of bacterial growth in liquid medium.

Consequences of exponential growth

amount of any given component of the cells increase at the same exponential rate; such growth is called *balanced growth,* which means the same as steady-state growth. The full reproductive potential of bacteria is exhibited during this phase: one cell gives rise to 2 in 1 generation, to 8 cells after 3 generations, to 1024 cells after 10 generations, and to about 1 million cells in 20 generations. For a bacterial species with a generation time of 20 min, therefore, it takes less than 7 hr in the exponential phase of growth to produce a million cells from one.

Using an equation for exponential growth it can be demonstrated that 2 days of growth at this rate would be sufficient to generate a mass of bacteria equal to 500 times the mass of the earth. Fortunately this never occurs, but not because the equation is faulty. Constant growth rate requires that there be no change in the supply of nutrients or the concentration of toxic by-products of metabolism (such as organic acids). This constancy can exist for only a short time (hours) in an ordinary culture vessel. Then growth becomes progressively limited (*decelerating phase*) and

Nutrient depletion or metabolite accumulation terminate exponential phase

eventually stops (*stationary phase*). Cells in the stationary phase are different than in the exponential phase. They are smaller, they have a different complement of enzymes (to deal with survival during starvation), and they have fewer ribosomes per unit mass. When an inoculum of such cells is placed into fresh medium, exponential growth cannot resume immediately, and hence the lag period is observed. Note that there is no lag phase if the inoculum consists of exponential-phase cells. Prolonged incubation of a stationary-phase culture leads to cell death for many bacterial species (such as the pneumococcus), though many (such as *E. coli*) are

Cultures of most species die slowly after the stationary phase

hardy enough to remain viable for days. During the *death phase* or *decline* of a culture, cell viability is lost by exponential kinetics as described in Chapter 11. As already noted, for those Gram-positive species that can sporulate, entry into the stationary phase usually triggers this event.

One way to maintain a culture in exponential, steady-state (balanced) growth for long periods of time is to use a device in which there is a continuous addition of fresh medium, but with the total volume of culture

Continuous exponential growth in chemostat

held constant by an overflow tube. One such constant-volume device is called a *chemostat;* it operates by infusing fresh medium containing a limiting nutrient at a constant rate, and the growth rate of the cells is set by

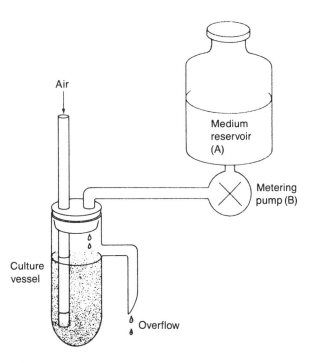

3.8 Schematic diagram of a chemostat. This continuous culture device consists of a constant volume growth chamber into which fresh sterile medium is fed at a constant rate by a pump. *(Reproduced with permission from Ingraham, J., Maaløe, O., and Neidhardt, F.C. 1983. Growth of the Bacterial Cell. Fig. 7, p. 24. Sinauer Associates. Sunderland, Mass.)*

the flow rate (Figure 3.8). A similar constant-volume device is the *turbidostat;* it operates by the infusion of fresh medium by a pump controlled indirectly by the turbidity of the culture. Although such devices may sound artificial, they mimic many situations of interest to medical microbiologists. Most of the places in which bacteria live on and within our bodies, in health and disease, provide conditions more closely resembling those of nutrient-limited continuous culture devices than of enclosed flasks (Chapters 9 and 10).

Regulation and Adaptation

Metabolic reactions must proceed in a coordinated fashion. It would not do to have them governed solely by the laws of "mass action" by which the concentration of reactants and products determine the rate of reactions. Furthermore, it would not do to have rates of individual reactions set at some fixed levels. Bacteria can do little to control their environment, and any change in environment (in its temperature, pH, nutrient availability, osmolarity, etc.) would disrupt the preset synchronization or render it inappropriate. Bacteria must, therefore, not just coordinate reactions, but must do so in a flexible, adjustable manner in order to make growth possible in a changing environment.

Flexible coordination of metabolic reactions in response to environmental changes

Bacteria have evolved many regulatory mechanisms. Some operate to control *enzyme activity;* some to control *gene expression.*

Control of Enzyme Activity

Although there are examples of covalent modification of enzymes (eg, by phosphorylation, methylation, or acylation) to alter their activity, by far the most prevalent means by which bacterial cells modulate the flow of material through fueling and biosynthetic pathways is by changing the

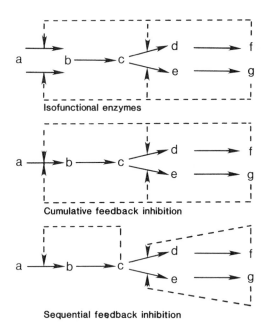

3.9 Sequential feedback inhibition. Patterns of end-product inhibition in branched biosynthesis pathways.

Most metabolic processes controlled by allosteric enzymes

Fueling pathway enzymes controlled by AMP, ADP, and ATP concentrations to maintain energy charge

Feedback inhibition control of biosynthetic pathways allows economy and efficiency

activity of *allosteric enzymes* through the reversible binding of low-molecular-weight metabolites (*ligands*). In fueling pathways it is common for AMP, ADP, and ATP to control the activity of enzymes by causing conformational changes of allosteric enzymes, usually located at critical branch points where pathways intersect. By this means, the flow of carbon from the major substrates through the various pathways is adjusted to be appropriate to the demands of biosynthesis. For example, the *energy charge* of the cell, defined as $(ATP + \frac{1}{2} ADP)/(ATP + ADP + AMP)$, is kept very close to 0.85 under all conditions of growth and nongrowth. In biosynthetic pathways, it is common for the end product of the pathway to control the activity of the first enzyme in the pathway. This pattern, called *feedback inhibition* or *end-product inhibition,* assures that each building block will be made at exactly the rate it is being used for polymerization. It also assures that building blocks supplied in the medium will not be wastefully duplicated by synthesis. Because many biosynthetic pathways are branched and have multiple end products, special arrangements must be made to produce effective regulation. These include the production of multiple isofunctional enzymes for the controlled step; the design of allosteric enzymes, which require the cumulative effect of all end products to be completely inhibited; and sequential inhibition of each subpathway by its last product (Figure 3.9).

Control of Gene Expression

To a far greater extent than eukaryotic cells, bacteria regulate their metabolism by changing the amounts of different enzymes. This is accomplished chiefly by governing their rates of synthesis, that is, by controlling gene expression. This works rapidly for bacteria because of their speed of growth; shutting off the synthesis of a particular enzyme will result in short order in the reduction of its cellular level due to dilution by the growth of the cell. Also, bacterial mRNA is degraded rapidly. With an average half-life of 2–3 min at 37°C, the mRNA complement of the cell

Changes in rate of transcription can rapidly change enzyme concentration

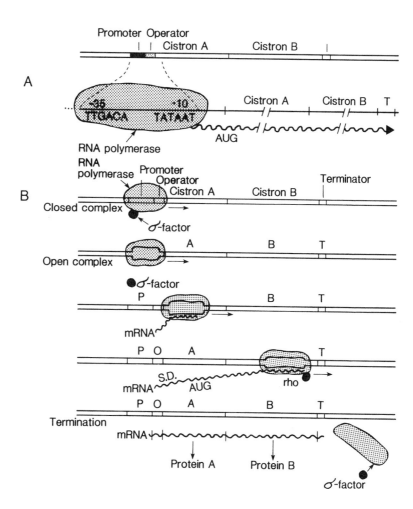

3.10 Control of transcription. Schematic representation of (**A**) a bacterial operon and (**B**) its transcription by RNA polymerase.

can be totally changed in a small fraction of a generation time. The synthesis of a given enzyme can therefore be rapidly turned on and just as rapidly turned off simply by changes in the rate of transcription of its gene.

Most, although not all, of the regulation of gene expression occurs at or near the beginning of the process: the initiation of transcription. That is, gene expression is not regulated by changing the rate of mRNA chain elongation; once started, transcription proceeds at a more or less constant rate. Regulation occurs by a decision of whether to initiate or not, or what amounts to the same thing, by setting the frequency of initiation.

Regulation frequently operates at initiation of transcription

A closer look at transcription is necessary to understand how it is controlled. Most of the genes we know about in bacteria are organized as *multicistronic operons*. A *cistron* is a segment of DNA encoding a polypeptide. An *operon* is the unit of transcription; the cistrons of which it is composed are cotranscribed as a single mRNA. The structure of a typical *operon* (Figure 3.10) consists of a *promoter* and an *operator* region in addition to its component cistrons and ends with a *terminator*. In the best-studied bacterium, *E. coli,* RNA polymerase, programmed by a removable subunit, *sigma-70,* recognizes the −35 and −10 regions of the promoter and binds to the DNA. Initially the binding is a *closed complex,* but this can be converted into an *open complex* in which the two strands of DNA are partially separated. Strand separation exposes the nucleotide bases and permits

Transcription steps

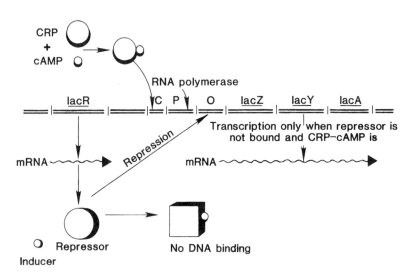

3.11 Schematic representation of the control of transcription initiation by repressor and activator proteins. The example chosen is the *lac* operon of *E. coli*. *lac R* (or i) = gene encoding the *lac* repressor protein; C = CAP region (binding site of cAMP receptor protein); P = promoter region (binding site of RNA polymerase); O = operator region (binding site of repressor); *lacZ* = gene encoding β-galactosidase; *lacY* = gene encoding permease for β-galactosides; *lacA* = gene encoding galactoside acetylase.

initiation of synthesis of a mRNA strand complementary to the sense strand of the DNA. In a simple case, transcription continues through the cistrons of the operon until the termination signal is reached. In some cases recognition of the termination signal requires another removable subunit of RNA polymerase, *rho*. This process is shown in Figure 3.10.

Near the promoter in many operons is an *operator* to which a specific *regulator protein* can bind. In some cases the binding of this regulator blocks initiation; in such a case of negative control, the regulator is called a *repressor*. Repressors are allosteric proteins, and their binding to the operator depends on their conformation, which is determined by the binding of ligands that are called *corepressors* if their action is to permit binding of the repressor and *inducers* if their action is to prevent binding. In some cases, the regulator protein is required for initiation of transcription, and it is then called an *activator*. The functioning of both types of regulator proteins on transcription initiation is illustrated in Figure 3.11 using the regulation of the *lac* operon as an example. This operon encodes proteins necessary for the utilization of lactose as a carbon and energy source.

Mechanisms of repression and induction of gene transcription

Once transcription is initiated it may continue uneventfully, but in some operons another site of control is quickly encountered. After transcription of a *leader region,* the RNA polymerase encounters a region known as an *attenuator*. Synthesis of mRNA is aborted at the attenuator; only a small percentage of the RNA polymerase molecules reaching the attenuator can successfully pass through it. However, the activity of the attenuator can be modified by a process that involves, not a regulator protein, but rather changes in the secondary structure of the mRNA. This regulatory process is illustrated in Figure 3.12 using the *His* operon, which encodes the enzymes necessary for the biosynthesis of the amino acid L-histidine, as an example. In enteric bacteria, attenuation is a common means of controlling biosynthetic operons. Note that it differs from the repression mechanism in that it requires no special regulatory gene or regulatory proteins.

Attenuation as a means of controlling biosynthetic operons

There are many instances known in which groups of genes that are independently controlled as members of different operons must cooperate to accomplish some response to an environmental change. When such a group of genes is subject to the control of a common regulator, the group is called a *regulon.* One such regulon, or global control system, is *catabolite*

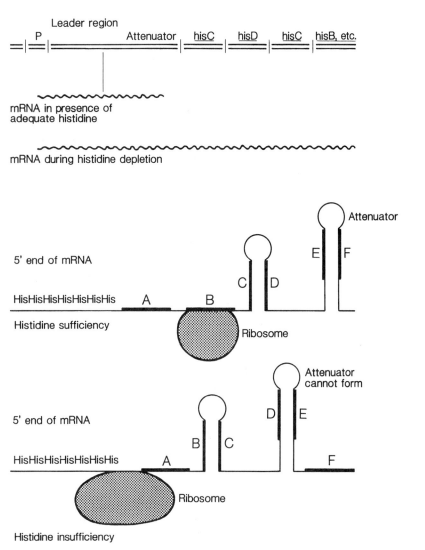

3.12 Schematic representation of the control of transcription by the process of attenuation. The example chosen is the *His* operon of *E. coli*. How attenuation works is fascinating. The leader region is always transcribed and translated into a small oligopeptide. The peptide near the attenuator site has a string of 7 *His* codons. Movement of the first ribosome coming behind the polymerase is drastically affected by the supply of charged *His* tRNA. If there is an adequate supply, the ribosome does not get delayed, and an attenuator loop forms in the mRNA, causing transcription to terminate. With a shortage of histidine, the first ribosome gets hung up over the *His* codons, and the attenuator loop is not formed, because alternate loops form. As a result, transcription proceeds, the complete *His* mRNA is made, and the biosynthetic enzymes can be made in large quantities.

The catabolite repression regulon ensures optimal use of preferred substrates

repression. Its function is to prevent the cell from responding to the presence of alternative carbon sources when the environment already provides a more than adequate supply from the preferred substrate, glucose. This control is brought about as follows. Operons that encode catabolic enzymes (those responsible for initiating the utilization of carbon sources, such as lactose, maltose, arabinose, and other sugars and amino acids) have weak promoters that need help to promote high-level initiation of transcription by RNA polymerase. The help is supplied by a regulator protein called CAP (catabolite activator protein) or CRP (cAMP receptor protein). This protein—if and only if cyclic AMP is bound to it—binds slightly upstream from the promoter and permits high-level expression if the operon is specifically induced (ie, and repressor has been removed by induction). Because cAMP levels are very low during growth on glucose or other favored substrates, there is insufficient cAMP–CRP complex to activate catabolic operons even if their inducers are present in the environment. As a result, the cells ignore the induction signal if they have an adequate supply of glucose.

Cell Survival

Cell Stress Regulons

The catabolite repression regulon is in essence a means by which the cell can optimize its synthesis of catabolic enzymes by making only those that will contribute to growth. But this regulon can also be viewed as a survival device, helping the cell to respond to the nutritional stress of running out of glucose. If an alternative source of carbon is present in the environment, the cell can redirect its pattern of gene expression to make a suitable adjustment to the nutritional stress.

From studies with *E. coli,* it is becoming appreciated that cells have many regulons involved in survival responses during difficult circumstances. One is the SOS system, a set of 17 genes that are turned on when the cell suffers damage to its DNA. The products of these genes are involved in several processes that repair damaged DNA and prevent cell division during the repair. Another is the heat-shock response, which is the expression of the HTP (high-temperature proteins) regulon. It encompasses 17 or more genes, which are transcriptionally activated by a shift-up in temperature. In the case of *E. coli,* the HTP regulator protein is a new subunit, called sigma-32, which replaces the sigma-70 subunit of RNA polymerase and reprograms this enzyme to recognize the special promoters of heat-shock genes. The specific functions of the heat-shock genes are not yet understood, but failure to induce them is lethal at even 42°C. Fever in humans can elevate body temperature sufficient to induce the heat-shock response, and it is suspected that this response may affect the outcome of various infections. Also, some viruses both of bacteria and humans utilize the heat-shock proteins of their host cells to promote their own replication.

Other regulons deal with cell survival in the face of such stresses as osmotic shock, high or low pH, oxidation damage, and the presence of toxic metal ions. Every bacterial culture exhibits a dramatic survival response at the end of the culture growth cycle; perhaps 100 or more changes occur that appear designed to foster survival in the stationary phase.

Perhaps the most elaborate bacterial survival responses are sporulation and chemotaxis. The former has been discussed in Chapter 2; the latter is presented here.

Motility and Chemotaxis

Motility in most bacterial species is the property of swimming by means of flagellar propulsion. The complex structure of a flagellum—its filament, hook, and basal body—has been presented in Chapter 2. The helical filament functions as a propeller, the hook possibly as a universal joint, and the basal body with its rod and rings as a motor anchored in the envelope. The flagellar motors turn the filaments using energy directly from the electrochemical gradient (protonmotive force) of the cell membrane rather than from ATP as energy. The filament can be rotated either clockwise or counterclockwise. Whatever the number of flagella on a cell and whatever their arrangement on the surface (polar, peritrichous, or lophotrichous), all are synchronized to rotate simultaneously in the same direction. Only counterclockwise rotation results in productive vectorial motion, called a *run*. Clockwise rotation of the flagella causes the cell to *tumble* in place. The flagella alternate between periods of clockwise and counterclockwise rotation according to an endogenous schedule. As a result, motile bacteria move in brief runs interrupted by periods of tumbling.

SOS system repairs damaged DNA and prevents multiplication during repair

Heat-shock genes are expressed at high temperature and allow cell survival

Flagellar motor uses protonmotive force energy

Direction of flagellar rotation determines a run or a tumble

Chemotaxis is directed movement toward chemical attractants and away from chemical repellents. It is accomplished by a remarkable molecular sensory system that possesses many of the characteristics that would be expected of behavioral systems in higher animals, including memory and adaptation. Beside the genes of the flagellar proteins (called *fla,* for *flag*-ella) over 30 genes (called *mot,* for *motility,* and *che,* for *che*motaxis) encode the proteins that make this system work: receptors, signalers, transducers, tumble regulators, and motors.

Whether a cell is moving toward an attractant or away from a repellent, chemotaxis is achieved by *biased random walks.* These result from alter-ations in the frequency of tumbling. When a cell is, by chance, progressing toward an attractant, tumbling is suppressed and the run is long; if it is swimming away, tumbling occurs sooner and the run is brief. It is sheer chance in what direction a cell is pointed at the end of a tumble, but by regulating the frequency of tumbles in this manner, directed progress is made.

The mechanism of chemotaxis is fairly well understood from work with *E. coli.* Small molecules diffuse through the pores of the outer membrane and bind to protein *receptors* in the cell membrane, either directly or after binding to specific *binding proteins* in the periplasm. Dozens of such chem-oreceptors are known. The stimulant—receptor complex interacts with one or another *methyl-accepting chemotaxis protein* (MCP). The MCPs relay the signal, depending on the extent of their methylation, to several cytosol proteins called the *tumble regulator complex.* As a result, a tumble regulator protein is released from the complex, binds to a flagellar motor protein, and causes the productive (counterclockwise) rotation of the flagella to be maintained. However, the MCP becomes methylated in this process. As a result, its activity as a signaler is reduced, and this causes *accommo*-*dation.* Accommodation results in the release of a different protein from the tumble regulator complex, which combines with another flagellar motor protein to cause clockwise rotation and, hence, tumbling. If by now the cell is in a higher concentration of stimulant, a new positive signal is generated faster than the endogenous schedule.

All this can be summarized as follows: binding of an attractant alters the endogenous routine schedule of runs and tumbles by prolonging the runs. Accommodation by methylation restores the endogenous schedule and resets the cell's sensitivity to the attractant to require a higher con-centration to prolong the run. This constitutes a molecular memory. The bacterial cell senses a concentration gradient not by measuring a difference between the concentration at each end of the cell, but by a molecular memory that enables it to compare the concentration now with what it was a short time ago. Escape from a repellent occurs in an analogous fashion.

Chemotaxis is both a survival device (for avoiding toxic substances) and a growth-promoting device (for finding food). It can also be a virulence factor in facilitating colonization of the human host by bacteria.

Special Attributes of the Colonizers of Humans

The ability to grow and to survive harsh conditions is possessed by most bacteria. Yet of the thousands of bacterial species, only a small percentage are associated with humans as part of the natural flora or as causative agents of disease. This fact generates the question that has been central to medical microbiology from the very start: what makes a bacterium pathogenic? The answer is not simple, because it turns out that many properties are

(margin notes)

Multiple genes required for chemotactic ability

Changes in duration of runs and tumbles determine chemotactic response

Molecular memory recognizes change in attractant concentration and ensures progress toward it

Chemotaxis serves survival, growth-promoting, and, sometimes, pathogenetic roles

Many bacterial structures and activities contribute to virulence

necessary for a bacterial cell to gain entrance to a human, evade its defense systems, and establish an infection. Virulence is a multigene property.

The structures and activities described in Chapter 2 and this chapter bear directly on virulence attributes of bacteria. They include the ability to colonize and penetrate epithelial surfaces, evade phagocytic and immunological attack, secrete toxic proteins, and survive adverse conditions both within and outside the body. These aspects will be considered further in Chapter 9.

Additional Reading

Ingraham, J.L., Maaløe, O., and Neidhardt, F.C. 1983. *Growth of the Bacterial Cell.* Sunderland, Mass.: Sinauer Associates, Inc. Chapters 2 and 3 of this book present bacterial metabolism in a manner similar to what was done here, but it is more detailed.

Lin, E.C.C., Goldstein, R., and Syvanen, M. 1984. *Bacteria, Plasmids,* and *Phages.* Cambridge, Mass.: Harvard University Press. A simplified account of bacterial metabolism and nutrition is presented in Chapter 3. Growth of bacterial cultures is presented with great clarity in Chapter 4. Gene expression and regulatory mechanisms are presented in Chapter 5 more fully than was done here.

Stanier, R.Y., Ingraham, J.L., Wheelis, M.L., and Painter, P.R. 1986. *The Microbial World.* 5th ed., Englewood Cliffs, N.J.: Prentice-Hall. This general textbook contains excellent descriptions of bacterial metabolism (Chapters 4 and 5) and growth (Chapters 7 and 8).

4

The Bacterial Cell:
Genetic Determinants of Growth, Survival, and Colonization

Frederick C. Neidhardt

Bacterial Variation and Inheritance

It was rather difficult to establish that many of the same rules of heredity apply to bacteria as well as to plants and animals. This may seem strange, because the most spectacular advances in molecular genetics have been achieved almost exclusively through work on *Escherichia coli* and its viruses. However, during the 1940s and early 1950s, serious experimental efforts were still being directed toward the question of whether mutations in bacteria were random or specifically directed by the environment.

The difficulty of establishing the basis of heredity in bacteria grew out of their inherent properties and their manner of growth. First, bacteria being *haploid,* the consequences of a mutation, even a recessive one, are immediately evident in the mutant cell. Because the generation time of bacteria is short, it does not take many hours for a mutant cell that has arisen by chance to become a significant component of a culture under appropriate selective conditions. This can lead to the false conclusion that the environment has directed a genetic change. Second, as was noted in Chapter 3, bacteria, to a far greater extent than animals and plants, respond to change in their chemical and physical environment by altering their pattern of gene function, thereby taking on previously unexpressed properties. For example, *E. coli* cells make the enzymes for lactose metabolism only when grown with this sugar as carbon source. Superficially this might suggest that lactose changes the cell's *genotype* (its complement of genes), when instead it is only the *phenotype* (the characteristics actually displayed by the cell) that has been changed by the environment. Finally, even when rather exceptional technical measures are taken to assure a pure culture, contamination can occasionally occur. With cultures containing more than one bacterial species, different conditions of growth can cause one or another species to predominate (by, for example, a million to one ratio), suggesting to the unwary observer that the characteristics of "the bacterium" under study are very unstable and dependent on the environment.

Mutations are rapidly expressed; mutants quickly predominate under selective conditions

Environment can influence phenotype expression of genotype

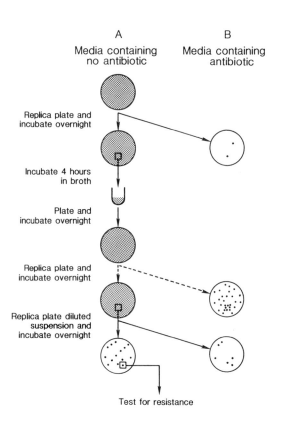

4.1 Lederberg technique for indirect selection of antimicrobic resistant mutants. Growth on plates in the left-hand column (**A**) is replicated to antimicrobic containing plates in the right-hand column (**B**). If resistant mutants arose in the absence of antimicrobic (**A**), the position of colonies on antimicrobic containing plates would indicate their position on the plates that do not contain antimicrobic. By selecting growth from this position and repeating the process with appropriate inoculum dilutions, resistant mutants that have never been exposed to antimicrobic can be directly selected (**A**).

Progress in bacterial genetics was rapid once it was recognized that mutation and selection can quickly change the makeup of a growing population, and that bacterial cells inherit genes that may or may not be expressed depending on the environment. Even so, it was not until the discovery in the 1980s of transposable genetic elements and insertion sequences (to be discussed later in this chapter) that certain examples of high-frequency variation—the so-called *phase transition* could be satisfactorily explained within the framework of classical genetic principles.

Several experiments were particularly important in establishing that mutations occur in nature as random events and are not guided by the environment. The most convincing introduced the technique of replica plating and was used to show how a population of cells totally resistant to an antimicrobic could be isolated from an initially sensitive population without ever exposing them to the toxic agent (Figure 4.1). This clarified the mechanism of an important clinical problem.

Proof of random occurrence of bacterial mutations

Mutation and Repair

The spontaneous development of mutations is a major factor in the evolution of bacteria. Mutations occur in nature at a low frequency (on the order of one mutation in every million cells for any one gene).

Kinds of Mutations

Mutations are heritable changes in the structure of genes. The normal, usually active, form of a gene is called the *wild-type allele:* the mutated, usually inactive, form is called the *mutant allele.* There are several kinds of mutations, based on the nature of the change in nucleotide sequence of the affected gene(s). *Replacements* involve the substitution of one base for another. *Microdeletions* and *microinsertions* are the removal or addition, respectively, of a single nucleotide (and its complement in the opposite strand). *Insertions* involve the addition of many base pairs of nucleotides at a single site. *Deletions* remove a contiguous segment of many base pairs.

Change in nucleotide sequence

By recalling the nature of genes and how their nucleotide sequence directs the synthesis of proteins, one can understand the immediate consequence of each of these biochemical changes. If a replacement mutation in a codon changes the mRNA transcript to a different amino acid, it is called a *missense mutation* [eg, an AAG (lysine) to a GAG (glutamate)]. The resulting protein may be enzymatically inactive or very sensitive to environmental conditions, such as temperature. If the replacement changes a codon specifying an amino acid to one specifying none, it is called a *nonsense mutation* [eg, a UAC (tyrosine) to UAA (STOP)], and the truncated product of the mutated gene is called a *nonsense fragment.* Microdeletions and microinsertions cause *frame shift mutations*—changes in the reading frame by which the ribosomes translate the mRNA from the mutated gene. Frame shifts usually result in polymerization of a stretch of incorrect amino acids until a nonsense codon is encountered, so the product is usually a truncated polypeptide fragment with an incorrect amino acid sequence at its *N*-terminus. Deletion or insertion of a segment of base pairs from a gene will shorten or lengthen the protein product if the number of base pairs deleted or inserted is divisible evenly by 3; otherwise it will also bring about the consequence of a frame shift. These mutations are summarized in Table 4.1.

One biochemical consequence of gene mutation that is unexpected is that many mutations, particularly if they occur near the end of a gene, prevent the expression of all genes downstream (away from the promoter) of the mutated gene. Such *polar mutations* are thought to exert their effect on neighboring genes by the termination of transcription of downstream genes when translation of the mRNA of the mutated gene is blocked by a nonsense codon.

There is a certain natural frequency of mutations, brought about by errors in replication, but various environmental and biological agents can increase the frequency greatly. Different types of mutations are increased selectively by different agents, as listed in Table 4.1.

Mutagenic agents

Mutations may also be classified according to their biological consequences. Some mutations change the susceptibility of a cell to an antimicrobic or other toxic agent; these *resistance mutations* might, for example, affect the structure of certain cell proteins in such a way that the agent cannot enter the cell or cannot inactivate its normal target. Some mutations, called *auxotrophic,* affect the production of a biosynthetic enzyme and result in a nutritional requirement of the mutant cell for the amino acid, nucleotide, vitamin, or other biosynthetic product it can no longer make for itself. The wild type from which the mutant was derived is said to be *prototrophic* for that nutrient. Some mutations affect a gene whose product is essential for growth and cannot be bypassed nutritionally; these are called *lethal mutations.* If the product of a mutated gene is active in some circumstances, but inactive under others (eg, high or low temperature), the mutation is called *conditional* (meaning *conditionally expressed*). The most common kind of conditional mutation is one in which the protein product of the mutated gene is inactive at a normally physiological temperature, but active at a higher or lower temperature, and these are called *temperature sensitive mutations.*

Table 4.1 Mutations

Type	Causative Agent	Consequence
Replacement		
Transition: pyrimidine replaced by a pyrimidine or a purine by a purine	Base analogs, UV, deaminating and alkylating agents, spontaneous	Transitions and transversions: nonsense codon formed, truncated peptide; missense codon formed, altered protein
Transversion: purine replaced by a pyrimidine or vice versa	Spontaneous	
Deletion		
Macrodeletion: large nucleotide segment deleted	HNO_2, radiation, bifunctional alkylating agents	Truncated peptide; other products possible, such as fusion peptides
Microdeletion: one or two nucleotides deleted	Same as macrodeletions	Frameshift, usually resulting in nonsense codon and truncated peptide
Insertion		
Macroinsertion: large nucleotide segment inserted	Transposons or IS elements	Interrupted gene yielding truncated product
Microinsertion: one or two nucleotides inserted	Acridine	Frameshift, usually resulting in nonsense codon yielding a truncated product
Inversion	IS or IS-like elements	Many possible effects

Reversion and Suppression of Mutations

Back mutations rare because highly specific corrections are needed

A *reversion*, or *back mutation*, is the conversion of a mutated gene back to its original wild-type allele. True back mutation can occur, but at a low frequency, because a very specific and improbable event is required. Much more commonly observed is the conversion of a mutant cell into one that is phenotypically identical to the original wild-type bacterium for the affected character, but which still retains the original mutation. These *suppressor* mutations can arise in several ways. Within the mutated codon a second mutation can create a new codon specifying the original amino acid. Alternatively, secondary mutations in other codons of the mutated gene can lead to a change in amino acid sequence that results in an active product despite the continued presence of the original amino acid error.

Suppressor mutations reestablish phenotype of mutated wild type

Suppressing mutations can even occur in genes other than the one that was originally mutated: for example, when two proteins interact to perform a function, the mutant form of one may be active when combined with a mutant form of the other. Another example involves tRNA molecules, the translators of the genetic code, which can themselves be altered by mutation; it is possible for a mutant tRNA to "mistake" a mutant codon and insert the original correct amino acid—a case of two wrongs making a right.

Repair of DNA Damage

Many mutagenic agents directly alter the structure of DNA, and some are ubiquitous components of our environment (heat, sunlight, acid, oxidants, and alkylating agents). It is not surprising, therefore, to learn that bacteria have evolved multiple biochemical mechanisms for repairing damaged DNA. In *E. coli,* for example, over 30 genes are known to be involved in DNA repair; many of these are members of the SOS response discussed in Chapter 3. Collectively these repair systems can remove thymine dimers produced by ultraviolet (UV) irradiation, can remove methyl or ethyl groups placed on guanine residues, can excise bases damaged by deamination or ring breakage and replace them with authentic residues, and can recognize and repair DNA depurinated by acid or heat. In large measure these repair systems utilize the fact that DNA is double stranded. Damage is recognized by the mispairing it causes, and the information on one strand is used to direct the proper repair of the damaged strand. Also, a *proofreading* process operates during DNA replication to detect any mismatch between each newly polymerized base and its mate in the template strand. Mismatches are excised to permit repolymerization with the properly matched nucleotide. Failures of this proofreading process can be detected and handled by an excision and resynthesis system similar to those that recognize and repair chemically damaged DNA.

One system bypasses DNA damaged by UV irradiation, when repair has failed, by directing replication to proceed across a region badly damaged by the formation of thymine dimers. This *error prone replication* is responsible for the mutations induced by UV light.

Genetic Exchange

Mutation and selection are important factors in bacterial evolution, but evolution proceeds far faster than it could by these processes alone. For instance, the probability that the process of random mutation alone can produce a cell that, let us say, requires five mutations for optimal growth in a new environment is terribly low. It is in fact the product of the individual mutation frequencies (eg, $10^{-6} \times 10^{-6} \times 10^{-6} \times 10^{-6} \times 10^{-6} = 10^{-30}$) that essentially precludes a natural population from ever acquiring the new property in this manner. Such alterations occur, however, because organisms exchange genetic material, thereby permitting combinations of mutations to be collected in individual cells.

Despite the fact that bacteria reproduce exclusively asexually, the sharing of genetic information within and between related species is now recognized to be quite common and to occur in at least three fundamentally different ways. All three processes involve a one-way transfer of DNA from a *donor cell* to a *recipient cell.* The molecule of DNA introduced into the recipient is called the *exogenote* to distinguish it from the cell's own original chromosome called the *endogenote.*

One process of DNA transfer, called *transformation,* involves the release of DNA into the environment by the lysis of some cells, followed by the direct uptake of that DNA by the recipient cells. By another means of transfer, called *transduction,* the DNA is introduced into the recipient cell by a nonlethal virus that has grown on the donor cell. The third process, called *conjugation,* involves actual contact between donor and recipient cell during which DNA is transferred as part of a plasmid (an autonomously replicating, extrachromosomal molecule of circular double-stranded DNA); in conjugation, donor and recipient cells are referred to

---

Multiple genes involved in DNA repair; damage recognized by mispairing of strands

Bacterial evolution is speeded by exchange of genetic material

Processes of genetic transfer

Transformation, transduction, and conjugation

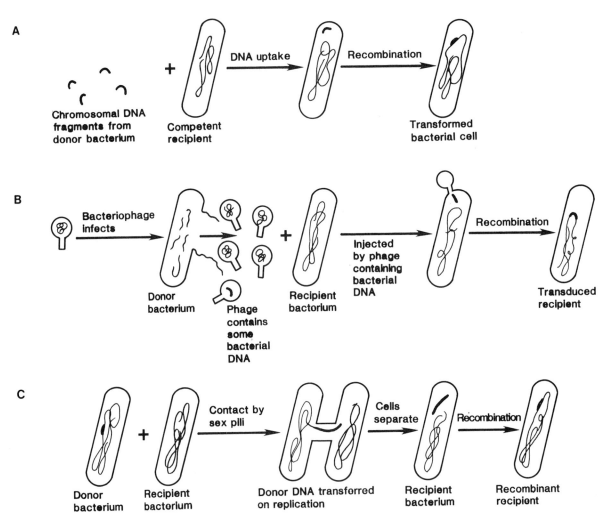

4.2 Chromosomal gene transfer mechanisms in bacteria. (**A**) Transformation. (**B**) Transduction. (**C**) Conjugation.

as male and female respectively. The three means of gene transfer are summarized in Figure 4.2.

Species of bacteria differ in their ability to transfer DNA, but all three mechanisms are distributed among both Gram-positive and Gram-negative species. However, only transformation is governed by bacterial chromosomal genes. Transduction is totally mediated by virus genes, and conjugation, by plasmid genes.

Transformation, transduction, and conjugation mediated by chromosomal, viral, and plasmid genes, respectively

Transformation

Transformation was first demonstrated in 1928 by F. Griffith (a British public health officer) who showed that virulent encapsulated *Streptococcus pneumoniae* (pneumococci) that had been killed by heat could confer on living avirulent nonencapsulated pneumococci the ability to make the polysaccharide capsule of the killed organisms and thus become virulent for mice. Subsequent work in 1944 by O. T. Avery, C. M. MacLeod, and

Early studies on pneumococcal transformation

M. McCarty at the Rockefeller Institute revealed that the "transforming factor" from the dead pneumococci was nothing other than DNA. This discovery had enormous impact on biology, because it was the first rigorous demonstration that DNA is the macromolecule in which genetic information is encoded. It opened the door to modern molecular genetics.

The ability to take up DNA from the environment is called *competence,* and in many species of bacteria, it is encoded by chromosomal genes that become active under certain environmental conditions. In such species, transformation can occur readily and is said to be *natural.* Other species cannot enter the competent state, but can be made permeable to DNA by treatment with agents that damage the cell envelope making an *artificial transformation* possible.

Natural transformation must be important in nature, judged by the variety of mechanism that different bacteria have evolved to accomplish it. Two of the best-studied systems are those of the Gram-positive pneumococcus and a Gram-negative rod, *Haemophilus influenzae.* Pneumococcal cells secrete a protein *competence factor* that induces many of the cells of a culture to synthesize special proteins necessary for transformation, including an autolysin that exposes a cell membrane DNA-binding protein. Any DNA present in the medium is bound indiscriminately—even salmon sperm DNA can be bound and taken up as readily as DNA from another *S. pneumoniae* cell. The surface-bound double-stranded DNA is cleaved into fragments of about 6–8 kilobases. One strand is degraded by a nuclease, while the complementary strand of each fragment is taken up by a process that seems to be driven by the protonmotive force of the cell membrane (see Chapter 3). The fate of the internalized DNA fragment then depends on whether it is homologous (the same or similar in base sequence) to a portion of the recipient cell's DNA, in which case recombination can occur (by a process described below), or heterologous (no similarity to the endogenote), in which case it is degraded and causes no heritable change in the recipient.

Transformation in *H. influenzae* is somewhat different. There is no competence factor, and cells become competent merely by growth in an environment rich in nutrients. Only homologous DNA (ie, DNA from the same or a closely related species of *Haemophilus*) is taken up, and it is taken up in double-stranded form. The selectivity is brought about by the presence of a special membrane protein that binds to an 11-base pair sequence (5′-AAGTGCGGTCA-3′) that occurs frequently in *Haemophilus* DNA and infrequently in other DNAs. Following binding to molecules of this protein, the homologous DNA is internalized by a mechanism that resembles membrane invagination, resulting in the temporary residence of the exogenote in cytoplasmic membrane vesicles. Although the DNA taken up is double stranded, only one of the two strands participates in the subsequent recombination with the endogenote.

The common use of *E. coli* as a host cell in which to clone genes on hybrid plasmids (see Genetic Engineering section of this Chapter) depends on procedures involving treatment with salt and temperature shocks to bring about artificial transformation; this organism has no natural competence mechanism.

Transduction

Transduction is virus-mediated transfer of genetic information from donor to recipient cell. To understand transduction and its several mechanisms, it is necessary to preview the nature of bacterial viruses, a topic dealt with more extensively in Chapters 5, 6, and 7.

Genes encoding competence activated by environmental conditions

Pneumococcal competence exposes a protein that binds any DNA

Portion of DNA strand combines with any homologous chromosomal DNA

H. influenzae endocytoses only homologous double-stranded DNA

Artificial transformation of *E. coli* for gene cloning

Viruses are capable of reproduction only inside living cells. Those that grow in bacteria are called *bacteriophages,* or simply *phages.* They are minimally composed of protein and nucleic acid, although some may have a very complex structure and composition. The individual virus particle or *virion* consists of a protein *capsid* enclosing genomic nucleic acid, which is either RNA or DNA, but never both. Virions infect sensitive cells by adsorbing to specific receptors on the cell surface and then, in the case of phages, injecting their DNA or RNA. Phages come in two functional varieties according to what happens after injection of the viral nucleic acid. *Virulent* (-lytic) phages cause lysis of the host bacterium as a culmination of the synthesis of many new virions within the infected cell. *Temperate* phages may initiate a lytic growth process of this sort or can enter a quiescent form (called a *prophage*) in which the infected host cell is permitted to proceed about its business of growth and division, but passes on to its descendents a prophage genome capable of being *induced* to produce phage in a process nearly identical to the growth of lytic phages. The bacterial cell that harbors a latent prophage is said to be a *lysogen* (capable of producing lytic phages), and its condition is referred to as *lysogeny.* Lysogens are immune to infection by virions of the type they harbor as prophage. Occasionally lysogens are spontaneously induced and lysed by the phage and release mature virions (as many as 75–150 or more per cell) into the environment. When triggered by UV irradiation or certain chemicals, an entire population of lysogens will be induced simultaneously to initiate reproduction of their latent virus followed by lysis of the host cells. Infection of a sensitive cell with the temperate phage can lead either to lysis or lysogeny. How this choice comes about is described in Chapter 7.

The prophage of different temperate phages exist in one of two different states. In one, the prophage DNA is physically integrated into a bacterial chromosome; in the second, it remains separate from the chromosome as an independently replicating, circularized, molecule of DNA. Prophages of this sort are in fact plasmids.

For the most part, transduction is mediated by temperate phage, and the two broad types of transduction result from the different physical forms of prophage and the different means by which the transducing virion is formed. These are termed *generalized transduction,* by which any bacterial gene stands an equal chance of being transduced to a recipient cell, and *specialized* or *restricted transduction,* by which only a few genes can be transduced.

Generalized Transduction.   Some phages package DNA into their capsids in a nonspecific way, the *headful mechanism,* in which any DNA can be stuffed into the capsid head until it is full. (The head is the principal structure of the virion to which, in some cases, a tail is attached. See Chapter 5.) An endonuclease then trims off any projecting excess. If fragments of host cell DNA are around during the assembly of mature virions, they can become packaged in place of virus DNA, resulting in *pseudovirions.* Pseudovirions are the transducing agents. They can adsorb to sensitive cells and inject the DNA they contain as though it were viral DNA. The result is the introduction of donor DNA into the recipient cell.

Any given gene has an equal probability of being transduced by this process. With the temperate phage P1 of *E. coli,* this probability is approximately one transduction event per 10^5 to 10^8 virions, because nearly 1 out of every 1000 phage particles made in a P1 lytic infection are pseudovirions, and the bacterial DNA fragments packaged are 1–2% of the length of the chromosome. Cotransduction of two bacterial genes by a single pseudovirion occurs only if they are located close together within

Bacteriophage structure, infection, and replication

Bacteria can be lysogenized with prophage from temperate phage

Prophage induction yields lytic phage

Some prophages integrate; others behave as plasmids

Transduction mediated by temperate phage

Occasional phages carry a random piece of host DNA to a recipient

Any gene has equal but low probability of being transduced

this small length of the chromosome, and this fact facilitates mapping the position of a newly discovered gene.

Once injected into the host cell, the transduced DNA will be lost by degradation unless it can recombine with the chromosome of the recipient cell, usually by homologous recombination (see Genetic Recombination section of this chapter) in which both strands of the exogenote cross into and replace the homologous segment of the recipient's chromosome. Sometimes, however, the exogenote can persist without degradation by assuming a stable circular configuration. In this interesting situation, called *abortive transduction,* there is only linear transmission of the exogenote to one of the two daughter cells of the transduced recipient, one of the four granddaughters, one of the eight greatgranddaughters, and so on.

Specialized Transduction. It has been noted that the prophage of some phages is integrated into the lysogen's chromosome. This integration does not occur haphazardly, but is restricted to usually one site, called *att (at-tachment)* site. When a lysogen carrying such a prophage is induced to produce virions, excision of the viral genome from the bacterial chromosome occasionally (eg, in 1 out of 10^5 to 10^6 lysogens) occurs imprecisely, resulting in a pickup of genes of the bacterium adjacent to the *att* site. The resulting virion may be infectious (if no essential phage genes are missing), or defective (if one or more essential genes are missing). In either case, adsorption to a sensitive cell and injection of the DNA can occur, and integration of the aberrant phage genome into the chromosome of the new host cell results in the formation of a lysogen containing a few genes that have been transduced as hitchhikers with the phage genome. Integration of the phage genome automatically accomplishes the recombinational event needed to guarantee reproduction of the transduced genes. Only genes that border the *att* site stand a chance of being transduced by this process, which is why it is called specialized or restricted transduction.

Because the original pickup event is rare, the first transducing process is termed *low-frequency transduction* (LFT). However, when a lysogenic transductant is, in turn, induced to produce phage, all of the new virions carry the originally transduced bacterial gene. The resulting mixture of lysed cells and virions now brings about *high-frequency transduction* (HFT) of the attached genes.

Bacterial geneticists have learned to move genes of interest near the phage integration site and thereby construct specialized transducing phages containing these genes. Such transducing phages are valuable aids to cloning and sequencing genes and to studying their function and regulation. Obviously a temperate phage that could form a prophage by integrating randomly at any site in the bacterial chromosome would be of special use. The temperate phage Mu of *E.coli* has this property.

Although both generalized and specialized transduction can be regarded as the result of errors in phage production, transfer of genes between bacterial cells by phage is a reasonably common phenomenom. It occurs at significant frequency in nature; for example, genes conferring antimicrobic resistance in staphylococci are often transduced from strain to strain in this way. Transduction is also used extensively as a tool in molecular biological research.

Conjugation

Conjugation leading to transfer of chromosomal genetic information from donor to recipient bacterial cell is plasmid mediated. Cell contact is required, and, hence, the process is frequently called *mating,* but all of the

---

Margin notes:

Generalized transduction involves homologous recombination

Specialized transduction involves prophage integration at specific site

Induction occasionally leads to incorporation of adjacent bacterial genes in phage

Hitchhiker genes cointegrated in chromosome with phage genes

All phages produced by lysogenic transductants carry original transduced gene

Value of specialized transduction in gene cloning and sequencing

Significance of transduction in nature

Conjugation is plasmid
encoded; requires cell contact

genes that govern it reside on plasmids resident within the donor (*male*) cells rather than on their chromosomes. Conjugation appears to differ between Gram-negative and Gram-positive species, as judged by its characteristics in two well-studied examples, *E.coli* and *Streptococcus faecalis*.

Conjugation among Gram-Negative Bacteria. Conjugation has been most studied in *E. coli* in which it is most often brought about by a plasmid called F (for fertility). These studies have been of particular importance because of the light they have thrown on the biology of plasmids generally.

E. coli F plasmid encodes sex
pilus, which binds F$^+$ to F$^-$
cell

Like all plasmids, the F plasmid consists of circular double-stranded DNA that is capable of replicating in the bacterial cell and being passed on to the daughter cells at the time of division. The F plasmid is also one of a class of plasmids called *conjugative* because they have the genetic ability to bring about their own transfer from one cell to another by conjugation. A cell harboring the F plasmid is designated F$^+$; one lacking it, F$^-$. Genes on this plasmid encode proteins that change the surface properties of the cell by producing a *sex pilus*. This structure, which is longer and thicker than a common pilus, facilitates the capture of an F$^-$ cell and the formation of a conjugation bridge through which DNA passes from the F$^+$ (called

F plasmid DNA passes from
F$^+$ to F$^-$ through conjugative
bridge

male) to the F$^-$ (called female) cell. This transfer of DNA is accomplished by a special replication of the F plasmid, called *transfer replication*. Transfer replication always begins at a point on the plasmid DNA called oriT (for *ori*gin of *t*ransfer). One strand directs synthesis of its complement within the donor (F$^+$, male) cell, while the other strand is driven through the conjugation bridge into the recipient (F$^-$, female) cell. Synthesis of a

Single DNA strand
transferred; complementary
strands resynthesized in
recipient and donor

strand complementary to the transferred strand occurs in the recipient cell while the transfer is in progress (Figure 4.3). The completed molecule circularizes, its genes are expressed, and it maintains itself by replication in the recipient cell, which is thus converted from F$^-$ (female) to F$^+$ (male). The recipient cell and all of its descendents than have the ability

F$^-$ recipient converted to F$^+$;
donor remains F$^+$

to conjugate with any F$^-$ cells they encounter. The original donor F$^+$ cell

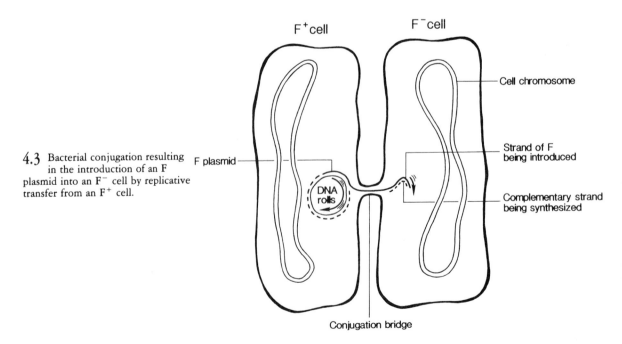

4.3 Bacterial conjugation resulting in the introduction of an F plasmid into an F$^-$ cell by replicative transfer from an F$^+$ cell.

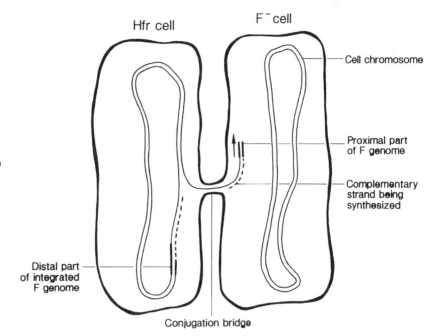

Hfr cell   F⁻ cell

Cell chromosome

Proximal part
of F genome

Complementary
strand being
synthesized

Distal part
of integrated
F genome

Conjugation bridge

4.4 Bacterial conjugation resulting in the introduction of chromosomal genes and a portion of the F plasmid genome into an F⁻ cell by replicative transfer from an Hfr cell.

remains F^+ because transfer replication has left an intact double-stranded F plasmid (Figure 4.3).

It is only the absence of the sex pilus that determines the mating behavior of the recipient cells, because if the sex pilus is lost from F^+ cells by physical shearing or by incubation of the cells for several hours in stationary phase, these genetically F^+ cells will behave as though they were F^-, that is, encounter with an F^+ cell will lead to conjugation. Cells that contain the F plasmid, but have lost their sex pilus are called F^- *phenocopies* (because their *pheno*typic behavior in mating *copies* that of genetically F^- cells).

Conjugation of an F^+ and an F^- cell thus normally leads to transfer of plasmid DNA, but does not involve chromosomal DNA. How do bacterial chromosomal genes get transferred?

F plasmid may integrate into chromosome to give Hfr cells

Transfer of chromosomal genes by conjugation is the result of encounters between F^- cells and rare cells in an F^+ culture, termed Hfr (*high frequency recombination*) cells that contain an F genome integrated into the chromosome. Integration occurs at a very low frequency at one of seven or eight chromosomal sites and results in linearization of the plasmid DNA as part of the giant circular chromosomal molecule. A cell with an integrated F factor resembles an F^+ male cell in many respects, including the synthesis of the sex pilus and the ability to form a conjugation bridge with an F^- cell. Transfer replication is initiated. However, this

DNA transfer from Hfr to F⁻ cells carries partial plasmid and chromosomal genes

process cannot readily transfer the complete F plasmid genome, because the F plasmid and the bacterial chromosome became integrated by a recombinational event that occurred at a site other than *oriT*. Thus, breaking the integrated plasmid DNA at *oriT* results in the formation of a linear strand in which the entire bacterial chromosome lies between two portions of the F genome (Figure 4.4). Transfer replication drives the leading segment of the F genome into the F^- cell, followed by bacterial genes one after the other. It would take about 100 min at 37°C for the entire bacterial genome to be transferred in this way. However, attachment between the mating cells is fragile and the conjugation bridge usually ruptures long before the entire bacterial chromosome with the trailing half of the F genome can be introduced into the F⁻ cell. As a result, only one part of the F genome and a variable length of the bacterial chromosome extending from the original site of integration of the F plasmid are transferred.

Hfr cells in the absence of F⁻ cells grow and divide normally, and every offspring of an Hfr cell has the same chromosomal configuration, with the F genome integrated at the same site and in the same clockwise or counterclockwise orientation. It is possible to select a colony derived from a single Hfr cell and thereby establish a pure culture in which every cell has an integrated F genome. In contrast to cultures of F⁺ strains, every cell in an Hfr culture has the ability to transfer chromosomal genes during mating. The process occurs identically in each mating pair and results in the transfer of bacterial chromosomal genes in a predictable linear order determined entirely by the site of integration of the original plasmid into the chromosome and the direction (clockwise or counterclockwise) of the integration. The longer the mating proceeds, the more distant genes transferred are found. Genes can thus be mapped as to their position on the chromosome by their time of entry into F⁻ cells. Distances on the chromosome of *E.coli* are therefore expressed in minutes. Different Hfr strains, formed by integration of the F plasmid at different sites and in different orientations, transfer bacterial chromosomal genes in different orders, as illustrated in Figure 4.5.

Conjugation between an Hfr and an F⁻ cell almost always leaves the recipient still F⁻, because of the unlikelihood of the complete F genome being transferred. The Hfr cell remains Hfr, because it retains a copy of the chromosome with its integrated F genome.

There is an additional wrinkle to chromosome transfer by conjugation in *E. coli*. It involves a process termed *sexduction* by which an F plasmid transfers from one cell to another a few bacterial chromosomal genes that it happens to contain. Here is how it comes about. The F genome in an Hfr cell can excise itself occasionally from the bacterial chromosome and

All Hfr offspring have F genome integrated at same site

Every cell in an Hfr culture can transfer genes in same sequence

Duration of mating determines number of chromosomal genes transferred

Incomplete transfer of F genome leaves recipient F⁻ in Hfr mating

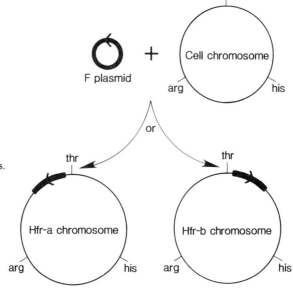

4.5 Integration of the F plasmid into the bacterial chromosome at two different sites, and with different orientations, resulting in the formation of two (or many possible) different Hfr chromosomes.

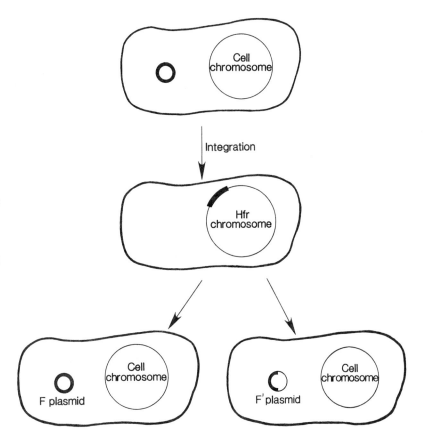

4.6 Integration of an F plasmid into a bacterial chromosome to form an Hfr chromosome, followed either by exact excision to reform the F plasmid or inexact excision to form an F′ plasmid containing some bacterial chromosome genes.

Excision of integrated F genome may include host genes in F′ plasmid

Sexduction involves transfer of F′ plasmid to F⁻ cell

S. faecalis coupling results from adhesin-receptor interactions

recircularize into plasmid form. Sometimes this excision is imperfect and leads to one or a few of the neighboring bacterial genes being included in the plasmid (Figure 4.6). The resulting hybrid plasmid is called F′ (F prime) to note its content of some bacterial DNA. The cell in which the F′ particle is formed is still haploid for all its genes, because the few incorporated into the F′ plasmid are missing from the chromosome. Transfer of the F′ plasmid into a normal F⁻ cell is called sexduction. The new F′ cell is designated a *secondary* F′ cell because it differs from the donor in being diploid for the genes introduced by the F′ plasmid. These cells are useful because they afford the opportunity of constructing mutations in one copy of an essential gene while maintaining one functional copy for cell survival. It is important to stress that part or all of these phenomena described for *E.coli* apply to other Gram-negative genera and species. They have simply been less well studied in detail. Furthermore, it must be understood that most transfers of genetic information by plasmids involve genes carried on the plasmid rather than on the chromosome. This will be considered later in the chapter.

Conjugation among Gram-Positive Bacteria. Conjugation in *S. faecalis* is mediated by plasmids, but there is also an involvement of chromosomal genes in the process. Donor and recipient cells do not couple by means of a sex pilus, but rather by the clumping of cells that contain a plasmid with those that do not. This clumping is the result of interaction between a proteinaceous *adhesin* on the surface of the donor (plasmid-containing) cell and a *receptor* on the surface of the recipient (plasmid-lacking) cell. Both types of cells make the receptor (possibly cell wall lipoteichoic acid), but only the plasmid-containing cell can make the adhesin, presumably because it is encoded by a plasmid gene. Interestingly, donor cells make the adhesin only when in the vicinity of recipient cells, because the recipients secrete small peptide *pheromones* that serve to notify the donor cells of the presence of recipients. Donor cells promptly make adhesin when they sense the pheromone, and, as a result, clumps are formed and plasmid DNA is transferred across conjugation bridges into the recipient cells held in the clumps. Pheromones are widely distributed among insects and other animals as sexual and other attractants.

Plasmid encoded *S. faecalis* adhesin is produced in response to recipient pheromone

All *S. faecalis* cells are genetically capable of making several (five or more) pheromones, each encoded by a chromosomal gene, but each specific for a different plasmid. Acquisition of a particular plasmid represses the synthesis of the pheromone specific for that plasmid. As a result, the cell containing a given plasmid no longer informs its neighbor that it is a potential recipient for that plasmid, but continues to send out pheromone signals for other plasmids that it could still receive by conjugation with a suitable donor. As a further guarantee that it and its neighbors will not respond to the pheromone specific for the plasmid already present in these cells, a competitive inhibitor is synthesized under the direction of a plasmid gene.

In addition to streptococcal species, species of *Bacillus, Staphylococcus,* and *Clostridium* have been found to contain conjugative plasmids. Conjugative transfer of genes has also been observed in a number of Gram-positive species in the absence of plasmid DNA, suggesting either that there has been an integration of plasmids into the chromosome, or that there is a method of conjugation independent of plasmids.

Plasmid transfer of resistance and virulence genes

Plasmids carrying genes encoding antimicrobic resistance, common pili and other adhesins, and some exotoxins are readily transferred by conjugation among Gram-positive bacteria in the natural environment as well as in the laboratory.

Genetic Recombination

However an exogenote is conveyed into a recipient cell, its effect depends on what happens after transfer. There are basically three possible fates. The exogenote DNA may be degraded by a nuclease, in which case no heritable change is brought about. It may be stabilized by circularization and remain separate from the endogenote. In this case, if it is unable to replicate, it will be unilinearly inherited (eg, abortive transduction), but if it is capable of self-replication, it will become established as an autonomous, inherited plasmid. The third possible fate is for recombination to occur between exogenote and endogenote, resulting in the formation of a partially hybrid chromosome with segments derived from each source. These possibilities are diagrammed in Figure 4.7.

Exogenote may be degraded, circularized, or integrated in recipient chromosome

In this section we shall examine some aspects of the third process, the formation of recombinant chromosomes following transformation, transduction, or conjugation.

Homologous Recombination

One mechanism by which an exogenote can recombine with the bacterial chromosome is called *homologous recombination*. Its name reflects one of the two requirements for this process; the exogenote must possess rea-

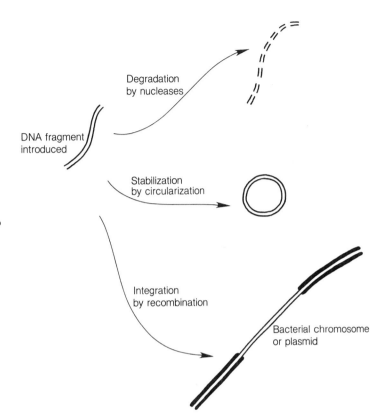

Degradation
by nucleases

DNA fragment
introduced

Stabilization
by circularization

4.7 Possible fates of a DNA
     fragment after transfer into
a bacterial cell.

Integration
by recombination

Bacterial chromosome
or plasmid

sonably large regions of nucleotide sequence identity or similarity to segments of the endogenote chromosome, because extensive base pairing
must occur between strands of the two recombining molecules.

The second requirement is that the recipient cell must possess the
genetic ability to make a set of enzymes that can bring about the covalent
substitution of a segment of the exogenote for the homologous region of
the endogenote. Not all the details are known, but the process includes
breaking one strand of each recombining molecule at a time and pairing
it with the unbroken, complementary strand of the other molecule. The
ends of the broken strands are partially digested, then repaired and joined
so that the rejoined strands are now continuous between the chromosomes. A protein known as RecA (*recombination*) controls the entire process. The same *breakage* and *reunion* process then links the second strand
of each recombining DNA molecule. This *crossover* event repeated further
down the chromosome results in the substitution of the exogenote segment between the two crossovers for the homologous segment of the
endogenote. This process is schematically presented in a very simplified
form in Figure 4.8.

Homologous recombination is responsible for integration of DNA fragments transferred by generalized transduction (eg, by phage P1), and by
plasmid-mediated conjugation (e.g., by Hfr-mediated conjugation). Recombination between the chromosome and DNA introduced by natural
transformation likewise requires homologous pairing of DNA strands, but
in this case it is only single-stranded exogenote DNA that pairs with the
appropriate region of the complementary strand of the endogenote. The
exogenote strand then displaces its nearly identical homologue, and break-

Recombination of double-
stranded DNA requires
nucleotide similarity and
crossover integration

Recombination of single-
stranded DNA produces
heterozygous chromosome

4.8 Homologous recombination.
(A) The central event in homologous recombination. Extensive base pairing between homologous regions of strands of two DNA molecules is illustrated. Events that accompany or follow this event include strand nicking, migration of the crossover point with partial digestion of the nicked strands, and resynthesis and ligation. Both strands of both recombining molecules must participate to effect a crossover event. **(B)** The result of homologous recombination. Two crossover events are necessary to achieve the exchange of segments shown.

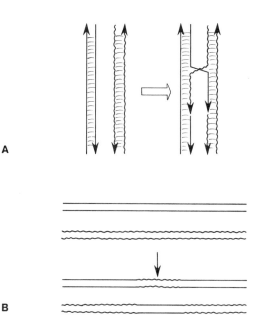

age and reunion results in the formation of a partially *heterozygous* chromosome in which, at the region of recombination, one strand is original and the other is derived from the exogenote. At the next round of DNA replication, one of the daughter chromosomes will therefore be a *homozygous* recombinant.

One daughter cell is homologous for transferred segment

Site-Specific Recombination

The second major type of recombination is actually a group of separate mechanisms that are RecA independent, that rely on only limited DNA sequence similarity at the sites of crossover, and that are mediated by different sets of specialized enzymes designed to catalyze recombination of only certain DNA molecules. Hence, one name for this group of mechanisms is *specialized recombination.* Its more common name, *site-specific recombination,* reflects the fact that these recombinational events are restricted to specific sites on one or both of the recombining DNA molecules.

RecA independent and occurs only at specific site

One good example of site-specific recombination has already been shown. The integration of some phage genomes into the chromosome occurs only at one site on the bacterial chromosome and one site on the phage chromosome. It was noted briefly that some phages, notably phage Mu, differ in being able to integrate almost anywhere in the bacterial chromosome. Because the site of recombination (the crossover site) in the Mu genome is the same in all cases, this, too, is a case of site-specific recombination.

The RecA-related set of enzymes apparently are sufficient only when extensive base pairing can occur. The enzymes that bring about site-specific recombination work on a different principle: unique DNA sequences are recognized and acted upon by specific recombination-generating enzymes. The unique DNA structures form the borders of the specific sites of integration or recombination; the specialized enzymes are usually encoded by genes on the exogenote.

Exogenote-encoded enzymes involved in site-specific integration

In addition to the special kind of recombination represented by pro-phage integration, a particular form of site-specific recombination occurs in other situations of enormous consequence to medical microbiology. These involve special genetic units called *transposable elements,* which have proven to be so important in the life of bacteria, particularly in their roles as agents of infectious disease, that a separate section must be devoted to their description.

Prophage and transposable element integration

Transposable Elements

Transposable elements are genetic units that are capable of mediating their own transfer from one chromosome to another, from one location to another on the same chromosome, or between chromosome and plasmid. This *transposition* relies on their ability to synthesize their own specific recombination enzyme.

Genetic units that move within and between chromosomes and plasmids

The three major kinds of transposable elements are *insertion sequence (IS) elements, transposons* (or Tn elements), and certain phages, such as Mu.

IS elements are segments of DNA of approximately 1000 base pairs. They encode enzymes for site-specific recombination and have distinctive nucleotide sequences at their termini. Different IS elements have different termini, but, as illustrated in Figure 4.9, a given IS element has the same sequence of nucleotides at each end, but in an inverted order. Only genes involved in transposition and in the regulation of its frequency are included in IS elements, and they are therefore the simplest transposable elements.

IS elements encode only their own insertion

Transposition, which occurs infrequently (approximately once every 10^5 to 10^7 generations), involves recognition by the transposition enzymes of the ends of the IS element and the selection of a target area into which a new copy of the IS element will be inserted. The original copy remains at its original site. Because transposition involves duplication of the IS element, the process is sometimes called *replicative recombination.* The molecular mechanism of transposition results in a duplication also of the nucleotide sequence of the chromosome at the site of insertion. Each IS element is, therefore, bounded by a short identical sequence (4–12 base pairs) on each end, and this duplicated sequence is different at each site of insertion of a particular IS element.

Transposition is by copy of original IS element; occurs at low frequency

IS elements bounded by identical sequence derived from site of insertion

Because IS elements contain only genes for transposition, their pres-

4.9 Structure of an insertion sequence (IS) element. The general features of bacterial IS elements are illustrated. As an example, IS2 has a total of 1327 base pairs (bp), of which there are terminal inverted repeat sequences of 41 base pairs flanking the central region that encodes the one or two proteins required for transposition of IS2. A direct repeat of 5 base pairs was created at the site of insertion of the element. Approximately five IS2 elements are found in the chromosome of many strains of *E.coli.*

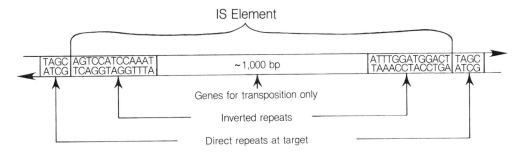

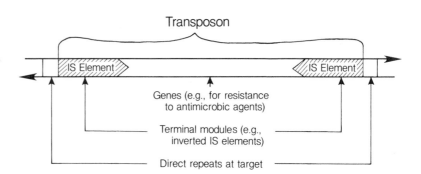

4.10 Structure of a transposon (Tn). The general features of bacterial transposons are illustrated. As an example, Tn9 has a total of 2500 base pairs. It consists of terminal direct repeat IS1 elements flanking a central region that contains a gene for chloramphenicol resistance and genes needed for transposition.

Insertion of IS element into a gene causes mutation

ence in a chromosome is not always easy to detect. If, however, an IS element transposes to a new site that is within a gene, this insertion is actually a mutation that alters or destroys the activity of the gene. Because most IS elements contain a transcription termination signal, the insertion also eliminates transcription of any genes downstream in the same operon. This property of IS elements led to their first recognition. Reversion of insertion mutations can occur by deletion, not transposition, because the latter does not delete the inserted element. The frequency of deletion is 100- to 1000-fold lower than insertion.

Numerous IS elements reside naturally at different locations in the *E. coli* chromosomes and in *E. coli* plasmids, for instance, and this has many consequences for the cell. Because their size is sufficient to permit strong base pairing between different copies of the same IS element, they can provide the basis for RecA-mediated homologous recombination. In this manner, the presence of particular IS elements in both the F plasmid and the bacterial chromosome provide a means for the formation of Hfr molecules by cointegration using IS sequence homology and the RecA system.

Base pairing between copies of IS elements can mediate homologous recombination

One of the major aspects of IS elements is that they are components of *transposons,* which are transposable segments of DNA containing genes beyond those needed for transposition. Transposons are as much as 10-fold larger than IS elements, because they are composite structures consisting of a central area of genes bordered by IS elements. The genes may code for such properties as antimicrobic resistance, substrate metabolism, or other functions. Some transposons are known in which the flanking regions are not exactly the same as independent IS elements, but strongly resemble them. A generalized transposon structure is shown in Figure 4.10.

Transposons comprise genes usually flanked by IS elements

Transposons can encode antimicrobic resistance

The IS or IS-like elements of a transposon are responsible for its transposability by replicative recombination. Beside the primary insertion reaction that was described for IS elements, all transposable units promote other types of DNA rearrangements, including deletion of sequences adjacent to a transposon, inversion of DNA segments, fusion of separate plasmids within a cell to form a cointegrate structure, similar fusions that integrate plasmids with cell chromosome, and repeated duplications that result in *amplification* of genes within transposons. All of these events have great significance for understanding the formation and spread of antimicrobic resistance through natural populations of pathogenic organisms. These subjects are dealt with in the description of plasmids in the next section.

Transposable units can produce genetic rearrangements, duplications, and amplification

The third type of transposable element is transposable prophage, such as that of bacteriophage Mu, which has the alternative of lytic growth or of lysogeny. During lysogeny the prophage of Mu can insert virtually anywhere in the *E. coli* chromosome and later can transpose itself from one location to another. It is, in fact, a transposon. When it integrates within a bacterial gene, it inactivates it in the same manner as any other transposable element. It was originally recognized as a virus that causes *mu*tation, hence, its name.

This concludes the discussion of the two main types of bacterial genetic recombination—homologous recombination and site-specific recombination—but it would not be complete without mention of the fact that a third sort of recombinational process exists. It has been called *illegitimate recombination* (because it does not obey the legitimate laws governing homologous and site-specific recombination). Little is known other than it results in some types of gene duplications and deletions.

Recombination Regulation of Gene Expression

A fascinating aspect of DNA rearrangements brought about by genetic recombination is that the expression of some chromosomal genes important in virulence are actually controlled by recombinational events. All the known cases involve *phase variation* of surface antigens. In *Neisseria gonorrhoeae,* the bacteria causing gonorrhoea, various genes encoding antigenically different pili are expressed depending on which one has been brought into a special expression site; the genes are otherwise silent because they lack effective promoters. Insertion of a pilin gene into the expression site and its replacement by another gene copy at a later time occurs by a process somewhat related to site-specific recombination. The whole process resembles the insertion of cassette tapes into a tape player and, therefore, is referred to as the *cassette mode* of gene regulation.

A different DNA rearrangement is responsible for the alternation of expression of antigenically distinct flagellins, H1 and H2, in *Salmonella* species. An *invertible element* of 995 base pairs lies between the two flagellin genes. The H2-encoding gene lies in an operon that also encodes a repressor for the H1-encoding gene. The latter gene is, therefore, active only if the former operon is inactive. Activity of the H2 operon, which lacks its own promoter, depends on a promoter within the invertible element. In one orientation, this promoter can initiate transcription of the H2-encoding gene; in the other orientation transcription, if it starts, proceeds in the opposite direction, and the H2-encoding gene is silent, allowing the H1-encoding gene to work. In this manner, excision of the invertible element and its reinsertion at the same site but in the opposite orientation leads to a shift from one flagellar form to the other (ie, to antigenic phase variation). The invertible element encodes its own site-specific *recombinase enzyme* that catalyzes the inversion in response to currently unknown signals.

The third example involves an invertible element too small to encode its own recombinase. It is a 314–base-pair segment located on the *E.coli* chromosome adjacent to the gene *fimA* encoding the structural protein for common pili (or *fim*briae). These pili function as an adhesin in mediating the binding of *E. coli* to eukaryotic cells, thereby aiding the early stages of colonization of various tissues by these bacteria. The *fimA* gene has no promoter other than one within the invertible element, therefore, the gene is turned off and on by inversion of the element.

It is believed that phase variation mediated by these site-specific DNA rearrangements provides a selective advantage to the bacteria in allowing invading populations to include individuals that can escape the developing immune response of the host and thus continue the infectious process. Similar strategies are employed by some eukaryotic parasites of humans, notably the trypanosomes (see Chapter 54).

More about Bacterial Plasmids

One of the unanticipated features of microbial genetics has been the revelation that many virulence factors and much clinically significant resistance to antibiotics are the result of the activities not of bacterial chromosomal genes, but of the accessory genomes present in plasmids. In a certain sense, the health professional treating infectious disease is frequently coping with autonomous self-replicating DNA molecules. Many of the properties of plasmids have already been touched on, but the information will now be consolidated and considered in more detail.

Properties of Plasmids

Plasmids are autonomous extrachromosomal elements composed of circular, double-stranded DNA. They are found in most species of Grampositive and negative bacteria and in most environments. A single organism can harbor several distinct plasmids. Like the chromosome, they have the property of governing their own replication by means of special sequences and regulatory proteins.

Many plasmids (the F plasmid of *E. coli* is an example) are able to bring about their own transfer by the products of a group of genes called *tra* (for *tra*nsfer); such plasmids are called *conjugative*. Other plasmids, called *nonconjugative*, lack this ability. Conjugative plasmids may facilitate the transfer of certain nonconjugative plasmids or, in the case of the F plasmid, may mobilize the cell's chromosome. Some plasmids, again including the F factor, can either replicate autonomously or as a segment of DNA integrated into the chromosome. These are sometimes termed *episomes*. Certain prophages can exist as plasmids, but most plasmids are not viruses, because at no point of their life cycle do they exist as a free viral particle. Most plasmids show little or no DNA homology with the chromosome and can, in this sense, be regarded as foreign to the cell.

Plasmids usually include a number of genes in addition to those required for their replication and transfer to other cells. Where their function has been established, these genes have been found to code for properties such as antimicrobic resistance or certain determinants of virulence that are not needed by the cell in all environments. In fact, they add a small metabolic burden to the cell, and in many cases a slightly reduced growth rate results. Thus, under conditions of laboratory cultivation where the properties coded by the plasmid are not required, there is a tendency for *curing* of a strain to occur because the progeny cells that have not acquired a plasmid (or have lost it) have a selective advantage during prolonged growth and subculture. Conversely, where the property conferred by the plasmid is advantageous (eg, in the presence of antimicrobic to which the plasmid determines resistance), selective pressure will favor the plasmid carrying strain.

The origin of plasmids remains uncertain. They could possibly be descendents of bacterial viruses that evolved a sophisticated means of selftransfer by conjugation and then lost their unneeded protein capsid. Alternatively, they may have evolved as separated parts of a bacterial chromosome that could provide both the means for genetic exchange and a

Margin notes:

Self-replicating plasmids found in most species

Conjugative plasmids can facilitate transfer of nonconjugatives

Some plasmids can integrate and replicate with chromosome

Most plasmids are nonhomologous with the chromosome

Many plasmid genes facilitate survival under certain conditions

Possible origins of plasmids

way to amplify certain genes of special value in a particular environment (eg, coding for an adhesin) or to dispense with them where they are superfluous.

Varieties of Plasmids

There are a great many bacterial plasmids known. Some show similarity with each other in nuceotide sequence; thus, plasmids can be classified by their degree of apparent relatedness. Unrelated plasmids can coexist within a single cell, but closely related plasmids become segregated during cell division and eventually all but one are eliminated. For this reason, a group of closely related plasmids that exclude each other is called an *incompatibility group*.

Plasmids show a great variety in size, in the mode of control of their replication, and in the number and kinds of genes they carry. Naturally occurring plasmids span the range from below 5×10^6 daltons to over 100×10^6 daltons, but even the largest are only a few percent of the size of the bacterial chromosome. The regulation of replication of a plasmid is said to be *stringent* if it is somehow closely tied to cell or chromosomal division so that few molecules of the plasmid exist per cell. Some plasmids are said to have *relaxed* regulations of replication, and many copies (even dozens) may be found in each cell with a consequent increase in the products of the genes that they carry. In general, small plasmids have relaxed regulation and large ones, stringent. Every plasmid, by definition, must have genes sufficient to govern its own replication (including, for example, a genetic region called *ori*, or origin of replication). In addition, a conjugative plasmid must have genes that mobilize its DNA and mediate its transfer into a recipient cell. Finally, plasmids may have one or many genes unrelated to these functions, but important to the cell under certain environmental conditions.

The variety of cellular properties associated with plasmids is very great, and includes: fertility (the capacity for gene transfer by conjugation), production of toxins, production of pili and other adhesins, resistance to some antimicrobics, resistance to other toxic chemicals, production of bacteriocins (toxic proteins that kill some other bacteria), production of siderophores for scavenging Fe^{3+}, and the production of certain catabolic enzymes important in biodegradation of organic residues.

R Plasmids

Plasmids that include genes conferring resistance to antimicrobics are of great significance to medicine. They are termed *R plasmids* or *R factors* (*resistance factors*). The genes responsible for resistance usually code for enzymes that inactivate antimicrobics or reduce the cell's permeability to them. In contrast, resistance conferred by chromosomal mutation usually involves modification of the target of the antimicrobics (eg, RNA polymerase or the ribosome).

R plasmids occupy center stage in approaches to chemotherapy because of the constellation of properties they possess. Those of Gram-negative bacteria can be transmitted across species boundaries and, at lower frequency, even between genera. Many encode resistance to several antimicrobics and can thus spread multiple resistance through a diverse microbial population under selective pressure of only one of those to which they confer resistance. Nonpathogenic bacteria can serve as a natural res-

Only unrelated plasmids can coexist within the cell

Difference in plasmid sizes and control of replication

Small plasmids often have many copies

Wide range of properties encoded by plasmids

R plasmids usually encode antimicrobic-inactivating enzymes or reduced permeability

Some R plasmids transmissible between species and genera; encode multiresistance

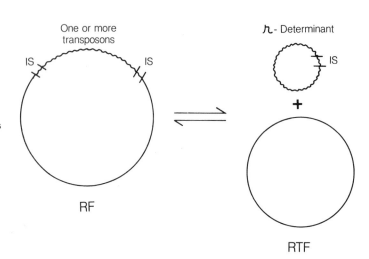

4.11 Structure and dissociation of an R factor (RF plasmid). The RF plasmid is shown with its two components: the r determinant, which contains one or more genes for antibiotic resistance (frequently present as transposons), and the resistance transfer factor (RTF), which contains the genes necessary for replication of the plasmid and its transfer to other cells.

ervoir of resistance determinants on plasmids that are available for spread to pathogens.

R plasmids evolve rapidly and can easily acquire additional resistance-determining genes from fusion with other plasmids or acquisition of transposons. Many have the capability of amplifying the number of copies of their resistance genes either by gene duplications within each plasmid or by increasing the number of plasmids (copy number) per cell. By these means resistance can be achieved to very high concentration of the antimicrobic. One process of gene amplification is based on the ability of some conjugative plasmids to dissociate their components into two plasmids, one (called the *resistance transfer factor*, or RTF) containing genes for replication and for transfer and another (called the *resistance* or *r* determinant) containing genes for replication and for resistance. Subsequent relaxed replication of the r determinant expands the cell's capacity to produce the resistance-conferring enzyme (Figure 4.11).

How are these remarkable properties to be understood? A decade ago, many of the molecular feats of R-factor plasmids were unexplainable on the basis of known genetic and evolutionary mechanisms. The discovery of transposable elements (insertion sequences and transposons) and their properties provide an explanation for much of the otherwise mysterious activities of R factors. Most plasmids, and all R factors, contain many IS elements and transposons. In fact, virtually all the resistance determinant genes on plasmids are present as transposons. As a result, these genes can be amplified by tandem duplications on the plasmid and can hop to other plasmids (or to the bacterial chromosome) in the same cell. Combined with the natural properties of many plasmids to transfer themselves by conjugation (even between dissimilar bacterial species), the rapid evolutionary development of multiple drug-resistance plasmids and their spread through populations of pathogenic bacteria during the past three decades can be seen as a predictable result of natural selection resulting from the widespread and intensive use of antimicrobics in human and veterinary medicine (see Chapter 13).

The properties of transposons can explain the present-day ubiquity and mobility of resistance genes, but not their origin. Two facts help point out at least a direction in which to search for an answer. First, R plasmids carrying the genes encoding antimicrobic-inactivating enzymes have been found in bacterial cultures preserved by lyophilization (freeze-drying)

New R genes acquired by plasmid fusion or from transposons

Gene amplification by increasing copy number

Resistance spread facilitated by transposition of R genes

Selective pressure of antimicrobic use

Resistance genes preexisted antimicrobic use

since before the era of antimicrobic therapy: an accelerated evolutionary development need not be invoked. Second, the enzymes themselves are remarkably similar to those found in certain bacteria (*Streptomyces* spp) that produce many clinically useful antimicrobics. Perhaps a long time ago there was a cross-genus transfer of genetic information (by transformation?) that became stabilized on plasmids under the selection pressure of antimicrobic released into the environment under natural conditions.

Detection of Plasmids

Rapid transfer of multiresistance indicates plasmid involvement

A number of physical, morphological, and functional tests can be used to reveal the presence of plasmids in a bacterial population. The rapid transfer of characteristics, such as resistance to antimicrobics from strain to strain, or alternatively the rapid loss of such traits, is a hallmark of plasmid-encoded characteristics. When several genetically distinct characteristics are transferred simultaneously in the laboratory into cells known not to have possessed them previously, the evidence is very strong that a plasmid is responsible.

Plasmid DNAs separable in density gradients or electrophoretically

Plasmids, including nonconjugative plasmids and those coding for no presently known trait, can be demonstrated more directly by physical means. Centrifugation of cell extracts through gradients of high salt concentrations can separate chromosomal DNA from plasmid DNA, because if the two kinds of DNA differ in density (which is a function of their respective content of GC relative to AT base pairs), they will form separate bands in the centrifuge tube. Cell extracts made with care so as not to fragment large DNA molecules can also be electrophoresed through semisolid (agarose) gels. DNA molecules move as a function of their size and shape, and, therefore, plasmid DNAs rapidly migrate through a gel that leaves most of the chromosomal DNA hung up at the origin. Plasmids of different size are frequently encountered in a single cell and can be detected and separated in this way. Figure 4.12 illustrates migration of plas-

4.12 Agarose gel electrophoresis of DNA to demonstrate the transfer of congugative plasmids between *Staphylococcus aureus* and *S. epidermidis.* In each of the lanes A–I the electrophoretic movement of the DNA is from top to bottom. *Lane A:* DNA from the recipient strain of *S. aureus* lacking plasmids. Only chromosomal DNA (band labeled Chr) is visible. *Lane B:* DNA from the donor strain of *S. epidermidis* showing three R-factor plasmids (pAM899-1, -2, and -3) in addition to the chromosomal DNA. *Lane C:* DNA from the recipient strain after conjugal transfer of all three plasmids from the donor. *Lanes D–I:* DNA from various strains derived by growing the plasmid-containing recipient of Lane C in the presence of ethidium bromide to "cure" it of one or more of the R-factors. (*Reproduced with permission from Forbes, B.A., and Schaberg, D.R. 1983. J. Bacteriol. 153:627–634.*)

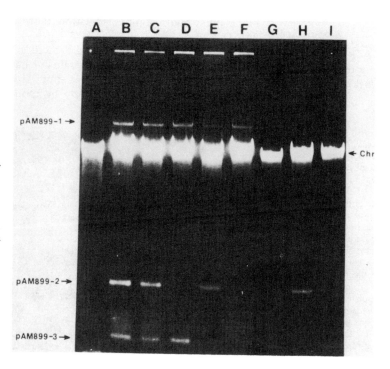

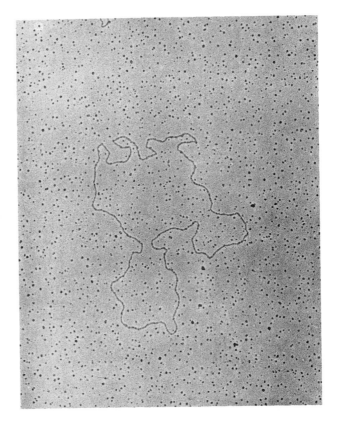

4.13 Electron micrograph of an R plasmid from *E.coli*. The plasmid is of 64 megadaltons, and contains about 40 kilobase pairs. (*Micrograph kindly supplied by Dr Jorge H. Crosa.*)

mid DNA in agarose electrophoresis. Electron microscopy can be used to visualize plasmids, to measure the length of their DNA, and to see the forms they take upon hybridization to other nucleic acid molecules (Figure 4.13).

Bacterial plasmids, including R factors, have become valuable markers for comparing closely related strains of bacteria in epidemiologic studies. In outbreaks, spread of an epidemic strain can sometimes be followed more easily and more accurately by monitoring the profile of plasmids

Methods for tracing plasmids epidemiologically

4.14 Agarose gel electrophoresis of various strains of staphylococci isolated from patients in a large metropolitan hospital. Each vertical lane displays the DNA of a separate isolate. The sharp bands visible in the upper half of most lanes are plasmids. The broad smear of DNA in the lower half is chromosomal DNA. The results illustrate the prevalence of multiple plasmids in freshly isolated bacterial strains. Most isolates contain more than one plasmid. (*Kindly provided by Dr D.R. Schaberg, University of Michigan.*)

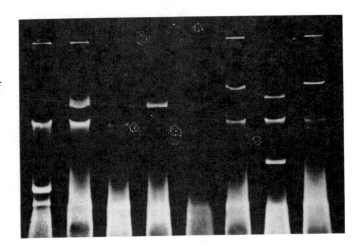

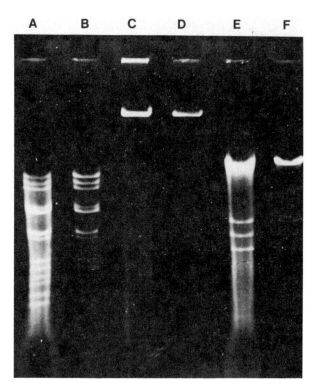

4.15 Use of agarose gel electrophoresis in molecular epidemiology. During an outbreak of bacteremia in infants in a neonatal intensive care unit, strains of *Klebsiella aerogenes* and *Enterobacter cloacae* were isolated that harbored R-factor plasmids of similar electrophoretic mobility and conferred resistance to some aminoglycosides, ampicillin, and chloramphenicol. To learn if an identical plasmid had established itself in both bacterial species, a restriction digest analysis was performed and the products separated by electrophoresis. Lanes C and D display the intact plasmid DNA isolated from *K. aerogenes* and *E. cloacae* respectively. Lanes A and B display the fragments produced by the action of the restriction enzyme BamH1 on the plasmids, and Lanes E and F display the fragments produced by the restriction enzyme EcoR1. For each pair of treated samples, the plasmid DNA from *K. aerogenes* is on the left (ie, Lanes A and E). The identical restriction patterns make it almost certain that the plasmids from the two bacterial species are identical, and raise the possibility that the epidemic itself was caused by the chance introduction and spread of this R plasmid. (*Kindly provided by Dr D.R. Schaberg, University of Michigan.*)

Fingerprinting plasmids

DNA restriction endonuclease enzymes common in bacteria

carried in strains isolated from different patients than by traditional typing methods (Figure 4.14). This approach is particularly useful in studying outbreaks of nosocomial (hospital-acquired) infections. Likewise, the spread of an R plasmid between different species can be followed by showing that they carry an identical plasmid conferring the same pattern of antimicrobic resistance. The plasmid comparison can be carried one step further in specificity by cutting the plasmid DNA with specific *restriction endonucleases* (see next section) and examining the resulting fragments by agarose gel electrophoresis (Figure 4.15). Variations of this procedure enable even the spread of specific genes among a variety of plasmids to be detected.

DNA Restriction and Genetic Engineering

The phenomena of *DNA modification* and *restriction* suggest that there is competition among the different replicons (prophages, plasmids, and chromosomes) for residence in a bacterial cell. Each of these genetic elements may possess genes for a restriction-modification system, which serves to attach protective groups to its own DNA and to degrade other unprotected DNA.

Restriction-modification systems are widespread in bacteria. Literally hundreds of bacterial *restriction enzymes* are now known. All are nucleotide-specific endonucleases that act upon double-stranded DNA. They fall into three broad categories. *Type I* systems are large enzymes of great biochemical complexity. They recognize specific, unprotected, nucleotide sequences, but cut the DNA molecule at variable distances from the recognized sequence. The enzymes have both endonuclease and methylating activity. They can modify DNA by methylating it at specific residues shortly after synthesis, thereby protecting it, but can cut mature DNA molecules that lack protection.

Type II systems are simpler enzymes. Each binds to and cuts at a specific nucleotide sequence. Some restriction enzymes of this type make a cut straight across the double-stranded DNA molecule, creating fragments with strands of equal length and therefore *blunt ended*. Others make a *staggered cut,* leaving single-stranded tails at the end of the fragment. These tails, being complementary to each other, can be reannealed under suitable conditions, making them exceptionally useful in *gene cloning* (Figure 4.16). Type II systems must always include a gene for an appropriate modifying methylase to protect the resident DNA.

Type III systems resemble type I in that methylase and endonuclease activities reside in one enzyme, and the endonucleolytic cut is made at a site distant from the specific sequence recognized by the enzyme; they differ from type I by making the cut at a fixed rather than variable number of residues from the recognized sequence.

Restriction enzymes of the type II variety are extremely useful in gene cloning and other aspects of genetic engineering. The fundamental procedure in *recombinant DNA technology* is the *splitting* and *recombining* of different DNA molecules in vitro. Before the discovery of type II restriction enzymes, such splicing was possible only by a somewhat laborious process involving attaching a tail of A residues to one molecule and T residues to another in order to create sticky or *cohesive ends* by which the two could be held together by *annealing* (base pairing) before covalently linking them by *DNA ligase*. Type II restriction endonucleases provided a shortcut, because many of these enzymes, by making staggered cuts, create cohesive ends on the fragments of DNA that they restrict. As a result, DNA fragments from any source can be readily spliced together if they have been restricted by the same type II endonuclease.

The application of this procedure to splice a fragment of foreign DNA into the DNA of a bacterial plasmid is illustrated in Figure 4.16. To clone a gene from any biological source (meaning to prepare multiple exact copies of it separate from its usual neighboring genes), it is customary to prepare suitable DNA fragments with a restriction endonuclease for which there is a recognition site in a particular *E. coli* plasmid or phage molecule, called a *vector*. The cohesive ends created by the action of the endonuclease on the foreign DNA and the vector DNA facilitate their annealing, and the action of DNA ligase creates a hybrid vector (ie, one containing a fragment of the foreign DNA). The vector can then be introduced into a recipient *E. coli* cell by artificial transformation (see Transformation). If the vector is an R factor, cells successfully transformed can be selectively grown, and nontransformed cells eliminated, by plating the mixture on solid media containing the antimicrobic against which the R factor has a resistance gene. Vectors with desirable restriction sites and genes for facilitating the recognition of desired recombinant molecules can be constructed by a multitude of powerful in vivo and in vitro techniques utilizing transposons and various enzymes that cut, extend, and ligate DNA molecules.

When combined with information about the mechanism of transcription of genes in bacteria, and how expression is regulated, recombinant DNA technology has made it possible to engineer *E. coli* cells to produce products from a variety of genetic sources. As a result medicine is now gaining the ability to produce efficiently large quantities of human enzymes and hormones, complex viral and bacterial products for vaccine production,

Many enzymes make staggered cuts in double-stranded DNA

Cohesive ends of different DNAs cut with the same enzymes can be spliced

Foreign genes can be spliced into plasmid or phage vector

Insertion of vector into bacteria by artificial transformation; selection and cloning

Some foreign gene products may be produced in bacteria

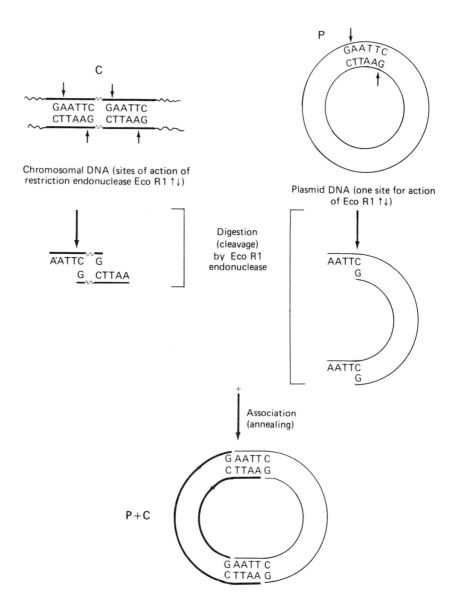

4.16 Construction of a recombinant DNA molecule. C = chromosomal fragments; P = plasmid.

and other useful biological products, many of which could only be obtained with great difficulty in the past and sometimes with significant risk to the recipient.

Bacterial Genetics and Classification

Bacteria are classified into genera and species according to a binomial Linnean scheme similar to that used for higher organisms. For example, in the case of *Staphylococcus aureus*, *Staphylococcus* is the generic name and *aureus* is the species designation. Some genera with common characteristics are further grouped into families. Bacterial classification, however, has posed many problems. Morphologic descriptors are not as abundant as in higher plants and animals, there is little readily interpreted fossil record to help establish phylogeny, and there is no elaborate developmental process (ontogeny) to recapitulate the evolutionary path from ancestral forms (phylogeny). These problems are minor compared to others: bacteria mutate and evolve rapidly, they reproduce asexually, and they exchange genetic material over wide boundaries. The single most important test of species—the ability of individuals within a species to reproduce sexually by mating and exchanging genetic material—cannot be applied to bacteria. As a result, bacterial taxonomy developed pragmatically by determining multiple characteristics and weighting them according to which seemed most fundamental; for example, shape, spore formation, Gram reaction, aerobic or anaerobic growth, and temperature for growth were given special weighting in defining genera. Properties such as ability to ferment particular carbohydrates, production of specific enzymes and toxins, and antigenic composition of cell surface components were often used in defining species. As presented in Chapter 14, such properties and their weighting continue to be of central importance in *identification* of unknown isolates in the clinical laboratory, and the use of *determinative keys* is based on the concept of such weighted characteristics. These approaches are much less sound in establishing taxonomic relationships based on phylogenetic principles.

Weighted classification schemes valuable for identification but not for taxonomy

The recognition that sound taxonomy ought to be based on the *genetic similarity* of organisms and reflect their *phylogenetic relatedness* has led in recent years to the use of new methods and new principles in taxonomy. The first approach was to apply *Adansonian* or *numeric taxonomy,* which gives equal weighting to a large number of independent characteristics and allocates bacteria to groups according to the proportion of shared characteristics as determined statistically. Theoretically, a significant correspondence of a large number of phenotypic characteristics could be considered to reflect genetic relatedness. A more direct approach available in recent years involves analysis of chromosomal DNAs from different organisms. Analysis can be somewhat crude, such as the overall ratio of A–T to G–C base pairs; differences of greater than 10% in G–C content are taken to indicate unrelatedness, but closely similar content does not imply relatedness. Closer relationships can be assessed by determining base sequence similarity, as by *DNA–DNA hybridization,* in which single strands of DNA from one organism are allowed to anneal with single strands of another. Some clinical laboratory tests have been devised based on the ability of DNA from a reference strain to undergo homologous recombination with DNA from an unknown isolate (see Chapter 14). Finally, the absence of a satisfactory fossil record by which to deduce phylogenetic relationships is now regarded as less of a drawback than previously, because comparison of nucleotide sequences of genes encoding ribosomal RNA, which are highly conserved in evolution, is providing some of the missing phylogenetic information.

Sound taxonomy based on degrees of genetic similarity

Phylogenetic relationships clarified by analyses of DNA base composition and base sequences

Additional Reading

Eisenstein, B.I., and Engleberg, N.C. 1986. Applied molecular genetics: New tools for the microbiologists and clinicians. *J. Infect. Dis.* 153:416–430. An easily read minireview on the nature and uses of gene cloning in medical microbiology.

Freifelder, D. 1987. *Molecular Biology.* 2nd ed. Boston: Jones & Bartlett Publishers,

Inc. Chapter 19 deals with plasmids in a clear yet comprehensive manner. Chapter 21 contains details on transposable elements, particularly on the mechanisms of transposition, not readily found elsewhere.

Lewin, B. 1987. *Genes.* 3rd ed. New York: John Wiley & Sons. Chapter 35 of this textbook on molecular biology is an excellent treatment of transposable elements.

Lin E.C.C., Goldstein R., and Syvanen, M. 1984. *Bacteria, Plasmids, and Phages.* Cambridge, Mass.: Harvard University Press. Chapters 6 through 12 deal, in somewhat more detail, with the same topics in bacterial genetics that have been covered here.

Stanier, R.Y., Ingraham J.L., Wheelis M.L., and Painter P.R. 1986. *The Microbial World.* 5th ed. Englewood Cliffs, N.J.: Prentice-Hall, Inc. Chapters 10 and 11 of this general microbiology textbook present elementary concepts of microbial genetics in clear and simple language and with excellent illustrations. Chapter 13, on the classification and phylogeny of bacteria, is particularly helpful and interesting.

5

Virus Structure

James J. Champoux

Overview of viruses

A virus is a set of genes, either DNA or RNA, packaged in a protein-containing coat. The resulting particle is called a *virion*. Viruses that infect humans are considered as part of the general class of animal viruses; viruses that infect bacteria are referred to as *bacteriophages,* or phages for short. Virus reproduction requires that a virus particle infect a cell and program the cellular machinery to synthesize the macromolecular constituents required for the assembly of new virions. Thus, a virus is considered an intracellular parasite. The infected host cell may produce hundreds to hundreds of thousands of new virions and usually dies. Tissue damage as a result of cell death accounts for the pathology of many viral diseases in humans. In some cases, the infected cells survive, resulting in persistent virus production and a chronic infection that can remain asymptomatic, produce a chronic disease state, or lead to relapse of an infection.

Viral latency

In some circumstances, a virus fails to reproduce itself and instead enters a latent state, often by integration into the host cell genome (called *lysogeny* in the case of bacteriophages), from which there is the potential for reactivation at a later time. A possible consequence of the presence of viral genes in a latent state is thus a new genotype for the cell. Some determinants of bacterial virulence and some malignancies of animal cells are examples of the genetic effects of latent viruses.

Apparently vertebrates have had to coexist with viruses for a long time because they have evolved the special nonspecific interferon system, which operates in conjunction with the highly specific immune system to control virus infections.

In the discussion to follow, the biologic and genetic bases for these phenomena will be provided. Three themes will be emphasized. The first is that different viruses can have very different structures, and this diversity is reflected in their replicative strategies. The second is that because of their small size viruses have achieved a very high degree of genetic economy. The third is that while viruses depend to a great extent on host cell

5.1 Schematic drawing of two
      basic types of virions.

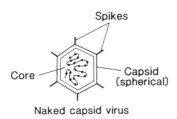

Naked capsid virus

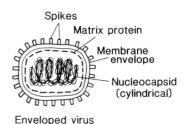

Enveloped virus

functions and, therefore, are difficult to combat medically, they do exhibit unique steps in their replicative cycles, which are potential targets for antiviral therapy.

Virion Size and Design

Size range from 20 to 300 nm

Viruses are approximately 100- to 1000-fold smaller than the cells they infect. The smallest viruses (parvoviruses) are approximately 20 nm in diameter (1 nm = 10^{-9} m), whereas the largest animal viruses (poxviruses) overlap the size of the smallest bacterial cells (*Chlamydia* and *Mycoplasma*), having a diameter of approximately 300 nm. This means that viruses generally pass through filters designed to trap bacteria and this property can, in principle, be used as evidence for a viral etiology.

Unenveloped viruses have nucleic acid genome within protein capsid

The basic design of all true viruses places the nucleic acid genome on the inside of a protein shell called a *capsid*. Some animal viruses are further packaged into a lipid membrane, or envelope, which is usually acquired from the cytoplasmic membrane of the infected cell during egress from the cell. Viruses that are not enveloped have a defined external capsid and are referred to as *naked capsid viruses*. Enveloped viruses contain a nucleic acid–protein complex called a *nucleocapsid* surrounded by a matrix protein that serves as a bridge between the nucleocapsid and the inside of the membrane. Protein or glycoprotein structures called *spikes* often emanate from the surface of virus particles. These basic design features are illustrated schematically in Figure 5.1 and in the electron micrographs shown in Figures 5.2 and 5.3.

Enveloped viruses have nucleocapsid of nucleic acid complexed to protein
Some viruses have surface protein or glycoprotein spikes

Cylindrical and spherical shapes

The protein shell forming the capsid or the nucleocapsid assumes one of two basic shapes, cylindrical or spherical. Some of the more complex bacteriophages combine these two basic shapes. Examples of these three structural categories can be seen in the electron micrographs in Figure 5.2.

Functions of outer shell

The functions of the outer shell of viruses are 1) to protect the nucleic acid genome from damage during the extracellular passage of the virus from one cell to another, 2) to aid in the process of entry into the cell, and 3) in some cases to package enzymes essential for the early steps of the infection process.

In general, the length of the viral nucleic acid genome is hundreds of times the longest dimension of the complete virion. It follows, therefore, that the viral genome must be extensively condensed during the process of virion assembly. For naked capsid viruses this condensation is achieved by the association of the nucleic acid with basic proteins to form what is called the *core* of the virus (Figure 5.1). The core proteins are usually encoded by the virus, but in the case of some DNA-containing animal viruses, the basic proteins are histones scavenged from the host cell. For

Genome of naked virus is condensed in core with basic proteins

Enveloped viral genome condensed in nucleocapsid

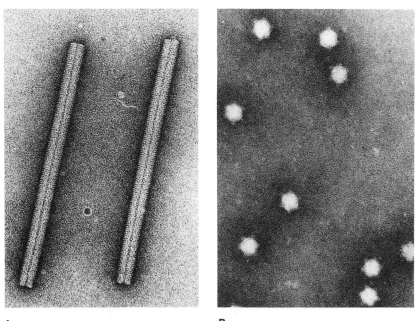

5.2 Three basic virus designs:
(A) tobacco mosaic virus;
(B) bacteriophage φX 174; (C)
bacteriophage T4. *(Electron
micrographs kindly supplied by Dr
Robley C. Williams.)*

A   **B**

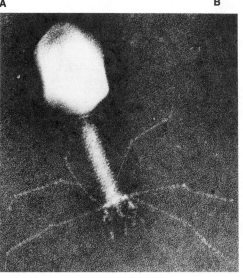

C

enveloped viruses, the formation of the nucleocapsid serves to condense
the nucleic acid genome.

Plant viroids are RNA
molecules lacking capsids
Prions appear to be infectious
proteins

Two classes of infectious agents exist that are structurally simpler than
viruses. Viroids are infectious circular RNA molecules that lack protein
shells; they are responsible for a variety of plant diseases. Prions, which
apparently lack any genes and are composed only of protein, are recently
reported agents that appear to be responsible for some chronic severe
neurological diseases such as Scrapie in sheep and Creutzfeldt–Jakob syndrome in humans.

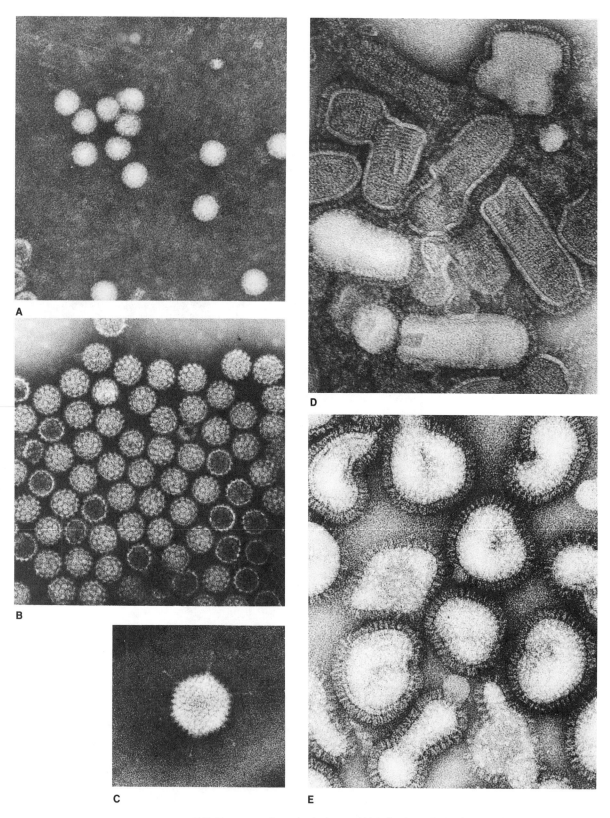

5.3 Representative animal viruses: **(A)** poliovirus; **(B)** SV40; **(C)** adenovirus; **(D)** vesicular stomatitis virus; **(E)** influenza virus. *(Electron micrographs kindly supplied by Dr Robley C. Williams.)*

Genome Structure

Genomes either of DNA or RNA

Structural diversity among the viruses is most obvious when the makeup of viral genomes is considered. Genomes can be made of RNA or DNA and be either double stranded or single stranded. For viruses with single-stranded genomes, the nucleic acid can either be of the same polarity (indicated by a +) or a different polarity (−) from that of the viral mRNA produced during infection. In the case of adeno-associated viruses, the particles are a mixture, about half of which contain (+)DNA, while the other half contain (−)DNA.

Positive- and negative-strand viruses

Genomes may be linear or circular and single or segmented molecules

The arenaviruses and bunyaviruses are unusual in apparently having an RNA genome, part of which has the same polarity as the mRNA and another part that is complementary to the corresponding mRNA. Both linear and circular genomes are known. In addition, whereas most viruses have a single nucleic acid molecule for their genome, in some cases several pieces of nucleic acid constitute the complete genome. Such viruses are said to have segmented genomes. One virus class (retroviruses) carries two identical copies of its genome and is, therefore, diploid. A few viral genomes (picornaviruses, hepatitis B, and adenoviruses) contain covalently attached protein on the ends of the polynucleotide chains. As will be shown in Chapter 6, the terminal protein molecules as well as other special genome structures found in other viruses play key roles in the replication process.

Capsid Structure

Subunit Structure of Capsids

The capsids or nucleocapsids of all viruses are composed of many copies of one or at most several different kinds of protein subunits. This fact follows from two fundamental considerations. First, all viruses code for their own capsid proteins, and it turns out that even if the entire coding capacity of the genome were to be used to specify a single giant capsid protein, the protein would simply not be large enough to enclose the nucleic acid genome. Thus, multiple copies are needed, and, in fact, the simplest spherical virus contains 60 identical protein subunits. Second, viruses are such highly symmetrical structures that it is not uncommon to visualize naked capsid viruses in the electron microscope as a crystalline array (eg, SV40 in Figure 5.3). However a polypeptide chain that constitutes the subunit is intrinsically irregular in shape. The only way to construct a regular symmetrical structure out of irregular subunits is to follow the rules of crystallography and form an aggregate involving many identical copies of the irregular subunits, where each subunit bears the same relationship to its neighbors as every other subunit.

Capsids and nucleocapsids are composed of multiple copies of protein molecule(s) in crystalline array

The presence of many identical protein subunits in viral capsids or the existence of many identical spikes in the membrane of enveloped viruses has important implications for adsorption, hemagglutination, and recognition of viruses by neutralizing antibodies (see Chapter 6).

Cylindrical Architecture

Cylindrical viruses have helical arrangement of genome and capsid protein molecules

A cylindrical shape is the simplest structure for a capsid or a nucleocapsid. The first virus to be crystalized and studied in structural detail was a plant pathogen, tobacco mosaic virus (TMV) (Figure 5.2). The capsid of TMV is shaped like a rod or a cylinder with the RNA genome wound in a helix

Table 5.1 Classification of RNA Animal Viruses

Family	Virion Structure	Genome Structure and Molecular Weight	Representative Members
Hepatitis δ	Cubic, enveloped	ss circular $(-)$ (6×10^5)	Human hepatitis δ virus
Picornaviruses	Cubic, naked	ss linear $(+)$ $(2-3 \times 10^6)$; protein attached	Human enteroviruses: poliovirus, Coxsackie virus, echovirus; rhinoviruses; bovine foot and mouth disease virus; hepatitis A
Arenaviruses	Helical, enveloped	2 ss linear segments $(+/-)$ (3×10^6)	Lassa virus; lymphocytic choriomeningitis virus of mice
Caliciviruses	Cubic, naked	ss linear $(+)$ (2.6×10^6)	Vesicular exanthema virus
Rhabdoviruses	Helical, enveloped	ss linear $(-)$ $(3-4 \times 10^6)$	Rabies virus; bovine vesicular stomatitis virus
Retroviruses	Cubic, enveloped	ss linear $(+)$, diploid $(3-4 \times 10^6)$	RNA tumor viruses of mice, birds, and cats; visna virus of sheep; human immunodeficiency viruses (human T-cell leukemia and acquired immunodeficiency syndrome)
Togaviruses	Cubic, enveloped	ss linear $(+)$ (4×10^6)	Alphaviruses: Sindbis virus and semliki forest virus; flaviviruses: dengue virus and yellow fever virus; rubella virus; mucosal disease virus
Orthomyxoviruses	Helical, enveloped	8 ss linear segments $(-)$ (5×10^6)	Types A, B, and C influenza viruses of humans, swine, and horses
Coronaviruses	Helical, enveloped	ss linear $(+)$ $(5-6 \times 10^6)$	Respiratory viruses of humans; calf diarrhea virus; swine enteric virus; mouse hepatis virus
Bunyaviruses	Helical, enveloped	3 ss linear segments $(+/-)$ (6×10^6)	Rift Valley fever virus; bunyamwera virus
Paramyxoviruses	Helical, enveloped	ss linear $(-)$ $(6-8 \times 10^6)$	Mumps; measles; Newcastle disease virus; canine distemper virus
Reoviruses	Cubic, naked	10 ds linear segments (15×10^6)	Human reoviruses; orbiviruses: Colorado tick fever virus, African horse sickness virus; human rotaviruses

Abbreviations: ss = single stranded; ds = double stranded.

inside it. The capsid is composed of many copies of a single kind of protein subunit arranged in a close-packed helix, which places every subunit in the same microenvironment. Because of the helical arrangement of the subunits, viruses that have this type of design are often said to have *helical symmetry*. Although less is known about the capsid structures of animal viruses with helical symmetry, it is likely their structures follow the same pattern as TMV. Thus, the nucleocapsids of influenza, measles, mumps, rabies, and poxviruses (see Table 5.1) are probably constructed with a helical arrangement of protein subunits in close association with the nucleic acid genome.

Table 5.2 Classification of DNA Animal Viruses

Family	Virion Structure	Genome Structure and Molecular Weight	Representative Members
Parvoviruses	Cubic, naked	ss linear $(1-2 \times 10^6)$	Minute virus of mice; adeno-associated satellite viruses
Hepatitis B	Cubic, enveloped	ds circular (2×10^6), gap in one strand; protein attached	Hepatitis B virus of humans; woodchuck hepatitis virus
Papovaviruses	Cubic, naked	ds circular $(3-5 \times 10^6)$	Papilloma viruses; polyoma virus (mouse); SV40 (monkey)
Adenoviruses	Cubic, naked	ds linear $(20-25 \times 10^6)$; protein attached	Human and animal respiratory disease viruses
Herpesviruses	Cubic, enveloped	ds linear $(80-130 \times 10^6)$	Herpes simplex virus, types 1 and 2; varicella–zoster virus cytomegalovirus; Epstein–Barr virus; human herpes virus type 6
Poxviruses	Helical, enveloped	ds linear $(160-200 \times 10^6)$	Smallpox; vaccinia; molluscum contagiosum; fibroma and myxoma viruses of rabbits

Abbreviations: ss = single stranded; ds = double stranded.

Spherical Architecture

The construction of a spherically shaped virus similarly involves the packing together of many identical subunits, but in this case the subunits are placed on the surface of a geometric solid called an *icosahedron*. An icosahedron has 12 vertices, 30 sides, and 20 triangular faces (Figure 5.4). Because the icosahedron belongs to the symmetry group that crystallographers refer to as *cubic*, spherically shaped viruses are said to have *cubic symmetry*. (Note that the term *cubic*, as used in this context, has nothing to do with the more familiar shape called the *cube*.)

When viewed in the electron microscope, many naked capsid viruses and some nucleocapsids appear as spherical particles with a surface topology that makes it appear that they are constructed of identical ball-shaped subunits (Figure 5.3). These visible structures are referred to as *morphological subunits*, or capsomeres. A capsomere is composed of either five or six individual protein molecules, each one referred to as a structural subunit or protomer. In the simplest case of a virus with cubic symmetry, five protomers are placed at each one of the 12 vertices of the icosahedron

Spherical viruses exhibit icosahedral symmetry

Capsomeres are surface structures composed of five or six protein molecules

The Icosahedron

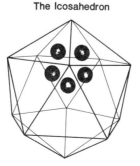

5.4 Diagram of an icosahedron showing 12 vertices, 20 faces, and 30 sides. The heavy dots indicate the position of protomers forming a capsomere on a spherical virus.

Table 5.3   Some Important Bacteriophages

Bacteriophage	Host	Genome Structure and Molecular Weight	Comments
MS2	*Escherichia coli*	ss linear RNA (1.2×10^6)	Lytic
Filamentous (M13, fd)	*Escherichia coli*	ss circular DNA (2.1×10^6)	No cell death
φx174	*Escherichia coli*	ss circular DNA (1.8×10^6)	Lytic
β	*C. diphtheriae*	ds linear DNA (23×10^6)	Temperate, codes for diphtheria toxin
λ	*Escherichia coli*	ds linear DNA (31×10^6)	Temperate
T4	*Escherichia coli*	ds linear DNA (108×10^6)	Lytic

Abbreviations: ss = single stranded; ds = double stranded.

as shown in Figure 5.4 to form a capsomere called a *pentamer*. Thus, the capsid is composed of 12 pentamers, or a total of 60 protomers. It should be noted that, as in the case of helical symmetry, this arrangement places every protomer in the same microenvironment as every other protomer.

To accommodate the larger cavity required by viruses with large genomes, the capsids contain many more protomers. These viruses are based on a variation of the basic icosahedron in which the construction involves a mixture of pentamers and hexamers instead of only pentamers. A detailed description of this higher level of virus structure is beyond the scope of this text.

Special Surface Structures

Many viruses have structures that protrude from the surface of the virion. In virtually every case these structures are important for the two earliest steps of infection, adsorption and penetration. The most dramatic example of such a structure is the tail of some bacteriophages (Figure 5.2), which, as will be described in Chapter 6, acts as a channel for the transfer of the genome into the cell. Other examples of surface structures include the spikes of adenovirus (Figure 5.3) and the glycoprotein spikes found in the membrane of enveloped viruses (see the influenza virus in Figure 5.3). Even viruses without obvious surface extensions probably contain short projections, which, like the more obvious spikes, are involved in the specific binding of the virus to the cell surface (see Chapter 6).

Importance of surface structures in adsorption and penetration

Classification of Viruses

Tables 5.1 and 5.2 present a classification scheme for animal viruses that is based solely on their structure. The viruses are arranged in the order of increasing genome size. It is important to bear in mind that phylogenetic relationships cannot be inferred from this taxonomic scheme. The tables should not be memorized, but instead used as a reference guide to virus structure. In general, viruses with similar structures exhibit similar replication strategies as will be shown in Chapter 6.

Representative and important bacteriophages are listed along with their properties in Table 5.3.

6

Virus Multiplication

James J. Champoux

Productive and nonproductive responses to viral infection

Transformation and hit and run changes in host cells

Lytic and virulent viruses destroy cells

Temperate viruses may enter latent state

A typical virus multiplication cycle is divided into discrete phases of 1) adsorption to the host cell, 2) penetration or entry, 3) uncoating to release the genome, 4) virion component production, 5) assembly, and 6) release from the cell. This series of events, sometimes with slight variations, describes what is called the *productive* or *lytic response*. However, this is not the only possible outcome of a virus infection. Some viruses can also enter into a very different kind of relationship with the host cell in which no new virus is produced, the cell survives and divides, and the viral genetic material persists indefinitely in a latent state. This outcome of an infection is referred to as the *nonproductive response*. The nonproductive response is called *lysogeny* in the case of bacteriophages and may involve oncogenic transformation by animal viruses. (This use of the term *transformation* is to be distinguished from DNA transformation of bacteria discussed in Chapter 4.) In addition, there may exist examples of viruses that can transiently infect a cell, cause some permanent change, and then be lost. Such an encounter between a virus and a cell is called a *hit and run infection*.

The outcome of an infection depends on the particular virus–host combination and on other factors such as the extracellular environment, multiplicity of infection, and the physiology and developmental state of the cell. Those viruses that can only enter into a productive relationship are called *lytic* or *virulent viruses*. Viruses that can undergo both the productive and nonproductive responses are referred to as *temperate viruses*. Some temperate viruses can be reactivated or "induced" to leave the latent state and enter into the productive response. Whether induction occurs depends on the particular virus–host combination, the physiology of the cell, and the presence of extracellular stimuli.

The remainder of this chapter will be concerned with the details of the steps of the lytic response. In Chapter 7 the topics of lysogeny and oncogenic transformation will be considered.

Growth and Assay of Viruses

Viruses are generally propagated in the laboratory by mixing the virus and susceptible cells together and incubating the infected cells until lysis occurs. After lysis, the cells and cell debris are removed by a brief centrifugation and the supernatant is called a *lysate.*

Mammalian cell culture procedures

The growth of animal viruses requires that the host cells be cultivated in the laboratory. To prepare cells for growth in vitro, a tissue is removed from an animal and the cells are disaggregated using the proteolytic enzyme, trypsin. The cell suspension is seeded into a plastic petri dish in a medium containing a complex mixture of amino acids, vitamins, minerals, and sugars. In addition to these nutritional factors, the growth of animal cells requires components present in animal serum. This method of growing cells is referred to as *tissue culture,* and the initial cell population is called a *primary culture.* The cells attach to the bottom of the plastic dish and remain attached as they divide and eventually cover the surface of the dish. When the culture becomes crowded, the cells generally cease dividing and enter a resting state. Propagation can be continued by removing the cells from the primary culture plate using trypsin and reseeding a new plate.

Normal cells cannot be propagated indefinitely

Immortalized cell lines useful for growing viruses

Cells taken from a normal (as opposed to cancerous) tissue cannot usually be propagated in this manner indefinitely. Eventually most of the cells die; a few may survive, and these cells often develop into a permanent cell line. Such cell lines are very useful as host cells for isolating and assaying viruses in the laboratory, but they rarely bear much resemblance to the tissue from which they originated. When cells are taken from a tumor and cultivated in vitro, they display a very different set of growth properties reflecting their tumor phenotype (see Chapter 7).

Cytopathic effects of viruses

When a virus is propagated in tissue culture cells, the cytological changes induced by the virus, which usually culminate in cell death, are often characteristic for a particular virus and referred to as the *cytopathic effect* of the virus. (See Figures 14.10 to 14.16.)

Quantitation of viruses

Viruses are quantitated by a method called the *plaque assay* (see below for detailed description of the method). Briefly, viruses are mixed with cells on a petri plate such that each infectious particle gives rise to a zone of lysed cells called a *plaque.* From the number of plaques on the plate, the titer of infectious particles in the lysate is calculated. Virus titers are expressed as the number of plaque-forming units per milliliter.

The One-Step Growth Experiment

A useful approach to describing an infection in temporal and quantitative terms is to perform a one-step growth experiment (Figure 6.1). The objective in such an experiment is to infect every cell in a culture so that the whole population proceeds through the infection process in a synchronous fashion. The ratio of infecting plaque-forming units to cells is called the *multiplicity of infection.* By infecting at a high multiplicity (eg, 10 as in Figure 6.1), it can be ensured that every cell will be infected.

High multiplicity of infection allows study of synchronous viral replication

The time course and efficiency of adsorption can be followed by the loss of infectious virus from the medium after removal of the cells (solid line, Figure 6.1). In the example shown, adsorption takes about a half-hour and all but 1% of the virus is adsorbed. If samples of the culture containing the infected cells are treated so as to break open the cells prior to assaying for virus (broken line, Figure 6.1), it can be observed that infectious virus initially disappears, because no particles are detectable

Shortly after infection, virus loses its identity (eclipse phase)

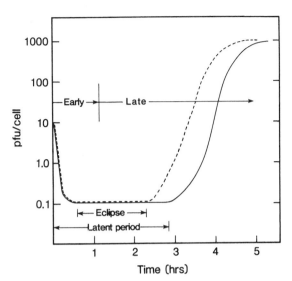

6.1 One-step growth
experiment. pfu = plaque-
forming units.

above the background of unadsorbed virus. The period of the infection where no infectious viruses are found is called the *eclipse phase* and serves to emphasize that the original virions lose their infectivity soon after entry into the cells. Infectivity is lost because, as will be shown below, the virus particles are dismantled as a prelude to their reproduction. Later, infec-

Reappearance of virus in high numbers

tious virus particles rapidly reappear in increasing numbers and are detected inside the cell prior to the time they are released to the medium (Figure 6.1). The length of time from the beginning of infection until progeny virions are found outside the cells is referred to as the *latent period*. Latent periods range from 15 min to hours for bacteriophages and from a few hours to many days for animal viruses.

Early and late phases of viral replication

The time in the infection at which genome replication begins has often been used to divide the infection operationally into early and late phases. In the early stages, viral gene expression is restricted to producing those proteins required for genome replication; later, the proteins synthesized are primarily those necessary for construction of the new virus particles.

The average number of plaque-forming units released per infected cell is called the *burst size* for the infection. In the example shown, the burst size is about 1000. Burst sizes range from less than 10 for some relatively inefficient infections to millions for some highly virulent viruses.

Adsorption

The first step in every viral infection is the attachment or adsorption of the infecting particle to the surface of the cell. A prerequisite for this interaction is a collision between the virion and the cell. Viruses do not have any capacity for locomotion and so the collision event is simply a random process determined by diffusion. Therefore, like any bimolecular reaction, the rate of adsorption is determined by the concentrations of both the virions and the cells.

Adsorption involves viral attachment proteins and cell protein receptors

Only a small fraction of the collisions between a virus and its host cell lead to a successful infection. This is because adsorption is a highly specific reaction that involves protein molecules on the surface of the virion called *virion attachment proteins* and certain cellular proteins on the surface of the cell called *receptors*. Typically there are 10^4–10^5 receptors on the cell surface. Receptors for some bacteriophages are found on pili, although the majority adsorb to receptors found on the bacterial cell wall. The receptors for animal viruses are usually glycoproteins located in the plasma membrane (also called *cytoplasmic membrane*), which carry out normal cellular functions. In the case of bacteriophages with tails, virion attachment proteins are found at the very end of the tails or the tail fibers (Figure 5.2). It appears that surface protrusions in general, such as the spikes found on adenoviruses and on virtually all of the enveloped animal viruses contain the virion attachment proteins.

Viral spikes and phage tails carry attachment proteins

Receptors for some animal viruses are also found on red blood cells of certain species and are responsible for the phenomena of hemagglutination and hemadsorption discussed below.

Viral hemagglutination and hemadsorption due to receptors on red blood cells

The repeating subunit structure of capsids and the multiplicity of spikes on enveloped viruses are probably important in determining the strength of the binding of the virus to the cell. The binding between a single virion attachment protein and a single receptor protein is relatively weak, but the combination of many such interactions leads to a strong association between the virion and the cell. The fluid nature of the animal cell membrane may facilitate the movement of receptor proteins to allow the clustering that is necessary for these multiple interactions.

Adsorption enhanced by multiplicities of attachment and receptor proteins

A particular kind of virus is only capable of infecting a limited spectrum of cell types called its *host range.* Thus, although a few viruses can infect cells from different species, most viruses are limited to a single species. For example, dogs do not contract measles, and humans do not contract distemper. In many cases, animal viruses only infect a particular subset of the cells found in their host organism. Clearly this kind of tissue tropism is very important in determining the pathology of the infection. In most cases studied, the host range of a virus and its associated tissue tropism is determined by the high specificity of adsorption at the level of the binding between the cell receptors and virion attachment proteins. Thus, these two protein components must possess complementary surfaces that fit together in much the same way as a substrate fits into the active site of an enzyme. It follows, therefore, that adsorption only occurs in that fraction of collisions that lead to a successful binding interaction between receptors and attachment proteins and that the inability of a virus to infect a cell type is usually due to the absence of the appropriate receptors on the cell. The exquisite specificity of these interactions is well illustrated by the case of a particular mouse reovirus, where it has been found that the tissue tropism and, therefore, the resultant pathology is altered by a point mutation that changes a single amino acid in the virion attachment protein. A few cases are known where the host range of a virus is determined at a step after adsorption and penetration, but these are the exceptions rather than the rule.

Differences in host range and tissue tropism due to presence or absence of receptors

Once a virus particle has penetrated to the inside of a cell, it is essentially hidden from the host immune system. Thus, if protection from a virus infection is to be accomplished at the level of antibody binding to the virions, it must occur before adsorption and prevent the virus from attaching to and penetrating the cell. It is not surprising, therefore, that most neutralizing antibodies, whether acquired as a result of natural infection or vaccination are specific for virion attachment proteins.

Neutralizing antibodies are usually specific for attachment proteins

Entry and Uncoating

The eclipse phase is a direct consequence of the fact that viruses are dismantled prior to being replicated. As will be shown below, the uncoating step may be simultaneous with entry or may occur in a series of

Viruses are dismantled before being replicated

6.2 Bacteriophage entry.

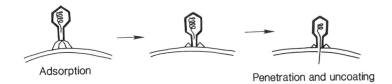

Adsorption   Penetration and uncoating

steps. Ultimately the nucleocapsid or core structure must be transported to the site or compartment in the cell where transcription and replication will occur.

The Bacteriophage Strategy

The processess of penetration and uncoating are simultaneous for all bacteriophages. Thus, the viral capsids are shed at the surface and only the nucleic acid genome enters the cell. In some cases, a small number of virion proteins may accompany the genome into the cell, but these are probably tightly associated with the nucleic acid or are essential enzymes needed to initiate the infection.

> Bacteriophage capsids are shed as the viral genome enters host cell

Bacteriophages with tails have evolved these special appendages to facilitate the entry of the genome into the cell. The process of penetration and uncoating for bacteriophage T4 is shown schematically in Figure 6.2. The tail fibers extending from the end of the tail are responsible for the attachment of the virion to the cell wall, and, in the next step, the end of the tail itself makes intimate contact with the cell surface. Finally the DNA of the virus is injected directly into the cell through the hollow tail structure. The process has been likened to the action of a syringe, but the energetics and the nature of the orifice in the cell surface through which the DNA travels are poorly understood.

> Tailed phages attach by tail fibers; DNA injected through tail

Enveloped Animal Viruses

There are two basic mechanisms for the entry of an enveloped animal virus into the cell. Both mechanisms involve fusion of the viral envelope with a cellular membrane, and the end result in both cases is the release of the free nucleocapsid into the cytoplasm. What distinguishes the two mechanisms is the nature of the cellular membrane that fuses with the viral envelope.

Figure 6.3 depicts the entry mechanism for paramyxoviruses such as the measles virus. The envelopes of these viruses contain protein spikes that promote fusion of viral envelopes with the plasma membrane of the cell, releasing the nucleocapsid directly into the cytoplasm. Because the viral envelope becomes incorporated into the plasma membrane of the infected cell and still possesses its fusion proteins, infected cells have a tendency to fuse with other uninfected cells. Cell–cell fusion is a hallmark of infections by paramyxoviruses and can be important in the pathology of a disease such as measles.

> Some enveloped viruses enter cell by membrane–envelope fusion

The mechanism for the entry of most of the remaining enveloped animal viruses, such as orthomyxoviruses (eg, influenza viruses), togaviruses (eg, rubella virus), rhabdoviruses (eg, rabies), and herpesviruses, is shown in Figure 6.4. Following adsorption, the virus particles are taken up by a cellular mechanism called *receptor-mediated endocytosis,* which is normally responsible for internalizing growth factors, hormones, and some nutrients. When it involves viruses, the process is referred to as *viropexis.*

> Other enveloped and naked viruses are endocytosed (viropexis)

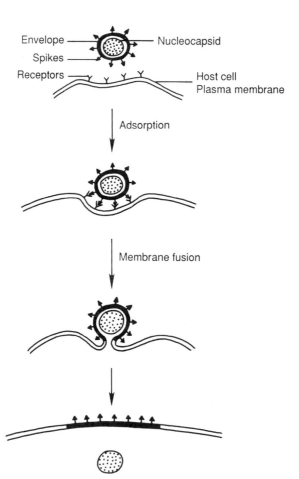

Envelope — Nucleocapsid
Spikes —
Receptors — Host cell
Plasma membrane

Adsorption

6.3 Paramyxovirus entry.

Membrane fusion

In viropexis the adsorbed virions become surrounded by the plasma membrane in a reaction that is probably facilitated by the multiplicity of virion attachment proteins on the surface of the particle. Pinching off of the cellular membrane by fusion encloses the virion in a cytoplasmic vesicle termed the *endosomal vesicle*. The nucleocapsid is now surrounded by two membranes, the original viral envelope and the newly acquired plasma membrane. The surface receptors are subsequently recycled back to the plasma membrane, and the endosomal vesicle is acidified by an unknown mechanism. The low pH of the endosome leads to a conformational change in a viral spike protein, which results in a fusion of the two membranes and release of the nucleocapsid into the cytoplasm. In some cases, the contents of the endosomal vesicle may be transferred to a lysosome prior to the fusion step that releases the nucleocapsid.

Acidified endosome releases nucleocapsid to cytoplasm

Naked Capsid Animal Viruses

Naked capsid viruses, such as poliovirus, reovirus, and adenovirus, also appear to enter the cell by viropexis. In this case, however, the virus cannot escape the endosomal vesicle by membrane fusion as described above for enveloped viruses. For poliovirus it appears that the viral capsid proteins in the low pH environment of the endosome expose hydrophobic domains, which result in the binding of the virions to the membrane and

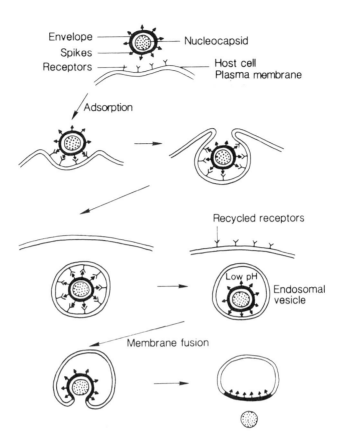

6.4 Viropexis.

release of the nucleic acid genome into the cytoplasm. In other cases the virions may escape into the cytoplasm by promoting the dissolution of the vesicle. This step is a potential target for antiviral chemotherapy, and recently drugs have been developed that bind to capsids of certain picornaviruses and prevent the release of the virus particles from the endosome.

Reovirus is unusual in that prior to release into the cytoplasm the contents of the endosome are transferred to a lysosome where the lysosomal proteases strip away part of the capsid proteins and activate virion-associated enzymes required for transcription.

Fate of Intracellular Particles

Even in the relatively simple bacterial cell, there is evidence that the entering nucleic acid must be directed to a particular cellular locus to initiate the infection process. Proteins known as *pilot proteins* have been described that accompany the phage genome into the bacterial cell and serve the function of "piloting" the nucleic acid to a particular target, such as a membrane site where transcription and replication is to occur.

The ultimate fate of internalized animal virus particles depends on the particular virus and on the cellular compartment where replication occurs. Most RNA viruses with the exception of influenza viruses and the retroviruses replicate in the cytoplasm, the immediate site of entry. Retroviruses and influenza viruses and all the DNA viruses except the poxviruses must move from the cytoplasm to the nucleus to replicate. The larger

Most RNA viruses replicate in cytoplasm

All DNA viruses except poxviruses replicate in nucleus

DNA viruses, such as herpesviruses and adenoviruses, must uncoat to the level of cores prior to entry into the nucleus. The smaller DNA viruses, such as the parvoviruses and the papovaviruses, enter the nucleus intact through the nuclear pores and subsequently uncoat inside. The largest of the animal viruses, the poxviruses, carry out their entire replicative cycle in the cytoplasm of the infected cell.

The Problems of Producing mRNA

From Genome to mRNA

Virus-specified mRNAs direct synthesis of viral proteins

An essential step in every virus infection is the production of mRNAs by transcription. The virus-specified mRNAs program the cellular ribosomes to synthesize viral proteins. Besides the structural proteins of the virion, viruses must direct the synthesis of enzymes and other specialized proteins required for genome replication, gene expression, and virus assembly and release. The production of the *first* viral mRNAs at the beginning of the infection is a crucial step in the takeover of the cell by the virus.

Most DNA virus mRNA synthesized by host polymerase

(+)-strand RNA virus genome serves as mRNA

For some viruses the presentation of mRNA to the cellular ribosomes poses no problems. Thus, the genomes of most DNA viruses are transcribed by the host DNA-dependent RNA polymerase to yield the initial mRNAs. The (+)-strand RNA viruses, such as the picornaviruses, the togaviruses, and the coronaviruses, possess genomes that can be utilized directly as mRNAs and are translated (at least partially, as will be discussed below) immediately upon entry into the cytoplasm of the cell.

However, for many viruses the production of mRNA starting from the genome is not so straightforward. The fact that poxviruses replicate in the cytoplasm means that cellular transcription enzymes are not available to transcribe the genome. Moreover, no cellular machinery exists that can utilize either single-stranded or double-stranded RNA as a template to synthesize mRNA. Therefore, these viruses must provide their own transcription enzymes to produce the initial mRNAs at the beginning of the infection process. This is accomplished by synthesizing the transcriptases in the later stages of viral development in the previous host cell and packaging the enzymes into the virions where they remain associated with the genome as the virus enters the new cell and uncoats. In general, the presence of a transcriptase in virions is indicative that the host cell is unable to utilize the viral genome as mRNA or as a template to synthesize mRNA. At later times in the infection of the cell, any special enzymatic machinery required by the virus, and not initially present in the cell, can be supplied among the proteins translated from the first mRNA molecules.

Other RNA viruses carry transcription enzymes to produce initial mRNAs

Pathways for synthesis of mRNA by different virus groups

The pathways for the synthesis of mRNA by the major virus groups are summarized in Figure 6.5 and related to the structure of viral genomes. The polarity of mRNA is designated as (+) and polynucleotide chains complementary to mRNA as (−). The heavy arrows denote synthetic steps for which host cells provide the appropriate enzymes whereas the thinner arrows indicate synthetic steps that must be carried out by virion enzymes. Several additional points need to be emphasized. The parvoviruses and some phages have single-stranded DNA genomes. Although the RNA polymerase of the cell requires double-stranded DNA as a template, these viruses need not carry special enzymes in their virions because host cell DNA polymerases can convert the genomes into double-stranded DNA. Note that the production of mRNA by the picornaviruses and similar (+)-strand viruses requires the synthesis of an intermediate (−)-strand tem-

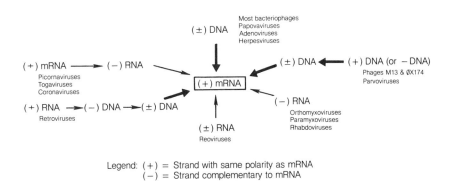

6.5 Pathways of mRNA synthesis for major virus groups.

plate. The enzyme required for this process is produced by translation of the genomic RNA at early times in infection of the cell.

The retroviruses are a special class of (+)-strand RNA viruses. Although their genomes are of the same polarity as mRNA and could in principle serve as mRNAs early after infection, their replication scheme apparently precludes this. Instead, the RNA genomes of these viruses are copied into (−)DNA strands by an enzyme carried within the virion called *reverse transcriptase*. The (−)DNA strands are subsequently converted by the same enzyme to double-stranded DNA in a reaction that requires the degradation of the original genomic RNA. The DNA product of reverse transcription is ultimately transcribed by the host RNA polymerase to complete the replication cycle as well as produce viral mRNA. The need to package reverse transcriptase in the virion apparently derives from the fact that translation of the genomic RNA to produce the enzyme at early times would prevent the use of the RNA as a template for reverse transcription (see Chapter 41).

The arenaviruses and bunyaviruses are not included in the scheme shown in Figure 6.5. These viruses possess unusual genomes, part of which is the same polarity as the mRNA and another part that is opposite in polarity to the corresponding mRNA. That region that is the same polarity as the mRNA is probably translated directly as shown in Figure 6.5 for picornaviruses and togaviruses; the other region must be transcribed into mRNA in a fashion similar to that shown for the (−)RNA viruses.

The Monocistronic mRNA Rule in Animal Cells

The ribosome requires input of information in the form of mRNA. In order for a viral mRNA to be recognized by the ribosome, its production must conform to the rules of structure that govern the synthesis of cellular mRNAs. Prokaryotic mRNA is relatively simple and can be polycistronic, which means it can contain the information for several proteins. Each cistron is translated independently beginning from its own ribosome binding site. In fact the genome of the well-studied *Escherichia coli* RNA phage is just such a polycistronic mRNA.

Eukaryotic mRNAs are more complex, containing a special 5'-cap structure and a 3'-poly(A) attachment. In addition their synthesis often involves removal of internal sequences by a process called *splicing*. Most importantly, virtually all eukaryotic mRNAs are monocistronic. Eukaryotic translation is initiated by the binding of the ribosome to the 5'-cap, fol-

Retroviral RNA copied to DNA by virion reverse transcriptase; host RNA polymerase transcribes DNA into more RNA

Prokaryotic mRNA (and, thus, phage RNA) can be polycistronic

lowed by movement of the ribosome along the RNA until the first AUG initiation codon is encountered. The corollary to this first AUG rule is that the eukaryotic ribosome cannot initiate translation at internal sites on a mRNA. Recent evidence indicates that this rule is occasionally broken with one or more AUG sites being skipped before initiation occurs. However, it is clear that efficient translation cannot occur by initiation at internal sites on a mRNA. Thus, animal viruses must program the synthesis of mRNAs that are translated to produce only a single polypeptide chain by initiation of translation near the 5'-end of the mRNA.

Animal virus mRNA must be monocistronic; variety of viral strategies used to accomplish this

Because most DNA animal viruses replicate in the nucleus, they adhere to the monocistronic mRNA rule by either having a promoter precede each gene or by programming the transcription of precursor RNAs that are processed by nuclear splicing enzymes into monocistronic mRNAs. The virion transcriptase of the cytoplasmic poxviruses must synthesize monocistronic mRNAs by initiation of transcription in front of each gene.

RNA-Containing animal viruses have evolved three different strategies to circumvent or conform to the monocistronic mRNA rule. The simplest strategy involves having a segmented genome. Each genomic segment of the orthomyxoviruses and the reoviruses corresponds to a single gene, and, therefore, the mRNA transcribed from a given segment constitutes a monocistronic mRNA. The orthomyxovirus virus, influenza A, unlike most RNA viruses, replicates in the nucleus and some of its monocistronic mRNAs are produced by splicing of precursor RNAs.

A second solution to the monocistronic mRNA rule is very similar to the strategy employed by cells and the DNA viruses. The paramyxoviruses, togaviruses, rhabdoviruses, and coronaviruses synthesize monocistronic mRNAs by initiating the synthesis of an mRNA at the beginning of each gene. In most cases, the transcriptase terminates mRNA synthesis at end of each gene so that each message corresponds to a single gene. For the coronaviruses, RNA synthesis initiates at the beginning of each gene and continues to the end of the genome so that a set of mRNAs is produced. Each mRNA, however, is functionally monocistronic and is translated to produce only the protein encoded near its 5'-end.

The picornaviruses have evolved yet a third strategy to deal with the monocistronic mRNA requirement (Figure 6.6). The (+)-strand genome contains just a single ribosome-binding site near the 5'-end and is translated into one long polypeptide chain called a *polyprotein*. The polyprotein is subsequently broken into the final set of protein products by a series of proteolytic cleavages. In fact, the required proteolytic activity resides within the polyprotein itself.

Several viruses employ more than one of these strategies to conform to the monocistronic mRNA rule. For example, the retroviruses and the togaviruses synthesize multiple mRNAs each one coding for a polyprotein.

Genome Replication

DNA Viruses

Cells obviously contain the enzymes and accessory proteins required for the replication of DNA. In bacteria these proteins are present continuously, whereas in the eukaryotic cell they are only present during the S phase of the cell cycle, and they are restricted to the nucleus. The extent to which viruses depend on cell replication machinery depends on the size of their genome and thus on their protein-coding potential.

The smallest of the DNA viruses, the parvoviruses, are so completely

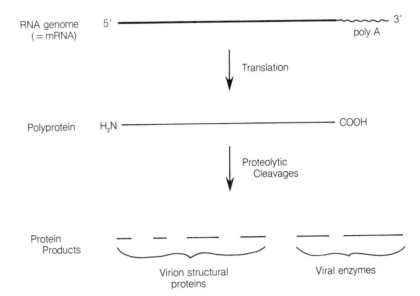

6.6 Poliovirus gene expression.

Smallest DNA viruses depend exclusively on host DNA replication machinery

Larger DNA viruses code for enzymes important for DNA replication

Virally encoded DNA polymerase is target for chemotherapy (eg acyclovir)

dependent on host machinery that they require the infected cells be dividing so that a normal S phase (DNA synthesis phase of cell cycle) will occur and replicate their DNA along with the cellular DNA. At the other end of the spectrum are the largest of the viruses, which are relatively independent of cellular functions. The largest bacteriophages, such as T4, degrade the host cell chromosome at an early time in infection and replace all of the host replication machinery with virus-specified proteins. The largest animal viruses, the poxviruses, are similarly independent of the host. Because they replicate in the cytoplasm, they must code for virtually all of the enzymes and other proteins required for replicating their DNA.

The remainder of the DNA viruses are only partially dependent on host machinery. For example, bacteriophages φX174 and λ code for proteins that direct the initiation of DNA synthesis to the viral origin. The actual synthesis of DNA, however, occurs by the complex of cellular enzymes responsible for replication of the *E. coli* DNA. Similarly the small DNA animal viruses, such as the papovaviruses, code for a protein that is involved in the initiation of synthesis at the origin, but the remainder of the replication process is carried out by host machinery. The slightly larger adenoviruses and herpesviruses, in addition to providing origin-specific proteins, also code for their own DNA polymerases and other accessory proteins required for DNA replication.

The fact that the herpesviruses code for their own DNA polymerase has important implications for the treatment of infections by these viruses and illustrates a central principle of antiviral chemotherapy. Certain antiviral drugs (adenine arabinoside and 5'-iododeoxyuridine) have been found to be effective against herpesvirus infections (see Chapter 37), because they are sufficiently similar to natural substrates that the virally encoded DNA polymerase mistakenly incorporates them into viral DNA resulting in an inhibition of subsequent DNA synthesis. The host cell enzyme is more discriminatory and fails to utilize the analogs in the synthesis of cellular DNA, and, thus, the drugs do not kill uninfected cells. The antiviral drug, acyclovir (acycloguanosine) preferentially kills herpesvirus–infected cells because the viral enzyme, thymidine kinase, unlike the cellular counterpart, phosphorylates the thymidine analog, converting it to a form which when incorporated into DNA by DNA polymerases inhibits further DNA synthesis. In principle, any viral process that is distinct from a normal cellular process is a potential target for antiviral drugs. As more becomes known about the details of viral replication, more drugs will become available that are targeted to those processes unique to the virus.

As noted above, with the exception of the poxviruses, all of the DNA animal viruses are at least partially dependent on host cell machinery for the replication of their genomes. However, unlike the parvoviruses, the other DNA viruses do not need to infect dividing cells for a productive infection to ensue. Instead, all of these viruses code for a protein expressed early in infection that induces an unscheduled cellular DNA replication (S phase). In this way, these viruses ensure that the infected cell makes all of the machinery required for the replication of their DNA. It is noteworthy that all of the DNA viruses except the parvoviruses are capable, in some circumstances, of transforming a normal cell into a cancer cell (see Chapter 7). This correlation suggests that the unlimited proliferative capacity of the cancer cells may be due to the continual synthesis of the viral protein or proteins responsible for inducing the unscheduled S phase in a normal infection. Therefore, the fact that these DNA viruses can induce oncogenic transformation of cell types that are nonpermissive for viral multiplication may simply be an accident related to the need to induce cellular enzymes required for DNA replication during lytic infection.

All DNA viruses except parvoviruses can transform host cells

All DNA polymerases, including those encoded by viruses, synthesize DNA chains by the successive addition of nucleotides onto the 3'-end of the new DNA strand. Moreover, all DNA polymerases require a primer terminus containing a free 3'-hydroxyl to initiate the synthesis of a DNA chain. In cellular replication, a temporary primer is provided in the form of a short RNA molecule. The priming RNA is synthesized by an RNA polymerase, and after elongation by the DNA polymerase it is removed. With circular chromosomes, such as those found in bacteria and many viruses, the unidirectional chain growth and primer requirement of the DNA polymerase pose no structural problems for replication. However, as illustrated in Figure 6.7, when a replication fork encounters the end of a linear DNA molecule, one of the new chains (heavy lines, Figure 6.7) cannot be completed at its 5'-end, because there exists no means of starting the DNA portion of the chain exactly at the end of the template DNA. Thus, after the RNA primer is removed, the new chain is incomplete at its 5'-end. This constraint on the finishing of DNA chains on a linear template is sometimes called the *end problem* in DNA replication.

The end problem in DNA replication

It is beyond the scope of this text to detail all of the strategies viruses have evolved to deal with this problem, but it is worthwhile pointing out some of the structural features found in linear viral genomes whose presence are related to the solutions to this problem. Some of these structures are diagrammed schematically in Figure 6.8. The linear double-stranded genome of bacteriophage λ possesses 12 base single-stranded extensions that are complementary in sequence to each other and thus called *cohesive ends*. Very early after entry into the cell, the two ends pair up to convert the linear genome into a circular molecule in preparation for replication. The linear double-stranded adenovirus genome contains a protein molecule covalently attached to the 5'-end of both strands. These proteins provided the primers required to initiate the synthesis of the DNA chains during replication. The need for RNA primers is circumvented, thus solving the end problem in replication.

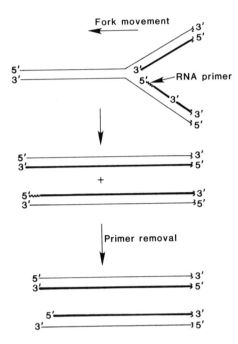

6.7 The end problem in DNA replication.

Protein is also found attached to the hepatitis B genome, presumably a vestige of chain initiation by this virus as well. The single-stranded parvovirus genome contains a self-complementary sequence at the 3'-end that causes the molecule to fold into a hairpin making it self-priming for DNA replication. The poxviruses contain linear double-stranded genomes in which the ends are continuous. In these latter two cases, the solution to the end problem creates additional problems that must be solved to produce replication products that are identical to the starting genomes.

RNA Viruses

RNA animal viruses generally replicate in the cytoplasm, since nuclear functions are designed for DNA metabolism. Influenza and the other orthomyxoviruses are an exception to this rule. They replicate in the nucleus using pieces of newly synthesized cellular mRNAs to prime their own mRNA synthesis. In addition, they utilize the nuclear RNA splicing enzymes in the synthesis of some of their mRNAs.

Cells do not have RNA polymerases that can copy RNA templates.

6.8 Some solutions to the end problem.

Phage λ–Cohesive ends

Adenovirus–"Protein" primers

Parvovirus–Hairpin end

Poxvirus–Continuous ends

RNA viruses must encode
their own transcriptases

Transcription and replication
separated for most RNA
viruses

Therefore, RNA viruses not only need to code for transcriptases as discussed above, but also must provide the replicases required to duplicate the genomic RNA. Furthermore, except in the cases of the RNA phage and the picornaviruses where transcription and replication are synonymous, the RNA viruses must temporally and functionally separate replication from transcription. This requirement is especially apparent for the rhabdoviruses, paramyxoviruses, togaviruses, and coronaviruses, where a complete genome or complementary copy of the genome is transcribed into a set of subgenomic monocistronic mRNAs at early times of infection. After replication begins, these same templates are used to synthesize full-length strands for replication.

Two mechanisms exist to separate the process of replication from transcription. First, in many cases, transcription is restricted to subviral particles and involves a transcriptase transported into the cell within the virion. Second, the replication process involves a somewhat different set of enzymes that make full-length copies of the genome template rather than the shorter length monocistronic mRNAs. In the case of reoviruses, the switch from transcription to replication appears to involve the synthesis of a replicase that converts the $(+)$mRNAs synthesized early in infection to the double-stranded genome segments.

Viral RNA polymerases, like DNA polymerases, synthesize chains in only one direction. However, RNA polymerases in general can initiate the synthesis of new chains without primers. Thus, there is no obvious end problem in RNA replication. There exists one exception to this general rule. The picornaviruses contain a protein covalently attached to the 5'-end of the genome called *Vpg*. It is clear that this protein is involved in priming the synthesis of new $(-)$ strands as well as new $(+)$RNA viral genomes by a mechanism that resembles the priming described above for adenoviruses.

Assembly of Naked Capsid Viruses and Nucleocapsids

The process of forming the capsid structure that surrounds the viral genome is called *encapsidation*. Four general principles govern the construction of capsids and nucleocapsids. First, the process generally involves self-assembly of the component parts. Second, assembly is stepwise and ordered. Third, individual protein structural subunits or protomers are preformed into capsomeres in preparation for the final assembly process. Fourth, assembly often initiates at a particular locus on the genome called a *packaging site*.

Capsids and nucleocapsids
self-assemble from preformed
capsomeres

Viruses with Helical Symmetry

The assembly of the cylindrically shaped tobacco mosaic virus (TMV) has been extensively studied and provides a model for the construction of helical capsids and nucleocapsids. For TMV, donut-shaped disks containing many individual structural subunits are preformed and added stepwise to the growing structure. Elongation occurs in both directions from a specific packaging site on the single-stranded viral RNA (Figure 6.9). The addition of each disk involves an interaction between the protein subunits of the disk and the genome RNA. The nature of this interaction is such that the assembly process ceases when the end of the RNA is reached. The structural subunits as well as the RNA trace out a helical path in the final virus particle.

The basic design features worked out for TMV probably apply in gen-

TMV as a model

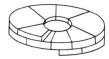

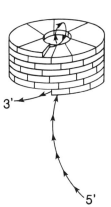

6.9 Tobacco mosiac virus assembly.

eral to the assembly of the nucleocapsids of enveloped viruses. Thus, it is likely that the protein subunits are intimately associated with the RNA and that the nucleoprotein complexes are assembled by the stepwise accretion of protein subunits. For influenza and the other viruses with segmented genomes, the various segments are assembled into nucleocapsids independently and then brought together by a mechanism that is as yet poorly understood. It is notable that virtually all of the animal RNA viruses with helical symmetry are enveloped.

Viruses with Cubic Symmetry

Icosahedral capsids are preassembled and genomes threaded in

For both phage and animal viruses, icosahedral capsids are preassembled and the nucleic acids genomes, usually complexed with condensing proteins, threaded into the empty structures. The construction of the hollow capsids appears to occur by a self-assembly process, sometimes aided by other proteins. The stepwise assembly of components involves the initial aggregation of structural subunits into pentamers and hexamers, followed by the condensation of the capsomeres to form the empty capsid. In some cases, it appears that the structurally significant intermediates in assembly involve dimers or trimers of the structural subunits rather than pentamers and hexamers.

Features Unique to Bacteriophages

Phage heads, tails, and tail fibers synthesized separately and then assembled

The morphogenesis of a complex bacteriophage such as T4 involves the prefabrication of each of the major substructures by a separate pathway, followed by the ordered and sequential construction of the final particle from its component parts. Figure 6.10 diagrams the assembly process for T4 showing how the head, tail, and tail fibers are assembled and then brought together to form the completed phage (many steps are omitted).

An intermediate in the assembly of a bacteriophage head is an empty structure containing an internal protein network that is removed prior to insertion of the nucleic acid. The constituents of this network are often appropriately referred to as *scaffolding proteins*. The scaffolding proteins

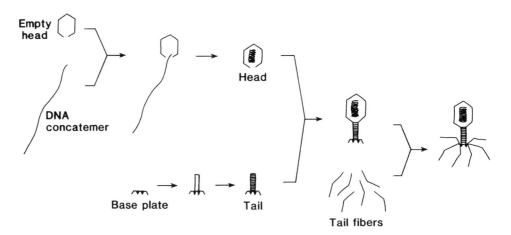

6.10 Assembly of bacteriophage T4.

apparently provide the lattice necessary to hold the capsomeres in position during the early stages of head assembly.

Phage DNA replicated as multigenomic molecules

For many DNA bacteriophages, the products of replication are long linear DNA molecules called *concatemers,* which are made up of tandem repeats of genome size units. During the packaging of the DNA into the preformed capsids, these concatemers are processed by nuclease cleavages to generate genome-size pieces.

Mechanisms for cutting phage DNA during packaging

There are two mechanisms for determining the correct sites for cleavage by the packaging nuclease. Bacteriophage λ typifies one type of mechanism in which the enzyme that makes the cuts is a site-specific nuclease. The enzyme sits poised at the orifice of the capsid as the DNA is being threaded into the head, and when the specific cut site is encountered, the DNA is cleaved. For λ, the breaks are made in opposite strands, 12 base pairs apart, to generate the cohesive ends. Bacteriophages T4 and P1 are examples of bacterial viruses that illustrate the second mechanism. For these phages, the nuclease does not recognize a particular DNA sequence, but instead cuts the concatemer when the capsid is full. Because the head of the bacteriophage can accommodate slightly more than one genome equivalent of DNA and packaging can begin anywhere on the DNA, the "headful" mechanism produces genomes that are terminally redundant (the same sequence is found at both ends) and circularly permuted. The fact that packaging is nonspecific with respect to DNA sequence explains why the P1 bacteriophage is capable of incorporating host DNA into phage particles, thereby promoting generalized transduction (see Chapter 4). T4 does not carry out generalized transduction, because the bacterial DNA is completely degraded to nucleotides early in infection.

Host DNA may be incorporated by headful mechanism, and generalized transduction results

Release

Bacteriophages

Phages encode lysozyme or peptidases that lyse bacterial cell wall

Most bacteriophages escape from the infected cell by coding for an enzyme (or enzymes) synthesized late in the latent phase that causes the lysis of the cell. The enzymes are either lysozymes or peptidases, which weaken the cell wall by cleaving specific bonds in the peptidoglycan layer. The weakened cells burst due to osmotic pressure.

Animal Viruses

Cell Death. Nearly all productively infected cells die (see below for exceptions), presumably because the viral genetic program is dominant and precludes the continuation of normal cell functions required for survival. The naked capsid animal viruses lack specific mechanisms for lysing the infected cell and apparently are released into the extracellular milieu simply as a consequence of cell death. Release may, therefore, be facilitated by the liberation of a variety of degradative lysosomal enzymes that aid in the dissolution of the dying cell.

Naked capsid viruses released with cell death and autolysis

Budding. With the exception of the poxviruses, all enveloped animal viruses acquire their membrane by budding through either the plasma membrane or, in the case of herpesviruses, through the nuclear membrane. Thus, for these viruses, release from the cell is coupled to the final stage of virion assembly. How the herpesviruses ultimately escape from the cell after budding through nuclear membrane is unclear; they may travel through channels in the endoplasmic reticulum to get from the nucleus to the outside. The poxviruses appear to program the synthesis of their own outer membrane. How the poxvirus envelope is assembled on the nucleocapsid is not known.

Most enveloped viruses acquire envelope during release by budding

Poxviruses synthesize their own envelopes

The membrane changes that accompany budding are just the reverse of the entry process described before for paramyxoviruses (compare Figures 6.3 and 6.11). The region of the cellular membrane where budding is to occur acquires a cluster of viral glycoprotein spikes. These proteins are synthesized by the pathway that normally delivers cellular membrane proteins to the surface of the cell by way of the golgi apparatus. The presence of hydrophobic leader sequences on the amimo terminus tags the proteins for transport to the plasma membrane. At the site of the glycoprotein cluster, the inside of the membrane becomes coated with a virion structural protein called the *matrix* or *M protein*. The accumulation of the matrix protein at the proper location is probably facilitated by the presence of a binding site for the matrix protein on the cytoplasmic side of the transmembrane glycoprotein spike. The matrix protein attracts the completed nucleocapsid that triggers the membrane fusions that enclose the nucleocapsid in the envelope and at the same time release the completed particle to the outside (Figure 6.11).

Membrane site for budding first acquires virus-specified spikes and matrix protein

For viruses that bud, it is important to note that the plasma membrane

6.11 Viral release by budding.

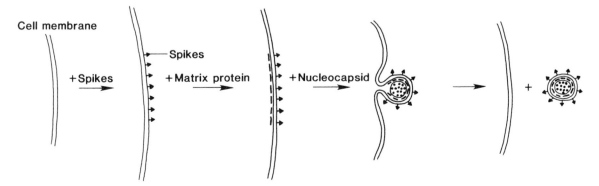

Cell membrane

+Spikes

Spikes
+Matrix protein

+Nucleocapsid

of the infected cell contains virus-specific glycoproteins that represent foreign antigens. This means that the infected cells become targets for the immune system. In fact, cytotoxic T cells that recognize these antigens can be a significant factor in combating a virus infection.

Budding process rarely causes cell death

The process of viral budding usually does not lead directly to cell death, because the plasma membrane can be repaired following budding. It is likely that cell death for most enveloped viruses, as for naked capsid viruses, is related to the loss of normal cellular functions required for survival. The causative agent of AIDS (acquired immunodeficiency syndrome) represents an exception to this generalization. The agent is a retrovirus (called *human immunodeficiency virus,* or HIV) that replicates in the T4 class of lymphocytes. It appears that the virus is latent in the host cell until triggered by external factors (see Chapter 73) to produce massive quantities of new virus. The cytotoxic nature of this virus, unlike most retroviruses, apparently results from permanent membrane damage that occurs during budding.

Most retroviruses (except HIV) reproduce without cell death

Cell Survival.   For retroviruses other than HIV and the filamentous bacteriophages, virus reproduction and cell survival are compatible. Retroviruses convert their RNA genome into double-stranded DNA, which integrates into a host cell chromosome and is transcribed just like any other cellular gene (see Chapter 41). Thus, the impact on cellular metabolism is minimal. Moreover, the virus buds through the plasma membrane without any permanent damage to the cell (see above for HIV exception).

Filamentous phages assemble during extrusion without damaging cells

Because the filamentous phages are nonenveloped viruses, cell survival is even more remarkable. In this case, the helical capsid is assembled onto the condensed single-stranded DNA genome as the structure is being extruded through both the membrane and the cell wall of the bacterium. How the cell escapes permanent damage in this case is unknown. As with the retroviruses, the infected cell continues to produce virus indefinitely.

Quantitation of Viruses

Hemagglutination Assay

For some animal viruses, red blood cells from one or more animal species contain receptors for the virion attachment proteins. Because both the receptors and attachment proteins are present in multiple copies on the cells and virions respectively, an excess of virus particles will coat the cells and cause them to aggregate. This aggregation phenomenon was first discovered with influenza virus and is called *hemagglutination.* The virion attachment protein on the influenza virion is appropriately called the *hemagglutinin.* Furthermore, the presence of the hemagglutinin in the plasma membrane of the infected cell means that the cells as well as the virions will bind the red blood cells. This reaction, called *hemadsorption,* is a useful indicator of infection by certain viruses (see Chapter 14).

Titer of hemagglutinin-containing virus can be measured by hemagglutination

Hemagglutination can be used to estimate the titer of virus particles in a virus-containing sample. Serially diluted samples of the virus preparation are mixed with a constant amount of red blood cells and the mixture allowed to settle in a test tube. If there is insufficient virus to agglutinate the red blood cells, they will settle to the bottom of the tube and form a tight pellet. However, the agglutinated red blood cells settle to the bottom to form a thin disperse layer of cells. The difference is easily scored visually and the end point of the agglutination used as a relative measure of the virus concentration in the sample.

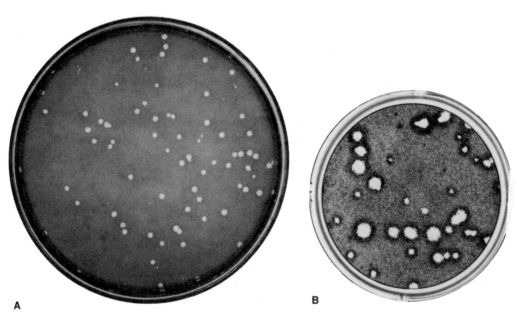

6.12 Plaque assays: (**A**) bacteriophage λ; (**B**) adenovirus.

Plaque Assay

Plaque assay: dilutions of virus added to excess cells; cells immobilized in agar

The plaque assay is a method of determining the titer of infectious virions in a virus preparation or lysate. The sample is diluted serially and an aliquot of each dilution added to a vast excess of susceptible host cells. For an animal virus, the host cells are usually attached to the bottom of plastic petri dish, while bacterial cells are infected in suspension. In both cases the infected cells are immersed in a semisolid medium, such as agar, which localizes the infection to a particular site on the petri dish. Because of the agar, the virus released from the initial and subsequent infections can only invade the cells in the immediate vicinity of the initial infected cell. The end result is an easily visible clearing of dead cells at each of the sites on the plate where one of the original infected cells was localized. (Visualization in the case of animal cells usually requires staining the cells.) The clearing is called a *plaque* (Figure 6.12). By counting the number of plaques and correcting for the dilution factor, the virus titer in the original sample can be calculated. The titer is usually expressed as the number of plaque-forming units per milliliter (pfu/ml).

Replicated virus infects neighboring cells; visible plaques result and can be counted

Interferons

Interferons from virally infected cells inhibit viral production in other cells

Interferons are host encoded, species specific, but not virus specific

Interferons are host-encoded proteins that provide the first line of defense against viral infections. Virus infection of all types of cells stimulates the production and secretion of an interferon that in turn acts on other infected cells to prevent virus production. Unlike immunity, interferon is not specific to a particular kind of virus. However, interferons usually act only on cells of the same species. Other agents stimulate the production of interferons by lymphoid cells. In this case interferon appears to play an important role in the immune system independent of any role as an antiviral protein (see Chapter 10).

The signal that leads to the production of interferon by an infected cell appears to be double-stranded RNA. This conclusion is based on the fact that treatment of cells with purified double-stranded RNA or synthetic double-stranded ribopolymers results in the production of interferon. It is not obvious why double-stranded RNA should be present in an infected cell except in the case of reovirus. However, for the other RNA viruses, transcription and replication require complementary RNA molecules as templates. It is likely that complementary strands occasionally combine during the infection to produce sufficient quantities of double-stranded RNA to induce interferon. In the case of DNA viruses, double-stranded RNA may accumulate because transcription of a particular region of DNA occasionally occurs in both directions producing complementary RNA strands. Alternatively, viral mRNAs may in general possess more secondary structure than the typical cellular mRNA.

The viral inhibitory effects of interferon are not yet well understood and what follows is at best an incomplete description of how interferon works. It appears that interferon acts to inhibit virus production at two different stages of protein synthesis. In the presence of interferon, the synthesis of two cellular enzymes are induced. The first is a protein kinase that phosphorylates and thereby inactivates one of the subunits of an elongation factor (eIF-2) necessary for protein synthesis. The second is 2',5'-oligo (adenylate) synthetase, which synthesizes chains of 2',5'-oligo (A) up to 10 residues in length. The 2',5'-oligo (A) in turn activates a constitutive ribonuclease that degrades mRNA molecules. The action of both of these enzymes requires the presence of double-stranded RNA, the intracellular signal that an infection is occurring. This requirement prevents interferon from having an adverse effect on protein synthesis in uninfected cells.

It is not clear whether this cascade of reactions can specifically prevent virus-specific protein synthesis in the infected cell without inhibiting cellular protein synthesis at the same time. Conceivably, the presence of double-stranded RNA in the vicinity of viral, but not host mRNAs, could locally activate the two inhibitory pathways, preventing only virus-specific protein synthesis. Alternatively, the role of interferon may simply be to prevent both viral and cellular protein synthesis in the infected cell. The result is cell death, but no virus production. If this is the case, then in the presence of interferon the infected cells are, in effect, "sacrificed" for the good of the whole organism.

Interferons produced in response to double-stranded RNA accumulating during viral synthesis

Interferons act by inhibiting viral protein synthesis and possibly cell protein synthesis

Additional Reading

Joklik, W.K., Ed. 1988. *Virology.* 3rd ed. Norwalk, Conn.: Appleton-Century-Crofts. An up-to-date overview of medical aspects of virology.

Notkins, A.L., and Oldstone, M.B.A., Eds. 1984. *Concepts in Viral Pathogenesis.* New York: Springer-Verlag, Inc. A collection of articles relating basic virology to pathogenesis.

7
Viral Genetics

James J. Champoux

In a typical lytic infection considered in Chapter 6, viruses invade a host cell and usurp the machinery of the cell for their own reproduction. The end result is usually cell death with the release of large numbers of new infectious virus particles, most of which are phenotypically identical to the original invading virus. This apparent homogeneity is deceptive, and in this chapter the methods used by viral genomes to change by mutation and recombination will be considered, and the medical consequences of some of these changes will be examined. The methods used by temperate viruses to enter, maintain, and sometimes leave the latent state will also be discussed. Further, the means by which both bacterial and animal cells can be permanently changed by viral latency will be examined in some detail.

Mechanisms of Genetic Change

For DNA bacteriophages, the ratio of infectious particles to total particles usually approaches a value of one. Such is not the case for animal viruses. Typically less than 1% of the particles derived from an infected cell are infectious in other cells. Although some of this discrepancy may be attributable to inefficiencies in the assay procedures, it is clear that many defective particles are being produced. The production of defectives arises from unusually high mutation rates for animal viruses and from the fact that many infections occur at high multiplicities, where defective genomes are complemented by nondefective viruses and therefore propagated.

Greater than 99% of animal virus particles from an infected cell are defective

Mutation

Many DNA viruses utilize the host DNA synthesis machinery for replicating their genomes and, therefore, benefit from the built-in proofreading and other error-correcting mechanisms used by the cell. However, the

Larger DNA viruses lack proofreading capabilities and have high error rates

largest animal viruses (adenoviruses, herpesviruses, and poxviruses) code for their own DNA polymerases and these enzymes lack efficient proofreading activities. The resulting high error rates in DNA replication endow the viruses with the potential for a high rate of evolution, but are also responsible for the high rate of production of defective viral particles.

Similar high error rates for RNA viruses produce genetically heterogenous populations

The replication of RNA viruses is also characterized by very high error rates, because neither viral nor cellular RNA polymerases possess proofreading capabilities. The result is that error rates for RNA viruses commonly approach one mistake for every 2500 to 10,000 nucleotides polymerized. Such a high misincorporation rate assures that, even for the smallest RNA viruses, virtually every round of replication introduces one or more nucleotide changes somewhere in the genome. Assuming errors are introduced at random, most of the members of a clone (for example, in a plaque) are different genetically from all other members of the clone. Because of the redundancy in the genetic code, some mutations are silent and not reflected in changes at the protein level, but many occur in essential genes and contribute to the large number of defective particles found with RNA animal viruses. The concept of genetic stability takes on a new meaning in view of these considerations and the virus population as a whole maintains some degree of homogeneity only because of the high degree of fitness exhibited by a small subset of the possible genome sequences. Thus, strong selective forces continually operate on a population to eliminate most mutants that fail to compete with the few very successful members of the population.

High mutation rates permit adaptation to changed conditions

Mutations produce diversity of rhinoviruses and antigenic drifts of influenza viruses

The high mutation rates found for RNA viruses endow them with a genetic plasticity that leads readily to the occurrence of genetic variants and permits rapid adaptation to new environmental conditions. The large number of serotypes of the rhinoviruses causing the common cold, for instance, may reflect the potential to vary by mutation. Although rapid genetic change occurs for most if not all viruses, no RNA virus has exhibited this phenomenon as conspicuously as influenza virus. Point mutations accumulate in the influenza genes coding for the two envelope proteins (hemagglutinin and neuraminidase) resulting in changes in the antigenic structure of the virions. These changes lead to new variants not recognized by the immune system of previously infected individuals. This phenomenon is called *antigenic drift* (see Chapter 32). Apparently, those domains of the two envelope proteins that are most important for immune recognition are not essential for virus reproduction and, as a result, can tolerate amino acid changes leading to antigenic variation. This feature may distinguish influenza from other human RNA viruses that possess the same high mutation rates, but do not exhibit such high rates of antigenic drift. Antigenic drift in epidemic influenza viruses from year to year requires continual updating of the strains used to produce immunizing vaccines.

Retroviruses use two error-prone polymerases; high mutation rates result

The retroviruses likewise show high rates of variation because they depend for their replication on two different polymerases, both of which are error prone. In the first step of the replication cycle, the reverse transcriptase that copies the RNA genome into double-stranded DNA lacks a proofreading capability. Once the proviral DNA has integrated into the chromosome of the host cell, the DNA is transcribed by the host RNA polymerase II, which similarly is incapable of proofreading. As expected these viruses exhibit a high rate of mutation in vitro and in vivo.

Retroviruses, such as HIV (human immunodeficiency virus, the causative agent of acquired immunodeficiency syndrome, AIDS), that exhibit high rates of antigenic variation pose particularly difficult problems for the development of effective vaccines. Attempts are being made to identify conserved, and therefore presumably essential, domains of the envelope proteins for these viruses, which might be useful in developing a genetically engineered vaccine. Success will depend on finding regions that are common to all virulent strains and are capable of eliciting a neutralizing immune response.

von Magnus Phenomenon and Defective Interfering Particles

In early studies with influenza virus, it was noticed that serial passage of virus stocks at high multiplicities of infection led to a steady decline of infectious titer with each passage. At the same time, the titer of noninfectious particles increased. As will be discussed below, the noninfectious genomes interfere with the replication of the infectious virus and so are called *defective interfering particles,* or DI particles. Later, these observations were extended to include virtually all DNA as well as RNA animal viruses. The phenomenon is now named after von Magnus, who described the initial observations with influenza virus.

The combination of two separate events lead to this phenomenon. First, deletion mutations occur at a significant frequency for all viruses. For DNA viruses, the mechanisms are not well understood, but deletions presumably occur as a result of mistakes in replication or by nonhomologous recombination. The basis for the occurrence of deletions in RNA viruses is better understood. All RNA replicases have a tendency to dissociate from the template RNA, but remain bound to the end of the growing RNA chain. By reassociating with the same or a different template at a different location, the replicase can "finish" replication, but in the process create a shorter or longer RNA molecule. A subset of these variants possess the proper signals for initiating RNA synthesis and continue replicating. Because the deletion variants in the population require less time to complete a replication cycle, they eventually predominate and constitute the DI particles.

Second, as their name implies, the DI particles interfere with the replication of nondefective particles. Interference occurs because the DI particles successfully compete with the nondefective genomes for the limited supply of replication enzymes. The virions released at the end of the infection are, therefore, enriched for the DI particles. With each successive infection, the DI particles can predominate over the normal particles as long as the multiplicity of infection is high enough so that every cell is infected with at least one normal infectious particle. If this condition is met then the normal particle can complement any defects in the DI particles and provide all of the viral proteins required for the infection. Eventually, however, as serial passage is continued, the multiplicity of infectious particles drops below one and the most of the cells are only infected with DI particles. When this happens the proportion of DI particles in the progeny virus decreases.

In good laboratory practice, virus stocks are passaged at high dilutions to avoid the problem of the emergence of high titers of DI particles. Nevertheless, the presence of DI particles is a major contributor to the low fraction of infectious virus found in all virus stocks.

In principle, the emergence of high titers of DI particles during infections in humans could form the basis for a long-term viral infection that is hidden from the immune system and result in the gradual release of infectious virus. Whether this form of latency actually occurs and is a contributing factor to slow viral diseases remains to be seen.

(margin notes)

Serial passage of viruses results in increasing proportion of DI particles

DI particles produced by deletion mutations compete successfully for replication enzymes

Recombination

Besides mutation, genetic recombination between related viruses is a major source of genomic variation. Bacterial cells as well as the nuclei of animal cells contain the enzymes necessary for homologous recombination of DNA. Thus, it is not surprising that recombinants arise from mixed infections involving two different strains of the same type of DNA virus. The larger bacteriophages such as λ and T4 code for their own recombination enzymes, a fact that attests to the importance of recombination in the life cycles of these viruses. The fact that recombination has also been observed for cytoplasmic poxviruses suggests that they too code for their own recombination enzymes.

As far as is known, cells do not possess the machinery to recombine RNA molecules. However, recombination among at least some RNA viruses has been observed by two different mechanisms. The first is unique to the viruses with segmented genomes (orthomyxoviruses and reoviruses) and involves reassortment of segments rather than true recombination. A mixed infection of two different influenza viruses yields progeny virus different from either one of the parents. The "recombinants" can be accounted for by the formation of new combinations of the genomic segments that are free to mix with each other at some time during the infection. Reassortment during mixed infections of human and certain animal influenza viruses is believed to account for the occasional drastic change in the antigenicity of the human virus. These dramatic changes are called *antigenic shifts* and produce strains to which much of the human population lacks immunity and can have enormous epidemiological and clinical consequences (see Chapter 32).

Genetic recombination between different forms of poliovirus has also been observed. Because the poliovirus RNA genome is not segmented, reassortment cannot be invoked as the basis for the observed recombinants. In this case, it appears that recombination occurs during replication by a "copy choice" type of mechanism. During RNA synthesis, the replicase dissociates from one template and resumes copying a second template at the exact place where it left off on the first. The end result is a progeny RNA genome containing information from two different input RNA molecules. Strand-switching during replication, therefore, generates a recombinant virus. Although not frequently observed, it is likely that most of the RNA animal viruses are capable of this kind of recombination.

A copy choice mechanism has also been invoked to explain a high rate of recombination observed with retroviruses. At early times after infection, the reverse transcriptase within the virion synthesizes a DNA copy of the RNA genome in the cytoplasm of the infected cell. The process of reverse transcription requires the enzyme to "jump" between two sites on the RNA genome (see Chapter 41). The propensity to switch templates apparently explains why the enzyme generates recombinant viruses. Because reverse transcription takes place in subviral particles, free mixing of RNA templates brought into the cell in different virus particles is not permitted. However, retroviruses are diploid; each particle carries two copies of the genome. This arrangement appears to be a situation ready-made for template switching during DNA synthesis and most likely accounts for retroviral recombination. In the absence of appealing alternative explanations, some virologists believe that the advantages conferred by the ability to reshuffle genetic material provided sufficient selective pressure to lead evolutionarily to the diploid genome structure for these viruses.

Margin notes:

Homologous recombination in DNA viruses

Genetic exchange between segmented genome RNA viruses involves reassortment of segments

Genomic reassortment probably accounts for antigenic shifts of influenza virus

Copy choice recombination of RNA viruses

Diploid nature of retroviruses permits template switching and recombination during DNA synthesis

Occasionally retroviruses package a cellular mRNA into the virion instead of a second RNA genome. This arrangement can lead to copy choice recombination between the viral genome and a cellular mRNA. The end result is sometimes the incorporation of a cellular gene into the viral genome. This mechanism is believed to account for the production of highly oncogenic retroviruses containing modified cellular genes (see below).

Occasional incorporation of host mRNA into retroviral particle may produce oncogenic virus

The Latent State

Temperate viruses can infect a cell and enter a latent state that is characterized by little or no virus production. The viral genome is replicated and segregated along with the cellular DNA when the cell divides. There exist two possible states for the latent viral genome. It can exist extrachromosomally like a bacterial plasmid, or it can become integrated into the chromosome like the bacterial F factor in the formation of an HFR strain (see Chapter 4). Because the latent genome is usually capable of reactivation and entry into the lytic cycle, it is called a *provirus* or, in the case of bacteriophages, a *prophage.* In many cases, viral latency goes undetected. However, limited expression of proviral genes can occasionally endow the cell with a new set of properties. For instance, lysogeny can lead to the production of virulence-determining toxins in some bacteria (lysogenic conversion). Latency by an animal virus may produce oncogenic transformation.

Latent state involves infection of the cell with little or no virus production

Latent genomes can exist extrachromosomally or be integrated

Latent virus may be silent, change cell phenotype, or reactivate to lytic cycle

Lysogeny

Infection of an *Escherichia coli* cell by bacteriophage λ can have two possible outcomes. A fraction of the cells (ranging up to 90%) enters the lytic cycle and produces more phage. The remainder of the cells enter the latent state by forming stable *lysogens.* The proportion of the population that lyses depends on as yet undefined factors including the nutritional and physiological state of the bacteria. In the lysogenic state, the phage DNA is physically inserted into the bacterial chromosome (see below) and thus replicates when the bacterial DNA replicates. Because λ can replicate either extrachromosomally as in the lytic cycle or as a part of the bacterial chromosome in lysogeny, it is an episome (see Chapter 4). The only phage gene that remains active in a lysogen is the gene that codes for a repressor protein that turns off expression of all of the prophage genes except its own. This means that the lysogenic state can persist for as long as the bacterial strain survives. Because the lysogen contains more repressor proteins than is required to occupy the prophage operators, and because the repressor will bind to the operators of any λ phage entering the cell, the lysogen is resistant to reinfection by λ. This phenomenon is called *superinfection immunity.* Environmental insults, most notably exposure to ultraviolet light, cause inactivation of the repressor, resulting in loss of repression and induction of all the bacteria to proceed through the lytic cycle.

E. coli phage λ as a model for integrated latency

When integrated silently, the only active gene encodes repressor for other phage genes

Loss of repressor causes induction and virus production

Once established, the perpetuation of the lysogenic state requires a mechanism to ensure that copies of the phage genes are faithfully passed on to both daughter cells during cell division. In the lysogenic state, bacteriophage P1 exists extrachromosomally as an autonomous single-copy plasmid. Its replication is tightly coupled to chromosomal replication and the two replicated copies are precisely partitioned to daughter cells. Bac-

Latent phage P1 exists as extrachromosomal plasmid

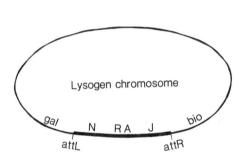

7.1 λ integration and excision. A, J, N, and R show the locations of some λ genes on the λ genome; gal and bio represent the *Escherichia coli* galactose and biotin operons, respectively.

Phage λ integrates by site-specific recombination

teriophage λ integrates into the *E. coli* chromosome to guarantee its replication and successful segregation during cell division.

Because of its mechanistic importance and relevance to lysogenic conversion and phage transduction (see Chapter 4), λ integration and the reverse reaction called *excision* will be described in some detail. Bacteriophage λ integrates by a site-specific, reciprocal recombination event as outlined in Figure 7.1. There exist unique attachment sites on both the phage and bacterial chromosomes where the crossover occurs. The phage attachment site is called *attP* and the bacterial site, which is found on the *E. coli* chromosome between the galactose and biotin operons, is called *attB*. The recombination reaction is catalyzed by the phage-encoded integrase protein in conjunction with two host proteins and occurs by a highly concerted reaction that requires no new DNA synthesis. Although most temperate phages integrate into one, or at most a few different sites in the bacterial chromosome, bacteriophage Mu can integrate (by transposition, see Chapter 4) randomly into the chromosome.

Excision after induction involves recombination at junctions between host DNA and prophage

Excision of the phage genome after induction of a lysogen by ultraviolet light is just the reverse of integration, except that excision requires, in addition to the integrase enzyme, a second phage protein called Xis. In this case the combined activities of these two proteins catalyze site-specific recombination between the two attachment sites called *attL* and *attR* that flank the prophage DNA (Figure 7.1). At early times after infection, when integration is to occur in some fraction of the infected cells, the synthesis of the Xis protein is blocked. Otherwise, the integrated prophage DNA would excise soon after integration and stable lysogeny would be impossible. However, after induction of a lysogen, both the integrase and the Xis proteins are synthesized and catalyze the excision event that releases the prophage DNA from the chromosome and leads to lysis.

At a very low frequency, excision involves sites other than the *attL* and *attR* borders of the prophage and results in the linking of bacterial genes to the phage genome. Thus, if a site to the left of the bacterial *gal* genes recombines with a site within the λ chromosome (to the left of the *J* gene, otherwise the excised genome is too large to be packaged), then the resulting phage can transduce the genes for galactose metabolism to another cell (see Chapter 4). Similarly, transducing particles can be formed that carry the genes involved in biotin biosynthesis. Because only those cellular genes adjacent to the attachment site can be picked up by an aberrant excision event, this process is called *specialized transduction* to distinguish it from generalized transduction in which virtually any bacterial gene can be transferred by headfull packaging (see Chapters 4 and 6).

Occasionally, one or more phage genes, in addition to the gene coding for the repressor protein, are expressed in the lysogenic state. If the expressed protein confers a new phenotypic property on the cell, then it is said that *lysogenic conversion* has occurred. Diphtheria, scarlet fever, and botulism are all caused by bacteria that have been "converted" by a temperate bacteriophage. In each case, the gene that codes for the toxin protein resides on a phage and is expressed along with the repressor gene in the lysogenic state. It remains a mystery as to how these toxin genes were acquired by the phage; it is speculated that they may have been picked up by a mechanism similar to specialized transduction.

Malignant Transformation

A tumor is an abnormal growth of cells. Tumors fall roughly into two categories called *benign* or *malignant,* depending on whether they remain localized or have a tendency to spread by metastasis. A malignant cell, therefore, has at least two defects. It fails to respond to controlling signals that normally limit the growth of nonmalignant cells, and it fails to recognize its neighbors and remain in its proper location. Malignant tumor cells, when grown in tissue culture in the laboratory, exhibit a series of properties that correlate with the uncontrolled growth potential associated with the tumor in the organism. These properties include 1) an altered cell morphology, 2) failure to grow in the organized patterns found for normal cells, 3) growth to much higher cell densities than normal cells under conditions of unlimited nutrients, 4) lower nutritional and serum requirements than normal cells, 5) capacity to divide in suspension, whereas normal cells require an anchoring substrate and grow only on surfaces (eg, on glass or plastic), and 6) ability to grow indefinitely in cell culture.

Many DNA animal viruses and some representatives of the retroviruses can convert normal cultured cells into cells that possess the properties listed above. This process is called *malignant transformation.* In addition to the listed properties, viral transformation usually, but not always, endows the cells with the capacity to form a tumor when introduced into the appropriate animal. Although the original use of the term *transformation* referred to the changes occurring in cells grown in the laboratory, current usage often includes the initial events in the animal that lead to the development of a tumor. In recent years, it has become increasingly clear that some, but not all of these viruses, also cause cancers in the host species from which they were isolated. The oncogenic potential of animal DNA viruses is summarized in Table 7.1.

All known DNA animal viruses with the exception of the parvoviruses are capable of causing aberrant cell proliferation under some conditions.

Mechanisms of specialized transduction

Lysogenic conversion results from expression of prophage gene that alters cell phenotype

Several bacterial exotoxins are encoded in temperate phages

Properties of malignant cells

Malignant transformation of cell cultures by DNA viruses and some retroviruses

Virally induced tumors in mammalian species

Table 7.1   Oncogenicity of DNA Viruses

Virus or Virus Group	Tumors in Natural Host[a]	Tumors in Other Species[b]	Transform Cells in Tissue Culture
Parvoviruses (rat, mouse, human)	No	No	No
Animal polyoma viruses (polyoma, SV40)	No	Yes	Yes
Human polyoma viruses (JC, BK)	No	Yes	Yes
Papilloma viruses (human, rabbit)	Yes, usually benign	?	No
Human hepatitis B virus	Possibly	?	No
Human adenoviruses	No	Yes	Yes
Human herpes viruses	Yes	Yes	Yes
Poxviruses (human, rabbit)	Occasionally, usually benign	Yes	No

[a] *Yes* means that at least one member of the group is oncogenic.
[b] Test usually done in newborns or immune-suppressed hosts.

For some viruses, transformation or tumor formation has only been observed in species other than the natural host. Apparently infections of cells from the natural host are so cytocidal that no survivors remain to be transformed. In addition, some viruses have been implicated in human or animal tumors without any indication that they can transform cells in culture.

Transformation is analogous to lysogenic conversion but recombination is nonhomologous

In nearly all cases that have been characterized, viral transformation is the result of the continual expression of one or more viral genes (see Chapter 6). In many respects, transformation is analogous to lysogenic conversion and requires that the viral genes become incorporated into the cell as inheritable elements. Incorporation usually involves integration into the chromosome (eg, polyoma viruses, the adenoviruses, and the retroviruses), although papilloma viruses and some herpesviruses are found in transformed cells as extrachromosomal plasmids. Unlike many temperate bacteriophages that code for the enzymes necessary for integration, polyoma viruses and adenoviruses integrate by nonhomologous recombination using enzymes present in the host cell. Therefore, the recombination event is nonspecific, both with respect to the viral DNA and with respect to the chromosomal locus at which insertion occurs. It follows that for transformation to be successful, the insertional recombination must not occur within any of the viral genes required for transformation.

Only part of transforming viral genome may be integrated; complete genome not recoverable

Furthermore, in many cases only that portion of the viral genome that carries these genes is found integrated into the transformed cell DNA and the complete genome is not recoverable. In summary, two events appear to be necessary for viral transformation: a persistent association of viral genes with the cell and the expression of certain viral "transforming" proteins.

Transformation by Retroviruses

Retroviral infection and virus production without cell death

DNA copy of viral genome is integrated, but not at specific site

Acquired oncogenes encode a protein causing transformation

Insertional mutagenesis causes inappropriate expression of a protooncogene adjacent to integrated viral genome

Two features of the replicative cycle of retroviruses are related to the oncogenic potential of this class of viruses. First, most retroviruses do not kill the host cell, but instead set up a permanent infection with continual virus production. Second, the DNA copy of the RNA genome is integrated into the host cell DNA. At least part of the enzymatic machinery for integration is encoded by the virus. However, unlike bacteriophage λ integration, the linear form of the proviral genome is the substrate for integration rather than a circular form. Furthermore, unlike λ, there does not appear to be a specific site in the cell DNA where integration occurs.

Retroviruses are known to transform cells by three different mechanisms. First, many animal retroviruses have acquired transforming genes called *oncogenes*. More than twenty such oncogenes have now been found since the original gene called *src* was identified in Rous sarcoma virus. Because normal cells possess homologs of these genes (called *protooncogenes*) it is generally assumed that viral oncogenes originated from host DNA. It is possible they were picked up by copy choice recombination involving packaged cellular mRNAs as described above. Most viral oncogenes have suffered one or more mutations that make them different from the cellular protooncogenes. These changes presumably alter the protein products so that they cause transformation. Although the mechanisms of oncogenesis are not well understood, it appears that transformation results from inappropriate production of an abnormal protein that interferes with the normal signaling processes within the cell. Uncontrolled cell proliferation is the result. Because tumor formation by retroviruses carrying an oncogene is efficient and rapid, these viruses are often referred to as *acute transforming viruses*. Although common in some animal species, this mechanism has not yet been recognized as a cause of any human cancers.

The second mechanism is called *insertional mutagenesis* and is not dependent on continued production of a viral gene product. Instead, the presence of the viral promoter and/or enhancer is sufficient to cause the inappropriate expression of a cellular gene residing in the immediate vicinity of the integrated provirus. This mechanism was first recognized in avian B-cell lymphomas caused by an avian leukosis virus, a disease characterized by a very long latent period. Tumor cells from different individuals were found to have a copy of the provirus integrated at the same place in the cell DNA. The site of the provirus insertion was found to be next to a cellular protooncogene called *c-myc*, where the *c* stands for cellular. The *myc* gene had previously been identified as a viral oncogene called *v-myc*. In this case, transformation occurs not because the *c-myc* gene is altered by mutation, but because the gene is turned on at the wrong time in development, and the gene product is overproduced. The disease has a long latent period, because, although the birds are viremic from early life, the probability of an integration occurring next to the *c-myc* gene is very low. Once such an integration event does occur, however, cell proliferation is rapid and a tumor develops. No human tumors are known to be the result of insertional mutagenesis caused by a retrovirus. However, human cancers are known where a chromosome translocation has placed an active cellular promoter next to a cellular protooncogene (Burkitt's lymphoma and chronic myelogenous leukemia).

The third mechanism was revealed by the discovery of the first human retrovirus. The virus is called *human T-cell lymphotropic virus 1* (HTLV-1) and is the causative agent of adult T-cell leukemia. HTLV-1 is found

Human T-cell leukemia
caused by transactivating
factor encoded in integrated
HTLV-1
Transactivating factor turns
on cellular genes causing cell
proliferation

integrated in the DNA of the leukemic cells and all the tumor cells from a particular individual have the proviral DNA in the same location. This observation implies that the tumor is a clone derived from a single cell. However, the sites of integration in tumors from different individuals are found to be different. Thus, HTLV-1 does not cause malignancy by promoter insertion near a particular cellular gene. Instead, the virus codes for a protein that acts in trans (ie, on other genomes in the same cell) to promote maximal transcription of the proviral DNA and also turns on one or more cellular genes to cause cell proliferation. The viral gene coding for this protein is called *tax* for transactivating factor. The *tax* gene is therefore an oncogene that is different from the oncogenes of the acute transforming retroviruses in being a viral gene rather than a gene derived from a cellular protooncogene.

8

An Overview of the Specific Immune Response

John C. Sherris and
C. George Ray

Recognition of nonself
threats

Complexity of system

Immunogical memory

The evolution and survival of our species has required a variety of mechanisms designed for defense against infection, while maintaining a state of balanced parasitism with our own microbial flora. Some of these defenses are permanently in place and are nonspecific in their effects, in that they are not directed against specific invaders.

Another major defense system, the adaptive immune response, is highly *specific* with regard to an infecting agent. The acquired immunity that it provides is brought about by a finely tuned system that is activated on recognition of foreign (nonself) threats to the integrity of the host. The development of specific immunity involves collaboration and feedback between different subsets of cells of the lymphocyte series and between lymphocytes, macrophages, and related cells of the reticuloendothelial system. The effector arms of the immune system involve soluble products that stimulate and activate nonspecific defense mechanisms, specific antibody activity against invading organisms or their products, activation of the complement system, and direct killing by certain specialized cells. The system is endowed with the property of *memory*, so that reexposure to the inciting agent in the future will usually bring about an enhanced response.

This chapter is an overview of immunology as it relates to medical microbiology and infectious disease. It is designed to allow readers who have not yet studied immunology to understand the details of host–parasite interactions and immune responses to specific infections that are given elsewhere in the text. All students in the biomedical sciences will be studying immunology in much more depth, because it is a vital and rapidly developing discipline with many facets of great biological and practical importance that have not been considered. Some excellent texts that provide comprehensive coverage are referenced at the end of the chapter.

Antigens and Epitopes

Complex antigens trigger immune response

The body reacts to the incursion of many foreign substances by the development of a specific immune response. The foreign substances that initiate an immune response are usually proteins or complex carbohydrates of molecular weight of over 10,000. They may be present in free molecular form, but more often as part of the structure of a larger particle such as a bacterium or a virus. The substance or particle that initiates an immune response is usually termed an *antigen* and will be so described in this chapter, although a more appropriate term often used is *immunogen.*

Response directed against small epitopes (antigenic determinants) on antigen

The critical determinant of specificity of the immune response is usually a small component of the antigen termed an *epitope* or *antigenic determinant,* which will not itself initiate an immune response.* In the case of a protein antigen, an epitope consists of small numbers (10–20) of amino acids folded in a particular three-dimensional configuration that is recognized by the immune system. Because of their complexity, many proteins may elicit immunological responses of several specificities directed against different epitopes on the same molecule. A complex structure, such as a bacterium, may thus elicit responses of very many different specificities.

To summarize, an immunizing antigen must generally be foreign to the host (nonself), include protein or complex carbohydrate components or both, and also have specific epitopes that can be recognized by the immune system.

The Processing of Antigen

Most antigens must be processed by certain accessory cells (antigen-processing cells) before their epitopes can be effectively recognized by the immune system. The majority of these cells are fixed or wandering phagocytic mononuclear cells. Others include Langerhans cells of the skin and dendritic and interdigitating reticulum cells of the lymphoid organs, which are adjacent to immunoresponsive cells. All will be considered as *macrophages* in what follows.

Role of macrophages in processing antigens and epitope presentation

Association of epitopes with MHC molecules

Macrophages break down complex particles, such as bacteria, to free up the antigenic molecules, but beyond this, most antigens must be further processed by the macrophage to yield molecules that contain both an immunologically recognized epitope and a site that binds to a specific glycoprotein on the surface of the macrophage. This glycoprotein is one of two classes of such molecules that determine the immunological individuality of the host (ie, whether a graft from another human, such as a transplanted kidney, will be accepted or rejected). They are encoded in the major histocompatibility genetic complex (MHC) of the host. The macrophage has class II MHC molecules on its surface, and this class is found primarily on macrophages, related accessory antigen-processing cells, and on cells of the lymphocyte series. Epitopes are only recognized by a key immunocompetent cell (T-helper cell) when they are associated with the class II molecule.

A similar situation applies to antigen generated within nonphagocytic cells, for example, epithelial cells infected by a virus. In this case, epitopes or larger particles of antigen associate on the cell surface with the other

---

* Another term that will be encountered is *hapten,* which refers to a molecule that bears one or more epitopes that will react with preformed antibody in the test tube in a detectable manner, but that will not initiate an immunological response unless coupled to a larger *carrier* molecule.

MHC molecules, termed class I (HLA-*A, HLA-B, and HLA-C in humans), which are expressed on essentially all cells of the body, in contrast to class II molecules (HLA-DR in humans). Specialized immunocompetent effector cells (T-cytotoxic cells) recognize epitopes when combined with a class I molecule. However, as will be discussed later, immunological activity in this case requires collaboration with T-helper cells.

Some polysaccharide antigens do not require macrophage processing

In the case of pure polysaccharide antigens with repeating sugar subunits, processing and presentation in association with MHC molecules is not necessarily needed, and the antigenic epitope can be recognized directly by certain immunocompetent cells.

The Immunoresponsive Cells

Cells involved in the specific recognition of antigenic determinants are of the lymphocytic series. There are two classes of immunoresponsive lymphocytes (immunocytes) termed *T cells* and *B cells,* respectively. Both are derived from the same bone marrow stem cells, but T cells have matured and differentiated in the thymus gland, whereas B cells have done so elsewhere, probably in the bone marrow. In avians, B cells differentiate and mature in the *bursa* of Fabricius from which they take their *B* designation.

T and B lymphocytes (immunocytes)

T cells mature in the thymus, B cells in bone marrow

T cells are responsible for 1) the initiation and modulation of immune responses (including B-cell responses), 2) cell-mediated immune processes that involve direct damage to antigen-bearing tissue or blood cells (eg, virally infected host cells expressing a viral antigen on their surfaces), and 3) stimulating and enhancing the nonspecific immune functions of the host (eg, the inflammatory reaction and antimicrobial activity of phagocytes). There are subsets of T cells responsible for some of these different functions.

Multiple roles of T-cell subsets in defense

B cells are responsible for humoral immunity due to antibody production. B cells can differentiate into cells producing different classes of antibody.

B cells differentiate to antibody-producing cells

T and B cells are widely dispersed throughout the body, where they play both a patrolling and a sentinel function. They exist in large numbers in the bone marrow, in specialized areas of the lymph nodes and spleen, in lymphoid structures adjacent to the alimentary and respiratory tracts (eg, Peyer's patches and adenoids), and throughout all the subepithelial tissues of the internal organs. They are continually replaced, and there is considerable circulation of B and T cells between the different areas of the body through the lymphatic and blood vascular circulations. The lymph nodes contain very many T and B cells and are strategically placed for filtering out invading microbes or their products. Lymph nodes contain fixed phagocytic macrophages that can break down complex particles, such as bacteria, and process antigen for presentation to adjacent immunoresponsive lymphocytes. The spleen and bone marrow also contain many fixed macrophages and large numbers of T and B lymphocytes, allowing rapid immunoresponse to microorganisms or their products that reach the bloodstream. The lymphoid tissues associated with the gut and respiratory tract play a similar role locally in response to microbial attack on these organs.

Wide strategic distribution of lymphoid cells and macrophages

---

* Human leukocyte antigen.

8.1 Schematic of epitope recognition by an immunoresponsive lymphocyte. Epitope B on the antigen binds to a complementary recognition site on the surface of the immunoresponsive cell. *Notes:* 1) Antigens may have multiple different epitopes, but an immunoresponsive lymphocyte has receptors of only one specificity. 2) In most cases, epitopes are recognized on the surface of macrophages that have processed the antigen.

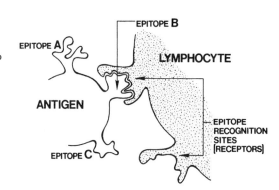

The Basis of Immunological Specificity

Immunocyte receptors specific for a particular epitope

The basis of specificity of the immune response is the complementary configuration of recognition sites (*receptors*) on the surface of B and T lymphocytes for the antigenic determinants. This allows them to bind together and stimulate an immunological response. There is an astounding heterogeneity of immunoresponsive lymphocytes with respect to their epitope recognition sites. Each lymphocyte expresses only a single specificity in its recognition sites, and it has been estimated that recognition sites for upward of 10^{10} different epitopes are represented, each on different cells of the B- and T-lymphocyte populations of a human. It is now known that the structure of these recognition sites is determined by multiple adjacent genes on a host chromosome—the immunoresponse genes. The tremendous diversity of recognition sites is created genetically by a series of excisions, crossovers, recombinations, and random mutations during the development and replacement of populations of lymphocytes. Thus, the unchallenged immune system has in place one or more lymphocytes of both B and T series that will react with almost any foreign antigen encountered in nature, and indeed, some synthetic products that do not occur naturally.

Up to 10^{10} immunocytes with different specificities

Immunocyte diversity derives from genetic rearrangements and mutations

Lock and key association of epitope and recognition site

The interaction of epitope with recognition site on the lymphocyte involves a mirror-image, three-dimensional association (see Figure 8.1) held together by noncovalent intermolecular forces. It can be visualized crudely as a lock and key fit, although it is important to recognize that small differences in epitope structures do not necessarily preclude binding to a single recognition site.

Clonal Expansion and Immunological Memory

Activation and amplification of specific immunocytes

When appropriately presented epitopes on an antigen molecule react with a complementary recognition site on an immunoresponsive lymphocyte, the lymphocyte is stimulated to divide and to produce an expanding clone of cells, each carrying recognition sites of the same specificity. This amplification process continues as long as a sufficient antigenic stimulus is available and is essential for the production of enough immunologically active cells to bring about the protective effect, which is the major function of the immune system. In the process of clonal expansion, there are continued somatic mutations in the immunoresponse genes with a selective

8.2 Primary and secondary immunological responses. The response to first inoculation of antigen becomes apparent in a week to 10 days. It is small, predominantly of IgM, and declines rapidly. Activation of memory cells by a second inoculation leads to a much greater, more rapid, and more long-lived IgG response.

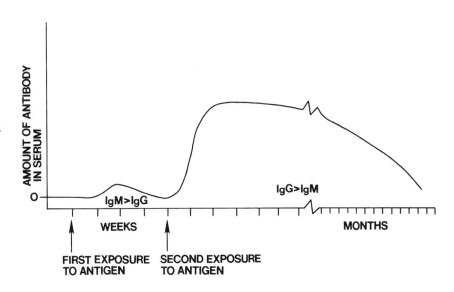

pressure toward cells whose recognition sites have the greatest affinity for the initiating epitope. In this way the already high specificity of the immune response is further enhanced.

With the elimination of antigen, the majority of the clone of immunoreactive lymphocytes will be lost over time by normal cell replacement. However, the speed with which antigen is lost is very variable and depends on such factors as excretion and enzymatic breakdown. Some polysaccharide antigens and bacterial cell wall peptidoglycans are so resistant to host enzymatic breakdown that they can persist for years, whereas many protein antigens are rapidly metabolized. Fortunately, the immune system has a recall ability in the case of protein antigens, because certain cells in the clone, termed *memory cells,* survive for long periods and probably slowly replicate to maintain a core population with the capacity to expand very rapidly if the antigen (or the same epitope on another antigen) is encountered again.

Memory cells provide rapid enhanced response to reexposure

Rates of elimination of antigen

Memory cells may be either T or B cells and are probably variants within the original clone having recognition sites with higher specific affinity for the relevant antigenic determinant and, thus, greater immunological efficiency. In consequence, the response to a second encounter with an antigen is more rapid than the first and quantitatively greater in its effect. It is referred to as a *secondary response* in contrast to the initial primary response. This is illustrated in Figure 8.2 using antibody production as a measure of immune response of B cells. Memory cells and the secondary response phenomenon account for the prolonged or lifelong immunity that follows many infections (such as measles), and the secondary response is exploited in scheduling doses of various vaccines to obtain the maximum and most long-lived immunity.

The T-Cell Response

The major roles of T cells in the immune response are

Range of T-cell functions

1. Recognition of epitopes presented with MHC molecules on cell surfaces. This is followed by activation and clonal expansion of T cells in the case of epitopes associated with class II MHC molecules.

2. Production of peptides termed *lymphokines* that act as intercellular signals and mediate the activation and modulation of various aspects of the immune response and of nonspecific host defenses.

3. The direct killing of foreign cells, of host cells bearing foreign surface antigens along with class I MHC molecules (eg, some virally infected cells), and of some immunologically recognized tumor cells.

These functions involve subsets of T cells and collaboration between them.

The T4 Helper/Inducer Lymphocyte.   This cell is responsible for much of the immune response, starting with its ability to recognize antigenic determinants presented by the macrophage. In addition to its epitope recognition site, it carries a surface molecule termed *CD4* by which it can be identified and which contributes to its ability to recognize the class II MHC/epitope molecules on the surface of the macrophage. When binding occurs between the recognition site on the T4 cell and the epitope on the macrophage surface, the previously quiescent T4 cell is activated under the influence of a cytokine, interleukin 1 (IL1),* produced by the macrophage. The activated T4 cell then produces a lymphokine, interleukin 2 (IL2), and expresses large numbers of IL2 receptors on its surface. Reaction of IL2 with these receptors leads to clonal proliferation of the activated T4 cell. Immunologically specific T4 cells thus increase dramatically at the site of the stimulus, which is frequently the site of infection, and also migrate widely throughout the lymphoid system.

The clone of activated immunologically specific T4 cells elaborates a number of lymphokines. Some are designated by terms that describe their effects. Others, of which the molecules have been fully characterized, are classified as numbered interleukins (IL1, IL2, etc).

The major activities of lymphokines produced by activated T4 cells are listed in Table 8.1. Their effects include stimulation of the activity and multiplication of other classes of T cells, stimulation of growth and differentiation of antigen specific B cells (and thus of antibody production), accumulation of macrophages at the site of infection, stimulation of macrophage antimicrobial and antigen-presenting activities, and the inhibition of viral replication. In these activities, the stimulus for activation of T4 cells, and thus of lymphokine production, is specific, but the effects of the lymphokines are non-specific.

The critical significance of T4 helper cells to the body is shown by the catastrophic effects of infection with the human immunodeficiency virus (the causative agent of acquired immunodeficiency syndrome, AIDS), which binds to the CD4 molecule, enters the cell, and interferes with its function or destroys it. As a result, the body becomes susceptible to a wide variety of bacterial, viral, protozoal, and fungal infections, both through loss of preexisting immunity and through failure to mount an effective immune response to newly acquired pathogens.

Cytotoxic T8 cells.   These are a second class of effector T cells. They are lethal to cells expressing the epitope against which they are directed when the epitope is in conjunction with class I MHC molecules. They too have specific epitope recognition sites, but are characterized by a cell surface

CD4 molecule contributes to epitope/MHC II recognition

Activation by macrophage IL1 and IL2-mediated clonal expansion

Other lymphokines produced by T4 cells

T4 cells and AIDS

Recognize epitopes associated with class I MHC molecules

---

* Cytokines are signaling peptides responsible for communication between a variety of cells. Lymphokines are cytokines produced by lymphocytes.

Table 8.1 Some Major Lymphokines and Cytokines Involved in Immune Responses

Agent	Source	Effects
Interleukin 1	Macrophages, T and B cells	Activates T cells; induces wide range of antimicrobial effects, including fever, PMN leukocytosis, macrophage activation, other lymphokine synthesis, inflammatory response, etc.
Interleukin 2	T4 lymphocytes	Growth factor for activated T cells; activates cytotoxic T cells
Interleukin 3	T lymphocytes	Growth factor for undifferentiated bone marrow progenitors of red and white blood cells and platelets; growth factor for mast cells
Interleukin 4	T4 lymphocytes	Growth factor for activated B cells, mast cells, and resting T cells
B-Cell differentiation factor[a]	T4 lymphocytes	Causes differentiation of activated B cells to antibody-producing plasma cells
Colony-stimulating factors	T4 lymphocytes	Stimulate bone marrow production and antimicrobial activation of macrophages and PMNs
Macrophage chemotactic factor	T4 lymphocytes	Attracts macrophages to site of infection
Migration inhibition factor	T4 lymphocytes	Holds macrophages at site of infection
Interferon gamma	T4 lymphocytes	Induces expression of MHC molecules on cell surfaces; activates macrophages; inhibits viral replication
Tumor necrosis factor	Macrophages	Overlaps manifestation of IL1, and stimulates IL1 production; contributes to septic shock and necrosis of some tumor cells; does not activate T cells

Abbreviations: PMN = polymorphonuclear leukocytes; MHC = major histocompatibility genetic complex; IL1 = interleukin 1.

[a] Identical to interferon beta-2.

marker that differs from that of T4 (CD4) cells and is termed *CD8*. They are thus referred to as cytotoxic T8 cells.

Lethal to many virally infected cells

These cells recognize the association of antigenic epitopes with class I MHC molecules on a wide variety of cells of the body. This recognition, however, does not itself lead to the necessary clonal expansion of T8 cells, which also requires the lymphokine IL2 to be produced by activated T4 lymphocytes. In the case of virally infected cells, cytotoxic T8 cells prevent viral production and release by eliminating the host cell before viral synthesis or assembly is complete.

T Suppressor Cells.   T suppressor lymphocytes also carrying the CD8 marker and epitope recognition sites are involved in modulating and terminating the immunological activities of both T and B cells, thus avoiding excessive or needlessly prolonged responses that could interfere with

Modulate and control immune response

other immunological activities. It is known that the suppression they produce may be antigen specific or it may be polyclonal (ie, affecting general immunological responses irrespective of the inciting antigen). The mechanisms of suppression and control are less well defined than are the activities of T4 helper cells. In AIDS, the proportion of T8 suppressor cells relative to helper T4 cells is substantially increased because T8 cells are not attacked by the virus. This imbalance, in addition to the depletion of T4 helper cells, may contribute to the immunosuppression that is characteristic of the disease.

Cell-mediated Immunity and Delayed-type Hypersensitivity.

Cell-mediated immunity is most dramatically expressed as a response to obligate or facultative intracellular pathogens. These include certain slow-growing bacteria, such as the mycobacteria, against which antibody responses are ineffective. In experimental infections, cell-mediated immunity can be passively transferred from one animal to another by T lymphocytes, but not by serum. (In contrast, short-term, antibody-mediated (B-cell) immunity can be passively transferred with serum.) The mechanisms of cell-mediated immunity are complex and involve a number of lymphokines and other cytokines with amplifying feedback mechanisms for their production. The initial processing of antigen is accompanied by sufficient IL1 production by the macrophages to stimulate activation of the antigen-recognizing T4 (helper) cell. Lymphokine feedback from the T4 cells to macrophages further increases IL1 production with all the effects listed in Table 8.1. IL2 produced by the T4 cells facilitates their clonal expansion and activates T8 (cytotoxic) lymphocytes. Other lymphokines from T4 cells chemotactically attract macrophages to the site of infection, hold them there, and activate them to greatly enhanced microbicidal activity.

Role in immunity to obligate and facultative intracellular pathogens

Amplifying effects of lymphokines on immune and inflammatory responses

The inflammatory cellular process that results from cell-mediated immune reactions develops slowly over days. It involves predominantly the T-cell clones and macrophages and is often associated with some tissue necrosis induced by hydrolytic enzymes liberated from phagocytic cells as well as by activities of specific cytotoxic T cells. Multiplication of fibroblasts and laying down of collagen occur as the infectious process continues or resolves.

Chronic inflammatory response and enhanced macrophage activity

The sum of these individual and collaborative activities of T cells, macrophages, and their products is a progressive mobilization of a range of nonspecific host defenses to the site of infection and greatly enhanced macrophage activity. In the case of viruses, interferon gamma inhibits replication, and T8 (cytotoxic) cells destroy their cellular habitat, leaving already assembled virions accessible to circulating antibody.

Delayed-type hypersensitivity reactions; role in pathogenesis of disease

With certain infections in which reaction to protein antigens is particularly strong (eg, tuberculosis), the cell-mediated responses are of such magnitude that they become major deleterious factors in the disease process itself. This degree of reaction is termed *delayed-type hypersensitivity* (type IV hypersensitivity) in contrast to class I, II, and III hypersensitivity in which antibody is involved. These are discussed later in the chapter. Type IV hypersensitivity can produce extensive areas of necrosis that can exacerbate a disease such as tuberculosis by erosion into blood vessels, bronchi, or other organs. Mechanical effects can occur from expansion of the lesion because of dense cellular infiltrates, areas of necrosis, and reactive fibrosis.

Tuberculin skin test reaction

Delayed-type hypersensitivity is so called because reexposure of the host to the antigen that elicited the immune response produces a maximum hypersensitive reaction only after a day or two when mobilization of immune lymphocytes and of phagocytic macrophages is at its peak. This is exemplified in the tuberculin skin test reaction, which only reaches its maximum after 2 or 3 days, in sharp contrast to the rapidly developing antibody-mediated anaphylactic hypersensitivity responses that are described later in the chapter.

The B-Cell and Antibody Responses

Maturation in bone marrow

B lymphocytes are the cells responsible for antibody responses. They develop from precursor cells in the yolk sac and fetal liver before birth and thereafter in the bone marrow before migrating to other lymphoid tissues. Each mature cell of this series carries a surface recognition site with specificity for a particular configuration of an epitope, just as do T4 helper cells. The specific epitope recognition site of the B lymphocyte is the antigen-recognizing (variable) region of antibody that will be produced subsequently by its progeny.

Activation of B cells; role of macrophages and T cells

There is more than one mechanism whereby B cells can be activated by antigen to clonal expansion. Antigenic epitopes that are often widely separated on the protein molecule will not provoke a B cell to respond simply by reacting with its receptor. First, the protein must be processed by a macrophage, then the epitope must be presented in conjunction with a class II MHC molecule and recognized by a T4 helper cell as described in the previous section, and finally contact must be established between the activated T4 helper cell and the B cell. The T4 cell elaborates lymphokines, in particular IL2, that initiate and maintain clonal expansion of the B cell and then bring about maturation to the antibody producing *plasma cells* (see Figure 8.3). The plasma cell has an extensive rough endoplasmic reticulum and is, in effect, a factory for the production and secretion of the antibody encoded by its B-cell progenitor. Some polysaccharide antigens with repeating sugar epitopes can activate B lymphocytes directly without T-cell involvement. These are called *T-independent antigens* and provoke primarily IgM antibody responses (see below). Memory cells do not result from the clonal expansion that follows. Immunological reactivity to such polysaccharides usually develops much more slowly after birth than does the T-cell–dependent response. This delay in responsiveness probably contributes to the increased susceptibility to some bacterial infections in early life.

Antibody production by plasma cells

T-independent antibody production to some polysaccharides

Classes of antibodies

Antibodies are specific proteins of the globulin class, which are termed *immunoglobulins*. There are five known broad classes (isotypes) of anti-

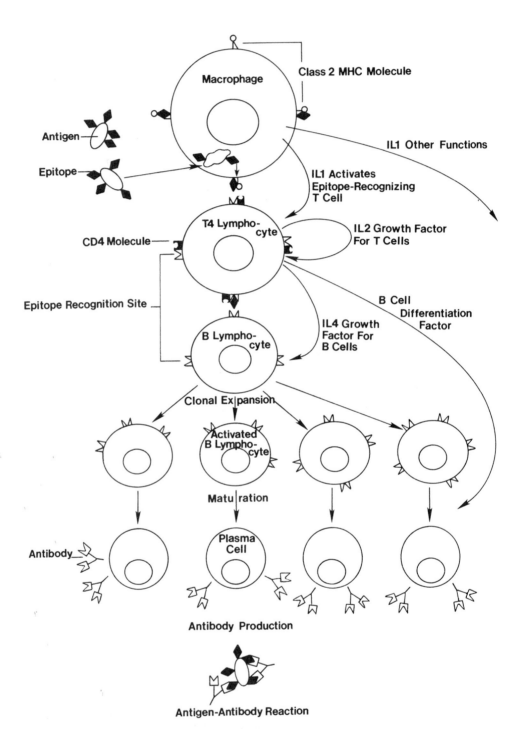

8.3 T-cell–dependent antibody synthesis.

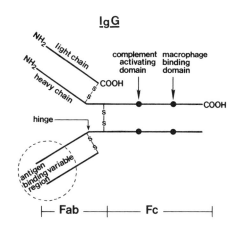

IgG

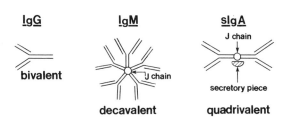

8.4 Schematic of antibody structure.

body, IgG, IgM, IgA, IgE, and IgD. Ig is the abbreviation for immunoglobulin and the other letters were variously allocated as knowledge of antibody structure and function developed and have no consistent logical basis. The structure of the first four is shown diagrammatically in Figure 8.4. Before activation, the B cell expresses a monomer of IgM on its surface that serves as an epitope recognition site. IgD is expressed during activation, but finally B cells express on their surface the particular class of antibody that will be produced by the plasma cells to which they differentiate (IgM, IgG, IgA, IgE). This process, which is termed *class switching,* involves a number of complex genetic recombinations, but retains throughout the immunological specificity of the original unactivated B cell.

B-Cell epitope recognition site is monomer of IgM

Class switching

IgG Antibody.   This is the most abundant immunoglobulin in health and provides the most extensive and long-lived antibody response to the various microbial and other antigens that have been encountered throughout the lifespan of the individual. Although at least four subclasses of IgG have been characterized, they will be grouped together for the purpose of this chapter.

Structure of IgG

The IgG molecule has a molecular weight of approximately 150,000. As shown in Figure 8.4, it consists of two pairs of amino acid peptide chains linked by disulfide bonds. One pair is larger than the other and its components are termed the *heavy chains.* The components of the smaller pair are not unreasonably termed the *light chains.* There is a hinge region of the molecule at the carboxy terminal end of the light-chain peptide that allows the two arms of the molecule to diverge flexibly. The amino terminal ends of the light and heavy chains on the two arms form the *variable regions* of the molecule and are the combining sites for epitopes. They are also termed the *Fab* (fragment antigen binding) portion of the molecule.

Functions of variable and constant regions

The antibody molecule is thus bivalent with two identical and specific combining sites. The rest of the molecule is the *constant region,* also termed *Fc,* which does not vary with differences in specificity of combining sites of different antibody molecules. The constant region has specific sites for binding to phagocytic cells and for reaction with the first component of complement (C1q). These sites are made available when the variable region of the antibody molecule has reacted with specific antigen.

IgG predominates in secondary response as IgM declines

IgG antibody is characteristically formed in large amounts during the secondary response to an antigenic stimulus (see Figure 8.2) and usually follows production of IgM (see below) in the course of a viral or bacterial infection. Memory cells are programmed for rapid IgG response when another antigenic stimulus of the same type occurs later.

Opsonic and neutralizing effects of IgG

IgG antibodies are the most significant antibody class for neutralizing soluble antigens (eg, exotoxins) and viruses. They act by blocking the sites on the antigenic molecule or virus that determine attachment to cell receptors. IgG also enhances phagocytosis of particulate antigens such as bacteria because the exposed Fc sites of antibody that is bound to the antigen have a specific affinity for receptors on the surface of phagocytic cells. As described later, the third component of complement also mediates attachment to phagocytes. Enhancement of phagocytosis by antibody, complement, or both is referred to as *opsonization.* Accelerated IgG responses from memory cell expansion frequently confers life-long immunity when directed against microbial antigens that are determinants of virulence. There is active transport of the IgG molecule across the placental barrier that allows maternal protective antibody to pass, and thus

Transplacental transport of IgG protects newborns

provides passive immune protection to the fetus and newborn pending development of a mature immune system. It is the only immunoglobulin class known to be placentally transferred. The half-life of passively transferred IgG within the same species is approximately a month, and thus the infant can be protected during a particularly vulnerable period of life.

IgM Antibody. IgM has a molecular weight of about 900,000. It is a pentamer with five subunits, each similar in size to a single IgG molecule. Each subunit has two epitope-combining sites. Monomers of IgM constitute the specific epitope recognition sites on B cells that will ultimately give rise to plasma cells producing one or other of the different immunoglobulin classes of antibody.

Large molecule of five subunits and 10 combining sites

Because of its multiple specific combining sites, IgM is particularly effective in agglutinating particles carrying epitopes against which it is directed (see Chapter 14). It also contains multiple sites for binding the first component of complement. These sites become available once the IgM molecule has reacted with antigen. IgM is particularly active in bringing about complement-mediated cytolytic damage to foreign antigen-bearing cells. It is not, itself, an opsonizing antibody because its Fc portion is not recognized by phagocytes. However, opsonization occurs through its activation of the complement pathway: this process is discussed later in the chapter.

Particularly effective in agglutination, complement activation, and cell lysis

IgM is usually the earliest antibody to appear after an antigenic stimulus, but it tends to decline rapidly and is often succeeded by IgG production from the same clone of cells. It is primarily intravascular, and does not cross the placental barrier to the fetus (in contrast to IgG). Thus, the presence of specific IgM against a potentially infecting agent in the blood of a neonate is a priori evidence of active infection rather than of passively acquired antibody from the mother. Antibody response to certain antigens, including the lipopolysaccharide O antigen of Gram-negative bac-

IgM is early intravascular antibody; does not pass placenta

teria, is characteristically IgM. Some universally occurring antibodies (natural antibodies), such as those directed against blood group antigens, are also of the IgM class.

IgA Antibody.   IgA is present in serum, usually as a monomer, at much lower concentrations than IgG. It has a special role as a major determinant of so-called local immunity in protecting epithelial surfaces from colonization and infection. Certain B cells in lymphoid tissues adjacent to or draining surface epithelia of the intestines, respiratory, and genitourinary tract are encoded for specific IgA production. After antigenic stimulus, the clone expands locally and some of the IgA-producing cells also migrate to other viscera and secretory glands. At the epithelia, two IgA molecules combine with another protein, termed the *secretory piece,* which is present on the surface of local epithelial cells. The complex, then termed *secretory IgA* (sIgA), passes through the cells into the mucus layer on the epithelial surface or into glandular secretions where it exerts its protective effect. The secretory piece not only mediates secretion, but also protects the molecule against proteolysis by enzymes such as those present in the intestinal tract.

    The major role of sIgA is to prevent attachment of antigen-carrying particles to receptors on mucous membrane epithelia. Thus, in the case of bacteria and viruses, it reacts with surface antigens that mediate adhesion and colonization and serves to prevent the establishment of local infection or invasion of the subepithelial tissues. It can agglutinate particles, but has no Fc domain for activating the classical complement pathway; however, it can activate the alternative pathway (see below). Reaction of IgA with antigen within the mucous membrane initiates an inflammatory reaction that helps mobilize other immunoglobulin and cellular defenses to the site of invasion. IgA response to an antigen is shorter lived than the IgG response.

IgE Antibody.   Immunoglobulin E is normally present in very small amounts in serum, and most IgE is bound firmly by its Fc portion to tissue *mast cells* and basophils, which are major producers of histamine. When IgE bound to mast cells reacts with specific antigen, the mast cells degranulate and release histamine and other factors that mediate an inflammatory reaction with dilatation of the capillaries, exudation of plasma components, and attraction of neutrophils and eosinophils to the site. Thus, IgE contributes to a rapid second line of defense if surface-protective mechanisms are breached. IgE also plays a significant indirect role in the immune response to a number of helminthic (worm) infections because of attraction of eosinophils to the site at which it reacts with antigen. The eosinophils bind to the Fc portions of IgG molecules that have reacted with surface antigens of the parasite and help bring about its destruction.

    Certain types of allergies, to be discussed under adverse effects of antigen-antibody reactions later in this chapter, are due to excessive production of IgE with specificity for a foreign protein. The pharmacological effects of histamine and the other vasoactive mediators released from mast cells largely account for the symptoms of the disorder.

IgD Antibody.   This antibody is highly susceptible to proteolytic enzymes in the tissues and is found only in very low concentrations in serum. Its role is not fully understood, although, as indicated earlier, it is present on the surface of some activated B cells and may serve as a recognition site for antigen.

Marginal notes:

IgA provides local immunity at mucosal surfaces

Dimer of IgA with attached secretory piece passes to epithelial surfaces

sIgA blocks microbial adherence, colonization, and invasion of epithelial surfaces

Other functions of IgA

IgE bound to mast cells; reaction with antigen releases vasoactive mediators; initiates inflammatory response

IgE attracts eosinophils to site of helminthic infection

Association with allergies

Antibody-Mediated Immunity

Antibodies provide immunity to infection and disease in a variety of ways.

Antitoxic and neutralizing effects; inhibition of colonization

1. They can neutralize the infectivity of a virus, the toxicity of an exotoxin molecule, or the ability of a bacterium to colonize. This is usually brought about by reaction between the antibody and an epitope that is required for attachment of the organism or toxin to a target host cell. IgA and IgG antibodies are particularly significant in neutralizing activity.

Inhibition of microbial nutrient uptake

2. Antibodies can inhibit essential nutrient assimilation by some bacteria. This occurs when a specific antigenic site or protein is involved in transport of the essential nutrient into the cell. For example, some siderophores (see Chapter 3) are antigenic, and antibody against them can prevent assimilation of the iron that is essential for growth.

Opsonization

3. IgG antibody can promote phagocytosis of extracellular bacteria by combining with capsules or other surface antigens that otherwise inhibit ingestion of the organism by phagocytes. When antigen–antibody reactions occur, the attachment sites for phagocytes on the Fc regions of the antibodies are exposed, the organism is bound to the phagocyte, and ingestion occurs. The significance of such opsonization is that many bacteria and some viruses are rapidly destroyed within the phagocytic cell.

Complement activation

4. Antigen–antibody reactions involving IgG and IgM activate the classical pathway of the complement cascade, which is described in the next section of this chapter. Complement components enhance a wide range of nonspecific host defense mechanisms, synergize antibody-mediated opsonization and lead to lysis of many Gram-negative bacteria with which antibody has reacted. A similar event occurs with blood and tissue cells carrying surface antigens recognized as foreign.

5. Antibodies that recognize foreign antigens on the surface of a host cell, such as a virally infected cell, will react with them and can mediate destruction of the cell by the process of antibody-dependent, cell-mediated cytotoxicity (ADCC) involving cells of uncertain lineage termed *natural killer* (NK) cells. NK cells have receptors for the exposed Fc portion of antibody and are bound in this way to the antibody-coated target cell that they kill on contact. Macrophages and related cells with Fc receptors may also be cytotoxic under these conditions. ADCC differs from the activity of cytotoxic T cells in that NK cells have no specific antigen recognition sites; thus, they can act nonspecifically against any antibody-coated target cells. NK cells are also active against some tumor cells that express altered surface molecules that are recognized as foreign.

Antibody-dependent, cell-mediated cytotoxicity; NK cells

The Complement System

Activation of system leads to cascade of activation reactions

The complement system plays a critical adjunctive role to the specific immune system. Complement consists of 20 major distinct components and several other precursors. It is a highly complex system, and focus will be placed on only nine major components for the purposes of this chapter. Some of the components are proenzymes, and all are present in the plasma of healthy individuals. When the complement system is triggered, a cascade of reactions occurs that activate the different components in a fixed

Several activated components contribute to host defenses

sequence. Several of these activated components have differing and important effects in defense against infection. Components of complement are designated by numbers, which, unfortunately for the student, reflect the order in which they were first described rather than the sequence in which they are activated. There is no immunological specificity in complement activation or in its effects, although specific antigen–antibody reactions are major initiators of activation, and some complement components enhance the effects of antigen–antibody interactions, for instance in opsonization.

The Classical Complement Pathway. This is summarized in Figure 8.5. It

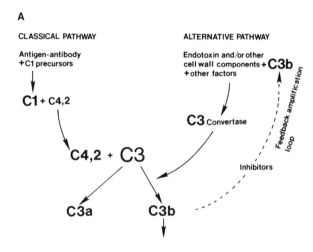

8.5 Schematic of the complement system. (**A**) Pathways for activation of C3. (*Note:* Both pathways converge at C3.) (**B**) Subsequent cascade and biological effects. Activated components shown in bold type.

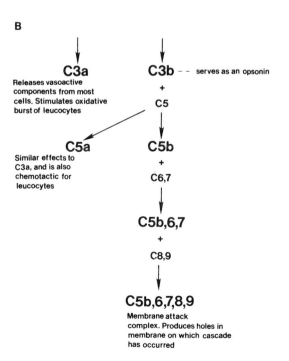

Activation of C1 by antigen–antibody reaction initiates cascade

is initiated by antigen–antibody reactions involving IgM or IgG. These reactions expose specific sites on the Fc portion of the immunoglobulin molecules that bind and activate the C1 component of complement. C1 then activates C4 and C2, and this complex splits C3 to two components, C3a and C3b. C3a liberates histamine and other vasoactive mediators from mast cells and stimulates the respiratory burst of phagocytes thus increasing their microbicidal power (see Chapter 9). C3b binds to the membrane of microorganisms or to cells such as tumor cells or red cells and to specific sites on Fc portions of IgM and IgG. Polymorphonuclear leukocytes (PMNs) and macrophages have receptors for C3b, which thus serves as an opsonin for microorganisms. The opsonic process is markedly enhanced when specific antibody has reacted with the organism.

C3a liberates mast cell vasoactive mediators and stimulates phagocytes

Opsonic activity of C3b

C5a has similar effects to C3a and is chemotactic for PMNs

C3b in association with activated C4,2, continues the cascade by splitting C5 to two components C5a and C5b. C5a stimulates release of histamine and other vasoactive mediators from mast cells, is a chemotactic factor for PMNs and enhances their metabolic antimicrobial activity. C5b binds to the membrane of cells on which an antigen–antibody reaction has occurred and inititiates activation of the terminal components C6–9. The insertion of the complex C5b, 6, 7, 8, 9 into the cell membrane produces functional holes and leads to the osmotic lysis of eukaryotic cells against which the antibody was directed. Some Gram-negative bacteria are similarly affected when there is an antibody response to accessible sites on the outer membrane. In this case, lysis (bacteriolysis) requires also the activity of lysozyme from phagocytes to break down the peptidoglycan layer of the cell wall.

C5b,6,7,8,9 damages cell membranes at site of initiating Ag:Ab reaction

The Alternative Pathway. This is a more primitive system than the classical pathway and does not require the presence of antibody. Instead, C3 can be activated by certain nonimmunological stimuli. These include endotoxin, other bacterial cell wall components, aggregated IgA, and feedback from the activation of the classical pathway. The alternative pathway is shown with the classical pathway in Figure 8.5. It produces the same inflammatory mediators (C3a, C5a) and increased phagocytic activity that result from activation of the classical pathway, but is not as efficient in cell lysis, because direction of complement components to the cell membrane by antibody is not involved. This pathway is particularly important in early response to infection.

C3 activated by endotoxin and some other nonimmunological stimuli; initiates cascade at C3 level
Main biological effects of alternative pathway are those of C3a, C3b, and C5a

Inherited deficiencies in complement components are often associated with increased susceptibility to bacterial infections. Most noticeable is the association of recurrent or unusually severe infections due to *Neisseria* (see Chapter 19) with individual complement component deficiencies (usually of C5, C6, C7, or C8).

Adverse Effects of Immunological Reactions

Immunological reactions in the body may result in excessive responses, sometimes far beyond those needed to remove or neutralize microbial pathogens or molecules contributing to disease. Such responses are classified as hypersensitivity reactions if they cause marked physiologic changes, tissue damage, and exacerbate disease processes. Several distinct classes of hypersensitivity reactions are recognized involving different immunological processes, but in each case they represent an extension of a normal defense mechanism.

Hypersensitivity reactions

Anaphylactic (Type I) Hypersensitivity. This has already been touched on

IgE determined; vasoactive
and other mediators liberated
from mast cells

briefly in relation to IgE antibody. Certain individuals produce particular IgE antibodies in response to some foreign antigens. Subsequent exposure to even minute amounts of the antigen leads within seconds to degranulation of the mast cells to which the IgE is bound and liberation of histamine, heparin, platelet-activating factor, and other factors attracting neutrophils and eosinophils to the site. When the reaction occurs locally, as in immunologically mediated asthma, the major manifestations include contraction of smooth muscle, increased mucus production, capillary vasodilatation, and increased vascular permeability. The latter results in exudation of plasma components from the blood vessels and edema. Other factors that prolong these effects (eg, leukotrienes and prostaglandins) are produced from arachidonic acid, which is liberated from the mast cell membrane as a result of activation of membrane phospholipases. These local responses can develop in some individuals in response to microbial antigens during the course of an infection.

Physiological effects

Systemic anaphylaxis; can
develop to some low-
molecular-weight haptens

When hypersensitivity is very marked, or antigen is introduced systemically, mast cells throughout the body degranulate, and systemic anaphylaxis results with constriction of the bronchi, edema of the larynx and other tissues, vascular collapse, and sometimes death. A generalized anaphylactic reaction rarely if ever occurs as a manifestation of an infection, but may occur following parenteral inoculation of an antigen to which the individual has been sensitized (eg, bee sting venom). It may also occur in individuals who have been sensitized to a low-molecular-weight hapten that binds to a tissue protein and becomes antigenic because of the size of the complex. An IgE response to hapten epitopes can then lead to anaphylactic-type hypersensitivity if the epitope is again encountered. A penicillin degradation product has this property, and occasional individuals develop severe anaphylactic reactions to penicillins, although this complication is very rare.

Rapid therapeutic intervention is critical in systemic anaphylaxis. It includes parenteral administration of epinephrine, which reverses the major manifestations of the syndrome by producing bronchodilatation, vasoconstriction, and raised blood pressure. Tracheostomy or intubation may be needed to overcome respiratory obstruction due to laryngeal edema.

Antibody-Mediated Cytotoxic (Type II) Hypersensitivity.   Opsonization, lysis of cells carrying foreign antigens, and the inflammatory effects of complement activation play important roles in defense, but can cause excessive damage to host cells under certain conditions. This is the case when antibodies reacting with a small peptide epitope on a microbial antigen cross-react with a similar amino acid sequence on a host cell or when they react with microbial antigen bound to the surface of host cells. In both these cases the body is attacked by its own immune system. Mechanisms such as these appear to be responsible for the tissue damage of rheumatic fever following a streptococcal infection, or some clinical manifestations of viral diseases, such as coxsackie B virus infection (see Chapter 35). These phenomena may involve not only antibodies, but also cytotoxic T cells.

Immunological damage to
host cells by cross-reacting
antibody or when microbial
antigen is bound to surface of
cell

Autoimmune disease

A more important mechanism of autoimmune phenomena is a breakdown in the self-recognition process of the immune system that allows it to attack certain host cells and tissues such as red cells. This subject, which is of great theoretical and practical importance, lies beyond the scope of our consideration.

Immune Complex Disease (Type III Hypersensitivity).   When IgG, which is

Lattice formation

bivalent with two epitope-binding sites, is mixed in appropriate proportions with multivalent antigen molecules (ie, bearing multiple epitopes), aggregates containing a lattice of many antigen and antibody molecules form. With appropriate concentrations of the two reactants, a macroscopic precipitate can develop (see Chapter 14). A similar situation applies to IgM, which is multivalent. When the epitope is present on the surface of a larger particle, such as a bacterium or red blood cell, the particles can be cross-linked by antibody, and microscopic or macroscopic agglutination results. These phenomena can occur in vivo when a sufficient amount of specific antibody and of free antigen from an infecting microorganism react locally or in the bloodstream to form an antigen–antibody lattice; the size of the immune complex depends on the relative properties of the two reactants. Large immune complexes are phagocytosed and usually broken down within the phagocyte. Smaller complexes, however, are deposited in small blood vessels and capillaries through which they do not pass, activate the complement system, and thus produce an acute inflammatory response mediated largely by C3a and C5a. This results in the manifestations of vasculitis. Phagocytes attracted chemotactically to the site release hydrolytic enzymes, and the sum of these effects is tissue damage that is acute and can become chronic depending on the survival of the antigen or on whether it is continually replaced. Acute glomerulonephritis following certain streptococcal infections is an example of an immune complex disease in which glomeruli of the kidney are damaged by the complexes, resulting in various manifestations of renal impairment. Inflammatory skin lesions can result from deposition of immune complexes in the cutaneous blood vessels in patients with infective endocarditis. Deposition in joints, the pericardium, or the pleura produces arthritis, pericarditis, and pleuritis or pleurisy, respectively.

Small complexes deposit in capillaries; initiate complement mediated inflammation

Examples of immune complex diseases

Serum sickness

A systemic form of immune complex disease, termed *serum sickness*, can follow the injection of foreign antigen. An example is the therapeutic use of diphtheria antitoxin that has been produced in horses. About 10 days after inoculation, sufficient antibody against horse proteins has been produced to form immune complexes made up of human antibody reacting against horse serum protein (including horse immunoglobulins). These complexes are deposited in various organs resulting in a syndrome of arthritis, nephritis, rash, urticaria, and fever. The disease usually resolves as the foreign antigen concentration decreases through immune clearance and catabolism of the antigen(s).

Delayed-Type (Type IV) Hypersensitivity. This has been described under "The T-Cell Response" in relationship to cell-mediated immunity and differs substantially in mechanisms and manifestations from the hypersensitivity reactions due to antibody.

Laboratory Production of Specific Antibodies

Specific antibodies are widely exploited in seroidentification of microorganisms, in basic studies of the immune response, as microchemical reagents in biological research, and as agents in prophylaxis and therapy. Various practical aspects of these uses are described in Chapter 14, but some principles of specific antibody production need to be described here.

Seroidentification procedures use antibodies to detect specific antigenic epitopes on microorganisms and thus aid in their identification. Antisera for this purpose are produced by inoculating one or more animals (usually rabbits, goats, or horses) with a known organism or purified antigens de-

Antibodies prepared by immunizing animals

rived from it. The inoculation schedule is designed to produce a maximum antibody response. When this is reached the animal is bled, the serum separated, and its antibody quantitated by testing the ability of increasing dilutions of serum (titration) to react with the inciting antigen in a particular test system (agglutination, neutralization, etc). It is important to recognize that such antisera are usually polyclonal, and contain antibodies of many different specificities. These can be against different molecules of the material injected into the animal and against different epitopes on the same molecule. Even when a single epitope is involved, antibodies of varying affinity will be produced.

In many cases, when the immunizing antigen was an organism of complex antigenic structure, such as a bacterium, some of the antibodies produced cross-react with the same, or closely similar, antigens on taxonomically distinct organisms. These antibodies can be removed by treating the antisera in vitro with cross-reacting organisms until all antibody to common antigens has reacted with them. The cross-reacting organisms and antibodies that have reacted with them are then removed by centrifugation, and the *absorbed serum* that remains has become a more specific seroidentification reagent. This is a very simplified account of what may be a complex process. Distinction between the hundreds of different salmonella bacteria, for example, involves discrimination of many different antigenic epitopes represented on flagella, capsules, and cell surface polysaccharide antigens. It requires dozens of absorbed antisera made specific for the different epitopes that exist in many different combinations. Obviously, the process is simplified when purified antigen is available for immunizing the animals, but this is often impossible because the precise nature of the antigen is unknown or it has not been separated from others.

Monoclonal Antibodies.   The heterogeneity of antibody responses in terms of specificity and affinity introduces problems in their use as precise tools for identifying specific epitopes. This has been overcome by the development of procedures that allow the almost unlimited production of antibody that was encoded in a single B cell. The process involves in vitro fusion of antigen-stimulated B cells with cells of a B-cell malignant tumor (myeloma) that synthesizes large amounts of a nonspecific immunoglobulin. The myeloma cell is capable of unrestricted growth in cell culture or in the animal from which it was derived. Genetic reassembly within the fused cells yields some that have the growth characteristics (immortality) and Ig synthesizing capability of the tumor but produce antibody with the specificity encoded in the nonmalignant B cell and thus for a single epitope. These are termed *hybridoma cells*.

Techniques have been developed that allow selection of clones of hybridoma cells that produce the desired antibody and can be grown continually in vitro or in vivo. The concept is outlined in Figure 8.6 Monoclonal antibody is homogeneous and highly specific for a single epitope and can be produced in almost limitless quantities. These antibodies are being used increasingly in seroidentification procedures and have the potential for use as therapeutic agents in instances in which critical antigens of a microorganism or a tumor cell are not recognized by the immune system of the host. The monoclonal antibody can also be combined with a substance that is lethal to the cell or organism carrying the antigen against which it is directed.

Monoclonal antibodies can be produced from hybridoma cells grown in vivo in the peritoneal cavity of mice or from in vitro cultures. Human monoclonal antibody production can result from fusion between human

Antisera usually contain antibodies of many different specificities

Absorption of cross-reacting antibodies

Fusion of antigen-stimulated B cells with immortal myeloma cells

Hybridoma cells produce homogeneous antibody and are immortalized

8.6 Concept of monoclonal antibody production. (A) B cells are each producing Ig against different epitopes and carrying gene α for production of enzyme A. B cells cannot be maintained in culture. (B) Mutant myeloma cells lack gene α and do not produce specific Ig. Myeloma cells can be propagated indefinitely. (C) Cell fusion enhanced with polyethylene glycol. (D) Incubate in selective medium that allows growth only of immortal (M) cells that produce enzyme A. These are antibody producing hybridoma cells. Clone individual hybrid cells, expand in culture, test for production of antibody of desired specificity, and propagate that clone as an epitope-specific hybridoma.

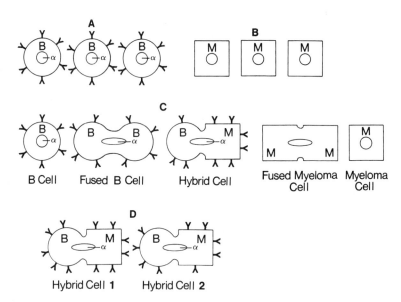

B cells and mouse myeloma cells, but the hybrids are less stable than when antigenically stimulated B cells of mice are used. A variety of approaches are being explored to facilitate the safe production of human monoclonal antibodies for therapeutic purposes.

Antigen Surrogates. A recently developed approach has the potential of allowing the use of antibodies as antigen surrogates in immunization. Antibodies are themselves antigenic in animal species to which they are foreign. The anti-antibodies that can be produced include some with specificity for unique epitope-reacting portions of the Fab variable region of the antibody against which they are directed as well as for epitope-recognizing sites on immunoresponsive B cells. These are termed *anti-idiotypic antibodies* and have the same three-dimensional geometry as would the epitope molecule.* Monoclonal antibodies that have this structure can be selected and produced in large amounts and may then act as antigens for the production of specific antibodies against the epitope of interest. Immunization with such anti-idiotype antibodies has promise for producing specific immunity against critical antigens that are impossible or uneconomical to produce in bulk. At present there are many problems to overcome before such procedures could begin to be applied to humans.

Additional Reading

Claman, H.N. 1987. The biology of the immune response. *J.A.M.A.* 258:2834–2840. This and subsequent articles in the same issue of the journal present a clinical perspective that is useful.

Cooper, M.D. 1987. B lymphocytes. Normal development and function. *N. Engl. J. Med.* 317:1452–1456. This is a concise review of B-cell ontogeny, metabolism, and function, including a description of isotype switching.

---

* Idiotype refers to the highly specific antigenic properties of an antibody molecule, which are conferred by the epitope recognizing site of the variable region. There are thus, potentially, hundreds of thousands of distinct idiotypes of antibody in any individual.

Cramer, D.V., and Gill, T.J., III. 1986. Genetic aspects of cellular interactions in the immune response. *Lab. Invest.* 55:126–137. A clear discussion is given of cell surface determinants regulating immune responses and cell-to-cell interactions.

Dinarello, C.A., and Mier, J.W. 1987. Lymphokines. *N. Engl. J. Med.* 317:940–945. A review of the current understanding concerning lymphokines and other cytokines.

Johnson, K.J., Chensue, S.W., Kunkel, S.L., and Ward, P.A. 1988. Immunopathology. In *Pathology.* Rubin, E., and Farber, J.L., Eds. Philadelphia: J.B. Lippincott Co., pp. 96–139. This chapter is an excellently illustrated review of immunology as viewed by the immunopathologist. The descriptions of hypersensitivity reactions, types I–IV, are particularly useful.

Nossal, G.J.V. 1987. The basic components of the immune system. *N. Engl. J. Med.* 316:1320–1325. A stimulating discussion of the six basic components of the natural defense system: encounter, recognition, activation, deployment, discrimination, and regulation.

Royer, H.D., and Reinherz, E.L. 1987. T lymphocytes: Ontogeny, function, and relevance to clinical disorders. *New Engl. J. Med.* 317:1136–1142. This review describes the structure and development of the T-cell receptor and the activation process, relating these to clinical medicine.

There are many excellent recent texts providing more detailed general coverage of immunology. They include the following:

Golub, E.S. 1987. *Immunology. A Synthesis.* Sunderland, MA, Sinauer Associates, Inc.

Hood, L.E., Weissman, I.L., Wood, W.B., and Wilson, J.H. 1984. *Immunology.* 2nd ed. Menlo Park, CA, and Reading, MA, Benjamin Cummings Publishing Co., Inc.

Roitt, I. 1988. *Essential Immunology.* 6th ed. Oxford: Blackwell Scientific Publications.

Sell, S. 1987. *Basic Immunology. Immune Mechanics in Health and Disease.* New York: Elsevier Science Publishing Co.

9

Normal
Microbial Flora

John C. Sherris

The term *normal* or *indigenous flora* is used to describe microorganisms that are frequently found in particular sites in normal, healthy individuals. The constituents and numbers of the flora vary in different areas of the body, and sometimes at different ages. They comprise microorganisms whose morphologic, physiologic, and genetic properties allow them to colonize and multiply under the conditions that exist in particular sites, to coexist with other colonizing organisms, and to inhibit competing intruders. Thus, each accessible area of the body presents a particular ecological niche, colonization of which requires a particular set of properties of the invading microbe.

Organisms of the normal flora can be classified as *parasites,** which live at the expense of the host: *symbionts,* which benefit the host; and *commensals,* which have a neutral relationship to the host. In many instances, however, not enough is known about the organism's interactions with the host to make such distinctions. They can also be categorized as *residents,* which are present invariably or for many weeks or months in a particular

Residents and transients

site, and *transients,* which may establish themselves briefly for colonization or infection without disease, but tend to be excluded by competition from residents or by the host's innate or immune defense mechanisms. The distinction between the transient and the *carrier state* is blurred when potentially pathogenic organisms are involved. For example, *Streptococcus pneumoniae* (the pneumococcus), isolated from the upper respiratory tract of many healthy people during the winter months, is often considered part of the transient normal flora. In contrast, the presence of *Neisseria*

Normal flora and the carrier state

meningitidis (the meningococcus) in the nasopharynx of healthy individuals during epidemics of meningococcal meningitis is usually regarded as carriage.

---

* The term *parasite* is also used to describe members of the animal kingdom that infect humans or animals. These organisms are discussed in Chapters 51–58.

It is important for students of medical microbiology and infectious disease to have a good grasp of the role of the normal flora, because of its significance both as a defense mechanism against infection and as a source of potentially pathogenic organisms. It is also important to know its sites and composition to avoid confusion between members of the normal flora and specific organisms of disease when interpreting laboratory results.

Origin of the Normal Flora

Initial flora acquired during and immediately after birth

The healthy fetus is sterile until the birth membranes rupture. During and after birth, the infant is exposed to the flora of the mother's genital tract, to the skin and respiratory flora of those handling it, and to organisms in the environment. During the infant's first few days of life, the nature of the flora often reflects chance exposure to organisms that can grow on particular sites in the absence of competitors. Subsequently, as the infant is exposed to the full range of human floral organisms, those best adapted to colonize particular sites become predominant. Thereafter, the flora generally resembles that of other individuals in the same age group and cultural milieu.

Factors Determining the Nature of the Normal Flora

Physiologic conditions

Bacterial adherence

Bacterial interactions

Local physiologic and ecologic conditions determine the nature of the flora. They are sometimes highly complex, differing from site to site, and sometimes vary with age. These conditions include the amounts and types of nutrients available, pH, oxidation-reduction potentials, and resistance to local antibacterial substances such as bile or lysozyme. Many bacteria have a remarkable affinity for receptors on specific types of epithelial cells to which they attach and on which they multiply. This adherence, which is mediated by pili or other surface component adhesins, permits the bacteria to colonize and multiply while avoiding removal by the flushing effects of surface fluids and peristalsis. Various microbial interactions also determine their relative prevalence in the flora. These interactions include competition for nutrients, inhibition by the metabolic products of other organisms (for example, by hydrogen peroxide or volatile fatty acids), and production of antibiotics and bacteriocins.

With a complex flora, it is difficult to determine the relative importance of these factors, but the importance of interbacterial interactions is clear and is illustrated by the dramatic distortions that can result from antibiotic therapy.

Normal Flora of Different Sites

The total normal flora of the body probably contains more than 100 distinct species of microorganisms. In this chapter the major members known to be important in preventing or causing disease will be indicated, as well as those that may be confused with etiologic agents of local infections. These organisms are summarized in Table 9.1, and most will be described in greater detail in subsequent chapters. The student should not attempt to memorize unfamiliar names at this point.

Blood, Body Fluids, and Tissues

Normally sterile in health

In health, the blood, body fluids, and tissues are normally sterile. Occasional organisms may transgress epithelial barriers as a result of trauma (including physiologic trauma such as the act of heavy chewing or during

Table 9.1 Predominant and Important Flora of Various Body Sites in Health

Body Site	Flora
Blood	Sterile; occasional transient low-level bacteremia from physiologic trauma (e.g., viridans streptococci)
Tissues; cerebrospinal fluid; urinary bladder; uterus and fallopian tubes; middle ear; paranasal sinuses	Sterile
Skin; distal urethra; external ear	*Propionibacterium acnes;* diphtheroids; *Staphylococcus epidermidis;* other coagulase-negative staphylococci
Mouth	
Tongue and buccal mucosa	Viridans streptococci; *Neisseria* spp.; *Branhamella;* occasional *Candida albicans*
Gingival crevices and tonsillar crypts	*Bacteroides* spp.; *Fusobacterium* spp.; *Peptostreptococcus* spp.; *Actinomyces;* other anaerobes
Nasopharynx	Oral organisms—transient carriage of *Streptococcus pneumoniae, Haemophilus* spp., and *Neisseria meningitidis;* oral anaerobes
Esophagus	Transient mouth flora
Stomach	Rapidly becomes sterile after meals
Small intestine	Scanty, variable, and ill-defined
Colon	
After weaning	*Bacteroides* spp; *Fusobacterium* spp.; *Clostridium* spp.; *Peptostreptococcus* spp.; *Escherichia coli; Proteus* spp.; other Enterobacteriaceae; *Pseudomonas aeruginosa;* numerous other bacteria and yeasts
During breast-feeding	*Bifidobacterium;* lactobacilli; aciduric streptococci
Vagina	
Prepubertal and postmenopausal stages	Skin and some colonic organisms
Childbearing years	Lactobacilli; aciduric streptococci and yeasts

Transient bacteremia can result from trauma

childbirth); they may be briefly recoverable from the bloodstream before they are filtered out in the pulmonary capillaries or removed by cells of the reticuloendothelial system. Such transient bacteremia may be the source of infection of damaged or abnormal heart valves that leads to bacterial endocarditis (Chapter 68).

Skin

Variation in different sites

The skin plays host to an abundant flora that varies somewhat according to the number and activity of sebaceous and sweat glands; variation between individuals may be substantial and consistent. The flora is most abundant on moist skin areas (axillae, perineum, and between toes). *Staphylococcus epidermidis* and members of the genus *Propionibacterium* occur all over the skin. Other coagulase-negative staphylococci may colonize certain sites, and facultative diphtheroids (corynebacteria) are found in moist areas. Propionibacteria are slim, anaerobic or microaerophilic Gram-positive rods that grow in subsurface sebum and break down skin lipids to fatty acids. They are thus most numerous in the ducts of hair follicles and of the sebaceous glands that drain into them (pilosebaceous units). They cannot be removed from skin sites bearing pilosebaceous units even by the most vigorous washing or application of antiseptics, and small numbers are often isolated from biopsy materials because of contamination from the skin during the operative procedure. Propionibacteria, *S. epidermidis*, and other coagulase-negative staphylococci are nonpathogenic, except in certain situations in which general or local host defenses are compromised or foreign bodies present. Organisms of the skin flora are resistant to the bactericidal effects of skin lipids and fatty acids, which inhibit or kill many extraneous bacteria.

Propionibacteria grow in pilosebaceous units

Stability of skin flora

Conjunctival Sac

In health, the conjunctivae have a very scanty flora of nonpathogenic corynebacteria and *S. epidermidis*. The low bacterial count is maintained by the high lysozyme content of lacrimal secretions, and by the flushing effect of tears.

Intestinal Tract

The *mouth* and *pharynx* contain large numbers of facultative and strict anaerobes. Many species of facultative streptococci are encountered, most of which are α-hemolytic or nonhemolytic (see Chapter 16). Different species of streptococci predominate on the buccal and tongue mucosa because of different specific adherence characteristics; one species, *Streptococcus mutans,* shows specific adherence to teeth and plays an etiologic role in caries. Gram-negative diplococci of the genera *Neisseria* and *Branhamella* make up the balance of the facultative organisms most commonly isolated. Strict anaerobes and microaerophilic organisms of the oral cavity have their niches in the depths of the gingival crevices surrounding the teeth and in sites such as tonsillar crypts, where anaerobic conditions can develop readily. Anaerobic members of the normal flora are major contributors to the etiology of periodontal disease (Chapter 62).

Abundant anaerobic and facultative flora including viridans streptococci

Although it varies from site to site, the total number of organisms in the oral cavity is very high. Saliva usually contains a mixed flora of about 10^8 organisms per milliliter, derived mostly from the various epithelial colonization sites.

The *stomach* contains few, if any, resident organisms in health because of the lethal action of gastric hydrochloric acid and peptic enzymes on bacteria.

Stomach has few residents

The *small intestine* has a scanty resident flora, except in the lower ileum, where it begins to resemble that of the colon. Many animal species have bacteria very closely associated with the epithelium, which have been grown in artificial culture with difficulty or not at all. The extent to which analogous situations may exist in humans is still unclear. These mucosa-associated organisms probably evolved as symbionts with the host species.

Resident flora scanty; increases toward lower ileum

The *colon* carries the most prolific flora in the body (Figures 9.1 and

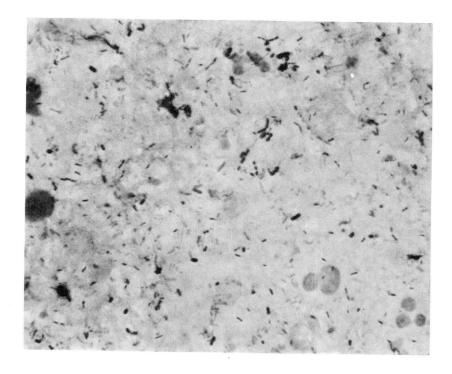

9.1 Gram-stained smear of feces, showing great diversity of microorganisms.

Adult colonic flora is mixed and predominantly anaerobic

Bifidobacteria are predominant flora of breast-fed infants

9.2) In the adult, feces are 25% or more bacteria by weight (about 10^{10} organisms per gram). More than 90% are anaerobes, predominantly members of the genera *Bacteroides* and *Fusobacterium,* although *Clostridium perfringens,* a major etiologic agent of gas gangrene, is invariably present. The remainder of the flora is composed of facultative organisms such as *Escherichia coli,* fecal streptococci (enterococci), yeasts, and numerous other species. There are considerable differences in adult flora depending on the diet of the host. Those whose diets include substantial amounts of meat have more *Bacteroides* and other anaerobic Gram-negative rods in their stools than those on a predominantly vegetable or fish diet.

The fecal flora of breast-fed infants differs from that of adults; up to 99% comprises anaerobic Gram-positive rods of the genus *Bifidobacterium*

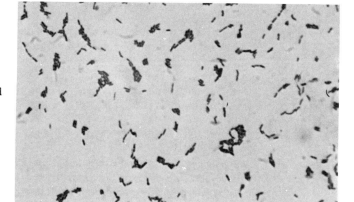

9.2 Gram-stained smear of stool of breast-fed infant. Note homogeneous flora of Gram-positive rods.

(Figure 9.2). Human milk is high in lactose and low in protein and phosphate, and its buffering capacity is poor compared to that of cow's milk. These conditions select for bifidobacteria, which ferment lactose to yield acetic acid and grow optimally under the acidic conditions (pH 5–5.5) that they produce in the stool. Infants fed cow's milk, which has a greater buffering capacity, tend to have less acidic stools and a flora more similar to that found in the colon of the weaned infant or of the adult. These findings also apply to infants fed some artificial formulas.

Effect of artificial feeding

Respiratory Tract

S. aureus carriage in anterior nares

The *anterior nares* is lined with squamous epithelium in its external 1cm and has a flora similar to that of the skin except that it is the predominant site of carriage of a pathogen, *Staphylococcus aureus*. About 25–30% of healthy people in the community carry this organism at any given time, 15% permanently and 15% transiently. The organism may spread to other skin sites or colonize the perineum; it can be disseminated by hand-to-nose contact, by desquamation of the epithelium, or by droplet spread during upper respiratory infection.

Often site of carriage of potential pathogens

The *nasopharynx* has a flora similar to that of the mouth; however, it is often the site of carriage of potentially pathogenic organisms such as pneumococci, meningococci, and *Haemophilus* species.

Lower tract is protected by mucociliary action

The *respiratory tract* below the level of the larynx is protected in health by the action of the epithelial cilia and by the movement of the *mucociliary blanket* (Chapter 10); thus, only transient inhaled organisms are encountered in the trachea and larger bronchi. The accessory sinuses are normally sterile and are protected in a similar fashion, as is the middle ear by the epithelium of the eustachian tubes.

Genitourinary Tract

Bladder and upper urinary tract are sterile in health

The *urinary tract* is sterile in health above the distal 1 cm of the urethra, which has a scanty flora derived from the perineum. Thus, in health the urine within and above the bladder is sterile.

Hormonal effects on vaginal flora

The *vagina* has a flora that varies according to hormonal influences at different ages. Before puberty and after menopause, it is mixed, nonspecific, and relatively scanty and contains organisms derived from the flora of the skin and colon. During the childbearing years, it is composed predominantly of anaerobic and microaerophilic members of the genus *Lactobacillus,* with smaller numbers of anaerobic Gram-negative rods, Gram-positive cocci, and yeasts that can survive under the acidic conditions produced by the lactobacilli. These conditions develop because glycogen is deposited in vaginal epithelial cells under the influence of estrogenic hormones and metabolized to lactic acid by lactobacilli. This process results in a vaginal pH of 4–5, which is optimal for growth and survival of the lactobacilli, but inhibits many other organisms. The consistency of the lactobacillary adult flora is seen in Gram-stained preparations of vaginal smears (Figure 9.3).

Utilization of epithelial glycogen by lactobacilli gives low pH

Role of the Normal Flora in Disease

Many species among the normal flora are opportunists in that they can cause infection if they reach protected areas of the body in sufficient numbers or if local or general host defense mechanisms are compromised. For example, certain strains of *E. coli* can reach the urinary bladder by

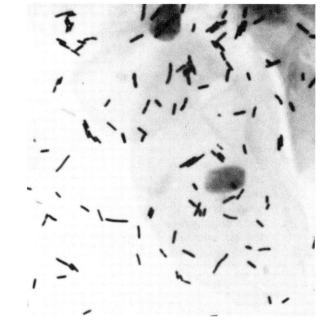

9.3 Gram-stained smear of normal adult vagina, showing lactobacillary flora and squamous epithelial cells.

Urinary tract and abdominal infections

ascending the urethra (Chapter 66) and cause acute urinary tract infection, usually in sexually active women. Perforation of the colon from a ruptured diverticulum or a penetrating abdominal wound will release feces into the peritoneal cavity; this fecal contamination may be followed by peritonitis, primarily caused by facultative members of the flora, and by intraabdominal abscesses, primarily caused by Gram-negative anaerobes. Viridans streptococci from the oral cavity may reach the bloodstream as a result of physiologic trauma or injury (for example, tooth extraction) and colonize a previously damaged heart valve, initiating bacterial endocarditis (Chapter 68). These and other diseases, such as actinomycosis (Chapter 28), result from displacement of normal flora into body cavities or tissues.

Bacterial endocarditis

Opportunistic infections in the immunocompromised

Reduced specific immunologic responses, defects in phagocytic activity, or weakening of epithelial barriers by vitamin deficiencies can all result in local invasion and disease by normal floral organisms. This source accounts for many infections in patients whose defenses are compromised by disease (for example, diabetes, lymphoma, or leukemia) or by cytotoxic chemotherapy for cancer. One specific local infection of this type is Vincent's angina of the oral mucosa, a local invasion and ulceration apparently caused by the combined action of oral spirochetes and members of the genus *Fusobacterium*. Death after lethal radiation exposure usually results from massive invasion by normal floral organisms, particularly those of the intestinal tract.

Fusospirochetal disease

Role in caries and periodontal disease

Caries and periodontal disease are both caused by organisms that may be considered members of the normal flora. They are considered in detail in Chapter 62.

Nonspecific adverse effects were often postulated in the past

Early in the 20th century, it was widely believed that the normal flora of the large intestine was responsible for many "toxic conditions," including rheumatoid arthritis, degenerative diseases, and a range of conditions now recognized as psychosomatic. Ritualistic purging and colonic lavage flourished, particularly at expensive mineral spas, and some patients were even subjected to colectomy as the ultimate cure. The concept was given respectability by Metchnikoff, who suggested that the longevity of Georgian peasants in Russia was attributable to their heavy consumption of yogurt, resulting in replacement of their colonic flora with lactobacilli to the general benefit of their health. These concepts fell into disrepute as the etiology of the "toxic" diseases was clarified and when it was found that lactobacillary replacement of flora of the adult colon did not occur under the conditions used.

More recently, however, attention has again been focused on the less specific contributions of the normal flora to health and disease. In patients with large or multiple blind-ended diverticula in the small intestine, heavy colonization by the anaerobic intestinal flora may occur. This colonization results in bacterial deconjugation of bile salts needed for absorption of fat and fat-soluble vitamins and also in competition for vitamin B_{12}. Similar situations sometimes occur in the elderly when the small intestine is invaded by colonic flora. If the primary cause (for example, Meckel's diverticulum) cannot be eliminated surgically, these conditions can be ameliorated with antibiotic therapy and fat-soluble vitamin supplements. An analogous situation occurs in tropical sprue, in which secondary colonization of the jejunum by facultative Gram-negative enteric bacteria leads to fat malabsorption and vitamin B_{12} and folic acid deficiencies. It has been postulated that the higher colon cancer rates in those consuming western as opposed to oriental diets may be a result of greater production by members of the normal flora of carcinogens such as nitrosamines or bile acid derivatives.

Under certain conditions, a "toxemia" can result from the action of the normal colonic flora. In severe hepatic cirrhosis, the portal circulation may be partially diverted to the systemic circulation. The detoxification by the liver of ammonia produced by bacterial action on protein residues is bypassed, and severe dysfunctions of the central nervous system (hepatic encephalopathy) can result. This problem can be ameliorated with a strict low-protein diet.

There is considerable evidence that cattle and poultry maintained under conditions of intensive husbandry may have slower growth rates than those kept under more stringent hygienic conditions and that this disparity is caused by differences in their normal flora. Addition of antibiotics to feed may improve growth; the resulting development of antibiotic-resistant flora, however, poses important ecologic and epidemiologic problems.

Beneficial Effects of the Normal Flora

Priming of Immune System

Organisms of the normal flora play an important role in the development of immunologic competence. Animals delivered and raised under completely aseptic conditions ("sterile," or gnotobiotic, animals) have a poorly developed reticuloendothelial system, low serum levels of immunoglobulins, and none of the antibodies to normal floral antigens that often cross-react with those of pathogenic organisms and confer a degree of protection against them. As long as they are maintained under sterile conditions, gnotobiotic animals are often larger and live longer than those exposed to the environment. However, when moved to normal conditions, they immediately become vulnerable, because many bacteria that are nonpathogenic to normal hosts can be lethal to them, presumably because immunologic priming has not occurred under the protection of maternally derived antibody.

Blind-loop syndrome of fat malabsorption and B_{12} deficiency

Colonization of jejunum in tropical sprue

Ammonia production and hepatic encephalopathy

Intensive husbandry and antibiotic feeds

Sterile animals have little immunity to microbial infection

Exclusionary Effect

Beneficial effect of breast-feeding and a bifidobacterial flora

The normal flora produces conditions that tend to block the establishment of extraneous pathogens and their ability to infect the host. The bifidobacteria in the colon of the breast-fed infant produce an environment inimical to colonization by enteric pathogens; this protective effect is aided by ingested maternal IgA. Breast-feeding has clearly been shown to help protect the infant from enteric bacterial infection.

Protective effect of normal vaginal flora

The normal vaginal flora has a similar protective effect. Before the introduction of antibiotic therapy, it was found that institutional outbreaks of fomite-transmitted gonococcal vulvovaginitis in prepubertal girls were controlled by synthetic estrogen therapy. This treatment led to glycogen deposition in the vaginal epithelium and establishment of a protective lactobacillary flora. The possible hazard of such therapy in this age group was not then recognized.

Superinfections may follow broad spectrum antibiotic therapy

Candidiasis

Antibiotic therapy, particularly with broad-spectrum agents, may so alter the normal flora of the gastrointestinal tract that antibiotic-resistant organisms multiply in the relative ecologic vacuum produced, sometimes causing significant infections, particularly in immunocompromised patients. The pathogenic yeast *Candida albicans*, a minor constituent of the normal flora, may multiply dramatically and cause diarrhea and superficial fungal infections in the mouth, vagina, or anal area. Certain resistant strains of *S. aureus* may largely replace the facultative flora of the colon during antibiotic therapy, particularly after gastrointestinal surgery, and produce a severe necrotizing enterocolitis that is often fatal. Fortunately, although the reasons are not clear, this disease is now rare. More recently, a non-staphylococcal pseudomembranous colitis associated with antibiotic therapy was shown to result from proliferation of a toxin-producing anaerobe, *Clostridium difficile*, which can be a minor constituent of the flora or acquired from an external source. It may be resistant to several antibiotics, particularly lincomycin and clindamycin, and can multiply and elaborate its toxin during and after therapy. The toxin is responsible for the damage to the colonic epithelium.

Staphylococcal enterocolitis

C. difficile pseudomembranous enterocolitis

The exclusionary effect of the flora in health has been demonstrated in numerous experiments on gnotobiotic and antibiotic-treated animals. For example, *C. albicans* attaches to oral epithelial cells of germ-free rats; however, prior colonization with certain viridans streptococci that attach to similar epithelial cells prevents establishment of *C. albicans*. In another experiment, the infecting oral dose for mice of streptomycin-resistant *Salmonella typhimurium* was shown to be approximately 10^5 organisms in untreated animals. Oral streptomycin treatment, which inhibits many members of the normal flora, reduced the infecting dose by approximately 1000-fold.

Production of Essential Nutrients

Vitamin production

In ruminants, the action of the extensive anaerobic flora in the rumen is essential to the nutrition of the animal. The flora digests cellulose to usable form and provides many vitamins, including 70% of the animal's vitamin B requirements. In humans, members of the vitamin B group and vitamin K are produced by the normal flora; however, except for vitamin K the amounts available or absorbed are small compared to those in a well-balanced diet. Bacterial vitamin production is reduced during broad-spectrum antibiotic therapy, and supplementation with vitamin B complex is indicated in malnourished individuals.

Manipulation of the Normal Flora

Attempts to manipulate the normal flora have usually been fruitless and have sometimes been dangerous. Manipulation has proved useful, however, in two situations. Patients whose immunologic defenses are massively compromised (for example, during whole body irradiation and bone marrow transplantation in the treatment of leukemia) may have their normal flora greatly reduced by judicious use of combined chemotherapy, reduction or exclusion of extraneous organisms by sterilization of food and supplies, and by aseptic nursing procedures. These conditions substantially reduce the risk of infection during a highly vulnerable period.

It has also been shown that nursery outbreaks of *S. aureus* infections, a major problem in the 1950s and 1960s, may be controlled by deliberate colonization of the infant's nares with *S. aureus* 502A, a strain of low virulence that tends to exclude more virulent strains of *S. aureus*. Unfortunately, some infections have also occurred with the 502A strain. As greater understanding of the complex ecology of the normal flora is gained, it is probable that other techniques for its manipulation will be developed to augment protection from infection.

Additional Reading

Gibbons, R.J., and Van Houte, J. 1975. Bacterial adherence in oral microbial ecology. *Annu. Rev. Microbiol.* 29:19–44. A pioneering review of the role of bacterial adherence in the oral cavity.

Noble, W.C. 1984. Skin microbiology: Coming of age. *J. Med. Microbiol.* 17:1–12.

Rosebury, T. 1970. *Life on Man.* New York: Berkeley Publishing Co. A delightful, wry, and instructive paperback. Highly recommended for recreational reading.

Savage, D.C., and Fletcher, M., Eds. 1985. *Bacterial Adhesion: Mechanisms and Physiological Significance.* New York/London: Plenum Press. A multiauthored book by leading contributors to the field that gives an up-to-date account of knowledge of the mechanisms and significance of adherence, including those of members of the normal flora.

Skinner, F.A., and Carr, J.G., Eds. 1974. *The Normal Microbial Flora of Man.* The Society for Applied Bacteriology Symposium No. 3. London: Academic Press. This and the Noble reference give excellent coverage of their topics and are good reference sources.

10

Pathogenesis of Bacterial and Viral Infections:
Initial Defenses, Infectivity, Virulence, and Host Responses

John C. Sherris and
C. George Ray

The factors that determine the initiation, development, and outcome of an infection involve a series of complex and shifting interactions between the parasite and the host, which can vary with different infecting organisms. They include

1. The host's primary physical barriers against invasion and the ways in which they can be breached.

2. The ability of an organism to evade destruction by local and tissue host defenses.

3. The manner in which an organism spreads in the body and causes disease.

4. The body's adaptive immunologic ability to control and eliminate invading parasites.

Despite the complexity of interactions between different parasites and hosts, several components of pathogenetic processes and principles have broad application to infectious diseases and will be described in this chapter with appropriate examples. More details of individual organisms and diseases will be given in subsequent chapters.

Basic mechanisms of specific immune responses have been discussed in Chapter 8 and will not be recapitulated here.

Species immunity and susceptibility

In considering this topic, it is essential to bear in mind that the ability of an organism to infect or cause disease depends on the susceptibility of the host and that there are remarkable species differences in host susceptibility to many infections. For example, dogs do not get measles, and people do not get distemper. Thus, the term *pathogenicity*, which is defined as the ability to cause disease, must be qualified according to the host species involved. In recent years, increasing numbers of infections have been caused by organisms previously considered nonpathogenic. These

Primary and opportunistic
pathogens

infections develop in patients whose immunologic or cellular defenses are compromised by genetic defects, disease, or therapy. Therefore, the concept of pathogenicity requires further qualification, and it is useful to consider organisms as *primary pathogens,* which may initiate disease in previously healthy individuals, and *opportunists,* which are frequent causes of disease in the immunocompromised host or when first-line defense barriers are breached. *Virulence,* as applied to infectious agents, is defined as the degree of pathogenicity. Thus, a pathogenic organism may be of high or low virulence for a particular host species, or particular strains of a pathogenic species of bacteria may have lost a critical determinant of virulence and be categorized as *avirulent.*

Virulence is degree of
pathogenicity

First-Line Defenses against Microbial Invasion

First-line defenses of the healthy individual are those that prevent colonization of certain body surfaces or block access of potentially pathogenic organisms to subepithelial tissues. They are summarized in Table 10.1 and will be considered in more detail according to the structures and processes involved.

Epithelial Barriers

Sites of penetration

Chemical defenses of the skin

Vaginal epithelial defenses

Conjunctival protection by
flushing and lysozyme

Skin, Vaginal, and Conjunctival Epithelium. A simple mechanical barrier to microbial invasion is provided by intact epithelia, the most effective of which is the multilayered stratified squamous epithelium of the skin with its superficial cornified anucleate layers. Organisms can only gain access to the underlying tissues by breaks, or by way of hair follicles, sebaceous glands, and sweat glands that traverse the stratified layers. The surface of the skin continuously desquamates and thus tends to shed contaminating organisms. It is also inhibitory to the growth of most extraneous microorganisms because of low moisture, low pH, and the presence of substances with antibacterial activity. These include lactic acid from sweat glands, free fatty acids, waxes, and alcohols from the secretions of sebaceous glands and products of metabolic activity of the indigenous microbial flora. Greater moisture (for example, beneath occlusive dressings) can increase the number of potential pathogens on the skin surface, and significant destruction of skin is invariably followed by infection, as in the case of severe burns. The vaginal epithelium, a modified squamous epithelium, is protected during childbearing years by the low pH and exclusionary effects produced by the normal bacterial flora discussed in Chapter 9. The conjunctiva is protected by the flushing effects of the tears, aided by a high concentration of lysozyme.

Mucociliary escalator

Respiratory Epithelium. The epithelium of the paranasal sinuses and of the respiratory tract from the level of the larynx to the alveoli is a less effective mechanical barrier but is protected by a mucus covering to which microorganisms adhere, aided by any secretory IgA (sIgA) secreted into the mucus, and by the epithelial cilia, which move the mucus away from the area at risk. In the respiratory tract, particles larger than 5 μm are trapped in this fashion, moved upward at a rate of about 1 cm/min to pass through the larynx, and are then swallowed and destroyed by the defenses of the alimentary tract. Interference with the action of cilia from toxic substances or from infections such as influenza or whooping cough can permit colonization and infection of the lower respiratory tract with pathogenic bacteria, leading to the development of bronchitis or pneumonia.

Table 10.1 Nonspecific Defenses against Colonization with Pathogens

Site	Mechanical Barrier	Ciliated Epithelium	Competition by Normal Flora	Mucus	sIgA	Lymphoid Follicles	Low pH	Flushing Effects of Contents	Peristalsis	Special Factors
Skin	+++	-	+	-	-	-	++	-	-	Fatty acids from action of normal flora on sebum
Conjunctiva	++	-	-	-	+	-	-	+++	-	Lysozyme
Oropharynx	+++	-	+++	-	+	Yes	-	++	-	
Upper respiratory tract	++	+	+++	++	++	Yes	-	+	-	Turbinate baffles
Middle ear and paranasal sinuses[a]	++	+++	-	++	?	-	-	+	-	
Lower respiratory tract[a]	++	+++	-	++	++	Yes	-	-	-	Mucociliary escalator, alveolar macrophages; cough reflex
Stomach	++	-	-	++	-	-	+++	+	+	Production of hydrochloric acid
Intestinal tract	++	-	+++	+++	+++	Yes	-	+	+++	Bile; digestive enzymes
Vagina	+++	-	+++	+	+	-	+++	-	-	Lactobacillary flora ferments epithelial glycogen
Urinary tract[a]	++	-	-	-	+	-	+	+++	-	

Abbreviations: +, ++, +++ = relative importance in defense at each site; - = unimportant.

[a] Sterile in health.

Gastrointestinal Epithelium.   Like the epithelium of the respiratory tract, that of the intestinal tract below the esophagus is a less efficient mechanical barrier than the skin, but there are other effective defense mechanisms.

Chemical defenses

The high level of hydrochloric acid and gastric enzymes in the normal stomach kill many ingested bacteria, and others are susceptible to pancreatic digestive enzymes or to the detergent effect of bile salts. Again like the respiratory tract, the intestinal epithelium (or mucous membrane)

Entrapment in mucus and removal by peristalsis

is coated with a film of mucus that traps many organisms directly or by reaction with specific sIgA secreted into it. The mucus and attached particles are continuously passed along and out of the alimentary tract by contractile peristaltic waves. Inhibition of these processes decreases the infecting dose of various pathogens or permits colonization of areas, such as the small intestine, that usually have a limited normal flora. The net result is an increased risk of infection. For example, the infecting dose of the cholera vibrio is lowered by several orders of magnitude in patients who have achlorhydria (absence of gastric hydrochloric acid) because of disease or malnutrition. Stagnation of intestinal contents from several causes is also associated with abnormal bacterial overgrowth (Chapter 9).

Urinary Tract.   The transitional epithelium of the urinary tract is multilayered and resistant to invasion, especially in the undistended state.

Urine as culture medium

Urine is a good culture medium for many bacteria, however, and if they reach the normally sterile bladder, they can multiply to very large numbers (for example, more than 10^5/ml), particularly if there is urinary stasis.

Protective effects of flushing and low pH

Primary mechanisms of defense are the flushing effect of urine and its relatively low pH, which tend to inhibit microbial growth. Urinary tract infections are much more common in women than men because the shortness of the female urethra allows easier passage of organisms to the bladder; such infections in women are often associated with sexual intercourse.

Stasis predisposes to infection

Infections are also common in any situation that produces urinary stasis, such as partial obstruction by an enlarged prostate or when passage of bacteria into the bladder is facilitated by the use of catheters.

Secreted Antimicrobial Products

Lysozyme and Lactoferrin.   In addition to some antimicrobial substances mentioned previously, most mucosal secretions and those of adjacent glands produce other nonspecific inhibitory substances, including lysozyme (Chapter 2), which disrupts the accessible cell wall peptidoglycan of some Gram-positive bacteria, and lactoferrin, which competes for the iron essential to microbial multiplication.

Role of sIgA in protecting mucosal surfaces

Secretory IgA.   Secretory IgA, which has been described in Chapter 8, plays a special role in protecting epithelial surfaces from colonization and infection, either by direct secretion through mucous membranes or from its presence in glandular secretions such as milk. Although the initial antigenic stimulus to production of secreted IgA is derived from a particular hollow viscus (eg, intestinal or respiratory tract), some of the IgA-producing B lymphocytes migrate to subepithelial regions of other viscera

Local antigenic stimulus leads to wide distribution of sIgA

and secretory glands where the pairs of IgA molecules acquire their secretory pieces and pass through the epithelial cells. Secretory IgA produced as a result of a local antigenic stimulus is thus widely distributed on mucosal surfaces and in glandular secretions.

Secretory IgA molecules react with specific antigens against which they are directed or with cross-reacting antigens. They interfere with the first

Specific sIgA can block attachment of microorganisms or toxins to cell receptors

stages of colonization or invasion by preventing attachment of viruses or bacteria to receptors on epithelia and, in some cases, by inhibiting motility. They also block the activity or absorption of soluble antigenic molecules such as toxins that could otherwise contribute to the initiation of infection or disease.

sIgA prevents initiation of some infections, but is not essential to immunity

Secretory IgA is not essential to immunity, because many patients with genetically determined absence of IgA can nonetheless mount effective IgG and IgM responses to invading organisms; however, it has been shown to be an important primary immune mechanism for preventing a variety of infections, such as cholera and giardiasis, and some respiratory virus diseases that depend on initial attachment to mucosal surface receptors.

Protective effect of sIgA in human milk

Secretory IgA in human milk plays an important role in protecting the infant from intestinal infections.

Secreted antimicrobial substances can probably act cooperatively, and it has been shown that sIgA can increase the speed of bacterial inactivation by lysozyme.

Normal Microbial Flora

The role of the normal microbial flora in protection against infection has been considered in Chapter 9. It is therefore sufficient to stress its great significance in competing with pathogenic intruders for particular ecologic niches and in priming the immune system.

Alveolar and Other Surface Macrophages

Alveolar macrophages ingest particles that reach alveoli

Phagocytic cells of the macrophage series are found free in the alveoli of the lungs and play a very important role in ingesting and destroying organisms that are inhaled in very small droplet nuclei (less than 5 μm) and escape the mucociliary defenses of the trachea and bronchial tree. Similarly, a few macrophages reach the surface of other mucous membranes, but are less significant in defense. The mechanisms of killing by phagocytes are discussed in the next section.

Microbial Infectivity

Ability to penetrate or colonize epithelia

To invade the tissues, an organism must be able to overcome the initial epithelial barriers. This process sometimes involves direct spread through wounds, human or animal bites, or bites of insect vectors. Often, however, a primary bacterial pathogen establishes itself locally by attaching to and then colonizing the epithelial surface before entering the tissues through the epithelium. Thus, a requirement for infectivity is an ability to survive

Resistance to local antimicrobial conditions

and, if necessary, multiply under conditions that exist on a surface epithelium or in a tissue into which they are deposited. Examples of ability to survive local conditions are the lysozyme insusceptibility of bacteria that cause conjunctivitis and the resistance of pathogens of the lower intestinal tract to the antibacterial effects of bile and the digestive enzymes. The ability of a bacterium to grow depends on the availability of suitable nutrients and appropriate physicochemical conditions. Ability to grow or

Temperature requirements

replicate at the body temperature of 37°C is also an obvious essential requirement for organisms that infect any area except the skin or nasal mucosal surfaces, which have a lower temperature. Some pathogenic organisms, such as the rhinoviruses of the common cold and the fungi that cause ringworm of the skin, grow poorly, if at all, at 37°C and thus cannot invade deeper tissues.

Adherence to cell receptors as a general prerequisite for colonization or infection

Bacterial adhesins are highly specific and often components of pili or capsules

Influence of mucolytic enzymes on adherence and colonization

Roles of bacterial IgA protease and antiphagocytic capsules

Mechanisms of penetrating epithelia; cytotoxic lesions, endocytosis, or passage within macrophages

Viral endocytosis

A general prerequisite for infection is the capacity to adhere to the surface of epithelial cells. Most viruses attach specifically to sites on target cells. For example, the influenza viruses attach specifically to neuraminic acid-containing glycoprotein receptors on the surface of respiratory cells before penetrating to the interior of the cell. With many bacteria, the attachment is also highly specific and mediated by an affinity of chemical groups on the microbial surface, termed *adhesins,* for receptors on the epithelial surface. For example, lipoteichoic acid associated with pili of group A streptococci (Chapter 16) binds to a particular component of fibronectin on the surface of certain epithelial cells. Adhesins are frequently structural components of pili, but may be other surface components such as capsules. Adherence facilitates colonization and subsequent penetration of epithelia, because it brings the organism into intimate contact with its target and prevents its removal by the flushing effects of visceral contents or secretions or, in the respiratory tract, by the action of cilia. Also, the activity of bacterial toxins on epithelial cells is enormously enhanced by this juxtaposition. For example, *Bordetella pertussis* adheres specifically to the cilia of respiratory epithelial cells, and one of its toxins directly inhibits ciliary action. In some bacterial and viral infections, mucolytic enzymes assist in penetration to the epithelial surfaces; in others, the penetration of mucus appears to require active motility of bacteria and possibly a chemoattractant response.

Microorganisms that reach mucosal surfaces will often encounter secretory IgA antibody, which can react with them and inhibit their adherence to epithelia and their growth. Some species, such as the gonococcus, the meningococcus, and *Haemophilus influenzae,* produce an IgA protease that may neutralize these effects. In the pulmonary alveoli, an organism immediately encounters phagocytic macrophages; however, many successful pulmonary pathogens, such as the pneumococcus and *Klebsiella pneumoniae,* possess capsules that inhibit their ingestion.

Penetration of organisms into subepithelial tissues or cells is accomplished in a variety of ways. Some produce exotoxins (described later) that destroy epithelial cells and thus open the way to the underlying tissues. Some, such as the *Shigella* of bacillary dysentery, are able to direct their own endocytosis into colonic epithelial cells and destroy or pass through them. Some epithelial cells, termed *M cells,* directly overlie lymphoid follicles, such as those of Peyer's patches, and are adapted to take up antigenic molecules and bring them into contact with cells of the immune system. Some pathogenic organisms, such as the typhoid bacillus, appear to take advantage of this special route of penetration of the epithelium. Other bacteria, such as the tubercle bacillus, are taken up by alveolar macrophages in which they can multiply and be carried by the macrophages through the alveolar membrane to regional lymph nodes. Viruses in general attach to specific epithelial cell receptors, are endocytosed by the mechanisms discussed in Chapter 6, and reach their initial intracellular replication sites in this way.

Second-Line Defenses Against Invasion

Once a microorganism has breached the surface epithelial barrier, it is subject to a series of nonspecific processes designed to remove, inhibit, or destroy it. These defenses are complex, dynamic, and interacting, but will be considered under the general headings of the initial environment, the inflammatory response, phagocytic activity, and some general host responses that tend to increase resistance to infection.

Initial Environment

Lysozyme in tissues

Effects of host's iron-binding proteins

Phagocytosis by tissue histiocytes

Lymph flow to regional nodes

Microorganisms that reach the subepithelial tissues are immediately exposed to the intercellular tissue fluids, which have some defined properties that act to inhibit multiplication of many bacteria. For example, most tissues contain lysozyme in sufficient concentrations to disrupt the cell wall of some Gram-positive bacteria, and other less well-defined inhibitors from leukocytes and platelets have been described. Tissue fluid itself is a suboptimal growth medium for most bacteria and deficient in free iron. Iron is essential for bacterial growth, but it is sequestered by the body's iron-binding proteins such as transferrin and lactoferrin and is thus inaccessible to organisms that do not themselves produce siderophores (see Chapter 3). Tissue macrophages (histiocytes), which are phagocytic cells derived from the monocytic series, can phagocytose and destroy many infectious agents even when the organisms are not specifically opsonized or the macrophages are activated by lymphokines. Furthermore, the natural turnover of tissue fluids from the blood capillary circulation to the lymphatic drainage system serves to move the occasional invading organism to a lymph node, in which fixed phagocytic cells can remove and destroy it. Pathogenic bacteria, almost by definition, can overcome these initial defenses, and, as they multiply, secondary nonspecific defenses come into play.

Inflammatory Response and Its Effects

Vasodilatation and fluid extravasation

Attraction of polymorphonuclear leukocytes

Mediators of inflammatory responses

When bacteria multiply in the tissues, the usual result is an inflammatory response. The blood-carrying capillaries dilate, which leads to local extravasation of fluid containing high levels of protein, including immunoglobulins and complement components. Polymorphonuclear leukocytes are attracted to the infected site and reach the tissue fluids by passing between the capillary endothelial cells. Mediators of the inflammatory response include histamine liberated from mast cells, serotonin from platelets, lysosomal enzymes from damaged leukocytes and tissue cells, and low-molecular-weight peptides termed *kinins* that are generated from precursor proteins in plasma and tissues. Many of these mediators are cross-activating. The process of inflammation can be initiated by the alternative complement pathway (or classical pathway when specific IgG or IgM is present), since C5a is tactic for leukocytes, and C3a and C5a cause mast cells to degranulate and release histamine and other vasoactive mediators. Prostaglandin derivatives of arachidonic acid from damaged host cell membranes are longer acting and serve to maintain the inflammatory response until the infection is controlled. As discussed below, many of these processes are stimulated or enhanced by macrophage-derived interleukin 1 (IL1) and tumor necrosis factor (TNF or cachectin). The end results are the classic inflammatory manifestations of swelling (tumor), vasodilatation of surface vessels with redness (rubor) and increased skin temperature (calor), pain from increased pressure and tissue damage (dolor), and loss of function because of reflex nerve inhibition or the pain caused by movement. The inflammatory response has several immediate defensive effects. It increases tissue fluid flow from the bloodstream to the lymphatic circulation and brings phagocytes, complement, and any existing antibody to the site of infection. Later, the deposition of fibrin may contribute to the walling off of the lesion before the healing process begins. A major effect of the increased lymphatic drainage serves to bring microbes or their antigens into contact with the cells in the local lymph nodes that mediate the development of specific immune response.

Local defensive role of inflammation

Interaction with immune system

A local inflammatory response can also produce important systemic effects largely mediated by IL1 and TNF. Polymorphonuclear leukocytes are mobilized from the bone marrow pool to increase the numbers of those present at the infected site and to replace those destroyed or at the end of their life span. Thus, polymorphonuclear leukocytosis, primarily involving neutrophils, is a common feature of most bacterial infections and serves to increase the immediately available phagocytic defenses. Fever, a frequent concomitant of inflammation, is primarily mediated by IL1 and TNF released by macrophages (for example, on exposure to bacterial endotoxin). These act upon the hypothalamus and increase the "setting" of the body's thermostatic mechanisms. The value of fever is not completely clear; however, it increases the effectiveness of several processes involved in phagocytosis and microbial killing and frequently reduces the multiplication or replication rate of bacteria or viruses below that occurring at 37°C.

IL1 has many other effects relating to defense against infection. It enhances release of lactoferrin and lysozyme from neutrophils at the site of infection; stimulates the oxidative antibacterial activity of phagocytes (see below); enhances chemotaxis of leukocytes to the infected area; increases prostaglandin production by monocytes and macrophages; enhances iron uptake by the liver, which effectively reduces its availability for infecting organisms; and stimulates production of a number of proteins (acute phase proteins) by the liver that appear to enhance defense against infection. IL1 is thus a major orchestrator of protective responses to infection.

Phagocytic Defenses

Phagocytic cells include polymorphonuclear leukocytes (particularly neutrophils), blood monocytes, macrophages, tissue histiocytes, and the fixed phagocytic cells of the reticuloendothelial system. All are derived from the same stem cells, and blood monocytes that reach the tissues assume the characteristics of macrophages when they reach inflammatory sites. Despite the differences between them, all of these cells share certain common mechanisms for ingesting and attempting to destroy invading microorganisms.

The Neutrophil. The neutrophil leukocyte is a short-lived (circulating half-life, 7 hr) cell with a multilobed nucleus and numerous cytoplasmic granules containing enzymes and other substances with antimicrobial action. The cell is metabolically active and demonstrates marked chemotaxis to some bacterial products, to the C5a component of complement, and to other products of the imflammatory process. These factors attract leukocytes to the sites of microbial invasion. Particles, including bacteria, that attach to the surface of polymorphonuclear leukocytes are ingested in a vacuole called the *phagosome,* which is bounded by the portion of the cytoplasmic membrane involved in their uptake. Once within the cell there are several mechanisms by which organisms can be killed. These are summarized in Table 10.2. One results from a burst of metabolic activity by the phagocyte with increased oxygen uptake leading to a fall in pH within the phagosome and to production of superoxide, hydrogen peroxide, singlet oxygen, and hydroxyl radicals, all of which, although often evanescent, are damaging to many bacteria and viruses.

A second oxygen-dependent system requires catalysis by the enzyme *myeloperoxidase,* which is discharged into the phagosome by one class of neutrophil granules. In the presence of peroxide and halide (chloride or

---

Leukocytosis and fever mediated by IL1 and TNF have antimicrobial effects

Diverse protective effects of IL1

Polymorphonuclear and mononuclear phagocytes derived from the same stem cells

Short-lived phagocyte that exhibits chemotaxis

Phagocytic process

Microbicidal effects of oxygen-dependent metabolic burst

The oxygen-dependent myeloperoxidase–halide system

Table 10.2 Microbicidal Responses of Phagocytes

A. Oxygen dependent
  1. Respiratory burst; generation of toxic superoxide, singlet oxygen, and other reactive radicals
  2. Halogenation of critical microbial components by myeloperoxidase system[a] (hydrogen peroxide, myeloperoxide, and halide)

B. Nonoxygen dependent
  Release of antimicrobial lysosomal contents to phagosome including
  1. Cationic proteins[a]
  2. Acid hydrolases
  3. Lysozyme
  4. Lactoferrin[a]
  5. Proteases

[a] Not represented in mature macrophages.

iodide), the enzyme catalyses the halogenation of peroxide. Thus, in the case of chloride, the highly bactericidal hypochlorous anion is produced.

$$H_2O_2 + Cl^- + H^+ \xrightarrow{\text{myeloperoxidase}} H_2O + HOCl$$

$$HOCl \rightleftharpoons H^+ + OCl^-$$

Oxygen-independent killing in phagolysosome

Intracellular killing of microorganisms by neutrophils also involves oxygen-independent mechanisms. When neutrophil granules fuse with the phagocytic vacuole, they discharge their lysosomal enzymes and other antibacterial substances to produce a *phagolysosome*. Any organisms ingested under anaerobic conditions, or organisms that have survived the effects of oxygen metabolites, are exposed to a pH of 3.0–4.0 and to lysozyme, phosphatases, and nucleases as well as to lactoferrin and antimicrobial cationic proteins. These all serve to produce an environment that is highly hostile to most organisms. Lysosomal enzymes, including collagenase and elastase, are damaging to tissues when released from the neutrophil and contribute to the enhancement of the inflammatory process.

Effects of liberated lysosomal enzymes on tissues

Macrophages are widely distributed in tissues and live longer than neutrophils

The Macrophages. Macrophages, which are derived from blood monocytes, play a wider and more continuing role than the neutrophil in defense against infection. They are widely distributed in the tissues, exhibit chemotaxis to C5a and to neutrophil lysates, and phagocytose microorganisms and cellular debris resulting from infection. Unlike the shorter-lived neutrophil, the macrophage can resynthesize its lysosomal granules and contained enzymes and repeat the process of phagocytosis and microbial destruction. Also, unlike the neutrophil, it does not possess myeloperoxidase, has a less dramatic respiratory burst, and lacks lactoferrin and antimicrobial cationic proteins. However, it has a much larger complement of lysosomal enzymes and can be activated by lymphokines to increase their synthesis and antimicrobial effectiveness. The phagocytic and debriding aspects of macrophage function are particularly significant in the later stages of infection and in the control of obligate or facultative intracellular pathogens.

Activation by lymphokines to increased microbicidal activity in phagolysosomes

Macrophages play key roles in local, systemic, and immunological responses to infection

Other contributions of macrophages to control infection are shown in Table 10.3. They include antigen processing and presentation to T cells as described in Chapter 8; synthesis of some complement proteins and precursors; production of tactic factors for neutrophils; synthesis of prostaglandins, transferrins, lysozyme, and interferons; production of pro-

Table 10.3 Contribution of Macrophages and Their Products to Control of Infection

A.   Inflammation and fever IL1, TNF, prostaglandins, complement factors, clotting factors, H_2O_2, acid hydrolases
B.   Lymphocyte activation Antigen processing, antigen presentation, IL1 production
C.   Tissue debridement, reorganization, and repair Elastase, collagenase, hyaluronidase, fibroblast-stimulating factor, angiogenesis factor
D.   Microbicidal activity Oxygen dependent, oxygen independent

Abbreviations: IL1 = interleukin 1; TNF = tumor necrosis factor.

teases, elastase, and collagenases; and synthesis of IL1 and TNF. Thus, macrophages contribute in a major way to the local and systemic response to infection and to the repair of the damage that ensues, quite apart from their contributions to the immune response.

In addition to tissue and alveolar macrophages, cells with similar function and derivation comprise those of the reticuloendothelial system. They are present, particularly in the lymph node sinuses and along small blood vessels and vascular sinuses of the liver, spleen, and bone marrow. Microorganisms that escape from a local lesion into the lymphatic circulation or bloodstream are rapidly cleared by reticuloendothelial cells or arrested in the small pulmonary capillaries and then ingested by phagocytic cells. This process is so efficient that when a million organisms are injected into a vein of a rabbit few if any will usually be recoverable in cultures of blood taken 15 min after injection, although the ultimate result of such clearance may not be a cure.

Clearing effects of reticuloendothelial cells

Phagocytosis.   The processes of phagocytosis that can occur when a microbe encounters a phagocyte are enhanced greatly by opsonization by antibodies directed against the infecting organism, as well as by activation of the classical complement pathway. Phagocytic cells have surface receptors for the Fc fraction of IgG and for the C3b derivatives of complement. Thus, bacteria and viruses with attached antibody are brought to the surface of phagocytic cells to facilitate ingestion, and this process is enhanced (or mediated in the case of IgM) by the C3b component of complement. Many bacterial products (particularly endotoxin) and viruses activate the alternative pathway of complement, which can lead to opsonization in the absence of antibody.

Enhancement of phagocytosis by antibody and complement opsonization

It must be remembered that phagocytosis and the mechanisms for intracellular killing are not always effective, because organisms have evolved that resist ingestion, that are insusceptible to lysosomal enzymes, that interfere with the fusion of lysosomal granules with the phagosome, or that escape the phagosome and multiply in the cytoplasm.

Failure of intracellular killing

Mechanisms of Virulence of Invasive Bacteria

Bacteria that can invade and cause disease possess a variety of mechanisms to avoid or subvert the defenses of the host and a range of means by which they produce pathologic lesions and systemic illness. First, however, they

Siderophores and hemolysins
as mechanisms for obtaining
iron

must have the ability to obtain the iron they require in an environment in which free iron is highly restricted by the host's iron-binding proteins. This requirement is satisfied by production of iron-chelating siderophores, such as enterochelin from pathogenic Enterobacteriaceae, or by their ability to utilize iron-containing compounds derived from hemoglobin. It is of interest that many nonspecific and immune defensive mechanisms will themselves reduce even further the amount of free iron in plasma and tissue fluids. Conversely, injection of iron compounds into infection sites will considerably increase the severity of disease.

Avoidance of Host Defense Mechanisms

Antiphagocytic effects of
capsules

Many important pathogenic bacteria are strict extracellular pathogens and are rapidly destroyed when phagocytosed. To multiply and cause disease they must avoid this situation. Several, such as *Streptococcus pneumoniae* and *Haemophilus influenzae*, produce polysaccharide capsules that protect the unopsonized organism from phagocytosis in tissue fluids and reduce phagocytic effectiveness on epithelial surfaces. The C3b component of complement generated by the alternative pathway may bind to the cell wall of encapsulated bacteria, but its attachment site for phagocyte receptors is "buried" within the capsule and is unavailable for opsonization. Consequently, extracellular multiplication proceeds until an effective opsonizing antibody response is mounted against the invader. Other organisms, such as *Streptococcus pyogenes*, *Staphylococcus aureus*, and *Clostridium perfringens*, produce extracellular toxic products that are lethal to polymorphonuclear leukocytes (and often other cells) and thus directly attack the host defense system.

Leukocidins

Intraphagocytic survival and
multiplication

In some cases already discussed briefly, microorganisms can survive the phagocytic process, and migration of macrophages may contribute to their spread. For example, *Coxiella burnetii*, an obligate intracellular parasite, can multiply under the seemingly hostile conditions that exist in the phagolysosome. Others, such as *Mycobacterium tuberculosis*, are ingested, but then inhibit lysosomal fusion by a mechanism that remains unclear. Some of the mechanisms employed by various bacteria and other agents to subvert the action of the phagocyte are summarized in Table 10.4.

Intracellular organisms are
protected from antibody

In addition to the production of enzymes that destroy secretory IgA, various mechanisms are available for avoiding or delaying the effects of the immune response. Bacteria that can survive or multiply within macrophages or tissue cells are protected from the direct effects of circulating antibody because of its poor intracellular penetration. These infections are primarily controlled by cellular immune defense systems that produce both lymphokines that activate and increase the microbicidal power of macrophages and cytotoxic T cells that recognize microbial antigens expressed on the surface of infected cells and destroy them. Bacteria liberated on destruction or death of cells then become directly accessible to antibody.

Deviation of opsonizing
antibody by free antigen

In other cases, protective antibodies against extracellular pathogens may be neutralized by bacterial products before they can reach the organism. For example, the antiphagocytic capsular polysaccharide of a pneumococcus is soluble and may be found in considerable amounts in body fluids during a pneumococcal infection. Extracellular capsular antigen molecules can react with anticapsular antibody, thus protecting the organism itself. Only when sufficient antibody is produced to neutralize the free carbohydrate can the organism be effectively opsonized. In fact, the outcome of an untreated pneumococcal infection is a race between production of

Table 10.4   Microbial Perturbations of Intraphagocytic Microbicidal Mechanisms

A. Inhibition of lysosome–phagosome fusion 　1. *Mycobacterium tuberculosis*[a] 　2. *Toxoplasma gondii* 　3. *Chlamydia psittaci* 　4. *Histoplasma capsulatum* 　5. *Neisseria gonorrheae*	D. Inhibition of phagocyte oxidative response 　1. *Legionella pneumophila*[b] 　2. *Listeria monocytogenes* 　3. *Salmonella typhi*
B. Resistance to lysosomal enzymes 　1. *Mycobacterium lepraemurium* 　2. *Leishmania mexicana* 　3. *Salmonella typhimurium*	E. Inhibition of phagocyte function by bacterial adenylate cyclase 　1. *Bordetella pertussis*
C. Exotoxin-induced cytotoxicity 　1. *Pseudomonas aeruginosa* 　2. *Staphylococcus aureus*	F. Inhibition of lysosome–phagosome fusion and phagocyte oxidative response 　1. Influenza A virus

Reproduced with permission from Quie, P. G. 1983. *J. Infect. Dis.* 148:189–193, copyright 1983 by University of Chicago, publisher.

[a] By bacterial sulfatide.
[b] By toxin.

capsular polysaccharide and of anticapsular antibody. Some organisms, exemplified by the *Borrelia* spirochetes that cause relapsing fever have ingenious methods of circumventing host humoral immune mechanisms. *Borrelia* possess repertoires of genes encoding several variants of a major virulence determining surface antigen and move these genes sequentially to a site that permits their expression. These variant antigens do not react with antibody developed against the previously expressed antigen. Thus, the organism changes the rules of the game, and the infection may relapse two or three times with successive antigenic variations (see Chapter 26). A similar situation obtains with some gonococcal surface antigens, and this may explain the poor and evanescent immunity to gonorrhoea (see Chapter 19).

Some pathogenic organisms prevent or reduce the ability of the host to recognize them as foreign either by absorbing host materials to their surface or by synthesizing surface antigens that resemble components of the host. These mechanisms have been described respectively for the syphilis spirochete (*T. pallidum*) and for a strain of *Escherichia coli* (KI) that is associated with infant meningitis. Both mechanisms apply to a number of the eukaryotic pathogens of parasitic disease.

Strains of *S. aureus* have a unique defense against opsonizing antibody. Their surface includes a protein, protein A, that reacts with the Fc portion of IgG, inverts the antibody, and thus prevents its attachment to Fc receptors on phagocytes.

Avoidance of antibody response by surface antigenic variation

Antigenic masking or mimicry can prevent recognition of an organism as foreign

Inversion of potentially opsonizing IgG by staphylococcal protein A

Bacterial Determinants of Disease

Direct cell damage by intracellular parasites

Disease resulting from inflammatory response

Obligate intracellular bacteria, such as the rickettsias and chlamydias, can kill the cells that they infect and produce inflammatory reactions by releasing the host cell's lysosomal enzymes. Other organisms, the best example of which is the pneumococcus, have little direct cytotoxic effect but produce a dramatic acute inflammatory response that is itself responsible for disease manifestations. Thus, in pneumococcal pneumonia, the

Table 10.5 Differential Characteristics of Endotoxins
and Exotoxins

Characteristic	Endotoxins	Exotoxins
Chemical nature	Lipopolysaccharide (lipid A component)	Protein
Part of Gram-negative cell outer membrane	Yes	No
Most from Gram-positive bacteria	No	Yes
Usually extracellular	No	Yes
Phage or plasmid coded	No	Many
Antigenic	WR	Yes
Can be converted to toxoid	No	Many
Neutralized by antibody	WR	Yes
Differing pharmacologic specificities	No	Yes
Stable to boiling[a]	Yes	No

Abbreviations: WR = weak reaction.

[a] Enterotoxin of *Staphylococcus aureus* withstands boiling.

lung alveoli become filled with exudate and polymorphonuclear leukocytes from the pulmonary capillaries, resulting in failure of respiratory
exchange, fever, and leukocytosis. If the patient survives, resolution of
the disease is rapid and recovery of the normal structure and function of
the lung is complete, because significant tissue death did not occur.

In many infections caused by Gram-negative organisms, the endotoxin
(Chapter 2) of the outer membrane is a significant component of the
disease process. The major characteristics of endotoxin are contrasted with
those of exotoxins in Table 10.5. Endotoxin in nanogram amounts causes
fever in humans by release of IL1 and TNF from macrophages. In larger
amounts, whether on intact Gram-negative organisms or cell wall fragments, it produces dramatic physiologic effects. These include hypotension, lowered polymorphonuclear leukocyte and platelet counts from increased margination of these cells to the walls of the small vessels,
hemorrhage, and sometimes disseminated intravascular coagulation from
activation of clotting factors. Rapid and irreversible shock may follow
passage of endotoxin into the bloodstream. This syndrome is seen when
materials that have become heavily contaminated are injected intravenously or when a severe local infection leads to massive bacteremia. The
role of endotoxin in more chronic disease processes is less clear, but some
manifestations of typhoid fever and meningococcal septicemia, for example, are fully compatible with the known effects of endotoxin in humans. It should be noted that endotoxins are considerably less active than
many exotoxins, incompletely neutralized by antibody against their carbohydrate component, and stable even to autoclaving. The latter characteristic is important, because materials for intravenous administration
that have become contaminated with Gram-negative organisms are not
detoxified by sterilization.

In contrast to endotoxins, exotoxins (Table 10.5) are strikingly diverse
proteins of very high toxicity with different specific activities against a
wide variety of cellular structures and functions. For example, tetanus
toxin acts on the nervous system by interfering with normal activity of
neuromotor synapses, and cholera toxin on the transport of fluids and
electrolytes across the epithelial cells of the small intestine. Exotoxins are

Endotoxin fever mediated by
IL1 and TNF released by
macrophages

Systemic effects of endotoxin
and endotoxic shock

Endotoxin is heat stable

Exotoxins: a diverse group of
highly toxic proteins

excreted into the surrounding fluid by the organisms that produce them or liberated on bacterial lysis. Many are composed of binding subunits, which attach to receptors on specific target cells, and toxic subunits which are liberated during or after receptor-mediated endocytosis. Exotoxins are antigenic and neutralized by the specific antibodies that they elicit, particularly antibodies to the binding subunits. Several, by treatment in vitro with formaldehyde or genetic manipulation, can be converted to toxoids, which retain the antigenicity of the toxin but lose its toxicity. Toxoids are highly valuable as immunizing agents against diphtheria and tetanus, in which the toxin is the major determinant of virulence and of the disease process. In some bacteria, production of exotoxin is determined by genes carried on temperate phages (diphtheria, scarlet fever, and some botulism toxins) or on plasmids (*E. coli* enterotoxins). In these cases, toxigenicity can be readily transferred from toxigenic to nontoxigenic strains. At present, there is no satisfactory explanation for the high frequency of association of exotoxin genes with such transmissible elements.

Some exotoxins are the primary determinants of disease caused by organisms that multiply on an epithelial surface (for example, diphtheria) or in a restricted local site in the tissues (for example, tetanus). In these cases the major effects of the toxins are in tissues remote from the infection, such as the heart muscle in diphtheria and the spinal cord and medulla in tetanus. Other exotoxins contribute to the capacity of an organism to invade and spread; the lecithinase α-toxin of *C. perfringens,* for example, disrupts the cell membranes of a wide variety of host cells, including the leukocytes that might otherwise destroy the organism, and produces the necrotic anaerobic environment in which it can spread. Still other exotoxins are produced outside the body in contaminated foods and cause disease when they are eaten. For example, the spores of *Clostridium botulinum* can survive inadequate food preservation processes and germinate under appropriate anaerobic conditions. Toxin synthesis follows as the vegetative cells grow. The toxins that cause such food poisoning are resistant to digestive enzymes. In the case of staphylococcal enterotoxins they are also resistant to boiling, so that disease may follow ingestion of contaminated foods in which the organism has already been killed. The term *enterotoxin* has been used widely for exotoxins that act directly or indirectly on the intestinal epithelium to produce diarrhea and vomiting. This terminology has caused some confusion; it is best to regard enterotoxins simply as exotoxins that have an effect on the intestinal tract.

Many bacteria produce one or more enzymes that are nontoxic per se, but facilitate tissue invasion or help to protect the organism against the body's defense mechanisms. For example, various bacteria produce collagenases or hyaluronidases or convert serum plasminogen to plasmin, which has fibrinolytic activity. Although the evidence is not conclusive, it is reasonable to assume that these substances facilitate spread of infection. Hemolysins, some of which are highly cytotoxic, are produced by many bacteria and may liberate necessary growth factors for some of them. Deoxyribonucleases, elastases, and many other biologically active enzymes are also produced by some bacteria, but again their function in the disease process or in providing nutrients for the invaders is uncertain. All are proteins and have most of the characteristics of exotoxins, but do not produce specific toxicity.

In recent years, the molecular mechanisms of action of many exotoxins have been determined, and in some cases, exotoxin genes have been cloned.

Toxoids are nontoxic derivatives of toxins that retain the toxin's antigenicity

Many exotoxins are encoded in temperate phages or plasmids

Remote effects of exotoxins

Some exotoxins contribute to invasion

Some exotoxins are produced in foods

Enterotoxins are exotoxins affecting the gastrointestinal tract

Some nontoxic enzymes contribute to virulence

Several toxins catalyse ADP ribosylate of critical enzymes or control proteins

Effects of ADP ribosylation depend on function of the protein involved

Many toxins activate adenylate cyclase

It is of interest that some common mechanisms of exotoxin action are widely distributed among different pathogenic species, although the clinical and pathological effects of the toxins differ according to the tissue cells and molecular targets that they attack. Several exotoxins catalyze ADP ribosylation of critical enzymes or control proteins within the cell. This applies to diphtheria and cholera toxins as well as to some clostridial toxins and the exotoxin A of *Pseudomonas*. Their effects, however, can be dramatically different. Diphtheria toxin, for example, ADP ribosylates elongation factor 2 (EF-2), which is the enzyme that adds amino acids to the peptide chain being assembled on the ribosome. This results in cessation of protein synthesis and death of the cell. Myocardial, neural, and various epithelial cells are particularly affected. In contrast, cholera toxin ADP ribosylates and inactivates a protein that regulates adenylate cyclase. Unimpeded activation of this enzyme leads to excessive production of cyclic AMP, which produces massive excretion of water and electrolytes from intestinal cells with consequent severe diarrhea. Activation of adenylate cyclase is a widely distributed effect of exotoxins and also occurs with pertussis toxin, *E. coli* LT toxin, and some other toxins of intestinal pathogens. Details of the mechanisms of action of various toxins will be considered in the chapters that describe the organisms producing them.

The function of exotoxins in the economy of bacterial cells remains obscure. As virulence determinants, they may facilitate survival and spread of organisms that are highly adapted to human or animal hosts, but such an explanation cannot apply to the highly toxic exotoxins of the soil organism *C. botulinum*, which usually causes disease by production of toxin in certain foodstuffs outside the body.

From the foregoing consideration of determinants of infectivity and pathogenicity, it is clear that virulence is multifactorial and involves many genes in any given organism, some of which may be plasmid borne, some on temperate phages, and some on transposable elements within the chromosome. Recent work has shown that many of the genes involved in virulence of some organisms are juxtaposed and under control of a single regulatory site in the chromosome. This allows them to be fully activated only when the conditions required for invasion and multiplication in the host are encountered and constitutes what is probably an important adaptive mechanism in the economy of the bacterial cell both within and outside the body.

Mechanisms of Viral Virulence and the Role of Interferons in Immunity

Some viruses can effect the function of host cells without cytolysis

Tissue damage can also result from released cellular enzymes, hypersensitivity, and autoimmune reactions

The pathogenesis of viral diseases differs in a number of respects from that of most bacterial infections because of the totally different modes of replication of viruses and their strict intracellular habitat. No viruses possess lipopolysaccharide (LPS) and animal viruses do not produce classical exotoxins, although some temperate bacteriophages encode exotoxins that are excreted by their bacterial hosts. Viral diseases result directly or indirectly from the effects of the virus on the cell that it infects, and these effects can range from lysis and destruction to subtle changes in cell function. A major component of many viral diseases is the inflammation and tissue damage that results from release of cellular enzymes by viral cytotoxicity or from immunological attack on the infected cell. Released viral antigens can also be involved in immune complex diseases, initiate autoimmune responses, or mediate delayed-type hypersensitivity reactions. These are considered in more detail in the next section of this chapter.

Viral latency

Many viral infections can become latent, either by assuming an altered episomal form in the cell, or because of integration of viral DNA or DNA transcripts into the host genome, and can cause relapses or increased severity of disease when complete virions are resynthesized at a later date. Latency is not a unique characteristic of viruses; it occurs, for instance, with the *Rickettsia* of typhus fever and with the tubercle bacillus. However, it is much commoner and more significant in viral infections.

Because of the intimate relationship between virus and cell, the basic mechanisms of these interactions have been detailed in Chapters 6 and 7, and this section will focus on those aspects directly related to the disease process.

Initiation of Infection

Acquisition of viral infections

Viruses are acquired by routes similar to those of other pathogenic organisms. Thus, the respiratory, alimentary and genital tracts, skin, oropharyngeal mucosa, and the conjunctiva may all be infected directly with specific viruses. Some viruses, such as many arboviruses, are transmitted by insect bites, and the rabies virus by bites of infected animals. Others, such as cytomegalovirus and hepatitis B virus, that infect white blood cells or otherwise reach the bloodstream can be acquired from blood either as a result of inadequate sterilization of needles and syringes or through blood transfusion.

Presence and distribution of cell receptors determines tissue tropism and host range of viruses

The central determinant of the ability of a virus to infect involves contact with a host cell that carries surface receptors for components of the viral envelope or capsid. Such receptors, many of which are glycoproteins, are often restricted to cells of particular tissues and species of animals, and this accounts to a considerable degree for the tissue tropism and host ranges of viruses, although other factors can involve their ability to replicate within a cell. Thus, receptors for the influenza virus occur on ciliated respiratory epithelial cells, those for the human immunodeficiency virus (HIV, the cause of acquired immunodeficiency syndrome) on T4 helper-inducer lymphocytes and macrophages of humans, whereas receptors for many arboviruses are widely distributed among mammals and mosquitos and, thus, determine a wider host range. Receptors for viruses are often

Viral receptors are often multifunctional

multifunctional and include hormone receptors and cell surface enzymes as well as structural surface components. In some cases, receptors are associated with histocompatibility antigens, and thus there may be genetic differences in susceptibility to infection among different individuals of the same species.

The mechanisms of receptor-mediated endocytosis and replication of both naked and enveloped DNA and RNA viruses have been described in Chapter 6. For a wider infection to develop, replication in the initially infected cell must occur followed by spread to other susceptible cells.

Viral Spread in the Body

Viruses have a variety of methods of spread in the body that can influence the duration of the incubation period, the disease syndromes produced, and the ability of the host to control the infection.

Local extension can be by cytolysis and infection of adjacent cells

Some viruses, such as those of influenza, spread directly from cell to cell in the affected epithelium as they are released by cytolysis. Thus, free virus becomes subject to neutralization by antibody when it is produced.

Many viruses multiply first at a primary site of infection, such as the intestinal or oropharyngeal epithelium, and on release from these cells reach the bloodstream to produce a primary viremia followed by infection of specific target cells in other tissues. An example is the virus of mumps, which initially infects the nasopharynx, but causes its major disease manifestations in the salivary glands and sometimes in the central nervous and endocrine systems. In this case, the initial infection and viremia may be subclinical and the incubation period much longer than with the influenza virus.

Viremic spread of some viruses to target organs

Viruses such as *Herpes simplex* are less prone to cause cytolysis, but pass from cell to cell through syncytial bridges caused by fusion of the membranes of different cells. They tend to produce many chronic and relapsing infections, probably associated with waxing and waning of cell-mediated immune responses and their cytotoxic effector mechanisms. *Herpes simplex* and some other viruses have a particular affinity for cells of the nervous system or are able to travel through axons and are thus protected from the host's immune system. The varicella zoster virus, after causing a childhood attack of chickenpox, may remain latent and protected in dorsal root ganglion cells, but reemerge decades later to produce shingles in the distribution of the affected nerve routes. The rabies virus can pass slowly to its target in the central nervous system by traveling up axons that innervate the area of the original bite and fail to stimulate an immune response during what can be a prolonged incubation period.

Some viruses cross syncytial bridges between cells

Viruses causing neuronal infections are immunologically protected and often latent

Unlike most bacteria (the spirochete of syphilis being an important exception), several viruses causing infection during pregnancy can traverse the chorionic barrier and chronically infect the developing fetus. Rubella and cytomegalovirus infections are classic examples, both of which can result in severe developmental abnormalities and noncytolytic alteration of cell function.

Congenital and teratogenic viral infections

Interferons

Interferons (IFN) are polypeptide cytokines produced by many mammalian cell types. The family includes IFN-α (of which there are several derived from leukocytes), IFN-β (derived from fibroblasts and many other cell types), and IFN-γ (a product of activated T lymphocytes). IFN-α and IFN-β are synthesized when the producing cell is exposed to a variety of stimuli, in particular viral and other infections. Production is also stimulated by endotoxin, some other bacterial products, and natural or synthetic double-stranded RNA. Production of IFN-γ by T cells is stimulated by reaction of the cells with the specific antigen to which they are responsive or by some mitogens. The antiviral action of interferons is, however, nonspecific.

Family of interferon cytokines

Viral infections and other stimuli directly initiate interferon α and β synthesis Interferon γ derived from activated T4 cells

Interferons inhibit replication of RNA and DNA viruses and some other intracellular pathogens. They do not effect adsorption or endocytosis of viruses, but act by inducing production of proteins within the cell that inhibit viral protein and nucleic acid synthesis and, thus, replication. Their production is blocked by inhibitors of these syntheses. The molecular mechanisms of action of interferons is described in more detail in Chapter 6.

Inhibition of viral protein and nucleic acid synthesis

In addition to their activity within the infected cell, interferons bind to surface receptors of adjacent uninfected cells, are taken into the cell, and produce what has been termed an *antiviral state* that prevents replication of any virus that infects it. The phenomenon of viral interference

Passage of interferon to uninfected cells

(inability of a virus to superinfect during another viral infection) is largely due to interferon produced in response to the first infection.

Nonspecific role in early control of viral infections

Interferons clearly play a critical nonspecific role in the early control of many acute viral infections pending the development of humoral and cellular immunity. Interferon γ also contributes to resistance to infection by inducing activation and proliferation of natural killer and cytotoxic T cells, by activating macrophages, and by increasing expression of MHC antigens on a variety of cell types, and thus of antigen presentation to T cells.

Adverse effects of interferons

Not all effects of interferons are beneficial. They inhibit normal cell growth and produce transient suppression of cell-mediated immunity by selective inhibition of protein synthesis, and in some instances IFN-γ may excessively enhance inflammatory processes through its action on natural killer and cytotoxic T-cell activity.

Host specificity of interferons and production of recombinant interferon

Several interferon genes have been cloned, and their products expressed, in bacteria and yeasts. This has greatly facilitated clinical studies, because interferons are generally specific for each animal species, and human interferons were previously extremely difficult to obtain. The present status of the role of recombinant interferons in the prophylaxis and treatment of viral diseases is considered in Chapter 13.

Avoidance of Host Defense Mechanisms

Virus freed from the cell can be neutralized by antibody

Viruses passing intercellular bridges are protected from antibody

Cells infected with latent virus may be immunologically unrecognized

Most acute viral infections are controlled to varying extents by the development of neutralizing antibody that blocks attachment of extracellular virus to receptors on susceptible cells, and by the action of interferons. Virus may be liberated from its intracellular habitat either by direct cytolysis or by the action of cytotoxic T cells or natural killer cells on the infected cell. Viruses that pass between intercellular bridges, those that are protected within neurons, and those that fail to lyse a cell or express viral antigens on its surface are variably protected from the immune system. Integration of the viral genome into that of the host cell or production only of incomplete virus in the cell may also be totally unrecognized immunologically and result in latency.

HIV is immunosuppressive through effects on T4 cells and macrophages and by polyclonal B-cell activation

Several viral infections are directly immunosuppressive. The receptor for HIV is the CD4 molecule on T4 helper-inducer cells and on monocytes and other cells of the macrophage series. Infection of T4 cells directly affects cell-mediated immunity, and nonlethal infection of macrophages leads to reduction of their chemotactic and microbicidal power as well as providing a reservoir of infectious virus. In addition, the gp 120 protein of HIV is homologous to a B-cell–activating lymphokine and produces polyclonal activation of B cells. This leads to excessive but nonspecific immunoglobulin production at the expense of specific antibody responses.

Effects of some other viruses on immunocytes, macrophages, and polymorphonuclear leukocytes predispose to secondary infections

Some other viruses, for example, the measles virus, can also infect immunocytes and reduce immune responses, and cytomegalovirus-infected monocytes and macrophages are partially crippled in their microbicidal activities. These viruses, and some others including influenza viruses, also cause alterations in the functions of polymorphonuclear leukocytes, including chemotactic, oxidative, and bactericidal activity. In each of these cases, the most severe or fatal results of infection are often due to secondary infections with other organisms that develop as a result of the compromised cellular defense mechanisms.

Tissue Damage from Immune Reactions

Tissue damage and the manifestations of disease may also result from interaction between the host's immune mechanisms and the invading organism or its products. Reactions between high concentrations of anti-

Immune complex diseases

body, soluble microbial antigens, and complement can deposit immune complexes in tissues and cause acute inflammatory reactions and immune complex disease. In poststreptococcal acute glomerulonephritis, for example, the complexes are sequestered in the glomeruli of the kidney, with serious interference in renal function from the resulting tissue reaction.

Damage from antibody cross-reacting with host tissues

Sometimes, antibody produced against microbial antigens can cross-react with certain host tissues and initiate an autoimmune process. Such cross-reaction is almost certainly the explanation for poststreptococcal rheumatic fever, and it may be involved in some of the lesions of tertiary syphilis. Some viruses have been shown to have small peptide sequences that are occasionally shared by host tissues. Thus, a virus-induced immune response may also generate antibodies that react with shared determinants on host cells, such as in the heart.

Pathologic changes from delayed-type hypersensitivity reactions

In some other infections, the pathologic and clinical features are largely due to delayed-type hypersensitivity reactions to the organism or its products. Such reactions are particularly significant in tuberculosis and other mycobacterial infections. The mycobacteria possess no significant toxins and, in the absence of delayed hypersensitivity, their multiplication elicits little more than a mild inflammatory response. The development of delayed-type, cell-mediated hypersensitivity to their major proteins leads to dramatic pathologic manifestations, which in tuberculosis are manifested as a chronic granulomatous response around infected foci with massive infiltration of macrophages and lymphocytes followed by central devascularization and necrosis. Rupture of a necrotic area into a bronchus leads to the typical pulmonary cavity of the disease, and rupture into a blood vessel can produce extensive dissemination or massive bleeding from the lung. Injection of tuberculoprotein into an animal with an established tuberculous lesion can lead to acute exacerbation and sometimes death. Thus, the body's defense mechanisms are themselves contributing to the severity of the disease process.

These examples illustrate processes that are probably involved to varying degrees in the pathology and course of most infections. Immune reactions are essential to the control of infectious diseases; however, they are potentially damaging to the host, particularly when large amounts of antigens are involved and the host response is unusually active.

Alterations in Virulence of Pathogenic Organisms

The property of virulence is polygenic

The properties that impart virulence to invasive microorganisms, whether they be bacteria or viruses, are multiple. For example, a bacterium may require adhesins, siderophore production, enzymes to facilitate its spread, and toxins to protect it from phagocytes and free up nutrients that it may need. Thus, multiple genes and their products are involved, some of which may be present on plasmids. Likewise, many genes are involved in the properties of a virion that determine virulence. Changes in the presence or degree of expression of these genes can significantly reduce virulence without, necessarily, altering the surface antigens that are the targets of the immune system. Such changes, usually toward lower virulence, may develop during prolonged epidemic or endemic associations of a pathogenic organism with a particular host species and contribute to a more balanced state of parasitism. Virulence may also be manipulated experimentally to yield *attenuated* organisms that retain the antigenic specificity

Attenuation is reduction in virulence with retained immunogenicity

of the wild type and the capacity to multiply in vivo, but lose the ability to cause serious disease. Many of the most successful "live" vaccines have been prepared in this way. Attenuation of many species for vaccine production was achieved pragmatically by passing the organism repeatedly

Loss of virulence determining
plasmids

Temperature-sensitive
mutants

Defective interfering particles

Genetically engineered
attenuation

through a host species that it normally does not infect or by growing it in vitro under suboptimal conditions, such as unphysiologic temperatures.

The mechanisms involved in such attenuation are now understood more clearly. For example, Pasteur's classic attenuation of the anthrax bacillus to provide an effective vaccine for cattle is now known to have resulted from loss of a plasmid coding anthrax toxin when the organism was grown at elevated temperature. Likewise, temperature-sensitive mutants that fail to produce the full complement of an essential metabolite or structure at body temperature can lose part or all of their virulence, as can defective interfering viral particles that have all of the structural proteins of the wild type, but lack an essential portion of the viral genome. It is now possible to approach attenuation or production of live vaccines more directly by methods such as deliberate excision of particular genes, insertional mutagenesis, and the production of hybrids that possess the desired immunizing capacity but lack the virulence of the pathogenic parent strain.

Conclusion

Host-parasite interactions are enormously complex and have evolved in a manner that has tended to produce a more balanced state of parasitism between well-established species and the microorganisms with which they frequently come into contact. In this chapter the components of these interactions have been discussed separately, but it is important to recognize the dynamic and shifting nature of their role in determining the course and outcome of an infection. The diversity of mechanisms by which a host controls infection can be particularly appreciated if one recognizes that they are all intimately interrelated. If even one of these is absent, either as a result of heredity or acquired loss, the ability to cope with one, several, or even many pathogens can be seriously, and sometimes fatally, impaired. Overlying the specific host defense factors discussed here and in Chapter 8 are broader determinants such as the general health, nutrition, and quite probably the psychologic status of the host. There is increasing evidence that hormonal and diurnal controls of various aspects of the immune processes may be important. Study of these factors offers considerable hope for the possibility of manipulating general host resistance mechanisms more effectively in the future.

Additional Reading

Abramson, J.S., and Mills, E.L. 1988. Depression of neutrophil function induced by viruses and its role in secondary microbial infections. *Rev. Infect. Dis.* 10:326–341. In vivo effects of viruses on leukocyte functions are well summarized and examples given.

Brubaker, R.R. 1985. Mechanisms of bacterial virulence. *Ann. Rev. Microbiol.* 39:21–50. An excellent overall review, which is extensively referenced.

Bullen, J.J. 1981. The significance of iron in infection. *Rev. Infect. Dis.* 3:1127–1138. A thorough review of this important topic.

Cassell, G.H., Ed. 1988. Microbial surfaces: Determinants of virulence and host responsiveness. *Rev. Infect. Dis.* 10(suppl. 2):S273–S456. The proceedings of a symposium comprising a series of papers by leaders in the field with particular emphasis on bacterial infection.

Finlay, B.B., and Falkow, S. 1989. Common themes in microbial pathogenicity. *Microbiol. Rev.* 53:210–230. A comprehensive review of the molecular biological basis of bacterial pathogenesis.

Middlebrook, J.L., and Darland, R.B. 1984. Bacterial toxins: Cellular mechanisms of action. *Microbiol. Rev.* 48:199–221. A very thorough review of bacterial exotoxins and their modes of action with extensive references.

Miller, J.F., Mekalanos, J.J., and Falkow, S. 1989. Coordinate regulation and sensory transduction in the control of bacterial virulence. *Science* 243:916–922. An important review of the molecular mechanisms involved in regulation of genes encoding pathogenicity in response to different environments.

Mims, C.A. 1987. *The Pathogenesis of Infectious Disease.* 3rd ed. London: Academic Press. A very readable and balanced account of the pathogenesis of infection.

Oldstone, M.B.A. 1989. Viruses can cause disease in the absence of morphological evidence of cell injury: Implication for uncovering new diseases in the future. *J. Infect. Dis.* 159:384–389. A consideration of the role of viruses in nonlethal modification of the function of host cells.

Quie, P.G. 1983. Perturbations of the normal mechanisms of intraleukocytic killing. *J. Infect. Dis.* 148:180–193. A succinct discussion of organism–phagocyte interactions.

Rouse, B.T., and Horohov, D.W. 1986. Immunosuppression in viral infections. *Rev. Infect. Dis.* 8:850–873. The four major modalities by which viral infections can alter immune responses are discussed clearly and thoroughly.

Sneller, M.C., and Strober, W. 1986. M cells and host defenses. *J. Infect. Dis.* 154:737–741. A review of the role of M cells in transmitting antigens to immunocytes and the manner in which some pathogens exploit this process to traverse the epithelium.

Urbaschek, B., Ed. 1987. Perspectives on bacterial pathogenesis and host defense. *Rev. Infect. Dis.* 9(suppl. 5):S431–S659. As with the Cassell symposium, this symposium comprises authoritative up-to-date papers bearing on the subject of the chapter. Endotoxin action and immunostimulation is very well covered.

11

Sterilization, Pasteurization, Disinfection, Sanitization, and Asepsis

John C. Sherris and
James J. Plorde

Definitions

Death, as it relates to microbial organisms, can be defined as a loss of ability to multiply under any known conditions. The complexity of the definition reflects the fact that organisms that appear to be irreversibly inactivated may sometimes recover when appropriately treated. For example, bacteria that have been inhibited by certain mercurial compounds, such as merthiolate, will fail to multiply because of inactivation of critical microbial–SH groups by free mercury ions. If they are placed in a medium containing compounds with free–SH groups, such as thioglycolate, the process can be reversed and viability restored. Similarly, ultraviolet (UV) irradiation of bacteria can result in the formation of thymine dimers in the DNA with loss of ability to replicate or of fidelity in replication. A period of exposure to visible light may then activate an enzyme that breaks the dimers and restores viability by a process known as *photoreactivation.* Mechanisms also exist for repair of the damage without light. Such considerations are of great significance in the preparation of safe vaccines from inactivated virulent organisms.

> Absence of growth does not necessarily indicate sterility

Sterilization involves complete killing, or removal, of all living organisms from a particular location or material. It can be accomplished by incineration, nondestructive heat treatment, certain gases, exposure to ionizing radiation, some liquid chemicals, and filtration.

Disinfection involves the destruction of harmful microorganisms by liquid chemical agents known as *disinfectants.* These agents usually have some degree of selectivity, and bacterial spores, or organisms with waxy coats (for example, mycobacteria), show considerable resistance to most disinfectants. *Antiseptics* are disinfectant agents that can be used on body surfaces, such as the skin or vaginal tract, to reduce the numbers of the normal flora and of pathogenic contaminants. They have lower toxicity than disinfectants used environmentally, but are usually less active in killing vegetative organisms.

171

Sanitization is similar in principle to disinfection, but only involves providing an acceptable level of microbial cleanliness on inanimate objects such as surfaces used in food preparation.

Pasteurization is the use of heat at a temperature sufficient to inactivate certain harmful organisms in a liquid such as milk, but below that needed to ensure sterilization. For example, heating milk at a temperature of 74°C for 3–5 sec or 62°C for 30 min kills most pathogenic bacteria that may be present without altering its quality. Obviously, spores are not killed at these temperatures.

Asepsis, which involves prevention of microorganisms from reaching a protected environment, is usually applied to procedures used in the operating room, in the preparation of therapeutic agents, and in technical manipulations in the microbiology laboratory. An essential component of aseptic techniques is the sterilization of all materials and equipment used.

Microbial Killing

Exponential kinetics of killing

Killing of bacteria by heat, radiation, or chemicals is usually exponential with time, that is, a fixed proportion of survivors is killed during each time increment. Thus, if 90% of a population of bacteria is killed during each 5 min of exposure to a weak solution of a disinfectant, a starting population of 10^6/ml will be reduced to 10^5/ml after 5 min, 10^3/ml after 15 min, and theoretically to 1 organism (10^0)/ml after 30 min. Exponential killing corresponds to a first-order reaction or a "single-hit" hypothesis, in which the lethal change involves a single target in the organism and the probability of this change is constant with time. Thus, plots of the logarithm of the number of survivors against time will be linear; however, the slope of the curve will vary with the effectiveness of the killing process, which is influenced by the nature of the organism, lethal agent, concentration (in the case of disinfectants), and temperature. In general, the rate of killing increases exponentially with arithmetic increases in temperature or in concentrations of disinfectant. The data for developing killing curves are obtained from colony counts (Chapters 3 and 14) made on samples removed at intervals from a microbial suspension subjected to the sterilization process.

Sterility as a probability

An important consequence of exponential killing with most sterilization processes is that sterility is not an absolute term, but must be expressed as a probability. Thus, to continue the example given previously, the chance of a single survivor in 1 ml is theoretically 10^{-1} after 35 min. If a chance of 10^{-9} were the maximum acceptable risk for a single surviving organism in a 1-ml sample (for example, of a therapeutic agent), the procedure would require continuation for a total of 75 min.

Exponential killing

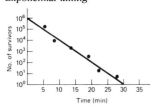

A simple single-hit curve often does not express the kinetics of killing adequately. In the case of some bacterial endospores, a brief period (activation) may elapse before exponential killing by heat begins. If multiple targets are involved, the experimental curve will deviate from linearity. More significant, is the fact that microbial populations may include a small proportion of more resistant mutants or of organisms in a physiologic state that confers greater resistance to inactivation. In these cases, the later stages of the curve are flattened, and extrapolations from the exponential phase of killing may seriously underestimate the time needed for a high probability of achieving complete sterility. In practice, materials that will come into contact with tissues are sterilized under conditions that allow a very wide margin of safety, and the effectiveness of inactivation of or-

Deviation from exponential killing

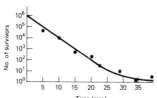

ganisms in vaccines is tested directly with large volumes and multiple samples before a product is made available for use.

Sterilization

The availability of reliable methods of sterilization has made possible the major developments in surgery and intrusive medical techniques that have helped to revolutionize medicine over the past century. Furthermore, sterilization procedures form the basis of many food preservation procedures, particularly in the canning industry.

Heat

Incineration

Dry heat: 160°C for 2 hr

The simplest method of sterilization is to expose the surface to be sterilized to a naked flame. This technique is used in microbiology to sterilize the platinum or nickel chromium wire loop used to transfer cultures or spread inocula on solid media. It can be used equally effectively for emergency sterilization of a knife blade or a needle. Disposable material is, of course, rapidly and effectively decontaminated by incineration. Carbonization of organic material and destruction of microorganisms, including spores, will occur after exposure to dry heat of 160°C for 2 hr in a sterilizing oven. This method is applicable to metals, glassware, and some heat-resistant oils and waxes that are immiscible in water and cannot, therefore, be sterilized in the autoclave. A major use of the dry heat sterilizing oven is in preparation of laboratory glassware.

Moist heat

Greater effectiveness of moist than dry heat

Boiling water fails to kill bacterial spores

Moist heat in the form of water or steam is far more rapid and effective in sterilization than dry heat, because reactive water molecules denature protein irreversibly by disrupting H bonds between peptide groups at relatively low temperatures. Most vegetative bacteria of importance in human disease are killed within a few minutes at 70°C or less, although many bacterial spores (Chapter 2) can resist boiling for prolonged periods. In the past, boiling water was widely used for sterilizing instruments; its effectiveness was often increased by adding sodium carbonate, which raised the temperature of boiling and the speed of killing and also helped to inhibit rusting. Currently, however, the use of boiling water has been replaced by the autoclave, which when properly used will ensure sterility by killing all forms of microorganisms.

Autoclave effective because of increased temperature of steam generated under pressure

Killing rate increases logarithmically with arithmetic increase in temperature

The *autoclave* is, in effect, a sophisticated pressure cooker (Figure 11.1). In its simplest form, it comprises a chamber in which the air can be replaced with pure saturated steam under pressure. Air is removed either by evacuating the chamber before filling with steam or by displacement through a valve at the bottom of the autoclave, which remains open until all air has drained out. The latter, which is termed a *downward displacement autoclave,* capitalizes on the heaviness of air compared to saturated steam. When the air has been removed, the temperature in the chamber is proportional to the pressure of the steam; autoclaves are usually operated at 121°C, which is achieved with a pressure of 15 psi. Under these conditions, spores directly exposed will be killed in less than 5 min, although the normal sterilization time is 10–15 min to account for variation in the ability of steam to penetrate different materials and to allow a wide margin of safety. As the velocity of killing increases logarithmically with arithmetic increases in temperature, a steam temperature of 121°C is vastly more effective than 100°C. For example, the spores of *Clostridium botulinum,* the cause of botulism, may survive 5 hr of boiling, but can be killed in 4 min at 121°C in the autoclave. The use of saturated steam in the autoclave

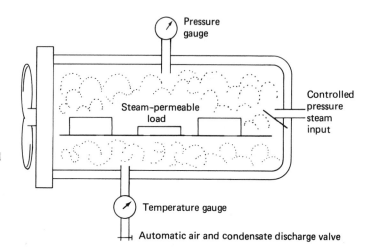

11.1 Simple form of downward displacement autoclave.

Role of condensation and latent heat in effectiveness of autoclave

Uses of autoclave

Need for access of pure saturated steam in autoclave

Causes of autoclave sterilization failures

has other advantages. Latent heat equivalent to 539 cal/g of condensed steam is immediately liberated upon condensation on the cooler surfaces of the load to be sterilized. The temperature of the load is thus raised very rapidly to that of the steam. Condensation also permits rapid steam penetration of porous materials such as surgical drapes by producing a relative negative pressure at the surface, which allows more steam to enter immediately. Autoclaves can thus be used for sterilizing any materials that are not damaged by heat and moisture, such as heat-stable liquids, swabs, most instruments, culture media, rubber gloves, and many others.

It is essential that those who use autoclaves understand the principles involved. Their effectiveness depends on absence of air, pure saturated steam, and access of steam to the material to be sterilized. Pressure per se plays no role in sterilization other than to ensure the raised temperature of the steam. A temperature of less than 121°C at the bottom of the chamber with a pressure of 15 psi indicates that air is still present. A temperature of more than 121°C at this pressure indicates that the steam is superheated and no longer at the phase boundary with water. Superheated steam behaves as a gas and is no more effective in sterilization than air at the same temperature. Failure can also result from attempting to sterilize the interior of materials that are impermeable to steam or the contents of sealed containers. Under these conditions, a dry heat temperature of 121°C is obtained, which may be insufficient to kill even vegetative organisms. Large volumes of liquids require longer sterilization times than normal loads, because their temperature must reach 121°C before timing begins. Thermocouples may be needed to measure the internal temperature of such containers. When sealed containers of liquids are sterilized, it is essential that the autoclave cool without being opened or evacuated; otherwise, the containers may explode as the external pressure falls in relation to that within.

Flash autoclave

"Flash" autoclaves, which are widely used in operating rooms, often use saturated steam at a temperature of 134°C for 3 min. Air and steam are removed mechanically before and after the sterilization cycle so that metal instruments may be available rapidly.

Quality control of autoclaves depends primarily on ensuring that the appropriate temperature for the pressure used is achieved and that packing and timing are correct. Biologic and chemical indicators of the correct conditions are available and are inserted from time to time in the loads.

Gas

A number of articles, particularly certain plastics and lensed instruments that are damaged or destroyed by autoclaving, can be sterilized with ethylene oxide. Occasionally formaldehyde gas is used to decontaminate larger areas.

Ethylene oxide sterilization of heat-labile materials

Ethylene oxide is an inflammable and potentially explosive gas. It is an alkylating agent that inactivates microorganisms by replacing labile hydrogen atoms on hydroxyl, carboxy, or sulfhydryl groups, particularly of guanine and adenine in DNA. Ethylene oxide sterilizers resemble autoclaves and expose the load to 10% ethylene oxide in Freon* or carbon dioxide at 50–60°C under controlled conditions of humidity. Exposure times are usually about 4–6 hr and must be followed by a prolonged period of aeration to allow the gas to diffuse out of substances that have absorbed

Need for aeration after ethylene oxide sterilization

it. Aeration is essential, because absorbed gas can cause damage to tissues or skin. Ethylene oxide is a mutagen, and special precautions are now taken to ensure that it is properly vented outside of working spaces. Used under properly controlled conditions, ethylene oxide is an effective sterilizing agent for heat-labile devices such as artificial heart valves that cannot be treated at the temperature of the autoclave.

Ultraviolet Light and Ionizing Radiation

Ultraviolet light in the wavelength of 240–280 nm is absorbed by nucleic acids and causes genetic damage, including the formation of the thymine dimers discussed previously. The practical value of UV sterilization is limited by its poor ability to penetrate. Apart from its use experimentally

UV light causes direct damage to DNA

Uses and limitations of UV light

as a mutagen, its main application has been irradiation of air in the vicinity of critical surgical sites and aiding in the decontamination of laboratory facilities used for handling particularly hazardous organisms. In these situations, single exposed organisms are rapidly inactivated. It must be remembered that UV light can cause skin and eye damage, and workers exposed to it must be appropriately protected.

Effects and uses of ionizing radiation

Ionizing radiation carries far greater energy than UV light. It, too, causes direct damage to DNA and produces toxic free radicals and hydrogen peroxide from water within the microbial cells. Cathode rays and gamma rays from cobalt-60 are widely used in industrial processes, including the sterilization of many disposable surgical supplies such as gloves, plastic syringes, specimen containers, some foodstuffs, and the like, because they can be packaged before exposure to the penetrating radiation. Ionizing irradiation does not always result in the physical disintegration of killed microbes. As a result, plasticware sterilized in this

Killed organisms may remain morphologically intact and stainable

way may carry significant numbers of dead, but stainable bacteria. If present in containers used to collect normally sterile body fluids such as cerebrospinal fluid, the bacterial bodies may produce a "false-positive" Gram-stained smear and result in inappropriate administration of antibiotics.

---

* It is probable that the use of fluorocarbons will soon be discontinued because of their effects on the global ozone layer.

Filtration

Membrane filters

Both live and dead microorganisms can be removed from liquids by positive- or negative-pressure filtration. Membrane filters, usually composed of cellulose esters (for example, cellulose acetate), are available commercially with pore sizes of 0.005–1 μm. For removal of bacteria, a pore size of 0.2 μm is effective because filters act not only mechanically but by electrostatic adsorption of particles to their surface.

Filtration is used for sterilization of large volumes of fluid, especially those containing heat-labile components such as serum.

Pasteurization

Pasteurization involves exposure of liquids to temperatures in the range of 55–75°C to remove all vegetative bacteria of significance in human disease. Spores are unaffected by the pasteurization process.

Pasteurization of milk, wine, and equipment for respiratory therapy

Pasteurization is used commercially to render milk safe and extend its storage quality. To the dismay of some of his compatriots, Pasteur proposed application of the process to winemaking to prevent microbial spoilage and vinegarization. This method was quickly adopted by the upstart California wine industry, and controlled experiments—an anathema to the finest palates—indicated no effect on the quality or bouquet of wine when the process was undertaken properly. Most wines currently available have been filter sterilized. Pasteurization in water at 70°C for 30 min has also been used for rendering respiratory equipment free of organisms that may otherwise multiply in mucus and humidifying water and cause respiratory infections.

Disinfection, Antisepsis, and Sanitization

Given access and sufficient time, disinfectants cause the death of pathogenic vegetative bacteria. Most are general protoplasmic poisons and are not currently used in the treatment of infections other than very superficial lesions, having been replaced by antimicrobics (see Chapter 13). Some, such as the quaternary ammonium compounds, alcohol, and the iodophors reduce the superficial flora and can eliminate contaminating pathogenic bacteria from the skin surface. Others, such as the phenolics, are valuable only for treatment of inanimate surfaces or for rendering contaminated materials safe. All are bound and inactivated to varying degrees by protein and dirt and lose considerable activity when applied to other than clean surfaces. Their activity increases exponentially with increases in temperature, but the relationship of increases in concentration to killing effectiveness is more complex and varies for each compound. Optimal in-use concentrations have been established for all available disinfectants. The major groups of compounds currently used are briefly discussed as follows.

Most agents are general protoplasmic poisons

Inactivation of disinfectants by organic material

Alcohols

Alcohols require some water for antibacterial effectiveness

The alcohols are protein denaturants that rapidly kill vegetative bacteria when applied as aqueous solutions in the range of 70–95% alcohol. They are inactive against bacterial spores and many viruses. Solutions of 100% alcohol dehydrate organisms rapidly and fail to kill, because the lethal process requires water molecules. Ethanol (70–90%) and isopropyl alcohol (90–95%) are widely used as skin decontaminants before simple invasive procedures such as venipuncture. Their effect is not instanta-

Uses of ethanol and isopropyl alcohol

neous, and the traditional alcohol wipe, particularly when followed by a vein-probing finger, is more symbolic than effective, because insufficient time is given for significant killing.

Isopropyl alcohol has largely replaced ethanol in hospital use because it is somewhat more active and is not subject to diversion to house staff parties.

Halogens

Effectiveness of tincture of iodine

Iodine is an effective disinfectant that acts by iodinating or oxidizing essential components of the microbial cell. It is commonly used as a tincture of 2% iodine in 50% alcohol. It kills more rapidly and effectively than alcohol alone, but has the disadvantage of sometimes causing hypersensitivity reactions and of staining materials with which it comes in contact. It is an excellent preparation for use on skin before drawing a blood culture, a procedure in which contamination must be excluded as much as possible. Tincture of iodine is applied and allowed to dry, and the iodine then removed with alcohol swabs. This procedure ensures an application time sufficient for adequate skin disinfection. Other preparations are available in which iodine is combined with organic compounds such as detergents in dissociable complexes. These agents, termed *iodophors,* cause less skin staining and dehydration than tinctures and are widely used in preparation of skin before surgery. Although less allergenic than inorganic iodine preparations, iodophors should not be used on patients with a history of iodine sensitivity.

Allergenicity

Iodophors

Chlorination of water and swimming pools

Chlorine is a highly effective oxidizing agent, which accounts for its lethality to microbes. It exists as hypochlorous acid in aqueous solutions that dissociate to yield free chlorine over a wide pH range, particularly under slightly acidic conditions. In concentrations of less than one part per million, chlorine is lethal within seconds to most vegetative bacteria, and it inactivates most viruses; this efficacy accounts for its use in rendering supplies of drinking water safe and in chlorination of water in swimming pools. Chlorine reacts rapidly with protein and many other organic compounds, and its activity is lost quickly in the presence of organic material. This property, combined with its toxicity, renders it ineffective on body surfaces; however, it is the agent of choice for decontaminating surfaces and glassware that have been contaminated with viruses or spores of pathogenic bacteria. For these purposes it is usually applied as a 5% solution of sodium hypochlorite.

Use of NaOCl as a decontaminating agent

Surface-Active Compounds

Hydrophobic and hydrophilic groups of surfactants

Surfactants are compounds with hydrophobic and hydrophilic groups that attach to and solubilize various compounds or alter their properties. Anionic detergents such as soaps are highly effective cleansers, but have little direct antibacterial effect, probably because their charge is similar to that of most microorganisms. Cationic detergents, particularly the quaternary ammonium compounds ("quats") such as benzalkonium chloride, are highly bactericidal in the absence of contaminating organic matter. Their hydrophobic and lipophilic groups react with the lipid of the cell membrane of the bacteria, alter its surface properties and its permeability, and lead to loss of essential cell components and death. These compounds have little toxicity to skin and mucous membranes, and thus have been used widely in concentrations of 0.1% for their antibacterial effects. They are inactive against spores and most viruses. Quats in much higher con-

Action on bacterial cell membrane

centrations than those used in medicine (for example, 5–10%) have been used for sanitizing surfaces.

Problems with contamination of "quats"

The greatest care is needed in the use of quats because they will adsorb to most surfaces with which they come in contact, such as cotton, cork, and even dust. As a result, their concentration may be lowered to a point at which certain bacteria, particularly *Pseudomonas aeruginosa*, can grow in the solutions and then cause serious infections. Many instances have been recorded of severe infections resulting from contamination of ophthalmic preparations or of solutions used for treating skin before transcutaneous procedures. It should also be remembered that cationic detergents are totally neutralized by anionic compounds. Thus, the antibacterial effect of quaternary ammonium compounds is inactivated by soap. Because of these problems, quats have been replaced by other antiseptics and disinfectants for most purposes.

Neutralization of cationic detergents by soaps

Phenolics

Phenol, one of the first effective disinfectants, was the primary agent employed by Lister in his antiseptic surgical procedure, which preceded the development of aseptic surgery. It is a potent protein denaturant and bactericidal agent. Substitutions in the ring structure of phenol have substantially improved activity, and a range of phenols and cresols that are effective environmental decontaminants are now widely used in hospital hygiene. They are less deviated by protein than are most other disinfectants, have a detergentlike effect on the cell membrane, and are often formulated with soaps to increase their cleansing property. They are too toxic to skin and tissues to be used as antiseptics.

Environmental decontamination with phenols and cresols

Two diphenyl compounds, hexachlorophene and chlorhexidine, have been extensively used as skin disinfectants. Hexachlorophene is primarily bacteriostatic. Incorporated in a soap, it builds up on the surface of skin epithelial cells over 1–2 days of use to produce a steady inhibitory effect on skin flora and Gram-positive contaminants, as long as its use is continued. It was a major factor in controlling outbreaks of severe staphylococcal infections in nurseries during the 1950s and 1960s, but was then found to produce neurotoxic effects in some premature babies and, when applied in excessive concentrations, in older children. It is now a prescription drug.

Skin decontamination with hexachlorophene and chlorhexidine

Toxicity of hexachlorophene

Advantages of chlorhexidine

Chlorhexidine has replaced hexachlorophene as a routine hand and skin disinfectant and for other topical applications. It has greater bactericidal activity than hexachlorophene without its toxicity but shares with hexachlorophene the ability to bind to the skin and produce a persistent antibacterial effect. It acts by altering membrane permeability of both Gram-positive and -negative bacteria. It is cationic and, thus, incompatible with soaps and anionic detergents that neutralize its action.

Glutaraldehyde and Formaldehyde

Glutaraldehyde and formaldehyde are alkylating agents highly lethal to essentially all microorganisms. Formaldehyde gas is irritative, allergenic, and unpleasant, properties that limit its use as a solution or gas. Glutaraldehyde is an effective sterilizing agent for apparatus that cannot be heat treated, such as some lensed instruments and equipment for respiratory therapy. Formaldehyde vapor, an effective environmental decontaminant under conditions of high humidity, is sometimes used to decontaminate laboratory rooms that have been accidentally and extensively contami-

Use of glutaraldehyde in decontamination of equipment

nated with pathogenic bacteria, including those, such as the anthrax bacillus, that form resistant spores. Such rooms are sealed for processing and thoroughly aired before reoccupancy.

There are numerous other disinfectant compounds, but those discussed herein remain the most important.

Asepsis

In addition to the procedures described above, aseptic techniques designed to prevent or reduce transmission of microorganisms are critical to the care of patients, to the work of the microbiology laboratory, and in the manipulation and dispensing of sterile materials. In clinical settings, aseptic procedures are directed at preventing the spread of potentially pathogenic microbes from patient to patient, from attendant to patient, or from the infected patient to the attendant. The complexities of procedures used range from complete microbiological isolation from the environment of a patient whose immune system has been inactivated by whole body irradiation to the day-to-day precautions used in changing a dressing or examining a patient with a minor wound. Aseptic techniques at any level require rigid adherence to routines such as the use of the surgical scrub, sterile gowns and masks, and the no-touch techniques of the operating room. These rituals are designed to assure that all details that can prevent infection of the patient are followed without deviation, just as the cockpit checklist routine of a jetliner safeguards the passengers. It is beyond the scope of this chapter to consider the various aseptic techniques and procedures to control cross-infection used in medicine because these are handled in more detail in Chapter 72. However, it is appropriate to stress that the simplest and most fundamental process is adequate hand washing before and after examining or caring for patients. This is the single most important procedure in infection control and, unhappily, the most often ignored, particularly in the hurly-burly of intensive care units. All of those attending patients have an absolute obligation to follow rigorous hand-washing procedures.

Within the microbiology laboratory, aseptic procedures are directed toward preventing contamination of specimens and cultures derived from them and to blocking transmission of pathogens to laboratory workers. Contamination of a patient specimen or the media on which it is cultured can mask the presence of a causative agent or produce a false-positive microbiologic result; either can lead to inappropriate treatment, occasionally with catastrophic effect. Transmission of disease to a laboratorian from a biologic specimen is at least equally unfortunate as it needlessly induces illness in a previously healthy individual.

Specimens are protected from bacterial contamination during transport to the laboratory in sterile, tightly sealed containers that are usually placed in a second leak-proof bag. On receipt, they are processed within the confines of a laminar airflow hood or next to an active bunsen flame, the updraft of which carries potential contaminants away from the specimen. The opening of the container is flame sterilized, and the necessary manipulations executed with sterile pipettes, swabs, or inoculating loops. The container opening is then again flamed and resealed. Subsequent manipulations of cultures are handled in a similar fashion to prevent contamination.

Many of the same measures used in clinical medicine are employed to minimize the risk of direct pathogen transfer from specimen to laboratorian with hand protection and washing being of primary importance.

Goals of asepsis in patient care

Importance of aseptic rituals

Central role of hand washing

Laboratory asepsis procedures to prevent specimen and media contamination

Laboratory asepsis precautions to protect workers

Additional techniques are required to prevent the acquisition of respiratory infection. Many laboratory manipulations, including opening containers and agitation or centrifugation of liquids, produce aerosols of small fluid droplets that may contain pathogenic organisms at their center. Droplets measuring less than 5 μm in diameter remain suspended in air for a significant length of time and, if inspired, reach the alveoli of the lung where they can initiate infection. A variety of simple procedures are used to minimize production of aerosols, but when handling materials known or suspected to be highly infectious, technologists don gloves, gowns, and masks and/or manipulate the specimens within a negative-pressure biologic safety hood. To avoid the risk of aerosol spread beyond the laboratory confines, air in the laboratory is maintained at negative pressure relative to the rest of the building in which it is situated and laboratory exhaust ducts, even when filtered, are kept remote from hospital ventilation intake openings.

These few examples serve to illustrate the point that prevention of undesired microbial acquisition requires rigid techniques and mechanical safeguards and, most importantly, conscientious personnel who understand the nature of microorganisms and how they are transmitted.

Additional Reading

Block, S.S., Ed. 1983. *Disinfection, Sterilization and Preservation.* 3rd ed. Philadelphia: Lea & Febiger.

Favero, M.S. 1985. Sterilization, disinfection and antisepsis in the hospital. In *Manual of Clinical Microbiology.* 4th ed. Lennette, E.H., Balows, A., Hausler, W.J., and Shadomy, H.J., Eds. Washington, D.C.: American Society for Microbiology. A good account of the practical use of disinfectants.

Perkins, J.J. 1983. *Principles and Methods of Sterilization in Health Sciences.* 2nd ed. Springfield, Ill.: Charles C. Thomas.

The Block and Perkins books are excellent standard texts and sources of reference.

12

Epidemiology of Infectious Diseases

Lawrence Corey

Epidemiology, the study of the distribution of determinants of disease and injury in human populations, is a discipline that includes both infectious and noninfectious diseases. Most epidemiologic studies of infectious diseases have concentrated on the factors that influence acquisition and spread, because this knowledge is essential for developing methods of prevention and control. Historically, epidemiologic studies, and the application of the knowledge gained from them, have been central to the control of the great epidemic diseases, such as cholera, plague, smallpox, yellow fever, and typhus, which were, and in some circumstances still remain, major threats to human life and health throughout the world.

An understanding of the principles of epidemiology and the spread of disease is essential to all medical personnel, even though their work may be with the individual patient rather than the community. Most infections must be evaluated in their epidemiologic setting; for example, what is the risk to the patient's family, schoolmates, and work or social contacts? Has the patient recently traveled to an area of special disease prevalence? Is there a possibility of nosocomial infection from recent hospitalization? Is the patient suffering from a reportable disease? The physician must never hesitate to enlist the help of public health authorities, who have the knowledge, organization, and responsibility to undertake the epidemiologic studies and control measures needed to protect the community.

Sources and Communicability

Infectious diseases of humans may be caused by exclusively human pathogens, such as the measles virus, by environmental organisms, such as *Legionella pneumophila,* or by organisms that have their primary reservoir in animals, such as the plague bacillus. They can generally be classified as noncommunicable or communicable.

Noncommunicable infections include 1) those caused by the patient's nor-

181

mal flora, such as peritonitis after rupture of the appendix; 2) those caused by the ingestion of preformed toxins, such as botulism and staphylococcal food poisoning; and 3) infections caused by certain organisms common in nature, such as gas gangrene and Legionnaires' disease contracted from the environment. Many zoonotic infections (diseases transmitted from animals to humans), such as rabies and brucellosis, are rarely, if ever, transmitted between humans under natural conditions, although readily communicable within their animal reservoir.

Noncommunicable infections may occur as epidemics that involve a common source of infection. For example, ingestion of a chicken salad heavily contaminated with an enterotoxin-producing *Staphylococcus aureus* can produce acute food poisoning within an hour or two in those who ate it, but the disease is not transmissible to others. Likewise, extensive dissemination of *Legionella* through an air-conditioning system may lead to many cases of pulmonary infection, particularly in immunocompromised hosts, but without secondary spread.

Communicable infections are transmissible from person to person. They can be *endemic*, which implies that the disease may be present at a low but fairly constant level, or *epidemic*, which involves a level of infection above that usually found in a community or population. Communicable infections may be widespread in a region and sometimes worldwide with high attack rates, in which case they are termed *pandemic*. A communicable infection requires that an organism be able to multiply in or on the body and to leave the body in a form directly infectious to others or indirectly infectious after development in an animate vector or in a suitable environment. An example of direct communicability is the respiratory spread of the influenza virus. In contrast, the malarial parasite requires a developmental cycle in a biting mosquito before another human can be infected.

Infection and Disease

An important consideration in the study of the epidemiology of communicable organisms is the distinction between infection and disease. Infection involves multiplication of the organism in or on the host. Disease represents a clinically apparent response of the host to infection. With many communicable microorganisms, infection is much more common than disease, and apparently healthy infected individuals play an important role in disease propagation. Inapparent infections are termed *subclinical*, and the individual is sometimes referred to as a *carrier*. The latter term is also applied to situations in which an infectious agent establishes itself as part of a patient's flora or causes low-grade chronic disease after an acute infection. For example, the clinically inapparent presence of *S. aureus* in the anterior nares is termed *carriage*, as is a chronic gallbladder infection with *Salmonella typhi* that can follow an attack of typhoid fever and result in fecal excretion of the organism for years. With some infectious diseases, such as measles, infection is invariably accompanied by clinical manifestations of the disease itself. These manifestations facilitate epidemiologic control, because the existence and extent of infection in a community is readily apparent. Organisms associated with long incubation periods or high frequencies of subclinical infection (e.g., the human immunodeficiency virus of AIDS or hepatitis B and D viruses) may propagate and spread in a population for long periods before the extent of the problem is recognized. This makes epidemiological control more difficult.

The inherent infectivity and virulence of a microorganism are properties discussed in Chapter 10. They are important determinants of attack

---

Noncommunicable indigenous, environmental, and zoonotic infections

Single-source epidemics of noncommunicable diseases

Endemic, epidemic, and pandemic spread of communicable diseases

Distinction between infection and disease; some infections may be subclinical

Some infections result in carrier state; others have no carriers

Subclinical infections and long incubation periods may obscure epidemic spread

Infectivity and virulence determine attack rates

rates of disease in a community, because, in general, organisms of high infectivity spread more easily and those of greater virulence are more likely to cause disease than subclinical infection. Some infectious agents, such as the chickenpox (varicella) virus, are of high infectivity but low virulence, and the disease they cause is quite mild; others, such as the leprosy bacillus, are of low infectivity but high virulence in established infections. The infecting dose of an organism also influences the chance of infection and development of disease. A large dose of an organism of low virulence is more likely to cause disease than a small dose.

Host factors such as age, race, genetic predisposition, and immune status can dramatically influence the manifestations of an infectious disease and are largely responsible, with differences in infecting dose, for the wide spectrum of disease manifestations that may be seen during an epidemic. For example, in an epidemic of measles in an isolated population in 1846, the attack rate for all ages averaged 75%; however, mortality was 90 times higher in children less than 1 year of age (28%) than in those 1–40 years of age (0.3%). Conversely, in one outbreak of poliomyelitis, the attack rate of paralytic polio was 4% in children 0–4 years of age and 20–40% in those 5–50 years of age. Infections caused by Epstein-Barr virus are asymptomatic when acquired in childhood, but will frequently result in infectious mononucleosis when primary infection occurs in early adulthood. Racial differences markedly influence the progression of a number of diseases. For example, in the fungal disease coccidioidomycosis, clinical disease and dissemination to organs such as bone and brain are more common in Filipino, black, and Asian subjects than in white subjects. Sex may also be a factor in disease manifestations; for example, the likelihood of becoming a chronic carrier of hepatitis B is twice as high in males as in females. Prior exposure to the organism itself or related organisms may alter immune status and the frequency of acquisition, subclinical infections, or severity of clinical disease. For example, prior herpes simplex virus (HSV)-1 infection ameliorates the severity and frequency of subsequent HSV-2 infections, because of cross-reacting immune responses between the two viruses.

Role of infecting dose

Host factors greatly influence manifestations of disease

Influence of age, race and sex on attack rates and severity

Effects of prior exposure to related organisms

Routes of Transmission

Horizontal direct and indirect spread

Vector spread

Various transmissible infections may be acquired from others by direct contact, by aerosol transmission of infectious secretions, or indirectly through contaminated inanimate objects or materials. Some, such as malaria, involve an animate insect vector. These routes of spread are often referred to as *horizontal transmission* in contrast to *vertical transmission* from mother to fetus. The major horizontal routes of transmission of infectious diseases are summarized in Table 12.1 and discussed below.

Respiratory Spread

Respiratory aerosols and droplet spread

Many infections are transmitted by the respiratory route, often by aerosolization of respiratory secretions with subsequent inhalation by others. The efficiency of this process depends in part on the extent and method of propulsion of discharges from the mouth and nose, the size of the aerosol droplets, and the resistance of the infectious agent to desiccation and inactivation by ultraviolet light. In still air, a particle 100 μm in diameter requires only seconds to fall the height of a room; a 10-μm particle will remain airborne for about 20 min, smaller particles even longer. When inhaled, particles with a diameter of 6 μm or more are usually trapped by

Table 12.1 Common Routes of Transmission[a]

Route of Exit	Route of Transmission	Example
Respiratory	Aerosol droplet inhalation	Influenza virus; tuberculosis
	Nose or mouth → hand or object → nose	Common cold (rhinovirus)
Salivary	Direct salivary transfer (e.g., kissing)	Oral-labial herpes; infectious mononucleosis
	Animal bite	Rabies
Gastrointestinal	Stool → hand → mouth and/or stool → object → mouth	Enterovirus infection; hepatitis A
	Stool → water or food → mouth	Salmonellosis; shigellosis
Skin	Skin discharge → air → respiratory tract	Varicella, poxvirus infection
	Skin to skin	Human papilloma virus (warts); syphilis
Blood	Transfusion or needle prick	Hepatitis B; cytomegalovirus infection; malaria; human immunodeficiency virus (AIDS)
	Insect bite	Malaria; relapsing fever
Genital secretions	Urethral or cervical secretions	Gonorrhea; herpes simplex; *Chlamydia* infection
	Semen	Cytomegalovirus infection
Urine	Urine → hand → catheter	Hospital-acquired urinary tract infection
	Urine → aerosol (rare)	Tuberculosis
Eye	Conjunctival	Adenovirus
Zoonotic	Animal bite	Rabies
	Contact with carcasses	Tularemia
	Arthropod	Plague; Rocky Mountain spotted fever; Lyme disease

[a] The examples cited are incomplete, and in some cases more than one route of transmission exists.

the mucosa of the nasal turbinates, whereas particles of 0.6–6.0 μm will attach to mucus sites at various levels along the upper and lower respiratory tract and may initiate infection. Respiratory secretions are often transferred on hands or inanimate objects (fomites) and may reach the respiratory tract of others in this way. For example, spread of the common cold often involves transfer of infectious secretions from nose to hand by the infected individual with transfer to others by hand to hand contact, and then from hand to nose by the unsuspecting victim.

Manual and fomitic spread of respiratory infections

Salivary Spread

Some infections, such as herpes simplex and infectious mononucleosis, can be transferred directly by contact with infectious saliva through kissing or through bites. Salivary transmission of infectious secretions among chil-

Significance in day-care centers

dren in day-care centers through shared toys and utensils often accounts for the rapid dissemination of agents such as respiratory syncytial virus, parainfluenza virus, *Haemophilus influenzae* type b, the meningococcus, and cytomegalovirus. Reinfections with respiratory syncytial virus are common, but, in general, are associated with reduced frequency of lower respiratory illness and less severe symptoms than the initial exposure.

Fecal-Oral Spread

Direct spread and indirect contamination of food and water

Properties of intestinal pathogens

Greater risk of infection in achlorhydric host

Hazards posed by intestinal carriers

Fecal-oral spread is an important means of transmission of a variety of bacterial, viral, and parasitic diseases. It is a route associated with poor hygiene and may involve direct or finger-to-mouth spread, the use of night soil as a fertilizer, or fecal contamination of food or water. Food handlers who are infected with an organism transmissible by this route constitute a special hazard. Some viruses disseminated by the fecal-oral route infect and multiply in cells of the oropharynx, then disseminate to other body sites to cause infection. Commonly, however, organisms that are spread in this way multiply in the intestinal tract and may cause intestinal infections. They must, therefore, be able to resist the acid in the stomach, the bile, and the gastric and small-intestinal enzymes. Many bacteria and enveloped viruses are rapidly killed by these conditions, but Enterobacteriaceae and unenveloped viral intestinal pathogens are more likely to survive. Even with these organisms, the infecting dose in patients with reduced or absent gastric hydrochloric acid is often much smaller than in those with normal stomach acidity, which accounts in part for the greater attack rates in malnourished hosts. The carrier of enteric pathogens poses a particular hazard to others, especially when involved in food preparation and when personal hygienic practices are inadequate (for example, failure to wash hands after defecation).

Skin-to-Skin Transfer

Direct and fomitic skin-to-skin spread

This occurs with a variety of infections in which the skin is the portal of exit. Examples are the spirochete of syphilis (*Treponema pallidum*), strains of group A streptococci that can cause impetigo, and the dermatophyte fungi that cause ringworm and athlete's foot. In most cases, an inapparent break in the epithelium is probably involved in infection. Other diseases may be spread through fomites such as shared towels or inadequately cleansed shower and bath floors. Skin-to-skin transfer usually occurs through abrasions of the epidermis, which may be unnoticed.

Blood-Borne Transmission

Transmission through insect vectors

Direct transmission with infected blood

Blood-borne transmission through insect vectors is an essential feature of some protozoal, bacterial, and viral diseases. In some instances the infectious agent requires a period of multiplication or alteration within an insect vector before it can infect another human host; such is the case with the yellow fever virus in the *Aedes aegypti* mosquito and with the malarial parasite. Direct transmission through blood has become increasingly important in modern medicine because of the use of blood transfusions and blood products and the increased use of self-administered illicit drugs by intravenous or subcutaneous routes, using shared unsterile equipment. Hepatitis B virus and the HIV viruses have been frequently transmitted in this way.

Genital Tract Transmission

Transmission between sex partners or to infants at birth

Disease transmission through the genital tract has emerged as one of the most common infectious problems in the latter half of the 20th century and reflects changing social and sexual mores. Spread can be between sexual partners or to the infant at birth. A major factor in these infections has been the persistence, high rates of asymptomatic carriage, and frequency of recurrence with organisms such as *Chlamydia trachomatis,* cytomegalovirus, herpes simplex virus, and *Neisseria gonorrhoeae.*

Significance of chronic, asymptomatic and recurrent infection

Urinary Tract Nosocomial Transmission

Numerous organisms can infect the urinary tract and be excreted in the urine. Spread by person-to-person contact, although possible, is only a significant problem in the hospitalized patient. Transmission between patients with indwelling urethral catheters, which is particularly important, has been shown to occur by way of the inadequately washed hands of medical attendants and staff members.

Eye-to-Eye Transmission

Infections of the conjunctiva may occur in epidemic or endemic form. Epidemics of *Haemophilus* conjunctivitis may occur in institutions and are highly contagious. The major endemic disease is trachoma, caused by *Chlamydia,* which remains a frequent cause of blindness in developing countries. These diseases may be spread by direct contact or by secretions passed manually or through fomites such as towels.

Zoonotic Transmission

Blind-ended infections

Transmission of zoonotic infection between humans

Some infections are spread from animals, where they have their natural reservoir, to humans. These infections are termed *zoonotic diseases.* Some zoonotic infections, such as rabies contracted from the bite of a rabid animal, are blind ended in humans in that infection is rarely, if ever, transferred from person to person. Others may be transferred between humans once the disease is established in a population. Plague, for example, has a natural reservoir in rodents. Human infections contracted from the bites of rodent fleas may produce pneumonia, which may then spread to other humans by the respiratory droplet route.

Vertical Transmission

Certain diseases can spread from the mother to the fetus through the placental barrier. This mode of transmission involves organisms that can be present in the mother's bloodstream and may occur at different stages of pregnancy with different organisms. Examples of transplacental spread include congenital rubella infection, congenital syphilis, and congenital toxoplasmosis.

Transplacental and perinatal transmission of infection

Another form of transmission from mother to infant occurs by contact with organisms during the birth process. Example of infections transmitted in the perinatal period by this route include group B streptococcal disease and infections due to herpes simplex virus, *Chlamydia trachomatis,* and hepatitis B virus.

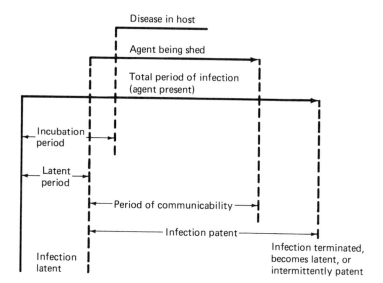

12.1 Schematic of stages of infection.

Incubation Period and Communicability

The incubation period is the time between exposure to the organism and the appearance of the first symptoms of disease. Generally, organisms that multiply rapidly and produce local infections, such as gonorrhea and influenza, are associated with short incubation periods (for example, 2–4 days). Diseases such as typhoid fever, which depend on hematogenous spread and multiplication of the organism in distant target organs to produce symptoms, often have longer incubation periods (for example, 10 days to 3 weeks). Some diseases have even more prolonged incubation periods because of slow passage of the infecting organism to the target organ, as in rabies, or slow growth of the organism, as in tuberculosis. Incubation periods may also vary widely depending upon route of acquisition and infecting dose; for example, the incubation period of hepatitis B infection may vary from 7 to more than 200 days.

The rapidity with which a disease is spread is also related to how soon the agent is shed from the host and the duration of communicability. These factors are not necessarily related to the development or duration of disease. For example, asymptomatic carriers of *Chlamydia* or gonococci in the uterine cervix can shed the agent for a longer time and be more infectious to others than those who are symptomatic and come to medical attention. Conversely, some agents, such as *S. aureus,* are more contagious from symptomatic infection than from asymptomatic carriers.

A common relationship of communicability to disease is illustrated in Figure 12.1, but there are substantial divergences from this model. For example, infectivity of a disease in which the organism is shed in secretions may occur primarily during the incubation period. In other cases, symptoms of disease may be related to host immune responses rather than to virulence determinants of the organism, and thus the disease process may extend far beyond the period in which the etiologic agent can be isolated. In other infections the disease course is short but the organisms can persist in the host for extended periods beyond resolution of the illness. For example, some organisms can persist in the host in immunologically protected sites and some viruses can integrate into the host genome or survive by replicating very slowly in the presence of an immune response. Such

(margin notes:)

Determinants of short and long incubation periods

Duration of shedding and communicability

Variations in relationship of time of communicability to disease manifestations

dormancy or latency is exemplified by the herpes viruses, and in each case the organism may emerge long after the original infection and potentially infect others.

Epidemics

The characterization of epidemics and their recognition in a community involve several quantitative measures and some specific epidemiologic definitions. *Infectivity,* in epidemiologic terms, equates to attack rate and is measured by the frequency with which an infection is transmitted when there is contact between the agent and a susceptible individual. The *disease index* of an infection can be expressed as the number of persons who develop the disease divided by the total number infected. The *virulence* of an agent can be estimated by the number of fatal or severe cases over the total number of cases. *Incidence,* the number of new cases of a disease within a specified period, is most often described as a rate in which the number of cases is the numerator and that in the population under surveillance is the denominator. *Prevalence,* which can also be described as a rate, is the total number of cases existing in a population at risk at a point in time or during a defined period.

Epidemics can be from a common source or propagated by spread from person to person. An example of the former would be an outbreak of *Salmonella* food poisoning in which a number of people consume a food heavily contaminated with *Salmonella enteritidis.* An example of a propagated epidemic would be an outbreak of influenza.

Common-source epidemics from preformed toxin in food, such as that causing botulism, are not associated with secondary spread. A secondary wave of propagated infections, however, may result from common-source outbreaks caused by transmissible organisms.

The prerequisites for a propagated epidemic are a sufficient degree of infectivity to allow the organism to spread, sufficient virulence for an increased incidence of disease to become apparent, and a sufficient level of susceptibility in the host population to permit transmission and amplification of the infecting organism. Thus, the extent of an epidemic and its degree of severity are determined by complex interactions between parasite and host.

The degree of susceptibility of a population to a potentially epidemic disease depends on genetic factors and on the level of acquired immunity. Prolonged and extensive exposure to a pathogen during previous generations will select for a higher degree of innate immunity in a population. For example, extensive exposure of Western urbanized populations to tuberculosis during the 18th and 19th centuries conferred a degree of resistance greater than that among the progeny of rural or geographically isolated populations. The disease spread rapidly and in severe form, for example, when it was first encountered by the North American Indian.

An even more dramatic example concerns the resistance to the most serious form of malaria that is conferred on peoples of West African descent by the sickle-celled trait (Chapter 52). These instances are clear cases of natural selection, a process that accounts for many differences in racial immunity.

Acquired immunity and its level in a population are often the major determinants of the frequency and duration of epidemics. For example, measles is highly infectious and attacks most susceptible members of an exposed population. Infection, however, gives solid lifelong immunity. Thus, in unimmunized populations in which the disease was maintained

Impact of degree of immunity on epidemic frequency

in endemic form, epidemics occurred at about 3-year intervals when a sufficient number of non-immune hosts had been born to permit rapid transmission between them. When a sufficient immune population was reestablished, epidemic spread was blocked and the disease again became endemic. When immunity is short lived or incomplete, epidemics can continue for decades if the mode of transmission is unchecked, thus accounting for the prolonged urban epidemic of tuberculosis during the last two centuries and the present epidemic of gonorrhea.

Pandemics of infection to which immunity is low or absent

Occasionally, an epidemic arises from an organism against which immunity is essentially absent in a population and that is either of enhanced virulence or appears to be of enhanced virulence because of the lack of immunity. When such an organism is highly infectious, the disease it causes may become pandemic and worldwide. A prime example of this is when a new major antigenic variant of influenza A virus arises against which there is little if any cross-immunity from recent epidemics with other strains. The 1918–1919 pandemic of influenza, for example, was responsible for more deaths (about 20 million) than World War I. Subsequent but less serious pandemics have occurred at intervals because of the development of strains of influenza virus with major antigenic shifts (Chapter 32).

Epidemics associated with unusual virulence

Some diseases of extraordinary severity and mortality, such as the sweating sickness of the 13th century, have appeared suddenly and disappeared equally suddenly, and their cause remains unknown. Possibly they involved a mutational or recombinational event that produced such enhanced virulence in a previously common pathogen that the variant was unable to maintain itself because of the death of so many of its victims. Similarly, epidemics of newly described agents appear to occur as humans change their ecological and social behavior. In the modern era, outbreaks of *Legionella* pneumonia and the recent epidemic of AIDS appear to be examples of this phenomenon.

Social and ecological determinants of epidemic diseases

A major feature of serious epidemic diseases is their frequent association with poverty, malnutrition, disaster, and war. The association is multifactorial and includes overcrowding, contaminated food and water, an increase in arthropods that parasitize humans and can carry some epidemic diseases, and the reduced immunity that can accompany severe malnutrition or certain types of chronic stress. Overcrowding and understaffing in day-care centers or institutes for the mentally impaired can similarly be associated with epidemics of infections.

Nosocomial epidemics with opportunistic pathogen

In recent years, increasing attention has been given to hospital (nosocomial) epidemics of infection. The hospital is not immune to the epidemic diseases that occur in the community; however, most nosocomial infections involve opportunistic organisms and result from the close association of infected patients with those who are unusually susceptible because of chronic disease; immunosuppressive therapy; or the use of bladder, intratracheal, or intravascular catheters and tubes. Control depends on the techniques of medical personnel, hospital hygiene, and effective surveillance. This topic is considered in greater detail in Chapter 72.

Control of Epidemics

The first principle of control is to recognize the existence of an epidemic. This recognition is sometimes immediate because of the high incidence of disease, but often the evidence is obtained from ongoing surveillance activities, such as routine disease reports to health departments and records of school and work absenteeism.

Importance of surveillance and recognition

The causative agent must be identified as soon as possible and characterized antigenically if more than one serotype exists. Studies to determine route of transmission (for example, in outbreaks of food poisoning) must be initiated immediately unless it is known from the organism's identity.

Measures must then be adopted to control the spread and development of further infection. These methods include 1) blocking the route of transmission if possible (for example, improved food hygiene or arthropod control); 2) identifying, treating, and, if necessary, isolating infected individuals and carriers if they are important contributors to maintenance of the epidemic; 3) raising the level of immunity in the uninfected population by immunization, where effective; 4) selective use of chemoprophylaxis for subjects or populations at particular risk of infection, as in epidemics of meningococcal infection; and 5) correcting conditions such as overcrowding or contaminated water supplies that have led to the epidemic or facilitated transfer.

General Principles of Immunization

Immunization is the most effective method of specific individual and community protection against many epidemic diseases. Recent developments in molecular biology and protein chemistry have brought greater sophistication to identifying and purifying specific immunizing antigens and in preparing and purifying specific antibodies for passive protection. Thus, immunization is being applied to a broader range of infections. Immunization can be active, with stimulation of the body's immune mechanisms through administration of a vaccine, or passive, through administration of plasma or globulin containing preformed antibody to the agent desired. Active immunization with living attenuated organisms generally results in a subclinical or mild illness that duplicates to a limited extent the disease to be prevented. These *live vaccines* generally provide both local and durable humoral immunity. Killed or subunit vaccines such as influenza, rabies, and typhoid vaccines or diphtheria or tetanus toxoids provide immunogenicity without infectivity. They generally involve a larger amount of antigen than live vaccines and must be administered parenterally with two or more spaced injections to give a satisfactory secondary response. Immunity usually develops more rapidly with live vaccines, but serious overt disease from the vaccine itself can result in patients with immunodeficiency syndromes or in those whose immune responses have been suppressed. Live attenuated virus vaccines are generally contraindicated in pregnancy because of the risk of infection and damage to developing fetus. Current vaccines and their uses are listed in appendix tables 12-A1 and 12-A2.

Prophylaxis or therapy of some infections can be accomplished or aided by passive immunization. This procedure involves administration of preformed antibody obtained from humans, derived from animals actively immunized to the agent, or produced by hybridoma techniques. Animal antisera induce immune responses to their globulins that result in clearance of the passively transferred antibody within about 10 days and carry the risk of hypersensitivity reactions such as serum sickness and anaphylaxis. Thus, human antibodies are preferable and are detectable in the circulation for several weeks. Two types of human antibody preparations are generally available. Immune serum globulin (gamma globulin) is the immunoglobulin G fraction of plasma, pooled from a large group of donors that contains antibody to many naturally occurring diseases. Hyperimmune globulins are purified antibody preparations from the blood of sub-

Appendix 12.A1 Vaccines for Use in Humans (Alphabetical Listing)[a]

Disease	Type of Vaccine	Administration and Frequency	Indications and Comments
Adenovirus infections	Live attenuated bivalent (types 4 and 7)	Oral once	Used only in military recruits
Anthrax	Inactivated bacilli	SC primary series + booster each 6 mo	Laboratory or industrial workers with special exposure
Cholera	Inactivated bacilli	SC primary series + booster approximately each 6 mo	For travel to cholera endemic areas; 50% effective in preventing disease; not effective in decreasing transmission
Diphtheria, tetanus	Toxoids	IM, childhood series, booster at least every 10 yr[b]	Routine use in all persons
Haemophilus influenzae type B	Purified polysaccharide	IM once	Routine use in children 18 mo of age or older
	Conjugate vaccine with diptheria toxoid		Gives better immune response in children 12–18 months of age
Hepatitis B	Inactivated, blood derived or recombinant	IM, 3-dose primary series	Groups at high risk for acquisition of hepatitis B (needlestick and IV exposure, household contacts of hepatitis B patients, patients requiring large volumes of clotting factors, homosexual men, selected medical and dental personnel, infants of infected mothers)
Influenza	Inactivated	IM yearly	Directed at reducing morbidity and mortality in those at risk of complications of influenza (ie, chronic heart and pulmonary disease patients, those over 65)
Measles (see Rubeola)			
Meningococcal infection (groups A and C)	Purified capsular polysaccharide	SC once	Military recruits; complement-deficient individuals; control of localized epidemics and adjunct to chemoprophylaxis in household contacts; travelers to epidemic areas
Mumps	Live attenuated	SC once[b]	Routine use in children; prevention of orchitis in susceptible seronegative male patients
Pertussis	Inactivated bacilli	IM, childhood series combined with diphtheria-tetanus toxoid[b]	Routine use in all children
Plague	Inactivated bacilli	SC, primary series, boosters every 2 yr	Agricultural workers in endemic areas; laboratory and field personnel with high exposure risk

(Continued)

Table 12.A1 Vaccines for Use in Humans (Alphabetical Listing)[a] (*continued*)

Disease	Type of Vaccine	Administration and Frequency	Indications and Comments
Pneumococcal infection	Purified multivalent polysaccharide	SC or IM once	Same population as influenza vaccination; also, patients with functional or surgical asplenia, cirrhosis, multiple myeloma, or nephrotic syndrome
Poliomyelitis	Live attenuated trivalent	Oral, primary series of 4 doses[b]	Preferred for routine use and during epidemics
	Inactivated trivalent	SC primary series	Selective use in unimmunized adults
Rabies	Human diploid inactivated	Dependent on risk	Exposed individual or workers with rabies virus
Rubella	Live attenuated	SC once[b]	Routine use in children and in adult women who are antibody (HI) negative if pregnancy can be prevented for 3 mo after vaccination; routine use in control of outbreaks
Rubeola	Live attenuated	SC once[b]	Routine use in all children and susceptible adults
Smallpox	Live vaccinia virus	Intradermally every 3–5 yrs	Not now recommended for use; no countries require vaccination certificates
Tetanus (see Diphtheria tetanus)			
Tuberculosis	Live attenuated BCG	SC or intradermally once	Considered for use in tuberculin negative subjects persistently exposed to positive sputum or in epidemic areas
Typhoid	Inactivated[c] *Salmonella typhi*	SC in two doses	Individuals living in or traveling to endemic areas. Potentially exposed laboratory workers. Household contacts of *S. typhi* carriers
Typhus	Inactivated *Rickettsia prowazekii*	SC in 2 doses	Administered only to persons in close contact with others where disease is endemic or epidemic
Varicella	Live attenuated	IM once	For selected immunosuppressed children at risk of varicella; selective use in nonpregnant susceptible adults
Yellow fever	Live attenuated	SC once every 10 year	For travel to yellow fever endemic areas; administered at yellow fever vaccination centers

Abbreviations: IM = intramuscularly; SC = subcutaneously; HI = hemagglutination inhibition.

[a] These are vaccines available at the time of writing. Most attenuated vaccines are contraindicated in pregnancy and in immunosuppressed individuals. Up-to-date recommendations and package inserts must be consulted before use.

[b] Recommended schedules are listed in Table 12.A2.

[c] Recently, an oral live attenuated vaccine has been licensed in the United States for use in individuals at risk.

Appendix 12.A2 Immunization for Normal Infants, Children and Adolescents

Recommended Age	Vaccines
2 months	DPT-1, OPV-1
4 months	DPT-2, OPV-2
6 months	DPT-3
15 months	MMR[a], DPT-4, OPV-3
18 months	HbCV[b]
4–6 years	DPT-5, OPV-4[c]
14–16 years	Td[d]

Source: Adapted with permission from Greer, T., and Lipsky, B. A. 1989. Immunization recommendations for 1989. *University of Washington Medicine* 15:10–12.

Note: These recommendations are based on those of the Immunization Practices Advisory Committee of the Public Health Service. For all products used, the recommendations given in the manufacturers product inserts must be followed.

Abbreviations: DPT = diphtheria pertussis tetanus vaccine; OPV = oral polio vaccine; MMR = mumps measles rubella vaccine; HbCV = *Haemophilus influenzae* type b conjugate vaccine; Td = adult diphtheria tetanus toxoid.

[a] Do not delay until 18 months. May be given with DPT, OPV.
[b] Conjugate vaccine is composed of *Haemophilus influenzae* b polysaccharide antigen conjugated to a protein carrier.
[c] Give before or at school entry.
[d] Repeat every 10 years throughout life.

Uses of immune serum globulin and hyperimmune globulin

jects with high titers of antibody to a specific disease that have resulted from natural exposure or hyperimmunization. Hepatitis B immune globulin, rabies immune globulin, and human tetanus immune globulin are examples of the latter. Details of the use of these globulins can be obtained from the chapters that discuss the diseases in question. Appendix table 12-A3 lists the diseases in which passive immunization has proved to be useful in preventing acquisition of disease. Passive antibody is most effective when given during the incubation period.

Appendix 12.A3 Passive Immunization

Disease	Preparation	Route	Comment
Diphtheria	Equine antiserum	IM or IV	Dose dependent on extent of pharyngeal membrane and degree of toxicity; has also been used to protect unimmunized household contacts
Herpes zoster	Human zoster immune globulin	IM	Prevention and amelioration of varicella in susceptible immunosuppressed hosts

(*continued*)

Appendix 12.A3 Passive Immunization *(continued)*

Disease	Preparation	Route	Comment
Hepatitis A	Human immune serum globulin	IM	Used in household contacts, those who have eaten food prepared or suspected to be contaminated, and travelers to areas of poor hygiene
Hepatitis B	Human hepatitis B immune globulin (HBIG)	IM	Prophylaxis for direct parenteral exposure (needle prick) or mucous membrane contact in susceptible hosts
	Human immune serum globulin		May prevent nonparenteral transmission if it contains antibody to hepatitis B surface antigen; HBIG preferable
Measles	Human immune serum globulin	IM	Used in susceptible household contacts, exposed susceptible pregnant women, and immuno-deficient hosts
Rabies	Human rabies immune globulin	Locally and IM	Used for postexposure prophylaxis
Rubella	Human immune serum globulin	IM	Used in exposed susceptible pregnant women who will not consider termination of pregnancy
Tetanus	Human tetanus immune globulin	IM	For immediate prophylaxis when potentially contaminated wounds in the unimmunized occur; when given with tetanus toxoid, use different syringes and sites

Abbreviations: IM = intramuscularly; IV = intravenously; HBIG = human hepatitis B immune globulin.

Additional Reading

American Academy of Pediatrics, Committee on Infectious Diseases Staff. 1988. *Report of the Committee on Infectious Diseases.* 21st ed. Evanston, Ill.: American Academy of Pediatrics. This reference manual provides synopses of the most important infectious diseases of children and recommended immunization procedures.

Benenson, A.S., Ed. 1985. *Control of Communicable Diseases in Man.* 14th ed. Washington D.C.: American Public Health Association. This excellent, authoritative, and inexpensive paperback provides the major features of infectious disease and methods for their identification and control.

Evans, A.S., Ed. 1989. *Viral Infections of Humans: Epidemiology and Control.* 3rd ed. New York: Plenum.

Evans, A.S. and Feldman, H.A., 1982. Eds. *Bacterial Infections of Humans: Epidemiology and Control.* New York: Plenum. These two compendia by Evans and Feldman are excellent sources of further information on the epidemiology of viral and bacterial diseases.

Mausner, J.S., and Kramer, S. 1985. Mausner and Bahn. *Epidemiology: An Introductory Text.* 2nd ed. Philadelphia: Saunders.

McNeill, W.H. 1976. *Plagues and Peoples.* Garden City, N.Y.: Anchor Press/Doubleday. This interesting book describes the impact of infectious diseases on the evolution of society and on the rise and fall of civilizations.

Recommendations of the Immunization Practices Advisory Committee. 1989.General recommendations on immunization. *MMWR* 38:205–227. An essential guide to routine immunization practices in the United States.

13

Antimicrobics and Chemotherapy of Bacterial and Viral Infections

John C. Sherris and
James J. Plorde

One of the major revolutions in medicine has been the introduction of a large range of clinically effective antimicrobial agents over the past half century. Natural materials with some activity against microbes were used in folk medicine in earlier times, such as the bark of the cinchona tree (containing quinine) in the treatment of malaria; however, rational approaches to chemotherapy began with Ehrlich's development of arsenical compounds for the treatment of syphilis early in the century. Many years then elapsed before the next major development, which was the discovery of the therapeutic effectiveness of a sulfonamide (prontosil rubrum) by Domagk in 1935. Penicillin, which had been discovered in 1929 by Fleming, could not be adequately purified at that time; however, this was accomplished later, and it was produced in sufficient quantities for its clinical effectiveness to be demonstrated by Florey and his colleagues in the early 1940s. Since then, numerous new antimicrobial agents have been discovered or developed, and many have found their way into clinical practice. These agents have played an important role in the extraordinary decline in morbidity and mortality from bacterial diseases particularly in developed countries.

ANTIBACTERIAL AGENTS

Major Principles and Definitions

Selective toxicity exploits differences between microbial and host cells

Clinically effective antimicrobial agents all exhibit selective toxicity toward the parasite rather than the host, a characteristic that differentiates them from the disinfectants (Chapter 11). In most cases, selective toxicity is explained by action on microbial processes or structures that differ from those of mammalian cells. For example, some agents act on bacterial cell wall synthesis, and others act on functions of the 70S bacterial ribosome, but not the 80S eukaryotic ribosome. Some antimicrobial agents, such as penicillin, are essentially nontoxic to the host, unless hypersensitivity has

197

Therapeutic index

developed. Others, such as the aminoglycosides, have a much lower therapeutic index, which is defined as the ratio of the dose toxic to the host to the effective therapeutic dose; as a result, control of dosage and blood levels must be much more precise.

Bactericidal and bacteriostatic activity

Some antimicrobial agents, such as the penicillins and aminoglycosides may be able to kill susceptible microorganisms without the intercession of humoral or cellular immune defenses. In the case of bacteria, this process is termed *bactericidal activity.* The effects of others, such as the sulfonamides or tetracyclines, reversibly inhibit essential metabolic processes, and metabolism can recommence when their level becomes subinhibitory. This process is termed *bacteriostatic activity,* and the ultimate destruction of an infecting organism depends on host defenses. Analogous terms for antifungal agents are *fungicidal* and *fungistatic activity,* respectively.

MIC and MLC or MBC are in vitro measures of activity

The basic measures of the in vitro activity of an antimicrobial agent against an organism are the minimum inhibitory concentration (MIC) and the minimum lethal concentration (MLC) or, in the specific case of bacteria, minimum bactericidal concentration (MBC). The MIC is the least amount that prevents growth of the organism under standardized conditions; the MLC is the least amount required to kill a predetermined portion of an inoculum (usually 99.9%) in a given time. The procedures for determining MICs and MLCs are considered in greater detail later in this chapter. For most clinically effective antimicrobial agents, the MICs for fully susceptible organisms range from 100 to 0.01 µg/ml or less, and successful therapy usually appears to require levels above the MIC at the site of the infection.

Clinical pharmacologic characteristics

The pharmacologic characteristics of antimicrobial agents are critical in deciding their use, their dosage, and the routes and frequency of administration. Among such characteristics are whether they are absorbed from the upper gastrointestinal tract, whether they are excreted and concentrated in active form in the urine, whether and how rapidly they are metabolized, and the duration of effective antimicrobial levels in blood and tissues. Most agents are bound to some extent to serum albumin, and the protein-bound form is usually unavailable for antimicrobial action. The amount of free to bound antibiotic can be described as an equilibrium constant that varies for different antibiotics. In general, high degrees of binding lead to more prolonged but lower serum levels of active antimicrobial agent after a single dose.

Protein binding

Antibiotics are derived from other organisms

There are three sources of antimicrobial agents. The true antibiotics are of biologic origin and probably play an important part in microbial ecology in the natural environment. Penicillin, for example, is produced by several molds of the genus *Penicillium,* and the prototype cephalosporin antibiotics were derived from other molds. The largest source of naturally occurring antibiotics is members of the genus *Streptomyces,* which are Gram-positive, branching bacteria found in soils and freshwater sediments. Streptomycin, the tetracyclines, chloramphenicol, erythromycin, and many others were discovered by the screening of large numbers of *Streptomyces* isolates from different parts of the world. A few antibiotics, mostly with low therapeutic indices, are derived from soil bacteria of the genus *Bacillus,* but because of their toxicity are now limited mostly to local application rather than systemic use. Antibiotics are mass produced by techniques derived from the procedures of the fermentation industry.

Chemotherapeutics are synthetic chemicals

The true chemotherapeutics are chemically synthesized antimicrobial agents. Most of the early chemotherapeutics were discovered among compounds synthesized for other purposes and tested for their therapeutic effectiveness in animals. The sulfonamides, for example, were discovered as a result of routine screening of aniline dyes. More recently, active compounds have been synthesized with structures tailored to be effective inhibitors or competitors of known metabolic pathways. Trimethoprim, which inhibits dihydrofolate reductase, is an excellent example.

Molecular manipulations of antibiotics and chemotherapeutics

The third source of new antimicrobial agents is by molecular manipulation of previously discovered antibiotics or chemotherapeutics to broaden their range and/or degree of activity against microorganisms or improve their clinical pharmacologic characteristics. This approach has been the major thrust of developments over the past 20 years, particularly with the antibiotics. Examples include the development of the penicillinase-resistant and broad-spectrum penicillins, as well as a large range of aminoglycosides and cephalosporins of increasing activity, spectrum, and resistance to inactivating enzymes.

Appropriateness of the term antimicrobic

The distinction between antibiotics and chemotherapeutics has become increasingly irrelevant, because some antibiotics, such as chloramphenicol and aztreonam, are now produced synthetically. The terms continue to be used, but the generic terms *antimicrobic* or *antimicrobial agent* to describe both classes of compounds are preferable, and the term *chemotherapy* is used to describe treatment with antimicrobics or antitumor compounds.

Spectra of antimicrobics

The range of activity of each antimicrobic is called its *spectrum,* a term used to describe the genera and species against which it has been shown to be active. Spectra overlap, but are usually characteristic for each broad class of antimicrobic. Some antibacterial antimicrobics are known as *narrow-spectrum agents;* for example, benzyl penicillin is highly active against many Gram-positive and Gram-negative cocci, but has little activity against enteric Gram-negative bacilli. Chloramphenicol and tetracycline, on the other hand, are *broad-spectrum agents* that inhibit a wide range of Gram-positive and Gram-negative bacteria, including some obligate intracellular organisms. Spectra relate to the general behavior of a genus or species at the time when the antimicrobic was introduced; resistant strains have since been selected within most species, and thus the spectrum of an antimicrobic often does not indicate or predict the behavior of an individual strain. For example, the spectrum of benzyl penicillin is considered to include *Staphylococcus aureus.* although most strains now are penicillin resistant.

Narrow-spectrum agents

Broad-spectrum agents

Mechanisms of bacterial resistance

Bacterial resistance to antimicrobics may be caused by 1) inability of the antimicrobic to traverse the cell envelope; 2) absence of the specific target site of the antimicrobic; 3) ability of the organism to bypass a blocked metabolic pathway; and 4) production by the organism of an enzyme that inactivates the antimicrobic. Resistance to an antimicrobic may be innate to all members of a species and involve any of the above mechanisms, or strains within a susceptible species may develop resistance. Such acquired resistance can be mutational or derived from another organism by one of the mechanisms of genetic exchange described in Chapter 4. Many resistance genes are grouped on plasmids (R plasmids), which can determine resistance to several different antimicrobics. Some of these genes are present on transposable elements that can move from plasmid to plasmid or between plasmid and chromosome. Resistant or multiresistant strains of many previously susceptible species are now encountered, sometimes as the predominant phenotype. Acquired resistance can involve all of the mechanisms responsible for innate resistance, but most frequently results from production of antimicrobic inactivating enzymes.

Innate resistance

Acquired resistance

R plasmid genes can encode resistance to many antimicrobics

Synergistic, additive and antagonistic effects of antimicrobic combinations

Combinations of different classes of antimicrobics may be synergistic, additive, or antagonistic. *Synergy* means that the combined effect is greater than the sum of its parts. For example, a penicillin and an aminoglycoside may kill an enterococcus far more effectively than either acting alone, because inhibition of cell wall synthesis by penicillin allows passage of the highly lethal aminoglycoside to its target in the cell. An *additive effect* means that the effect of the combination is no greater than the sum of its parts. *Antagonism* means that one antimicrobic, usually that with the least important properties, partially prevents the second from expressing its activity. Antagonism occurs with certain combinations of bacteriostatic antimicrobics with a β-lactain antimicrobic, such as penicillin. Penicillin exerts its bacterial effect only on dividing cells, and inhibition of growth by a bacteriostatic antimicrobic may prevent the lethal activity of penicillin.

Use of combinations to prevent resistance

One particular indication for combined therapy with different classes of antimicrobics is a large population of infecting organisms with a relatively high frequency of mutational resistance. If a lesion contains 10^9 organisms, and the frequency of resistant mutants to two antimicrobics, A and B, is 10^{-6} for each, the chance of relapse by selection of a resistant mutant is high with single therapy. The chance of a double mutant, however, is only 10^{-12}, and combined therapy will usually prevent this development. Pulmonary tuberculosis is an example, and established tuberculosis is always treated with two or more effective antimicrobics to reduce the risk of emergence of resistance.

Double resistance mutants are extremely rare

These aspects of antimicrobics, chemotherapy, and resistance will now be considered in more detail under the headings of the modes of action and major groups of antimicrobial agents. Principles will be stressed using antimicrobics commonly employed as examples. Details on specific antimicrobic use, dosage, and toxicity should be sought in one of the specialized texts or handbooks written for that purpose.

Antimicrobics Acting against Cell Wall Synthesis

Review of bacterial cell wall synthesis

Synthesis of the murein sac has been considered in some detail in Chapter 3. It will be recalled that an *N*-acetyl muramic (NAM) acid residue bearing its tetrapeptide with an additional terminal D-alanine is first synthesized in the cytoplasm. This is attached to a carrier molecule, bactoprenol, in the cell membrane where *N*-acetyl glucosamine (NAG) is added. Finally, the NAM–NAG disaccharide with attached peptide is added to the growing glycan chain of the cell wall, and cross-links are established by transpeptidation using energy derived from release of the terminal "excess" D-alanine. These processes have been shown in Figure 2.9. They are unique to bacteria and offer targets that have been points of attack of two of the most important groups of antimicrobics, the β-lactams and the glycopeptides (vancomycin and teicoplanin).

β-Lactam Antimicrobics

Activity of all classes of β-lactams depends on intact β-lactam ring

The β-lactam antimicrobics comprise the penicillins, cephalosporins, carbapenems, and monobactams. The first member of this class of antimicrobics, penicillin, was derived from molds of the genus *Penicillium*. Penicillin and all subsequent natural, semisynthetic, and synthetic β-lactams share possession of a β-lactam ring that is essential to their antibacterial activity.

Pharmacologic properties, activity, and spectra determined by side chains

The basic structural formulas of each of the four major classes of β-lactams is shown in Figure 13.1. Differences in side chains of the basic molecules influence pharmacologic properties and spectra by determining permeability into the bacterial cell, affinity for enzymes involved in cell

13.1. Basic structure of β-lactam antibiotics. a, Different side chains determine degree of activity, spectrum, pharmacologic properties, resistance to β-lactamases; b, β-lactam ring; c, thiazolidine ring; c′, dihydrothiazine ring; d, site of action of β-lactamases; e, site action of amidase.

Penicillins

6-Aminopenicillanic acid

Cephalosporins

7-Aminocephalosporanic acid

Carbapenems

Monobactams

β-Lactams interfere with transpeptidation reactions in cell wall synthesis

Penicillin binding proteins are targets of β-lactam antimicrobics

Role of PBPs in cell wall synthesis

Bactericidal action of β-lactams are usually due to cell lysis

Cell wall-deficient and nongrowing cells not killed by β-lactams

Antimicrobic tolerance

Mechanism of inherent resistance to β-lactams

wall synthesis, and susceptibility or resistance to inactivation by β-lactamases.

The β-lactam antimicrobics interfere primarily with the transpeptidation reactions that seal the peptide cross-links between glycan chains. Their activity is probably due to stereochemical similarity to the D-analyl-D-analine end of the pentapeptide. β-Lactams thus prevent the completion of the murein sac in growing cells.

The target enzymes of the β-lactams occur on the cytoplasmic membrane. They are described as penicillin-binding proteins (PBPs) because they were first detected with penicillin, although many of them bind other β-lactam antimicrobics avidly. Several distinct PBPs occur in any one bacterium, are usually species specific, and vary in their ability to react with different β-lactam antimicrobics. There are also functional differences between PBPs. Some appear to be responsible for forging the peptidoglycan linkages that give an organism its shape, and others are particularly involved in synthesizing the cross-walls that separate newly formed cells. Yet others, not all of which are necessary enzymes, have no known function. A β-lactam that is active primarily on a PBP that determines shape will result in rounding up and swelling of a susceptible organism before lysis occurs. One that acts primarily on cell separation and division can produce long cells with multiple nucleoids that can stretch from one side of a microscopic field to the other.

β-Lactam antimicrobics are usually highly bactericidal to susceptible bacteria. Killing involves attenuation and disruption of the developing peptidoglycan "corset," liberation or activation of autolytic enzymes that further disrupt weakened areas of the wall, and finally osmotic lysis from passage of water through the cytoplasmic membrane to the hypertonic interior of the cell. As would be anticipated, cell wall-deficient organisms, such as *Mycoplasma,* are insusceptible to β-lactam antimicrobics, nongrowing cells are not killed, and osmotically stabilized protoplasts remain viable in the presence of the antimicrobic. Mutations that reduce or eliminate the activity of autolytic enzymes result in diminished lysis and killing by β-lactams and can, in effect, change the action of the antimicrobics from bactericidal to bacteriostatic agents. This phenomenon is termed *tolerance.*

Inherent resistance to β-lactam antimicrobics is sometimes due to lack of susceptible PBPs or to failure to traverse outer membrane porin channels of Gram-negative bacteria because of charge, degree of hydrophobicity, or general molecular configuration. In some cases, inherent resistance is due to chromosomally encoded β-lactamases that open the β-lactam ring and inactivate the antimicrobic. Some chromosomal genes encoding β-lactamase production are under repressor control and subject to induction by certain β-lactam antimicrobics. This leads to increased production of β-lactamase, which usually results in phenotypic resistance to the inducer and to some other β-lactams to which the organism would otherwise be susceptible. Various other chromosomally encoded enzymes with β-lactamase activity are found in very low concentrations in almost all bacterial species, including those highly susceptible to β-lactam antimicrobics. They are believed to be involved in cell wall synthesis and turnover.

Mutational resistance due to change in permeability or PBPs

Acquired resistance to β-lactam antimicrobics can be mutational in which case it usually involves changes in PBPs or alterations in outer membrane proteins and permeability. Because mutations occur at low frequency and are often associated with other effects that are disadvantageous to the cell, strains that are resistant by these mechanisms have tended to evolve slowly. Much more commonly, acquired resistance is due to acquisition of genetic elements encoding β-lactamases. These are often transposable and usually found on plasmids, but may become chromosomal. In nature, they are most frequently acquired by conjugation and sometimes by transduction. Multiple β-lactamases have been described that have different specificities for different antimicrobics. One, the inducible penicillinase of *S. aureus*, now predominates among clinical isolates all over the world. Another, termed *TEM*, is encoded in a transposable element and is particularly significant among Gram-negative organisms in mediating resistance to some important β-lactams. It probably originated in Gram-negative rods of the normal intestinal flora, and has transposed to plasmids of a variety of organisms important in human diseases including enteric Gram-negative pathogens, *Haemophilus influenzae* and *Neisseria gonorrhoeae*. As new β-lactams are developed that are unaffected by most known β-lactamases, genes encoding enzymes with different specificities tend to appear and spread, thus producing further problems of antimicrobic resistance.

Plasmid-determined β-lactamase resistance

Multiple β-lactamases with different antimicrobic specificities

Spread of plasmid genes encoding β-lactamases through different species

Most of the search for new β-lactams has been driven by the need for broader spectra, greater activity, and resistance to commonly occurring β-lactamases. It has, however, also lead to the discovery of β-lactams that inactivate some β-lactamases, but have little or no useful antimicrobic action. Thus, for example, clavulanic acid is a potent inhibitor of some β-lactamases and, when used in combination with certain penicillins that are susceptible to these enzymes, extends their activity to organisms that would otherwise be resistant.

Nonantimicrobic β-lactamase inhibitors

Penicillins. All penicillins are derivatives of 6-aminopenicillanic acid, the basic structure of which is a β-lactam ring linked to a thiazolidine ring (Figure 13.1). Side chains of the molecule confer antibacterial activity and determine the pharmacologic properties and spectrum of the penicillin.

6-Aminopenicillanic acid nucleus

The prototype penicillin is benzyl penicillin (penicillin G), from which earlier semisynthetic penicillins were derived. The action of an enzyme, amidase, breaks the bond between the β-lactam ring and the side chain, allowing other side chains to be added.

Benzyl penicillin and derivatives

Examples of commonly used penicillins, their side chains, and their major properties are shown in Table 13.1. They can be classified conveniently as narrow-spectrum penicillins, narrow-spectrum penicillins re-

Table 13.1 Differential Characteristics of Some Representative Penicillins

Class	Compound	Side Chain	Route of Administration		Resistance to Staphylococcal β-Lactamase	Activity against Some Enterobacteriaceae	Activity against Some Pseudomonas
			Parenteral	Oral			
Narrow spectrum	Benzyl penicillin G	phenyl–CH_2–	+	−	−	−	−
	Penicillin V	phenyl–O–CH_2–	−	+	−	−	−
Narrow spectrum, penicillinase resistant	Nafcillin	naphthyl (OC_2H_5, CH_3 substituents)	+	±	+	−	−
	Dicloxacillin	dichlorophenyl-isoxazolyl (Cl, Cl, N, O, CH_3)	−	+	+	−	−
Broad spectrum	Ampicillin	phenyl–CH(NH_2)–	+	+	−	+	−
	Carbenicillin[a]	phenyl–CH(COOH)–	+	−	−	+	+
Extended spectrum	Piperacillin[b]	phenyl–CH(NH–)– with piperazinedione (C_2H_5–N, N–C=O, O, O)	+	−	−	+	+

[a] Carbenicillin is primarily used in *Pseudomonas* infections.
[b] Piperacillin combines the advantageous properties of ampicillin and carbenicillin, but with greater activity.

sistant to staphylococcal penicillinase, broad-spectrum penicillins, and extended-spectrum penicillins.

Narrow-spectrum penicillins fail to penetrate envelope of most Gram-negative bacteria

The narrow-spectrum penicillins are active mainly against Gram-positive organisms, some Gram-negative cocci, and some spirochetes including the spirochete of syphilis. They have little action against most Gram-negative bacilli, because the outer membrane prevents passage of these antibiotics to their sites of action on cell wall synthesis. Penicillin G is the least toxic and least expensive of all the penicillins. However, it is unstable in acid and, when given by mouth, may be largely destroyed by gastric hydrochloric acid. The modification of the molecule in penicillin V confers acid resistance, and this preparation is used orally.

Acid instability of benzyl penicillin G

Penicillinase-resistant penicillins active against β-lactamase-producing staphylococci

The penicillinase-resistant penicillins also have narrow spectra, but are active against a β-lactamase-producing *S. aureus*. They appear to owe their insusceptibility to the enzyme to steric hindrance resulting from the configuration of their side chain. They are, however, not resistant to other β-lactamases.

Broader-spectrum agents add activity against some Gram negatives

The broader-spectrum penicillins owe their expanded activity to the ability to traverse the outer membrane of some Gram-negative bacteria. Some, such as ampicillin, have excellent activity against a range of Gram-negative pathogens, but are ineffective against an important opportunistic pathogen, *Pseudomonas aeruginosa*. Others, such as carbenicillin, are active against many *Pseudomonas* strains when given in very high dosage, but are less active than ampicillin against some other Gram-negative organisms. It should be noted that broader-spectrum penicillins are all inactivated by staphylococcal penicillinase.

Extended-spectrum penicillins have widest range against Gram-negative rods including *Pseudomonas*

Extended-spectrum penicillins, such as the ureido penicillin piperacillin, are more active than ampicillin and carbenicillin against enteric bacteria and *Pseudomonas* and have a wider spectrum of activity against Gram-negative bacteria.

Mutational and β-lactamase-mediated resistance acquired by many species

Varying proportions of strains resistant to some or most of the penicillins are now encountered among the majority of species that were originally susceptible. In most cases, resistance involves plasmid-mediated β-lactamases, but PBP mutants of increased resistance have been selected among gonococci and pneumococci and probably account for resistance of some staphylococci (methicillin-resistant staphylococci) to the penicillinase-resistant penicillins. Likewise, some permeability mutants have occurred among Gram-negative bacteria. Fortunately, some species that were originally susceptible to penicillin, such as the spirochete of syphilis and group A streptococcus, have thus far retained their susceptibility over the more than four decades of use of the antimicrobic.

Some species (eg, *Treponema pallidum*) have retained original susceptibility

Very low toxicity: hypersensitivity to penicillins

The penicillins are among the least toxic agents used in therapy. Very high concentrations may be associated with convulsions, but doses on the order of 10–30 g a day of benzyl penicillin or carbenicillin are usually well tolerated. Occasionally, hypersensitivity develops to the penicillins. This reaction may be manifested as an anaphylactic type of response (which may sometimes be very severe) or more commonly as serum sickness, fever or skin rash.

Origin and nomenclature

Cephalosporins. The first cephalosporin antimicrobics were derived from cultures of *Cephalosporium* molds. Some members of the group, obtained from cultures of a genus of branching bacteria related to the *Streptomyces*, have been termed the *cefamycins.* Their basic chemical structure is the same, however, and herein we will refer to all of them as cephalosporins.

β-Lactam ring

The cephalosporins resemble the penicillins in possessing a β-lactam ring, the integrity of which is essential to their activity. They differ from

7-aminocephalosporanic acid nucleus

Resistance to staphylococcal β-lactamase

Later cephalosporins resist many Gram-negative β-lactamases

Range of cephalosporins

First-generation cephalosporins

the penicillins in that the five-membered thiazolidine ring is replaced by a six-membered dihydrothiazine ring. The nucleus of the cephalosporins, 7-aminocephalosporanic acid, like 6-aminopenicillanic acid, has little antibacterial action. Activity, pharmacologic properties, and spectra are conferred on the molecule by side chains in the positions indicated in Figure 13.1. The structure of the cephalosporins confers substantial or complete resistance to hydrolysis by staphylococcal penicillinase (β-lactamase), but the β-lactam ring of the earlier members of the group was opened by β-lactamases of many Gram-negative bacilli. The more recently introduced cephalosporins are much more resistant to such enzymatic inactivation, which accounts in part for their wider spectrum.

As with the penicillins, many semisynthetically produced cephalosporins are now available with extended spectra, varying pharmacologic properties and increased resistance to β-lactamases. New compounds continue to be introduced, while others decline in popularity. It would thus be quite unrewarding for the student to attempt to learn the specific details of those currently available. Even for the clinician, it is best to become familiar with two or three cephalosporins and learn to use them well. For these reasons, we will consider only a few representatives of the group, ranging from those with the narrowest to those with the broadest spectrum.

Six cephalosporins are considered in Table 13.2. Those designated first-generation agents have a more restricted spectrum than those developed subsequently. Their spectrum against Gram-positive organisms resembles that of the penicillinase-resistant penicillins, but they are also active against some Gram-negative bacilli (Appendix). They continue to have therapeu-

Table 13.2 Cephalosporins

Class	Compound	Route of Administration		Spectrum
		Parenteral	Oral	
First generation	Cefazolin	+	−	*Staphylococcus aureus* (penicillinase producing and nonproducing) and streptococci (other than enterococci); *Escherichia coli*; *Klebsiella* species; *Proteus mirabilis*
	Cephalexin	−	+	
Second generation[a]	Cefamandole	+	−	First-generation spectrum moderately expanded to include additional Gram-negative species.
	Cefotetan	+	−	Similar to cefamandole plus *Proteus,* and many Gram-negative anaerobes
Third generation[a]	Cefotaxime	+	−	Expanded spectrum against enteric and other Gram-negative rods.
	Cefoperazone	+	−	High activity against *Haemophilus influenzae* and *Neisseria gonorrhoeae*, including β-lactamase-producing strains; active against *Pseudomonas aeruginosa* and many Gram-negative anaerobes

[a] Second- and third-generation cephalosporins have less activity than first-generation agents against Gram-positive organisms. Each agent has specific advantages in activity against particular organisms.

tic value because of their high activity against Gram-positive organisms and because a broader spectrum may be unnecessary and is more likely to predispose the patient to the problem of superinfection. Of the two first-generation cephalosporins listed in Table 13.2, cefazolin must be given parenterally, but the side chains of cephalexin confer acid stability and absorbability and make it an effective oral preparation.

Second-generation cephalosporins

Second-generation cephalosporins are resistant to chromosomally or plasmid-determined β-lactamases of some Gram-negative organisms that inactivate first-generation compounds. For example, cefotetan is active against many strains of *Bacteroides fragilis* and *Serratia* species that are resistant to first-generation compounds and also resists breakdown by the TEM-type β-lactamase.

Third-generation cephalosporins

Third-generation cephalosporins, such as cefotaxime, have an even wider spectrum and are active against Gram-negative organisms in extremely low concentrations. They are resistant to many β-lactamases. Both second- and third-generation cephalosporins are generally less active against Gram-positive cocci than those of the first generation or the penicillins.

Resistance mechanisms

As with the penicillins, resistance to cephalosporins may result from failure to permeate the cell membrane, absence of high-affinity PBPs, lack of cell wall, or plasmid- or chromosomally determined β-lactamases. Many chromosomal β-lactamases of Gram-negative bacilli are cephalosporinases, which inactivate all first-generation compounds. The newer agents are progressively more resistant to such attack, as well as to enzymes that are plasmid encoded. Mutational resistance to several cephalosporins occurs at relatively high frequency ($10^{-6}-10^{-8}$), particularly among *Enterobacter, Citrobacter, Serratia,* and *Pseudomonas* species. Resistance results from mutational depression of a chromosomally encoded cephalosporinase.

Cephalosporinase β-lactamases

Toxicity and hypersensitivity

The cephalosporins now in use are of low toxicity and can be given in large doses for complex infections. Hypersensitivity may develop, but cross-sensitivity to the penicillins is unusual.

Carbapenems. Like the penicillins, carbapenems have a β-lactam ring fused with a second five-membered ring: their name (*carbapen-*) derives from the substitution of a carbon atom for the sulfur of the thiazolidine ring of the penicillins (Figure 13.1). Thienamycin, the parent compound of this category of β-lactam antibiotics, was derived from a species of *Streptomyces,* but is not in use clinically because it is chemically unstable. The only carbapenem currently available in the United States, imipenem, is a stable semisynthetic amidine derivative. Imipenem is rapidly hydrolyzed by a renal tubular dehydropeptidase and is, therefore, coadministered with an inhibitor of this enzyme (cilastatin), which greatly improves its urine levels and other pharmacokinetic characteristics.

Imipenem is administered with inhibitor of renal dehydropeptidase

The mode of action of the carbapenems is similar to that of other β-lactams. They readily penetrate bacterial cells, including Gram-negative bacilli, and the conformation of their side chains renders them highly resistant to β-lactamases of both staphylococci and of most Gram-negative bacilli except *Pseudomonas maltophilia* and *P. cepacia.* Accordingly, carbapenems have the broadest spectrum of all β-lactam antibiotics. They are active against streptococci, more active than cephalosporins against staphylococci, highly active against both β-lactamase positive and negative strains of gonococci and *H. influenzae,* as active as third-generation cephalosporins against Gram-negative rods, and effective against obligate anaerobes. Carbapenems are potent inducers of chromosomal β-lactamases of Gram-negative bacilli, even though they are unaffected by the enzymes.

Carbapenems are highly resistent to most β-lactamases

Very wide spectrum of activity

Combinations of carbapenems with other β-lactams may thus render the latter inactive.

Strains of *P. aeruginosa* frequently develop mutational resistance to imipenem during the course of therapy, probably because of mutational loss of an outer membrane porin leading to impaired penetration. No cross-resistance has been demonstrated with other β-lactam agents. Adverse reactions are uncommon and similar to those of the other β-lactams: cross-hypersensitivity to the penicillins can occur.

Monobactams. Monobactams are naturally occurring substances produced by a variety of soil bacteria. Aztreonam, the first monobactam licensed in the United States, is a natural product of *Chromobacterium violaceum,* but the commercial preparation is produced synthetically.

As their name suggests, monobactams, are monocyclic compounds (see Figure 13.1), a feature that distinguishes them from the other β-lactams. A sulfonic acid group, instead of a fused ring, serves to activate the β-lactam ring. Side chains identical to those found in third-generation cephalosporins are utilized to impart stability and enhanced activity against Gram-negative bacilli, including *P. aeruginosa.* The mode of action is similar to other β-lactam agents, but the spectrum of aztreonam is limited to aerobic and facultatively anaerobic Gram-negative bacteria including *Enterobacteriaceae, P. aeruginosa, Haemophilus,* and *Neisseria.*

Monobactams have poor affinity for the PBPs of Gram-positive organisms and anaerobes and thus little activity against them. They are highly resistant to hydrolysis by plasmid and chromosomally mediated β-lactamases of Gram-negative bacilli and do not induce production of chromosomally encoded enzymes, suggesting they can be used effectively in combination with other β-lactams. Emergence of resistant bacteria has been uncommon and appears to be chromosomally mediated; cross-resistance with other antimicrobial agents is rare. Untoward effects have been similar to those of other β-lactam antimicrobial agents; although hypersensitivity reactions, including anaphylaxis, have been reported, there appears to be little cross-sensitivity with penicillins and cephalosporins. Anaerobic superinfections and major distortions of the bowel flora are less common with aztreonam therapy than with other broad-spectrum β-lactam antimicrobics, presumably because aztreonam does not produce a general suppression of gut anaerobes.

β-Lactamase Inhibitors. A number of β-lactams with little or no antimicrobic activity are capable of binding irreversibly to β-lactamase enzymes and, in the process, rendering them inactive. Two such compounds, clavulanic acid (a clavam, see marginal figure) and sulbactam (a penicillanic acid sulfone), are referred to as *suicide inhibitors,* because they must first be hydrolyzed by a β-lactamase before becoming effective inactivators of the enzyme. Both are highly effective against staphylococcal penicillinases and TEM-type broad-spectrum β-lactamases; their capacity to inhibit cephalosporinases is significantly less. Combinations of one of these inhibitors with an appropriate β-lactam antimicrobic protects the therapeutic agent from destruction by many β-lactamases and significantly enhances its spectrum. Three such combinations are now available in the United States: amoxicillin/clavulanate, ticarcillin/clavulanate, and ampicillin/sulbactam. They all expand the spectrum of their contained penicillin to one roughly approximating that of the second-generation cephalosporins. Bacteria producing chromosomally encoded cephalosporinases that are inducible are not susceptible to the combinations. Whether these three com-

Pseudomonas aeruginosa may develop resistance during therapy

Monocyclic β-lactams

Active against wide range of aerobic and facultative Gram-negative bacteria

Little activity against Gram-positive organisms and anaerobes

Resistant to action of most β-lactamases

Bowel superinfections uncommon with aztreonam

Clavulanic acid

Active against staphylococcal and TEM β-lactamases

Combinations with some penicillins extends their spectra

Little or no activity against cephalosporinases

binations offer therapeutic or economic advantages compared to the β-lactamase stable antibiotics now available remains to be determined.

Clinical Use. The β-lactam antibiotics are usually the drugs of choice for infections by susceptible organisms because of their very high therapeutic index and bactericidal action. They have also proved of great value in the prophylaxis of many infections. They are excreted by the kidney and achieve very high urinary levels. Penicillins reach the cerebrospinal fluid when the meninges are inflamed and are used in the treatment of meningitis due to susceptible organisms. First- and most second-generation cephalosporins show poor penetration even with inflammation and are not appropriate for the treatment of meningitis. In contrast, the third-generation cephalosporins, carbapenems and monobactams, penetrate much better, and their marked activity makes them agents of choice in the treatment of meningitis caused by some Gram-negative organisms.

Glycopeptide Antimicrobics

Two agents, vancomycin and teicoplanin, fall in this group. At the time of writing, teicoplanin has not been approved by the Food and Drug Administration for use in the United States. Each of these antimicrobics inhibits the use of lipid-linked cell wall intermediates in the assembly of the linear peptidoglycan molecule. Both agents are primarily bactericidal and active against Gram-positive organisms. They are particularly useful against strains of *S. aureus* and coagulase-negative staphylococci that are resistant to the penicillinase-resistant penicillins and cephalosporins. They are also useful in the treatment of penicillin-resistant enterococcal endocarditis when used in combination with an aminoglycoside. Neither agent is absorbed by mouth, and both have been used orally to treat *Clostridium difficile* infections of the bowel (Chapter 18), but their main use has been against multiresistant Gram-positive infections and those involving prosthetic devices. Vancomycin is administered intravenously because it is toxic to tissues on local injection. Teicoplanin can also be administered intramuscularly.

Initially, it appeared that resistance to these agents did not occur or was very rare. It has now been shown that mutational resistance in one species of coagulase-negative staphylococci can occur during therapy and plasmid-encoded resistance has been encountered in enterococci. These agents have been of great value when held in reserve for use in infections that are not responsive to β-lactam antimicrobics.

Antimicrobics Acting on the Outer and Cytoplasmic Membranes

The Polymyxins

A number of polypeptide antimicrobics are produced by bacteria of the genus *Bacillus,* which are aerobic, Gram-positive, spore-forming rods living primarily in soil. All the polypeptide antimicrobics are relatively toxic, but two, polymyxin B and polymyxin E (colistin), were used parenterally in the past largely because of activity against *P. aeruginosa* and other Gram-negative rods that were resistant to antimicrobics then available.

The polymyxins have a cationic detergentlike effect. They bind to the cell membranes of susceptible Gram-negative organisms, alter their permeability, and lead to loss of essential cytoplasmic components and

---

Marginal notes (left column):

Agents of choice for susceptible infections

Bactericidal to most Gram-positive organisms

Clinical indications

Resistance although rare, can occur

Activity against *P. aeruginosa*

Detergentlike effect on cell membranes

Toxicity limits usefulness to
topical application

bacterial death. They react to a lesser extent with cell membranes of the host, resulting in nephrotoxicity and neurotoxicity. These agents are now essentially limited to topical applications and have the advantage that resistance to them rarely develops.

Inhibitors of Protein Synthesis at the Ribosomal Level

Aminoglycoside—Aminocyclitol Antibiotics

Origin and structure

The aminoglycoside-aminocyclitol antibiotics are a group of bactericidal agents characterized by combinations of six-membered aminocyclitol rings with varying side chains which determine their spectra and degrees of resistance to inactivating enzymes. The structure of tobramycin is shown in the marginal figure. Streptomycin and other earlier members of the group were produced from species of *Streptomyces*. The newer members are semisynthetic derivatives.

Tobramycin

The most important and commonly used members of the group are listed in Table 13.3, together with some key properties. Streptomycin is now rarely used, except for treatment of tuberculosis or in combination with penicillin for treatment of bacterial endocarditis, because high-level and stable resistant mutants are frequently selected during therapy. Similarly, kanamycin use has declined in relationship to the newer agents. Neomycin, the most toxic aminoglycoside, is used as an oral preparation to reduce the facultative flora of the large intestine before certain types of intestinal surgery. It is very poorly absorbed, and most of its activity is expressed in the bowel. Gentamicin, tobramycin, amikacin, and netilmicin have extended spectra that include activity against many strains of *P. aeruginosa*. Of these, amikacin is the most resistant to aminoglycoside-inactivating enzymes and may thus act on some gentamicin- and tobramycin-resistant strains.

Irreversible inhibition of
protein synthesis

Bactericidal effect

Streptomycin inhibits protein synthesis by combining with the bacterial ribosomal protein designated S12 of the 30S ribosomal subunit. With the newer and more active aminoglycosides, a similar process involves other binding sites on both 30S and 50S subunits, resulting in a broader spectrum of activity that includes many streptomycin-resistant strains. In sufficient concentrations, aminoglycosides bind to the ribosome irreversibly, block initiation complexes, and prevent elongation of polypeptide chains, resulting in a rapid bactericidal effect. Lower concentrations lead to distortion of the site of attachment of messenger (m)RNA, misreading of

Table 13.3 Characteristics of Commonly Used Aminoglycosides

Compound	Single-Step High Mutational Resistance	Anti-Pseudomonas Activity	Susceptibility to Aminoglycoside-Inactivating Enzymes[a]
Streptomycin	+	−	+ + +
Neomycin	+	−	+ + +
Kanamycin	±	−	+ +
Gentamicin	−	+	+
Tobramycin	−	+	+
Amikacin	−	+	±

[a] Number of plus signs indicates the degree of susceptibility to enzymatic attack.

the message, and failure to produce the correct proteins with dramatic effects on growth and bacterial structure.

Active transport into bacterial cells

The aminoglycosides are actively transported into the bacterial cell by a mechanism that involves oxidative phosphorylation. Thus, they have little or no activity against strict anaerobes or facultative organisms that only metabolize fermentatively (for example, streptococci). It appears highly probable that aminoglycoside activity against facultative organisms is similarly reduced in vivo when the oxidation-reduction potential is low.

Inactivity under anaerobic conditions

Eukaryotic ribosomes are resistant to aminoglycosides, and the antimicrobics are not actively transported into eukaryotic cells. These properties account for their selective toxicity and also explain their ineffectiveness against intracellular bacteria such as *Rickettsia* and *Chlamydia*.

Broad spectra other than against anaerobes

The newer aminoglycosides, gentamicin, tobramycin, amikacin and netilmicin have a broad spectrum of bactericidal action against many aerobic and facultative Gram-positive and Gram-negative rods, including *P. aeruginosa*. Their detailed spectrum is given in the appendix. It merits restressing that all anaerobes are resistant to their action and that they have little activity against streptococci, except when cell penetrability is increased by simultaneous action of a β-lactam antibiotic.

Mutational resistance

High-level mutational resistance to streptomycin can occur in a single step because of its single target protein. With more than one molecular target, mutational resistance to the newer aminoglycosides is much less common and of lower level. When it does occur, it usually involves permeability changes across the outer membrane, thus leading to increased resistance to all aminoglycosides.

Plasmid-determined enzymatic resistance

The most common cause of bacterial resistance involves production of one of more of a range of enzymes that can acetylate, adenylate, or phosphorylate various critical groups on the aminoglycoside molecule. This mechanism abrogates or greatly reduces antibacterial activity. Production of these enzymes is determined by transposable genes that are usually plasmid borne. Aminoglycosides have been successively developed with fewer sites susceptible to such inactivation, and amikacin and netilmicin are currently among the most resistant. In many hospitals, plasmids encoding resistance to gentamicin and tobramycin have been selected and have spread to a number of Gram-negative pathogens under the pressure of antimicrobic use. Nevertheless, these antimicrobics have retained a broad range of clinical usefulness.

Newer compounds increasingly resistant to inactivation

Toxicity to auditory and vestibular functions of eighth cranial nerve

All of the aminoglycoside antimicrobics are toxic to varying degrees to the vestibular and auditory branches of the eighth cranial nerve. Kanamycin and amikacin primarily affect hearing, whereas streptomycin and gentamicin are most toxic to vestibular function. The damage can lead to complete and irreversible loss of hearing and balance. These agents may also be toxic to the kidneys. Toxicity to the eighth cranial nerve greatly limits dosage, and even the most recent aminoglycosides have a very low therapeutic index for infections with *P. aeruginosa*. For example, the maximum safe blood level for gentamicin is approximately 9 μg/ml, whereas its MIC for many strains of *P. aeruginosa* is 2–4 μg/ml. Monitoring blood levels during therapy is often essential to ensure adequate, yet nontoxic dosage, especially when renal impairment diminishes excretion of the antimicrobic. The mechanism of toxicity appears to involve concentration in the inner ear fluids and destruction of the critical sensory cells mediating hearing and balance.

Need for blood level monitoring

Clinical uses

The clinical value of the aminoglycosides resides in their rapid bactericidal effect, their broad spectrum, the slow development of resistance to the agents now most often used, and their action against *Pseudomonas* strains that resist many other antimicrobics. They cause fewer disturbances of the normal flora than most other broad-spectrum antimicrobics, probably because of their lack of activity against the predominantly anaerobic flora of the bowel, and because they are only used parenterally for systemic infections. The β-lactam antibiotics often act synergistically with the aminoglycosides, probably because they facilitate aminoglycoside penetration into the bacterial cell. This effect has been exploited in treatment of bacterial endocarditis using combinations of penicillins and aminoglycosides and of severe *P. aeruginosa* infections using carbenicillin or a related analog and one of the aminoglycosides. Synergism is apparent in both in vitro bactericidal studies and in clinical trials. Unexpectedly, it has been found that carbenicillin can slowly inactivate gentamicin in solution. Therefore, these agents are never mixed in the same intravenous bottle.

The aminoglycosides are often used in combination with a β-lactam antibiotic in the initial treatment of life-threatening infections of unknown etiology until the results of cultures are available to allow more specific therapy. Their use has, however, declined with the advent of β-lactams of increasing activity, spectrum, and resistance to β-lactamases.

Tetracyclines

The tetracyclines are a group of antimicrobics of which the prototype, chlortetracycline, was derived from a species of *Streptomyces*. The newest agents are produced semisynthetically. All are absorbed orally and have similar and broad spectra (Appendix), with relatively inconsequential differences in ranges of activity. Acquired resistance to one generally confers resistance to all. Chemically, the tetracyclines are polycyclic compounds that differ from each other in their side groups.

Two classes of compound are now in common use, tetracycline, which produces relatively short therapeutic levels after single doses and is about 65% protein bound, and longer-acting tetracyclines, which are more highly protein bound but are better absorbed and give higher and more prolonged blood levels. In general, they also have a slightly expanded spectrum. Minocycline and doxycycline are examples of longer-acting agents.

Like the aminoglycosides, the tetracyclines are inhibitors of protein synthesis. They are taken into the cell by an energy-dependent process, bind to the 30S subunit of the ribosome, and block attachment of aminoacyl transfer (t)RNA to the mRNA-ribosome complex. Unlike the aminoglycosides, their effect is reversed on dilution; thus, they are bacteriostatic rather than bactericidal.

The tetracyclines are broad-spectrum agents with a range of activity that encompasses most common pathogenic species, including Gram-positive and -negative rods and cocci and both aerobes and anaerobes. They are active against cell wall–deficient organisms such as *Mycoplasma* and L forms and against some obligate intracellular bacteria, including members of the genera *Rickettsia* and *Chlamydia*. There are a few minor differences in spectrum between members of the group. For example, doxycycline has some activity against tetracycline-resistant anaerobic Gram-negative rods of the genus *Bacteroides,* and minocycline has greater activity than tetracycline against meningococci and *Nocardia*.

Tetracycline resistance, whether innate, mutational, or plasmid determined, appears to involve failure of the antimicrobics to permeate the cell. Inactivating enzymes do not appear to play a role. Resistant strains

Synergistic activity with β-lactam antimicrobics

Orally absorbed agents

Tetracycline

Longer-acting tetracyclines

Reversible inhibition of protein synthesis: bacteriostatic activity

Broad-spectrum includes obligate intracellular bacteria

Resistance involves failure to permeate

of most pathogenic species are now common and have been selected by the extensive use of these antimicrobics.

Absorption and excretion

The tetracyclines are chelated by divalent cations, and their absorption and activity reduced. Thus, they should not be taken with dairy products or many antacid preparations. Tetracyclines are excreted in the bile and urine in active form.

Discoloration of developing teeth

The tetracyclines have a strong affinity for developing bone and teeth, to which they give a yellowish color and are avoided in children up to 8 years of age. Common complications of tetracycline therapy are gastrointestinal disturbance due to alteration of the normal flora and superinfection

Gastrointestinal superinfections

with tetracycline-resistant organisms and vaginal or oral candidiasis (thrush) due to the opportunistic yeast *Candida albicans*.

Clinical uses

Because of their broad spectrum, the tetracyclines have been used extensively in the treatment of polymicrobial infections or infections of unknown etiology derived from the respiratory or gastrointestinal tracts. They have been widely used in the treatment of otitis media and sinusitis, because the most common etiologic agents are usually susceptible. In many cases, however, they have been used in the treatment of viral infections, against which they are quite inactive.

Tetracyclines are agents of choice in the treatment of infections caused by the obligate intracellular parasites *Rickettsia* and *Chlamydia* and by *Mycoplasma*. They have been used as alternates to penicillin in the treatment of the spirochete of syphilis and of the gonococcus, although many strains of gonococci are now relatively resistant. They were used in the past as primary agents in the treatment of infections caused by intestinal anaerobes, but many are now resistant. Probably no group of antimicrobics has been more overprescribed, and thus has contributed significantly to the overall problem of resistance.

Chloramphenicol

Chloramphenicol is a broad-spectrum, orally adsorbed antimicrobic originally derived from a culture of *Streptomyces*. Its relatively simple structure allowed its chemical synthesis, and it has since been produced commercially in this way.

Chloramphenicol

Bacteriostatic protein synthesis inhibitor

Chloramphenicol acts at the level of the 50S ribosomal subunit by inhibiting peptidyl transferase and thus prevents protein synthesis. Its action is reversed by dilution, and it is thus bacteriostatic. It has little effect on eukaryotic ribosomes, which explains its selective toxicity. Chloramphenicol is a broad-spectrum antibiotic that, like tetracycline, has a wide range of activity against both aerobic and anaerobic species (Appendix). It permeates readily into mammalian cells and is active against *Rickettsia* and

Permeability into cells and across blood-brain barrier

Chlamydia. It also crosses the blood-brain barrier and attains excellent levels in the cerebrospinal fluid. Its use is restricted, however, by its occasional severe toxicity.

Resistance by plasmid-encoded chloramphenicol acetylase

Acquired resistance to chloramphenicol is usually determined by plasmid genes encoding production of the enzyme chloramphenicol acetyl transferase. This enzyme acetylates and inactivates the antimicrobic. It is of interest that chloramphenicol resistance is much less common than tetracycline resistance, which probably reflects the less frequent use of chloramphenicol because of its toxicity.

Absorption and metabolism; urine levels low

Chloramphenicol is readily adsorbed from the upper gastrointestinal tract. It is conjugated in the liver to the glucuronide form, which has no antimicrobial activity. Little of the dose is excreted in the urine or bile.

Unlike those of most antimicrobics, urine levels of chloramphenicol are low, and it is not useful in urinary tract infections.

Bone marrow aplasia

High and prolonged doses of chloramphenicol result in some inhibition of blood-forming cells in the bone marrow (marrow hypoplasia). This inhibition is reversed on cessation of therapy and probably results from the action of the antimicrobic on host mitochondrial ribosomes. Occasionally, and probably by a different mechanism, progressive bone marrow aplasia with aplastic anemia and agranulocytosis develops even after low dosages and it is often fatal. The development of this complication in about 1 in 50,000 patients restricted the use of the antimicrobic to a limited number of highly specific indications. Chloramphenicol may also produce gray syndrome in the neonate, with abdominal, circulatory, and respiratory dysfunction. This syndrome, which can be fatal, results from excessive levels of active antibiotic because of failure of the infant liver to conjugate chloramphenicol to the glucuronide. Use of the drug is usually avoided in infants less than 1 month of age.

Aplastic anemia and agranulocytosis are serious complications

Gray syndrome

Clinical uses

Chloramphenicol is now largely restricted to treatment of severe infections for which its spectrum and diffusibility make it particularly valuable. These infections include typhoid fever, ampicillin-resistant *H. influenzae* meningitis, pyogenic coccal meningitis infections when the penicillins are contraindicated, intraabdominal anaerobic Gram-negative infections, and some cases of cerebral abscess. It is also an alternative to tetracycline in the treatment of *Rickettsia* infections. As with the tetracyclines, it is now much less used because of the availability of new β-lactams with equivalent spectra.

Erythromycin and Lincosamide Antibiotics

Macrolides and lincosamides

Erythromycin is the most commonly used of a group of antimicrobics termed the *macrolides*. The lincosamides, lincomycin and clindamycin (7-chlorolincomycin), are chemically unrelated to the macrolides but have similar modes of action and spectra and are thus considered with them.

Protein synthesis inhibitors

Predominantly bacteriostatic effect

Spectra

Erythromycin and lincomycin are derived from different species of *Streptomyces*. Both act on protein synthesis at the ribosomal level by binding to the 50S subunit and blocking the translocation reaction. The effect on sensitive bacteria is primarily bacteriostatic, but a higher proportion of the population is killed than is the case with chloramphenicol. Erythromycin has a spectrum of activity that is close to that of benzyl penicillin, but also includes penicillinase-producing *S. aureus, Legionella pneumophila, Mycoplasma pneumoniae,* and *Chlamydia trachomatis*. Lincomycin has a generally similar spectrum. Clindamycin, a more active compound, is highly effective against many Gram-negative and Gram-positive anaerobic bacteria (Appendix).

Mutational and plasmid-determined resistance

Mutational and plasmid-determined resistance occurs with both erythromycin and lincomycin. The former sometimes develops during therapy and may decrease permeability or affect the ribosomes so that the antimicrobics are not bound. Plasmid-determined resistance involves methylation of ribosomal RNA, which is induced by erythromycin and prevents its binding. Interestingly, induction with erythromycin leads to clindamycin resistance, although the reverse is unusual.

Absorption and excretion

Oral and intravenous preparations of both erythromycin and the lincosamides are available. Both classes of antimicrobics are eliminated by the liver, in the bile, and, to a much lesser extent, through the kidney.

Erythromycin in the estolate form can cause a reversible hepatitis, but is otherwise of low toxicity. Clindamycin can also be mildly hepatotoxic,

Clindamycin associated
pseudomembranous
enterocolitis

but the most serious complication of treatment is pseudomembranous enterocolitis as a result of inhibition of most of the anaerobic flora of the bowel and overgrowth by the clindamycin-resistant *C. difficile,* which elaborates both a cytotoxin and enterotoxin. These toxins are discussed in more detail in Chapter 18.

Therapeutic uses

Erythromycin is the drug of choice in treating Legionnaires' disease and, in the event that they need treatment, *Campylobacter* intestinal infections. It is effective in some *Chlamydia* and *Mycoplasma* infections. Clindamycin has displaced lincomycin in therapy, and its major role is in treating serious anaerobic Gram-negative infections.

Inhibitors of Nucleic Acid Synthesis and Replication

The Quinolones

The quinolones (see Figure 13.2) have a nucleus of two fused six-membered rings and are produced synthetically. The first antimicrobic of this class was nalidixic acid, which had limited clinical value because therapeutic levels were only attained in the urine, and high-level, single-step mutational resistance developed rapidly. More recently, a series of fluoroquinolones have been developed that give excellent levels of bactericidal activity against a wide range of organisms, have low protein binding, can be administered orally, and are much less prone to the development of resistance.

Broad-spectrum bactericidal
activity of fluoroquinolones

Fluorine atom enhances
Gram-negative activity and
adds Gram-positive spectrum

The fluoroquinolones differ from nalidixic acid in the presence of fluorine and piperazine substitutes at the 6- and 7-positions, respectively. Fluorine enhances activity against Gram-negative organisms and adds activity against Gram positives. Piperazine improves tissue concentrations and provides activity against *P. aeruginosa.* Two fluoroquinolones, norfloxacin and ciprofloxacin, have been approved for use in the United States at the time of writing, and their formulas are shown in Figure 13.2 with that of nalidixic acid.

Norfloxacin and ciprofloxacin

Inhibit DNA gyrase

Like nalidixic acid, the primary target of the fluoroquinolones appears to be bacterial DNA gyrase, which is the enzyme responsible for supercoiling, nicking, and sealing bacterial DNA. Four genes encode four subunits of the enzymes, only one of which is the target of nalidixic acid. This explains the occurrence of high-level, single-step mutations to resistance to this agent. It appears that the fluoroquinolones have more than one target on the enzyme, which greatly reduces the chance of such an occurrence. Resistant strains can, however, be selected in vitro and have

13.2. Examples of structures of quinolones and fluoroquinolones.

Permeability mutations can cause resistance

also been described in clinical isolates. The most significant appear to be permeability mutants. Neither enzymatic inactivation of fluoroquinolones nor plasmid-mediated resistance have been observed.

The fluoroquinolones are highly active and bactericidal against a wide range of aerobes and facultative anaerobes. However, streptococci, *Chlamydia,* and *Mycoplasma* are only marginally susceptible, and anaerobes are generally resistant. Ciprofloxacin is a particularly useful agent against *P. aeruginosa.*

Wide spectrum includes *P. aeruginosa,* little or no activity against anaerobes

Oral administration and excellent pharmocologic properties

In addition to their broad spectrum, fluoroquinolones possess a number of favorable pharmacological properties. These include oral administration, low protein binding, good distribution to all body compartments, penetration of phagocytes, and a prolonged serum half-life that allows once or twice a day dosing. Blood levels with accepted dosage are lower than those achieved with most antimicrobics, but this is offset by much lower MICs against most susceptible organisms. Both norfloxacin and ciprofloxacin are excreted by hepatic and renal routes, resulting in high drug concentrations in the bile and urine.

Adverse effects with the fluoroquinolones are relatively uncommon with recommended dosage. The antimicrobics concentrate in and damage cartilage of young animals and consequently are not recommended for use in children and in pregnant or nursing women.

Metabolic Inhibitors

Folate Inhibitors

The use of metabolic inhibitors as antimicrobics must exploit pathways that are present in microorganisms, but not in the host. The major successes in this field have been with agents that interfere with synthesis of folic acid by bacteria, because mammalian cells are unable to accomplish this feat and use preformed folate from dietary sources.

Many bacteria must synthesize folate; mammalian cells use dietary folate

Functions of folic acid

Folic acid is derived from *para*-aminobenzoic acid (PABA), glutamate, and a pteridine unit. In its reduced form it is an essential coenzyme for the transport of one-carbon compounds in the synthesis of purines, thymidine, and some amino acids and, thus, indirectly of nucleic acids and proteins. The major inhibitors of the folate pathway are the sulfonamides, trimethoprim, *para*-aminosalicylic acid, and the sulfones. The two latter are of significance only in mycobacterial infections and will be considered in Chapter 27.

Origin and structure

NH$_2$ NH$_2$

SO$_2$NHR   COOH

Sulfonamides   p-Aminobenzoic acid

Sulfonamides. Shortly after Domagk demonstrated the chemotherapeutic effectiveness of Prontosil Rubrum in 1935, Trefouel in Paris showed that the active portion of the molecule was *para*-aminobenzene sulfonamide, which was termed *sulfanilamide.* Subsequently, numerous compounds were synthesized with substitutions of the amide group. These compounds provided increased activity and special pharmacologic properties, such as higher or more prolonged blood levels, greater solubility in urine, or failure to be absorbed from the intestinal tract.

Competitive inhibition of PABA metabolism and effect on folate synthesis

Sulfonamides are structural analogs of PABA and compete with it for the enzyme (dihydropteroate synthetase) that combines PABA and pteridine in the initial stage of folate synthesis. Differences in the activity of the various sulfonamides largely reflect their ability to compete with PABA for this enzyme system.

Sulfonamides are bacteriostatic

The effect of sulfonamides is exclusively bacteriostatic, and addition of PABA to a medium that contains them neutralizes the inhibitory effect and allows growth to resume. This quality is exploited in the clinical laboratory by adding PABA to blood cultures drawn from patients on sulfonamide therapy.

Spectrum

Originally, the more active sulfonamides had a very broad spectrum that included pathogenic streptococci, pneumococci, a number of enteric Gram-negative rods (especially *Escherichia coli*), the gonococcus and meningococcus, and *Chlamydia*. They also had some activity against pathogenic staphylococci and anaerobes. Unfortunately, resistance developed and spread quickly, and their activity is now unpredictable without laboratory tests for measuring susceptibility.

Mutational and plasmid-determined resistance

Both mutational and R plasmid—mediated resistances are common in susceptible species. Resistance encoded in R plasmids usually involves decreased permeability to sulfonamides. Mutational resistance can involve decreased affinity for sulfonamides of the enzyme handling PABA, decreased permeability, or occasionally enhanced PABA production.

Absorption and excretion

Sulfonamides are well absorbed by the oral route, except those specifically designed to act only within the intestinal tract. They penetrate readily into host cells and across the blood-brain barrier. They are excreted in the urine, predominantly in active form, and very high urine levels are achieved.

Sulfonamide toxicity

Most toxic effects of the sulfonamides are hypersensitivity phenomena. They include fever, rashes, and a serum-sicknesslike syndrome. Occasionally, bone marrow depression occurs, which may progress to agranulocytosis or aplastic anemia.

Clinical uses

Sulfonamides combined with trimethoprim are still among the agents of choice for treatment of uncomplicated primary urinary tract infections, because most strains of *E. coli* encountered in the community have retained their susceptibility. Sulfonamides are also used in the treatment of some *Chlamydia* infections, in prophylaxis of meningococcal infections during epidemics caused by susceptible strains, and in the treatment of *Nocardia* infections (Chapter 28). They have little or no activity in abscesses or markedly purulent exudates, because disintegrating inflammatory cells provide many of the end products of folate activity that, like PABA, can neutralize the effects of sulfonamides. They have limited clinical value compared to the more powerful antibiotics, but their range of utility is considerably extended when combined with trimethoprim.

Competitive inhibitor of bacterial dihydrofolate reductase

Trimethoprim. Trimethoprim is a synthetic structural analog of the pteridine portion of the folic acid molecule. It competitively inhibits the activity of bacterial dihydrofolate reductase, which catalyzes the conversion of folate to its reduced active coenzyme form. Trimethoprim has little activity against the mammalian enzyme. As would be expected, this effect is not neutralized by PABA, but can be reversed by end products of essential reactions for which tetrahydrofolate serves as a coenzyme, particularly by thymidine. Trimethoprim is primarily bacteriostatic. When combined with a sulfonamide, the sequential blockade of the pathway leading to production of tetrahydrofolate often results in synergistic bacteriostatic or bactericidal effects. This quality is exploited in therapeutic preparations combining both agents in concentrations designed to give optimum synergy in vivo.

Synergism and bactericidal effects of mixtures with sulfonamides

Spectrum

Trimethoprim inhibits a considerable range of Gram-positive and Gram-negative facultative bacteria (Appendix), including those causing enteric and urinary tract infections. It is also active against some eukaryotic pathogens, including the malarial parasite and *Pneumocystis carinii* (Chapter 50).

Mutational and plasmid-
determined resistance

Absorption, excretion, and
toxicity

Acquired resistance can be mutational or plasmid mediated. The latter involves production of large amounts of a plasmid-encoded dihydrofolate reductase for which trimethoprim has a lower affinity.

Trimethoprim is readily absorbed by mouth and is excreted in the urine, yielding very high levels. Combinations with sulfonamides have a range of toxicities similar to that of the sulfonamides themselves. The most important potential side effect of trimethoprim is folate deficiency. Despite its poor affinity for mammalian dihydrofolate reductase, those on the verge of folate deficiency may become deficient during trimethoprim therapy. For this reason, trimethoprim is avoided in the newborn and during pregnancy.

Clinical uses

Trimethoprim-sulfonamide combination is widely and effectively used in the treatment of many urinary tract infections and in the treatment of otitis media and sinusitis (partly because of activity against *H. influenzae*), prostatitis, typhoid fever, and bacillary dysentery. It is the agent of choice in the treatment of pneumonia due to *P. carinii*.

The major characteristics of the antimicrobics discussed above are summarized in Table 13.4.

Other Clinically Valuable Antibacterial Agents

Several other effective antimicrobics are in use for special types of infections such as tuberculosis, urinary tract infections, and anaerobic infections. It is beyond the scope and intent of this book to provide comprehensive coverage of all available agents, if only because the field is rapidly changing. Table 13.5 lists a number of the commonly used agents that are not discussed herein, together with their more important properties and uses.

Laboratory Tests in Chemotherapy

Range of laboratory tests

The discovery of the great majority of effective antimicrobics and the characterization of their spectra were based on in vitro tests in the laboratory, and similar tests have become increasingly important in clinical work. Susceptibility tests to determine the responsiveness of individual strains of a species are often needed when resistance has become common through widespread use of the antimicrobic. Tests to determine bactericidal activity are sometimes used because infections in immunocompromised patients may only be controlled by agents or combinations that will kill the infecting strain in the absence of host defense factors. Measurements of levels of antimicrobics in blood or other fluids have become routine with agents such as the aminoglycosides for which the toxic and therapeutic levels are relatively close. It is, therefore, important to understand the principle of these tests.

Antimicrobic susceptibility
tests

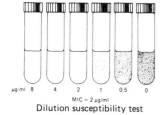

μg/ml   8   4   2   1   0.5   0

MIC = 2 μg/ml

Dilution susceptibility test

Manual antimicrobic susceptibility tests, which are used to determine the inhibitory activity of an antimicrobic against a particular strain, are of two broad classes termed *dilution* and *diffusion tests*. Dilution susceptibility tests are the most direct. In a typical macrodilution test, twofold dilutions of the antimicrobic are prepared in 1-ml amounts of broth in test tubes to span a clinically significant range of concentrations. A control tube without antimicrobic is included. One-milliliter quantities of broth containing 10^5–10^6 bacteria to be tested are then added to each tube, thus diluting the original antimicrobic concentration in half. The tubes are incubated overnight and examined for turbidity from bacterial growth. The least amount of antimicrobic to prevent any visible growth is taken as the MIC of the organism. Macrodilution tests such as that described are cum-

Table 13.4 Summary of Activity of Some Antibacterial Antimicrobics

Agents	Mode of Action	Basis of Selective Toxicity	Major Mechanisms of Acquired Resistance	Spectrum[a]	Effect
A. Cell Wall–Active Compounds					
β-Lactams (penicillins, cephalosporins, etc)	Inhibit final transpeptidation reaction in cross-linking peptidoglycan (3rd stage of murein synthesis)	Absence of peptidoglycan in mammalian cells	β-Lactamase production (P, M); permeability alteration (M); alteration of penicillin-binding proteins (M)	G+G−	Cidal
Vancomycin	Inhibits utilization of lipid-linked intermediate (2nd stage of murein synthesis)	Absence of peptidoglycan in mammalian cells	Very rare (M, P)	G+	Cidal
Cycloserine	Structural analog of D-analine; inhibits alanine racemase, preventing formation of pentapeptide (1st stage of murein synthesis)	Absence of peptidoglycan in mammalian cells	?	G+G− Primarily mycobacteria	Cidal
B. Outer and Cytoplasmid Membrane–Active Compounds					
Polymyxins	Cationic surfactants bind to and disrupt outer and cytoplasmic membranes	Lower toxicity to mammalian cell membranes	None	G−	Cidal
C. Inhibitors of Protein Synthesis at Ribosomal Level					
Streptomycin	Binds to 30S subunit; causes misreading and irreversible inhibition of protein synthesis	Differences between bacterial (70S) and mammalian (80S) ribosomes	Ribosomal and permeability alterations (M); antibiotic-modifying enzymes (P)	G+G−	Cidal
Other aminoglycosides	Similar to streptomycin but other targets on ribosomes	Differences between bacterial (70S) and mammalian (80S) ribosomes	Ribosomal and permeability alterations (M);	G+G−	Cidal

Agent	Mechanism of action	Basis of selective toxicity	Mechanism of resistance	Spectrum	Cidal/Static
	30S and 50S subunits		antibiotic-modifying enzymes (P)		
Tetracyclines	Reversibly bind to 30S subunit, inhibits binding of aminoacyl tRNA	Differences between bacterial (70S) and mammalian (80S) ribosomes	Permeability and uptake change (P)	G + G −	Static
Chloramphenicol	Reversibly binds to 50S subunit; inhibits peptidyl transferase and peptide bond formation	Differences between bacterial (70S) and mammalian (80S) ribosomes	Antibiotic-modifying enzyme (P)	G + G −	Static
Erythromycin and lincomycin	Bind to 50S subunit; inhibit peptidyl transferase and translocation reactions	Differences between bacterial (70S) and mammalian (80S) ribosomes	Inducible methylation of ribosomal RNA (P); alteration of 50S binding site (M)	G + (G − and G + anaerobes in case of clindamycin)	Static in most cases

D. Nucleic Acid Synthesis and Replication

Agent	Mechanism of action	Basis of selective toxicity	Mechanism of resistance	Spectrum	Cidal/Static
Quinolones (derivatives of nalidixic acid)	Inhibit DNA gyrase and thus replication	Analogous mammalian enzymes insensitive	Target alteration (M)	G − G +	Cidal
Rifampin	Inhibits DNA dependent RNA polymerase (transcription)	Mammalian enzyme insensitive	Target alteration (M)	G + and mycobacteria	Cidal

E. Metabolic Inhibitory

Agent	Mechanism of action	Basis of selective toxicity	Mechanism of resistance	Spectrum	Cidal/Static
Sulfonamides	Competive inhibitors of enzyme handling PABA in folate synthesis pathway	Mammalian cells require preformed folate	Altered enzyme with poor affinity for sulfas (P, M); decreased permeability (P, M)	G + G −	Static
Trimethoprim	Competitive inhibitor of dihydrofolate reductase	Mammalian enzyme essentially unaffected	Altered enzyme with poor affinity for trimethoprim (P)	G + G −	Static

Abbreviations: Mechanism of resistance, P = usually plasmid or transposon coded; M = mutational. Spectrum, G + = Gram positive; G − = Gram negative. PABA, *para*-aminobenzoic acid.

[a] Not all species in these classes are inhibited by an agent.

Table 13.5 Some Other Antibacterial Antimicrobics

Compound	Route of Administration		Mechanism	Major Spectrum	Clinical Usage	Special Properties
	Parenteral	Oral				
Nitrofurantoin	−	+	?	Enteric Gram-negative rods and enterococci	Urinary tract infections	Absent blood levels
Spectinomycin	+	−	Protein synthesis inhibition	Gonococcus	Penicillin-resistant gonorrhea	Unique aminoglycoside
Rifampin	−	+	Blocks initiation of transcription	Gram-positive bacteria, Neisseria, and Mycobacteria	Tuberculosis meningococcal carriage	High mutation rate to resistance
p-Aminosalicylic acid	−	+	PABA antagonist	Mycobacteria	Tuberculosis	Gastrointestinal disturbances
Isoniazid	−	+	? Inhibition of lipid synthesis	Mycobacteria	Tuberculosis	Neurotoxicity and nephrotoxicity
Ethambutol	−	+	?	Mycobacteria	Tuberculosis	Visual disturbances
Sulfones	−	+	PABA antagonists	M. leprae; some protozoa	Leprosy	Anemia; hypersensitivity reactions
Metronidazole	−	+	Interference with anaerobic metabolism	Anaerobic Gram-negative rods; some protozoa	Anaerobic infections	? Teratogenic

Abbreviations: PABA = *para*-aminobenzoic acid; ? = mechanisms yet to be fully determined.

bersome, and mechanized microdilution test procedures have been developed for routine use.

Automated procedures can determine MICs indirectly

Automated instruments are now available that measure bacterial growth turbidimetrically and indirectly determine MICs to individual antimicrobial agents by comparing the differences in the organism's growth in control and antimicrobic-containing compartments. Results are based on computer-analyzed algorithms and are usually available within several hours.

Results of susceptibility test procedures are influenced by a variety of methodological factors; however, reference procedures and standard control strains of defined performance have allowed the different procedures to give reasonably comparable results. With certain defined exceptions, results of automated early-read procedures correlate well with those of overnight dilution tests. In most clinical situations, successful treatment requires that the MIC of an antimicrobic for an organism should be substantially below the level achieved at the site of infection.

Diffusion susceptibility tests are less direct, but are simple, economic, and flexible for routine use. A standardized inoculum of the organism to be tested is seeded onto the surface of an agar plate, and filter paper discs containing defined amounts of antimicrobics are applied. The plates are then incubated overnight. The antimicrobic diffuses from each disc into the medium at a rate dependent on its chemical and physical characteristics. Zones of inhibition of growth of the organism develop, the diameter of which is determined by the susceptibility (MIC) of the organism, its growth rate, and the diffusibility of the antimicrobic. For common pathogenic bacteria such as the Enterobacteriaceae, *Pseudomonas*, staphylococci, and enterococci, differences in growth rate are relatively unimportant, and there is an inverse linear relationship between log MIC of such organisms and zone diameter. Thus, semiquantitative susceptibilities can be determined by a standardized procedure. The National Committee for Clinical Laboratory Standards (Kirby–Bauer) method used in the United States is such a standardized diffusion procedure. The diameters of the zones of inhibition obtained with the various antibiotics are measured and converted to "sensitive," "resistant," and "intermediate" categories by reference to a table. *Sensitive* implies that the organism is readily inhibited by the concentrations of antibiotic attainable in the blood (or urine, in the case of those agents only active in the urinary tract) with doses appropriate for treatment of uncomplicated systemic infections caused by the infecting organism. *Resistant* implies that the organism is not inhibited by normally attainable levels. Organisms in the *intermediate* range should be specially studied if therapy with that agent is to be used. The categories were developed by comparisons of zone diameter, MIC, and blood level data and from studies on the distribution of zone diameters (susceptibilities) of many species of known clinical responsiveness.

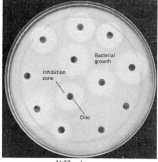

diffusion test

Interpretation of categories of susceptibility

Qualifications to definitions of resistance and sensitivity

Resistance and sensitivity are not always absolute. For example, relatively nontoxic antimicrobial agents, such as the penicillins or cephalosporins, can be administered in massive doses and may thereby inhibit some pathogens that would normally be considered resistant in vitro. Furthermore, in urinary infections, urine levels of some antimicrobics may be very high, and organisms that are seemingly resistant in vitro may be eliminated. When such therapy is considered, dilution tests are often needed for guidance. Diffusion tests with slow-growing organisms and with very poorly diffusing antimicrobics such as the polymyxins must be interpreted with caution. Resistance is significant, but sensitivity may need checking by a dilution test if systemic infections are to be treated. Obviously, diffusion tests do not measure bactericidal effects.

Tests of Bactericidal Activity

Methods for determining rate of killing by antimicrobics

Broth dilution tests can be adapted to determine the bactericidal or bacteriostatic effects of the antimicrobic on the organism tested. The number of viable organisms in the inoculum is measured, and samples are removed at intervals from tubes containing antimicrobic for viable counts (Chapter 3). Such counts can indicate the rate of killing if precautions are taken to ensure that the entire inoculum is exposed to antimicrobic and that antimicrobic carried over to the counting medium is either sufficiently diluted or neutralized to prevent any inhibition on the agar plate. A more commonly used procedure is simple measurement of the MBC, which is defined as the least amount of antimicrobic to kill 99.9% of an inoculum under standardized conditions after overnight incubation. Unfortunately, this measurement is subject to a series of technical problems that make it considerably less valuable than the more complex study of the rate of killing.

MBC tests

Limits of Sensitivity Tests

Other factors influencing effectiveness and selection of antimicrobics

In selecting therapy, the results of laboratory tests cannot be taken alone, but must be considered with information about the clinical pharmacology of the agent, the cause of the disease, the site of infection, and the pathology of the lesion. All of these factors will be taken into account in selecting the appropriate antimicrobic from those to which the organism has been reported as sensitive. Obviously, if the agent cannot reach the site of infection, it will be ineffective. For example, it must reach the subarachnoid space and cerebrospinal fluid in the case of meningitis. Similarly, therapy may be ineffective for an infection that has resulted in abscess formation unless the abscess is surgically drained. In some instances (for example, bacterial endocarditis or agranulocytosis), it is necessary to use an agent that is bactericidal, and an ordinary sensitivity test will not indicate this property. Previous clinical experience is also critical. In typhoid fever, for instance, chloramphenicol is effective and aminoglycosides are not, even though the typhoid bacillus may be sensitive to both in vitro. This finding appears to result from the failure of aminoglycosides to achieve adequate concentrations inside infected cells.

Antimicrobic Assays

Physical, chemical, and immunologic procedures are used

Bioassay

Levels of antimicrobic in blood and body fluids may be measured biologically, but, increasingly, physical, chemical, and immunological techniques, such as high-pressure liquid chromatography or radioimmunoassay, are used. Most bioassays use diffusion techniques in which zones of inhibition of a highly susceptible standard assay strain are measured around wells in an agar plate that have been filled with the material to be assayed and with different known concentrations of the relevant antimicrobic. A curve is plotted relating zone diameters to the known concentrations, and the concentration of antimicrobic in the unknown preparation is determined by relating the zone diameter it has produced to this curve. It is important for the laboratory to know whether more than one antimicrobic is being used to treat a patient, so that steps are taken to ensure that only the activity of the agent under consideration is being measured. For example, if gentamicin levels are to be measured in the presence of carbenicillin, a β-lactamase preparation can be added to inactivate the penicillin.

Other Tests

Tests of serum activity against infecting strain

Sometimes it is desirable to determine directly the effectiveness of antimicrobic levels in the patient's serum against the infecting organism. Dilutions of the patient's serum can be made in normal serum and equal amounts of broth added containing 10^5/ml of the infecting organism. After incubation, the inhibitory activity and, if desired, the lethal activity are measured as in MIC and MBC tests and expressed according to effective dilutions of the patients' serum. Tests of the activity of combinations of antimicrobial agents are sometimes important. These tests are made by inoculating the infecting organism into broth containing clinically relevant amounts of the antibiotics being studied, both alone and in combination. The tubes are incubated and quantitative counts made at intervals. This approach will indicate whether the effects of the combinations are synergistic, additive, or antagonistic.

Tests of antibiotic combinations

Selection and Administration of Antibacterial Antimicrobics

This topic is largely beyond the scope of the book, but a few principles merit stressing. Most bacterial infections are now potentially curable by chemotherapy alone or as an adjunct to surgical or other treatment, but the plethora of antimicrobics available to the physician makes the selection of the most appropriate agent(s) a particular challenge. Ideally the cause of the infection and its susceptibility to relevant antimicrobics would be known before treatment is initiated. This may be possible in subacute or chronic infections or in localized infections in which delay will not jeopardize the patient. However, in most cases of serious infection, the time required to obtain these data is unacceptable and a decision must be made as to which agents to use pending more specific information. The factors involved in this decision include

Treatment must often begin empirically

Factors influencing choice before definite diagnosis

1. Clinical signs and tests that indicate the most probable infection and infectious agent(s). In some cases these may be diagnostic, for example, when the clinical picture and cerebrospinal fluid cytology indicate bacterial meningitis, and the direct Gram smear shows an organism resembling a meningococcus. In others they are less specific, as when a computed tomographic scan indicates an abscess derived from the colon suggesting an infection with aerobes and anaerobes derived from the intestinal flora. In others, a very wide range of etiologic possibilities may exist, for example, when clinical findings suggest the development of bacteremia in a patient with agranulocytosis.

2. Previous experience from the literature as to the effectiveness of particular agents against the range of etiologic possibilities. For example, penicillin may be expected to be effective in the case of meningococcal meningitis, whereas antimicrobial therapy covering both aerobic and anaerobic intestinal flora will be needed for a paraintestinal abscess. In the case of possible bacteremia in agranulocytosis, broad-spectrum bactericidal antimicrobics covering the commonest organisms shown to be associated with this condition will be needed.

3. Account must be taken of recent data concerning the proportions of susceptible and resistant organisms among each species that may be etiologically involved. This is particularly important in hospital-acquired infections, and most clinical laboratories make updated information available from at regular intervals.

In all serious or potentially serious infections, it is essential that the appropriate specimens be obtained from the patient *before the initiation of therapy* so that a specific diagnosis may be made and the susceptibility of the etiologic agent(s) definitively established as soon as possible. This will allow appropriate changes in treatment to be made if the patient is not responding to the initial empiric therapy, change to an agent with a narrower spectrum and lesser potential for superinfection, or replacement with an equally effective but less costly agent.

In many common community-acquired bacterial infections, treatment is based on extensive studies of treatment of the particular infection, and bacteriologic diagnosis may not be sought. For example, this often applies to first attacks of cystitis in young women, to early middle ear infection in a child, or to "walking pneumonia" in a teenager with radiological evidence compatible with a *Mycoplasma* infection.

Although a source of discomfort to the clinical microbiologist, this approach is clinically justified as long as immediate steps to obtain a specific diagnosis are taken in the absence of a prompt response. What is unacceptable is the use of broad-spectrum antimicrobics for infections that have a high probability of a viral etiology in an otherwise healthy individual. This practice is sometimes based on the assumption that it will prevent bacterial superinfection, but is more often simply the result of a desire to let the patient feel that something is being done. Any needless or inappropriate antimicrobic therapy contributes to the resistance problem, to unpleasant superinfections, and to the cost of medical care. Furthermore, it may obscure the diagnosis of a really serious infection by interfering with recovery of the etiological agent in culture without curing the infection.

ANTIVIRAL AGENTS

Because the method of replication of viruses is so intimately associated with the metabolism of the host cell (Chapter 6), there is less opportunity for the development of nontoxic agents that attack the processes of viral synthesis than for agents that inhibit bacterial or fungal growth. Nevertheless, viral attachment, penetration, replication, and assembly are rather unique processes and offer potential sites of attack.

At present, antiviral agents have been most applicable to infections caused by the larger, more complex viruses, such as the herpes group, or to infections that become rapidly apparent because they affect body surfaces or the respiratory tract. The principal agents in current use are considered below according to their modes of action.

Inhibitors of Attachment

Attachment of a virus to a cell receptor is a specific event, and blocking of this process is the mechanism of viral neutralization by antibody. Until now, no clinically effective antiviral agent has been found that acts in this way, although the use of a recombinant CD4 molecule alone or linked to antibody has been shown to block attachment of the human immunodeficiency (HIV) virus to T4 cells and macrophages under experimental conditions. Similar approaches are being explored with other viruses.

Inhibitors of Cell Penetration and Uncoating

Two related synthetic amines, *amantadine* and *rimantadine,* are believed to act similarly at an early stage of infection by certain RNA viruses, either by prevention of virus uncoating after cell entry, inhibition of initial viral

RNA transcription, or both. They are active against influenza A viruses, but influenza B viruses are uniformly resistant. Naturally occurring influenza A viruses that are resistant to both agents have been shown to emerge during treatment and could become an increasing problem in the future. Development of resistance appears to require only a single amino acid change in the transmembrane portion of the viral M2 matrix protein. Amantadine and rimantadine are taken by mouth, have low toxicity, and have been used to provide temporary protection during acute epidemics to particularly susceptible subjects, such as nursing home residents. The agents also reduce the severity of the disease if given within the first few hours of development of symptoms.

Prophylaxis of influenza infection

Inhibitors of Nucleic Acid Synthesis

Most antivirals interfere with synthesis of, or are incorporated in, viral nucleic acid

At present, most antiviral agents are nucleoside analogs that either interfere with viral DNA and RNA synthesis or serve as chain terminators after incorporation into nucleic acids. Those that are most effective act on virus-specified nucleic acid polymerases or transcriptases and have much less activity against host nucleic acid synthesis. One investigational agent with this category of activity, trisodium phosphonoformate, is not a nucleotide.

Idoxuridine

Idoxuridine (5-iodo-2'-deoxyuridine), IUdR, is a halogenated pyrimidine that blocks nucleic acid synthesis through incorporation into DNA in place of thymidine to produce a nonfunctional molecule. Systemically it has considerable toxicity, but can be used locally as an effective treatment for herpetic infection of the cornea (keratitis). *Trifluorothymidine* is another pyrimidine analog effective in the treatment of herpetic infections of the cornea, including those caused by some strains that fail to respond to IUdR.

Trifluorothymidine

Adenine arabinoside

Adenine arabinoside (vidarabine) is a purine that inhibits DNA polymerase and has some selective action, in that herpes group viral polymerases are about 15–30 times more susceptible than the host cell enzyme. When given intravenously, adenine arabinoside reduces the mortality of herpes encephalitis, and it has been shown useful in the treatment of neonatal herpes simplex infection and herpes zoster in immunocompromised patients. It is used topically for treatment of herpetic infections of the eye, in which it has approximately the same effectiveness as IUdR. It is less toxic than IUdR, but can lead to destruction of blood-forming elements in the bone marrow with high dosages.

Acyclovir

Acyclovir (acycloguanosine) is very active against replicating *Herpes simplex* virus (HSV), but progressively less so for the varicella–zoster (VZV) and Epstein–Barr viruses. It is first phosphorylated to its monophosphate by virally specified thymidine kinase (but not cellular kinases). It is then further phosphorylated by cellular kinases to its triphosphate form, which is a potent inhibitor of the viral DNA polymerase. Because of its mode of action, acyclovir has little toxicity for host cells. Because cytomegalovirus (CMV) does not encode a viral thymidine kinase, it is resistant to this agent. Acyclovir is available in topical, oral, and intravenous preparations; it is effective in reducing the severity and duration of primary genital herpes simplex attacks, and of disseminated herpes simplex and VZV infections in immunocompromised and burn patients. It is the drug of choice in the treatment of disseminated neonatal herpes infections and adult herpes encephalitis. Prophylactic use suppresses recurrences of genital herpes and serious herpes recurrences in immunosuppressed patients. Acyclovir has been shown in vitro to act synergistically with zidovudine

Mode of inhibition via virus-specified thymidine kinase

Use of acyclovir in herpes virus infections

(AZT) against HIV and is currently undergoing clinical trials in acquired immunodeficiency syndrome (AIDS) patients.

Development of resistance

Resistant isolates of HSV and VZV sometimes emerge after long-term administration. This is usually the result of development of thymidine kinase–deficient mutants; other mechanisms include alterations in viral DNA polymerase or the substrate specificity of thymidine kinase. Adverse effects are uncommon and generally mild, although more serious central nervous system dysfunctions may occur.

Ganciclovir is more toxic than acyclovir; use in CMV infections

Ganciclovir (DHPG) is an acyclovir analog that inhibits growth of all human herpes viruses including CMV. It is phosphorylated to the active form by host cell thymidine kinase; however, it possesses significant toxicity for uninfected host cells, producing suppression of spermatogenesis, bone marrow precursors, and gut mucosal cells. It has been used to treat severe CMV infections in immunodeficient patients including those suffering from AIDS. It seems to be most effective in treating CMV retinitis and appears to be somewhat useful in CMV pneumonia and enteritis. However, elimination of the virus often does not occur, relapses of infection are common when the drug is stopped, and resistant strains can develop.

Ribavirin

Ribavirin is a synthetic triazole nucleoside that is active in vitro and in vivo in experimental animals against a range of DNA and RNA viruses. The exact mechanism of antiviral effect is unclear, but it inhibits the synthesis of guanosine 5'-phosphate, which is required for synthesis of viral nucleic acid. It shows some promise for use as an aerosol in the prevention and treatment of some respiratory viral infections, especially influenza A and B, and respiratory syncytial viral infection. Oral and intravenous preparations have been effective in the treatment of Lassa fever, a serious infection due to an arenavirus, and should be useful for postexposure prophylaxis. Ribavirin also suppresses HIV in vitro and appears to delay progression of AIDS-related complex (ARC) to AIDS. Unfortunately, it interferes with the action of zidovudine (see below) in vitro and should probably not be used in this combination.

Use as an aerosol

Zidovudine (AZT) inhibits reverse transcriptase

Zidovudine (azidothymidine, AZT) is a thymidine analog that inhibits HIV replication in vitro. It is phosphorylated in vivo by cellular enzymes to the 5'-triphosphate form, which inhibits viral reverse transcriptase and terminates viral DNA elongation. Controlled studies in patients with AIDS and ARC have demonstrated that the drug decreases mortality, reduces the frequency of opportunistic infections, and transiently increases T4 lymphocyte counts. There is also some evidence that it may reverse AIDS-related neuropsychiatric dysfunction, at least temporarily. In low doses, it has been found to delay onset of ARC and AIDS in asymptomatic HIV-infected patients with low T4 lymphocyte counts. It has significant toxicity for the bone marrow, producing severe anemia in 80% of patients. Severe headaches, myalgia, insomnia, seizures, and encephalopathy have all complicated treatment. Toxicity is significantly less when AZT is given in low dose to asymptomatically infected patients.

Use in HIV infections

Bone marrow toxicity

Inhibitors of Viral Assembly and Release

Although, clearly a potential target, no antiviral with these specific sites of action is in clinical use, although, one, methisazone, acts as a specific inhibitor of poxvirus infections by blocking late viral protein synthesis. It thus leads to production of incomplete virus. It has been proved effective in the prophylaxis of poxvirus infections, but, because of the elimination

Methisazone inhibits poxvirus protein synthesis

of smallpox from the world, it now is only of historic interest in human medicine.

Interferons

The human interferons and their role in defense against viral infections have been considered in Chapters 6 and 10. Definition of their place in the therapy and prophylaxis of viral infections has become feasible now that recombinant DNA techniques have allowed relatively inexpensive large-scale production of interferons by some bacteria and yeasts.

Recombinant α-interferon in viral prophylaxis, chronic hepatitis B, and HIV infections

α-Interferon has been shown to have a definite role in the prophylaxis and treatment of herpes zoster and CMV infections, particularly in immunocompromised patients. It has also proved beneficial in the treatment of chronic active hepatitis B liver infection. It is active against HIV in vitro and synergistic with zidovudine and has induced remissions in some patients with Kaposi's sarcoma.

Topical use in herpes keratitis and papilloma virus infections

Topical interferon application has been shown to be beneficial in the treatment of herpes keratitis and human papilloma virus infections. Under experimental conditions, it has been shown some effect in preventing colds caused by at least one type of rhinovirus, but it is still unclear whether this approach will have practical clinical application.

Unfortunately, the interferon preparations that have been tested clinically all show some toxicity in the doses used, partly because of their effect on host cell protein synthesis. It remains to be determined whether other interferons will prove more effective and less toxic for therapy and prophylaxis.

Use of interferon inducers

The use of interferon inducers in therapy was initially unsatisfactory because of their toxicity. Recently, a mismatched double-stranded RNA compound, Ampligen®, has been developed that is believed to augment immune mechanisms by triggering release of lymphokines and activating "natural" antiviral pathways. Clinical studies have demonstrated that it can influence HIV replication and restore some immunologic function. Improvement has been seen in patients with ARC and with generalized lymphadenopathy. Ampligen displays syngeristic activity with zidovudine against HIV in vitro, but more data are needed before its role in therapy of the disease can be established.

EPIDEMIOLOGY OF ANTIMICROBIC RESISTANCE

Development of Increased Resistance

When each antimicrobic was first introduced, its activity against individual isolates of a species was almost completely predictable from studies of its spectrum of activity. Some species were uniformly naturally resistant, and others were susceptible with few, if any, exceptions. With the use of most antimicrobics, resistant strains of many previously susceptible species became increasingly common—sometimes very rapidly—with serious clinical and epidemiologic consequences. For example, most strains of S. aureus were fully susceptible to penicillin when it was first introduced in 1944. By 1950, only about 30% of hospital isolates remained susceptible; the current figure is about 15%, and many isolates are multiresistant to several previously active antimicrobics. Similarly, many enteric Gram-negative rods developed resistance to antimicrobics such as ampicillin, cephalosporins, tetracycline, chloramphenicol, and aminoglycosides, with many strains becoming multiresistant to as many as 15 agents. Fortunately, these

Some species retain
predictable susceptibility

developments have not been universal, and the spirochete of syphilis, and the group A streptococcus, for example, have thus far retained their susceptibility to penicillin. Even this list may change, however, because 10 years ago it would have included the pneumococcus, but resistant strains of this organism have now been isolated in many countries. Resistance to antiviral agents may develop during the course of therapy, and this has been seen with both acyclovir and zidovudine.

Origin of Resistant Strains

Selection of preexisting
resistant strains

Resistant mutants

Plasmid-determined resistance

Transposable elements

Origin of plasmid genes

Resistant strains were occasionally found in a very small proportion of members of a species before introduction of an antimicrobic, and their frequency was greatly increased by its use. This situation was unusual, but partly explains the origin of penicillinase-producing *S. aureus*. In other cases, resistance involved the mutational or recombinational events discussed in Chapter 4. Most resistant mutants are genetically unstable in the absence of the selecting agent, but some, such as low-level penicillin-resistant gonococci and pneumococci and isoniazid-resistant mycobacteria, retain their virulence and can undergo epidemiologic spread. More important, plasmids carrying resistance markers have little, if any, adverse influence on the capacity of most organisms to survive, spread, and infect, and they frequently confer multiresistance. Transposable resistance genes introduce considerable genetic plasticity, and resistance determinants to new antimicrobics can be added to plasmids very quickly.

The origin of plasmid-carried determinants of resistance remains somewhat obscure. Some known to have preexisted the clinical use of the antimicrobic may have played a role in nature by protecting an organism against another that produced the agent. Some may have been derived from antibiotic-producing *Streptomyces,* in which they served to protect the cell from its own antibiotic. Some may have been chromosomal genes transposed to plasmids, and some may have been plasmid genes that mutated to provide altered specificity.

Enhancement and Spread of Resistance

Effect of antimicrobics on
susceptibility to infection
with resistant strains

Ecologic vacuum

Amplification of resistance
with R plasmid transfer

Example of acquisition and
spread of plasmid-borne
resistance determinants

The central factors involved in increasing incidences of resistance are the selective effect of the use of antimicrobics, the spread of infection in human populations, and the ability of plasmids to cross species and even generic lines. Therapeutic or prophylactic use of antimicrobics, particularly agents with a broad spectrum of activity, produces a relative ecologic vacuum in sites with a normal flora or on lesions prone to infection and allows resistant organisms to colonize or infect with less competition from others. Treatment with a single antimicrobic may select for strains that are also resistant to many other agents. Thus, chemotherapy can both enhance the opportunity for acquiring resistant strains from other sources and increase their numbers in the body. The amplifying effect of antimicrobic therapy on resistance is also apparent with the transfer of resistance plasmids to previously susceptible strains. This effect occurs primarily in the lower intestinal tract, where the antimicrobic may reduce the flora and also produce an increased oxidation–reduction potential that favors plasmid transfer to the same or other species.

As an example, consider a patient harboring as a very small part of his facultative intestinal flora a strain of *E. coli* carrying a plasmid with genes encoding resistance to tetracycline, ampicillin, chloramphenicol, and the sulfonamides. He develops an infection with a *Shigella* dysentery bacillus susceptible to all of these antimicrobial agents and is treated with tetracycline. Most of the normal flora and the *Shigella* are inhibited, and the resistant *E. coli* becomes predominant because its multiplication is not impeded and competition is removed. Plasmid transfer occurs between the resistant *E. coli* and some surviving *Shigella;* the latter then multiply, causing a relapse of the disease with a strain that is now multiresistant. Any endemic or epidemic spread of dysentery from this patient to others will now be with the multiresistant *Shigella* strain, and its ability to infect will be enhanced if the recipient is on prophylaxis or therapy with any of the four antimicrobics to which it is resistant.

Such occurrences are commonplace and involve both virulent organisms and members of the normal flora, especially enteric Gram-negative rods. They account for the much higher incidence of resistance and multiresistance that characterizes hospital-acquired as opposed to community-acquired strains. The procedures described in Chapter 4 allow resistance plasmids or even individual transposable elements to be "fingerprinted." It has thus been possible to trace their "epidemic" spread through different species and genera of bacteria.

Characterization and tracing of the spread of R plasmids and transposable elements

Major Selective Factors

The hospital remains the major source and reservoir of resistant organisms that affect humans, although similar selection and spread occur in the community. Isolates of group A β-hemolytic streptococci and pneumococci are frequently resistant to tetracycline and reflect what was widespread and often inappropriate community use of that agent. Most strains of gonococci now show substantially higher resistance to penicillin than was the case when the antibiotic was introduced to a considerable extent because of suboptimal therapy.

Central role of hospital in antimicrobic resistance

Community-acquired resistance

There are selective factors other than use of antimicrobics in human therapy and prophylaxis. Antimicrobic contamination of the hospital environment, as with antimicrobic from aerosols produced during administration or from high concentrations in urine, may be sufficient to inhibit the susceptible normal flora of the anterior nares of personnel and increase the carriage rate of resistant *S. aureus*. This contamination has been shown to occur in human and veterinary hospitals and in an antibiotic processing plant; its significance merits further study. Much attention has been paid to the use of antimicrobics in animal feeds both prophylactically and for their growth-promoting effects, which are economically important but involve mechanisms not yet fully characterized. Cattle or poultry that consume feed supplemented with antimicrobics rapidly develop a resistant enteric flora that spreads throughout the herd. Resistance is largely plasmid determined and has been shown capable of spreading to the flora of farmers and of those living in close proximity to cattle-rearing farms. *Salmonella* species, which commonly infect intensively raised cattle and poultry, usually acquire the resistance plasmids, and multiplication of the bacteria in contaminated food products can result in individual infections or epidemics of food poisoning caused by multiresistant *Salmonella*. Patients on treatment with antibiotics to which the organisms are resistant may become clinically infected with numbers of *Salmonella* well below those that will usually cause disease in healthy individuals. As a consequence, many countries have banned or controlled addition to animal feeds of antimicrobics that are useful for systemic therapy in humans. Important theoretic concerns are that stabilization of plasmids may occur under such intensive pressure and that they may then persist and spread in the absence of the selective effect of antimicrobics and acquire other undesirable genetic traits, such an enhanced virulence.

Environmental contamination and animal feed supplementation

Resistant zoonotic Salmonella infections

Concern of stabilization of R plasmids

Despite these various sources of resistant strains, by far the most significant problem in human medicine remains the large-scale use of antimicrobics for treating actual or assumed infections and epidemiologic spread of resistant strains both in hospitals and in the community under the selective pressure of antimicrobic use.

Control of Resistance

Loss of resistance on withdrawal of selective agent

In the past, numerous examples in the literature showed that the extent of resistance in a hospital directly reflects the extent of usage of an antimicrobic, and that withdrawal or control can lead to rapid reduction of the incidence of resistance. Obviously such measures will have little impact on the level of resistance in the community, and they can rarely be applied in practice. It is also possible that some resistance determinants have now become so stabilized that they are less likely to be lost in the absence of the selective agent. Experience and our understanding of the mechanisms and spread of resistance, however, indicate certain principles that can help to keep the problem under control, can sometimes reverse it, and are compatible with good therapeutic practice:

Principles for controlling resistance

1. Conservative and specific use of antimicrobics in therapy.

2. Adequate dosage and duration of therapy to eliminate the infecting organism and reduce the risk of selecting resistant variants.

3. Whenever possible, selection of antimicrobics according to the proved or anticipated known susceptibility of the infecting strain.

4. Use, when possible, of narrow rather than broad-spectrum antimicrobics when the specific etiology of an infection is known.

5. Use of antimicrobic combinations known to prevent emergence of resistant mutants in diseases like tuberculosis.

6. Prophylactic use of antimicrobics only in situations in which it has been proved valuable and for the shortest possible time to avoid selection of a resistant flora.

7. Avoidance of environmental contamination.

8. Application of careful, standard aseptic and hand-washing procedures to help to prevent spread of resistant organisms.

9. Use of containment isolation procedures for patients infected with resistant organisms that pose a threat to others and of protective precautions for those who are highly susceptible.

10. Epidemiologic monitoring for resistant organisms or determinants in an institution and the application of enhanced control measures if a problem develops.

11. Restriction of the use of therapeutically valuable antimicrobics for nonmedical purposes.

Behavioral aspects of problem of antimicrobic resistance

The problem of antimicrobic resistance and its spread has a considerable behavioral component. Needless and excessive therapy, failure to observe basic rules for preventing spread of infection to others, and lack of understanding of the process all serve to increase the problem. Conversely, intelligent, conservative, and specific use of chemotherapy with adequate precautions to prevent cross-infection provides the best chance of retaining the value of many of the agents we now possess.

Appendix 13.1　Usual Susceptibility Patterns of Common Bacteria to Some Commonly Used Bacteriostatic and Bactericidal Antimicrobics

Antimicrobic	Bactericidal	Bacteriostatic	Staphylococcus aureus	Enterococci	Other streptococci	Neisseria	Haemophilus	Legionella	Mycoplasma	Escherichia coli	Proteus mirabilis	Other Proteus spp.	Klebsiella	Enterobacter	Serratia	Pseudomonas aeruginosa	Bacteroides fragilis	Other Gram-ve anaerobes	Clostridium	Rickettsia	Chlamydia	
Benzyl penicillin	+		①C	②	①	①												①	①				Narrow-spectrum agents
Penicillinase-resistant penicillins	+		①		②																		
Erythromycin	±	+	②	②	②		①	①													②		
Clindamycin	±	+	②														①	①					
Vancomycin	+		②	①	②														①				
Ampicillin	+		②	①	②	①	①			①	①								①				Broad-spectrum agents
Piperacillin	+										①	①	①	①	①	①	②	①				
Cephalothin	+		②		②																	
Cefotetan	+				①	①				①	①	①	①			②						
Cefaperazone	+									①	①	①	①	②	②							
Imipenem	+		②	②	②	①	①			①	①	①	①	①	①	①	①	①				
Aztreonam	+					①	①			①	①	①	①		①	①						
Gentamicin	+		C							①	①	①	①	①	①	①						
Amikacin	+		C							①	①	①	①	①	①	①						
Tetracycline		+					②	①											①	①		
Chloramphenicol		+					②									①	②		①			
Ciprofloxacin	+					②				①	①	①	①	①	①	②						
Sulfamethoxazole + trimethoprim	±	+					①			①											③	

Proportions of susceptible and resistant strains: ◯ = 100% susceptible; ◖ = 25% resistant; ● = 100% resistant; ▨ = intermediate susceptibility.

Abbreviations: − = no present indication for therapy or insufficient data; 1 = antimicrobic of choice for susceptible strains; 2 = second-line agent; 3 = *C. trachomatis* sensitive, *C. psittaci* resistant; C = useful in combination of a β-lactam and an aminoglycoside.

These data reflect results in a single institution. Proportions of resistant strains may vary in different locations.

Additional Reading

Allan, D.J., Jr., Eliopoulos, G.M., and Moellering, R.C., Jr. 1987. Antibiotics: Future directions by understanding structure-function relationships. In *Contemporary Issues in Infectious Diseases: New Surgical and Medical Approaches in Infectious Diseases*. Root, R.K., Trunkey, D., and Sande, M.A. Eds. New York: Churchill Livingstone. A valuable account of newer developments in chemotherapeutics and the chemical determinants of their special properties.

Gilman, A.G., Goodman, L.S., Rall, T.W., and Murad, F., Eds. 1985. *Goodman and Gilman's The Pharmacological Basis of Therapeutics*. 7th ed. New York: Macmillan. A standard reference text with excellent sections on antibiotics and chemotherapy.

Knight, V., and Gilbert, B.E. 1987. *Antiviral Chemotherapy: Infectious Disease Clinics of North America*. Vol. 1(No. 2). Philadelphia: W.B. Saunders. An excellent series of chapters by experts in the field.

Peterson, P.K., and Verhoef, J., Eds. 1987. *The Antimicrobial Agents Annual 2*. Amsterdam/New York: Elsevier. An up-to-date series of chapters emphasizing particularly the clinical pharmacology and application of antimicrobials. It includes all of those considered in this chapter.

Pratt, W.B., and Fekety, R. 1986. *The Antimicrobial Drugs*. New York: Oxford University Press. An exceptionally informative account of the basis of antibacterial and antiviral chemotherapy, the characteristics of antimicrobics, and their clinical application.

Sanders, C.C., and Weidemann, B., Eds. 1988. New developments in resistance to β-lactam antibiotics among nonfastidious Gram-negative organisms. *Rev. Infect. Dis.* 10:677–914. Proceedings of a symposium that covers all aspects of β-lactam resistance with particular emphasis on β-lactamases.

Tyrell, D.A.J. 1987. Interferons and their clinical value. *Rev. Infect. Dis.* 9:243–249. An excellent overview of the present status of interferons in medicine.

14

Laboratory Diagnosis of Infectious Diseases

Kenneth J. Ryan and
C. George Ray

Diagnosis of microbial infections

The diagnosis of a microbial infection begins with an assessment of clinical and epidemiologic features, leading to the formulation of a diagnostic hypothesis. Anatomic localization of the infection with the aid of physical and radiologic findings (for example, right lower lobe pneumonia, subphrenic abscess) is usually included. This clinical diagnosis suggests a number of possible etiologic agents based on knowledge of infectious syndromes and their courses (Chapters 59–73). The specific etiologic diagnosis is then established by the application of the methods described in this chapter. A combination of science and art on the part of both the clinician and the laboratory worker is required: The clinician must select the appropriate tests and specimens to be processed and, where appropriate, suggest the suspected etiologic agents to the laboratory. The laboratory worker must design a battery of methods that will demonstrate the probable agents and be prepared to explore other possibilities suggested by the clinical situation or the findings of the laboratory examinations. The best results are obtained when communication between the clinic and the laboratory is maximal.

The Specimen

General Considerations

Critical nature of specimen

The prime interface between the clinic and the diagnostic laboratory is the specimen submitted for processing. If it is not appropriately chosen and/or collected, no degree of laboratory skill will rectify the error. Failure at the level of specimen collection is the most common reason for failure to establish an etiologic diagnosis, or worse, for suggesting a wrong diagnosis. In the case of bacterial infections, the primary problem lies in distinguishing normal floral organisms and surface contaminants from those causing the infection. Specimens may be divided into three cate-

233

14.1 Specimens for the diagnosis of infection. (**A**) Direct specimen. The pathogen (O) is localized in an otherwise sterile site, and a barrier such as the skin must be passed to sample it. This may be done surgically or by needle aspiration as shown. The specimen collected contains only the pathogen. Examples: deep abscess, cerebrospinal fluid. (**B**) Indirect sample. The pathogen is localized as in **A** but must pass through a site containing normal flora (*) in order to be collected. The specimen contains the pathogen, but is contaminated with the nonpathogenic flora. The degree of contamination is often related to the skill with which the normal floral site was "bypassed" in specimen collection. Examples: expectorated sputum, voided urine. (**C**) Sample from site with normal flora. The pathogen and nonpathogenic flora are mixed at the site of infection. Both are collected and the nonpathogen is either inhibited by the use of selective culture methods or discounted in interpretation of culture results. Examples: throat, stool.

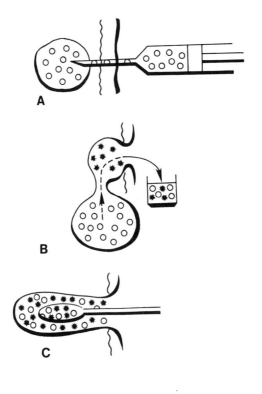

gories on the basis of probability of contamination with normal flora (Figure 14.1). Details for individual specimens are provided in Chapters 59–73.

Direct Tissue or Fluid Samples. Direct specimens (Figure 14.1A) are collected from normally sterile tissues (lung, liver) and body fluids (cerebrospinal fluid, blood). The methods range from needle aspiration of an abscess to surgical biopsy. In general, such collections require the direct involvement of a physician and may carry some risk for the patient. The results are always useful, because positive findings are diagnostic and negative findings can exclude infection at the suspected site.

Indirect Samples. Indirect samples (Figure 14.1B) are specimens of inflammatory exudates (expectorated sputum, voided urine) that have passed through sites known to be colonized with normal flora. The site of origin is usually sterile in healthy persons; however, some assessment of the probability of contamination with normal flora during collection is necessary before these specimens can be reliably interpreted. This assessment requires knowledge of the potential contaminating flora as well as the probable pathogens to be sought. Indirect samples are usually more convenient for both physician and patient, but carry a higher risk of misinterpretation. For some specimens, such as expectorated sputum and voided urine, specific guidelines to assess the probability of specimen contamination by the normal flora have been developed by correlation of clinical and microbiologic findings (Chapters 64 and 66).

Samples from sites with a normal flora. Frequently the primary site of infection is in an area known to be colonized with many organisms (pharynx, large and small intestine) (Figure 14.1C). In such instances, examinations are made only for organisms known to cause infection that are not normally found in the infected site. The laboratory workup is thus directed toward isolation and identification of a limited number of organisms. For example, *Salmonella, Shigella,* and *Campylobacter* may be sought in a stool specimen or group A β-hemolytic streptococci in a throat swab. It is neither practical nor relevant in these circumstances for the laboratory to describe the normal flora. Samples from sites with a normal flora are only useful for diagnosis of infections at remote sites when the organism sought is not encountered in health. For example, detection of *Streptococcus pneumoniae* in a throat swab is useless in the diagnosis of pneumonia, because the organism is often found in the throat in healthy persons. The specimen must have been derived from the lung to be useful. On the other hand, isolation of influenza virus from the throat is useful in the diagnosis of influenzal pneumonia, because the virus is not normally present in the respiratory tract.

Importance of seeking specific pathogens in normal floral sites

Types of Specimens

The sterile swab is the most convenient and most commonly used tool for specimen collection; however, it provides the poorest conditions for survival and can only absorb a small volume of inflammatory exudate. The worst possible specimen is a dried-out swab; the best involves collection, when possible, of 5–10 ml or more of the infected fluid or tissue, because infecting organisms present in small numbers may not be detected if too small a sample is taken. Furthermore, a sample of several milliliters will serve as its own transport medium. Swabs should be used only when fluid or tissue collection is not possible, and they should be processed quickly or placed in a suitable transport medium designed to maintain the viability of the infecting organisms. Swabs are unacceptable for diagnosis of diseases such as tuberculosis in which the numbers of organisms may be very small.

Limitation of swabs

Best specimens are of infected fluids or tissue

Specimen Transport

Specimens should be transported to the laboratory as soon after collection as possible, because some microorganisms survive only briefly outside the body. For example, unless special transport media are used, isolation rates of the bacteria that cause whooping cough (*Bordetella pertussis*) and gonorrhea (*Neisseria gonorrhoeae*) are decreased when processing is delayed beyond a few minutes. Likewise, many respiratory viruses survive poorly outside the body. On the other hand, some bacteria survive well and may even multiply after the specimen is collected. The growth of enteric Gram-negative rods in specimens awaiting culture may in fact compromise specimen interpretation by altering the numbers and relative proportions of different organisms, and thus interfere with the isolation of more fastidious organisms. Significant changes are associated with delays of more than 3–4 hr.

Various transport media have been developed to minimize the effects of the delay between specimen collection and laboratory processing. In general, they are buffered fluid or semisolid media containing minimal nutrients and are designed to prevent drying, maintain a neutral pH, and

Rapid loss of viability of some bacteria

Problems of overgrowth after *specimen collection*

Transport media

minimize growth. Other features may be required to meet special requirements, such as an oxygen-free atmosphere for obligate anaerobes.

Diagnostic Methods

The general approaches to laboratory diagnosis vary with different microorganisms and infectious diseases. The types of methods, however, will usually be some combination of the following:

1. *Direct examination.* Of the infectious agents discussed in this book, only some of the parasites are large enough to be seen with the naked eye. Bacteria can be seen clearly with the light microscope when appropriate methods are used; individual viruses can be seen only with the electron microscope, although aggregates of viral particles in cells (viral inclusions) may be seen by light microscopy. Various stains are used to visualize and differentiate bacteria in smears and histologic sections. The sensitivity and specificity of microscopic examinations can be improved by combination with a unique visible marker. The most common example of this is immunofluorescent staining, which employs a specific antibody linked to a fluorescent dye. The antibody binds only to the target antigen on the organism, which is then visualized by virtue of the fluorescent tag.

2. *Culture.* Growth and identification of the infecting agent in vitro is usually the most sensitive and specific means of diagnosis and is thus the method most commonly used. Most bacteria can be grown in a variety of artificial media, but strict intracellular bacteria (eg, *Chlamydia*, *Rickettsia*) and human and animal viruses can be isolated only in cultures of living eukaryotic cells.

3. *Antibody detection (serologic diagnosis).* Detection and quantitation of specific antibodies formed by the host in response to an infection can provide evidence of present or previous infection with a particular infectious agent. Numerous methods are employed using antigens prepared from a wide range of infectious agents.

4. *Detection of microbial components or metabolites.* Isolation and direct examination methods require living or morphologically intact organisms. In recent years, highly sensitive methods, including gas and liquid chromatography, have been developed that can detect structural components or metabolic products of microorganisms. In some cases these procedures can be applied directly to body fluids or tissues of patients (eg, blood, cerebrospinal fluid, and urine) and a diagnosis made rapidly. Specific antigenic proteins or polysaccharides of microorganisms may be detected by immunologic techniques (antigenic detection), including by counterimmunoelectrophoresis, latex agglutination, and radioimmunoassay procedures that are described later in the chapter. Genetic methods such as DNA–DNA hybridization can be used on tissue sections or smears of potentially infected material.

5. *Genome detection.* It is now possible to use cloned DNA or in vitro synthesized nucleic acid probes to detect genomes specific for a variety of infectious agents. Cloned DNA is currently most commonly used and has been successfully applied to the diagnosis of bacterial, viral, and mycoplasmal infections. Molecular analysis of nucleic acids can also be applied to epidemiologic studies.

Gas and liquid chromatography

Sensitive immunological techniques

Nucleic acid probes

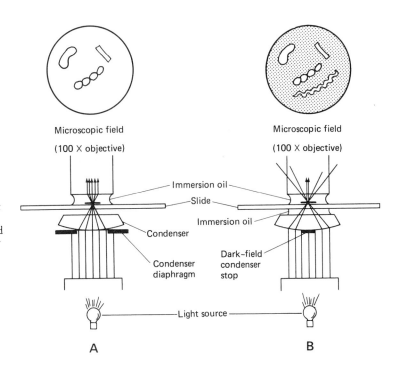

14.2 Bright- and dark-field illumination for light microscopy. (**A**) Bright-field illumination properly aligned. The purpose is to focus light directly on the preparation for optimal visualization against a bright background. (**B**) In dark-field illumination, a black background is created by blocking the central light. Peripheral light is focused so that it will be collected by the objective only when it is reflected from the surfaces of particles (for example, bacteria). The microscopic field shows bright halos around some bacteria and reveals a spirochete too thin to be seen with bright-field illumination.

In this chapter, we shall consider these principles in their application to the diagnosis of diseases caused by most bacteria and viruses. Many of the methods to be described can also be applied, with certain variations, to the diagnosis of diseases caused by fungi, *Mycoplasma, Rickettsia, Chlamydia,* and parasites; however, because of the special features of each of these groups, the specific approaches to their isolation and identification will be discussed in subsequent chapters. As the serologic diagnosis of all infectious diseases utilizes common basic concepts, this topic will be considered separately in the last section of this chapter.

Diagnosis of Bacterial Infections

Direct Examination

Limits of resolution of light microscope

Dark-field microscopy

Direct examination of stained or unstained preparations by light microscopy is particularly useful for detection of bacteria. Even the smallest bacteria (0.15 μm wide) can be visualized, although some require special lighting techniques. As the resolution limit of the light microscope is near 0.2 μm, the optics must be ideal if the organisms are to be seen clearly by direct transmission microscopy. These conditions may be achieved with a 100× oil immersion objective, a 5–10× eyepiece, and optimal lighting, as shown in Figure 14.2. Some bacteria, such as *Treponema pallidum,* the cause of syphilis, are too slim to be visualized with the usual bright-field illumination. They can be seen by use of the *dark-field* technique. With this method, a condenser that focuses only diagonal light on the specimen is used, and only light reflected from particulate matter such as bacteria reaches the eyepiece (Figure 14.2). The angles of incident and reflected light are such that the organisms are surrounded by a bright halo against a black background. This type of illumination is also used in other microscopic techniques, in which a high light contrast is desired, and for

Fluorescence microscopy

observation of fluorescence. Fluorescent compounds, when excited by light of one wavelength, emit light of a longer wavelength and thus a different color. Fluorescence microscopy involves the use of illumination sources that produce light in or near the ultraviolet range, combined with dark-field illumination. Barrier filters permit visualization of emitted light, but protect the observer from ultraviolet light. When the fluorescent compound is conjugated with an antibody as a probe for detection of specific antigen, the technique is called *immunofluorescence,* or fluorescent antibody microscopy. *Phase contrast* is another form of microscopy in which differences in refractive index in the specimen are converted to differences in intensity of light in the image. This allows better visualization of structures in unstained specimens (eg, within eukaryotic cells) than is possible with bright- or dark-field illumination. It is primarily used to view host cells, fungi, and parasites.

Phase-contrast microscopy

Stains

Bacteria may be stained by a wide variety of dyes, including methylene blue, crystal violet, carbol–fuchsin (red), and safranin (red). The two most important methods, the *Gram* and *acid-fast* techniques, employ staining, decolorization, and counterstaining in a manner that helps to classify as well as stain the organism.

Gram and acid-fast techniques assist bacterial classification

Gram Stain. The differential staining procedure described in 1884 by the Danish physician Hans Christian Gram has proved one of the most useful in microbiology and medicine. The procedure (Figure 14.3) involves the addition of a solution of iodine in potassium iodide to cells previously stained with certain acridine dyes, such as crystal violet. This treatment produces a mordanting action in which purple insoluble complexes are formed with the cell's ribonucleic acid. The difference between Gram-positive and Gram-negative bacteria is in the permeability of the cell wall to these complexes upon treatment with alcohol or mixtures of acetone and alcohol. Gram-negative bacteria lose the purple iodine-dye complexes, whereas Gram-positive bacteria retain them. An intact cell wall is necessary for a positive reaction; Gram-positive bacteria may fail to retain the stain if the organisms are old, dead, or damaged by antimicrobial agents. No similar conditions cause a Gram-negative organism to appear Gram positive. The stain is completed by the addition of safranin, a red counterstain taken up by bacteria that have been decolorized. Thus, cells stained purple are Gram positive, and those stained red are Gram negative. As indicated in Chapter 2, Gram positivity and negativity correspond to major structural differences in the cell wall.

When the Gram stain is applied to clinical specimens, the purple or red bacteria are seen against a Gram-negative (red) background of leukocytes, dried exudate, and debris. Retention of the purple dye in tissue or fluid elements, such as the nuclei of polymorphonuclear leukocytes, is an indication that the smear has been inadequately decolorized. In smears of uneven thickness, judgments on the Gram reaction can be made only in well-decolorized areas.

Etiologic bacteria often seen in direct Gram smears of specimens

In many bacterial infections, the etiologic bacteria are readily seen on stained Gram smears of pus or fluids. This information, combined with the clinical findings, may guide the management of infection before culture results are available. Interpretation requires knowledge of the probable etiologic agents for the clinical syndrome, of their morphology and Gram reaction, and of any organisms normally present in health at the infected

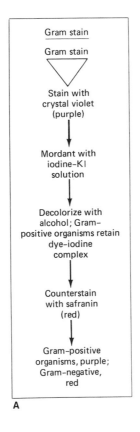

14.3 Gram stain and acid-fast stain for bacteria.

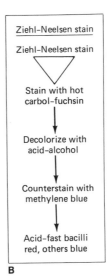

site. An accurate reading of the Gram smear requires considerable experience.

Acid-fast stain. Acid fastness is a property of the mycobacteria (for example, *Mycobacterium tuberculosis*) and related organisms (for example, some species of *Nocardia*). Acid-fast organisms generally stain very poorly with dyes, including those used in the Gram stain. They can, however, be stained with prolonged application, more concentrated dyes, and heat treatment. Their unique feature is that once stained, acid-fast bacteria resist decolorization by concentrations of mineral acids and ethanol that remove dyes from other bacteria. This combination of weak initial staining and strong retention once stained is probably related to the high lipid content of the mycobacterial cell wall. Acid-fast stains are completed with a counterstain to provide a contrasting background for viewing the stained bacteria (Figure 14.3).

The classic acid-fast procedure is the Ziehl–Neelsen stain in which the slide is flooded with carbol–fuchsin (red), heated, and then decolorized with a 3% solution of hydrochloric acid in alcohol. When counterstained with methylene blue, acid-fast organisms appear red against a blue background. A variant of this method is the Ponder–Kinyoun (cold) acid-fast stain, in which a more concentrated fuchsin is used and heating is omitted. Another variant is the fluorochrome stain, which uses a fluorescent dye, auramine, or an auramine-rhodamine mixture followed by decolorization with acid–alcohol. Acid-fast organisms retain the fluorescent stain, which allows their visualization with fluorescence microscopy. Fluorescing or-

Marginal notes:

Acid-fast bacteria stain with difficulty, but resist decolorization once stained

Acid-fastness related to cell wall lipid content

Ziehl–Neelsen classic technique

Fluorescent method

ganisms can be detected at lower magnification ($\times 250$), which increases the speed with which smears may be read.

Culture

Almost all medically important bacteria can be cultivated outside the host in artificial culture media. Usually, a single bacterium placed in the proper culture medium and environment will multiply to numbers that are often sufficient to cause changes detectable by the naked eye. Beginning with those of Louis Pasteur and Robert Koch, growth medium formulations of increasing sophistication have been developed to match the growth requirements of pathogenic bacteria.

Defined and undefined media

Media are of two basic types, defined and undefined. Defined media are prepared from chemically known ingredients. Undefined media are essentially recipes prepared from digests of animal or vegetable protein, often supplemented with substances such as glucose yeast extract, serum, or blood, to meet the metabolic requirements of the organism. Their chemical composition is therefore complex, and their success depends on the similar nutritional requirements of most heterotrophic living things.

Most diagnostic media are undefined

Most diagnostic bacteriology methods utilize undefined media because of their lower cost and ability to support growth of a broad range of pathogenic organisms. Defined media are useful for characterization of the biochemical activities of organisms and in research requiring tight control of all variables.

Growth in broth medium

Growth media are initially prepared in the fluid state to which bacteria or clinical specimens may be added directly. They are termed *broths*. The presence of bacteria in broth medium will not be apparent to the naked eye until they attain numbers sufficient to produce turbidity or macroscopic clumps. Turbidity results from reflection of transmitted light by the bacteria; depending on the size of the organism, more than 10^6 bacteria per milliliter of broth are usually required. Some strictly aerobic bacteria may grow as a film on the surface; other bacteria grow as a sediment.

Agar media

Special properties of agar

The addition of a gelling agent to a broth medium allows its preparation in solid form: as *plates* when poured into petri dishes and as *slants* in tubes. The universal gelling agent for diagnostic bacteriology is *agar,* a polysaccharide extracted from certain types of seaweed. Agar has the convenient property of becoming liquid at about 95°C, and thus during sterilization, but not returning to the solid state as a gel until cooled to less than 50°C. This allows the addition of a heat-labile substance, such as blood, to the medium before it sets. At the temperatures used in the diagnostic laboratory (37°C or lower) broth–agar exists as a smooth, solid, nutrient gel; its firmness depends on the agar concentration. This medium, usually termed "agar," may be qualified with a description of any supplement (for example, blood agar).

Plate streaking for isolation

Separation of bacteria may be accomplished by spreading a small sample over the surface of an agar plate in a structured form with a sterile wire loop. This procedure is termed *plate streaking.* Bacteria well separated from others grow as isolated colonies, often reaching 2–3 mm in diameter after overnight incubation in the case of rapidly growing organisms. The

Bacterial colonies

time of appearance and size of macroscopic colonies, which contain billions of organisms, depends on the generation time of the organism. Well-streaked plates will yield isolated colonies regardless of the numbers in the specimen (Figure 14.4).

For diagnostic work, growth of bacteria on solid media has advantages

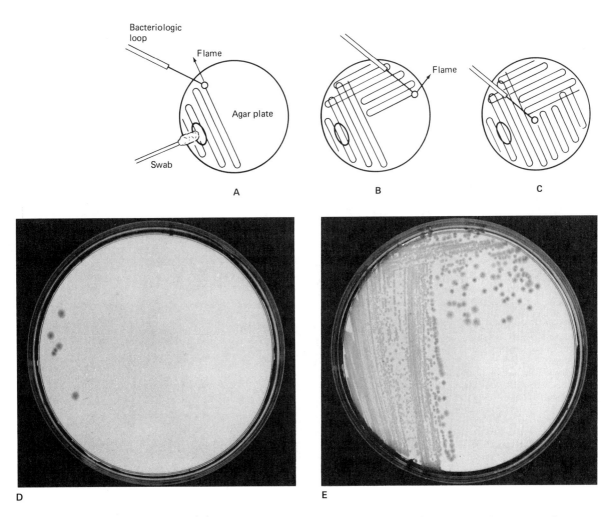

14.4 Bacteriologic plate streaking. Plate streaking is essentially a dilution procedure. The specimen is placed on the plate with a swab, loop, or pipette, and evenly spread over approximately one-fourth of the plate surface with a sterilized bacteriologic loop. (A) The loop is flamed to remove residual bacteria. (B) A secondary streak is made, overlapping the primary streak initially but finishing independently. (C) The process is repeated in a tertiary streak. (D) and (E) Two plates streaked in a similar manner. (D) Only a few bacteria grew. (E) A large number of bacteria grew. In each case, however, isolated colonies were produced for further study.

Use of plates in isolating pure cultures

Differences in colonial morphology aid in identification

over the use of broth cultures. It allows isolation of bacteria in pure culture, because a colony well separated from others can be assumed to arise from a single organism or an organism cluster (colony-forming unit). Colonies vary greatly in size, shape, texture, color, and other features. For example, colonies of organisms possessing large polysaccharide capsules are usually mucoid, those that fail to separate after division are frequently granular, and colonies of highly motile organisms may tend to spread on the surface of the medium. Colonies from different species or genera often differ substantially, whereas those derived from the same strain are usually consistent. Differences in colonial morphology are very useful for separating bacteria in mixtures and as clues to their identity. Experienced bacteriologists learn to recognize subtle differences in colonial morphology, in-

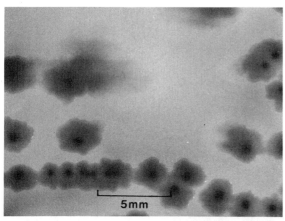

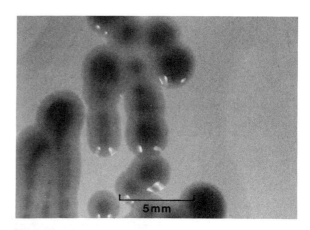

A   B

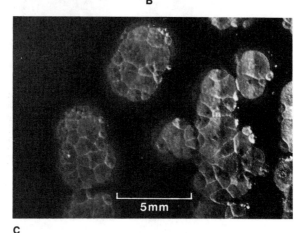

C

14.5 Bacterial colonial morphology. The colonies formed on agar plates by three different Gram-negative bacilli are shown at the same magnification. Each is typical for its species but variations are common. (**A**) *Escherchia coli* colonies are flat with an irregular scalloped edge. (**B**) *Klebsiella pneumoniae* colonies with a smooth entire edge and a raised glistening surface. (**C**) *Pseudomonas aeruginosa* colonies with an irregular reflective surface suggesting hammered metal.

Other methods of detecting bacterial growth in culture

cluding those seen with growth on different bacteriologic media. Some examples of different colonial morphology are shown in Figure 14.5.

New methods that do not depend on visual changes in the growth medium or colony formation may also be used to detect bacterial growth in culture. These techniques include release of radiolabeled products of bacterial metabolism, changes in the electrical impedance of the medium, bioluminescence and chromatographic detection of bacterial metabolic products in the medium. The only one of these methods currently used in a significant number of clinical laboratories is a radioisotopic method that measures ^{14}C-labeled carbon dioxide released from labeled substrates in nutrient broth. This approach, which has been automated, can detect bacterial growth before the development of turbidity or colony formation. Once detected, bacteria are stained, subcultured, and identified in the usual way.

Bacteriologic Media

Over the past 100 years, countless media have been developed by bacteriologists to aid in the isolation and identification of medically important bacteria. Only a few have found their way into routine use in clinical laboratories. These media may be classified as nutrient, selective, or indicator media. Most of those now used in clinical laboratories are purchased commercially in dehydrated form.

Nutrient Media.   The nutrient component of a medium is designed to satisfy the growth requirements of bacteria to permit growth and isolation. For medical purposes, the ideal isolation medium would allow rapid growth of all bacteria. No such medium has been and probably cannot be developed; however, several undefined media suffice for good growth of most medically important bacteria. These media are prepared with enzymatic or acid digests of animal or plant products such as muscle, milk, or beans. The digest reduces the native protein to a mixture of polypeptides and amino acids termed *peptone,* which also includes trace metals, coenzymes, and various undefined growth factors. For example, one common broth contains a pancreatic digest of casein (milk curd) and a papaic digest of soybean meal. To this nutrient base, salts, vitamins, or body fluids such as serum may be added to provide pathogens with the conditions needed for optimum growth.

Bacteriologic "peptones" are enzymatic digests of protein

Selective Media.   Selective media are used when specific pathogenic organisms are sought in sites with an extensive normal flora (for example, *N. gonorrhoeae* in specimens from the uterine cervix or rectum). In these cases, other bacteria may overgrow the suspected etiologic species in simple nutrient media, either because the pathogen grows more slowly or because it is present in much smaller numbers. Selective media usually contain dyes, other chemical additives, or antibiotics at concentrations inhibitory to contaminating flora, but not the suspected pathogen. Selective fluid media are called *enrichment broths,* because they allow small numbers of pathogens to outgrow inhibited organisms before subculture on plates.

Used when specific pathogens are sought among normal flora

Enrichment broths

Indicator Media.   Indicator media contain indicator systems designed to demonstrate features characteristic of specific pathogens or of groups of organisms that include pathogens. The addition to the medium of one or more carbohydrates and a pH indicator is frequently employed. A color change in the colony indicates the presence of acid products and thus of fermentation or incomplete oxidation of the carbohydrate. Other indicator media may enhance the production of a pigment or other changes useful for early recognition of certain bacteria. The addition of red blood cells to plates allows the hemolysis produced by some organisms to be used as a differential feature (see Chapter 16).

Detection of pH changes, hemolysis, etc.

In practice, nutrient, selective, and indicator properties are often combined to various degrees in the same medium. It is possible to include an indicator system in a highly nutrient medium and also make it selective by adding appropriate antibiotics. Culture media commonly used in diagnostic bacteriology are listed in Appendix 14.1, and more details of their constitution and application are provided in Appendix 14.2.

Cultural Conditions

Once inoculated most cultures are placed in an incubator with temperature maintained at 35–37°C. Slightly higher or lower temperatures are used occasionally to selectively favor a certain organism or organism group. For example, *Listeria monocytogenes* (Chapter 17) will outgrow most competitors at 4°C as will *Campylobacter jejuni* (Chapter 21) at 42°C.

Incubation usually at 35–37°C

CO$_2$ required by some species, enhances growth of others

Candle jar for CO$_2$ production

Growth of anaerobes in presence of reducing agents

Anaerobic jars and chambers for plated media

Need to maintain continuous anaerobiosis

Routines differ according to specimen and organism sought

Responsibility of clinician to provide information on possible diagnosis

Need for a pure culture

Classes of identification tests

Most bacteria that are not obligate anaerobes will grow in air; however, CO$_2$ is required by some and enhances the growth of others. Incubators that maintain a concentration of CO$_2$ in air of 2–5% are frequently used for primary isolation, because this level is not harmful to any bacteria and improves isolation of some. A less expensive method is the *candle jar,* in which a lighted candle is allowed to burn to extinction in a sealed jar containing plates. This method adds 1–2% CO$_2$ to the atmosphere.

Anaerobic incubation is a special case: strictly anaerobic bacteria will not grow under the conditions described previously, and many will die if exposed to atmospheric oxygen or high oxidation-reduction potentials. Most medically important anaerobes will grow in the depths of liquid or semisolid media containing any of a variety of reducing agents, such as cysteine, thioglycolate, ascorbic acid, or even iron filings. Growth is also facilitated by prior boiling to remove dissolved oxygen. Plates of solid medium are incubated in anaerobic jars or large chambers from which all oxygen is removed or excluded. The latter can be achieved by replacing air with a gas mixture containing 10% hydrogen and 5% CO$_2$ in 85% nitrogen and allowing the hydrogen to react with residual oxygen on a palladium catalyst to form water. A convenient commercial system generates hydrogen and CO$_2$ from a packet to which water is added before the jar is sealed. Anaerobiosis takes 2–4 hr to develop, but the system is adequate for medically important anaerobes, which are rarely exquisitely oxygen sensitive. Specimens suspected to contain significant anaerobes are transmitted to the laboratory and processed under conditions designed to minimize exposure to atmospheric oxygen at all stages.

Routine laboratory systems for processing specimens differ because no single medium or atmosphere is ideal for all bacteria, and selection of combinations depends on the nature of the specimens and the organisms sought. Thus, routines for different types of specimens vary; some examples are shown in Table 14.1. They include combinations of broth and solid plated media and aerobic, CO$_2$, and anaerobic incubation. Broths are most sensitive for detecting very small numbers of bacteria because a larger volume of specimen can be added; plates, however, facilitate rapid isolation of pure cultures and can give early indications of identity from colony structure and reactions on indicator media. Established routines may vary between laboratories, but for practical reasons, specialized media for rare organisms are seldom included (for example, those for *Leptospira* or *Corynebacterium diphtheriae*). For detection of these organisms, the laboratory must be informed of the clinical possibility of their presence. To be certain that appropriate media and procedures are employed, the physician should always indicate any suspicion of less common organisms in the request.

Bacterial Identification

Once growth is detected in any medium, the process of identification begins. Identification involves the use of methods to obtain pure cultures from single colonies, followed by tests designed to characterize and identify the isolate.

Positive broth cultures are Gram stained and subcultured to plated media. Representative colonies on these or on primarily seeded solid media are stained to determine the morphology and Gram reaction of the organism and are subcultured for any additional cultural, motility, biochemical, or serologic characterization that may be needed. The exact tests and their sequences vary with different groups of organisms, and the level

Table 14.1 Routine Use of Gram Smear and Isolation Systems for Selected Clinical Specimens[a]

Medium (Incubation)	Specimen							
	Blood	Cerebrospinal Fluid	Wound, Pus	Genital, Cervix	Throat	Sputum	Urine	Stool
Gram smear		X	X	X		X	X	
Soybean–Casein digest broth (CO_2)	X	X	X					
Selenite F broth (air)								X
Blood agar (CO_2)		X	X	X		X	X	
Blood agar (anaerobic)			X		X[b]			
MacConkey agar (air)			X	X		X	X	X
Chocolate agar (CO_2)		X	X	X		X		
Thayer–Martin agar (CO_2)				X				
Hektoen agar (air)								X
Campylobacter agar (CO_2, 42°C)[c]								X

[a] The added sensitivity of a nutrient broth is used only when contamination by normal flora is unlikely. Exact media and isolation systems may vary between laboratories.
[b] Anaerobic incubation used to enhance hemolysis by β-hemolytic streptococci.
[c] Incubation in a reduced oxygen atmosphere.

Levels of identification in clinical practice

of identification to be achieved varies according to the clinical usefulness of the information. Identification for genus, species, or occasionally subspecies or serotype level may be required. In other cases, only a general description or the exclusion of particular organisms is important in the management of a patient. For example, the report of "mixed oral flora" in a sputum specimen or "no *N. gonorrhoeae*" in a cervical specimen may provide all of the information needed.

Cultural Characteristics. Cultural characteristics beyond the basic observations of bacterial morphology, Gram reaction, motility, and patterns of growth in culture media have great taxonomic significance. They include the demonstration of properties such as unique nutritional requirements, pigment production, and the ability to grow in the presence of certain potentially inhibitory substances (sodium chloride, bile) or on different media (MacConkey, nutrient agar). Demonstration of the ability to grow at a particular temperature or to affect certain natural substances, such as milk, egg yolk, or meat, is often useful. The nature and pattern of hemolysis can also be considered a cultural characteristic.

Nutritional requirements, growth characteristics, and sensitivity to inhibitors

Biochemical Characteristics. These characteristics, which include the ability to attack various substrates or to produce particular metabolic products, have the broadest application to the identification of bacteria. Most of these tests are carried out in a simple peptone-based medium, unless this substrate will not support growth of the organism. The most common properties examined are listed in Appendix 14.3.

Table 14.2 Biochemical Reactions for Differentiation of
Certain Salmonellas

Test	Salmonella Species Reaction		
	S. choleraesuis	S. typhi	S. enteritidis
Indole production	−	−	−
Citrate utilization	(+)	−	+
Urease production	−	−	−
Lysine decarboxylase production	+	+	+
Ornithine decarboxylase production	+	−	+
Fermentation of			
Glucose	+	+	+
Gas from glucose	+	−	+
Lactose	−	−	−
Dulcitol	v	− or (+)	+
Inositol	−	−	v
Trehalose	−	+	+
Arabinose	−	−	+
Rhamnose	+	−	+
Hydrogen sulfide production	v	+^{w}	+

Data published by the Centers for Disease Control, Atlanta, Georgia.

Abbreviations: − = less than 10% of strains positive; (+) = delayed reaction, requiring 3 or more days; + = more than 90% of strains positive; v = variable, 10–90% of strains positive; w = weak.

Biochemical and cultural tests for bacterial identification are analyzed with reference to tables that show the reaction patterns characteristic for individual species. An example is shown in Table 14.2. Such tables, which represent the sum of testing with many strains of each species, are published in books, pamphlets, and scientific papers and by institutions such as the Centers for Disease Control in Atlanta. Shortened versions are often used in routine practice. Given the phenotypic variation possible with bacterial species, the results with an unknown isolate may not match those in the table precisely; a final decision may therefore require further testing.

Automation and computer analysis in bacterial identification

In recent years, instrumentation, automation, and computer analysis have been applied to speciation and identification of bacterial families such as the Enterobacteriaceae, which show a great diversity of biochemical activity. These systems employ the same biochemical principles, but use miniaturized reaction cuvettes, automatic readers, and a computerized data base to determine the most probable identification for the observed test pattern. Identification and taxonomic classifications derived from a range of such phenotypic characteristics are satisfactory procedures, but increased use of the more direct analyses of the bacterial genome that are described later in the chapter can be expected in the future.

Demonstrations of Toxin Production and Pathogenicity. These are sometimes needed to confirm a clinical diagnosis. In laboratory animals, a localized or lethal infection with a characteristic pattern of lesions may develop after inoculation with some species. The organisms should be demonstrated in the lesions to confirm the diagnosis. In diseases caused by production of a specific bacterial toxin, the presence of the toxin may be detected in vivo in experimental animals or in vitro through cell cultures or immunologic methods. In either case, neutralization of the toxic effect with specific antitoxin should be demonstrated to confirm its nature.

Susceptibility or Resistance to Antimicrobics.   Response to these or chemical substances is sometimes helpful in the identification of bacteria, but involves properties that may be variable. Such tests are usually considered presumptive or ancillary to methods that determine the final identification.

Serologic Identification.   As discussed in Chapter 2, bacteria possess many structures that may be antigenic, such as capsular polysaccharides, flagellar proteins, and several cell wall components. Serology involves the demonstration of specific antigen-antibody interactions in vitro and, in bacterial identification, uses antibodies of known specificity to detect antigens present on whole bacteria or free in bacterial extracts (soluble antigens). Several methods are used for demonstrating antigen-antibody reactions.

Optimum antigen-antibody ratios needed for precipitate formation

PRECIPITIN TESTS. When soluble antigen and antibody combine in the proper proportions, a visible precipitate is formed (Figure 14.6A). Optimum antigen-antibody ratios are produced by allowing one (or both) to diffuse slowly into the other. This test may be done in capillary tubes, where the antigen and antibody solutions are placed in direct contact, or with immunodiffusion procedures, where they diffuse through agar. In capillary tubes the precipitate is formed at or near the interface. In immunodiffusion, one or more precipitin lines are formed between the antigen and antibody wells; the number of lines depends on the number of different antigen-antibody reactions occurring. Counterimmunoelectrophoresis (CIE) is immunodiffusion carried out in an electrophoretic field. The pH and other conditions are adjusted so that the negatively charged antigen migrates to the anode while the less charged antibody is swept toward the cathode with the flow of buffer ions. The net effect is that antigen and antibody are rapidly brought together in the space between the wells to form a precipitin line. Both the speed and the sensitivity of immunodiffusion are improved by CIE.

Agglutination involves particulate antigens

AGGLUTINATION. The amount of antigen and antibody necessary to produce visible reaction can be reduced if either is on the surface of a relatively large particle. This condition, which may occur with whole bacterial cells, can be produced by coating soluble antigens or antibody onto the surface of red blood cells or microscopic latex particles (Figure 14.6B). The relative proportions of antigen and antibody thus become less critical, and antigen-antibody reactions are more easily detectable by clumping when immune serum and particulate antigen are mixed in test tubes or on a slide. When bacteria serve as the antigen, the process is termed *bacterial agglutination.* When red cells or latex particles serve as antigen or antibody carriers, the test is termed *passive hemagglutination* or *latex agglutination.* A variant of this procedure, *coagglutination,* utilizes the unique ability of protein A on the surface of *Staphylococcus aureus* to bind the Fc fragment of IgG, leaving the Fab portions free to react with homologous antigen. Thus, *S. aureus* cells can become a diagnostic reagent when antibody with specificity to any of a variety of antigens is attached to their surface protein.

Bacterial agglutination, hemagglutination, and latex agglutination

S. aureus as passive antibody carrier in coagglutination

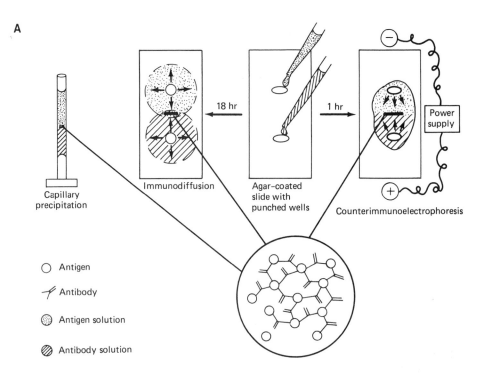

14.6 Precipitin formation and agglutination. **(A)** Three methods are shown for demonstrating antigen–antibody interaction with formation of a precipitate. In the capillary tube procedure, the antigen and antibody solutions are layered on each other. As they diffuse at the interface, an antigen–antibody complex is formed. In both immunodiffusion and counterimmunoelectrophoresis, the test is begun by adding the antigen and the antibody to separate wells cut in an agar gel; the precipitate forms as a line(s) where the antigen and antibody meet. In immunodiffusion, both antigen and antibody diffuse radially, with overlap between the wells; in counterimmunoelectrophoresis, the electrophoretic field concentrates both in the same area. The precipitate, composed of a lattice of antigen and antibody, is the same regardless of the method used and develops at an optimum antigen–antibody ratio. **(B)** Agglutination requires a particulate antigen small enough to produce smooth diffuse turbidity, but large enough to show visible aggregates when linked by specific antibody. The antigen may be 1) on the surface of the organism itself (simple agglutination); or 2) coated on the surface of the red blood cell or latex particle (hemagglutination or latex agglutination). Coagglutination, **(B3)** is more complex. The antibody is bound by its Fc receptor end to the protein A on the surface of a dead *Staphyloccus aureus.* Visible agglutination is produced when these particles combine with a soluble antigen or another particulate antigen.

Immunofluorescence procedures

RIA and ELISA procedures

LABELING METHODS. Detection of antigen-antibody interactions may be enhanced by attaching a label to one (usually the antibody), then measuring the label after removal of unbound reagents. The most common method of this type in diagnostic microbiology is *immunofluorescence,* in which the antibody is labeled with a fluorescent dye, usually fluorescein isothiocyanate, that can then be detected by fluorescence microscopy. Fluorescence localizes the position of the antibody and thus of the antigen to which it is bound. Two newer methods, radioimmunoassay (RIA) and enzyme-linked immunosorbent assay (ELISA), are now being used increasingly. The principles of these techniques are described and illustrated later in the sections on serologic detection of viruses, although they are equally applicable to other microorganisms.

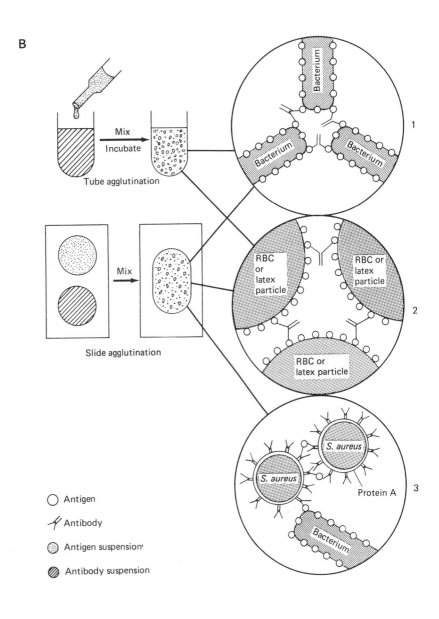

Antigenic analysis

Immunization of laboratory animals and cross-testing with homologous and heterologous strains

The application of these techniques to the development of systems for serologic identification of microorganisms is described in Chapter 8. It begins with selection of strains to be differentiated. Whole inactivated cells or antigens prepared from them by physical, chemical, or enzymatic treatment are injected repeatedly into animals (usually rabbits) to produce high antibody titers. After several weeks the animals are bled, the blood is allowed to clot, and the serum is separated. These immune sera (antisera) are cross-tested against homologous and heterologous strains using one of the antigen-antibody tests discussed previously, and the pattern of reactions is analyzed to determine the relatedness of the strains. An example of the process, taken from Dr. Rebecca Lancefield's work with streptococci, is shown in Table 14.3. This procedure involved extraction of cell

Table 14.3 Lancefield Serologic Classification of β-Hemolytic Streptococci[a]

Strain from Which Antigen Prepared			Precipitin Formation When Reacted with Rabbit Antiserum Prepared with Strain						Serologic Group Assignment
Strain	Source	Disease	C203	K96	K107	K126	K155	C6	
C203	Human	Scarlet fever	+	+	−	−	−	−	A
K96	Human	Pneumonia	+	+	−	−	−	−	A
K107	Cow	Mastitis	−	−	+	+	−	−	B
K126	Cow	None	−	−	+	+	−	−	B
K155	Horse	Pleuropneumonia	−	−	−	−	+	−	C
C6	Cheese	None	−	−	−	−	−	+	D

[a] Data from one of Dr. Lancefield's studies (*J. Exp. Med.* 57:571–595, 1933) are presented as an example of the development of a serologic system. Note that extract from each strain produces a precipitin reaction with rabbit antiserum prepared with extract from the same strain, indicating that the product is antigenic. The two human strains (C203, K96), which react with each other but not with the nonhuman isolates, were assigned to group A. Strains K107 and K126, which also react with each other but not with the other strains, were assigned to group B. Strains K155 and C6 are serologically unique and were assigned the new groups C and D. New Isolates may be classified in one of the existing groups or assigned a new one, depending on their reaction with known antisera. Continued application of these methods to streptococci has led to the recognition of groups A through T.

wall carbohydrate antigens for precipitin testing with antisera prepared against homologous and heterologous strains. The method allowed recognition of many distinct Lancefield groups of streptococci of greatly differing significance in human and animal disease.

The development of serologic classification schemes to detect specific antigens is often greatly complicated by the presence of some common and cross-reacting antigens in related organisms. If the specific antigens cannot be purified for immunization of the experimental animal, the mixture must be used. The antisera that develop thus contain both specific and cross reacting antibodies. The latter must be removed by adding the heterologous organism to the antiserum, allowing the cross-reacting antibody to adsorb to its surface, and removing both organism and unwanted antibody by centrifugation. The process is repeated until only the strain-specific antibody is left in the serum. Serologic classifications become enormously complex when multiple antigens are present in species with numerous distinct but overlapping serotypes, such as *Salmonella* (Chapter 20). Classification schemes of this complexity have been developed through the dedicated work of a few individual microbiologists, and thus their availability is uneven among the different bacterial groups.

In most cases, serotyping serves to subclassify organisms below the genus level. With some genera and species, the serologic detection of antigens allows fundamental taxonomic differentiation, as with the β-hemolytic streptococci (Chapter 16), or provides the most rapid means of diagnosis, as with *Legionella* (Chapter 25). With others, it is of primary value for epidemiologic and research purposes.

DNA–DNA Homology.   This is a powerful tool that has been applied increasingly to establish taxonomic relationships and to test and sometimes change those proposed by classical methods. DNA homology techniques compare the total genomic DNA of one organism to that of another in a manner demonstrated in Figure 14.7. Closely related species show homology in the 80–90% range, whereas strains with increasing taxonomic divergence show progressivily less homology. Thus, strain, species, genus, and higher taxonomic groupings can now be made by objective methods that can be applied to all microorganisms regardless of morphological and growth characteristics that are subject to phenotypic variation.

Marginal notes:

Adsorption techniques for removing cross-reacting antibody

Complexity of some serologic classifications

Compares genomic DNA of different organisms

REFERENCE DNA   TEST DNA

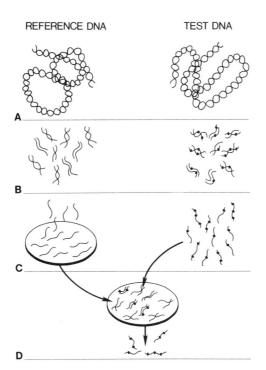

14.7 DNA–DNA homology.
(A) Double-stranded chromosomal DNA from a test strain is to be compared with a reference strain of the same or another species. (B) Both DNAs are fragmented and denatured. The test DNA is labeled ($-\bullet-$) with a radioisotope or some other marker. (C) The denatured (single-stranded) reference DNA is bound to a support matrix such as a nitrocellulose or nylon filter, thus leaving the nucleotide bases available for pairing. (D) The labeled test DNA is reacted with the material on the filter allowing homologous sequences to pair (hybridize) with the reference DNA. Nonhomologous DNA is washed away, and the amount of bound label measured. The percentage homology of the test to the reference DNA is determined from the ratio of bound to unbound label.

Use of DNA probes in diagnosis and identification

Nucleic Acid Probes.   A nucleic acid "probe" is usually a fragment of DNA that has been selected and cloned from a genomic or plasmid source. The probe may contain an important gene of known function or simply contain sequences empirically found to be unique for the organism in question. In some cases the probe is synthesized as a single chain of nucelotides (oligonucleotide probe) from known sequence data. A diagnostic probe procedure (Figure 14.8) detects by hybridization the homologous sequence of bases in DNA extracted from the entire organism. To date, a number of probes have been developed that will reliably detect organisms in culture or in some cases directly in clinical specimens. For example, probes that contain the gene for production of the heat-labile (LT) and heat-stable (ST) toxins of *Escherichia coli* have been used to detect toxigenic strains in stools without the need for culture.

RNA probes and targets

Although less commonly used, RNA can be the probe or target in hybridization reactions. Another approach to the use of probes is to digest the nucleic acid of the test strain and separate the fragments by electrophoresis. The fragments may then be transferred to filters where hybridization with a labeled probe is possible. This often gives information not available when the probe is hybridized with the total cellular DNA in one spot as shown in Figure 14.8. When the nucleic acid analyzed is DNA, this procedure is called a *southern blot;* when it is RNA, it is called a *northern blot.*

Southern and northern blots

Technical and cost considerations make many nucleic acid probe techniques impractical for clinical laboratory use at present, but these difficulties will probably be overcome soon.

Antigen Detection.   Theoretically, any of the methods described for detecting antigen–antibody interactions could be applied directly to clinical

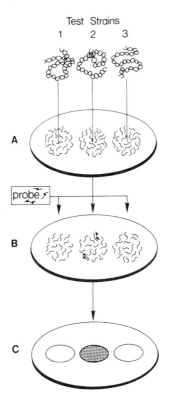

Test Strains

14.8 DNA probe detection.
(A) Chromosomal and/or
plasmid DNA from three
unknown strains is fragmented,
denatured, and bound to filters.
(B) The probe ($-\bullet-$) is a small
DNA fragment labeled with a
radioactive or other marker. It is
allowed to react with the single-
stranded test DNAs on the filter
and binds wherever homologous
sequences are found. (C) Probe
that has hybridized with test
DNA is detected on the filter by
an appropriate test for the
marker. Test strain 2 contained
sequences homologous to the
probe and thus gives a positive
reaction.

Importance of free specific antigen

specimens to detect free antigen, thus offering the possibility of bypassing direct examination, culture, and biochemical identification tests to achieve a diagnosis. Success with this approach requires a highly specific antibody, a sensitive detection method, and the presence of the homologous antigen in an accessible body fluid. The latter is an important limitation, because not all organisms are known to release free antigen in the course of infection. Furthermore, the antigen should not cross-react serologically with antigens from other possible infecting organisms. At present, diagnosis by antigen detection is limited to bacteria with polysaccharide capsules, such as *Haemophilus influenzae,* and to certain viruses and fungi. The techniques of CIE, latex agglutination, coagglutination, RIA, and ELISA can

Antigen detection techniques

detect free antigen in serum, urine, cerebrospinal fluid, and joint fluid. As live bacteria are not required for antigen detection, these tests are useful when the causative organism has been eliminated by antimicrobial therapy. Antigen detection procedures have the advantage of speed: they can yield results within an hour or two, sometimes within a few minutes. This feature is attractive for office practice, because it allows diagnostic decisions to be made during the patient's visit. A number of commercial products detect group A streptococci in sore throats with over 90% sensitivity. However, because these tests are less sensitive than culture, negative results must be confirmed.

Diagnosis of Viral Infections

Specimen Selection and Transport

The selection of specimens for viral diagnosis is based primarily on the clinical history to determine which etiologic agents should be considered. Some selected situations are illustrated in Table 14.4. For example, it can

Table 14.4   Some Appropriate Specimens for Viral Isolation[a]

Agent	Throat	Stool	Cerebrospinal Fluid	Urine	Vesicle Fluid	Other
Meningitis and encephalitis						
Mumps	+ + + +	−	+ +	+	−	−
Enteroviruses	+ + +	+ + + +	+ +	−	−	−
Herpes simplex	±	−	±	−	+	+ + + + (Brain biopsy)
Arboviruses[b]	−	−	+	−	−	+ + (Brain) + (Blood)
Respiratory diseases						
Influenza and parainfluenza viruses	+ + + +	−	−	−	−	
Adenoviruses	+ + + +	+ + + +	−	−	−	
Exanthems						
Measles	+ + + +	−	−	+	−	
Rubella[b]	+ + + +	−	−	+	−	
Varicella	−	−	−	−	+ + + +	
Herpes simplex	+ +	−	−	−	+ + + +	
Cytomegalovirus	+ +	−	−	+ + + +	−	+ (Leukocyte tissue biopsy)

Abbreviations: − = no yield; ± to + + + + = relatative yield (low to high).

[a] In general, it should be remembered that virus shedding often diminishes rapidly after onset of acute illness; it is therefore important to attempt specimen collection as early as possible.

[b] Because it is frequently very difficult to isolate these agents from the disease in question, it is emphasized that serologic tests are particularly important to ensure a diagnosis.

be seen that mumps and enteroviruses are among the more common viruses involved in acute infection of the central nervous system. Specimens that might be expected to yield these agents on culture would include throat, stool, and cerebrospinal fluid. On the other hand, the diagnosis of herpes simplex encephalitis may require brain biopsy, and the arbovirus-caused illnesses often require serologic study for confirmation. Specimens for culture should be processed and inoculated as soon after collection as possible, because many viruses in the extracellular habitat are labile on prolonged exposure to temperatures above 4°C or on freezing.

Viral Isolation Methods

There are several common methods of viral isolation, including inoculation of cell culture (most frequently used), of embryonated hen's eggs and of experimental animals.

Cell cultures in monolayers

Cell cultures from a variety of sources are used, each of which can support the replication of some viruses but not others. The preparation of cell culture monolayers is illustrated in Figure 14.9. The cells are derived from a tissue source by outgrowth of cells from a tissue fragment (explant) or by dispersal with proteolytic agents such as trypsin. They are allowed to grow in the presence of nutrient media on a glass or plastic surface until a confluent layer one cell thick (monolayer) is achieved. In some circumstances, a tissue fragment with a specialized function (for example, fetal trachea with ciliated epithelial cells) is cultivated in vitro and used for viral detection. This procedure is known as *organ culture.*

Organ cultures

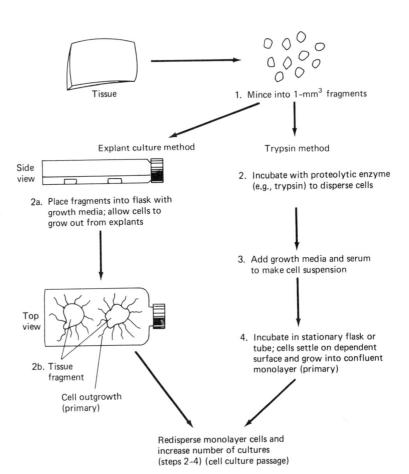

14.9 Preparation of cell culture monolayers.

Tissue

1. Mince into 1-mm³ fragments

Explant culture method

Side view

2a. Place fragments into flask with growth media; allow cells to grow out from explants

Top view

2b. Tissue fragment

Cell outgrowth (primary)

Trypsin method

2. Incubate with proteolytic enzyme (e.g., trypsin) to disperse cells

3. Add growth media and serum to make cell suspension

4. Incubate in stationary flask or tube; cells settle on dependent surface and grow into confluent monolayer (primary)

Redisperse monolayer cells and increase number of cultures (steps 2–4) (cell culture passage)

Primary and secondary cell cultures of limited viability

Three basic types of cell culture monolayers are used in diagnostic virology. The primary cell culture, in which all cells have a normal chromosome count (diploid), is derived from the initial growth of cells from a tissue source. Redispersal and regrowth produces a secondary cell culture, which usually retains characteristics similar to those of the primary culture (diploid chromosome count and virus susceptibility). Examples of primary and secondary cultures commonly used are monkey and human embryonic kidney cell cultures.

Transformed haploid or heteroploid lines may multiply indefinitely

Further dispersal and regrowth of secondary cell cultures usually leads to one of two outcomes: the cells eventually die, or they undergo spontaneous *transformation,* in which the growth characteristics change, the chromosome count varies (haploid or heteroploid), and the susceptibility to virus infection differs from that of the original. These cell cultures have characteristics of "immortality"; that is, they can be redispersed and regrown many times (serial cell culture passage). They can also be derived from cancerous tissue cells or produced by exposure to mutagenic agents in vitro. Such cultures are commonly called *cell lines.* A common cell line in diagnostic use is the Hep-2, derived from a human epithelial carcinoma.

Diploid cell lines

A third type of culture is often termed a *cell strain.* This culture comprises diploid cells, commonly fibroblastic, that can be redispersed and regrown a finite number of times; usually 30–40 cell culture passages can be made before the strain dies out or spontaneously transforms. Human

Effect of viral growth on cells

Cytopathic effect

Syncytia

Hemadsorption and
hemagglutination

embryonic tonsil and lung fibroblasts are common cell strains in routine diagnostic use.

Viral growth in susceptible cell cultures can be detected in several ways. The most common effect is seen with lytic or cytopathic viruses; as they replicate in cells, they produce alterations in cellular morphology (or cell death) that can be observed directly by light microscopy under low magnification ($\times 30$ or $\times 100$). This *cytopathic effect* (CPE) varies with different viruses in different cell cultures. For example, enteroviruses often produce cell rounding, pleomorphism, and eventual cell death in various culture systems, whereas measles and respiratory syncytial viruses cause fusion of cells to produce multinucleated giant cells (syncytia). The microscopic appearance of some normal cell cultures and the CPE produced in them by different viruses are illustrated in Figures 14.10–14.16.

Other viruses may be detected in cell culture by their ability to produce hemagglutinins. These hemagglutinins may be present on the infected cell membranes, as well as in the culture media as a result of release of free, hemagglutinating virions from the cells. Addition of erythrocytes to the infected cell culture, followed by a period of incubation under proper temperature conditions (which vary according to the virus sought), will result in adherence of the erythrocytes to the cell surfaces, a phenomenon known as *hemadsorption*. Influenza, parainfluenza, and mumps viruses are common examples of agents that can be detected in this fashion. If sufficient numbers of virions have been released into the fluid media of the

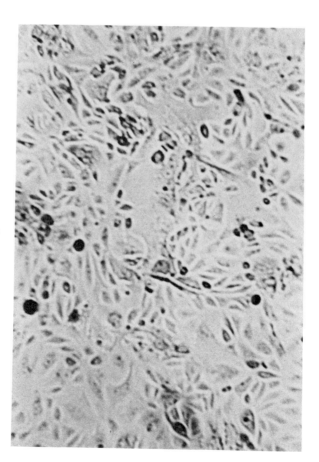

14.10 Normal monkey kidney cell culture monolayer (original magnification $\times 40$).

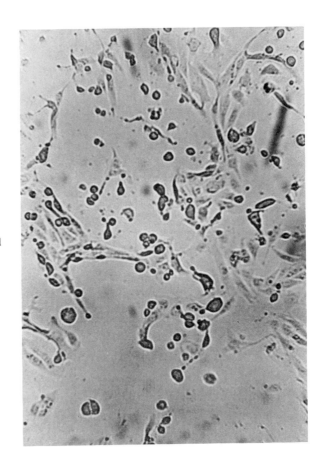

14.11 Enterovirus cytopathic effect in a monkey kidney cell monolayer. Note cell lysis and monolayer destruction (original magnification ×40).

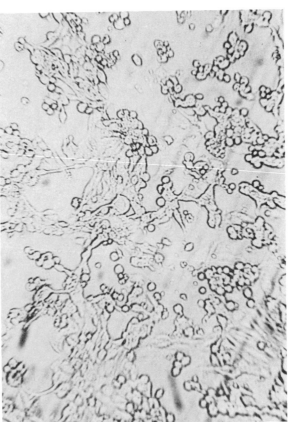

14.12 Adenovirus cytopathic effect in a monkey kidney cell monolayer. Note cell rounding and "lacy" appearance (original magnification ×40).

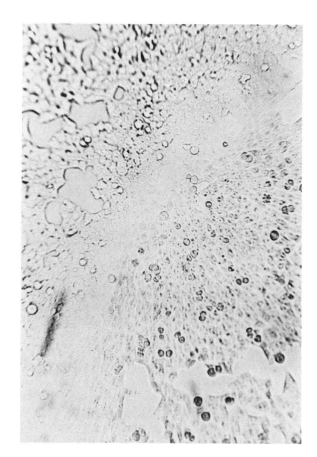

14.13 Normal heteroploid cell (Hep-2) monolayer (original magnification ×40).

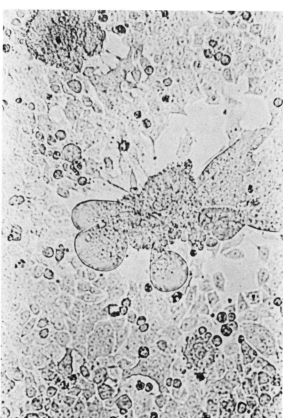

14.14 Respiratory syncytial virus cytopathic effect in Hep-2 cell monolayer. Note giant syncytial cell formation (original magnification ×40).

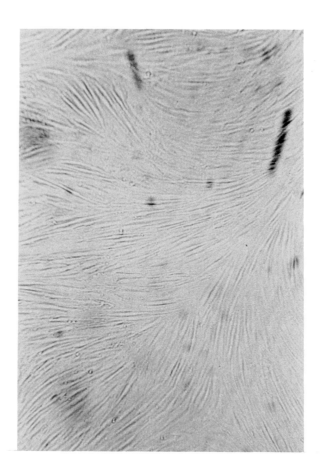

14.15 Normal human diploid fibroblast cell monolayer (original magnification ×40).

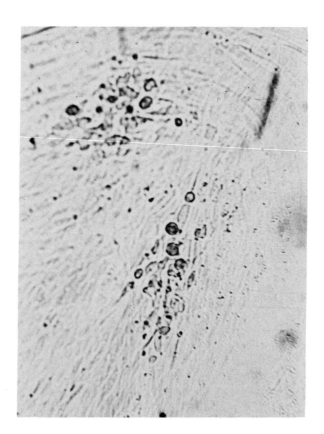

14.16 Cytomegalovirus cytopathic effect in human diploid cell monolayer. Note rounded, swollen cells in a focal area (original magnification ×40).

culture, they may be detected by the presence of hemagglutination when erythrocytes are mixed with the fluid and incubated.

Detection of virus by interference

Another method of viral detection in cell culture is by *interference*. In this situation, the virus that infects the susceptible cell culture produces no CPE or hemagglutinin, but can be detected by "challenging" the cell culture with a different virus that normally produces a characteristic CPE. The second, or *challenge*, virus fails to infect the cell culture because of interference by the first virus, which is thus detected. This method is obviously cumbersome, but has been applied to the detection of rubella virus in certain cell cultures, such as those derived from African green monkey kidney.

For some agents, such as Epstein–Barr virus (EBV) or human immunodeficiency virus (HIV), even more novel approaches may be applied. Both EBV and HIV will replicate in vitro in proper circumstances in suspension cultures of normal human lymphocytes such as those derived from neonatal cord blood. Their presence may be determined in a variety

Detection by immunologic or nucleic acid probes

Detection of retrovirus reverse transcriptase

of ways; for example, EBV-infected B lymphocytes and HIV-infected T lymphocytes will express virus-specified antigens and viral DNA, which can be detected with immunologic or genomic probes. In addition, HIV-infected cultures will produce reverse transcriptase, which can be detected with specific assay methods.

Immunologic and nucleic acid probes can also be utilized to detect virus in clinical specimens or in situations where only incomplete, noninfective virus replication has occurred in vivo or in vitro. An example is the use

In situ hybridization

of in situ cytohybridization, whereby specific labeled nucleic acid probes are used to detect and localize papillomavirus genomes in tissues where neither infectious virus nor its antigens can be detected.

In vivo methods for isolation are also sometimes necessary. These methods can include animal inoculation or the use of embryonated hen's eggs; each has special uses, which will be considered briefly.

Growth of virus in embryonated hen's egg

The embryonated hen's egg (Figure 14.17) is still used by many laboratories for the initial isolation and propagation of influenza A virus. It is also required for isolation of influenza C virus, which grows poorly in cell cultures. Several routes of inoculation are available, depending upon the agent sought. Virus-containing material is inoculated on the appropriate membrane, and the egg is incubated to permit viral replication and recognition.

Animal inoculation is used for some viruses. The usual animal host for

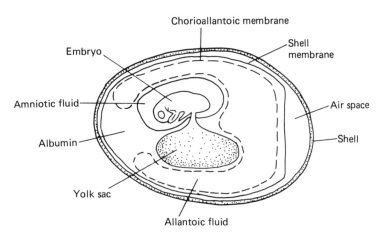

14.17 Inoculation of embryonated hen's egg for isolation of viruses, *Rickettsia*, or *Chlamydia*. Routes of inoculation include amniotic fluid (influenza virus); allantoic fluid (paramyxoviruses); chorioallantoic membrane (poxviruses, herpes simplex); and yolk sac (*Rickettsia*, *Chlamydia*).

Viral isolation in experimental animals: use of suckling mouse

viral isolation is the mouse; suckling mice in the first 48 hr of life are especially susceptible to many viruses. Intracerebral, subcutaneous, or intraperitoneal inoculation is used, depending upon the virus. Evidence for viral replication is based on the development of illness, manifested by such signs as paralysis, convulsions, poor feeding, or death. The nature of the infecting virus can be further elucidated by histologic and immunofluorescent examination of tissues or by detection of specific antibody responses. Many arboviruses, group A Coxsackie viruses, and rabies virus are best detected in this system.

With this background of viral isolation in mind, it is now possible to summarize the usual steps involved in this process. First, the viruses believed most likely to be involved in the illness are considered, and appropriate specimens are collected. Next, the specimens are processed; a schematic example is shown in Figure 14.18). Antibiotics and centrifugation or filtration are frequently required with respiratory or fecal specimens to remove organic matter, cellular debris, bacteria, and fungi, which can interfere with viral isolation. The specimens are then inoculated into the appropriate cell culture systems and observed. The time between inoculation and initial detection of viral effects varies; for most viruses, however, positive cultures are usually apparent within 5 days of collection. With proper collection methods and application of the diagnostic tools discussed subsequently, many infections can be detected within hours or a few days. On the other hand, some viruses may require culture for a month or more before they may be detected.

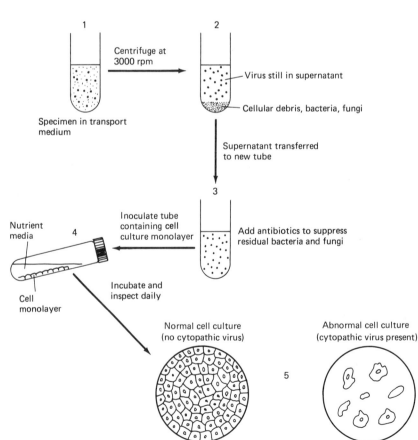

14.18 Preparation and inoculation of a specimen for isolation in cell culture (cytopathic virus).

Viral Identification

Effect on Cell Cultures.   Upon isolation, a virus can usually be tentatively identified with regard to family or genus by its cultural characteristics (for example, type of CPE produced). Confirmation and further identification of the isolate may require enhancement of viral growth to produce adequate quantities for testing. This result may be achieved by inoculation of the original isolate into fresh culture systems (viral passage) to amplify replication of the virus, as well as improve its adaptation to growth in the in vitro system.

Serologic Detection.   Of the several ways to identify the isolate, the most common is to neutralize its infectivity by mixing it with specific antibody to known viruses before inoculation into cultures. Figure 14.19 illustrates the use of this method for identification of a cytopathic virus. Other methods of identification include demonstration of specific attachment of fluorescein-labeled antiviral antibody to viral antigens in infected cells (Figure 14.20) and specific antibody inhibition of other viral properties such as hemagglutination (hemagglutination inhibition).

Viral passage

Neutralization, immunofluorescence, and hemagglutination inhibition

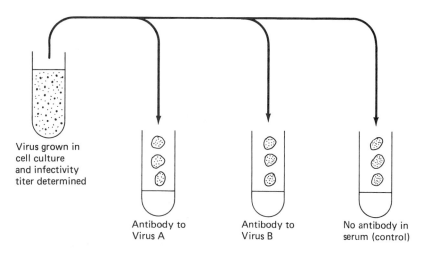

Virus grown in cell culture and infectivity titer determined

Antibody to Virus A

Antibody to Virus B

No antibody in serum (control)

14.19 Identification of a virus isolate (cytopathic virus) as "Virus B."

Virus aliquot added to tubes containing antibody to known viruses and to control, incubated for 1 hr, then each inoculated into cell culture tubes, incubated, and observed daily

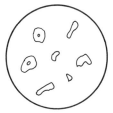

Antibody to A + virus: Cytopathic effect (not Virus A)

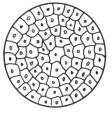

Antibody to B + virus: No cytopathic effect (confirms Virus B)

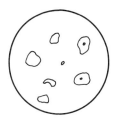

Serum control + virus: Cytopathic effect in control

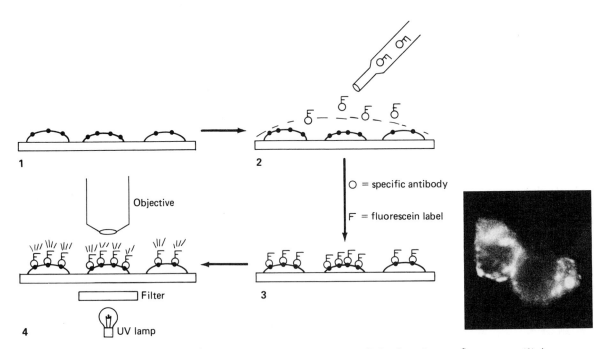

14.20 Detection of viral antigen in cells by direct immunofluorescence. (1) Acetone-fixed cells on slide. (2) Add fluorescein-conjugated antiserum and incubate. (3) Unattached antibody removed by washing. (4) Examine for fluorescence under UV illumination (the actual wavelength of light used is that which excites the fluorochrome). Illumination may be from below, using a dark-field condenser, or from above, through the objective (epifluorescence). Respiratory syncytial virus antigen in the cytoplasm of cells in culture is shown.

Other Methods of Viral Detection. Some viruses (for example, human rotaviruses, hepatitis A and B viruses) grow poorly or not at all in the laboratory culture systems currently available. These viruses have been demonstrated in some instances by inoculation of susceptible human volunteers, and some will replicate and cause disease in subhuman primates such as chimpanzees. Obviously, such methods of cultivation cannot be used in routine diagnosis. The use of nucleic acid probes has been already described; alternative methods for rapid detection of these and other viruses are summarized as follows.

Direct examination

ELECTRON MICROSCOPY. Direct examination of fluids and tissues from affected body sites, using negative staining techniques, has sometimes enabled visualization of viral particles. When the virions are present in sufficient numbers, they may be further characterized antigenically by specific agglutination of viral particles upon mixture with type-specific antiserum. This technique, *immune electron microscopy,* can be used to identify viral antigens specifically or to detect antibody in serum using viral particles of known antigenicity.

Immune electron microscopy

Direct and indirect immunofluorescence, RIA and ELISA techniques

LABELED ANTIBODY PROCEDURES. The principles of application of immunofluorescence, RIA, and ELISA to viral antigen detection are illustrated in Figures 14.20–14.22. Variations on direct immunofluorescence include

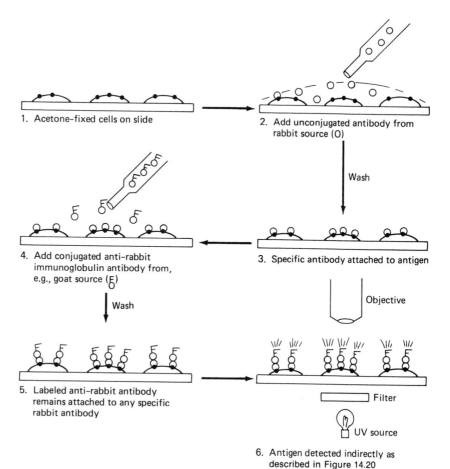

14.21 Detection of viral antigen in cells by indirect immunofluorescence.

1. Acetone–fixed cells on slide

2. Add unconjugated antibody from rabbit source (O)

Wash

3. Specific antibody attached to antigen

4. Add conjugated anti-rabbit immunoglobulin antibody from, e.g., goat source (F)

Wash

5. Labeled anti-rabbit antibody remains attached to any specific rabbit antibody

Objective

Filter

UV source

6. Antigen detected indirectly as described in Figure 14.20

1) *indirect methods,* whereby the antigen is first reacted with an unlabeled, specific antibody, which is then detected with a labeled antibody from a different species directed against the immunoglobulins that comprise the specific antibody (labeled anti-antibody) (Figure 14.21); and 2) *sandwich methods,* whereby the antigen adsorbs to a specific antibody, which has been attached to a surface. A second layer of labeled, specific antibody is used to detect the "trapped" antigen (Figure 14.22). These extremely sensitive techniques will be discussed further with regard to antibody detection.

Other methods of viral antigen detection include complement fixation, immunoprecipitation, thin-layer chromatography, and the like. Some are currently used primarily as research tools; details of others will be provided later in this chapter.

Intranuclear and cytoplasmic inclusions

CYTOLOGY AND HISTOLOGY. In some instances, viruses will produce specific cytologic changes in infected host tissues that aid in diagnosis. Examples include specific intranuclear inclusions, which can be seen in some herpes-virus and adenovirus infections (Figures 14.23 and 14.24); cytoplasmic inclusions; and cell fusion, which results in multinucleated epithelial giant cells (Figure 14.25). Although such findings are useful when seen, their overall diagnostic sensitivity and specificity are usually considerably less than that of the other methods outlined herein.

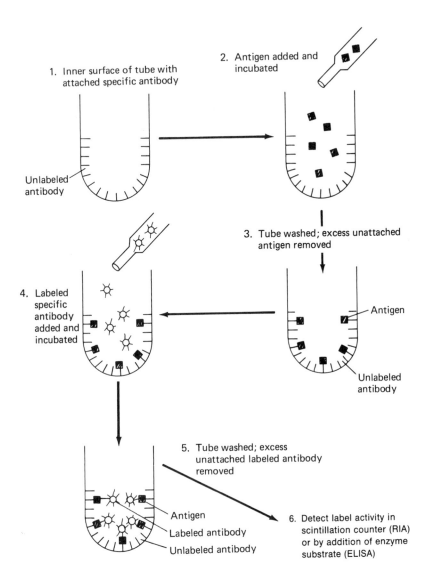

14.22 Detection of extracellular antigen by "sandwich" method.

1. Inner surface of tube with attached specific antibody

Unlabeled antibody

2. Antigen added and incubated

3. Tube washed; excess unattached antigen removed

Antigen

Unlabeled antibody

4. Labeled specific antibody added and incubated

5. Tube washed; excess unattached labeled antibody removed

Antigen
Labeled antibody
Unlabeled antibody

6. Detect label activity in scintillation counter (RIA) or by addition of enzyme substrate (ELISA)

Serologic Diagnosis of Infection

In infection, whether viral, bacterial, fungal, or parasitic, the host normally responds with the formation of antibodies, which can be detected by various methods. An example of temporal patterns of development and increase in quantities of specific antiviral antibodies measured by different tests are illustrated in Figure 14.26. These responses can be utilized to detect evidence of recent or past infection. Several basic principles must be emphasized:

1. In an acute infection, the antibodies usually appear early in the illness, then rise sharply over the next 10–21 days. Thus, a serum sample collected shortly after the onset of illness (acute serum) and another collected 2–3 weeks later (convalescent serum) can be compared quantitatively for changes in specific antibody content.

Comparison of amount of antibody in acute and convalescent sera

2. Antibodies can be quantitated by several means. The most common method is to dilute the serum serially in appropriate media and de-

Quantitation of antibody

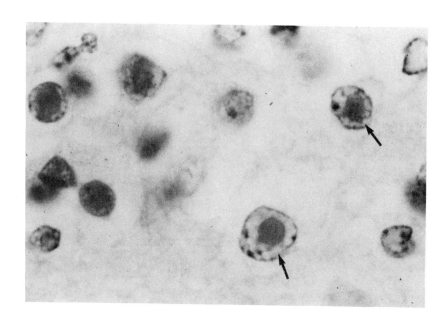

14.23 Brain biopsy from a patient with herpes simplex encephalitis. Arrows indicate infected neuronal nuclei with marginated chromatin and typical intranuclear inclusions. The cytoplasmic membranes are not clearly seen in this preparation (hematoxylin–eosin stain; original magnification ×400).

termine the maximal dilution that will still yield detectable antibody in the test system (for example, serum dilutions of 1:4, 1:8, 1:16, and so on). The reciprocal of the highest dilution that retains specific activity is called the *antibody titer*.

Antibody titer

3. The interpretation of significant antibody responses (evidence of specific, recent infection) is most reliable when definite evidence of *seroconversion* is demonstrated; that is, detectable specific antibody is absent from the acute serum (or preillness serum, if available) but present in the convalescent serum. Alternatively, a fourfold or greater increase

Seroconversion and significant titer increases

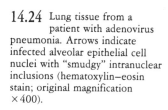

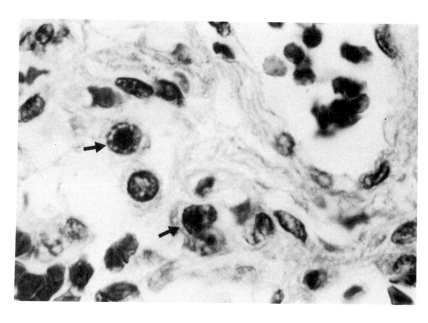

14.24 Lung tissue from a patient with adenovirus pneumonia. Arrows indicate infected alveolar epithelial cell nuclei with "smudgy" intranuclear inclusions (hematoxylin–eosin stain; original magnification ×400).

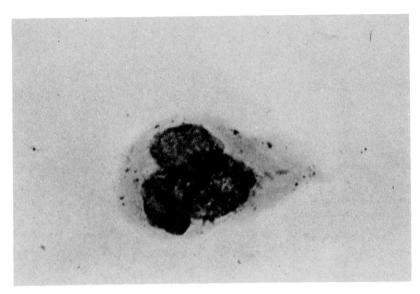

14.25 Multinucleated epithelial cells from a vesicle scraping of a patient with chickenpox. Cell fusion of this type can be seen with both varicella-zoster and herpes simplex infections (Wright's stain; original magnification ×400).

in antibody titer supports a diagnosis of recent infection; for example, an acute serum titer of 4 and a convalescent serum titer of 16 or greater would be significant.

4. In instances in which the average antibody titers of a population to a specific agent are known, a single convalescent antibody titer significantly greater than the expected mean may be used as supportive or presumptive evidence of recent infection. This finding, however, is considerably less valuable than those obtained by comparing responses of acute and convalescent serum samples. An alternative and somewhat

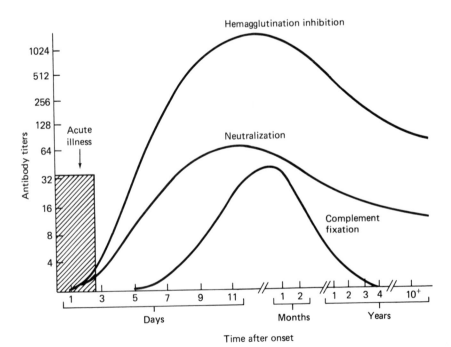

14.26 Examples of patterns of antibody responses, measured by three different methods, to an acute infection.

Value of determining
presence of specific IgM

more complex method of serodiagnosis is to determine which major immunoglobulin subclass constitutes the major proportion of the specific antibodies. In primary infections, the IgM-specific response is often dominant during the first days or weeks after onset, but is replaced progressively by IgG-specific antibodies; thus, by 1–6 months after infection, the predominant antibodies belong to the IgG subclass. Consequently, serum containing a high titer of antibodies of the IgM subclass would suggest a recent, primary infection.

Serodiagnostic methods

The immunologic methods that can be used to identify a bacterial or viral agent have been discussed in relation to serologic identification of bacteria and viruses. Most of these methods can also be applied to serologic diagnosis by simply reversing the detection system: that is, using a known rather than an unknown antigen to detect the presence of an antibody. The methods of serologic diagnosis to be employed are selected on the basis of their convenience and applicability to the antigen in question. As shown in Figure 14.26, the temporal relationships of antibody response to infection vary according to the method used. Of the methods for measuring antigen-antibody interaction discussed previously, those now used most frequently for serologic diagnosis are agglutination, hemagglutination, RIA, and ELISA. In the remainder of this chapter, some of the additional tests and test modifications used primarily in serologic diagnosis (antibody detection) will be considered briefly.

NEUTRALIZATION. Neutralization is commonly employed in serodiagnosis of viral infection. The principle is relatively simple in concept: some observable function of the agent (for example, cytopathic effect) is neutralized by first reacting the agent with antibody, then placing the antigen-antibody mixture into the test system. In viral neutralization, a single antibody molecule can bind to surface components of the extracellular virus and interfere with one of the initial events of the viral multiplication cycle, such as adsorption, penetration, or uncoating. Neutralizing antibodies often persist for the life span of the patient, and they correlate well with resistance to reinfection.

Blocking the effect of virus
with antibody

AGGLUTINATION. In the agglutination test, the known antigen may be a suspension of whole infectious particles, such as bacteria, or represent antigenic material adsorbed and fixed (for example, with glutaraldehyde) to the surface of a particulate carrier (for example, latex particles or erythrocytes). The presence of specific antibody results in immune aggregation of the particles, which can be read microscopically (or macroscopically in some systems) as agglutination (Figure 14.6).

HEMAGGLUTINATION INHIBITION. Some antigens will react with naturally occurring receptors on cell membranes; for example, influenza viruses will agglutinate erythrocytes from certain animal and avian species. This phenomenon can be utilized in the hemagglutination inhibition test (Figure 14.27). First, the known antigen is reacted with serum; then the erythrocytes are added. If the antigen has reacted with adequate amounts of specific antibody, its ability to agglutinate the erythrocytes is abrogated (or "neutralized"), and agglutination is inhibited.

Complement bound if
antigen–antibody reactions
occur in test system

COMPLEMENT FIXATION. Complement fixation assays depend on two properties of complement. The first is the ability to cause hemolysis of sheep red blood cells (RBCs) coated with anti-sheep RBC antibody (sensitized

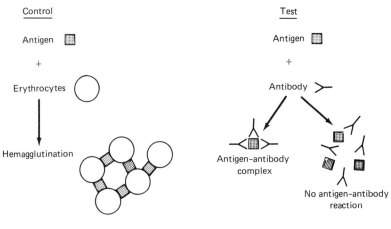

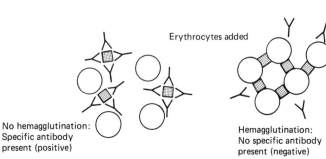

14.27 Hemagglutination inhibition for antibody detection (used when antigen agglutinates erythrocytes).

Unbound complement detected in sheep RBC: anti-sheep RBC indicator

Absence of hemolysis indicates positive test

RBCs). The second, under the proper conditions, is fixation (inactivation) of complement upon formation of antigen-antibody complexes. Complement fixation assays are performed in two stages: The *test system* reacts the antigen and antibody in the presence of complement; the *indicator system,* which contains the sensitized RBCs, detects residual complement. Hemolysis indicates that complement was present in the indicator system and therefore that antigen-antibody complexes were *not* formed in the test system. Primarily used to detect and quantitate antibody, complement fixation is gradually being replaced by simpler methods. The principles involved are shown in Figure 14.28.

INDIRECT IMMUNOFLUORESCENCE. Indirect immunofluorescence was detailed previously as one way to detect and identify antigens. In serodiagnosis, the known antigen is reacted with dilutions of the test serum, and the specific antibody that remains attached is detected by the addition of labeled anti-human immunoglobulin antibody.

IMMUNOASSAYS. Figure 14.29 outlines the basic steps involved in antibody detection by solid-phase immunoassays. In essence, the known antigen is chemically fixed to the surface of a tube or latex bead (solid phase); succeeding steps involve reaction with the test serum, followed by incubation with specifically labeled antibody to human immunoglobulins. The result is measured by counting radioactivity (RIA) or by addition of a substrate for the enzyme label that will undergo a color change in the presence of specific binding (ELISA).

The western blot immunoassay is another technique that is now commonly employed to detect and confirm the specificity of antibodies to a variety of epitopes. Its greatest use has been in the diagnosis of human

Western blot immunoassay

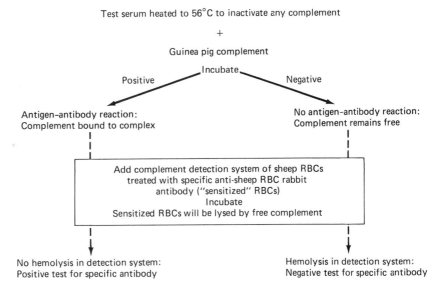

Antigen

+

Test serum heated to 56°C to inactivate any complement

+

Guinea pig complement

Incubate

Positive   Negative

Antigen–antibody reaction: No antigen–antibody reaction:
Complement bound to complex   Complement remains free

Add complement detection system of sheep RBCs
treated with specific anti-sheep RBC rabbit
antibody ("sensitized" RBCs)
Incubate
Sensitized RBCs will be lysed by free complement

No hemolysis in detection system: Hemolysis in detection system:
Positive test for specific antibody   Negative test for specific antibody

14.28 Complement fixation test.

immunodeficiency virus infections (see Chapter 73) in which virions are electophoresed in a polyacrylamide gel to separate the protein and glycoprotein components and then transferred onto nitrocellulose. This is then incubated with patient serum and antibody to the different viral components detected by using an anti-human globulin IgG antibody conjugated with an enzyme label.

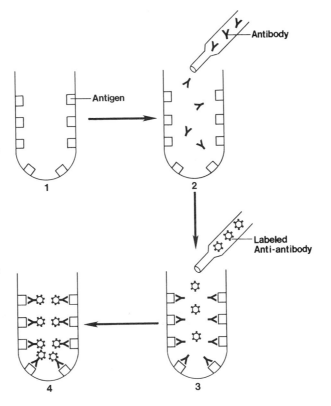

14.29 Solid-phase immunoassay for antibody detection. (1) Tube with known antigen attached to interior surface. (2) Add antibody-containing serum and incubate. (3) Specific antibody binds to antigen, wash and add labeled anti-antibody from different species, and incubate. (4) Wash off excess anti-antibody and measure activity of label.

Antibody

Antigen

Labeled Anti-antibody

1

2

3

4

Appendices

Appendix 14.1 Some Media Used for Isolation
of Bacterial Pathogens

Medium	Uses
General Purpose Media	
Nutrient broths (eg, Soybean–Casein digest broth)	Most bacteria, particularly when used for blood culture
Thioglycolate broth	Anaerobes, facultative bacteria
Blood agar	Most bacteria (demonstrates hemolysis)
Chocolate agar	Most bacteria, including fastidious species (eg, *Haemophilus*)
Selective Media	
MacConkey agar	Nonfastidious gram-negative rods
Hektoen-enteric agar	*Salmonella* and *Shigella*
Selenite F broth	*Salmonella* enrichment
Special Purpose Media	
Löwenstein–Jensen medium Middlebrook agar	*Mycobacterium tuberculosis* and other mycobacteria (selective)
Thayer–Martin medium	*Neisseria gonorrhoeae* and *Neisseria meningitidis* (selective)
Fletcher medium (semisolid)	*Leptospira* (nonselective)
Tinsdale agar	*Corynebacterium diphtheriae* (selective)
Charcoal agar	*Bordetella pertussis* (selective)
Charcoal–yeast extract agar	*Legionella* species (nonselective)
Campylobacter (Skirrow) blood agar	*Campylobacter fetus* (selective)
Thiosulfate-citrate-bile-sucrose agar (TCBS)	*Vibrio cholerae* and *Vibrio parahemolyticus* (selective)

Appendix 14.2 Characteristics of Commonly Used Bacteriologic Media

1. *Nutrient broths.* Some form of nutrient broth is used for culture of all direct tissue or fluid samples from sites that are normally sterile to obtain the maximum culture sensitivity. Selective or indicator agents are omitted to prevent inhibition of more fastidious organisms.

2. *Blood agar.* The addition of defibrinated blood to a nutrient agar base enhances the growth of some bacteria, such as streptococci. It often yields distinctive colonies and provides an indicator system for hemolysis. Two major types of hemolysis are seen: a) β-hemolysis, a complete clearing of red cells from a zone surrounding the colony; and b) α-hemolysis, which is incomplete (that is, intact red cells are still present in the hemolytic zone), but shows a green color caused by hemoglobin breakdown products. The net effect is a hazy green zone extending 1–2 mm beyond the colony. A third type, α'-hemolysis, produces a hazy, incomplete hemolytic zone similar to that caused by α-hemolysis, but without the green coloration.

3. *Chocolate agar.* If blood is added to molten nutrient agar at about 80°C and maintained at this temperature, the red cells are gently lysed, hemoglobin products are released, and the medium turns a chocolate brown color. The nutrients released permit the growth of some fastidious organisms, such as *H. influenzae,* that fail to grow on blood or nutrient agars. This quality is particularly pronounced when the medium is further enriched with vitamin supplements. Given the same incubation conditions, any organism that grows on blood agar will also grow on chocolate agar.

4. *Thayer-Martin medium.* A variant of chocolate agar, Thayer-Martin medium is a solid medium selective for the pathogenic *Neisseria* (*N. gonorrhoeae* and *N. meningitidis*). Growth of most other bacteria and fungi in the genital or respiratory flora is inhibited by the addition of antimicrobics. A current formulation includes vancomycin, colistin, trimethoprim, and anisomycin.

5. *MacConkey agar.* MacConkey agar is both a selective and an indicator medium for Gram-negative rods, particularly members of the family Enterobacteriaceae and the genus *Pseudomonas.* In addition to a peptone base, the medium contains bile salts, crystal violet, lactose, and neutral red as a pH indicator. The bile salts and crystal violet inhibit Gram-positive bacteria and the more fastidious Gram-negative organisms, such as *Neisseria* and *Pasteurella.* Gram-negative rods that grow and ferment lactose produce a red (acid) colony often with a distinctive colonial morphology.

6. *Hektoen enteric agar.* The Hektoen medium is one of many highly selective media developed for the isolation of *Salmonella* and *Shigella* species (Chapter 20) from stool specimens. It has both selective and indicator properties. The medium contains a mixture of bile, thiosulfate, and citrate salts that inhibits not only Gram-positive bacteria, but members of the Enterobacteriaceae other than *Salmonella* and *Shigella* that appear among the normal flora of the colon. The inhibition is not absolute; recovery of *E. coli* is reduced 1000- to 10,000-fold relative to that on nonselective media, but there is little effect on growth of *Salmonella* and *Shigella.* Carbohydrates and a pH indicator are also included to help to differentiate colonies of *Salmonella* and *Shigella* from those of other enteric Gram-negative rods.

7. *Anaerobic media.* In addition to meeting atmospheric requirements, isolation of some strictly anaerobic bacteria (Chapter 18) on blood agar is enhanced by reducing agents such as L-cysteine and by vitamin enrichment. Sodium thioglycolate, another reducing agent, is often used in broth media. Plate media are made selective for anaerobes by the addition of aminoglycoside antibiotics, which are active against many aerobic and facultative organisms but not against anaerobic bacteria. The use of selective media is particularly important with anaerobes because they grow slowly and are commonly mixed with facultative bacteria in infections.

8. *Highly selective media.* Media specific to the isolation of almost every important pathogen have been developed. Many will allow only a single species to grow from specimens with a rich normal flora (for example, stool). The most common of these media are listed in Table 13.1; they are discussed in greater detail in following chapters.

Appendix 14.3 Common Biochemical Tests for Microbial Identification

1. *Carbohydrate breakdown.* The ability to produce acidic metabolic products, fermentatively or oxidatively, from a range of carbohydrates (for example, glucose, sucrose, and lactose) has been applied to the identification of most groups of bacteria. Such tests are crude and imperfect in defining mechanisms, but have proved useful for taxonomic purposes. More recently, gas chromatographic identification of specific short-chain fatty acids produced by fermentation of glucose has proved useful in classifying many anaerobic bacteria.

2. *Catalase production.* The enzyme catalase catalyzes the conversion of hydrogen peroxide to water and oxygen. When a colony is placed in hydrogen peroxide, liberation of oxygen as gas bubbles can be seen. The test is particularly useful in differentiation of staphylococci (positive) from streptococci (negative), but also has taxonomic application to Gram-negative bacteria.

3. *Citrate utilization.* An agar medium that contains sodium citrate as the sole carbon source may be used to determine ability to utilize citrate. Bacteria that grow on this medium are termed *citrate positive.*

4. *Coagulase.* The enzyme coagulase acts with a plasma factor to convert fibrinogen to a fibrin clot. It is used to differentiate *aureus* from other, less pathogenic staphylococci (Chapter 15).

5. *Decarboxylases and deaminases.* The decarboxylation or deamination of the amino acids lysine, ornithine, and arginine is detected by the effect of the amino products on the pH of the reaction mixture or by the formation of colored products. These tests are used primarily with Gram-negative rods.

6. *Hydrogen sulfide.* The ability of some bacteria to produce H_2S from amino acids or other sulfur-containing compounds is helpful in taxonomic classification. The black color of the sulfide salts formed with heavy metals such as iron is the usual means of detection.

7. *Indole.* The indole reaction tests the ability of the organism to produce indole, a benzopyrrole, from tryptophan. Indole is detected by the formation of a red dye after addition of a benzaldehyde reagent. A spot test can be done in seconds using isolated colonies.

8. *Nitrate reduction.* Bacteria may reduce nitrates by several mechanisms. This ability is demonstrated by detection of the nitrites and/or nitrogen gas formed in the process.

9. *O-Nitrophenyl-β-D-galactoside (ONPG) breakdown.* The ONPG test is related to lactose fermentation. Organisms that possess the β-galactoside necessary for lactose fermentation but lack a permease necessary for lactose to enter the cell are ONPG positive and lactose negative.

10. *Oxidase production.* The oxidase tests detect the *c* component of the cytochrome-oxidase complex. The reagents used change from clear to colored when converted from the reduced to the oxidized state. The oxidase reaction is commonly demonstrated in a spot test, which can be done quickly from isolated colonies.

11. *Proteinase production.* Proteolytic activity is detected by growing the

organism in the presence of substrates such as gelatin or coagulated egg.

12. *Urease production.* Urease hydrolyzes urea to yield two molecules of ammonia and one of CO_2. This reaction can be detected by the increase in medium pH caused by ammonia production. Urease-positive species vary in the amount of enzyme produced; bacteria can thus be designated as positive, weakly positive, or negative.

13. *Voges-Proskauer test.* The Voges-Proskauer test detects acetylmethylcarbinol (acetoin), an intermediate product in the butene glycol pathway of glucose fermentation.

Additional Reading

Cowan, S.T. 1974. *Cowan and Steel's Manual for the Identification of Medical Bacteria.* 2nd ed. New York: Cambridge University Press. This book is essentially a series of taxonomic tables linked by a scholarly (and sometimes entertaining) discussion of their application to bacterial identification. Media, reagents, and tests are also covered in greater detail than in the present chapter.

The CUMITECH Series. Washington, D.C.: American Society for Microbiology. Cumulative Techniques and Procedures in Clinical Microbiology (CUMITECH) is a series of 10- to 25-page pamphlets, each of which covers important topics related to diagnostic microbiology (blood cultures, urinary tract infections, antimicrobial susceptibility testing, and the like). Each pamphlet is jointly written by at least three authors representing the clinical as well as the laboratory viewpoint and includes clinical, specimen collection, isolation, and identification recommendations for all agents pertinent to the topic.

Lennette, E.H., Balows, A., Hausler, W.J., Jr., and Shadomy, H.J., Eds. 1985. *Manual of Clinical Microbiology.* 4th ed. Washington, D.C.: American Society for Microbiology. A widely used comprehensive text for clinical microbiology and virology.

15

Staphylococci

John C. Sherris and
James J. Plorde

Gram-positive cocci in
clusters

Staphylococcus

Facultative; catalase
producers

Pathogenic significance and
carriage of *S. aureus*

S. aureus is coagulase positive

Members of the genus *Staphylococcus* (commonly called staphylococci) are round, Gram-positive cocci that can divide in any plane and tend to be arranged in grapelike clusters (from the Greek *staphyle,* bunch of grapes). Some single cells and pairs are also seen. Occasional short chains, which can occur as a chance feature of the organisms' mode of division, should not be confused with the regular occurrence of chains among the streptococci. Staphylococci have a typical Gram-positive cell wall structure. Like all medically important cocci, they are nonflagellate, nonmotile, and non-spore forming.

Staphylococci grow best aerobically, but are facultatively anaerobic. They can oxidize or ferment various carbohydrates. Unenriched nutrient broth or nutrient agar supports their growth, and their doubling time (mean generation time) can be as short as 20 min. In contrast to streptococci, staphylococci produce catalase.

There are 12 species of staphylococci that colonize humans (Table 15.1); three are of major medical importance: *Staphylococcus aureus, Staphylococcus epidermidis,* and *Staphylococcus saprophyticus.*

Staphylococcus aureus colonizes the anterior nares and sometimes other skin sites of about 30% of people in the community; more may be colonized in hospitals. The species is pathogenic and can cause a variety of infections in many otherwise healthy individuals. It can also colonize or infect some animal species. Its name (*aureus,* gold) was suggested by the golden color that develops in older colonies of many, but not all, strains grown on agar plates. The primary distinguishing characteristic of *S. aureus* is its production of the enzyme *coagulase,* which leads to coagulation of plasma. It also produces a number of toxins and extracellular enzymes known or believed to contribute to disease processes; however, many gaps remain in our understanding of the pathogenesis of staphylococcal infections.

Staphylococcus epidermidis is a member of the normal skin (epidermal)

Table 15.1   Human Staphylococcal Species

Species	Frequency of Infection	Coagulase Production	Common Human Habitat
S. aureus	Common	Positive	Anterior nares, perineum
S. epidermidis	Common	Negative	Anterior nares, head, axilla, arms and legs
S. saprophyticus	Common	Negative	Urinary tract
S. hemolyticus	Uncommon	Negative	Axilla, pubes (apocrine glands)
S. hominis	Uncommon	Negative	Axilla, pubes (apocrine glands)
S. simulans	Uncommon	Negative	—
S. auricularis	Rare	Negative	Ear canal
S. capitis	Rare	Negative	Scalp, forehead (sebaceous glands)
S. cohnii	Rare	Negative	—
S. saccharolyticus	Rare	Negative	—
S. warneri	Rare	Negative	—
S. xylosis	Rare	Negative	—

S. epidermidis and *S. saprophyticus* are coagulase negative; may cause opportunistic infections

flora of essentially all humans and many animals. Its colonies often show white pigmentation, and it does not produce coagulase. The organism causes disease only in those whose local or systemic defenses are compromised; such individuals constitute an increasing proportion of hospital populations, however, and more infections have been seen in the past few years.

Staphylococcus saprophyticus is free living in nature, but may also colonize the skin. Like *S. epidermidis,* it is coagulase negative and rarely causes infections in healthy individuals, although it can cause primary urinary tract infections in women. In contrast to *S. aureus* and *S. epidermidis,* it is resistant to the antibiotic novobiocin. Many diagnostic laboratories do not routinely differentiate coagulase-negative species and simply report them as coagulase-negative staphylococci.

Staphylococcus aureus

Morphology and Staining

In young cultures and untreated lesions, the cells of *S. aureus* are quite regular in size, with a diameter of approximately 1 μm. They fit together in their clusters with the precision of a collection of pool balls and are rather uniformly Gram positive. In older cultures, in resolving lesions, and in the presence of some antibiotics the cells often become more variable in size, and many lose the Gram positivity. The typical morphology of staphylococci in culture is shown in the marginal figure shown earlier and in pus from a staphylococcal abscess in Figure 15.1.

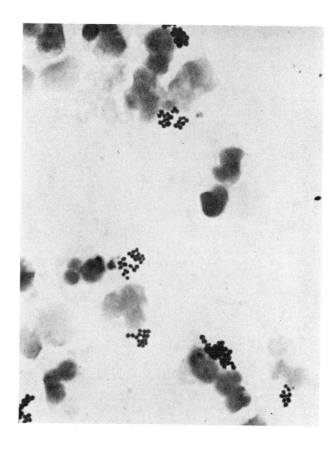

15.1 *Staphylococcus aureus* in pus. (*Reproduced with permission of Schering Corporation, Kenilworth, N.J., the copyright owner. All rights reserved.*)

Cell Wall and Other Surface Structures

Peptidoglycan interspersed with teichoic acid

Surface protein A binds to Fc portion of IgG

The cell wall of *S. aureus* consists of a typical Gram-positive peptidoglycan (Chapter 2). The peptidoglycan is interspersed with molecules of a ribitol-teichoic acid, which is antigenic and relatively specific for *S. aureus*. In most strains, the peptidoglycan of the cell wall is overlaid with surface proteins; one protein, protein A, is unique in that it has a strong affinity for the Fc portion of IgG molecules, which are firmly bound to the staphylococcal cell, leaving the antigen-reacting Fab portion directed externally. The significance of this phenomenon in test systems for detecting free antigens is discussed in Chapter 14. It probably contributes to the virulence of *S. aureus* by interfering with opsonization. Rare strains of *S. aureus* have a large external morphologic capsule with a marked antiphagocytic effect. These strains are virulent to mice and have been used extensively in experimental studies. Most infections in humans are caused by strains with small or absent polysaccharide capsules, and their mechanisms of virulence and immunity differ from those of the encapsulated strains in mice.

Cultural Characteristics

Rapid growth

Under aerobic conditions, *S. aureus* grows rapidly and diffusely in liquid medium. After overnight incubation on blood agar, it produces soft, regular, low, convex colonies approximately 2–3 mm in diameter. Most, but

Variable hemolysis on blood agar

not all, strains show a rim of β-hemolysis surrounding the colony. The buff-golden color of the colonies, when present, can be seen when they are drawn up into a small pile with a bacteriologic loop. Occasional strains require the addition of 2–10% carbon dioxide to the atmosphere for growth. In contrast to other staphylococci, *S. aureus* grows well on agar medium containing 7.5% sodium chloride and is able to ferment mannitol to yield organic acids and an acidic reaction. These characteristics have been exploited in a selective medium, mannitol salt agar, which incorporates a pH indicator (phenol red) to detect acid from mannitol fermentation. This medium is used in environmental and public health studies when it is necessary to detect potential *S. aureus* colonies among many contaminating organisms.

Mannitol salt agar as a selective medium

Tests for Identification and Subtyping

Test for free coagulase

The single most important test used to distinguish *S. aureus* from other staphylococci demonstrates production of coagulase, which exists in two distinct forms, free and bound. Free coagulase is demonstrated by inoculating staphylococcal growth from solid medium into diluted rabbit or human plasma and incubating at 35–37°C. Coagulase production results in development of a fibrin clot, usually within 4 hr. Coagulase activates prothrombin or a prothrombin derivative that initiates the terminal clotting sequence: thrombin + fibrinogen → fibrin. Bound coagulase can be demonstrated by a simple procedure, the slide coagulase or slide clumping test. A dense emulsion of staphylococcal colonies is made in a drop of water, mixed with undiluted plasma, and stirred with the loop. Immediate dense clumping enhanced by stirring denotes a positive test. In this test, the cell-bound coagulase leads to deposition of fibrin on the surfaces of the staphylococci, which renders them "sticky" and results in clumping. There is a 95% correspondence with the results of tests for free coagulase. Recently, commercial latex agglutination tests that simultaneously detect the presence of cell-bound coagulase and protein A have been marketed. The sensitivity and specificity of these tests in identifying *S. aureus* exceeds that of the slide coagulase test while retaining its simplicity.

Mechanism of coagulase action

Slide test for bound coagulase

Bacteriophage typing for epidemiologic purposes

Strains of *S. aureus* can be subdivided by bacteriophage typing and thus "fingerprinted" for epidemiologic purposes. The procedure depends on differing subjectivity to lysis of different strains by bacteriophages. It employs an international set of more than 20 bacteriophages derived originally from lysogenic strains of *S. aureus*. The bacteriophages are propagated on special strains of *S. aureus*, which also serve as controls for the specificity of the bacteriophages. The phages are dropped onto a plate seeded with the strain to be tested, using a template and an orientation marker. The pattern of lysis is read after overnight incubation (Figure 15.2). Most strains of *S. aureus* are lysed by more than one phage in the typing set. A phage type may be reported, for example, as 52/52A/80/81. Mutation or lysogenization during the course of an epidemic may occasionally change the reaction of a staphylococcus to particular phages. Thus, interpretation of phage typing results requires assistance from those familiar with the test. In general, typing patterns can be grouped together to reflect some common characteristics; four such groups (I, II, III, and IV) are recognized. Grouping is insufficiently precise to determine whether staphylococcal isolates have a common source; it has been helpful in pathogenic studies, however, because certain diseases are usually associated with a particular group (for example, bullous impetigo with phage group II strains). Bacteriophage typing of an isolate from an infected pa-

Variations in phage types

Phage groups

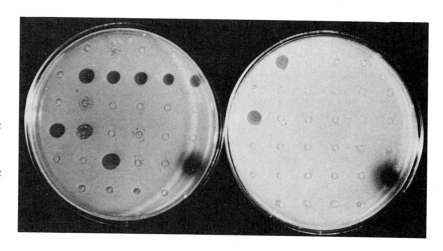

15.2 Bacteriophage typing of two strains of *Staphylococcus aureus:* results after overnight incubation. Lysis is indicated by absence of growth at the site of deposition of individual phages to which the strain is susceptible. The test shows that the two strains are not of common origin.

tient has no diagnostic or therapeutic significance in contrast to its epidemiologic value.

Antigenic structure

Like all bacteria, *S. aureus* has many antigenically active components. Although strains can be subdivided serologically on the basis of surface protein and cell wall structural antigens, serotyping has not proved as valuable for epidemiologic studies as bacteriophage typing.

Toxins and Biologically Active Extracellular Enzymes

Strains of *S. aureus* produce a wide range of substances that contribute or possibly contribute to their virulence. The most important of these substances appear to be the following.

α-Hemolysin (α-toxin).   α-Hemolysin is a chromosomally encoded, antigenic protein exotoxin of low molecular weight that is lethal to many cells in low concentrations. It hemolyzes red cells, destroys platelets, kills leukocytes, causes necrosis of skin (dermonecrosis) when injected intradermally, and is lethal to experimental animals when sufficient amounts are injected intravenously. Although α-hemolysin can be converted to toxoid, neither toxoid nor anti-α-hemolysin has proved of significant value in the treatment or prevention of chronic staphylococcal infection. Other hemolysins (β, γ, and δ) have been less extensively studied.

Exotoxin active against a wide range of blood and tissue cells

Leukocidin.   Leukocidin is an exotoxin, distinct from the α-hemolysin, that is lethal to polymorphonuclear leukocytes by partially disrupting their membranes.

Produces pores in leukocyte membrane

Enterotoxins.   Certain strains of *S. aureus* (particularly those of phage groups III and IV) produce one of several antigenically distinct exotoxins that cause acute gastrointestinal symptoms, usually within 2–5 hr of ingestion. These toxins are thus termed *enterotoxins.* They are low molecular weight proteins that retain activity after 30 min of boiling and are resistant to gastric and jejunal enzymes. Production of some has been shown to be encoded in temperate bacteriophages. Ingestion of sufficient preformed toxin in food results in staphylococcal food poisoning. The toxin appears to act on neural receptors in the upper gastrointestinal tract, leading to stimulation of the vomiting center in the brain.

Resistance to boiling and upper G.I. enzymes

Exfoliatins. Certain strains of *S. aureus* belonging to phage group II produce exfoliatin, an exotoxin that leads to separation and loss of the most superficial layers of the epidermis. Two distinct exfoliatins, one chromosomally and the other plasmid mediated, have been described. Individual strains of staphylococci can produce either one, both, or neither. Sufficient toxin may be produced at a local site of infection to cause marked epithelial desquamation at remote sites of the body (Ritter's disease, or scalded skin syndrome). The toxins are antigenic, and circulating antibody confers immunity to their effects.

Separates superficial layers of epidermis locally or remotely

Toxin Associated with Toxic Shock Syndrome. It is now clear that toxic shock syndrome is usually caused by a staphylococcal exotoxin distinct from all of those mentioned previously. It is termed *toxic shock syndrome toxin 1* (TSST-1). This toxin induces production of interleukin 1 (IL1) and tumor necrosis factor (TNF) by macrophages, is pyrogenic, enhances the susceptibility of the human host to the effects of bacterial endotoxin, and appears to be capable of producing widespread organ damage through other, as yet poorly defined, mechanisms. The end result may be severe toxic shock. Production and release of the toxin in vitro is increased when growth conditions for the organism are suboptimal (eg, limited availability of magnesium ions).

TSST-1 has multiple effects leading to severe toxic shock

Coagulase. Although free and bound coagulase are not toxins, they probably play some role in the pathogenesis of staphylococcal infections and in determining their characteristics. Staphylococci coated with fibrin are resistant to phagocytosis, and fibrin deposition in the area of a staphylococcal infectious focus may help to localize the lesion.

Other extracellular products. Strains of *S. aureus* produce several other extracellular, biologically active substances, including hyaluronidase, nuclease, lipase, protease, and a plasminogen activator. Their roles in the pathogenesis of staphylococcal infection remain obscure.

Other Probable Contributors to Virulence

Staphylococcal teichoic acid binds specifically to fibronectin on the surface of host cells and to subendothelial tissues and clots. It thus mediates adherence of the organism and contributes to the initiation of infection. *Staphylococcus aureus* surface components also bind to collagen.

Adherence by teichoic acid–fibronectin binding

Two surface components of the organism interfere with phagocytosis. The small polysaccharide capsule possessed by some strains blocks peptidoglycan-mediated complement activation or "buries" C3b so that it is not available to its receptor site on the phagocyte. In nonencapsulated strains, protein A binds the Fc portion of IgG making it also unavailable to its receptor site on the phagocyte. Interestingly, if a nonencapsulated strain of *S. aureus* reaches the bloodstream, exposed peptidoglycan may produce massive complement activation, leukopenia, thrombocytopenia, and a clinical syndrome of septic shock.

Capsules can prevent opsonization by alternative complement pathway

Protein A interferes with opsonization by IgG

Once phagocytosed, *S. aureus* strains are much more resistant to lysosomal killing than are coagulase-negative staphylococci, and they may multiply within and kill the phagocyte. Furthermore, *S. aureus* can multiply in fresh human serum, whereas the growth of many coagulase-negative strains is partially or completely inhibited.

Multifactorial nature of virulence

Thus, *S. aureus* has a variety of characteristics and products that may contribute to its virulence, although no single factor has been identified as the major contributor to its ability to multiply and cause lesions in tissues. Not all strains that cause infection possess all of the putative virulence factors discussed previously, and a single candidate for an effective immunizing vaccine appears unlikely.

Resistance

Like all medically important non–spore-forming bacteria, *S. aureus* is rapidly killed by temperatures above 60°C. It is also susceptible to all disinfectants and antiseptics commonly used. Unlike many pathogenic vegetative organisms, however, it can survive long periods of drying; for example, recurrent skin infections can result from use of uncleaned clothing contaminated with pus from a previous furuncle.

Resistant to drying

Antibiotic Susceptibility

When penicillin was first introduced, most strains of *S. aureus* were highly susceptible to it. Now, because of β-lactamase penicillinase production encoded by plasmid genes, most isolates from the community as well as from hospitals are penicillin resistant.

Most isolates produce penicillinase

Most penicillin-resistant strains of *S. aureus* are fully susceptible to the penicillinase-resistant penicillins and cephalosporins, but resistance or multiresistance to other antistaphylococcal antimicrobics is common, particularly in hospitals. Vancomycin is the exception, and resistance to it is very rare. Most staphylococcal resistance is plasmid determined, and strains may carry several R plasmids. Resistance may be acquired by transduction between strains of *S. aureus* or by conjugative transfer from other strains of *S. aureus,* coagulase-negative staphylococci, or even enterococci. Conjugative transfer does not involve sex pili and appears to be facilitated by conditions on the surface of the skin. It should be noted that transduction may be accompanied by lysogenization with a new bacteriophage, and this can lead to alteration of the phage type of the lysogenized strain.

Most are susceptible to penicillinase-resistant penicillins and cephalosporins

Most resistances are plasmid encoded and can be acquired by transduction or conjugation

Some multiresistant strains are also resistant to the penicillinase-resistant penicillins and cephalosporins and have caused epidemics of hospital infection in many parts of the world. These strains have been widely referred to as *methicillin-resistant Staphylococcus aureus* (MRSA), and we will use this terminology despite the fact that resistance applies also to other β-lactam antimicrobics. MRSA have also been described as *heteroresistant,* because most cells in a population are relatively susceptible to penicillinase-resistant penicillins and cephalosporins, but a decreasing proportion show progressively increasing resistance to quite high levels. This type of resistance is not due to penicillinase production and is chromosomally mediated. It is probably mutational in origin and involves production of a particular penicillin-binding protein, PBP-2', which is believed to be a peptidoglycan transpeptidase with a low affinity for β-lactam antimicrobics. The clinical significance of methicillin resistance has been clearly established.

"Methicillin-resistant" (MRSA) strains are resistant to penicillinase-resistant penicillins and cephalosporins

Heteroresistance

Methicillin resistance due to expression of unusual chromosomally encoded PBP

There are some problems in detecting MRSA. Tests are made with oxacillin (a penicillinase-resistant penicillin) under special conditions that facilitate expression of the resistance. Oxacillin-resistant strains are considered to be of increased resistance to all other penicillinase-resistant penicillins and cephalosporins, irrespective of the results of susceptibility tests made under other conditions. Multiresistant strains and particularly MRSA can produce serious therapeutic problems, although vancomycin remains effective against almost all of them. The extent of multiresistance

MRSA detected with oxacillin using special culture conditions

Multiresistant strains usually hospital acquired; value of vancomycin

in a population or hospital reflects the extent of antibiotic use and of cross-infection.

Susceptibility data from an American hospital are illustrated in the appendix of Chapter 13; it must be realized, however, that very different, and often higher, proportions of resistant strains may be encountered in other institutions and populations.

Staphylococcal Infections

Pyogenic, suppurative lesions

Staphylococcal infections are characterized by intense suppuration, necrosis of local tissues, and a tendency for the infected area to become walled off with the formation of a pus-filled local abscess.

Furuncle. The prototypic, and most common, infection is the furuncle or boil, a superficial skin infection that develops in a hair follicle, sebaceous gland, or sweat gland. Blockage of the gland duct with inspissation of its contents causes predisposition to infection; thus, furunculosis is often a complication of acne vulgaris. Infection at the base of the eyelash gives rise to the common stye. The infected patient is often a carrier of the offending staphylococcus, usually in the anterior nares. The course of the infection is usually benign; no specific treatment is needed, and the infection resolves upon drainage of pus.

Association with acne

Stye

Chronic Furunculosis. Some individuals are subject to chronic furunculosis, in which repeated attacks of boils are caused by the same phage type of *S. aureus*. There is little, if any, evidence of acquired immunity to the disease; indeed, delayed-type hypersensitivity to staphylococcal products appears responsible for much of the inflammation and necrosis that develops. Chronic staphylococcal disease may be associated with factors that depress host immunity, especially in patients with diabetes or congenital defects of polymorphonuclear leukocyte function (Chapter 71). In most instances, however, predisposing disease other than acne is not present.

May indicate defects in leukocyte function

Carbuncle. Infection may spread from a furuncle to the subcutaneous tissues, with the development of one or more abscesses extending to subcutaneous tissues known as *carbuncles*. These abscesses occur most often on the back of the neck, but may involve other skin sites. They are serious lesions that may result in bloodstream invasion (bacteremia).

Bullous impetigo. Certain strains of *S. aureus*, especially of phage type 71, can cause *bullous impetigo*, a highly communicable superficial skin infection characterized by large blisters containing many staphylococci in the superficial layers of the skin. Bullous impetigo is seen most often in infants and children under conditions in which direct spread can occur (for example, sharing of contaminated towels). The strains produce exfoliatin, and the disease can thus be considered a localized form of scalded skin syndrome.

Paronychia. Another common *S. aureus* infection is paronychia, which involves the soft tissue around the nails. Paronychia may result from autoinfection or from an external source.

Deep lesions. Staphylococcus aureus can cause a wide variety of infections of deep tissues, by bacteremic spread from a skin lesion that may be unnoticed. These infections include osteomyelitis (usually of the meta-

Osteomyelitis; abscesses; bacteremia and endocarditis

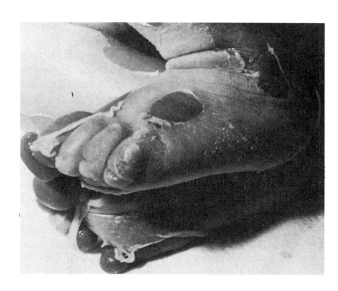

15.3 Staphylococcal scalded skin syndrome in a neonate. The staphylococcal infection was a breast abscess in the infant

physis of the long bones in children); arthritis; cerebral, pulmonary, and renal abscesses; and breast abscesses in the nursing mother. Bacteremia and endocarditis can develop. All are serious infections that constitute acute medical emergencies. The organism can also cause bacterial pneumonia, which is always secondary to some other insult to the lung or tracheobronchial tree, such as influenza, aspiration of gastric contents, or severe pulmonary edema. If untreated, multiple pulmonary abscesses develop. In all of these situations, diabetes, leukocyte defects, or general reduction of host defenses by alcoholism, malignancy, old age, or steroid or cytotoxic therapy can be a predisposing factor. Severe *S. aureus* infections, including endocarditis, are particularly common in drug abusers using injection methods. Occasionally a severe and life-threatening enterocolitis may develop when certain strains of *S. aureus* replace much of the normal colonic flora after a broad-spectrum antibiotic treatment to which the staphylococcus is resistant.

Wound Infections. The organism is also a major cause of wound infection. The source may be the patient's own carrier state, other carriers (for example, physicians or nurses), or other infected patients. Cross-infection of the umbilical stump of the newborn infant can lead to extensive contamination of the infant and its environment. Spread to other infants and mothers in the hospital can result in a variety of staphylococcal infections, such as furuncles, conjunctivitis, breast abscess, and other deep infections. Surgical wound infections can be very severe, and infections at the site of intravenous lines can result in bacteremia and metastatic infection.

Diseases Caused by Staphylococcal Toxins

Scalded skin syndrome (Ritter's disease) results from the production of exfoliatin in a staphylococcal lesion, which can be quite minor (for example, conjunctivitis). The toxin is absorbed into the bloodstream, and erythema and intraepidermal desquamation may occur at remote sites from which *S. aureus* cannot be isolated (Figure 15.3). The disease is most common in neonates and in children less than 5 years old. The face, axilla, and groin tend to be affected first, but the erythema, bullous formation and

Staphylococcal pneumonia

Endocarditis in I.V. drug abusers

Staphylococcal enterocolitis

Auto infections

Surgical, neonatal and cross-infections

Due to remote effects of exfoliatin

subsequent desquamation of epithelial sheets can spread to all parts of the body. The disease occasionally occurs in adults, particularly those who are immunocompromised.

Milder versions of what is probably the same disease are staphylococcal scarlet fever, in which erythema occurs without desquamation, and bullous impetigo, in which local desquamation occurs.

Toxic shock syndrome is a serious disease associated with *S. aureus*. It has been most commonly seen in young women during or immediately after menstruation and associated with the use of highly absorbent intravaginal tampons. In such cases, *S. aureus* grows in large numbers in and around the tampon with apparent liberation of TSST-1 and probably other toxins. Release of toxin may be facilitated by binding of magnesium to the fibers of certain high-absorbancy tampons. Magnesium deficiency slows growth of the organism and increases toxin release.

The disease is characterized by the development of high fever, vomiting, diarrhea, sore throat, and muscle pain. Within 48 hr, it may progress to severe shock with evidence of renal and hepatic damage. A skin rash may develop, followed by exfoliation at a deeper level than in scalded skin syndrome. Blood cultures are usually negative. To what extent the disease is a response to IL1 and TNF production or to other effects of the toxin remains uncertain. It is clear that toxins other than TSST-1 can be involved, because strains that do not produce TSST-1 have been associated with the rare instances in which the disease follows extragenital infections, particularly after surgery.

In contrast to others in the same age group, most of those who develop menstruation-associated toxic shock syndrome have low or absent antibody levels to TSST-1, and often fail to mount significant antibody response during the disease. Repeated attacks have been recorded and also suggest a genetic predisposition. With removal of certain high-absorbancy tampons from the market, the incidence of toxic shock syndrome has declined greatly.

Staphylococcal food poisoning results from production of staphylococcal enterotoxin in food before ingestion. It is an intoxication, not an infection. Characteristically, the food is moist and highly nutritious to *S. aureus*, as well as to people. Potato salads and creamy dishes are often involved. The food is contaminated by a carrier or, more often, by a preparer with a staphylococcal lesion. If the food is not refrigerated or refrigeration is inadequate, staphylococcal multiplication can result in 10^5 or more *S. aureus* per gram. If the strain produces enterotoxin, the food becomes toxic. Because of the heat resistance of the toxin, toxicity persists even if the food is subsequently heated to boiling.

Ingestion of the food results in acute vomiting and diarrhea within 1–5 hr. There is prostration, but usually no fever. Recovery is rapid, except sometimes in the elderly and in those with another disease. Staphylococcal food poisoning has been an unhappy and embarrassing sequel to innumerable group picnics and wedding parties in which gastronomic delicacies have been exposed to temperatures that allow bacterial multiplication.

Infectivity, Pathogenesis, and Immunity

There is excellent epidemiologic evidence that strains of *S. aureus* differ considerably in infectivity and virulence, although the mechanisms involved are not understood. Multiresistant strains of phage type 80/81, prominent in the 1950s and 1960s, were associated with unusually serious outbreaks of staphylococcal disease in hospital patients. Many family out-

Margin notes (left column):

Staphylococcal scarlet fever

Toxic shock syndrome

Association with tampons

Clinical manifestations of toxic shock

Can be caused by toxins other than TSST-1

Staphylococcal food poisoning

Conditions for multiplication

Resistance of toxin to boiling

Short incubation

Rapid recovery

Variations in virulence

breaks also occurred when carriers of the hospital strains returned home. Fortunately, this problem has diminished greatly (for reasons that are quite unclear), and present isolates of type 80/81 appear no more virulent than those of other phage types.

Influence of local conditions on infectivity

In general, strains of *S. aureus* are of quite low infectivity unless local conditions provide special opportunities for multiplication in the body. Experiments in medical student volunteers in the 1950s showed that intradermal injection of approximately 10^5-10^6 organisms was needed to initiate a small, local, infected lesion; in the presence of a suture, however, less than 10^2 organisms were required. Needless to say, these experiments were performed under conditions in which effective antibiotic therapy was immediately available to control complications, although none occurred. Similar situations, involving foreign material or local reduction in blood supply, play a role in many naturally occurring infections.

Once infection is initiated, the pathogenesis of staphylococcal disease becomes extremely complex and obscure. Some of the parameters and the different toxins, enzymes, and structures involved have been discussed

Acute inflammatory response

above. There is an acute inflammatory response, initiated by microbial products and by tissue and leukocyte damage. The lesion tends to be localized, perhaps in part because of fibrin deposition through the action

Survival in leukocytes

of staphylococcal coagulase. The organisms may multiply within and destroy leukocytes; in addition, various mechanisms, including production of protein A, serve to protect them from phagocytosis. Staphylococcal α-hemolysin and delayed hypersensitivity responses to staphylococcal proteins contribute to the necrosis of the lesions.

Resolution of infection

The resolution of staphylococcal infection in the absence of medical intervention usually results from an abscess "pointing" to the skin, with superficial necrosis followed by drainage of pus and healing by granulation and fibrosis. This process can occur with a small lesion, such as a furuncle, or with a large subcutaneous abscess. Immune mechanisms are undoubt-

Uncertain role of immune mechanisms

edly involved; however, the relative roles of humoral and cellular immune mechanisms are again uncertain, and attempts to induce immunity artificially with various staphylococcal products have been disappointing at best. The natural history of staphylococcal infections indicates that immunity is of short duration and incomplete. Chronic furunculosis, for example, can recur over many years; staphylococcal osteomyelitis, if not effectively treated in its early stages, is notorious for its chronicity and is often associated with sinuses that drain the infected site to the skin surface for long periods. This chronicity, however, results in part from the poor vascularity of the affected bone.

Multiple factors influencing pathogenesis and immunity

It seems likely that the imprecision of our understanding of staphylococcal infection and immunity reflects its multifactorial nature, in which different toxins, biologically active enzymes, antigens, and immune responses have a different constellation of roles in different cases.

Epidemiology

Nasal carriage

The basic habitat of *S. aureus* is the anterior nares. About 30% of individuals in the community carry the organism in this site at any given time. Nasal carrier rates among hospital personnel and patients may be much higher when staphylococcal infections both result from and contribute to the staphylococcal environmental load. Some individuals have extensive colonization of the perineum. They, and some nasal carriers, may disseminate the organism extensively with desquamated epithelial cells and thus constitute a source of infection to others.

Community infections

Most *S. aureus* infections acquired in the community are autoinfections with strains that the subject has been carrying in the anterior nares, on the skin, or both. Community outbreaks of bullous impetigo in children are usually associated with poor hygiene and fomite transmission from case to case.

Hospital infections

Hospital epidemics caused by a single phage type of *S. aureus* are a continuing and recurrent problem. Outbreaks are usually associated with patients who have undergone surgical or other invasive procedures or with nurseries. The initial source of the outbreak may be a patient with an overt

Routes of cross-infection

or inapparent (for example, decubitus ulcer) staphylococcal infection; spread to other patients can occur through fomites, occasionally through air transmission, but is usually through the hands of personnel. A nasal or perineal carrier among medical, nursing, or other hospital staff may be the source of an outbreak, especially if carriage is heavy and numerous organisms are disseminated. A more serious source is the medical attendant with a staphylococcal lesion (for example, a furuncle on the wrist), whose hands may become heavily contaminated with *S. aureus* of proved pathogenicity.

Increased carriage rate

Hospital outbreaks of *S. aureus* infection can be self-perpetuating: infected patients and those who attend them frequently become carriers, and the total environmental load of the causative staphylococcus is increased. The principles of control of epidemics in general and of hospital outbreaks are described in Chapters 12 and 72.

In *S. aureus* outbreaks, it is critical to define the extent of infection with the responsible strain and to detect carriers who may have initiated or contributed to continuation of the outbreak. For these purposes, phage typing and determination of patterns of resistance to antimicrobics (antibiograms) are critical epidemiologic tools.

Laboratory Diagnosis

Direct Gram smear

In general, laboratory procedures to assist in diagnosis are quite simple. Most staphylococcal lesions contain numerous polymorphonuclear leukocytes and large numbers of *S. aureus*. These findings are readily demonstrated by a direct Gram smear of pus (Figure 15.1) unless the patient has been treated with antibiotics. This method is also applicable to properly collected sputum samples from cases of staphylococcal pneumonia and to stool specimens from patients with staphylococcal enterocolitis.

Cultures, coagulase, and susceptibility tests

The organism can usually be grown aerobically on blood agar, and typical colonies 2 mm or more in diameter develop overnight. Coagulase tests can be performed directly from these colonies. Antibiotic susceptibility tests are usually indicated because of the unpredictability of staphylococcal susceptibility patterns.

Blood cultures

Blood cultures from untreated bacteremic patients are usually positive after overnight incubation. The organism produces colonies in the sedimented blood layer of unshaken blood culture bottles, probably because fibrin deposited on the surface by coagulase prevents separation and diffuse growth.

Serodiagnostic procedures and limitations

Possible deep staphylococcal infection, such as osteomyelitis or perirenal abscess, poses special diagnostic problems when the lesion cannot be aspirated. Antibodies to staphylococcal hemolysin, nuclease, and cell wall ribitol–teichoic acid can be detected by a variety of immunologic techniques, including counterimmunoelectrophoresis and radioimmunoassay. Unfortunately, the sera of many individuals without deep staphylococcal infections may also contain such antibodies, and overlap is considerable in antibody titers of infected and uninfected subjects. Thus, these procedures are ancillary at best: their results must be interpreted with caution, and they are not generally available in clinical laboratories.

Prevention

Control of carriage and reinfection

In patients subject to recurrent infection, such as chronic furunculosis, preventive measures are aimed at controlling reinfection and, if possible, eliminating the carrier state. Clothes and bedding that may cause reinfection should be washed at a sufficiently high temperature to destroy staphylococci (70°C or higher) or dry-cleaned. In adults, the use of chlorhexidine or hexachlorophene soaps in showering and washing increases the bactericidal activity of the skin (see Chapter 11). In such individuals, or in medical personnel found to be a source of infection to patients, anterior nasal carriage can be reduced and often eliminated with nasal creams containing antimicrobics not used for systemic infections (eg, neomycin and bacitracin) used in conjunction with oral therapy with antimicrobics that are concentrated within phagocytes and nasal secretions (eg, rifampin or ciprofloxacin). Attempts to reduce nasal carriage more generally among medical personnel in an institution are usually fruitless and encourage replacement of susceptible strains with those that are multiresistant.

Chemoprophylaxis is usually considered mandatory in surgical procedures such as hip and cardiac valve replacements, in which infection with coagulase-positive or -negative staphylococci can have devastating consequences for the prosthesis and for the patient. Brief high-dose chemoprophylaxis is given around the time of surgery with the intention of preventing the super-infections that often complicate longer periods of antibiotic administration.

Treatment

Simple drainage usually suffices for superficial staphylococcal lesions and is also an important component of treatment of chronic lesions.

Antimicrobic therapy

Acute, serious staphylococcal infections (for example, pneumonia or bacteremia) require immediate antibiotic therapy. A penicillinase-resistant penicillin or cephalosporin would normally be used pending the results of a susceptibility test. Infections proved to be caused by strains susceptible to benzyl-penicillin are thus best treated with that antibiotic. Severe infections caused by strains resistant to the penicillinase-resistant penicillins (methicillin-resistant staphylococci) are usually treated with vancomycin.

Combination therapy

There is synergy between cell wall–active antibiotics and the aminoglycosides when the staphylococcus is sensitive to both. Such combinations are often used in severe systemic infection, particularly in the compromised host, when effective and rapid bactericidal action is needed.

Some chronic or recurrent infections of the compromised host can be controlled by administration over months or years of an oral preparation of one of the penicillinase-resistant penicillins.

Coagulase-Negative Staphylococci

Distribution of coagulase-negative staphylococci on human skin

Staphylococcus epidermidis and most other species of coagulase-negative staphylococci are normal commensals of the skin, anterior nares, and ear canals of humans. Their large numbers and ubiquitous distribution result

Significance in infection of prosthetic devices and implanted equipment

in frequent contamination of specimens collected from or through the skin, making these organisms among the most frequently isolated in the clinical laboratory. In the past, they were rarely the cause of significant infections, but with the increasing use of implanted catheters and prosthetic devices, they have emerged as important agents of hospital-acquired infections. Immunosuppressed or neutropenic patients have been particularly affected.

Adherence to foreign material initiates infection

Organisms may contaminate prosthetic devices during implantation, seed the device during a subsequent bacteremia, or gain access to the lumina of shunts and catheters when they are temporarily disconnected or manipulated. The outcome of the bacterial contamination is determined by the microbe's capacity to attach to the surface to the foreign body and to multiply there. Initial adherence is facilitated by the hydrophobic nature of the synthetic polymers and the natural hydrophobic nature of many coagulase-negative staphylococci. Following attachment, some strains (generally of *S. epidermidis*) produce a viscous extracellular polysaccharide slime or biofilm. This biofilm provides additional adhesion, completely covers the bacteria, and serves as a mechanical barrier to antimicrobial agents and host defense mechanisms; it is also believed to enhance nutrition of the microbes by functioning as an ion-exchange resin. The resistance of many coagulase-negative staphylococci to multiple antimicrobic agents contributes further to their persistence in the body. Infections are generally low grade, but unless controlled, they can proceed to serious tissue damage or a fatal outcome.

Protective effect of extracellular polysaccharide

Interpretation of blood culture isolates of coagulase-negative staphylococci

The interpretation of blood cultures that grow coagulase-negative staphylococci is fraught with difficulty. In most cases, the finding is attributable to skin contamination, although it can indicate infection when a patient has implanted devices, or his defenses that are otherwise compromised. The repeated isolation of organisms with similar antibiograms and biochemical characteristics strongly indicates the presence of an infection. The probability is strengthened if the isolated strains are shown to be slime-producing *S. epidermidis*, although *S. hominis*, *S. hemolyticus*, or *S. simulans* are responsible for 5–20% of coagulase-negative staphylococcal infections. Unfortunately, there is, at present, no standardized phage-typing procedure for coagulase-negative staphylococci that can establish the identity of repeated isolates. A number of molecular procedures, including plasmid pattern analysis, restriction endonuclease analysis of plasmid, or chromosomal DNA, and DNA hybridization techniques, can do this, but are not yet generally in clinical laboratories.

Molecular procedures can establish the identity of different isolates

S. saprophyticus causes some primary urinary tract infections

Staphylococcus saprophyticus, which is widely dispersed in the environment, has a similar, but restricted ability to cause opportunistic infection in the compromised host. It is the etiologic agent in 10–20% of primary urinary tract infections in young women.

Many strains are multi-resistant

Most coagulase-negative staphylococci now encountered are resistant to penicillin, either because of penicillinase production or because of intrinsic resistance. Many are also resistant to the penicillinase-resistant penicillins (such as methicillin and cloxacillin), as well as to other antimicrobics with spectra of activity that include many Gram-positive cocci. Many resistance determinants are plasmid encoded. Strains resistant to the penicillinase-resistant penicillins often show varying degrees of resistance to the cephalosporins; this resistance may be detectable only with dilution tests. Treatment of coagulase-negative staphylococcal infections of prosthetic devices frequently requires removal of the device, as well as chemotherapy to prevent recurrence.

Some are resistant to penicillinase-resistant penicillins

Micrococci

Micrococcus

A genus related to *Staphylococcus* is *Micrococcus*. The micrococci comprise commensal, free-living, Gram-positive cocci that are often larger than *S. aureus* and often arranged in regular packets of four or eight, depending on whether they divide in two or three planes before separation. They are coagulase negative and, like the staphylococci, produce catalase. In contrast to the staphylococci, micrococci metabolize oxidatively only and cannot grow anaerobically. Their pathogenic significance is similar to that of the coagulase-negative staphylococci.

Additional Reading

Arbuthnott, J., Bergdoll, M.S., Best, G.K., et al, Eds. 1989. International symposium on toxic shock syndrome. *Rev. Infect. Dis.* 11 (suppl I):S1–S333. A detailed account of present knowledge of this disease by experts in the field.

Elek, S.D., and Conan, P.E. 1957. The virulence of *Staphylococcus pyogenes* for man. A study of the problems of wound infections. *Br. J. Exp. Pathol.* 38:573–586. A classic study of the factors influencing the development of staphylococcal wounds infections in humans.

Elias, P.M., Fritsch, P., and Epstein, E.H., Jr. 1977. Staphylococcal scalded skin syndrome. *Arch. Dermatol.* 113:207–219.

Espersen, F. 1987. Interactions between human plasma proteins and cell wall components of *Staphylococcus aureus*. *Dan. Med. Bull.* 34:59–69. An excellent review of biologically active surface structures of *S. aureus* and their role in virulence.

Lyon, B.R., and Skurray, R. 1987. Antimicrobial resistance of *Staphylococcus aureus:* Genetic basis. *Microbiol. Rev.* 51:88–134.

Peters, G. 1988. New considerations in the pathogenesis of coagulase-negative staphylococcal foreign body infections. *J. Antimicrob. Chemother.* 21 (suppl C):139–148.

Pfaller, M.A., and Herwaldt, L.A. 1988. Laboratory, clinical and epidemiological aspects of coagulase-negative staphylococci. *Clin. Microb. Rev.* 1:281–299. This and the Peters paper above review the epidemiologic and pathogenetic factors influencing the emergence of coagulase-negative staphylococci as important nosocomial pathogens.

Sheagren, J.N. 1984. *Staphylococcus aureus:* The persistent pathogen. *N. Eng. J. Med.* 310:1368–1373, 1437–1442. A good general review of the epidemiology, clinical syndromes, and prevention of staphylococcal infections.

16
Streptococci

Kenneth J. Ryan

The genus *Streptococcus* comprises species of Gram-positive spherical or oval cocci that tend to be arranged in chains. Most grow best in enriched bacteriologic media. Streptococci form a significant portion of the indigenous microflora of humans and animals; most of these species are found in the respiratory tract, but some inhabit the intestinal tract. Although most species rarely cause disease, the genus includes three of the most important pathogens of humans: *Streptococcus pyogenes*, the group A streptococcus, causes a variety of acute infections and can stimulate the post-streptococcal sequelae of rheumatic fever and acute glomerulonephritis. *Streptococcus agalactiae*, the group B streptococcus, is one of the most important causes of neonatal sepsis and meningeal infection. *Streptococcus pneumoniae* is a major cause of both acute bacterial pneumonia and acute purulent meningitis.

Group Characteristics

Morphology

Streptococci stain readily with common dyes, demonstrating coccal cells 0.5-1 μm in diameter. In contrast to staphylococci, streptococcal cells are generally smaller and ovoid in shape. They are usually arranged in chains with oval cells touching end to end because they divide in one plane and tend to remain attached. Length may vary from a single pair to continuous chains of over 30 cells, depending on the species and growth conditions. The Gram reaction is positive, although some cells in older cultures or purulent discharges may lose their ability to retain the crystal violet – iodine complex and thus appear Gram negative.

Medically important streptococci are not acid fast, do not form spores, and are nonmotile. Some members form capsules composed of polysaccharide complexes or hyaluronic acid.

Arrangement in chains

Gram positivity

Streptococcus

291

Cultural and Biochemical Characteristics

Enriched media

Blood agar

Catalase-negative facultative anaerobes

α- and β-hemolysis

Nonhemolytic streptococci

Lactic fermentation

Biologically active extracellular products

Streptococci grow best in media enriched with digests of animal tissues, serum, or defibrinated blood. The plating medium most commonly used is blood agar, which consists of a simple nutrient broth to which agar and animal blood are added. Sheep blood is preferred by most bacteriologists because of its clear demonstration of streptococcal hemolytic patterns. Medically important species grow best at temperatures of 35–37°C. Streptococci metabolize fermentatively, fail to produce catalase, but can grow under atmospheric conditions ranging from aerobic to strictly anaerobic. Growth of many strains is enhanced by the presence of 2–10% carbon dioxide. Strictly anaerobic strains, previously called *anaerobic streptococci*, are now classified in the genus *Peptostreptococcus* (Chapter 18).

After incubation for 18–24 hr on blood agar plates, small colonies ranging from pinpoint size to 0.5–2 mm in diameter are produced. A distinctive feature of streptococcal growth on blood agar is the production by many species of α (green)- or β (clear)-hemolysis of the erythrocytes suspended in the agar (Chapter 14). Hemolysis is dependent on several cultural features and the species of blood used. Nonhemolytic variants of typically hemolytic species may be seen, and some species are inherently nonhemolytic. The term γ-*hemolytic*, sometimes used to describe the latter, is confusing and should be abandoned.

Streptococci are biochemically active, attacking a variety of carbohydrates, proteins, and amino acids. Glucose fermentation yields mostly lactic acid. Extracellular enzymes with substrates such as hyaluronic acid and DNA are produced by certain species and may contribute to virulence. Although circulating exotoxins are not prominent among the streptococci, at least one, the erythrogenic toxin, is produced by some group A strains.

Classification

Hemolytic and biochemical characteristics

Lancefield antigenic groups

Some α- and nonhemolytic streptococci contain Lancefield group antigens

Initially, streptococci were classified simply on the basis of the presence and type of hemolysis that they showed (β-hemolytic, α-hemolytic, nonhemolytic) and by certain biochemical tests. It was known that hemolytic strains were often, but not always, associated with important infections in humans and animals, but the significance could not be predicted. Taxonomy was put on a sounder basis by the studies of Rebecca Lancefield on β-hemolytic streptococci. She demonstrated specific carbohydrate antigens (now known also to have included teichoic acid antigens) in cell wall extracts that allowed classification into groups correlating well with known bacteriologic, epidemiologic, and pathogenic features. Later, it was shown that some non-β-hemolytic streptococci had the same cell wall antigens and pathogenic significance as the β-hemolytic strains. Thus, Lancefield grouping became an essential component of taxonomy of the genus. From a practical point of view, type of hemolysis and certain biochemical reactions remain valuable for the initial recognition and presumptive classification of streptococci, and as an indication of what subsequent taxonomic tests to perform. Thus, β-hemolysis indicates that the strain has one of the Lancefield group antigens, but strains of some Lancefield groups may be α-hemolytic or nonhemolytic. The streptococci will be considered as follows: 1) pyogenic streptococci (Lancefield groups); 2) pneumococcus; 3) viridans streptococci; and 4) other, principally nonhemolytic, streptococci. This classification scheme is illustrated in Table 16.1.

Comprise Lancefield groups A–T; most strains β-hemolytic

Pyogenic streptococci.   Streptococci with cell wall antigens of Lancefield

Table 16.1   Classification of Streptococci by Hemolytic and Serologic Reactions

Group	Common Terms	Hemolysis	Taxonomically Useful Antigens			Disease Associations
			Lancefield Cell Wall	Surface Protein	Surface Polysaccharide	
Pyogenic						
S. pyogenes	Group A streptococcus	β	A	70 + M protein	—	Pyogenic, scarlet fever, rheumatic fever, glomerulonephritis
S. agalactiae	Group B streptococcus	β, occasionally α or nonhemolytic	B	—	Ia, Ib, Ic, II, III	Pyogenic, neonatal sepsis, meningitis
S. faecalis S. faecium S. durans	Enterococci	α or nonhemolytic (rarely β)	D	—	—	Pyogenic, urinary infection
S. bovis S. equinus	Nonenterococcal group D streptococci	α or nonhemolytic	D	—	—	Low virulence, endocarditis
Other species		β, occasionally α or nonhemolytic	C, E–T	—	—	Pyogenic
Pneumococcus (S. pneumoniae)	Pneumococcus	α	—	—	80+	Pneumonia, meningitis
Viridans and nonhemolytic S. sanguis S. salivarius S. mitis S. milleri S. mutans Other species	Viridans streptococci or nonhemolytic streptococci (depending on hemolytic reaction)	α or nonhemolytic	—	—	—	Low virulence, endocarditis; S. mutans associated with dental caries

groups A–T frequently cause pyogenic infections in humans or animals and are thus termed *pyogenic streptococci*. The primary characteristic of pyogenic streptococci is the presence of one of the Lancefield antigens, designated as *groups A–T*. The most common Lancefield groups of streptococci isolated from humans are A, B, C, D, F, and G, and of these, groups A, B, and D are of greatest pathogenic significance. Some of these group designations correlate with species names previously assigned on the basis of cultural, biochemical, and pathogenic features, such as *S. pyogenes* (group A) and *S. agalactae* (group B). The importance of the serologic definition is emphasized, however, by the common description of isolates according to their group (for example, group A β-hemolytic streptococci strains) rather than by the species name. To recapitulate, not all strains possessing Lancefield group antigens are β-hemolytic, especially in group D; however, all that are β-hemolytic are included among the pyogenic streptococci.

Antigenic polysaccharide capsule, but no Lancefield group antigen; α-hemolytic

Pneumococcus. The pneumococcus group contains a single species, *S. pneumoniae*. Its distinctive feature is the presence of a polysaccharide capsule. Differences in the chemical composition and, thus, the antigenic specificity of the capsule of different pneumococci has defined more than 80 immunotypes. Although the pneumococcal cell wall shares some common antigens with other streptococci, it does not possess any of the Lancefield group antigens. The pneumococcus is α-hemolytic.

α-Hemolytic; several species among normal flora

Viridans streptococci. Viridans streptococci are α-hemolytic and lack both the group carbohydrate antigens of the pyogenic streptococci and the capsular antigens of the pneumococcus. The term encompasses several species, including *Streptococcus salivarius* and *Streptococcus mitis*. Viridans streptococci comprise members of the normal respiratory flora of humans. They almost never demonstrate invasive qualities, although some species (*Streptococcus milleri*) have been associated with deep tissue abscesses and several with bacterial endocarditis.

Other streptococci (nonhemolytic). A variety of other streptococci may be encountered that lack the features of the pyogenic streptococci or pneumococci; they would be classified with the viridans group, except they are not α-hemolytic. Such strains are usually assigned descriptive terms such as *nonhemolytic streptococci* or *microaerophilic streptococci*. They have been less thoroughly studied, but generally have the same biologic behavior as the viridans streptococci. The usual hemolytic biochemical and cultural reactions of commonly encountered streptococci are summarized in Table 16.2.

Streptococcus pyogenes (Group A)

Growth Characteristics

Group A β-hemolytic streptococci typically appear in purulent lesions or broth cultures as spherical or ovoid cells in chains of short to medium length (4–10 cells). On blood agar plates, colonies are usually compact, small, and surrounded by a 2- to 3-mm zone of β-hemolysis that is easily seen and sharply demarcated (Figure 16.1) Strains that produce marked

Table 16.2 Usual Hemolytic, Biochemical, and Cultural Reactions of Common Streptococci[a]

	Susceptibility to		Bile Solubility	Bile/Esculin Reaction[b]	Growth in 6.5% NaCl
	Bacitracin	Optochin			
β-Hemolytic					
Lancefield group A	+	−	−	−	−
Lancefield groups B, C, F, G	−	−	−	−	−
α-Hemolytic					
S. pneumoniae	−	+	+	−	−
Viridans group	−	−	−	−	−
Nonhemolytic	−	−	−	−	−
Variable hemolysis (β, α, nonhemolytic)					
Lancefield group D					
Enterococcal	−	−	−	+	+
Nonenterococcal	−	−	−	+	−
Other Lancefield groups	−	−	−	−	−

[a] All are tests commonly substituted for serological identification in clinical laboratories.
[b] Tests for the ability to grow in bile and reduce esculin.

β-Hemolysis by streptolysins S and O

hyaluronic acid capsules may produce mucoid colonies. β-Hemolysis is caused by two hemolysins, streptolysin S and the oxygen-labile streptolysin O, both of which are produced by most group A strains. Occasional strains lack streptolysins S, and β-hemolysis by streptolysin O then occurs only under anaerobic conditions. This feature is of practical importance, because such strains would be missed if incubated only under the usual aerobic conditions.

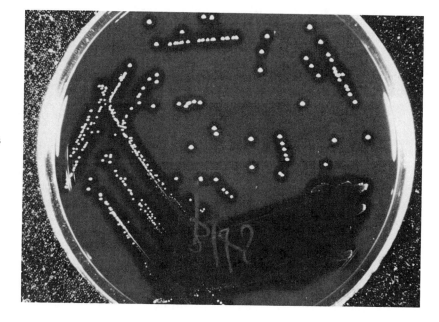

16.1 β-hemolytic streptococcus grown on blood agar medium. The colonies are surrounded by a clear area of hemolysis.

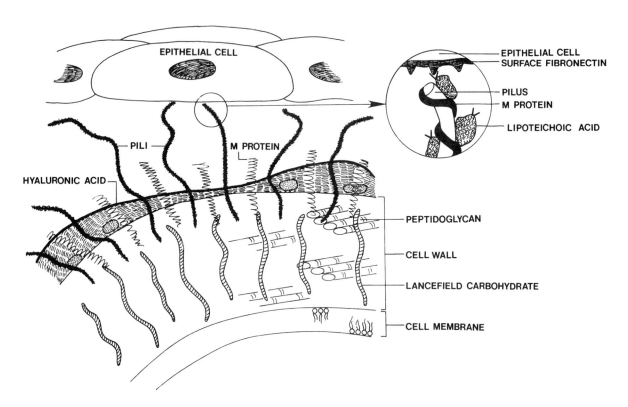

16.2 Antigenic structure of *Streptococcus pyogenes*, and adhesion to an epithelial cell. The location of peptidoglycan and Lancefield carbohydrate antigen in the cell wall is shown in the diagram. M protein and lipoteichoic acid are associated with the cell surface and the pili. Lipoteichoic acid mediates binding to fibronectin on the host surface. The term *fimbriae* is often used to describe the very thin, somewhat diffuse pili.

Structure

Cell wall Lancefield group A antigen

M protein type-specific antigens

The structure of group A streptococci is illustrated in Figure 16-2. The cell wall is built upon a peptidoglycan matrix that provides rigidity, as in other Gram-positive bacteria. Within this matrix lies the group-specific antigen, which is composed of rhamnose and *N*-acetylglucosamine. By definition all group A streptococci possess this antigen. The M protein is a surface component extending beyond the limits of the cell wall in association with hairlike pili (Figure 16.3). Group A streptococci are divided into more than 70 serotypes based on antigenic differences in the M protein. The M protein itself is a fibrillar molecule with its carboxy terminal attached to the peptidoglycan of the cell wall and the amino terminal regions extending toward the surface. There is evidence that the antigenic specificity of M protein lies in the amino-terminal portion because it is the most variable part of the molecule and the most available to immune surveillance. A more recently studied surface structural component, lipoteichoic acid (LTA), is associated with the pili and M protein. LTA and M protein form complexes that are probably important to the contribution each makes to the pathogenesis of group A streptococcal infections. Figure 16.2 shows the M protein providing structural support for the LTA ligand that binds to epithelial cells; conversely, this arrangement of M protein plays a role in resistance to phagocytosis. Some strains have an overlying nonantigenic hyaluronic acid capsule.

Pili contain M protein and LTA antigens

Variable hyaluronic acid capsule

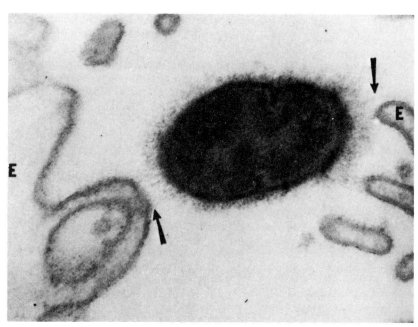

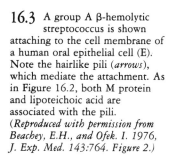

16.3 A group A β-hemolytic streptococcus is shown attaching to the cell membrane of a human oral epithelial cell (E). Note the hairlike pili (*arrows*), which mediate the attachment. As in Figure 16.2, both M protein and lipoteichoic acid are associated with the pili. (*Reproduced with permission from Beachey, E.H., and Ofek. I. 1976, J. Exp. Med. 143:764. Figure 2.*)

Toxins, Hemolysins, and Biologically Active Extracellular Products

Various exotoxins, hemolysins, and other biologically active extracellular products are produced, primarily by the group A streptococci. Some other pyogenic streptococci may produce similar extracellular products.

Oxygen-labile antigenic hemolysin
Cytotoxic activity

Streptolysin O.   One of two hemolysins responsible for hemolysis on blood agar plates is streptolysin O. It is an antigenic protein that is only active in the reduced form, hence its designation O for oxygen lability. Streptolysin O is a general cytotoxin, lysing leukocytes, tissue cells, and platelets. The toxin does not appear to have enzymatic activity, but inserts directly into the host cell membrane, forming circular transmembrane pores in the cell surface. This injury is similar to that produced by complement and by staphylococcal α-toxin. Antibodies against streptolysin O

Antistreptolysin O

are often formed as a result of *S. pyogenes* infection, and inhibition of hemolysis by these antibodies is the basis of the antistreptolysin O test.

Streptolysin S.   Another hemolysin, streptolysin S, is a nonantigenic low-molecular-weight peptide. It is oxygen stable and is responsible for the hemolysis seen around colonies of group A streptococci on blood agar plates incubated aerobically. It is also toxic to leukocytes.

Fibrinolysis by activating serum plasminogen

Streptokinase.   Filtrates of most strains of *S. pyogenes* cause lysis of fibrin clots through production of streptokinase. The action is not direct, but through conversion of plasminogen in normal plasma to a protease, plasmin. Streptokinase is antigenic, and antistreptokinase antibodies appear after group A streptococcal infection.

Deoxyribonuclease (DNA-ase).   Various antigenic nucleases with activity against DNA and, to a lesser extent, RNA are formed by group A streptococci. Of the several immunologically distinct classes described, the most important is DNA-ase B. This enzyme is that produced most consistently in group A streptococcal infections.

Hyaluronidase. Because of its solubilizing action on the ground substance of mammalian connective tissues, hyaluronidase has been called the spreading factor. It is tempting to associate this enzyme with the diffuse, spreading lesions characteristic of streptococcal cellulitis, but its precise role in pathogenesis is not known. Many *S. pyogenes* have hyaluronic acid capsules, including some that produce hyaluronidase; however, the two features usually do not coexist.

Spreading factor

Erythrogenic toxin. Some group A strains form erythrogenic toxin. It has no clear role in the pathogenesis of invasive streptococcal disease; however, it is responsible for the rash seen in scarlet fever. It is a protein exotoxin complexed with a carrier molecule and appears in three immunologically distinct forms. Only strains lysogenized with particular temperate bacteriophages produce toxin. The rash of scarlet fever is probably caused by a combination of the direct effect of the erythrogenic toxin on the skin and delayed-type hypersensitivity to toxin.

Association with scarlet fever

Production determined by temperate phages

Pathogenesis of Infection

The first event in streptococcal infection in individuals with intact epithelia is attachment of group A streptococcal cells by their pili to epithelial cells, usually of the pharynx. Although both M protein and LTA are required for epithelial cell attachment, blocking studies indicate that the specific binding is between the glycolipid end of the streptococcal LTA and lipid-binding regions of a surface-associated glycopeptide, fibronectin, which covers the surface of the target epithelial cell. Upon attachment and multiplication, local epithelial damage occurs. In many *S. pyogenes* infections, however, invasion occurs through epithelial breaks.

Attachment by pilus LTA to host cell surface fibronectin

After these initial events, M protein plays the key role in allowing the streptococcal infection to become established. Strains containing M protein can resist phagocytosis by polymorphonuclear leukocytes and grow readily in tissue fluids and serum. Strains lacking M protein do not exhibit these features and are avirulent. The mechanism of resistance to phagocytosis involves failure of C3b generated by the alternative pathway of complement to recognize the surface of M protein-producing streptococci. In the presence of M type-specific antibody, opsonophagocytosis proceeds, and the streptococci are rapidly killed. It has long been known that, in humans, antibody directed against a particular M type is protective only for subsequent infection with other strains of the same type. Unfortunately there are many M types. The precise role of other factors in the pathogenesis of infection is uncertain, but the combined effect of streptokinase, DNA-ase, and hyaluronidase may prevent effective localization of the infection while the streptolysins produce tissue injury. Antibodies against these components are formed in the course of streptococcal infection, but are not known to be protective.

M proteins protect against nonimmune phagocytosis

Anti-M antibody provides type-specific opsonization and immunity

Possible effects of extracellular enzymes

Antimicrobic Susceptibility

Group A streptococci are highly susceptible to penicillin G. Concentrations as low as 0.01 μg/ml have a bactericidal effect, and penicillin resistance is so far unknown. Numerous other antimicrobics are also active, including other penicillins, cephalosporins, tetracyclines, chlorampheni-

Penicillin susceptibility

col, and erythromycin, but not aminoglycosides. Tetracycline resistance has been found in 5–10% of strains, and erythromycin resistance also occurs when that agent is widely used.

Diseases

The group A streptococcus is unique in its ability to cause a variety of acute pyogenic infections and two nonsuppurative diseases that can follow streptococcal infection but do not involve the live organism. The latter diseases, acute rheumatic fever and glomerulonephritis, are known as *post-streptococcal sequelae*, or nonsuppurative complications of streptococcal infection.

A. Infections

Streptococcal pharyngitis.   One of the most common bacterial infections is streptococcal pharyngitis. Although it may occur at any age, it is most

Most common in childhood

frequent between 5 and 15 years. The illness is characterized by acute sore throat, malaise, fever (38.9–40°C), and headache. Infection typically involves the tonsillar pillars, uvula, and soft palate, which become red, swollen, and covered with a yellow-white exudate. The cervical lymph nodes that drain this area may also become swollen and tender. No single finding or combination of clinical features is sufficient to make or exclude

Diagnosis requires laboratory confirmation

a diagnosis of group A streptococcal pharyngitis in an isolated case, because the condition can be indistinguishable from viral pharyngitis. Streptococcal pharyngitis can only be diagnosed by demonstrating the presence of the organism with laboratory tests.

Group A streptococcal pharyngitis is usually self-limiting. Typically, the fever is gone by the third to fifth day, and other manifestations subside

Suppurative complications

within a week. Occasionally the infection may spread beyond the pharynx to produce peritonsillar or retropharyngeal abscesses, otitis media, suppurative cervical adenitis, and acute sinusitis. Rarely, more extensive spread occurs, producing meningitis, pneumonia, or bacteremia with metastatic infection in distant organs. In the preantibiotic era, these suppurative complications were responsible for a mortality of 1–3% from acute streptococcal pharyngitis. Such complications are much less common now, and fatal infections are rare.

Impetigo.   Group A streptococcal infection of healthy skin usually produces a localized skin disease known as *impetigo*. Invasion is through minor trauma, such as skin abrasions or insect bites. The primary lesion of streptococcal impetigo is a small (up to 1 cm) vesicle surrounded by an area of erythema. The vesicle enlarges over a period of days, becomes pustular, and eventually breaks to form a yellow crust. The lesions usually appear

Skin infection, usually in children

in 2- to 5-year-old children on exposed body surfaces, typically the face and lower extremities. Multiple lesions may coalesce to form deeper ulcerated areas. Streptococcal impetigo is often caused by nephritogenic strains, especially in the tropics. An early vesicle yields a pure culture of group A streptococci; an older, crusted lesion, however, often becomes

Secondary colonization with *S. aureus*

secondarily colonized with *Staphylococcus aureus*. There is no evidence that staphylococci play any role in the natural history of streptococcal impetigo, although it should be recalled that *S. aureus* can produce its own clinically distinct form (bullous impetigo). The presence of staphylococci that produce penicillinase does not appear to compromise the effectiveness of penicillin therapy.

Erysipelas.   Erysipelas is a distinct form of streptococcal infection of the skin and subcutaneous tissues, primarily affecting the dermis. It is characterized by a spreading area of erythema and edema with rapidly advancing, well-demarcated edges, pain, and systemic manifestations, including fever and lymphadenopathy. Infection usually occurs on the face, and a previous history of streptococcal sore throat is common. Erysipelas is a serious disease that requires immediate antimicrobic therapy, usually with penicillin.

Dermal infection with spreading erythema and edema

Wound and burn infections.   Although less common than in the past, group A streptococcal infections of wounds and burns can develop and spread rapidly to adjacent tissues, with the risk of sepsis and bacteremia. Burn infections are associated with failure of skin grafts. Burn and wound infections in hospitalized patients carry a substantial risk of cross-infection to other patients with similar conditions.

Failure of skin grafts

Risk of cross-infection

Puerperal infection.   Infection of the endometrium at or near delivery is a life-threatening form of group A streptococcal infection. Fortunately, it is now relatively rare, but in the 19th century the clinical findings of "childbed fever" were characteristic and common enough to provide the first clues to the transmission of bacterial infections in hospitals (see Chapter 72). Spread to other pelvic organs and the bloodstream via the lymphatic vessels produces a rapidly progressive infection, which can be fatal unless appropriate antimicrobic therapy is initiated early in its course. The disease is highly contagious, and special precautions are needed to prevent its spread to other hospitalized patients.

Life-threatening, contagious, postpartum infection

B. Disease Due to Erythrogenic Toxin

Scarlet fever.   Infection with strains that elaborate the erythrogenic toxin may superimpose the signs of scarlet fever on a streptococcal pharyngitis in subjects with no circulating antibody to the toxin. In scarlet fever, the buccal mucosa, temples, and cheeks are deep red, except for a pale area around the mouth and nose (circumoral pallor). Punctate hemorrhages appear on the hard and soft palates, and the tongue becomes covered with a yellow-white exudate through which the red papillae are prominent (strawberry tongue). A diffuse red rash appears on the second day of illness, spreading from the upper chest to the trunk and extremities. Close examination of the skin shows the rash to consist of multiple, discrete, red pinpoint elevations, which impart an irregular "sandpaper" feel to the skin. For unknown reasons, scarlet fever is both less frequent and less severe than earlier in the century. The disease can occur with any type of *S. pyogenes* infection caused by an organism that produces erythrogenic toxin.

Localized infection; remote effects of toxin

Circumoral pallor

Strawberry tongue and rash

C. Delayed, Nonsuppurative, Noninfectious Complications

Rheumatic fever.   Rheumatic fever is a nonsuppurative inflammatory disease characterized by fever and inflammation of the joints, heart, subcutaneous tissue, and central nervous system. The major clinical manifestations are carditis, subcutaneous nodules, chorea, and migratory polyarthritis. Attacks typically begin 3 weeks (range 1–5 weeks) after a group A streptococcal pharyngitis, and in the absence of antiinflammatory therapy last 2–3 months. During this period the clinical manifestations vary in severity at different times. The most serious manifestation of rheumatic fever and the only one with a major potential to produce long-range

Complication of streptococcal pharyngitis

Carditis, chorea, and arthritis

disability is carditis, which involves the connective tissue and the endocardium, particularly of the valves. Cardiac enlargement, valvular murmurs, and effusions are seen clinically and reflect endocardial, myocardial, and epicardial damage, which can lead to heart failure either acutely or through the production of chronic lesions. Acute rheumatic fever also has a marked predilection for recurrence with subsequent streptococcal infections as new M types are encountered. The first attack usually occurs between the ages of 5 and 15 years. The risk of recurrent attacks after subsequent group A streptococcal infections continues into adult life and then decreases. Repeated attacks lead to progressive damage to the endocardium and heart valves, with scarring and valvular stenosis or incompetence (rheumatic heart disease).

The association between group A streptococci and rheumatic fever is based on epidemiologic studies demonstrating prior episodes of streptococcal pharyngitis and marked immune responses to streptococcal products. Rheumatic fever does not follow nonrespiratory infections or infections with streptococci other than *S. pyogenes* (group A). Although some strains may be more likely to cause initial attacks, the events involved in recurrent rheumatic fever and the subsequent cardiac damage indicate that the pathogenesis of the disease is group (A) rather than M type-specific, because recurrences can be caused by many M protein types. Prophylactic penicillin therapy is used to prevent recurrent rheumatic fever by preventing subsequent streptococcal infections.

Several theories have been advanced to explain the role of group A streptococci in rheumatic fever: 1) an autoimmune mechanism caused by similarities between streptococcal and human tissue antigens; 2) a serum sickness-like state mediated by antigen-antibody complexes; 3) residual toxicity of streptococcal products such as streptolysin S or O; and 4) persistence of the organisms in tissues (for example, as cell wall defective forms).

Of these theories, the first has the most experimental support. Patients with rheumatic fever have higher levels of various antistreptococcal antibodies than those with streptococcal infections who do not develop rheumatic fever. Some of these antibodies have been shown to react with both heart tissues and streptococcal antigens. For example, antibodies directed against streptococcal cell wall and cell membrane components cross-react with cardiac sarcolemmal sheaths, smooth muscle of vessel walls, and cells of the endocardium. Just which of the many cell wall components are stimulating these antibodies is a matter of intense interest. Fragments of M protein from a serotype strongly associated with rheumatic fever have been shown to possess epitopes that cross-react with human heart sarcolemma membranes. Studies of genetic homology between different M types of group A streptococci suggest that conserved domains of the M protein molecule may be responsible for its heart cross-reactivity, while variable domains confer its specific antiphagocytic properties. Identifying and separating these components is crucial both to understanding rheumatic fever and to approaches to its prevention through immunization. Cross-reactions between the group A polysaccharide and a glycoprotein isolated from heart valves have also been described. These observations correlate with the long-known heightened humoral immune response of patients with rheumatic fever to a variety of streptococcal products. Such patients also show greater cell-mediated immunity to streptococcal antigens. A cellular reaction pattern consisting of lymphocytes and macrophages aggregated around fibrinoid deposits is found in human hearts.

Marginal notes

Recurrences with subsequent *S. pyogenes* infections

Valvular damage

Role of *S. pyogenes* in pathogenesis; not type-specific

Antimicrobic prophylaxis

Possible pathogenetic mechanisms

Probable autoimmune etiology

Possible role of conserved M protein epitopes

This lesion, called the *Aschoff body*, is characteristic of rheumatic carditis.

Genetic and socioeconomic predisposing factors

Genetic factors are probably also important in rheumatic fever, because only a small proportion of individuals infected with group A streptococci develop the disease. Attack rates have been highest among those of lower socioeconomic status and vary among those of different racial origins. The gene for an alloantigen found on the surface of B lymphocytes occurs among rheumatic fever patients at a frequency fourfold to fivefold greater than the general population. This further suggests a genetic predisposition to hyperreactivity to streptococcal products.

Recent outbreaks of disease

Rheumatic fever declined dramatically in the United States during the past few decades. Recently, however, there have been several sharp outbreaks of the disease, particularly in the intermountain area of the country. In contrast to earlier experience, these have also affected children of higher socioeconomic status. The outbreaks have been associated with mucoid encapsulated strains of group A streptococci of a limited number of M types.

Acute glomerulonephritis.

Course usually benign

Glomerulonephritis is primarily a disease of childhood, characterized clinically by edema, hypertension, hematuria, and proteinuria and pathologically by diffuse proliferative lesions of the glomeruli. The clinical course is usually benign, with spontaneous healing over weeks to months. Occasionally a progressive course leads to renal failure and death. The frequency with which acute glomerulonephritis leads to chronic nephritis is not conclusively established, except that it is much more common in adults than children. There are a number of causes of the disease other than group A streptococci and a significant proportion of cases have no known etiology.

May follow respiratory or skin infection by specific M types (nephritogenic strains)

Poststreptococcal glomerulonephritis may follow either respiratory or cutaneous group A streptococcal infection. It involves only certain strains, known on epidemiologic grounds as *nephritogenic*. The average latent period between infection and glomerulonephritis is 10 days from a respiratory infection, but generally about 3 weeks from a skin infection. Nephritogenic strains are of a few M protein serotypes only, such as type 12 (respiratory) and type 49 (skin). Second attacks require infection with a nephritogenic strain of another M type; this event is rare, however, and recurrences are unusual.

Role of immune complexes

As in rheumatic fever, the pathogenesis of acute glomerulonephritis appears to involve immunologic mechanisms. Immunoglobulins, complement components, and antigens that react with antibodies against group A streptococci have been identified in the diseased glomerulus. The renal injury may be caused by cross-reactions between renal tissue and antistreptococcal antibodies, but more likely simply by deposition in the glomerulus of preformed antigen-antibody complexes with complement activation and consequent inflammatory reaction. Such complexes have been identified in the serum during acute disease and, together with complement components, as discrete deposits in the glomerulus.

Epidemiology

Group A Streptococcal Pharyngitis.

Direct or droplet spread

This is spread by respiratory secretions. Acquisition can be by direct contact with the mucosa or secretions or through large droplets produced by coughing, sneezing, or even conversation. Droplet transmission is most efficient at short distances (2–5 feet).

Influence of crowding

Spread is common in families and may be accentuated by crowding in institutions such as schools and military barracks. Food, although a less common vehicle of transmission, has been the source of many outbreaks. Environmental sources and fomites are not important means of spread, although group A streptococci survive for some time in dried secretions.

Role of carriers

The acute case of streptococcal pharyngitis is the most important source of the organism. Without treatment, the organism is often present for 1–4 weeks after symptoms have disappeared. Asymptomatic carrier rates are usually very low; however, rates of more than 10% have sometimes been documented in children. Carriage may be both pharyngeal and nasal and occasionally anal. The epidemiologic importance of asymptomatic and convalescent carriers is clearly less than that of acute cases. Nasal carriers have greater infectivity than those who carry S. pyogenes in the throat only.

"Ping-pong" infections

Recurrent infections are sometimes seen in families when prompt antimicrobial therapy has prevented the development of type-specific immunity. This situation allows reinfection from other infected or colonized siblings when antimicrobic treatment is stopped. Such "ping-pong" infection-reinfection cycles sometimes require simultaneous treatment of the entire family to prevent continued transmission.

Usually disease of childhood

Transmission by contact or fomites

Impetigo.   Impetigo caused by S. pyogenes has an earlier peak age incidence (2–5 years) than streptococcal pharyngitis. Clinical impetigo is often preceded by skin colonization, which is favored by poor hygiene. Minor trauma of colonized skin (for example, insect bites) then leads to development of the lesions. Transmission involves direct contact or shared fomites such as towels. Certain flies have been shown to serve as vectors. Impetigo is most common among lower socioeconomic groups, in hot climates, and at times when insect bites are frequent. The M protein types of S. pyogenes most commonly associated with impetigo are different from those causing respiratory infection, and some are nephritogenic. Multiple cases of acute glomerulonephritis have occurred in association with epidemics of impetigo.

Nosocomial Wound and Puerperal Infections.   Group A streptococci were once a leading cause of nosocomial postoperative wound and puerperal infections (Chapter 72). The primary mode of transmission from patient to patient was by the hands of physicians or other medical attendants and through poor hygienic practices. The potential for hospital spread, however, is still present. Infections may be derived from staff or patients ill with pharyngitis or carrying the organism in the pharynx or nose. Contaminated particles or epithelial cells from nonrespiratory carriage sites can also be a source of infection. For example, some nosocomial outbreaks of group A streptococcal infections have been traced to anal carriers who disseminated the organisms widely in operating rooms.

Outbreaks associated with anal carriage of S. pyogenes

Treatment and Prevention

Continued universal susceptibility to penicillin

Prevention of rheumatic fever

Streptococcus pyogenes remains universally highly susceptible to penicillin G, the antimicrobic of choice. Patients allergic to penicillin are usually treated with erythromycin if the organisms are susceptible or with a cephalosporin if cross-allergy is absent. Adequate penicillin treatment of streptococcal pharyngitis within 10 days of onset will prevent rheumatic fever by removing the antigenic stimulus; its effect on the duration of the pharyngitis is less, because of the short course of the natural infection. Penicillin does not prevent the development of acute glomerulonephritis.

Penicillin prophylaxis with long-acting preparations is used to prevent recurrences of rheumatic fever during the most susceptible ages (5–15 years). Patients with a history of rheumatic fever or known rheumatic heart disease usually receive antimicrobial prophylaxis while undergoing procedures known to cause transient bacteremia, such as dental extraction.

Attempts to develop an M protein vaccine resulted in some postimmunization cases of rheumatic fever. Research is now centering on seeking epitopes of the M protein molecules of common serotypes that stimulate antistreptococcal immunity without risking the nonsuppurative complications of the disease.

Laboratory Diagnosis

Direct Gram smears unhelpful in diagnosis of pharyngitis

Culture on blood agar

A typical clinical picture with demonstration of the organism in the infected site is the usual means by which active *S. pyogenes* infection is diagnosed. In pharyngitis, a swab of the posterior pharynx and tonsils is taken to include all inflamed areas. A direct Gram-stained smear is unhelpful because of the many other streptococci in the normal pharyngeal flora. Direct Gram smears from normally sterile sites will usually demonstrate streptococci. (Figure 16.4) Blood agar plates are seeded and incubated at 35–37°C. When *S. pyogenes* alone is sought (throat swabs), many laboratories use anaerobic incubation because of its favorable effect on the demonstration of β-hemolysis.

Presumptive differentiation of S. pyogenes from other β-hemolytic streptococci with bacitracin

After overnight incubation, β-hemolytic colonies are Gram stained to confirm that they are streptococci, then identified according to Lancefield group. Although definitive speciation is primarily through immunologic techniques, nonimmunologic methods can be used because of their good correlation with the definitive test. The *bacitracin test* (see Table 16.2) is based on the exquisite susceptibility of group A strains to bacitracin and the relative resistance of strains of other groups (Table 16.2). When a disc containing a small amount of bacitracin (0.02 U) is placed on a plate streaked from an isolated colony, more than 99% of group A strains show a zone of inhibition, whereas 90–95% of non-group A strains do not. The low rate of false-negative results has made this method a valuable presumptive test in hospital laboratories. Definitive identification of *S. pyogenes* requires demonstration of the group A-specific antigen by precipitin, immunofluorescence, or agglutination procedures. Direct detection of group A antigen in throat swabs is now possible, but is not as sensitive as culture. M typing may be done for epidemiologic purposes;

Serologic detection of group A antigen

Epidemiologic subtyping

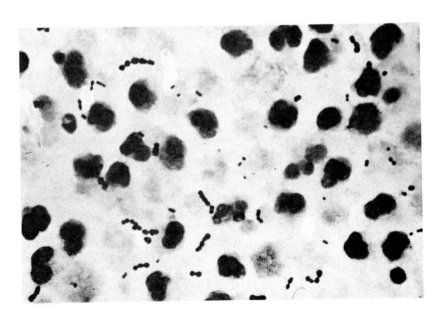

16.4 Gram stain of pus from a streptococcal suppurative lesion. Reproduced with permission of Schering Corporation, Kenilworth, N.J., the copyright owner. All rights reserved.

the procedure is serologic, using precipitin techniques with type-specific antisera.

Several serologic tests have been developed to aid in the diagnosis of poststreptococcal sequelae. They include the antistreptolysin O, anti-DNA-ase B, antistreptokinase, and antihyaluronidase tests. As characteristically high titers of antistreptolysin O are usually found in sera of patients with rheumatic fever, that test is used most widely.

Serologic test results in rheumatic fever

Streptococcus agalactiae (Group B)

Larger colonies than group A strains
β-hemolysis less distinct

In broth culture and in purulent lesions, group B streptococci produce short chains and occasional pairs of spherical or ovoid Gram-positive cells. β-Hemolysis is less distinct than with group A streptococci and may be absent, particularly under aerobic conditions. In addition to their Lancefield antigen, group B streptococci possess polysaccharide capsular antigens. This characteristic forms the basis of a serologic typing system for strains within the group. The type antigens are designated Ia, Ib, Ic, II, and III. Sialic acid is a component of all five capsules. Sialic acid has been shown to allow group B streptococci to resist opsonophagocytosis in the absence of type-specific antibody. As with M protein of group A streptococci, this is accomplished by blocking the opsonic effects of activation of the alternative pathway of complement. Specific antibody is required for recognition of the streptococci by phagocytes, and opsonization is then enhanced by C3b. Although extracellular products and hemolysins have been identified in group B streptococci, their association with virulence has not been studied extensively.

Capsules inhibit phagocytosis in absence of antibody

Penicillin susceptibility less than in group A

Group B streptococci are susceptible to the same antimicrobics as group A organisms; however, they are less susceptible to penicillin G (MIC, 0.2–1.0 μg/ml) and less readily killed by the antibiotic. They are more frequently resistant to tetracycline than group A strains.

Diseases

Neonatal pneumonia, sepsis, and meningitis

Group B streptococci are a leading cause of pneumonia, sepsis, and meningitis during the first 2 months of life. The incidence of group B infections in this age group has been estimated at 1–3 cases per 1000 births, and the mortality is between 30 and 60% of infected cases. Most cases, which develop in the immediate perinatal period, result from contamination of the infant with group B streptococci from the female genital tract. As group B streptococci are present in the vagina in one-third of all normal women, factors other than simple exposure must be involved in infection. Type-specific antibody has been shown to be protective; therefore, it is probable that only those infants who have not received specific transplacental IgG from their mothers are susceptible. A "late onset" syndrome may also occur 3–8 weeks after birth. These cases usually involve type III strains and have a lower mortality than those with early onset. Most cases with late onset have fever with no obvious primary site or meningitis. Some are examples of nosocomial cross-infection; others acquire the organisms after leaving the hospital.

Probable protection by transplacental IgG

Late onset syndrome in infants

Other group B streptococcal infections

Group B streptococci may also colonize the throat in children and adults, in whom they have been associated with a variety of pyogenic infections at nonrespiratory sites. Prominent examples are puerperal fevers and infections associated with gynecologic manipulations or surgery. As indicated by the species name *agalactiae*, these organisms cause mastitis in cattle; however, pasteurization of milk has eliminated this source as an important link to human disease. Group B streptococci are not associated with rheumatic fever or acute glomerulonephritis.

Because the organisms' susceptibility to penicillin is somewhat less than that of many other streptococci, group B streptococcal infections are often treated with combinations of penicillin and an aminoglycoside.

The laboratory diagnosis of group B infection is by culture on blood agar medium both aerobically and anaerobically, the latter to demonstrate hemolysis more clearly. Definitive identification involves serologic determination of the Lancefield group; however, certain biochemical and cultural identification tests show a high degree of correlation with Lancefield grouping and are commonly used in clinical laboratories.

Group D and Other Pyogenic Streptococci

The terms *group D streptococci* and *enterococci* are often used interchangeably, because the first demonstration of the group D antigen was in several species commonly found in the gastrointestinal tract. This usage is not correct, because enterococci are a subset of species within group D (Table 16.1). Enterococci* are found in the intestinal tract and have many biochemical and cultural features that reflect their habitat, such as the ability to grow in the presence of high concentrations of bile salts and sodium chloride. Several different species are biochemically distinct (see Table 16.2). Some are β-hemolytic, but most produce nonhemolytic or α-hemolytic colonies that are larger than those of other streptococci.

The enterococci are the most resistant of the streptococci to antimicrobics. They require 4–16 μg/ml penicillin for inhibition and much higher concentrations for bactericidal effect. Enterococci are consistently resistant to aminoglycosides and sulfonamides, often resistant to tetracycline, and occasionally resistant to erythromycin and chloramphenicol. Ampicillin is the antimicrobial agent most consistently active. Despite their resistance to aminoglycosides, many, but not all, strains of enterococci are inhibited and rapidly killed by combinations of low concentrations of penicillin and aminoglycosides. Under these conditions, the action of penicillin on the cell wall allows the aminoglycoside to enter the cell, reach its ribosomal receptor site, and kill the cell. Some strains show exceptionally high resistance to aminoglycosides, which are usually plasmid encoded and which abrogate synergistic effects.

Since the original Lancefield classification was developed, the teichoic acid group D antigen has been found in some streptococcal species previously considered ungroupable. These organisms, termed *nonenterococcal group D streptococci*, resemble the viridans streptococci more than the enterococci in their cultural, biologic, and antimicrobic susceptibility features.

Streptococci of groups C, G, and F may be isolated from humans and other animals. These organisms can cause pyogenic infection, but do so much less frequently than those of groups A, B, or D. In general, their susceptibility to antimicrobial agents is similar to that of groups A and B streptococci.

Diseases

Enterococci cause opportunistic urinary tract infections, and occasionally wound and soft tissue infections, in much the same fashion as members of the Enterobacteriaceae. Infections are often associated with urinary tract

Margin notes:

Combination therapy

Laboratory diagnosis

Resistance of enterococci to bile salts and NaCl

Relative resistance to penicillin

Synergistic effects of penicillin and aminoglycosides on enterococci

Nonenterococcal group D streptococci

Pathogenicity of groups C, G, and F streptococci

Enterococcal infections

---

* Recently, it has been proposed that enterococci be included in a genus *Enterococcus* separate from the streptococci.

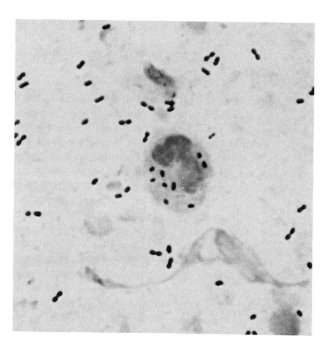

16.5 *Streptococcus pneumoniae* in sputum of patient with pneumonia. Note the marked tendency to form oval diplococci.

manipulations, malignancies, biliary tract disease, and gastrointestinal disorders. There is often an associated bacteremia, which can result in the development of endocarditis on previously damaged cardiac valves.

Treatment of enterococcal infection depends on its site and severity. Ampicillin is effective in most urinary tract and minor soft tissue infections. More severe infections, particularly endocarditis, are usually treated with combinations of a penicillin and an aminoglycoside.

For technical reasons, biochemical and cultural tests, such as growth in bile and esculin hydrolysis, are usually substituted for serologic identification of group D streptococci in the clinical laboratory. Occasionally further biochemical tests are used to separate the enterococcal from the nonenterococcal species (Table 16.2).

Infections caused by pyogenic streptococci of other groups

The other pyogenic streptococci occasionally produce various respiratory, skin, wound, soft tissue, and genital infections, which may resemble those caused by groups A and B streptococci. None has been clearly associated with poststreptococcal sequelae. The role of pyogenic streptococci other than those of group A in acute pharyngitis is unestablished. A few case reports of food-borne outbreaks have shown some strains of groups C and G streptococci to cause pharyngitis, but the evidence is not yet strong enough to draw this conclusion in individual cases.

Streptococcus pneumoniae

Morphology

Encapsulated, Gram-positive, lanceolate diplococci

In clinical material or culture, cells of *S. pneumoniae* appear as Gram-positive, oval diplococci with their axes end to end (Figure 16.5). They sometimes form short chains. The adjacent ends of a pair tend to be rounded, the distal ends more pointed, giving the individual cell a bullet or lancet shape. Older cells or those exposed to antimicrobial agents may appear Gram negative and show morphologic distortion. Virulent strains

Virulence associated with capsule

are encapsulated, but the capsules are not apparent in Gram-stained preparations.

Cultural Characteristics

Pneumococci are fastidious organisms, requiring a relatively complex medium for isolation. Rapid growth is frequently followed by autolysis. Initially turbid broth may clear on continued incubation; once formed, colonies begin to lyse in the center and even disappear. This behavior is caused by their susceptibility to autolytic enzymes and to peroxides produced during growth. Autolysis can be hastened with surfactants such as detergents and bile; this quality forms the basis of the bile solubility test.

Autolysis and bile solubility

On blood agar, encapsulated pneumococci produce round, glistening colonies (0.5–2 mm in diameter after 18 hr) surrounded by a zone of α-hemolysis. Because of autolysis, the colonies often develop a dimpled, then a craterlike appearance. Pneumococcal colonies may, however, be indistinguishable from those of viridans streptococci, particularly in young cultures.

α-hemolysis and colony morphology

Virulence and the Pneumococcal Capsule

The structural features of pneumococci are similar to those of other streptococci; the important exception is their surface capsules, which are composed of high-molecular-weight complex polysaccharides forming hydrophilic gels. They are antigenic and there are more than 80 distinct serotypes of capsule (types 1,2, . . . 24, and so on) forming the basis of a pneumococcal serotype classification system. The chemical structure of the polysaccharides has been determined for a few types and shows unique features for each. It is of interest that antibodies against capsules of certain serotypes are known to cross-react with polysaccharides produced by other bacteria (*Haemophilus, Klebsiella*) and even with human blood group B isoantigen.

More than 80 antigenic types of pneumococcal polysaccharide capsules

The polysaccharide capsule of the pneumococcus inhibits its engulfment by phagocytes and is the major determinant of virulence. Unencapsulated mutants are avirulent in experimental infections. Thus, specific anticapsular antibody, whether produced by active or passive immunization, opsonizes capsulate strains and confers type-specific immunity to infection. While the antiphagocytic effect of the capsule has long been attributed to its physical size and electrostatic charge, the amount of capsular material does not correlate well with virulence. Recent studies, again, suggest that the capsule interferes with the opsonizing activity of the alternative complement pathway. When antibody binds to the capsule, C3b generated by the classical pathway also attaches and the opsonized organisms are phagocytosed and killed. Capsule production and virulence can be conferred on noncapsulate strains by transformation with DNA extracted from a capsulate strain. Thus, an avirulent noncapsulate mutant of a type II pneumococcus can be transformed to a virulent capsulate type III strain with DNA from another type III strain.

Antiphagocytic effect of capsule

Type-specific anticapsular antibody opsonizes organism and confers immunity

Alternative complement pathway opsonization inhibited by capsule

Transformation of capsule type

Toxins and Extracellular Enzymes

A pneumolysin, a neuraminidase, and a substance that causes purpura and dermal hemorrhage in experimental animals have been isolated from pneumococci. The pneumolysin has some properties similar to those of streptolysin O, including toxicity in experimental animals, and the neuraminidase may contribute to invasiveness by splitting membrane glycoproteins and glycolipids. There is no convincing evidence, however, that these substances play an important role in pneumococcal infection. Virulence is largely attributable to the antiphagocytic properties of the capsule, and disease, to the acute inflammatory response to infection; however, these findings do not fully explain some of the clinical features of infection with *S. pneumoniae*, such as the abrupt onset, the toxicity, and the fulminant course and disseminated intravascular coagulation seen in some cases. For these reasons, interest in toxins continues, but their role is presently inconclusive.

Antimicrobial Susceptibility

Usually susceptible to penicillin

Recent development of penicillin resistance

Pneumococci generally follow the pattern of group A streptococci in their susceptibility to antimicrobics. They are usually highly susceptible to penicillin and other β-lactam agents. Tetracycline resistance is common (3–30%), but resistance to erythromycin or chloramphenicol is rare. Aminoglycosides are not effective. In recent years, pneumococci resistant to penicillin and other antimicrobics were first reported from South Africa and now from many other countries, including the United States. These strains require penicillin concentrations of 0.12–4.0 μg/ml for inhibition, whereas fully susceptible strains are inhibited by 0.01–0.05 μg/ml. Patients with pneumonia and meningitis caused by the more resistant strains respond poorly or not at all to penicillin therapy. The mechanism of resistance appears to be mutational and involves alterations of penicillin-binding proteins, rather than penicillinase production. Resistant strains are still uncommon in most areas of the United States.

Diseases

Predisposing factors

Pneumococcal pneumonia. *Streptococcus pneumoniae* is by far the most common cause of bacterial pneumonia. As with other bacterial pneumonias, viral respiratory infection and underlying chronic disease are important predisposing factors. Although infection may occur at any age, the incidence and mortality of pneumococcal pneumonia increase sharply after 50 years. Alcoholism, diabetes mellitus, chronic renal disease, and some malignancies are all associated with more frequent and serious pneumococcal pneumonias. In the preantibiotic era, the mortality in hospitalized patients was 20–30%; it has now been reduced to 5–10%. Although these mortality estimates are probably higher than those for cases in the community, the disease remains an important cause of death.

Pneumococcal pneumonia begins with aspiration of respiratory secretions containing pneumococci. This event must be common, as 10–30% of normal people carry one or more serologic types of *S. pneumoniae* in the throat. Aspirated organisms are normally cleared rapidly by the defense mechanisms of the lower respiratory tract, including the cough and epiglottic reflexes, the mucociliary "blanket," and phagocytosis by alveolar macrophages. Events that impair the combined efficiency of these defenses can allow pneumococci to reach and multiply in the alveoli. They include the chronic illnesses mentioned previously, damage to bronchial epithelium from smoking or air pollution, and respiratory dysfunction from alcoholic intoxication, narcotics and other drugs, anesthesia, and trauma.

Normal host defenses and factors that impair them

Type-specific immunity and course of infection

In immune individuals with a sufficient level of circulating antibody against the capsular polysaccharide of organisms that reach the alveoli, the infection is controlled rapidly; in nonimmune individuals, however, al-

Consolidation caused by inflammation: interference with gas exchange

Lobar distribution

Effect of free capsular polysaccharide

Absence of structural damage

Clinical manifestations

Crisis associated with effective levels of opsonizing antibody

Predisposing factors and age of incidence

Sinusitis and otitis media

veolar multiplication is followed by a profuse outpouring of serous edema fluid, which facilitates growth and spread of pneumococci to adjacent alveoli and interferes with gas exchange. The fluid outpouring is quickly followed by an influx of polymorphonuclear leukocytes and erythrocytes, the latter as a result of capillary fragility. By the second or third day of illness, the lung segment has increased three- to fourfold in weight through accumulation of this cellular, hemorrhagic fluid. By the fourth or fifth day, neutrophils predominate in the consolidated alveoli, which usually affect a single lobe of the lung. Although some surface phagocytosis and destruction of pneumococci occurs in the absence of opsonizing antibody, it is outpaced by multiplication of the organism, and bacteremia is common. Even when formation of anticapsular antibody begins, it may be neutralized by free soluble capsular polysaccharide in the exudate and bloodstream. If antibody production is sufficient to overcome this neutralization, however, the pneumococci are readily phagocytosed and destroyed. When actively growing pneumococci are no longer present, macrophages replace the granulocytes and resolution of the lesion ensues. A remarkable feature of pneumococcal pneumonia is the lack of structural damage to the lung, which usually leads to complete resolution on recovery.

Clinically, pneumococcal pneumonia begins abruptly with a shaking chill and high fever. Cough with production of sputum pink to rusty in color (indicating the presence of red blood cells) and pleuritic chest pain are common. Physical findings usually indicate pulmonary consolidation. Children and young adults typically demonstrate a lobar consolidation on chest radiography, whereas older patients may show a less localized bronchial distribution to the infiltrates. Without therapy, sustained fever, pleuritic pain, and productive cough continue until, in patients who recover, a "crisis" occurs 5–10 days after onset of the disease. The crisis involves a sudden decrease in temperature and of improvement in the patient's condition. It is associated with effective levels of opsonizing antibody reaching the lesion.

Pneumococcal meningitis. With *Neisseria meningitidis* and *Haemophilus influenzae, S. pneumoniae* is one of the three leading causes of bacterial meningitis. The signs and symptoms are similar to those produced by other bacteria (Chapter 67). Acute purulent meningitis may follow pneumococcal infection at another site or appear with no apparent antecedent infection. It may also develop after trauma involving the skull. All ages are affected, however, in later life, pneumococcal meningitis is the most common form of the disease. The mortality and frequency of sequelae are slightly higher with pneumococcal meningitis than with other forms of pyogenic meningitis.

Upper Respiratory Tract Infections. Pneumococci are common causes of sinusitis and otitis media. The latter frequently occurs in children in association with viral infection. Chronic infection of the mastoid or respiratory sinus sometimes extends to the subarachnoid space to cause meningitis. Pneumococci do not cause pharyngitis or tonsillitis.

Other infections. Pneumococci may also cause endocarditis, arthritis, and peritonitis, usually in association with bacteremia. Patients with ascites caused by diseases such as cirrhosis and nephritis may develop spontaneous pneumococcal peritonitis.

Treatment and Prevention

Penicillin therapy for susceptible strains

Pencillin is the antimicrobic of choice because the great majority of pneumococci are fully sensitive to it. Infections caused by the more resistant strains encountered recently may require treatment with erythromycin or chloramphenicol. The therapeutic response to treatment of pneumococcal pneumonia is often (but not always) dramatic. Reduction in fever, respiratory rate, and cough can occur in 12–24 hr, but may occur gradually over several days. Chest radiography may yield normal results only after several weeks.

Polyvalent capsular polysaccharide vaccine

A vaccine has been prepared from capsular polysaccharide extracted from the 23 types of *S. pneumoniae* most commonly encountered. This vaccine, which is protective against these 23 types, is presently recommended for patients particularly susceptible to pneumococcal infection because of age, underlying disease, or immune status.

Laboratory Diagnosis

Direct Gram smears

Need for adequate specimens

Gram smears of material from sites of pneumococcal infection usually show typical Gram-positive, lancet-shaped diplococci (Figure 16.5). A properly collected sputum sample comprising inflammatory exudate from the affected lung segment will usually reveal the typical appearance. Sputum collection may be difficult, however, and specimens contaminated with respiratory flora are useless for diagnosis. Other types of lower respiratory specimens may be needed for diagnosis (Chapters 14 and 64).

Culture

Streptococcus pneumoniae grows well overnight on blood agar medium incubated aerobically. Supplementation with carbon dioxide often enhances growth. Colonies are surrounded by a zone of α-hemolysis. The pneumococcal capsule, which is not seen on Gram staining can be demonstrated by the quellung (capsular swelling) reaction. When capsulate pneumococci are mixed with type-specific antisera, the opsonized capsule absorbs water, becomes increasingly refractile and visible under the light microscope, and appears swollen. This test is made practicable by the commercial availability of a polyvalent antiserum containing antibodies for over 80 capsular types (Omniserum).

Quellung reaction

Distinguishing factors from viridans streptococci

The pneumococcus is distinguished from viridans streptococci by several tests (Table 16.2) including:

1. Susceptibility to the synthetic chemical ethylhydrocupreine (Optochin), which can be demonstrated by a disc diffusion test; viridans streptococci are resistant.

2. Bile solubility; viridans streptococci are insoluble.

3. Presence of a capsule.

4. Virulence for mice.

5. Capsular swelling reaction with type-specific or pooled polyvalent sera against the pneumococcal capsule.

Blood culture

Bacteremia is common in pneumococcal pneumonia and meningitis, and blood cultures are valuable supplements to cultures of local fluids or exudates.

Detection of pneumococcal antigen in clinical material

Pneumococcal capsular antigen can frequently be demonstrated in body fluids, serum, and urine using counterimmunoelectrophoresis, latex agglutination, or coagglutination methods (Chapter 14). This is particularly valuable when cultures are negative due to previous antimicrobic therapy.

Viridans Streptococci

α-hemolytic organisms

The viridans group comprises all α-hemolytic streptococci that remain after the criteria for defining pyogenic streptococci and pneumococci have been applied. Characteristically members of the normal flora of the oral and nasopharyngeal cavities, they have the basic bacteriologic features of streptococci, but lack the specific antigens, toxins, and virulence of the other groups. Although the viridans group includes several species (Table 16.1), they are usually not characterized in clinical practice because there is little difference among them in medical significance. Viridans streptococci generally produce small (0.5–1.0 mm) colonies surrounded by a zone of α-hemolysis. They lack the autolytic properties of pneumococci, even in the presence of surface-active agents such as bile salts. The procedures for distinguishing viridans streptococci from pneumococci have been described previously.

Bile insoluble, optochin negative, noncapsulate

Subacute bacterial endocarditis

Although their virulence is very low, viridans strains can cause disease when they are protected from host defenses. The prime example is subacute bacterial endocarditis. In this disease, viridans streptococci reach previously damaged heart valves as a result of transient bacteremia associated with manipulations, such as tooth extraction, that disturb their usual habitat. Protected by fibrin and platelets, they multiply on the valve, causing local and systemic disease that is fatal if untreated. Extracellular production of glucans, complex polysaccharide polymers, may enhance their attachment to cardiac valves in a manner similar to the pathogenesis of dental caries by *Streptococcus mutans* (Chapter 62). The clinical course of viridans streptococcal endocarditis is subacute, with slow progression over weeks or months (Chapter 68). It is effectively treated with penicillin, but uniformly fatal if untreated. The disease is particularly associated with valves damaged by recurrent rheumatic fever. The decline in the occurrence of rheumatic heart disease has reduced the incidence of this particular type of endocarditis.

Adhesion to damaged heart valve endocardium

Additional Reading

Fischetti, V.A. 1989. Streptococcal M protein: Molecular design and biologic behavior. *Clin. Microbiol. Rev.* 2:285–314. This in-depth review addresses aspects of M-protein structure, immunochemistry, and genetics which are important for designing a vaccine to prevent group A streptococcal disease.

Kasper, D.L. 1986. Bacterial capsule—old dogmas and new tricks. *J. Infect. Dis.* 153:407–415. Current concepts concerning how the group B streptococcal and pneumococcal capsules interfere with opsonophagocytosis are discussed.

Lancefield, R.C. 1933. A serological differentiation of human and other groups of hemolytic streptococci. *J. Exp. Med.* 57:571–595. The classic study that changed streptococcal classification.

Unny, S.K., and Middlebrooks, B.L. 1983. Streptococcal rheumatic carditis. *Microbiol. Rev.* 47:97–120. This review covers all aspects of the pathogenesis of rheumatic myocarditis and valvulitis including the evidence for immunologic cross-reactions.

Wannamaker, L.W. 1970. Differences between streptococcal infections of the throat and of the skin. *N. Engl. J. Med.* 282:23–31. Some important clinical, epidemiologic, and immunologic features are summarized in greater detail than in the present chapter.

17

Corynebacteria and Other Aerobic and Facultative Gram-Positive Rods

Kenneth J. Ryan

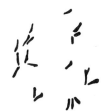

Corynebacterium diphtheriae

This chapter includes a variety of Gram-positive rods, some of which are highly pathogenic, but none of which are currently common causes of human disease in the United States. Their importance to the student lies in the lessons in pathogenesis, epidemiology, and prevention learned when they were more common and in the continued threat that their existence poses. *Corynebacterium diphtheriae*, the cause of diphtheria, is a prototype for causing toxigenic disease, and *Bacillus anthraciss*, the cause of anthrax, has virulence and environmental survival characteristics that still cause concern about its potential use in bacterial warfare. *Listeria monocytogenes* has long been recognized as a sporadic cause of meningitis and other infections in the fetus and immunocompromised and has now been shown to cause epidemic foodborne disease.

Corynebacteria

Group Characteristics

The genus *Corynebacterium* includes many species of aerobic and facultative gram-positive rods. Corynebacteria (from the Greek *koryne*, club) are small and pleomorphic, and in some species tend to have clubbed ends. The cells often remain attached after division, forming "Chinese letter" or palisade arrangements. Spores are not formed. Some species contain polyphosphate granules that stain red-purple with methylene blue (metachromatic granules). Growth is generally best under aerobic conditions, but many strains will grow under microaerophilic or anaerobic conditions on media enriched with blood or other animal products.

Colonies on blood agar are usually small (1–2 mm); however, some strains of *Corynebacterium diphtheriae* may produce colonies 3 mm in diameter after incubation for 24 hr. Most are nonhemolytic. Catalase is produced, and many strains form acid (usually lactic acid) through carbohydrate fermentation.

313

The type species *C. diphtheriae* produces a powerful exotoxin, which is responsible for the disease diphtheria and which usually results from a pharyngeal infection. Some corynebacteria, which are primarily pathogenic to animals, produce other toxins. Others are nonpathogenic commensal inhabitants of the pharynx, nasopharynx, distal urethra, and skin; they are collectively designated as *diphtheroids*.

Corynebacterium diphtheriae

Growth and Identification.   Because it is clinically important to distinguish *C. diphtheriae* rapidly from members of the respiratory flora, several media and methods have been developed to demonstrate this organism.

Tellurite selective media

Most selective media contain potassium tellurite, which inhibits many members of the normal oral flora. *Corynebacterium diphtheriae* also reduces the potassium tellurite to produce gray or black colonies, the morphology of which differs with each of three types of the organism: *gravis, mitis,* and *intermedius*. Differentiation of *C. diphtheriae* from other corynebacteria depends on several biochemical reactions, including carbohydrate fermentation tests.

Diphtheria exotoxin is protein synthesis inhibitor

Pathogenicity.   Virulence is determined by production of diphtheria exotoxin, a protein with potent cytotoxic features. It inhibits protein synthesis in cell-free extracts of virtually all eukaryotic cells, from protozoa and yeasts to higher plants and humans. However, it is only toxic to the intact cells of certain mammals. The diphtheria toxin molecule (DT) contains both an active subunit A that catalyzes the toxic activity and a subunit B that mediates receptor binding and membrane insertion. The B subunit attaches to the cell membrane by a receptor that is probably a glycolipid. The toxin traverses the membrane either directly or by receptor-mediated endocytosis as shown in Figure 17.1. At some point the A and B subunits separate. Separation is required for full activity of the A subunit on its target, elongation factor 2 (EF-2), which transfers polypeptidyl-transfer RNA from acceptor to donor sites on the ribosome of the host cell. The specific action of the A subunit is to catalyze the transfer of the adenine ribose phosphate portion of nicotinamide adenine dinucleotide (NAD) to EF-2, an enzymatic reaction called *ADP-ribosylation*. This inactivates EF-2 and shuts off protein synthesis. The extraordinary potency of diphtheria toxin is demonstrated by experiments showing that a single molecule is able to inhibit protein synthesis in a cell within a few hours. ADP-ribosylation is now known to be the mechanism of action for a number of toxins including those which act on EF-2 (diphtheria toxin, *Pseudomonas aeruginosa* exotoxin A) and those with other target proteins (cholera toxin, *Escherichia coli* LT, pertussis toxin).

B subunit of toxin binds to cell receptor

The A subunit catalyses ADP-ribosylation of EF-2 to inactive form

Toxin coded by temperate phage
Nontoxigenic strains

Lysogenic conversion

The structural gene for the diphtheria toxin molecule is contained in a bacteriophage (β phage), and only strains of *C. diphtheriae*, which are lysogenic for this phage, produce toxin. Nontoxigenic strains of *C. diphtheriaea* can produce pharyngitis, but not the toxic manifestations of diphtheria. They can be converted to toxicity by lysogenization in vitro with β phage, and this process can probably occur in vivo.

Toxin is antigenic and neutralized by antibody

Immunity.   Diphtheria toxin is antigenic, stimulating the production of antitoxin antibodies during natural infection. Formalin treatment of toxin produces *toxoid*, which retains the antigenicity but not the toxicity of native toxin and is used in immunization against the disease. It is clear that this process functionally inactivates fragment B. Whether it also in-

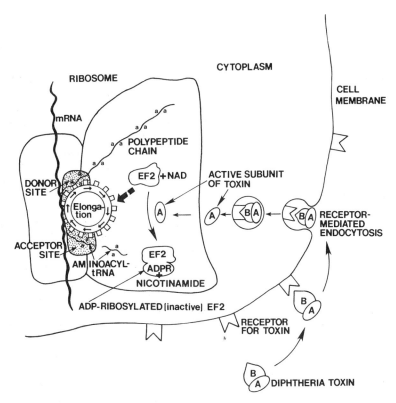

17.1 Action of diphtheria toxin. The toxin-binding (B) portion attaches to the cell membrane, and the complete molecule enters the cell. In the cell, the A subunit dissociates and catalyzes a reaction that ADP-ribosylates and thus inactivates elongation factor 2 (EF-2). This factor is essential for ribosomal reactions at the acceptor and donor sites, which transfer triplet code from messenger RNA (mRNA) to amino acid sequences via transfer RNA (tRNA). Inactivation of EF-2 stops building of the polypeptide chain.

activates fragment A or prevents its ability to dissociate from fragment B is not known. Recent studies of the A subunit structure and action suggest that another approach to producing a toxoid may be through genetic engineering. For example, substitution of a single amino acid located in the NAD-binding site of the A subunit of DT can completely detoxify, but retain the immunogenic specificity of the toxin. Although this may not be used for diphtheria immunization, it could have great importance for other ADP-ribosylating toxins for which toxoids are not available.

Diphtheria

Usually localized pharyngeal or upper respiratory infection

Diphtheritic membrane

Cervical lymphadenitis

Respiratory obstruction

After an incubation period of 2–4 days, diphtheria usually presents as pharyngitis or tonsillitis. Typically, malaise, sore throat, and fever are present, and a patch of exudate or membrane develops on the tonsils, uvula, soft palate, or pharyngeal wall. The gray-white membrane is caused by the action of the diphtheria toxin on the epithelium at the site of infection. It is composed of a coagulum of fibrin, leukocytes, cellular debris, and bacteria; adheres to the mucous membrane; and may extend from the oropharyngeal area down to the larynx and into the trachea. Associated cervical adenitis is common, and in severe cases cervical adenitis and edema produce a "bullneck" appearance. In uncomplicated cases, the infection gradually resolves and the membrane is coughed up after 5–10 days.

The complications and mortality of diphtheria are caused by respiratory obstruction or by the systemic effect of diphtheria toxin absorbed at the site of infection. Mechanical obstruction of the airway produced by membrane, edema, and hemorrhage can be sudden and complete and can lead to suffocation death, particularly if large sections of the membrane separate from the tracheal or laryngeal epithelial surface. Diphtheria toxin absorbed into the circulation causes damage to various organs, the most serious of which is to the heart. Diphtheritic myocarditis appears during the second or third week in severe cases of respiratory diphtheria. It is manifested by cardiac enlargement and weakness, arrhythmia, and congestive heart failure with dyspnea. Paralyses caused by involvement of cranial and peripheral nerves later in the course of disease, most often involve the soft palate, oculomotor (eye) muscles, or motor paralysis of select muscle groups. Paralysis is reversible, and it is generally not serious unless respiratory muscles such as the diaphragm are involved.

Remote effects of toxin on heart

Neurologic manifestations

Corynebacterium diphtheriae may produce nonrespiratory infections, particularly of the skin. The characteristic lesion ranges from a simple pustule to a chronic, nonhealing ulcer and is most common in tropical and hot, arid regions. Cardiac and neurologic complications from these infections are infrequent, suggesting that the efficiency of toxin production or absorption is low compared to that in respiratory infections.

Cutaneous diphtheria produces ulcerative lesion

It is important to remember that the manifestations of diphtheria are produced by multiplication of the organism and toxin production at the local site of infection. The organism has little invasive capacity, but the toxin causes tissue damage at both local and distant sites. Thus, *C. diphtheriae* is not isolated from the blood or from remote sites during the disease. The disease resolves with the formation of antitoxin antibody.

Little invasive capacity

Epidemiology. *Corynebacterium diphtheriae* is transmitted by droplet spread, by direct contact with cutaneous infections, and, to a lesser extent, by fomites. Some subjects become convalescent pharyngeal or nasal carriers and continue to harbor the organism for weeks to months or even for a lifetime. Other carriers have no history of the disease. Carriers represent the major reservoir for infection of nonimmune subjects. Diphtheria still occurs significantly in developing countries, but is rare where immunization is widely used. In the United States, for example, only zero to five cases per year have been reported since 1979, because of the routine practice of active immunization. Cases appear sporadically and as small outbreaks in populations who have not received adequate immunization, such as migratory workers, transients and those who refuse immunization on religious grounds.

Droplet and fomitic spread

Carriers

Rarity in United States

Treatment. Treatment of diphtheria is directed at neutralization of the toxin with concurrent elimination of the organism. The former is accomplished by administering a diphtheria antitoxin produced in horses. This must be done as soon as possible because, whereas antitoxin neutralizes free toxin and that being produced, it has no effect on toxin already fixed to cells. Hypersensitivity and serum sickness reactions frequently can complicate this mode of therapy. *Corynebacterium diphtheriae* is susceptible to a variety of antimicrobics, including penicillins, cephalosporins, erythromycin, and tetracycline. Of these, erythromycin has been most effective in eliminating the carrier state, but plasmid-determined erythromycin resistance has been associated with small outbreaks of the disease. The complications of diphtheria are managed primarily by supportive measures such as tracheostomy, cardiac monitoring and electric pacing, and drugs such as digitalis and antiarrhythmic agents.

Antitoxin therapy

Adjunctive antimicrobic therapy

Diagnosis. The initial diagnosis of diphtheria is entirely clinical. There

Primary diagnosis is clinical

Direct smears unreliable

Culture

Virulence tests

are presently no rapid laboratory tests of sufficient value to influence the decision regarding antitoxin administration. Direct smears of infected areas of the throat are not reliable diagnostic tools. Definitive diagnosis is accomplished by isolating and identifying *C. diphtheriae* from the infected site and demonstrating its toxigenicity. Isolation is usually achieved with Tinsdale agar, which is a selective medium containing potassium tellurite. Toxigenicity (virulence) tests can be performed by injecting two guinea pigs with the organism and protecting one with diphtheria antitoxin. Death of the test animal, with autopsy findings characteristic of the effects of diphtheria toxin, establishes the toxigenicity of the strain. Tissue culture and immunodiffusion methods for demonstrating toxigenicity are used in reference laboratories.

It should be acknowledged that while this diagnosis could be made and confirmed with great confidence in the past it is now more difficult because experience with the disease is rare. Most younger clinicians have never seen a case of diphtheria, and many bacteriologists have never isolated the organism. As most routine throat culture procedures will not isolate *C. diphtheriae*, the physician must advise the laboratory *in advance* of the suspicion of diphtheria. Generally, 2 days are required to exclude *C. diphtheriae* (that is, they are not isolated on Tinsdale agar); however, more time is needed to complete identification and virulence testing of a positive culture.

Toxoid immunization

Prevention. The mainstay of diphtheria prevention is immunization. Three to four doses of diphtheria toxoid produce immunity by stimulating antitoxin production. The initial series is begun in the first year of life (Chapter 12). Booster immunizations at 10-year intervals will maintain immunity. This vaccine is high effective. Fully immunized individuals may become infected with *C. diphtheriae*, because the antibodies are directed only against the toxin, but the disease is mild. Serious infection and death occur only in unimmunized or incompletely immunized individuals.

Other Corynebacteria

C. ulcerans and diphtheria toxin
Other diseases caused by corynebacteria

Corynebacteria other than *C. diphtheriae* are often called *diphtheroids*; some are commonly found in the normal flora of the skin and other body sites. The term actually encompasses several well-defined species, some of which have definite but unusual disease associations. Some species, such as *Corynebacterium ulcerans*, may carry the β-phage, produce a small amount of diphtheria toxin and cause infections with mild toxic manifestations. Different toxins with dermonecrotic and/or hemolytic action may be produced also by *C. ulcerans, Corynebacterium hemolyticum*, and some other species, and many of them cause infection in animals and are occasionally the source of human disease. Clinical syndromes in humans include pharyngitis, pneumonia, granulomatous lymphadenitis, and skin infections. Corynebacteria may also produce disease in settings similar to those of *Staphylococcus epidermidis* (Chapter 15), the most common of which is endocarditis.

Group JK strains in immunosuppressed patients

One currently unnamed corynebacterium, group JK, has been increasingly associated with nosocomial infections in immunosuppressed patients. They include bacteremia, which is often associated with intravascular devices such as catheters and prosthetic heart valves. A striking feature of the JK corynebacterium is the extent of its antimicrobic resistance, which typically includes all common agents except vancomycin.

Other diphtheroids

Diphtheroids are not usually speciated in clinical laboratories, because the vast majority of isolates represent colonization or contamination rather than disease. When circumstances suggest that a diphtheroid isolate may be significant, further identification can be accomplished with several standard bacteriologic tests.

Listeria

Gram-positive rod

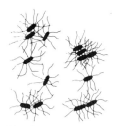

Listeria monocytogenes

Meningitis and sepsis

Intrauterine infections

Food-borne listeriosis

Treatment

Listeria monocytogenes is a Gram-positive rod with some bacteriologic features that resemble those of corynebacteria. In stained smears of clinical and laboratory material, the organisms resemble diphtheroids. In culture, a small, smooth colony surrounded by a narrow rim of β-hemolysis is produced. *Listeria* species are catalase positive, which distinguishes them from streptococci, and produce a characteristic tumbling motility in fluid media at 25°C that distinguishes them from corynebacteria.

Members of *Listeria* are widespread in nature. They can colonize or infect a wide variety of animals; human exposure usually involves transient colonization without disease. Resistance to infection involves cell-mediated as well as humoral immunity. Serious infections can occur and are seen most commonly in neonates and in immunocompromised individuals.

The most common human infections are meningitis and sepsis. Neonatal and puerperal infections, associated with vaginal colonization by *Listeria*, appear in settings similar to those of infections with group B streptococci. Intrauterine infection results in the clinical syndrome of granulomatosis infantiseptica, in which the fetus is often stillborn with disseminated abscesses and/or granulomas.

Until recently the source for most human infections could not be determined or was assumed to be related to transient colonization from an animal source. Following a 1983 report of an outbreak throughout the Maritime Provinces of Canada traced to contaminated coleslaw, it has now become clear that foodborne transmission is important in listeriosis. A widely publicized 1985 California outbreak involved Mexican-style cheeses and included 86 cases and 29 deaths. Fifty-eight of the cases were among mother–infant pairs. An interesting feature of the Canadian epidemic was the importance of bacterial growth at refrigerator temperatures, a long-known characteristic of *L. monocytogenes*. In outbreaks involving dairy products, the *L. monocytogenes* strains appeared to be relatively resistant to pasteurization. Thus, for at least some strains of *Listeria* there may be enhanced ability to survive two of the major means of preventing foodborne infection: pasteurization and refrigeration. Diagnosis of listeriosis is usually by culture of blood, cerebrospinal fluid, or focal lesions. *Listeria monocytogenes* is susceptible to penicillin G, ampicillin, erythromycin, and chloramphenicol, all of which have been used effectively.

Erysipelothrix

Environmental and zoonotic sources

Erythematous spreading lesion

Erysipelothrix rhusiopathiae is a Gram-positive rod with features similar to those of both corynebacteria and *Listeria*. This organism is widely distributed among animals and in decaying organic matter. Traumatic inoculation of *E. rhusiopathiae* into the skin produces *erysipeloid*, an occupational disease of fishermen, butchers, veterinarians, and others who handle animal products. Erysipeloid is a painful, slow-spreading, erythematous swelling of the skin. Penicillin is the treatment of choice, although the organism is also susceptible to erythromycin and tetracycline.

Lactobacillus

Acidophilic Gram-positive
non-spore forming rods

Lactobacilli are Gram-positive, non–spore-forming rods. They are typically nonmotile and nonacid fast. The cells, which are usually long and slender with squared ends, are often arranged to form chains. They are aerobic and facultatively anaerobic and grow optimally at about pH 6. Lactobacilli actively ferment carbohydrates, forming lactic acid as the primary metabolic product. Numerous species have been described, of which the most commonly occurring in humans is *Lactobacillus acidophilus*.

Member of the normal flora

Lactobacilli are important members of the normal human oral, gastrointestinal, and vaginal flora. Their reputation as beneficial members of the intestinal flora is responsible for the popularity of certain "natural" foods, such as yogurt, that contain lactobacilli and their fermentation products (Chapter 9). Lactobacilli are not pathogenic for humans or animals, although *L. acidophilus* has, from time to time been believed to play some role in the pathogenesis of dental caries.

Propionibacterium

Bacteria of the genus *Propionibacterium* resemble corynebacteria morphologically. Members are anaerobes or microaerophiles and are a major and significant part of the normal skin flora (Chapter 9). Like most normal floral organisms, propionibacteria can be an occasional cause of bacterial endocarditis or of other infections in the severely immunocompromised.

Bacillus

Group Characteristics

Gram-positive spore-forming
rods

The genus *Bacillus* includes many species of aerobic or facultative, spore-forming, Gram-positive rods. With the exception of one species, *Bacillus anthracis*, they are low-virulence saprophytes widespread in air, soil, water, dust, and animal products. *Bacillus anthracis* causes the zoonosis *anthrax*, a disease of animals that is occasionally transmitted to humans.

Morphology and Staining. The genus comprises rod-shaped organisms approximately 0.7 μm wide and 3–10 μm long. The rods can thus vary from coccobacillary to rather long filaments, and they may be arranged in chains. The ends may be rounded or sharply truncated. Motile strains have peritrichous flagella. Formation of round or oval spores, which may be central, subterminal, or terminal depending on the species, is characteristic of the genus. Spores may be larger than the diameter of the bacillus, but usually are not. *Bacillus* species are Gram positive; however, positivity is

Loss of Gram positivity

often lost, depending on the species and the age of the culture. With some strains only very young (3–6 hr) cultures stain as Gram positive.

Growth and Resistance. Growth is obtained with ordinary media incubated in air and is reduced or absent under anaerobic conditions. Aerobic

Aerobic growth

conditions are required for sporulation. The frequent development of a surface pellicle in broth cultures also reflects the aerobic preference. Colonies vary from 1 to 5 mm in diameter, and morphology ranges from mucoid to dry and pigmented. Some strains are β-hemolytic. The spores

Heat resistance of spores

survive boiling for varying periods and are sufficiently resistant to heat that those of one species are used as a biologic indicator of autoclave efficiency. Spores of *Bacillus anthracis* survive in soil for decades. A small

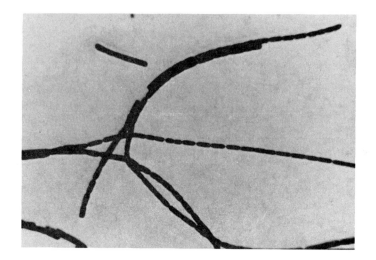

17.2 *Bacillus anthracis*. Large Gram-positive bacilli in chains are typical of this species. Other *Bacillus* species vary greatly in shape.

island contaminated during bacteriological warfare studies in the 1940s is still considered uninhabitable.

Metabolism. Most species are metabolically active, producing acid but not gas from oxidation of glucose and various other sugars. They are catalase positive and produce proteolytic enzymes such as gelatinase. Many other biochemical reactions are variable among species and thus taxonomically useful.

Antigenic Structure. Multiple antigenic types have been described, primarily using agglutination reactions with antibody to cell wall or spore antigens. These procedures, however, are not used in routine diagnostic work.

Bacillus Anthracis, Anthrax and Other Bacillus Infections

The isolation of *B. anthracis*, the proof of its relationship to anthrax infection, and the demonstration of immunity to the disease are among the most important events in the history of science and medicine. Robert Koch rose to fame in 1877 by growing the organism in artificial culture using pure culture techniques. He defined the stringent criteria needed to prove that the organism caused anthrax (Koch's postulates), then met them experimentally. Louis Pasteur made a convincing field demonstration at Pouilly-le-Fort to show that vaccination of sheep, goats, and cows with an attenuated strain of *B. anthracis* prevented anthrax. He was cheered and carried on the shoulders of the grateful farmers of the district, an experience now, unhappily, largely restricted to successful football coaches.

Experiments of Koch and Pasteur on anthrax

Morphological and cultural characteristics

Bacillus anthracis. In the clinical laboratory, *B. anthracis* is recognized by its tendency to form very long chains of rods with elliptic central spores. This appearance has sometimes been likened to that of bamboo rods (Figure 17.2). In infected tissues, chains are shorter and capsules are prominent, but spores do not develop. Colonies, which consist of parallel interlacing chains of bacilli, are characterized by a rough uneven surface with multiple curled extensions at the edge resembling a "Medusa head." *Bacillus anthracis* is nonmotile and nonhemolytic; these characteristics

Medusa head colonies

Table 17.1 Some Characteristics of *Bacillus* Species

| Organism | Bacteriologic Features | | Toxin Production | Distribution | Human Disease |
	Capsule	Motility			
B. anthracis	+	−	Exotoxin (EF, PA, LF)	Animals and contaminated soil where disease is enzootic	Anthrax
B. cereus	−	+	Enterotoxin; pyogenic toxin	Ubiquitous	Food poisoning; opportunistic infections (rare)
Other species	−	+	—	Ubiquitous	Opportunistic infections (rare)

Abbreviations: EF = edema factor; PA = protective antigen; LF = lethal factor.

combined with other important bacteriologic features, help to differentiate the organism from other *Bacillus* species (Table 17.1).

The anthrax bacillus differs from other *Bacillus* species in several important features. Of prime importance for virulence are its capsule and production of exotoxin. The capsule is a D-glutamic acid polypeptide of a single antigenic specificity. It has antiphagocytic properties and is required for full virulence. The exotoxin(s) produces extensive edema and death in a variety of animals. This activity has been separated into at least three components: edema factor, protective antigen, and lethal factor. These factors are proteins or protein-carbohydrate complexes; their ability to produce pathologic lesions experimentally and stimulate immunity varies with the relative proportions of each. It now appears the edema factor has adenylate cyclase activity in the presence of calmodulin, a regulatory protein found in mammalian cells. This is similar to the adenylate cyclase activity of *Bordetella pertussis* (Chapter 23). Strains repeatedly subcultured at 42°C become avirulent. This characteristic was the basis of Pasteur's attenuated vaccine and has been shown to be due to loss of a plasmid required for toxin production. Capsule production is also plasmid determined but this plasmid is present in avirulent as well as virulent strains.

The specific mechanisms of immunity against *B. anthracis* are not known. Experimental evidence favors antibody directed against the toxin complex, but the relative role of the three toxin components is not clear. The capsular glutamic acid is not immunogenic.

Anthrax. Anthrax is usually acquired through unrecognized breaks in skin or mucous membranes to which spores of *B. anthracis* gain access. The spores germinate to yield vegetative cells, which multiply and produce either localized or systemic infection depending on the animal species infected and the site inoculated. Herbivores such as horses, sheep, and cattle are most commonly affected and develop fatal septicemic disease. The disease is spread by spores in pastures contaminated with exudates of live or dead infected animals. Humans are usually infected by contact with infected animals or animal products. Because of the long survival of the spores, infection may result from contaminated hides, wool, bone, and

Marginal notes:

Antiphagocytic effect of D-glutamic acid capsule

Exotoxins

Attenuation of virulence with loss of plasmid

Infection through small epithelial lesions

Spread of disease in herbivores and occasionally to humans

even imported processed items such as fertilizer containing bone meal. The disease is now rare in developed countries, although animal anthrax persists in the southern United States. The incidence in humans in the United States has decreased from more than 100 cases annually in the 1920s to only a few reported cases each year. This dramatic reduction is associated with the control of animal anthrax through quarantine, sacrifice of infected herds, and immunization and with improved industrial hygiene. In the past, farmers, veterinarians, and meat handlers were infected most frequently; now, however, the rare case in the United States is usually related to contaminated imported materials.

Control of animal anthrax

Cutaneous anthrax usually begins 2–5 days after inoculation of spores in an exposed part of the body, typically the forearm or hand. Scalp lesions have been associated with headgear contaminated with spores. The initial lesion is an erythematous papule, which may be mistaken for an insect bite. This papule usually progresses through vesicular and ulcerative stages over 7–10 days to form a black eschar (scab) surrounded by edema. This complex is known as the *malignant pustule,* although it is neither malignant nor a pustule. Associated systemic symptoms are usually mild, and the lesion typically heals after the eschar separates. Less commonly, the disease progresses with massive local edema, toxemia and bacteremia, and a fatal outcome if untreated.

"Malignant pustule"

Pulmonary anthrax, contracted by inhalation of spores, can develop when contaminated hides, hair, wool, and the like are handled in a confined space. The infection was thus termed *woolsorter's disease*, as it was quite common among these workers at the turn of the century. Pulmonary anthrax has also developed following laboratory accidents. More ominously, it has been considered as a means of biologic warfare, which is now outlawed by international treaty. After 1–5 days of nonspecific malaise, mild fever, and nonproductive cough, progressive respiratory distress and cyanosis ensue with massive edema of the neck, chest, and mediastinum. If untreated, progression to a fatal outcome is usually very rapid once edema has developed. Enormous numbers of organisms are found in the lungs, blood, and all organs. A gastrointestinal form of anthrax results from ingestion of raw or inadequately cooked meat containing *B. anthracis* spores. Infections at other sites, such as the meninges, may follow bacteremia in the course of cutaneous or pulmonary anthrax.

Woolsorters disease

Rapid fatal pneumonia

The anthrax bacillus is sensitive to penicillin, and penicillin therapy is indicated as soon as possible in the disease.

Penicillin therapy

Other Bacillus Infections. As spores are widespread in the environment, isolation of one of the more than 20 *Bacillus* species other than *B. anthracis* from clinical material usually represents contamination of the specimen. Occasionally *Bacillus cereus, Bacillus subtilis*, and some other species produce genuine infections, including infections of the eye, soft tissues, and lung. Bacteremia and endocarditis may also result. Infection is usually associated with immunosuppression, trauma, an indwelling catheter, or contamination of complex equipment such as an artificial kidney. The relative resistance of *Bacillus* spores to disinfectants aids their survival in medical devices that cannot be heat sterilized.

Bacillus infections in immunocompromised hosts

Bacillus cereus deserves special mention. It is the species most likely to cause opportunistic infection, which suggests a virulence intermediate between that of *B. anthracis* and the other species. A strain isolated from an abscess has been shown to produce a destructive pyogenic toxin. *Bacillus cereus* can also cause food poisoning by means of enterotoxins. One enterotoxin acts by stimulating adenyl cyclase production and fluid ex-

Food poisoning from *B. cereus*

cretion in the same manner as toxigenic *E. coli* and *Vibrio cholerae* (Chapters 20 and 21). One interesting strain has been shown to cause vomiting rather than diarrhea, but only with cultures grown on rice. It was isolated in association with an outbreak of nausea and vomiting that occurred 1–5 hr after consumption of cooked rice in a Chinese restaurant.

Diagnosis.   Diagnosis of *Bacillus* infections follows the principles outlined in Chapter 14. The organisms are readily grown on a variety of media. *Bacillus anthracis* may be distinguished from other species by the characteristics listed in Table 17.1, by its virulence to experimental animals, and by other biochemical and cultural features. The appropriate tests may not be performed unless the suspicion of anthrax is communicated to the clinical laboratory. Isolates of other *Bacillus* species are usually contaminants; the rare situation in which they play a pathogenic role is suggested by multiple isolations, large numbers of organisms in fresh specimens, and the special circumstances of the case. Again, to ensure retention of the strain for further study, the laboratory must be advised that infection is suspected.

Susceptibility of *B. anthracis* to penicillin

Treatment.   As *B. anthracis* is susceptible to penicillin, anthrax is treated with this agent. Antimicrobial therapy for other species must be guided by in vitro testing, because susceptibilities to penicillins, cephalosporins, aminoglycosides, tetracycline, and chloramphenicol are not predictable. Other modes of management of opportunistic *Bacillus* infections, such as removal of indwelling catheters, may be equally important.

Additional Reading

Collier, R.J. 1975. Diphtheria toxin: Mode of action and structure. *Bacteriol. Rev.* 39:54–85. All aspects of diphtheria toxin are reviewed in detail, including the experimental evidence supporting current concepts of its biologic activity.

Koopman, J.S. and Campbell, J. 1975. The role of cutaneous diphtheria infections in a diphtheria epidemic. *J. Infect. Dis.* 131:239–244. This study shows that cutaneous diphtheria may be more contagious than respiratory infection.

McCloskey, R.V., Eller, J.J., Green, M., Mauney, C.U., and Richards, S.E.M. 1971. The 1970 epidemic of diphtheria in San Antonio. *Ann. Intern. Med.* 75:495–503. A clear and informative description of a modern diphtheria outbreak is provided. The clinical features are given in detail, including color photographs of diphtheritic membranes.

Melling, J., Capel, B.J., Turnbull, P.C.B., and Gilbert, R.J. 1976. Identification of a novel enterotoxigenic activity associated with *Baccillus cereus*. *J. Clin. Pathol.* 29:938–940.

Mikesell, P., Ivins, B.E., Ristroph, J.D., and Dreier, T.M. 1983. Evidence for plasmid-mediated toxin production in *Bacillus anthracis*. *Infect. Immun.* 39:371–376. These investigators repeated Louis Pasteur's attenuation experiments but with molecular studies to explain why his strains lost virulence.

Schlech, W.F., Lavigne, P.M., Bortolussi, R.A., Allen, A.C., et al. 1983. Epidemic listerosis-evidence for transmission by food. *N. Engl. J. Med.* 308:203–206. This epidemiological study nicely traces events beginning on a Halifax farm to 34 cases of listerosis.

Turnbull, P.C.B. 1976. Studies on the production of enterotoxins by *Bacillus cereus*. *J. Clin. Pathol.* 29:941–948. This report suggests possible virulence mechanisms for intestinal and extraintestinal infections caused by *Bacillus cereus*.

18

Clostridia, Gram-Negative Anaerobes, and Anaerobic Cocci

John C. Sherris and
James J. Plorde

Energy generated by
fermentation

Anaerobes inhibited or killed
by oxygen

Explanations for anaerobiosis

Many anaerobes are members
of the normal flora

The bacteria discussed in this chapter are known as *obligate anaerobes*, or simply *anaerobes*. They generate energy solely by fermentation (see Chapter 3) and not only lack the capacity to utilize oxygen as an electron acceptor, but are damaged by it to varying degrees. Some are sensitive to oxygen concentrations as low as 0.5% and are killed by even brief exposures to air. Most can survive in 3 to 5% oxygen. A few actually grow, although poorly, in the presence of air and are often referred to as *aerotolerant anaerobes*.

Several explanations have been proposed for obligate anaerobiosis and oxygen toxicity. Anaerobes lack the cytochromes required to use oxygen as a terminal hydrogen acceptor in energy-yielding reactions. Most, but not all, lack catalase and peroxidase enzymes, but possess flavoproteins; thus, in the presence of oxygen they may produce hydrogen peroxide, which is toxic to many of them. Some anaerobes, which lack or only produce low concentrations of the enzyme superoxide dismutase, may be inhibited or killed by other peroxides and toxic oxygen radicals. Certain critical enzymes (for example, fumarate reductase) of some anaerobes must be in the reduced state to be active; thus, aerobic conditions create a metabolic block. It therefore seems probable that no single characteristic is responsible for obligate anaerobic requirements or oxygen toxicity; some of those indicated previously, rather than being its cause, may have been selected *because* of the anaerobic nature of the organism.

Despite our constant immersion in air, anaerobes are able to colonize the many oxygen-deficient or oxygen-free microenvironments of the body. Often these are created by the presence of facultative organisms whose growth reduces oxygen and decreases the local oxidation–reduction potential. Such sites include the sebaceous glands of the skin, the gingival crevices of the gums, the lymphoid tissue of the throat, and the lumina of the intestinal and urogenital tracts (Table 18.1). The anaerobic flora of these sites normally live in a harmless commensal relationships with the

Table 18.1   Usual Locations of Opportunistic Anaerobes in the Human Body

Organism	Mouth or Pharynx	Intestine	Urogenital Tract	Skin
Bacteroides				
fragilis group		+		
melanogenicus	+	+	+	
Clostridia		+		
Fusobacterium	+	+		
Peptostreptococci	+	+	+	
Propionibacterium				+

Infections can result when anaerobes are introduced into damaged or devitalized tissues

Infections are often polymicrobial

host. However, they may cause life-threatening infections when introduced into tissues devitalized by trauma, malignancy, inflammation, or impaired blood supply.

Anaerobic infections are frequently polymicrobic, containing a number of different anaerobic and facultative species. Exquisitely oxygen-sensitive anaerobes are seldom involved, probably because they are inactivated by even the small amounts of oxygen dissolved in tissue fluids. Except for infections with some environmental clostridia, the organisms are almost always derived from the patient's normal flora. Case-to-case transfer is very rare except with some hospital-acquired *Clostridium difficile* infections.

The major groups of clinically significant anaerobes are as follows:

Gram-positive spore formers

Clostridia.   The clostridia are Gram-positive, spore-forming motile or non-motile bacilli. Some species are potentially highly pathogenic to humans or animals and produce potent exotoxins associated wtih particular disease syndromes. Others are nonpathogenic. Clostridia are found in soil (particularly soil fertilized with animal excreta) and in the lower intestinal tract of humans and animals. They are generally highly susceptible to penicillin.

Gram-negative rods

Bacteroides.   Members of the genus *Bacteroides* are Gram-negative, non–spore-forming rods. Some are markedly pleomorphic, but others are quite uniform. They are distinguished from *Fusobacterium* by the organic acids that constitute their metabolic end products. *Bacteroides* species occur among the normal flora of the oral cavity and colon in humans and animals.

Fusiform Gram-negative rods

Fusobacteria.   Fusobacteria are also Gram-negative, non–spore-forming rods. Their morphology is fusiform with pointed ends, and they are distinguished from *Bacteroides* by metabolic end-product analysis. Their habitat is the same as that of *Bacteroides*.

Gram-positive cocci

Peptostreptococci.   Peptostreptococci, commonly, but erroneously, known as *anaerobic streptococci*, are Gram-positive, nonmotile organisms that generally occur in chains. They are part of the normal flora of the upper alimentary and respiratory tracts and lower intestinal tract in humans and animals. Anaerobic Gram-positive cocci forming clusters rather than chains were previously referred to as peptococci. Recent studies of their DNA content has revealed a close taxonomic relationship to peptostreptococci, and they have now been reassigned to that genus. They rarely play a pathogenic role.

Some other genera and species of anaerobic organisms (for example, *Actinomyces israelii*) are considered elsewhere in this text. Many others are not included in this chapter because they rarely cause disease, and because those discussed herein serve as satisfactory models for both specific and mixed anaerobic infections.

Clostridia

Many clostridia are of great significance as causes of disease in livestock and wildlife; however, these organisms are beyond the scope of this text. Discussion is limited to those that cause disease in humans, which may be categorized as follows:

Medically important species

1. The gas gangrene group, of which the most important is *Clostridium perfringens*. In addition to its role in gas gangrene, *C. perfringens* can cause anaerobic cellulitis, anaerobic puerperal sepsis, and a form of food poisoning.

2. *Clostridium tetani*, the cause of tetanus.

3. *Clostridium botulinum*, the cause of botulism.

4. *Clostridium difficile*, cause of toxic enterocolitis.

Clostridium perfringens

Subtypes are based on toxin production

Importance of type A

Clostridium perfringens produces a remarkable number of exotoxins and extracellular enzymes with specific biologic activity. The species has been subdivided on the basis of these products into seven types (A–G), which have different pathogenic significance in different animal species. Type A is by far the most important in humans and is found consistently in the colon and often in soil.

Clostridium perfringens

Morphologic, Cultural, and Metabolic Characteristics. *Clostridium perfringens* is a large, Gram-positive, nonmotile encapsulated rod with squarish ends. Spores are rarely seen in culture or during infection, but develop in the natural habitat. The organism grows very rapidly overnight on blood agar medium or in broth under anaerobic conditions. Its mean generation time can be as short as 7 min. Incubation overnight on sheep or horse blood agar (usually used in diagnostic laboratories) produces round, smooth colonies about 2–3 mm in diameter; they are surrounded by a zone of complete hemolysis caused by θ-toxin and a wider zone of in-complete hemolysis caused by α-toxin (Figure 18.1). If the plate is re-frigerated and rewarmed, the outer zone of hemolysis becomes complete. In broth containing fermentable carbohydrate, growth of *C. perfringens* is accompanied by the production of large amounts of hydrogen and carbon dioxide, which can result in markedly increased pressure in a sealed con-tainer. Much gas is also produced in vivo in necrotic tissues, hence the term *gas gangrene*.

Hemolytic activity of α- and θ-toxins

Much gas produced from carbohydrates

Resistance. Spores of *C. perfringens* are resistant to all disinfectants and to boiling for brief periods. The spores of some strains that cause food poisoning are often more heat resistant: they can withstand temperatures of 100°C for an hour or more, which accounts for their survival in cooked food. The vegetative cells are readily killed by disinfectants. They are susceptible to penicillin and many other antimicrobics, except the ami-noglycosides.

Heat-resistant spores of food poisoning strains

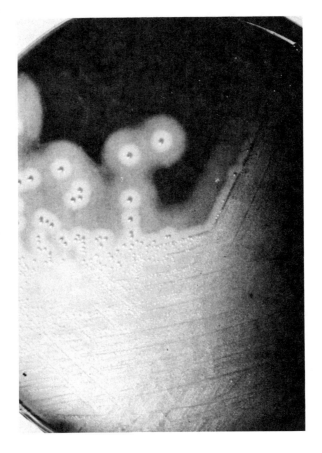

18.1 *C. perfringens* colonies on a blood agar plate showing double zone of hemolysis.

Toxins and Biologically Active Extracellular Enzymes. Clostridium perfringens can produce several exotoxins and biologically active extracellular proteins that may contribute to virulence. The most important is the α-toxin, a phospholipase *C* that hydrolyzes lecithin and sphingomyelin and, thus, disrupts the cell membranes of various host cells, including erythrocytes, leukocytes, and muscle cells. α-Toxin production can be detected in vitro on a lecithin-containing agar mediuum because breakdown products of lecithin (phosphoryl choline and diglycerides) precipitate in the immediate vicinity of a streak of growth of *C. perfringens*. The reaction can be neutralized by anti-α toxin antibody (antitoxin), which provides a useful test for identifying the organism (Figure 18.2). The median lethal dose (LD_{50}) of the toxin for experimental animals is approximately 5 μg/kg.

Lecithinase and cytotoxic activity of α-toxin

θ-Toxin is an oxygen-labile hemolysin that also alters capillary permeability and is toxic for heart muscle. It is closely related to streptolysin O (Chapter 16) and is responsible for the complete β-hemolysis seen after overnight incubation on blood agar plates.

θ-toxin alters capillary permeability; related to streptolysin O

An enterotoxin produced by some strains of *C. perfringens* type A is responsible for a common and benign form of bacterial food poisoning. This low-molecular-weight protein is a component of the bacterial spore and is released into the upper gastrointestinal tract when ingested vegetative forms undergo sporulation. It causes diarrhea by reversing the flow

Enterotoxin of C. perfringens type A is liberated during sporulation

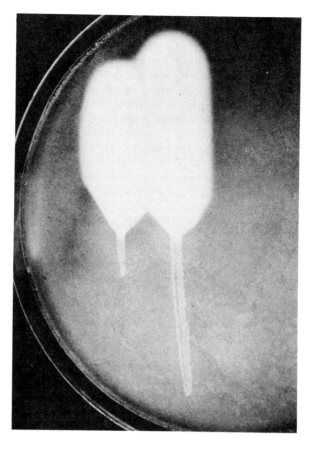

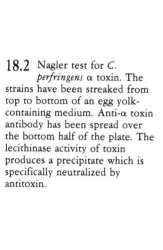

18.2 Nagler test for *C. perfringens* α toxin. The strains have been streaked from top to bottom of an egg yolk-containing medium. Anti-α toxin antibody has been spread over the bottom half of the plate. The lecithinase activity of toxin produces a precipitate which is specifically neutralized by antitoxin.

of water and electrolytes in the small intestine. The precise mechanism by which it brings this about has not yet been defined.

Another enterotoxin, β-toxin, is produced by some strains of *C. perfringens* type C as they proliferate in the small bowel, resulting in a rare but severe necrotizing enteritis (enteritis necroticans). The toxin appears to induce intestinal paralysis, inflammation, and gangrenous necrosis.

β-toxin of type C can cause necrotizing enteritis

Other biologically active extracellular products include a collagenase, a deoxyribonuclease, a hyaluronidase, and proteases. All may contribute to invasive pathologic processes, but none shares the central role of the α-toxin.

Diseases Caused by Clostridium perfringens

Open wounds with muscle damage predispose to gas gangrene

Other clostridia may cause the disease

Postsurgical gas gangrene

Gas Gangrene.   Gas gangrene can develop in severe traumatic open lesions, such as compound fractures or bullet wounds, when there is muscle damage, contamination with dirt, clothing, or other foreign material, and if *C. perfringens* or, less commonly, one of the other gas-gangrene–causing clostridia (for example, *Clostridium novyi* or *Clostridium septicum*) is introduced. The disease is most often seen in war wounds, but occasionally follows severe trauma in civilian life. It can develop within a few hours of wounding. As *C. perfringens* is sometimes present in bile in cholecystitis, gas gangrene of the abdominal muscles is an occasional complication of gallbladder or bile duct surgery, particularly when bile is spilled.

Conditions for multiplication

α-toxin production kills cells locally

Muscle necrosis and gas production

θ-toxin and oxygen deprivation contribute to shock

Major role of α-toxin in initiating disease

Central role of early surgical debridement in prevention

Aggressive surgery with chemotheraphy and hyperbaric oxygen

Septicemia and intravascular hemolysis; central role of α-toxin

If the oxidation-reduction potential in a wound is sufficiently low, *C. perfringens* spores can germinate and the organism can multiply very rapidly. Infections are always mixed; the presence of numerous facultative species contributes to the reducing conditions. *Clostridium perfringens* elaborates its α-toxin, which passes along the muscle bundles killing all cells, including inflammatory cells, and producing additional necrotic areas into which the organism can grow. Fermentation of muscle carbohydrate by *C. perfringens* produces gas in the subcutaneous tissues that can be felt when palpated (crepitation) and seen on radiography. As the disease progresses, increased vascular permeability and shock cause severe systemic disease. θ-Toxin and oxygen deprivation due to the metabolic activities of *C. perfringens* are probable contributors. Ultimately, *C. perfringens* bacteremia develops. Untreated gas gangrene is always fatal.

The critical role of anaerobiosis and of α-toxin production in the development of the infection has been clearly demonstrated in animal experiments. *Clostridium perfringens* cells washed free of toxin and inoculated intramuscularly into guinea pigs cause no lesion. When substances causing muscle necrosis or actively metabolizing aerobic organisms are introduced, however, gas gangrene develops. Active immunization with α-toxin or passive immunization with anti-α-toxin antibody will prevent the disease.

Rapid and adequate surgical debridement with removal of dead tissue is the most important preventive measure. It is supplemented if possible with high doses of penicillin as soon after wounding as possible in an attempt to inhibit accessible clostridia and delay infection with other organisms that may promote clostridial disease. Antimicrobic prophylaxis cannot replace surgical debridement, and the disease may develop in cases receiving such treatment because the antimicrobics fail to reach the organism in devascularized tissues.

Treatment must be initiated immediately. Excision of all devitalized tissue and massive doses of penicillin are most important. Recent studies have indicated that other antimicrobics may be equally or more effective. Frequently, amputation of a limb is required to prevent further spread of the infection. Placing the patient in a hyperbaric oxygen chamber increases the tissue level of dissolved oxygen and has been shown to slow the spread of disease, probably by inhibiting bacterial growth and toxin production and by neutralizing the activity of θ-toxin. This measure also appears to reduce the "toxicity" of the patient. In the past, gas gangrene polyvalent antitoxin was administered intravenously in large amounts to neutralize free toxin. It may help prevent hemolysis, but is of doubtful benefit in halting the gangrene.

Anaerobic cellulitis. Anaerobic cellulitis is a clostridial infection of wounds and surrounding subcutaneous tissue in which there is marked gas formation (more than that in gas gangrene), but in which the pain, swelling, and toxicity of gas gangrene are absent. It is much less serious than gas gangrene and can be controlled with less rigorous methods.

Clostridial Endometritis. If *C. perfringens* gains access to necrotic products of conception retained in the uterus, it may multiply and infect the endometrium (Figure 18.3). Necrosis of uterine tissue and septicemia with massive intravascular hemolysis due to α-toxin may then follow. Clostridial uterine infection was seen more commonly in the past, usually after an incomplete illegal abortion with inadequately sterilized instruments. The disease is extremely serious and may require emergency hysterectomy and hemodialysis for renal shutdown resulting from hemoglobinemia.

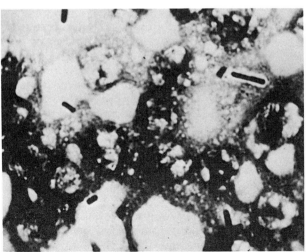

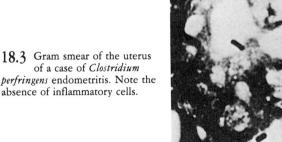

18.3 Gram smear of the uterus of a case of *Clostridium perfringens* endometritis. Note the absence of inflammatory cells.

Clostridial Food Poisoning.   *Clostridium perfringens* can cause food poisoning if large numbers of an enterotoxin-producing strain are ingested.

Incubation 8–24 hr; diarrhea without fever

The incubation period of 8–24 hr is followed by nausea, abdominal pain, and diarrhea. There is no fever, and vomiting is rare. Recovery is usual within 24 hr. The disease is caused by the enterotoxin, which is liberated from the organism during sporulation in the small intestine. Outbreaks of the disease usually involve meat dishes such as stews, soups, or gravy.

C. perfringens grows rapidly in meat dishes at warm temperatures

Heat-resistant spores of *C. perfringens* may survive the initial cooking and the organism multiplies rapidly if cooling and storage at room temperature are prolonged or if the food is rewarmed. Prevention involves good cooking hygiene and adequate refrigeration. There is growing evidence that enterotoxin-producing strains of *C. perfringens* may also be responsible for some cases of antimicrobic-induced diarrhea.

Enteritis necroticans is a more serious form of food poisoning now seen most often in poor countries and particularly in malnourished children following the ingestion of large quantities of pork or other meats at feasts.

Association with malnutrition and pork or other meat products

It is caused by the formation of β-toxin by strains of *C. perfringens* type C that have multiplied in the food. It has been hypothesized that decreased production of pancreatic trypsin in the malnourished, combined with the concomitant ingestion of food rich in trypsin inhibitors, such as sweet potatoes, interferes with trypsin-mediated destruction of the β-toxin. The

High mortality

toxin produces segmental intestinal paralysis, inflammation, hemorrhage, and necrosis. The patient experiences a sudden onset of abdominal cramps, bloody diarrhea, and shock. The mortality rate is high.

Diagnosis of Serious C. perfringens Infections

Diagnosis is primarily clinical

Diagnosis is based ultimately on clinical observations. Bacteriologic studies are adjunctive. It is quite common, for example, to isolate *C. perfringens* from contaminated wounds without evidence of clostridial disease. The organism can also be isolated from the postpartum uterine cervix of healthy women or from those with only mild fever. Occasionally, *C. perfringens* is even isolated from blood cultures of patients who do not develop serious clostridial infection.

Gram smears from cases of gas gangrene show many clostridia and other organisms (for example, Enterobacteriacie) that multiply in the necrotic tissue. Pieces of necrotic muscle may be seen, and the absence of inflammatory cells is noteworthy. The appearance of smears from the endometrium in clostridial endometritis or of aspirates from skin blebs surrounding gas gangrene lesions is similar, although in these cases *C. perfringens* is usually the only organism present.

Absence of inflammatory cells in gas gangrene and clostridial endometritis

In clostridial food poisoning, isolation of more than 10^5 *C. perfringens* per gram of the ingested food in the absence of any other cause is usually sufficient to confirm the etiology of a characteristic food poisoning outbreak.

Clostridium tetani

Clostridium tetani spores exist in many soils, especially if they are manured, and the organism is sometimes found in the lower intestinal tract of humans and animals.

Primary reservoir in soil

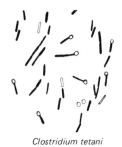

Clostridium tetani

Swarming growth on agar

Morphology.   *Clostridium tetani* is a slim, Gram-positive rod; it may be predominantly Gram negative in very young or old cultures. It forms spores readily in nature and in culture, yielding a typical round terminal spore that gives the organism a drumstick appearance before the residual vegetative cell disintegrates. The organism is flagellate and motile.

Cultural Characteristics.   *Clostridium tetani* requires strict anaerobic conditions. Because of its motility, it spreads over the surface of anaerobic blood agar plates in a thin veil of growth. Its identity is suggested by cultural and biochemical characteristics, but definite identification depends on demonstrating its neurotoxic exotoxin.

Spores are highly resistant

Resistance.   *Clostridium tetani* spores remain viable in soil or culture for many years. They are resistant to most disinfectants and withstand boiling for several minutes. They are killed by autoclaving at 121°C for 15 min.

Tetanospasmin exotoxin

Toxin is convertible to toxoid

Toxin Production.   The most important product of *C. tetani* is its neurotoxic exotoxin, tetanospasmin, which is found extracellularly. It is a heat-labile antigenic protein readily neutralized by antitoxin and rapidly destroyed at 65°C and by intestinal proteases. Treatment with formaldehyde yields a nontoxic product, toxoid, that retains the antigenicity of toxin and thus stimulates production of antitoxin. The LD_{50} of the toxin for mice is on the order of 10^{-4} µg; less than 1 µg would probably be lethal to humans.

Tetanus

Predisposing Conditions.   Spores of *C. tetani* may be introduced into wounds with contaminated soil or foreign bodies. The predisposing wounds are often quite small, for example, a puncture wound containing a splinter. In contrast to those in gas gangrene, infected wounds often do not extend below the subcutaneous tissues. Occasionally, the disease may follow severe burns; it has also occurred as a complication of chronic otitis media, probably when the organism gains access to the middle ear through a perforated eardrum. In many less developed countries, the majority of tetanus cases occur in recently delivered babies and their mothers. The uterus of the new mother may be infected by inexpert removal of the

May result from small contaminated wounds or splinters

placenta. The neonate suffers infection when the umbilical cord is severed or bandaged in an uncleanly manner. Similarly, tetanus may follow an unskilled abortion, scarification rituals, female circumcision, and even surgery performed with unsterile instruments or dressings.

The usual predisposing factor for tetanus is an area of very low oxidation-reduction potential in which tetanus spores can germinate. This can be provided by a large splinter, an area of necrosis from introduction of soil, or necrosis after injection of contaminated illicit drugs. Infection with facultative or other anaerobic organisms can contribute to the development of an appropriate anaerobic nidus for spore germination.

Pathogenesis.   Tetanus bacilli multiply locally and neither damage nor invade adjacent tissues. Tetanospasmin is elaborated at the site of infection and reaches the central nervous system mainly by ascending the motor nerves. In the spinal cord, it acts at the level of the anterior horn cells by blocking postsynaptic inhibition of spinal motor reflexes. Thus, an afferent stimulus produces spasmodic contractions of both protagonist and antagonist muscles, initially in the area of the causative lesion. In the more serious forms of the disease toxin extends up and down the spinal cord, and generalized spasms can result from minor stimuli, such as a sound or a draft.

Clinical Presentation.   The incubation period of the disease is from 4 days to several weeks. The shorter incubation period is usually associated with wounds in areas supplied by the cranial motor nerves, probably because of a shorter transmission route for the toxin to the central nervous system. In general, shorter incubation periods are associated with more severe disease.

Although tetanus may be localized to muscles innervated by nerves in the region of the infection, it is usually more generalized. The masseter muscles are often the first to be affected, resulting in inability to open the mouth properly (trismus); this effect accounts for the use of the term *lockjaw* to describe the disease. As other muscles become affected, intermittent spasms can become generalized to include muscles of respiration and swallowing. In extreme cases, generalized convulsions produce opisthotonus, caused by massive contractions of the back muscles. Risus sardonicus (sardonic smile) is a late sign in which trismus combined with facial spasm leads to separation of the lips over clenched teeth. The untreated patient with tetanus retains consciousness and is aware of his plight, in which small stimuli can trigger massive contractions. In fatal cases, death results from exhaustion and respiratory failure. All of these results are attributable to very small amounts of tetanospasmin produced at the site of what is often a small, sometimes unrecognized local lesion. The amount of toxin is so small that unimmunized patients often do not have an antibody response. Untreated, the mortality caused by the generalized disease varies from 15 to more than 60%, according to the lesion, incubation period, and age of the patient. Mortality is highest in the neonate and in the elderly.

Treatment.   Specific treatment of the disease involves neutralization of any unbound toxin with large doses of human tetanus immune globulin (TIG), which is derived from the blood of volunteers hyperimmunized with toxoid. In countries where TIG is unavailable, horse antitoxin is still used. Most important in treatment are nonspecific supportive measures, including maintenance of a quiet dark environment, sedation, and pro-

---

Neonatal and postpartum tetanus in developing countries

Low Eh in wound allows spores to germinate

Local multiplication only

Toxin ascends motor nerves to anterior horn cells

Variable incubation period

Masseter muscles often involved first

Severe tetanus with generalized muscle spasms

Spasms triggered by minor stimuli

Mortality

Antitoxin given to neutralize unbound toxin

Supportive measures and curarelike drugs

vision of an adequate airway. In severe cases, curarelike drugs are used to block nerve impulses at the neuromuscular junctions. These patients require artificial ventilation to maintain oxygenation because of respiratory paralysis. Such measures have resulted in a substantially reduced mortality.

Active immunization with tetanus toxoid

Prevention. Routine active immunization with tetanus toxoid, combined with diphtheria toxoid and pertussis vaccine (DPT) for primary immunization in childhood, can completely prevent the disease. It has reduced the incidence of tetanus in the United States to less than 50 reported cases per year. Five doses of DPT are now recommended, to be given at the ages of 2, 4, 6, and 18 months, and once again between the ages of 4 and 6 years. Thereafter a booster of adult-type tetanus diphtheria toxoid should be given every 10 years (see Chapter 12). Unfortunately, routine childhood immunization is not administratively and economically feasible in many less well-developed countries, where as many as a million cases of tetanus occur annually. In such settings, immunization efforts have been focused on the pregnant woman, because transplacental transfer of antibodies to the fetus also prevents the highly lethal neonatal tetanus.

Active immunization of a pregnant woman protects the infant

Passive immunization for potentially exposed unimmunized subjects

Prophylactic booster doses for immunized subjects

Unimmunized subjects with tetanus-prone wounds should be given passive immunity with a prophylactic dose of TIG as soon as possible. This immunization provides immediate protection. Those who have had a full primary series of immunizations, and appropriate boosters, are given toxoid for tetanus-prone wounds if they have not been immunized within the previous 10 years in the case of clean minor wounds or 5 years for more contaminated wounds. If immunization is incomplete or the wound has been neglected and poses a serious risk of disease, TIG is also given.

Penicillin therapy is a prophylactic adjunct in serious or neglected wounds, but in no way alters the need for specific prophylaxis. All those who have not been actively immunized should be given a first dose of toxoid as soon as possible and followed up for a complete immunization series. If toxoid and TIG are given in opposite arms with different syringes there is no significant interference between them. Recommended immunization schedules change from time to time, and those responsible for their administration should be familiar with current recommendations.

Clostridium botulinum

Environmental natural habitat

Spores of *C. botulinum* are found in soil, pond, and lake sediments in many parts of the world, including the United States. The major characteristic of medical importance is that strains of *C. botulinum* elaborate one of seven antigenically distinct neurotoxins of extraordinary toxicity: the estimated lethal dose for humans is less than 1 μg. Production of toxin is determined by carriage of temperate phage by the organism. *Clostridium botulinum* is classified into groups A–G based on the antigenic specificity of the toxin. Groups A, B, E, and F are most often associated with human disease.

Neurotoxin production

Type differentiation by toxins

Toxins are heat labile; act on neuromuscular junctions

Clostridium botulinum neurotoxins are heat labile and destroyed rapidly at 100°C. They are resistant to the enzymes of the gastrointestinal tract and are readily absorbed by this route. They act on neuromuscular junctions by inhibiting release of acetylcholine, resulting in muscular paralysis. Both the voluntary and autonomic cholinergic nervous systems are affected.

Heat-resistant spores

Germination and multiplication in food

Spores of *C. botulinum* resist boiling for long periods, but are rapidly destroyed by moist heat at a temperature of 121°C. Germination of spores and growth of *C. botulinum* can occur in a variety of alkaline or neutral foodstuffs when conditions are sufficiently anaerobic. Occasionally, under

Methods of toxin detection and typing

the same conditions, the organism can multiply in wounds or in the lower intestinal tract of infants.

Clostridium botulinum is identified by its morphologic, cultural, and biochemical characteristics, particularly its toxin production. Toxin is detected by injecting culture supernatants into unprotected mice and into mice protected with antitoxins against the different serotypes of toxin. Unprotected mice and mice given heterologous antitoxin die of paralytic disease within 3 days. Mice protected against the specific serotype of toxin survive.

Botulism

Association with home canning of alkaline foods

Other sources

Botulism is usually associated with home-canned alkaline vegetables, such as green beans or mushrooms, that have not been heated at temperatures sufficient to kill *C. botulinum* spores. The organism multiples on storage, often with no change in food taste or odor, and elaborates its toxin. If the food is ingested without cooking, botulism will result. Other sources include vacuum-packed freshwater fish and occasionally inadequately sterilized or faulty commercial canning. Acidic foods such as canned fruit do not support the growth of *C. botulinum*. The disease often occurs in small epidemics among those who have eaten the toxic food uncooked.

Muscular paralyses

Effects on autonomic cholinergic nerve endings

After an incubation period of 18–96 hr, signs of paralysis develop, first involving the ocular, pharyngeal, laryngeal, and respiratory muscles. There may be extensive paralysis of voluntary muscles. Dry mouth, constipation, and urinary retention occur through the action of the toxin on the autonomic cholinergic nervous system. The mortality caused by the disease is over 20%, even with treatment.

Antitoxin treatment

Treatment.   Specific treatment involves the use of large doses of horse *C. botulinum* antitoxin to neutralize any free toxin. Supportive measures are designed to maintain respiration and a clear adequate airway.

Adequate cooking inactivates toxin

Prevention.   Adequate pressure cooking or autoclaving in the canning process will kill spores. Heating food at 100°C for 10 min before eating will destroy the toxin. Food from damaged cans or those that present evidence of positive inside pressure should not even be tasted because of the extreme toxicity of the *C. botulinum* toxin.

Wound Botulism.   Very rarely, wounds infected with other organisms may allow *C. botulinum* to grow. Disease similar to that from food poisoning can develop.

Toxin can be produced in infant's colon

Infant Botulism.   In recent years, a syndrome associated with *C. botulinum* has been recognized in infants between the ages of 3 weeks and 8 months. It is now the most commonly diagnosed form of botulism. The organism is apparently introduced on weaning or with dietary supplements, especially honey, and multiplies in the infant's colon, with absorption of small amounts of toxin. The infant shows constipation, poor muscle tone, lethargy, and feeding problems and may have ophthalmic and other paralyses similar to those in adult botulism. Infant botulism may contribute to the sudden infant death syndrome.

Other.   Botulism without an obvious food or wound source is occasionally reported in individuals beyond infancy. It is possible that some such cases result from ingestion of spores of *C. botulinum* with subsequent in vivo production of toxin in a manner similar to that in infant botulism.

Laboratory Diagnosis.   Toxin can frequently be demonstrated in blood, intestinal contents, or remaining food, by inoculation into mice. Unprotected mice die, whereas those protected with specific antitoxin survive. *Clostridium botulinum* may also be isolated from stool or from foodstuffs apparently responsible for botulism.

Clostridium difficile

Clostridium difficile was first isolated from the stools of healthy newborn children over three decades ago, but its role as an enteric pathogen was more recently documented. The organism appears to be widespread in the environment and occurs in the intestinal flora of 2–4% of healthy adults in the community. Asymptomatic carriage in the stools of hospital-delivered neonates and outbreaks of *C. difficile*-induced diarrhea in hospitalized adults suggests that many hospitals are heavily contaminated with the spores of this organism. Once in this environment, they may persist for many months and be passed from patient to patient.

Medically important strains produce two distinct large polypeptide toxins, A and B, which are encoded in linked chromosomal genes and released during stationary or poststationary growth phases of the vegetative organism, perhaps at the time of cell lysis. Highly virulent strains produce up to a million times as much toxin as weakly virulent members of the species.

Toxin A is primarily an *enterotoxin* with cholera toxinlike activity (see Chapter 21), but unlike the latter, also causes extensive mucosal damage, resulting in the formation of a hemorrhagic fluid rich in albumin.

Toxin B is a highly potent cytotoxin, which decreases cellular protein synthesis and disrupts the microfilament system of cells in a fashion similar to that of diphtheria toxin (see Chapter 17). Animal studies suggest that toxin A-induced mucosal damage allows absorption of toxin B from the gut lumen.

Clostridium difficile received its name because of the difficulty early investigators had in isolating this relatively slow-growing organism in culture. Fortunately, this problem was overcome with the development of media capable of selectively suppressing more abundant and rapidly growing bowel flora. The organism can be identified on the basis of the morphologic, biochemical, and/or chromatographic characteristics of its metabolic products. Both toxins may be detected in stool, toxin B by tissue culture assays, and toxin A with antibody-based tests currently under development.

Clostridium difficile and Antimicrobic-Associated Diarrhea.   Diarrhea is a frequent side effect of antimicrobic treatment. In some patients, it may progress to a severe, occasionally lethal inflammation of the colon. When this is accompanied by the formation of an overlying "pseudomembrane" composed of fibrin, leukocytes, and necrotic colonic cells, the clinical syndrome is referred to as pseudomembranous colitis (PMC). It is now known that *C. difficile* is responsible for most PMC and, perhaps, many of the milder cases of antimicrobic-associated diarrhea (AAD).

The fastidious *C. difficile* is seldom able to establish itself in the colon of individuals with normal gut flora, although newborn children, who lack the complex flora of adults, frequently become colonized during their brief

---

Occurrence in the environment, in healthy individuals, and in hospitals

Enterotoxin and cytotoxin production

Enterotoxin has some cholera toxinlike properties

Cytotoxin acts by inhibiting protein synthesis

C. difficile as a cause of antimicrobic-associated pseudomembranous colitis and diarrhea

Newborns are often colonized, but rarely diseased

stay in a hospital nursery. Newborns rarely suffer clinical consequences, possibly because toxin receptors within their gut are immature or unavailable. On the other hand, alteration of the colonic flora of the adult with antimicrobics (particularly with ampicillin, cephalosporins, and clindamycin) or antineoplastic agents can result in overgrowth of the organism with diarrhea or PMC. The diarrhea may be mild and watery or bloody and accompanied by abdominal cramping, leukocytosis, and fever. It is estimated that *C. difficile* is responsible for 25% of all reported cases of AAD and for the overwhelming majority of those with PMC. Interestingly, the rate of colonization of newborns within a hospital nursery closely parallels the incidence of clinically manifested *C. difficile* disease in adult patients, suggesting newborn colonization rates reflect the level of environmental contamination with *C. difficile* within a hospital.

Predisposing effects of antimicrobic therapy in adults

Diagnosis. Endoscopic examination of the colon is the most definitive procedure for establishing the presence of a pseudomembrane. The isolation and identification of *C. difficile* and the direct detection of toxins A and/or B in the stool of a patient with AAD establishes this organism as the likely etiologic agent.

Detection of toxin in stool

Treatment. Usually, discontinuing the implicated antimicrobic will result in the resolution of clinical symptoms. If patients are severely ill or fail to respond to drug withdrawal, they are treated with oral antimicrobics, such as vancomycin or metronidazole. Relapses requiring retreatment occur in as many as 20% of patients. *C. difficile* is susceptible to the penicillins and cephalosporins in vitro, but they are ineffective and may predispose to the disease, because they are destroyed by β-lactamases produced by other intestinal organisms.

Discontinuation of antimicrobic usually suffices; oral vancomycin or metronidazole therapy

Prevention. Antimicrobial therapy should be limited to the treatment of infectious diseases known to be susceptible to such agents. Affected patients should be isolated and efforts made to minimize the transmission of organisms from patient to patient by careful implementation of the infection-control procedures discussed in Chapters 11 and 72.

Anaerobic Gram-Negative Rods and Anaerobic Cocci

Two large and important groups of organisms, anaerobic Gram-negative rods and anaerobic cocci, are considered together because they share many features in terms of habitat, diseases produced, and methods used in identification. They are more common causes of disease than the clostridia; those associated with human infections are opportunists, however, and their determinants of pathogenicity are more obscure. All are members of the normal flora of the upper alimentary and respiratory tracts, the female genital tract, or the colon.

Opportunistic members of normal flora

Presumptive laboratory identification depends on morphologic and staining characteristics, biochemical tests, and, in some circumstances, the detection of characteristic organic acid metabolic end products by gas chromatography.

Autoinfections from transgression of epithelial barriers

Diseases caused by these organisms are almost invariably examples of autoinfection: the normal flora transgress epithelial barriers through trauma or pathologic conditions (for example, a ruptured appendix or colonic diverticulum) or because of compromised immune defenses. The result is usually abscess formation. The great majority of infections caused by the non–spore forming anaerobes are mixed; that is, two or more

Most infections mixed; association with abscess formation

anaerobes are isolated, often in combination with facultative bacteria such as *Escherichia coli* (Figure 18.4). In some cases the components of these mixtures synergize each other's growth.

Multiplication of these opportunistic pathogens in abscesses is facilitated by inhibition of oxygen-dependent leukocyte bactericidal functions under the anaerobic conditions in the lesions. Many, but not all, anaerobic infections are associated with foul-smelling lesions, and thrombophlebitis is a common complication. The more aerotolerant anaerobes may occasionally cause endocarditis. The most commonly isolated genera, species, and subspecies of these organisms and the sites of infections with which they are usually associated are listed in Table 18.2. The student should not attempt to commit the names of the individual species to memory.

Bacteroides

B. fragilis complex are the most commonly involved pathogens

Minority members of colonic flora

Antiphagocytic properties of *B. fragilis* and extracellular enzyme production

Penicillin resistance of *B. fragilis*

The *Bacteroides fragilis* complex comprises the most common opportunistic pathogens of the genus *Bacteroides*. They are slim, pale-staining, capsulate, Gram-negative rods that form colonies overnight on blood agar medium and are relatively tolerant to atmospheric oxygen. The implication of fragility in the name is misleading, because they are actually among the hardier and more easily grown anaerobes. Although *B. fragilis* constitutes less than 10% of *Bacteroides* species in the normal colon, it predominates among Gram-negative infections in the abdominal cavity. Its polysaccharide capsule confers resistance to phagocytosis, stimulates abscess formation when injected into experimental animals, and may inhibit macrophage migration. Bacteroides species produce a number of extracellular enzymes that may contribute to pathogenicity including collagenase, IgA protease, heparinase, and DNA-ase. *Bacteroides fragilis* is almost always resistant to penicillin and many other β-lactams in part because of chromosomally encoded β-lactamase. Resistance to tetracycline is common, but most strains are susceptible to chloramphenicol, clindamycin, and metronidazole, although increasing resistance has been reported. Plasmids carrying resistance determinants have been demonstrated in *B. fragilis*.

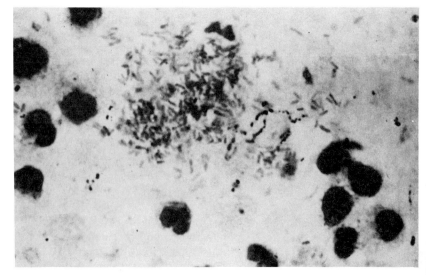

18.4 Gram smear of pus from an abdominal abscess showing polymorphonuclear leucocytes and large numbers of Gram-negative anaerobes and some peptostreptococci. (*Reproduced with permission of Schering Corporation. Kenilworth, N.J., the copyright owner. All rights reserved.*)

Table 18.2 Anaerobic Gram-Negative Rods and Anaerobic Cocci

Organism Groups	Percentage of All Anaerobic Isolates	Frequency within Group	Isolation Site				
			Ororespir-atory	Intestinal	Genital	Soft Tissue	Bone
Bacteroides fragilis complex	35		±	+ + + +	+ +	+ +	+
B. f. fragilis		Common					
B. f. thetaiotaomicron		Occasional					
B. f. vulgatus		Rare					
B. f. distasonis		Rare					
B. f. uniformis		Rare					
B. f. ovatus		Rare					
Bacteroides melaninogenicus complex	10		+ + + +	−	+ +	+	+ +
B. asaccharolyticus		Common					
B. intermedius		Occasional					
B. melaninogenicus		Rare					
B. gingivalis		—					
Fusobacterium spp.	5		+ + +	+ +	+ +	−	+
F. nucleatum		Common					
F. necrophorum		Rare					
F. mortiferum		Rare					
F. varium		Rare					
Peptostreptococcus spp.	25		+ + +	+ + +	+ + +	+ + +	+
P. magnus		Common					
P. anaerobius		Common					
P. asaccharolyticus		Common					

Numbers of +'s indicate frequency of occurrence.

B. melaninogenicus found in mouth, upper alimentary, and respiratory tracts

Penicillin-sensitive organisms that possess potent endotoxin

The *B. melaninogenicus–asaccharolyticus* complex is the second most common cause of human infection in this genus. *Bacteroides melaninogenicus* derives its name from the characteristic black colonies it forms as a result of production of a black pigment from hemoglobin derivatives. Organisms of this group are found in the oral cavity, upper alimentary and respiratory tracts, and colon. In contrast to that of the *B. fragilis* complex, the cell wall has powerful endotoxic properties, and the organisms are usually susceptible to penicillin. Infections with *B. melaninogenicus* are usually derived from the oral flora; they include dental and sinus infections, pulmonary infections and abscesses, and infections of human bites. The latter tend to be serious and refractory unless treated adequately with debridement and antibiotics. This group of organisms is also encountered in abdominal and pelvic lesions.

Several other designated species of *Bacteroides* comprise the predominant organisms in the adult colon. Their pathogenic potential is less than that of the *B. fragilis* and pigmenting bacteroides groups.

Fusobacterium nucleatum

Fusobacterium

Fusobacterium nucleatum is the most common species of the genus in human infection. It is a spindle-shaped, slow-growing, Gram-negative, anaerobic rod that inhabits the oral cavity, the colon, and sometimes the female genital tract. It is less virulent than the species of *Bacteroides* discussed previously and usually appears in mixed infections. It is sensitive to penicillin.

Other fusobacteria contribute to chronic ulcerative lesions of the gums, to abscesses deriving from the oral cavity and pharynx, and to a necrotic ulcerative lesion of the pharynx called *Vincent's angina* (Chapters 26 and 62).

Peptostreptococcus and Microaerophilic Streptococci

The taxonomy of this group of organisms has been shifting and has thus been a source of considerable confusion. Some clinically important species, previously designated as peptostreptococci, although primarily anaerobic can grow slowly in reduced oxygen or increased CO_2 concentrations and have been reassigned to the genus *Streptococcus*. They have pathogenic potential similar to that of the peptostreptococci and will be considered here as microaerophilic streptococci.

These organisms are usually small, Gram-positive cocci that tend to occur in long chains in clinical material and to lose their Gram positivity easily. They are members of the normal flora of the oral cavity, the colon, and the female genital tract. They are opportunists and are often found in lesions with other anaerobic and facultative organisms. Sometimes, anaerobic or microaerophilic streptococci are the sole etiologic agents in cerebral and other abscesses and in puerperal infections and pelvic peritonitis. They can cause anaerobic cellulitis and are often associated with septic thrombophlebitis, which may result in metastatic abscesses. Peptostreptococcal lesions tend to be foul smelling and to show gas production.

Microaerophilic streptococci can cause a form of spreading, *synergistic*, subcutaneous gangrene (Meleney's ulcer) in association with *Staphylococcus aureus*, usually after serious abdominal surgery. The infection arises in a suture line.

Peptostreptococci and microaerophilic streptococci are sensitive to penicillin and usually to other antimicrobics active against Gram-positive cocci, with the exception of the aminoglycosides.

Other Nonclostridial Anaerobic Organisms

Many other anaerobic species of Gram-negative and non–spore-forming Gram-positive rods have been described. Their role in infection is usually only subsidiary, so they will not be discussed here. It is important to remember, however, that they probably play an important adjunctive role in lesions such as periodontal disease, the single major cause of tooth loss and oral sepsis. The genus *Veillonella*, which comprises small anaerobic Gram-negative cocci, merits special mention, because it may be confused with *Neisseria* on Gram staining. It is often present in anaerobic lesions, but plays little role in infection.

Laboratory Diagnosis

The key to detection and identification of anaerobes is a good specimen, preferably pus or fluid exudate from the infected site. It should be collected in special anaerobic transport tubes or in a syringe from which all air is excluded. These measures prevent loss of viability from contact with atmospheric oxygen. Specimens should, whenever possible, be taken to the microbiology laboratory immediately after collection for prompt placement in culture.

A direct Gram-stained smear of clinical material is often helpful. Nu-

Causes of some abscesses, puerperal infectious, and thrombophlebitis

Subcutaneous tissue infections and synergistic gangrene

Adequate specimens collected under anaerobic conditions

Direct Gram stain helpful

merous pale-staining Gram-negative rods are usually seen in anaerobic Gram-negative infections. They are often slim or fusiform and are frequently associated with some Gram-positive bacteria. Numerous polymorphonuclear leukocytes are usually seen (Figure 18.4). These findings are highly suggestive of anaerobic Gram-negative infection, especially if little or no growth occurs on overnight aerobic culture.

Anaerobic cultures and taxonomic tests

Cultural identification often requires special procedures. Media maintained under reduced or anaerobic conditions are used throughout, and exposure to atmospheric oxygen is kept to a minimum. Specific identification procedures, which vary according to species, include toxin detection among clostridia and biochemical characterization, or end-product detection by gas chromatography among the Gram-negative rods and Gram-positive coccal species.

Clinical Manifestations and Treatment

Organisms are opportunistic members of normal flora

As indicated previously, *Bacteroides, Fusobacterium,* and peptostreptococci are opportunists, gaining access to tissues through trauma or other breakdown in normal host defenses. Those with the greatest virulence are selected out and multiply under conditions of sufficiently low Eh. Alone or together with other facultative or obligate anaerobes, the more virulent species are responsible for the overwhelming majority of localized abscesses or empyemas within the cranium, peridontium, thorax, peritoneum, liver, and female genital tract. In addition, they appear to play major causal roles in chronic sinusitis, chronic otitis media, aspiration and necrotizing pneumonia, bronchiectasis, cholecystitis, septic arthritis, osteomyelitis, decubitus ulcers, and soft tissue infections of patients with diabetes mellitus. They account for approximately 10% of positive blood cultures; the mortality rate of bacteremias arising from nongenital sources is 20–40%, which is equivalent to the rates with bacteremias due to staphylococci or Enterobacteriaceae.

Responsible for many localized abscesses and empyemas

Surgical drainage and chemotherapy

In most cases, treatment requires detection of abscesses and drainage of the purulent material, in addition to appropriate chemotherapy. Frequently, chemotherapy alone is ineffective because of failure to penetrate the site of infection. Anaerobic organisms derived from the oral flora are usually susceptible to penicillin and are the most common cause of infection above the diaphragm. Fecal anaerobes, particularly *B. fragilis,* are usually resistant to penicillin and are the etiologic agents of most abdominal infections. They are most likely to respond to chloramphenicol, clindamycin, metronidazole, or an appropriate third-generation cephalosporin. It merits further emphasis, however, that surgical drainage is often essential to therapeutic success.

Additional Reading

Arnon, S.A. 1986. Infant botulism: Anticipating the second decade. *J. Infect. Dis.* 154:201–206. A well-referenced update of knowledge of this disease.

Finegold, S.M. 1989. *Anaerobic Infections in Human Disease.* San Diego, Calif.: Academic Press. A recent and comprehensive text with particular emphasis on clinical syndromes, significance, and therapy.

Lyerly, D.M., Krivan, H.C., and Wilkins, T.D. 1988. *Clostridium difficile:* Its disease and toxins. *Clin. Microbiol. Rev.* 1:1–18. An excellent review of the pathogenesis of *C. difficile* infections and of its toxins.

Schofield, F. 1986. Selective primary health care: Strategies for control of disease in the developing world. XXII. Tetanus. A preventable problem. *Rev. Infect.*

Dis. 8:144–156. A very important review with particular emphasis on prevention of neonatal tetanus.

Smith, L.D.-S., and Williams, B.S. 1984. *The Pathogenic Anaerobic Bacteria*, Publication 1064, American Lecture Series. Springfield, Ill.: Charles C Thomas. An authoritative review of the subject.

Stevens, D.L., Maier, K.A., and Mitten, J.E. 1987. Effects of antibiotics on toxin production and viability of *Clostridium perfringens. Antimicrob. Ag. Chemother.* 31:213–218. Evidence is presented that protein-synthesis–inhibiting antimicrobics may be more effective than penicillin in inhibiting toxin production.

19

Neisseria *Including* Branhamella

Kenneth J. Ryan

Neisseria

Neisseria are Gram-negative diplococci. The genus contains two pathogenic and many commensal species, most of which are normal inhabitants of the upper respiratory and alimentary tracts. The pathogenic species are *Neisseria meningitidis* (meningococcus), a major cause of meningitis and bacteremia, and *Neisseria gonorrhoeae* (gonococcus), the cause of gonorrhea.

Morphology

Gram-negative bean-shaped diplococci

The organisms are Gram-negative cocci that typically appear in pairs with the opposing sides flattened. A "kidney bean" appearance, with the long axes of the cells parallel, is thus produced. This morphology is seen in cultured bacteria and in clinical specimens, although the typical features may not be demonstrable with every pair. Both gonococci and meningococci are readily phagocytosed by polymorphonuclear leukocytes (PMNs); cells containing 10 or more pairs of gonococci may be seen in Gram smears of pus. *Neisseria* are nonmotile, non–spore forming, and are non–acid fast. Their cell walls are typical of Gram-negative bacteria with a peptidoglycan backbone and endotoxic lipopolysaccharide complexed with protein in an outer membrane. Capsules and pili may be demonstrated by ultrasturcture or by immunologic techniques.

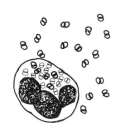

Neisseria gonorrhoeae in WBC

Pathogenic species more fastidious than commensals

Cultural Characteristics

The gonococcus and the meningococcus require an aerobic atmosphere with added carbon dioxide and enriched media for optimal growth. The gonococcus grows more slowly and is more fastidious than the meningococcus, which can grow on routine blood agar. Both grow only at temperatures of 30–37°C. Other *Neisseria* are generally less fastidious and can also grow at temperatures as low as 22–25°C.

Table 19.1 Differential Bacteriologic Features of *Neisseria* and *Branhamella*

Organism	Growth			Acid Production from Carbohydrates			
	Blood Agar	Room Temperature	Special Medium[a]	Glucose	Sucrose	Maltose	Lactose
N. gonorrheoae	−[b]	−	+	+	−	−	−
N. meningitidis	+	−	+	+	−	+	−
Other *Neisseria*	+	+	−[d]	v	v	v	v
Branhamella	+	+	−	−	−	−	−

[a] Modified Thayer–Martin or similar selective medium.
[b] Poor growth may occur with some strains.
[c] Reaction varies with different strains and species.
[d] *N. lactamica* is an exception.

Classification

Oxidase positive

Neisseria are oxidase positive (Chapter 14). Some of the bacteriologic and biochemical features used to distinguish the various species of the genus are illustrated in Table 19.1.) Gonococci and meningococci may also be differentiated from the other *Neisseria* by immunologic methods such as slide agglutination, coagglutination, precipitin reactions, and immunofluorescence. There is increasing use of monoclonal antibodies in such tests.

Neisseria meningitidis and meningococcal infections

Growth and Structure

Meningococci grow on most nonselective routine laboratory media, and produce about 1.5-mm-diameter colonies after overnight incubation on blood agar. Carbon dioxide enhances growth, but is not required. Most isolates produce a small capsule that is not seen by routine microscopic methods.

Growth enhancement by CO_2

Antigenic Structure

Serogroups on basis of capsular polysaccharide

Meningococci are divided into nine serogroups, largely on the basis of polysaccharide capsules. The most important serogroups are A, B, C, W-135, and Y. Not all strains can be grouped with currently available antisera, and it is likely other antigens remain to be identified. The chemical structure of the group-specific polysaccharide has been identified for most serogroups. Purified polysaccharides of groups A, C, W-135, and Y are immunogenic and are used as vaccines. In contrast, the polysaccharide of group B meningococci lacks the immunogenicity of those in the other groups, although the reasons for this are not clear. In addition to the group antigens, several serotypes have been identified within group B and C meningococci. The serotypes within Group B are based on differences in outer membrane proteins. Further study is necessary to determine whether different serotypes within the serogroups are associated with predictable virulence or epidemiologic features.

Pathogenesis and Immunity

Exclusively human parasite

The meningococcus is an exclusively human parasite; like other pyogenic cocci (*Staphylococcus aureus*, *Streptococcus pneumoniae*), it can either exist as an apparently harmless member of the normal flora or produce acute

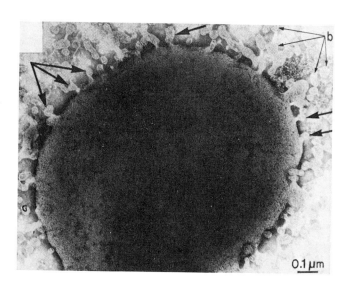

19.1 *Neisseria meningitidis.* Cell wall is shown shedding multiple "blebs" (*arrows*) containing LPS-endotoxin. Note the typical trilamellar Gram-negative cell wall structure in the wall and the blebs. (*Reproduced with permission from Devoe, I.W. and Gilcrist, J.E. 1973. J. Exp. Med. 138 (5):1160, Figure 3.*)

0.1 μm

Nasopharyngeal carriage

disease. Carrier rates of meningococci in the upper respiratory tract are usually between 5 and 15% in healthy adults and children, higher colonization rates are found occasionally in closed populations such as military recruit camps and boarding schools. The carrier state is associated with the development of group specific antibodies and immunity, but before this develops, meningococci may sometimes spread from the nasopharynx to produce bacteremia, endotoxemia, and meningitis. The initial events of infection have been studied using human nasopharyngeal organ cultures. The meningococci appear to attach selectively to the nonciliated columnar epithelium, but damage the ciliated cells, possibly by direct action of the meningococcal lipopolysaccharide. The specific attachment mechanisms are not clear, although piliated meningococci adhere more readily than nonpiliated strains. Viable meningococci also interact with the microvilli of the nonciliated cells entering and passing through these cells to the submucosa. The polysaccharide capsule is probably important in resisting phagocytosis, and the potent endotoxic activity of the cell wall is responsible for some of the clinical manifestations. *Neisseria meningitidis* strains like gonococci have been shown to readily release endotoxin-containing blebs from the cell surface (Figure 19.1). The organism does not produce a significant exotoxin. It is unclear whether certain meningococcal strains are more virulent than others.

Meningococci attach to nonciliated cells, but damage ciliated cells

Antiphagocytic effect of capsule

Endotoxin activity

Immunity by opsonizing and bactericidal effects of antibody

Immunity to meningococcal infections is related to circulating group-specific opsonizing and bactericidal antibody, and antibody against endemic serogroups is present in many but not all adults. The peak incidence of serious infection is between 6 months and 2 years of age, which corresponds to the time between loss of transplacental antibody and the appearance of naturally acquired antibody (Figure 19.2). Infections later in life appear when populations carrying virulent strains mix with susceptible individuals lacking specific antibody. Examples of this process include outbreaks of meningococcal disease among young adults in military recruit camps. In these outbreaks, *N. meningitidis* spreads among newly exposed recruits readily, but disease develops only in those lacking group-specific antibody.

Populations at risk

Acquisition of protective antibody

Protective antibody is usually acquired through subclinical or overt infection and through the carrier state, which produces immunity within

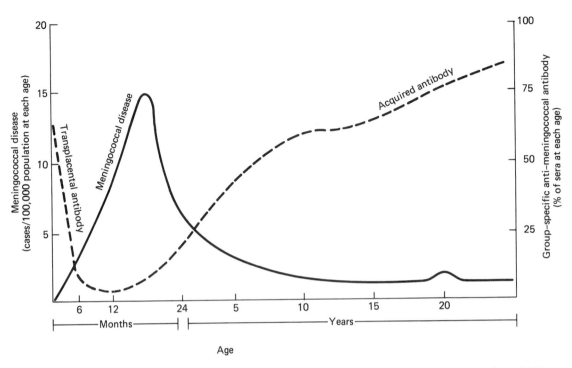

19.2 Immunity to the meningococcus. The inverse relationship between bactericidal meningococcal antibody and meningococcal disease is demonstrated. The "blip" in the disease curve around age 20 is attributable in part to military and other closed-population outbreaks. (*Adapted from Goldschneider et al. 1969.*)

a few weeks. However, natural immunization may not require infection or colonization with every serogroup or even with *N. meningitidis*, because antibody may be produced in response to cross-reacting antigens on other *Neisseria* species and even on other genera. For example, the K1 surface antigen of some *Escherichia coli* strains is chemically and immunologically identical to the group B meningococcal polysaccharide.

Epidemiology

Meningococcal infections must be reported by law in the United States, and usually more than 3000 cases per year are recorded. Currrently about half of all cases are caused by serogroup B and another 20–25% by serogroup C. The remainder are primarily serogroup Y and serogroup W-135, which has emerged as an important cause of disease since 1975. All occur primarily as isolated cases, as sporadic small epidemics, or in small family or closed-population (school or day-care center) outbreaks. Group A strains are more ominous and have the potential to cause widespread epidemics, which in the past have appeared in 8- to 12-year cycles. In the interim, group A meningococci curiously disappear with only 1–2% per year of reported cases of meningococcal infection due to this group. It has been more than 40 years since such an epidemic has occurred in the United States, although serious group A epidemics have occurred in Brazil and South Africa in recent years.

Transmission of meningococci is by respiratory droplets and requires both close contact and susceptibility (lack of antibody). This combination

Most endemic disease now due to groups B, C, Y, and W-135

Epidemic potential of group A meningococci

Route and conditions for transmission

is most likely to occur in family members of an index case, particularly children. The attack rate of meningococcal infections among family members is 1000-fold higher than in the general population; prophylactic chemotherapy is indicated. Despite their contact with meningococcal infections, hospital employees have not shown an increased frequency of infection, probably because of the lack of prolonged close contact in a largely immune adult population.

Clinical Manifestations

Meningitis

Meningococcemia and rash

The most frequent form of meningococcal infection is acute purulent meningitis with clinical and laboratory features similar to those of other causes of meningitis (Chapter 67). A distinguishing feature of meningococcal meningitis is the appearance of scattered skin petechiae, which may evolve into ecchymoses or a diffuse petechial rash. These features are manifestations of meningococcal bacteremia (meningococcemia) and thrombocytopenia, which develops with evolution of the disseminated intravascular coagulation (DIC) syndrome. Many of these features are similar to those of experimental endotoxic shock. Meningococcemia sometimes occurs without meningitis, and may progress to fulminant DIC and shock with bilateral hemorrhagic destruction of the adrenal glands (Waterhouse-Friderichsen syndrome). It is not always fulminant, however, and some patients have only low-grade fever, arthritis, and skin lesions that develop slowly over a period of days to weeks. The finding of *N. meningitidis* in the blood or even the cerebrospinal fluid (CSF) of patients with chronic meningococcemia is often unexpected from the clinical severity of the illness. Meningococci may also cause pneumonia, but this disease is uncommon and is not associated with the more common manifestations of meningococcal infection.

Waterhouse-Friderichsen syndrome

Chronic meningococcal bacteremia

Diagnosis

Direct gram smears

Culture and serogrouping

Direct Gram smears of CSF in meningitis may demonstrate the typical bean-shaped, Gram-negative diplococci. Definitive diagnosis is by culture of CSF, blood, or skin lesions. Although reputed to be somewhat fragile, the organism requires no special handling for isolation from presumptively sterile sites such as blood and CSF; *N. gonorrhoeae*, in contrast, is more fragile and fastidious. Good growth develops on blood or chocolate agar after 18 hr of incubation. If sufficient growth is present, confirmation and serogrouping may be done directly from the primary plates by slide agglutination methods. Speciation is based on carbohydrate degradation patterns (Table 19.1).

Antigen detection in clinical material and latex agglutination

For rapid diagnosis and in cases in which cultures are negative because of previous antimicrobic therapy, meningococcal polysaccharide antigen may be detected by methods such as counterimmunoelectrophoresis and latex agglutination (Chapter 14). Meningococcal antigen has been detected in CSF, blood, and urine; false-negative results are common, however, particularly with serogroup B strains.

Treatment

Penicillin or chloramphenicol treatment

Penicillin is the treatment of choice for meningococcal infections because of its antimeningococcal activity and because it can penetrate inflamed meninges. Patients with penicillin hypersensitivity are treated with chloramphenicol. Although *N. meningitidis* is susceptible in vitro to a wide range of antimicrobics, relatively few are considered appropriate because of poor clinical results or lack of clinical experience. For example, cephalothin gives inconsistent clinical results despite good in vitro susceptibility. Some of the newer cephalosporins, however, may serve as alternatives to penicillin. Sulfonamides, although effective in the past, have been discarded in favor of penicillin and chloramphenicol.

Rare increased resistance to penicillin

Although strains of increased resistance to penicillin have been described, they are presently extremely rare, and chloramphenical resistance has not been reported. In comparison to gonococci, meningococci typically carry few plasmids, which may partially explain their continued susceptibility to commonly used anitmicrobics except sulfonamides.

Prevention

Chemoprophylaxis

Sulfonamide-resistant strains

In the past, the primary means of preventing secondary cases and further spread of meningococcal infection was chemoprophylaxis with sulfonamides. This approach was effective for populations ranging from individual family members to whole military camps. The development and spread of sulfonamide-resistant meningococci in the 1960s changed this situation. Currently, 40–50% of group C meningococci (one of the most common serogroups) are resistant to sulfonamides with lower incidences of resistance among group B and group Y strains. Sulfonamides are still the preferred prophylactic agents for susceptible strains, but in individual cases, sulfonamide susceptibility must be demonstrated before sulfonamides can be used. Rifampin is currently used for prophylaxis against sulfonamide-resistant meningococci or in situations in which the susceptibility is unknown. Penicillin is *not* effective as a prophylactic agent, probably because of inadequate penetration to the surface of the uninflamed nasopharyngeal mucosa. Selection of cases to receive prophylaxis is based on epidemiologic assessment of risk (see "Epidemiology"). Typically, family members are given prophylaxis but hospital employees are not, unless close contact such as mouth-to-mouth resuscitation has occurred. Culture findings play no role in these decisions, because they do not accurately predict risk of serious infection.

Rifampin in chemoprophylaxis

Indications for prophylaxis

Meningococcal vaccines

Purified polysaccharide meningococcal vaccines have been shown to prevent group A and C disease in military and civilian populations, and a quadrivalent vaccine containing A, C, Y, and W-135 polysaccharides is now licensed for use in the United States. Unfortunately, its effectiveness in preventing disease in a major susceptible group is compromised by a poor antibody response to polysaccharides in the first year of life. This resembles the situation with *Haemophilus influenzae* type b (Chapter 23). Meningococcal vaccines are currently used in populations of those at particular risk, such as in military recruit camps, and in control of epidemics. Routine immunization of children is not recommended unless there are predisposing factors such as deficiencies of the terminal complement components or asplenia. Polysaccharide–protein conjugate vaccines, such as that against *H. influenzae*, may be developed that are more effective producers of immunity in young children. The lack of an effective serogroup B vaccine remains a problem.

Neisseria gonorrhoeae and gonorrhoea

Growth

Fastidiousness of gonococci and CO_2 requirement

Neisseria gonorrhoeae grows well only on chocolate agar and on similar specialized media enriched to ensure its growth. It requires CO_2 supplementation. Small colonies appear after 18–24 hr of incubation and are

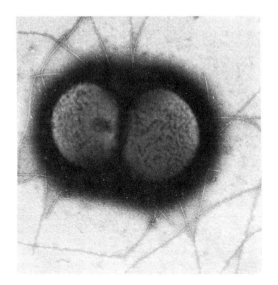

19.3 *Neisseria gonorrhoeae.* Surface pili are asssociated with virulence and may mediate initial attachment to epithelial surfaces. (*Kindly provided by Dr. John Swanson.*)

well developed (2–4 mm) after 48 hr. The colonies are smooth and non-pigmented. Under specialized growth and illumination conditions, four colony types have been recognized, designated T1 to T4. In general, T1 and T2 colonies are seen on primary isolation, are associated with virulence, and are able to produce experimental infections. Larger T3 and T4 colonies tend to appear on continued subculture and are avirulent. The ability to grow on defined media lacking specific nutrients has been used to develop an auxotyping scheme for gonococci. Over 30 types, some of which have been associated with particular clinical or epidemiologic features, can be separated with these procedures.

T1–4 colony types and association with virulence

Different auxotypes

Structure

In addition to the typical Gram-negative cell wall structure, gonococci possess numerous pili that extend through and beyond the peptidoglycan and outer membrane (Figure 19.3). In general, the T1 and T2 colony types typical of fresh virulent isolates have pili, but others do not. The pili are polymers of repeating protein subunits that are antigenically diverse among different gonococcal strains. The gonococcal outer membrane is composed of phospholipids, lipopolysaccharide, and several distinct outer membrane proteins (OMP). Of the outer membrane protein classes, OMP I and OMP III are found in all gonococci. OMP I is the principle structural protein of the outer membrane and is the major antigen used in serotyping gonococci. OMP II is actually a group of six to eight proteins of which none, one, or several may be expressed by any single strain. As with pili, OMP II expression can be correlated with changes in colonial morphology. Gonococcal strains have been shown to possess surface polysaccharide and capsules, but the pathogenic significance of these structures is not yet known.

Pili on T1 and T2 colony types

Outer membrane proteins

Antigenic Variation

Neisseria gonorrhoeae is one of a number of microorganisms under intensive study to determine the occurrence, mechanism, and significance of antigenic variation within the same strain. The structures of major interest in gonococci are the surface pili and OMP II, both of which have demonstrated antigenic variation in vitro and in vivo.

Gonococcal pili are particularly variable. They contain a highly conserved region in which the amino acid sequence is the same for each type and a variable terminal region that is immunodominant and accounts for the serological diversity seen in clinical isolates. Under different conditions cells of the same strain may produce or fail to produce pili (phase variation) or the pili undergo antigenic variation; a single cell, however, produces only one antigenic type of pilus at a time. Genetically, there appear to be multiple pilin genes in each strain, some of which are transcriptionally active and others that are "silent." The antigenic variation is due to the recombination of pilin DNA sequences from silent to active loci within the cell. By transformation, extracellular DNA may accomplish the same conversion of active genes with variant pilin sequences. A single gonococcal cell may thus gain the genetic capacity to produce multiple antigenically distinct pili.

As with pili, OMP II production can be switched on or off, but a single cell may express more than one antigenically distinct protein. These changes have been studied in vitro. It seems likely that they also occur in vivo, because clinical isolates from the uterine cervix tend to be OMP II+, but those from the fallopian tubes or during menses are generally OMP II−.

The genetic mechanism for gonococcal OMP antigenic variation appears to differ from that described for pili. Multiple copies of OMP genes are present and constitutively transcribed in each strain. Their expression, however, is regulated at the translational level. This occurs through variations in the number of repeats of a five nucleotide sequence (CTCTT) immediately preceding each gene that place the translation either in or out of the protein reading frame. When out of frame, the gene expresses only a short nonfunctional peptide. In frame, the complete OMP is expressed. Because there are multiple genes, none, one, or several antigenically distinct OMPs may be expressed on a single strain.

Pathogenesis and Immunity

Gonococci are *not* normal inhabitants of the respiratory or genital flora. When introduced onto a mucosal surface by sexual contact with an infected individual, the organisms attach to mucosal epithelium, enter, and multiply within the epithelial cells and pass to the submucosa resulting in an acute inflammatory response. Pili are the primary mediators of adherence to urethral and vaginal epithelial and to non-ciliated fallopian tube cells, as well as to sperm and neutrophils. OMP II is also involved in adherence and in increased adhesion between gonococcal cells contributing to the formation of large clusters of gonococci. These "sticky" clusters could be the primary infectious unit for transmission of gonorrhea. The fate of gonococci once they encounter phagocytes is not entirely clear. Pili facilitate attachment to neutrophils, but may reduce ingestion. The extent of intracellular killing of phagocytosed gonococci is a matter of current debate. There is evidence that killing by neutrophils is sufficiently retarded to explain prolonged survival of gonococci in mucosal and submucosal locations.

Spread beyond the local site to the fallopian tubes may be facilitated by pilus-mediated attachment to sperm and then to nonciliated fallopian tube cells. The gonococci are able to enter and pass through these cells and at the same time injure the ciliated cells. This is similar to the mech-

---

Variable region of pilus

Phase variation

Antigenic variation of pili by genetic rearrangement

Variation in OMP II proteins

Translational regulation of OMP II expression

Attachment, penetration of cells, multiplication, and acute inflammatory response
Pili are primary mediators of adherence

Attachment of neutrophils, but possibly delayed phagocytosis

Attachment to sperm and nonciliated fallopian tube cells

anism of infection by *N. meningitidis*, although gonococcal injury seems to be mediated by fragments of the cell wall peptidoglycan, as well as by lipopolysaccharide. Gonococci are unique among Gram-negative bacteria in their rapid turnover of peptidoglycan during periods of exponential growth and for their ability to release peptidoglycan fragments into the local environment. This injury mechanism presumably may operate at sites other than the fallopian tube. Infection also extends to deeper structures by progressive infection of mucosal and glandular epithelial cells. These structures include the lining of the paracervical and paraurethral glands and of the fallopian tubes in women and the prostate and epididymis in men. Extension along the fallopian tubes from an initial cervical infection can lead to seeding of the pelvic cavity. In most cases the disease remains localized although bacteremia and hematogenous extension occur in a small proportion of cases. This is termed *disseminated gonococcal infection* (DGI). The strains involved in cases of DGI differ from other gonococci in possessing a greater resistance to the bactericidal effects of normal human serum and in commonly being of a single auxotype. Both DGI and salpingitis tend to begin during or shortly after completion of menses. This may relate to changes in the cervical mucus during menses with influx of blood into the fallopian tubes.

The apparent lack of immunity to gonococcal infection has long been a mystery. Among sexually active persons with multiple partners, repeated infections are the rule rather than the exception. Recent studies of antigenic variation strongly suggest it may be the prime mechanism by which the gonococcus avoids immune surveillance. Antigenic variation of pili is particularly likely to be important. Outbreaks have been traced to a single strain that demonstrated multiple pilin variations in repeated isolates from the same person or from sexual partners. In experimental models, passive administration of antibody directed against one pilin type has been followed by emergence of new pilin variants. Changes in OMP II may also occur as suggested by differences in its expression in mucosal versus tubal isolates. The emerging pattern is that immunity to gonococcal infection is present, but is complicated by the ability of the organism to change structure during the course of infection. The presence or absence of pili or OMP II and their antigenic makeup has different significance at different stages of the disease and the ability to regulate these changes gives the gonococcus a major edge against the immune system.

Marginal notes:
Cell wall fragments in tissue injury

Direct extension to other sites

Disseminated infection associated with one auxotype

Immunity to reinfection is weak because of antigenic variation

Gonococci change or lose pili and OMP II during infection

Epidemiology

Gonorrhea is a major worldwide public health problem. In the United States the number of reported cases increased rapidly during the 1960s and 1970s. Since 1977, the number first stabilized, and then began to decline slowly. In 1986, the number of reported cases per 100,000 of the population was about 375, although many more were probably unreported. No truly effective means of control is yet in sight. The reasons for our inability to control gonorrhea are complex and include changed sexual mores and practices, lack of an effective means to detect asymptomatic cases, decreased susceptibility of *N. gonorrhoeae* to penicillin (see "Therapy"), and, to some extent, lack of public appreciation of the importance of this disease. The latter is evidenced by failure of patients to seek medical care and of physicians to report cases to public health authorities to protect the privacy of their patients. In the minds of many, syphilis is dreaded and "unclean," whereas gonorrhea is only "the clap" (clap: archaic French, *clapoir*, a rabbit warren; later, a brothel).

Marginal notes:
Recent epidemic of gonorrhea

Difficulties in controlling the disease

Major reservoir is
asymptomatic infections

The major reservoir for continued spread of gonorrhea is the asymptomatic patient. Screening programs and case contact studies have shown that almost 50% of infected women are asymptomatic or at least do not have symptoms usually associated with venereal infection. Most men (95%) have acute symptoms with infection. Many who are not treated become asymptomatic but remain infectious. Asymptomatic male and female patients can remain infectious for months. The attack rates for those engaging in genital intercourse with an infected patient are not known, but are estimated to be 20–50%. The organism may also be transmitted by oral-genital contact or by rectal intercourse. When all of these factors operate in a sexually promiscuous population, it is easy to explain the high prevalence of gonorrhea.

Rarity of fomitic transfer

Although gonococci can survive for brief periods on the proverbial toilet seat, nonsexual transmission is extremly rare. Fomite transmission of a purulent vulvovaginitis in prepubescent girls has been reported, but currently most isolations of gonococci in children can be traced to sexual abuse by an infected adult.

Genital Gonorrhea

Urethritis and endocervicitis

In men, the primary site of infection is the urethra. Symptoms begin 2–7 days after infection and consist primarily of purulent urethral discharge and dysuria. Although uncommon, local extension can lead to epididymitis or prostatitis. The endocervix is the primary site in women, in whom symptoms include increased vaginal discharge, urinary frequency, dysuria, abdominal pain, and menstrual abnormalities. As mentioned previously, symptoms may be mild or absent in either sex, particularly in women.

Other Local Infections

Rectal infection

Rectal gonorrhea occurs after rectal intercourse or, in women, after contamination with infected vaginal secretions. This infection is generally asymptomatic but may cause tenesmus, discharge, and rectal bleeding. Pharyngeal gonorrhea is caused by orogenital sex and, again, is usually asymptomatic. Sore throat and cervical adenitis may occur. Infection of other structures near primary infection sites, such as Bartholin's glands in women, may lead to abscess formation.

Pharyngeal infection

Conjunctivitis and ophthalmia
neonatorum

Inoculation of gonococci into the conjunctiva produces a severe, acute, purulent conjunctivitis. Although this infection may occur at any age, the most serious form is gonococcal ophthalmia neonatorum acquired by an infant from an infected mother. The disease was formerly a common cause of blindness, and for this reason eye prophylaxis is used at birth. Gonococcal ophthalmia neonatorum had all but disppeared in the United States in the 1950's but with the increase in gonococcal infections, and antimicrobic resistance, it is now being encountered again (Chapter 69).

Pelvic Inflammatory Disease

Salpingitis and pelvic
peritonitis

The clinical syndrome of pelvic inflammatory disease (PID) includes fever, lower abdominal pain, adnexal tenderness, and leukocytosis with or without signs of local infection. These features are caused by spread of organisms along the fallopian tubes to produce salpingitis and into the pelvic cavity to produce pelvic peritonitis and abscesses. Although defined previously as a gonococcal disease, PID is now known to develop when other potential pathogens in the genital flora ascend by the same route. These

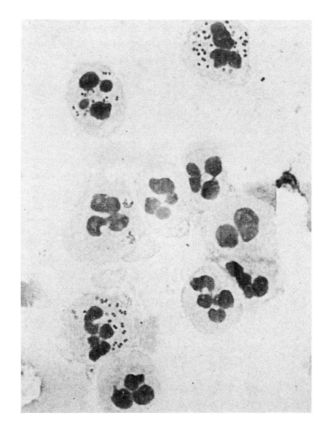

19.4 Gram smear of urethral exudate of an acute case of gonorrhoea in a male. Note typical intracellular diplococci in polymorphonuclear leukocytes. The gonococci are Gram negative.

organisms include anaerobes and *Chlamydia trachomatis*, which may appear alone or mixed with gonococci. The most serious complication of PID is infertility, which can result from a single attack and is common after multiple attacks, regardless of the microbial etiology.

Disseminated Gonococcal Infections

Skin rash, arthralgia, and arthritis

Any of the local forms of gonorrhea or their extensions such as PID may lead to bacteremia. In the bacteremic phase the primary features are fever, migratory polyarthralgia, and a petechial, maculopapular, or pustular rash. These features may be immunologically mediated, as gonococci are infrequently isolated from the skin or joints at this stage despite their presence in the blood. The bacteremia may lead to infections such as endocarditis or meningitis, but the most common is purulent arthritis. The arthritis typically follows the bacteremia and involves large joints such as elbows and knees. Gonococci are readily cultured from the pus.

Further consideration of gonorrhea is given in Chapter 70.

Diagnosis

Use and limitations of direct smear

Gram smear.   The presence of multiple pairs of bean-shaped, Gram-negative diplococci within a neutrophil is highly characteristic of gonorrhea when the smear is from a genital site (Figure 19.4). Unfortunately, other bacteria in the female genital flora may have a similar appearance. This finding, combined with the more acute exudate generally found in men has given the direct Gram smear a reputation for sensitivity and specificity in men, but insensitivity and nonspecificity in women; however, skilled microscopists, such as those in venereal disease clinics, who regularly see many cases can achieve a diagnostic accuracy in women that approaches that in men. The student or harried intern, however, cannot necessarily apply the same criteria with equal results despite published statistics, and cultural confirmation should be obtained. Cases in which the findings are unexpected or have particular social or medicolegal implications should always be confirmed by culture.

Culture.   Attention to detail is necessary for isolation of the gonococcus, as it is a fragile organism often mixed with hardier members of the normal flora. Success requires proper selection of culture sites, protection of specimens from environmental exposure, culture on appropriate media, and definitive laboratory identification. In men the best specimen is of urethral exudate or urethral scrapings (obtained with a loop or special swab). In women cervical swabs yield most positive results. Gonococci may also be isolated from the urethra and vagina, but the rate of positive results is significantly below that of cervical culture. The highest diagnostic yield in women is with the combination of a cervical and an anal canal culture, because some patients with rectal gonorrhea will have negative cervical cultures. Throat and rectal cultures in men are needed only if indicated by the patient's sexual practices.

Swabs may be streaked directly onto culture media or transmitted to the laboratory in a suitable transport medium if the delay is not more than 4 hr. Laboratory requests must always specify the suspicion of gonorrhea, as specialized, selective media are required. These media satisfy the nutritional requirements of the gonococcus and inhibit competing normal flora, which may interfere with isolation. The most common is Thayer-Martin agar, an enriched selective chocolate-type agar. The exact formulation has changed over the years, but includes antimicrobics active against Gram-positive bacteria (vancomycin), Gram-negative bacteria (colistin, trimethoprim), and fungi (nystatin, anisomycin) at concentrations that do not inhibit *N. gonorrhoeae*.

Colonies appear after 1–2 days of incubation in CO_2 at 35°C. They may be identified as *Neisseria* by demonstration of typical Gram-stain morphology and a positive oxidase test. Speciation is made by carbohydrate degradation pattern (Table 19.1), immunofluorescence, or coagglutination. *Neisseria* other than *N. gonorrhoeae* are unusual in genital specimens, but speciation is the only way to be certain of the diagnosis.

Serology.   Attempts to develop a serologic test for gonorrhea have not yet achieved the needed sensitivity and specificity. A test that would detect the disease in asymptomatic patients would be very useful in control of this disease.

Treatment

Penicillin was, for a long time, the primary treatment for gonorrhea, although two changes in the susceptibility of the organism have influenced its use. The first has been a slowly decreasing susceptibility of gonococci to penicillin, which has been noted since the 1950s. Older strains were uniformly inhibited by less than 0.1 μg/ml penicillin, whereas up to 25%

Selection of culture sites

Immediate culture or use of transport media

Thayer-Martin selective medium

Identification of Neisserial isolates

Penicillin susceptibility

Increasing mutational resistance

of recent isolates in several U.S. cities require 0.5–2.0 μg/ml. This resistance is mutational, involving changes in cell wall penicillin-binding proteins; the strains do not produce penicillinase and most can still be treated with a penicillin at high doses. Many of the more resistant isolates are also resistant to other antimicrobics.

Plasmid-coded penicillinase production

In the late 1970s, penicillinase-producing *N. gonorrhoeae* (PPNG) appeared throughout the world, originating primarily in the Far East. These strains produced a plasmid-coded TEM-type β-lactamase identical to that of members of the Enterobacteriaceae and ampicillin-resistant *H. influenzae*. These gonococci are inhibited, if at all, only by high concentrations of penicillin and do not respond to penicillin therapy. Initially, most cases in the United States could be traced to the Far East through military or other contacts. There is now sustained disease transmission with PPNG in endemic foci throughout the United States. Gonorrhea due to strains that do not produce penicillinase is usually treated with high-dose penicillin, ampicillin, or amoxicillin in combination with probenecid to block renal tubular excretion of the antimicrobics and thus boost serum levels. Erythromycin and tetracycline are also effective against susceptible strains. For PPNG strains or for patients who are hypersensitive to the penicillins, spectinomycin or ceftriaxone is preferred. Concurrent treatment of co-existing chlamydial infections is also recommended (Chapter 70).

Use of penicillin and probenecid for susceptible strains

Spectinomycin and ceftriaxone for PPNG strains

Prevention

Methods to block direct mucosal contact (condoms) or inhibit the gonococcus (vaginal foams, douches) have not been studied extensively, but it is likely that they provide protection against gonorrhea if used regularly. The classic public health methods of case-contact tracing and treatment have become more difficult with the increasing size of the primary reservoir. The availability of a good serologic test would greatly aid control, as it has for syphilis. The development of a gonococcal vaccine awaits further understanding of the immunology and epidemiology of gonorrhea.

Other Neisseria

Oral and upper respiratory tract commensals

Many other *Neisseria* species exist primarily as normal inhabitants of the oral cavity and upper respiratory tract. Some have been shown to cause mild to serious infections, including meningitis, but only rarely. With the exception of *Neisseria lactamica*, these other *Neisseria* generally fail to grow on Thayer-Martin agar (Table 19.1). They are distinguished from *N. gonorrhoeae* and *N. meningitidis* by biochemical and serologic tests. They can grow at 22–25°C and frequently produce dry, wrinkled, or pigmented colonies, which are readily distinguished from those of pathogenic species.

Branhamella

Branhamella may cause respiratory tract infections

Organisms in the genus *Branhamella* were previously classified as *Neisseria*, because, as oxidase-positive Gram-negative diplococci, they superficially resembled them. Studies of DNA homology have shown clear differences, however, and some clinical studies indicate that *Branhamella* may have a greater potential to produce respiratory tract infections than do true *Neisseria*.

Branhamella species are found in the indigenous flora of the oral and nasal cavities as are commensal *Neisseria*. Clinical studies show *Branha-*

mella to be an uncommon cause of lower respiratory tract infection and otitis media. Many strains produce β-lactamase.

Additional Reading

Britigan, B.E., Cohen, M.S., and Sparling, P.F. 1985. Gonococcal infection: A model of molecular pathogenesis. *N. Engl. J. Med.* 312:1683–1694. This review covers what is known about the virulence factors of the gonococcus and how they correlate with the clinical manifestations of gonorrhea.

Goldschneider, I., Gotschlich, E.C., Liu, T.Y., and Artenstein, M.S. 1969. Human immunity to the meningococcus I-V. *J. Exp. Med.* 129:1307–1395. This series of five papers defines the basis of immunity to *Neisseria meningitidis* and the development of vaccines from the polysacchharide capsule.

McGee, Z.A., et al. 1983. Mechanisms of mucosal invasion by pathogenic *Neisseria. Rev. Inf. Dis.* 5:S708–S714. An electron microscope study demonstrating the attachment and invasive properties of gonococci and meningogococci using human organ cultures.

Roberts, M., Elwell, L.P., and Falkow, S. 1977. Molecular characterization of two beta-lactamase-specifying plasmids isolated from *Neisseria gonorrhoeae. J. Bacteriol.* 131:557–562. This molecular study shows the mechanism of penicillinase production by gonococci and the relation of these plasmids to others, such as those found in *Haemophilus influenzae.*

Seifert, H.S., and So, M. 1988. Genetic mechanisms of antigenic variation. *Microbiol. Rev.* 52:327–366. The genetics of antigenic variation are nicely explained and the evidence for the importance of these changes in clinical gonorrhea is discussed.

20

Enterobacteriaceae

Kenneth J. Ryan

Enterobacteriaceae

Gram-negative facultative rods

The Enterobacteriaceae are a large and diverse family of Gram-negative rods, members of which are found free living in nature and as part of the indigenous flora of humans and animals. They grow rapidly under aerobic and anaerobic conditions and are metabolically active, attacking a variety of substrates. Many species are motile, but none forms spores or demonstrates acid fastness. Most species are opportunistic pathogens; some, however, are highly and specifically pathogenic, particularly in the intestinal tract.

Habitat

Many are present in normal flora of colon

Occurrence in respiratory tract of hospitalized patients

Most Enterobacteriaceae are primarily inhabitants of the lower gastrointestinal tract of humans and animals. Many survive readily in nature, and many are found free living where water and minimal energy sources are available. In humans they include the main facultative portion of the bacterial content of the colon. They are also found in the female genital tract and as transient colonizers of the skin. Enterobacteriaceae are occasionally present in small numbers in the respiratory tract of healthy persons; however, they appear in increased numbers in hospitalized patients, particularly those with chronic debilitating diseases. *Escherichia coli* is the most common species of Enterobacteriaceae found among the indigenous flora, followed by *Klebsiella, Proteus,* and *Enterobacter* species. *Salmonella, Shigella,* certain *E. coli* strains, and *Yersinia* species are primarily pathogenic and not part of the normal flora.

Morphology

The Enterobacteriaceae are among the larger bacteria that colonize humans. They are usually 2–4 μm in length and 0.4–0.6 μm in width with parallel sides and rounded ends: the length is variable, however, producing

357

forms that range from large coccobacilli to an elongated, filamentous appearance. Motile strains have peritrichous flagella, which have a regular wavelength and extend 1–5 μm beyond the cell wall. Many also have surface pili. Some species (for example, *Klebsiella*) are typically encapsulated. Most have extracellular surface slime layers, that are often poorly circumscribed and readily released into the surrounding medium. The cell wall, cell membrane, and internal structure, which are morphologically similar for all Enterobacteriaceae, are as described in Chapter 2 for Gram-negative bacteria.

Peritrichous flagella of motile strains

Pili, capsules, and slime layers

Growth

Enterobacteriaceae grow readily on simple media, often with only a single carbon energy source. Growth is rapid under both aerobic and anaerobic conditions, producing 2- to 5-mm colonies on agar media and diffuse turbidity in broth after 12–18 hr of incubation. Their simple growth requirements and relative resistance to many substances, such as bile salts and some bacteriostatic dyes, are exploited in selective media and in identification methods. Conversely, their ability to grow under almost any conditions may interfere with the isolation of more fastidious bacteria when clinical specimens also contain Enterobacteriaceae.

Rapid growers

Characteristics exploited in selective media

Colonies of Enterobacteriaceae formed on media such as MacConkey agar (Chapter 14) are distinctive for the group and often characteristic for genera. For example, *Klebsiella* typically produces a large, round, pink (acid), mucoid colony on MacConkey agar through its production of a polysaccharide capsule and its fermentation of lactose. These colonial features are useful guides in clinical microbiology laboratories, but are not intrinsically diagnostic because exceptions are common.

Antigenic Structure

The cell wall, capsular slime layer, and flagellar antigens are valuable in identification and in subtyping for epidemiologic purposes. The extent to which these features have been studied and classified varies greatly among the genera. *Escherichia* and *Salmonella* have been divided into hundreds of types based on the presence of various combinations of antigens, whereas other common genera such as *Proteus* have fewer described antigens. The difference in the number of serotypes within different species is probably attributable to the extent to which they have been studied as much as to biologic differences.

Multiple serotypes

Flagella are composed of proteins, and their antigenic determinants are designated *H antigens*. Cell surface antigens are generally polysaccharides and are termed *K antigens* (from the Danish *Kapsel,* capsule) regardless of whether they form a well-defined capsule. Specialized designations are given to surface polysaccharides of certain species, such as the Vi antigen of *Salmonella typhi*. The pili are proteins with a repeating subunit structure, and, although antigenic, they are not part of any formal typing scheme. The cell wall lipopolysaccharide (LPS) is described as the *O antigen*. The antigenic specificity of the O antigen is determined by the composition and linkage of the sugars that form the polysaccharide side chains. The remaining portion of the LPS is a conserved core polysaccharide backbone linked to the lipid A (see Chapter 2 for details). These core antigens are common to other members of the Enterobacteriaceae and to some other Gram-negative bacteria. Their use as immunogens has demonstrated some cross-immunity between species.

Flagellar H antigens

Polysaccharide surface K antigens

Cell wall O antigen

Core antigen

Classification

Genera classified by differences in motility and major biochemical characteristics

Species identified by battery of biochemical tests

Because they are among the most metabolically diverse of bacteria, the Enterobacteriaceae have been classified into genera according to their many cultural and biochemical characteristics. All are facultative, all ferment glucose and reduce nitrates to nitrites, and all are oxidase negative. The currently recognized tribes, genera, and species of significant medical importance and their major characteristics are shown in the appendix. Species designations are based on a battery of physiologic characteristics, including most of those discussed in Chapter 14. They include the ability to ferment various carbohydrates, indole production from tryptophan, citrate utilization, amino acid breakdown, and hydrogen sulfide production from sulfur-containing amino acids. These and many other characteristics, including presence or absence of motility, are used to construct probability tables for assignment of individual isolates to genera and species.

Subspecies classified by antigenic structure

Bacteriophage and bacteriocin typing

Within species, differences in the antigenic structure are used for further subdivision into serotypes. For some species, panels of bacteriocins or bacteriophages have been used to establish typing systems in place of, or in addition to, serotyping systems. None of these subtyping systems alone can identify unknown organisms, because cross-reactions are common with organisms from genera other than that for which the system was devised.

For practical reasons, only a portion of the diagnostic tools available for classifying the Enterobacteriaceae are used in clinical laboratories. A battery of 6–12 biochemical reactions is often sufficient to assign a genus identification, and a few more reactions will allow accurate species identification. In some instances, serologic reactions are used to confirm or extend the biochemical identification.

Significance of lactose fermentation

Rapid fermentation of lactose as demonstrated by acid (pink) colonies on MacConkey agar is a useful characteristic for initial differentiation of Enterobacteriaceae. The most common members of the intestinal flora, *Escherichia coli, Klebsiella,* and *Enterobacter,* ferment lactose promptly in more than 90% of cases, whereas many other genera, including the intestinal pathogens *Salmonella* and *Shigella,* are rarely positive.

Toxins

Endotoxin in all species

Some produce exotoxins

All Enterobacteriaceae possess the LPS endotoxin, the structure and functional effects of which are discussed in Chapters 2, 10, and 68. Many of the effects of endotoxin such as fever, leukopenia, and activation of blood coagulation factors are seen in human infections, particularly when organisms enter the bloodstream to produce bacteremia. In addition to LPS endotoxin, some Enterobacteriaceae also produce exotoxins, including enterotoxins and cytotoxins. These toxins will be discussed with the individual species, although it is now clear they may be found in a wide range of Enterobacteriaceae (Table 20.3). The genes for many are coded on plasmids that may be exchanged among the various genera.

Pathogenicity

Some cause specific diseases

Some species of Enterobacteriaceae are primary pathogens in that they have unique pathogenic features that may allow them to produce gastrointestinal or systemic infections in previously healthy individuals. Examples are bacillary dysentery, caused by *Shigella,* and typhoid fever, caused by *S. typhi.* Certain strains of species that are usually considered normal flora may also possess specific virulence factors that make them primary pathogens. These infections will be discussed as they relate to particular species. Species that are resident members of the normal flora, or that exist in the environment, can act as opportunistic pathogens if they are displaced from their normal site or if local or systemic defense mechanisms are damaged. They can produce a variety of infections, the characteristics of which are primarily determined by the organ involved. The most common are urinary tract infections, of which Enterobacteriaceae are the leading causes (Chapter 66), and wound infections (Chapter 59); however, spread beyond the local site may produce more extensive infection, including bacteremia and Gram-negative shock (Chapter 68).

Many are opportunists

Antimicrobic Susceptibility

Combinations of chromosomal and plasmid-determined resistance (Chapter 13) render Enterobacteriaceae the most variable of all bacteria in their susceptibility to antimicrobial agents. They are usually resistant to high concentrations of penicillin G, erythromycin, and clindamycin, but may be susceptible to the broader-spectrum β-lactams, aminoglycosides, tetracycline, chloramphenicol, sulfonamides, quinolones, nitrofurantoin, and the polypeptide antibiotics. As the probability of resistance varies among genera and in different epidemiologic settings, the susceptibility of any individual strain must be determined by in vitro tests. Typical frequencies of resistance for the more common Enterobacteriaceae appear in the appendix to Chapter 13.

Marked variation in susceptibility between and within species

Frequent need for in vitro tests

Escherichia coli

Escherichia coli is the most commonly encountered member of the Enterobacteriaceae in the normal colonic flora and a common cause of opportunistic infections. Most strains ferment lactose rapidly and produce indole. When grown on blood agar, many strains isolated from infections are hemolytic, a feature uncommon in other Enterobacteriaceae. The hemolysin, an antigenic protein encoded by plasmid genes, has been shown to be toxic in tissue culture and animal experiments. Serotyping systems have been established based on O and K antigens and using agglutination tests. There are over 150 somatic O antigens (for example, O55, O111, O144). The *E. coli* K antigens are also designated by number. Thus, the antigenic structure of individual strains is described by designations such as O111:K58 and O18:K76. In distinguishing O and K antigens, the heat stability of the LPS antigen is exploited: it can withstand boiling for an hour or more, whereas surface K antigens are either destroyed or removed by heating. Approximately 40 flagellar H types have also been defined for *E. coli*, but are used less frequently than O and K antigen types in diagnostic and epidemiologic studies.

Member of normal colonic flora; motile; lactose positive

Escherichia coli

Multiple serotypes based on O and K antigens

Pili are frequently present on the surface of *E. coli* strains and, as with group A streptococci (Chapter 16), play a role in virulence as mediators of attachment to human epithelial surfaces. *Escherichia coli* pili are classified according to the host cell types and specific receptors (if known) to which they bind (Table 20.1). Most *E. coli* possess pili that bind to the D-mannose residues present on the surface of a wide variety of cells. Experimentally, this binding is blocked by addition of mannose and they are thus called *mannose-sensitive* (MS) *pili*. Other terms for these are common pili or type 1 pili. Pili with other receptors and that are not blocked by mannose are called *mannose resistant* (MR). The receptor for some MR pili is known,

Pathogenic significance of pili

Mannose-sensitive common (type 1) pili

Many mannose-resistant pili with affinity for different receptors

Table 20.1 Adherence Characteristics of *Escherichia coli* Strains

Strain	Epithelial Cell Type	Adhesin		Epithelial Cell Receptor	Genetic Control
		Class	Pili		
General (common)	Various	MS	Type 1	D-Mannose	Chromosomal
Uropathic	Bladder, kidney	MR	P (Gal–Gal)	Galactopyranosyl–galactopyranoside (P blood group)	Chromosomal
ETEC (human)	Enterocyte (human)	MR	CFA	Unknown	Plasmid
ETEC (animal)	Enterocyte (pigs, calves)	MR	K88, K99	Unknown	Plasmid

Abbreviations: MS = mannose sensitive; MR = mannose resistant; ETEC = enterotoxigenic *E. coli*; CFA = colonizing factor antigens, CFA I, CFA II, others (see text).

for example, for some of the uropathic and enteropathic strains described below. Knowing the chemical nature of the receptor has increased understanding of pathogenic mechanisms and is important to the development of immunization strategies aimed at preventing attachment.

Variation in expression of pili; genetics and significance

The genetics of pilin expression is complex. Pili of different types may coexist on the same bacterium, and their expression may vary under different environmental conditions. Type 1 pilin expression can be turned on or off by inversion of a chromosomal DNA sequence containing the promoter responsible for initiating transcription of the pilin gene. Other genes control the on/off orientation of the "switch." Although not quite as complex as the situation with gonococci (Chapter 19), this is another example of the ability of a successful pathogen to produce a surface protein for a useful purpose (attachment) and then shed it when it may be a disadvantage (immune surveillance).

Urinary Tract Infections

E. coli from intestinal flora commonest cause of urinary tract infection

Escherichia coli is the most common cause of infections of the urinary bladder, renal pelvis, and kidney (Chapter 66). This finding is explained in part by the large numbers of *E. coli* commonly found in the large intestine and by contamination of the perineum and urethra, particularly in women. Relatively minor trauma or the mechanical effect of sexual intercourse may allow *E. coli* and other organisms from the perineum to gain access to the bladder. *Escherichia coli* can grow rapidly in urine, typically producing more than 10^5 bacteria per milliliter of urine in clinical infections. The attack rate is highest in sexually active women, and more than 90% of urinary tract infections developing outside hospitals are caused by *E. coli*.

Predominance in women during childbearing years

Certain serotypes predominate in urinary infections

In addition to the presence of the organism in the fecal flora, some determinants of virulence appear to be important in the pathogenesis of *E. coli* urinary infections; less than 20 of the 150 serotypes are responsible for most cases. A number of virulence factors have statistical association with urinary infection. These include adherence to uroepithelial cells, hemolysin production, amount and type of K antigen, siderophore production, and resistance to serum bactericidal activity. Type 1 pili are probably important in periurethral colonization as well as mediating attachment

Properties associated with virulence

to uroepithelial cells, but the binding is not as strong as by some of the MR pili.

Pili that bind to a galactopyranosyl galactopyranoside (Gal–Gal) receptor on human uroepithelial cells exhibit tighter binding than type 1 pili, and their presence is associated with ascending urinary tract infections. These pili are called *Gal–Gal* or *P pili,* because the receptor is present in the P blood antigen on the surface of human erythrocytes. Antibody against Gal–Gal pili blocks adherence, suggesting that this could be an approach to prevention of certain urinary tract infections. Factors that provide more ready access or delay the exit of *E. coli* from the bladder, such as urinary catheters or urinary obstruction by an enlarged prostate gland, are also associated with infection.

Urinary tract infections vary from asymptomatic to involvement of the entire tract, including the kidney; there are no clinical differences, however, between those caused by *E. coli* and those caused by other organisms (Chapter 66). The most common symptoms are dysuria and urinary frequency. When the renal pelvis and kidney are involved (pyelonephritis), fever and flank pain are common and bacteremia may develop. The duration of symptoms is quite variable, but response to antimicrobial therapy is usually prompt in uncomplicated cases.

Intestinal Infections

It had long been suspected that certain strains of *E. coli* could produce diarrhea, but the association was difficult to prove because multiple strains are present in virtually every stool specimen. When serotyping procedures became available, it was found that the presence of one or another of a small number of serotypes of *E. coli* was strongly associated with nursery outbreaks of diarrhea and, later, that their presence was also statistically associated with endemic disease in infants, children, and adults, particularly in developing countries. Subsequently, numerous studies showed that diarrhea in travelers to these areas was associated with the acquisition of serotypes of *E. coli* not represented before the disease developed. The serotypes involved, however, were generally different from those described in nursery outbreaks. From the mid-1960s to the present, the correlation of virulence factors (adherence, toxins, invasion) with epidemiologic data has clarified our understanding of how and when *E. coli* produces intestinal disease as a primary pathogen.

The major pathogenic classes of *E. coli* are enterotoxigenic *E. coli* (ETEC), enteroinvasive *E. coli* (EIEC), enterohemorrhagic *E. coli* (EHEC), and a group that includes most of the originally described serotypes, but that appear to owe their virulence to firm adherence to intestinal cells and local damage to the cell surface. These are now usually termed *enteropathic E. coli* (EPEC), a term that hopefully will be changed when their pathogenic mechanism is fully understood. The properties of these classes are summarized in Table 20.2.

Enterotoxigenic E. coli (ETEC). The ETEC strains elaborate two distinct enterotoxins that act on the intestinal mucosa to cause fluid outpouring and thus diarrhea. They are differentiated by whether or not they are stable to heat (boiling) and by their mechanism of action. ETEC strains may produce either heat-labile toxin (LT) or heat-stable toxin (ST) but most often produce both. The genes for both toxins are plasmid borne, usually on the same plasmid.

Heat-labile toxin is inactivated by boiling and acts by stimulating aden-

Margin notes

Roles of type 1 and P pili

Symptoms

Epidemiologic association of serotypes with nursery and traveler's diarrhea

Classes of pathogenic *E. coli*

Plasmid coded heat-labile and -stable toxins

Table 20.2 Features of Intestinal Infection by *Escherichia coli*

Feature	ETEC	EIEC	EHEC	EPEC
Primary pathogenic mechanism	Enterotoxin LT and/or ST	Invasion of enterocytes	Shigalike cytotoxin	Adherence to enterocytes
Primary site	Small intestine	Large intestine	Large intestine	Small intestine[a]
Mucosal pathology	Intact, hyperemia	Necrosis, ulceration, inflammation	Destruction of microvilli, cell death	Destruction of microvilli
Genetic control	Toxin genes on plasmid	Invasive genes on plasmid	Lysogenic phage	Plasmid associated
Epidemiology	Traveler's diarrhea, childhood diarrhea[b]	Sporadic, uncommon	Hemorrhagic colitis; hemolytic–uremic syndrome	Infantile and childhood diarrhea[b]
Fever	Absent	Common	Absent	Common
Stools				
Nature	Copious, watery	Scanty, purulent	Copious, bloody	Copious, watery
Blood	Absent	Common	Prominent	Absent
Pus (WBCs)	Absent	Prominent	Absent	Absent

Abbreviations: ETEC = enterotoxigenic *E. coli*; EIEC = enteroinvasive *E. coli*; EHEC = enterohemorrhagic *E. coli*; EPEC = enteropathogenic *E. coli*; LT = heat-labile toxin; ST = heat-stable toxins; WBCs = white blood cells.

[a] In experimental animals EPEC strains produce lesions in the large intestine as well.

[b] These are much more common in developing countries. ETEC strains are rare in the United States.

LT acts like cholera toxin

ST also causes fluid loss

Role of colonizing factor antigens (pili)

Plasmid genes code for pili and toxins

Significance of ETEC in developing world

ETEC produce afebrile watery diarrhea

ylate cyclase in mucosal cells. This produces an accumulation of cyclic AMP, which interferes with transport of sodium and chloride ions by the intestinal epithelial cells. The net effect is the transfer of electrolytes and water from the mucosa to the intestinal lumen. The structure and mechanism of action of the toxin are similar to cholera toxin, which is considered in more detail in Chapter 21. Heat-stable toxin produces effects similar to LT, but through stimulation of guanylate cyclase (Table 20.3).

Toxin production alone is not sufficient for ETEC strains to produce disease, and pilin-mediated attachment to intestinal epithelial cells must occur. The ETEC pili are called *colonizing factor antigens* (CFA) and are assembled from various combinations of protein subunits of which six have been described. The pili are MR, but their specific receptor is not known. In contrast to type 1 and Gal–Gal pili, the genes for the CFAs are located on plasmids. In fact, in individual strains the same plasmid usually carries the genes for CFA, LT, and/or ST.

When the *E. coli* enterotoxins were discovered, it was expected that they would be the mechanisms of disease in the earlier epidemiologic studies of *E. coli* diarrhea. This has only been partially borne out, although ETEC are the most common cause of traveler's diarrhea and an important cause of infant diarrheas in the developing world.

Clinically, they cause an afebrile, watery diarrhea that resolves in a few days. ETEC strains have not, however, been recovered in the majority of hospital nursery epidemics and, aside from occasional outbreaks, are rarely found in the United States or other developed countries.

Enteroinvasive E. coli (EIEC).   The EIEC strains produce disease by mech-

Table 20.3 Exotoxins Produced by *Enterobacteriaceae*

Toxin	Target	Enzymatic Activity	Primary Action	Effect	Genetic Control
Escherichia coli LT	G regulatory protein	ADP-ribosylation	Adenylate cyclase stimulation	Fluid loss	Plasmid
Escherichia coli ST	Unknown	Unknown	Guanylate cyclase stimulation	Fluid loss	Plasmid
Shigella dysenteriae, type 1 Shiga toxin	60S ribosome	Unknown	Inhibits protein synthesis	Cell death	Chromosomal
Shigalike toxins[a]	? 60S ribosome	Unknown	Inhibits protein synthesis	Cell death	Temperate phage[b] or chromosomal
Candidate toxins					
Salmonella enterotoxin	Unknown	Unknown	Adenylate cyclase stimulation	Fluid loss	Unknown
Salmonella cytotoxin	Unknown	Unknown	Unknown	Cell death	Unknown
Yersinia ST	Unknown	Unknown	Guanylate cyclase stimulation	Fluid loss	Unknown

Abbreviations: LT = heat-labile toxin; ST = heat-stable toxin; EHEC = enterohemorrhagic *E. coli*; EPEC = enteropathogenic *E. coli*.

[a] Produced by other *Shigella* species, EHEC, and some EPEC.

[b] Phage conversion shown for strains of EHEC and EPEC, others chromosomal or unknown.

anisms entirely analogous to *Shigella,* which are described below. They penetrate epithelial cells and multiply within them, leading to cell death. As with *Shigella,* these features are associated with a large plasmid and result in a dysenteric illness characterized by fever and blood and pus in the stool. Epidemiologic studies have shown EIEC to be a relatively rare cause of diarrhea, although outbreaks occur, including foodborne outbreaks.

EIEC produce dysentery by same mechanism as *Shigella*

Enterohemorrhagic E. coli (EHEC).   This is the most recently recognized class of diarrhea-producing *E. coli.* Its detection derives from a 1982 multistate outbreak of hemorrhagic colitis traced to a strain of the 0157:H7 serotype. The disease was characterized by copious bloody diarrhea without pus in the stool. This strain, and others of the same serotype from similar cases, were later shown to elaborate a potent cytotoxin distinct from LT and ST. The toxin has been given a variety of names, but is now termed Shigalike toxin because it acts in a manner apparently identical to that produced by *Shigella dysenteriae type 1* (see below). At least one other serotype has been included in the EHEC class, and there may be a second form of the Shiga toxin. The hemolytic–uremic syndrome is also strongly associated with toxin-producing 0157:H7 strains.

EHEC commonly of 0157:H7 serotype

Produces potent cytotoxin

Cause of bloody diarrhea and hemolytic–uremic syndrome

Enteropathogenic E. coli (EPEC).   These strains belong to many of the serotypes described in the early investigations of nursery outbreaks of diarrhea. Recent studies, including human volunteer studies, show that

EPEC show firm adherence to Hep-2 cells

they are primary pathogens. Enteropathogenic *E. coli* adhere to a continuous line of human laryngeal carcinoma cells (Hep-2). This property is associated with a large plasmid characteristic of classical EPEC serotypes but which is rare in ETEC, EIEC, or other *E. coli*. In addition, a distinctive histopathologic lesion has been noted in human intestines. The EPEC bacteria adhere tightly to the small bowel mucosa with destruction of the enterocyte microvilli. The precise mechanisms of pathogenesis have not been established and are being actively investigated.

Destruction of enterocyte microvilli

Febrile diarrhea and vomiting; severe in infants

Clinically, EPEC produce diarrhea with malaise, vomiting, and often fever. The stools contain mucus, but not gross blood. In infants, the illness may be prolonged and life-threatening with severe dehydration. Enteropathogenic *E. coli* are important causes not only of nursery outbreaks, but of other infant and childhood diarrheas in developing countries.

It is clear also that the virulence factors described above are not strictly limited to their respective groups. Shigalike toxin, for example, is produced by some EPEC strains and plasmid-mediated toxins (LT and ST) and adherence factors can be transmitted and expressed in different *E. coli* strains or even other members of the Enterobacteriaceae.

Precise diagnosis involves detecting virulence factors or genes

The diagnosis of *E. coli* diarrhea requires detection of one or more of the virulence factors and is not yet a routine clinical laboratory procedure. Determining that the strain falls into one of the serotypes that have been associated with disease is, at best, only presumptive evidence in suspected outbreaks. Gene probes for ETEC (LT and ST) have been successfully applied to clinical isolates and direct stool specimens, and an EHEC probe has been shown to detect EHEC strains of both 0157:H7 and other serotypes. These hybridization methods are not yet used for routine diagnosis in the United States due to their cost in relation to the relatively small number of infections. In short, despite great advances in our knowledge, it is still not practicable for hospital laboratories to separate the *E. coli* strains capable of producing diarrhea from all the others.

Meningitis

Common cause of neonatal meningitis

Escherichia coli is one of the most common causes of neonatal meningitis (Chapters 67 and 69). This infection results from *E. coli* colonization of the vagina and contamination of amniotic fluid, failure of protective maternal immunoglobulin M (IgM) antibodies to cross the placenta, and the special susceptibility of newborns. Fully 75% of cases are caused by strains possessing the K1 surface polysaccharide antigen, which appears in less than 10% of normal fecal isolates. Interestingly, it is chemically and antigenically identical to the group B meningococcal polysaccharide, but the genes coding for the two show no homology. A significant proportion of blood isolates are also K1 strains. The mechanism for enhanced virulence of these *E. coli* strains is not known.

Association with K1 antigen

Opportunistic Infections

Predisposing factors

With the exception of urinary tract infections, extraintestinal *E. coli* infections are uncommon. If there is a significant breach in host defenses, however, *E. coli* and other members of the Enterobacteriaceae are potent opportunists. Opportunistic infection may follow mechanical damage, such as a ruptured intestinal diverticulum or intestinal trauma, or involve a generalized impairment of immune function.

The particular diseases that result depend on the sites involved and include many of the syndromes covered in Chapters 59–73. Because of the underlying diseases, opportunistic infections are commonly associated with hospitalized patients and often involve strains resistant to multiple antimicrobics.

Antimicrobial Susceptibility

Community-acquired strains often susceptible

In the community, *E. coli* strains are commonly susceptible to all agents with potential activity against the Enterobacteriaceae. Sulfonamides and/ or trimethoprim are frequently used in uncomplicated urinary tract infections in the community because of the high probability that a susceptible *E. coli* is the cause. Antimicrobial therapy of complicated and opportunistic infections must be guided by susceptibility testing; because of the frequent occurrence of R plasmids, strains acquired in hospitals may be resistant to any combination of potentially effective antimicrobics.

Hospital isolates often resistant through R plasmids

Shigella

Shigella species are closely related to *E. coli* biochemically and antigenically. Most fail to ferment lactose or to produce gas when fermenting glucose, and all are nonmotile. They are strict pathogens that cause bacillary dysentery, a common disease with worldwide distribution. They do not appear as members of the normal flora, although they may be carried for days or weeks during convalescence.

Nonmotile; lactose negative

Shigella

Classification

The genus *Shigella* is divided into four species, or groups, on the basis of differences in O antigens and some biochemical reactions. They are *Shigella dysenteriae* (group A), *Shigella flexneri* (group B), *Shigella boydii* (group C), and *Shigella sonnei* (group D), as shown in the appendix. All but *S. sonnei* are further subdivided into a total of more than 30 individual serotypes. *Shigella dysenteriae* type 1, also known as the *Shiga bacillus,* is the cause of classic tropical bacillary dysentery, a disease more serious than those produced by other *Shigella* strains.

Four species; 30 serotypes

Pathogenesis

Strict human pathogens

All *Shigella* species can be considered strict human pathogens. Significant nonhuman reservoirs do not exist, except in laboratory-maintained primates, and the organism does not survive long after excretion. The organism itself is highly communicable: less than 100 bacteria can initiate infection in healthy persons. Transmission is usually by contaminated fingers, food, or water. Multiplication to high numbers (10^8-10^9 bacteria/ ml) in the distal small intestine requires 12 hr or less. Within 1–4 days, the organism invades the large intestine. The primary mechanism of disease production is penetration of colonic epithelial cells, subsequent multiplication both within the cells and in the lamina propria, and then superficial tissue destruction. This process, which occurs mainly in the lower colon, produces acute inflammation and shallow ulcers scattered along the mucosal surface. Invasion beyond the intestinal mucosa or local lymph nodes is rare, and the organisms are rarely found in deeper tissues or the bloodstream. The Shiga bacillus (*S. dysenteriae* type 1) is more likely than other species to produce bacteremia.

Low infecting dose

Multiplication in small intestine

Penetration and ulceration of colonic epithelium

Invasiveness

Shigella virulence plasmid

Under experimental conditions, virulent shigellae are able to penetrate and multiply in a wide variety of cell types both in animal models and in cell culture. Invasiveness requires the presence of a large "virulence" plasmid, and if this plasmid is lost or altered, the organism is no longer virulent. One region of the virulence plasmid of *S. flexneri* has been shown to contain genes for a series of proteins that are required for invasiveness. These, and the plasmid that encodes them, are also features of invasive *E. coli*. In fact, the EIEC virulence plasmids are at least 80% homologous with their *Shigella* counterparts.

Endocytosis and multiplication within cells

The invasive process involves the ability of the organism to induce its endocytosis by epithelial cells. Subsequent stages are lysis of the endocytic vacuole, multiplication in the cytoplasm, cell destruction, infection of adjacent cells, and spread to the connective tissue of the intestinal villus. The first two steps appear to be mediated by the plasmid-encoded invasive proteins, but at least three chromosomal loci are also required for full expression of virulence and are probably important for survival of shigellae when they have escaped the cell. A siderophore aids multiplication by scavenging scarce iron in tissues, and Shiga toxin (see below) surely contributes to cell death.

Shiga and Shigalike Toxins

Neurocytotoxin

Binding and toxic subunits of toxin

The Shiga bacillus has long been known to produce an exotoxin with enterotoxic, cytotoxic, and neurotoxic properties. Recently the structure and action of Shiga toxin have been discovered. It has an A/B structure with one active (A) and five binding (B) subunits. The B subunits bind to a glycoprotein receptor on the cell membrane, and the toxin enters by receptor-mediated endocytosis. Once in the cell, the A subunit is modified prior to or during the course of leaving the vacuole to act on its target. These events are similar to those with diphtheria toxin (Chapter 17). The

Ribosomal target; inhibits protein synthesis

target of Shiga toxin is the 60S ribosome to which it binds and inhibits protein synthesis, leading to cell death. The genes for Shiga toxin appear to be chromosomal.

Shigalike toxins in other *Shigella* spp. and pathogenic *E. coli*

Until recently, the Shiga bacillus was felt to be the only organism producing Shiga toxin. It is now clear that other species of *Shigella*, EHEC strains of *E. coli,* and some EPEC strains of *E. coli* produce toxin(s) very similar if not identical to Shiga toxin. One definite difference between *Shigella* and both EPEC and EHEC strains of *E. coli* is that in *E. coli* the toxin is encoded in specific temperate bacteriophages.

Responsible for colonic cell necrosis

The watery diarrhea often seen in the early stages of shigellosis while the organisms are still in the small intestine may be due to other enterotoxins, but Shiga and Shigalike toxins appear responsible for the cell death and necrosis of colonic epithelium. The unusual severity of *S. dysenteria* type 1 may be due to production of larger amounts of Shiga toxin than is the case with the other species.

Immunity

Immunity short-lived, apparently IgA dependent

Shigellosis is usually self-limiting, and infection produces relatively short-lived immunity to reinfection with homologous serogroups. The exact mechanism is not known; however, local IgA production in the intestinal wall is probably more important than humoral immunity. The development of herd immunity through infection and exposure to one serogroup may be responsible for shifts in serogroup prevalence. This hypothesis is suggested by the cyclic patterns of prevalence and serogroup distribution seen over 20- to 30-year periods.

Epidemiology

Fecal–oral spread

Like other diarrheal infections, shigellosis is strongly associated with poor sanitary practices and poor nutrition. Its fecal-oral mode of spread, from contaminated hands, food, or fomites, usually involves close contact with infected cases; however, flies can be passive vectors.

High infectivity

The low infecting dose and short incubation period facilitate efficient transmission through a population by direct contact. In the past, major outbreaks often occurred during military infantry campaigns through stress and lack of washing or sanitary facilities, and sometimes proved effective peacemakers. Transmission through water and food is responsible for most focal outbreaks. In the United States, 15,000–20,000 cases of shigellosis are reported yearly. Most of these cases are *S. sonnei* infections in children under 10 years of age, with the peak at age 2. Once a case is introduced into a household or day-care center, the secondary attack rate by simple hand-to-mouth spread among toddlers may exceed 50%. Organisms are present in stools up to 1 month after an untreated infection. Prolonged carriage is uncommon, but may be the source of a food-borne outbreak.

Outbreaks of *S. sonnei* infection in small children

The most common *Shigella* species in developed countries is *S. sonnei,* followed by *S. flexneri* and *S. boydii. Shigella dysenteriae,* particularly the Shiga bacillus, is rare where hygiene is good, but is endemic in tropical, underdeveloped countries. In the mid-1970s, an extensive epidemic of Shiga dysentery occurred in Central America, with occasional cases imported into the United States.

Clinical Features

Fever, bloody mucoid stools, and cramping

Shigellosis is an acute diarrheal illness marked by painful passage of bloody, mucoid stools with cramping (dysentery). The stools may initially be watery and voluminous, but quickly become mucoid, bloody, and of smaller volume as the disease localizes in the colon. The typical picture comprises frequent, small stools (squirts) with urgency and tenesmus. Although fever is considered a useful feature in differentiating shigellosis from other infectious diarrheas, it is present in less than one-half of cases.

Most infections self-limiting

The disease is almost always self-limiting; symptoms last a few days to a month, although most cases recover in less than a week without treatment. Except with Shiga dysentery, fatal infections and complications are rare, unless serious underlying disease and/or malnutrition are present. Dysentery caused by the Shiga bacillus is typically more severe; it may occasionally extend beyond the gastrointestinal tract to produce bacteremia.

Shiga dysentery most severe; may be fatal

The illness may prove fatal in previously healthy persons, and mortality in epidemics has been as high as 10–20%. With the speed of modern travel, imported cases of Shiga dysentery are possible despite the short incubation period.

Diagnosis

Shigellosis should be suspected in any patient with a diarrheal illness associated with fever, toxemia, or other systemic symptoms. The presence of blood and pus in the stool is suggestive, but not specific; other invasive pathogens (for example, enteroinvasive *E. coli, Campylobacter*), as well as some noninfectious diseases, can also produce this finding. Furthermore, absence of macroscopic or microscopic blood and pus does not exclude shigellosis.

Stool culture on selective media

The only definitive laboratory test is the stool culture. Stool specimens or rectal swabs will yield the organism if promptly plated on appropriate indicator (MacConkey agar) and selective media (Hektoen agar). Enrichment culture techniques are less effective with *Shigella* than with *Salmonella*. Specimens collected early in the course of illness are more likely to be positive, because the organisms are much more numerous.

Specimens must be cultured promptly to avoid loss of viability

Prompt plating of specimens is important, as the organisms do not survive well outside the body. Non–lactose-fermenting colonies are screened with biochemical tests, and identification is confirmed with antisera specific for each of the four serogroups (A–D). Typing within the groups is usually available only in reference facilities.

Treatment

Treatment may shorten illness and period of excretion

Several antimicrobics have proved effective in the treatment of shigellosis. Because the disease is usually self-limiting, the beneficial effect of treatment is in shortening the illness and the period of excretion of organisms; however, resistance may develop by plasmid transfer. The original discovery of in vivo plasmid transfer involved cases of shigellosis in which the infecting strain acquired multidrug resistance during therapy from an *E. coli* present simultaneously in the bowel. Resistance rates of 5–50% to ampicillin, once considered the treatment of choice, have caused a shift to trimethoprim-sulfamethoxazole in many areas. Tetracycline and the quinolones have also been effective against susceptible strains. Mild cases are usually not treated, particularly in adults, who are already improving by the time the organism is isolated. As the diarrhea is not voluminous, fluid replacement can usually be accomplished orally. Antispasmodic agents to control diarrhea may make the patient worse and are not indicated in shigellosis or other invasive diarrheas.

R plasmid-determined resistance

Fluid replacement

Prevention

Sanitation, insect control, hand washing, cooking

Standard sanitation practices such as sewage disposal and water chlorination are important in preventing the spread of shigellosis. In certain circumstances insect control may also be important, because flies can serve as passive vectors when open sewage is present. Good individual sanitary practices, such as hand washing and proper cooking of food, are highly protective.

Vaccines

Killed parenteral vaccines lead to serum antibody responses, but have not been effective in preventing the disease. Orally administered live attenuated strains are proving more promising. These strains include *Shigella* mutants and *E. coli-Shigella* hybrids that fail to penetrate the mucosa or to multiply after penetration. The most recent interest is in construction of plasmids containing selected *Shigella* virulence factors that can then be transformed into an otherwise avirulent *E. coli*. Such strains used as live vaccines could, for example, immunize against the invasive proteins but lack the other determinants necessary to produce disease.

Klebsielleae

Members of colonic flora or free living

Although neither as frequent nor as numerous as *E. coli*, the Klebsielleae, or *Klebsiella-Enterobacter-Serratia* group, are commonly found among the gastrointestinal flora. Many are found free living in nature. Members of

Most ferment lactose

Opportunists

the group share similar biochemical features (appendix). With the exception of *Serratia* species, they are usually characterized by prompt lactose fermentation. All can be considered opportunistic pathogens, but do not characteristically produce exotoxin or invade healthy individuals. They are usually associated with nosocomial infections, particularly pneumonia and urinary tract infections. The group as a whole is resistant to ampicillin, and multiresistant strains are common.

Klebsiella

Nonmotile, encapsulated

Multiple capsular types

Association with disease

The most distinctive bacteriologic features of the genus *Klebsiella* are the absence of motility and the presence of a polysaccharide capsule. The latter gives colonies a glistening, mucoid character and forms the basis of a serotyping system. Seventy-two capsular types have been defined; they can be differentiated by precipitin, agglutination, and quellung reactions, although the antisera are usually available only in reference laboratories. Cross-reactions occur between certain *Klebsiella* polysaccharide capsular antigens and those of other encapsulated pathogens, such as *Streptococcus pneumoniae* and *Haemophilus influenzae*. These cross-reactions suggest parallels in the mechanisms of pathogenesis and immunity; the relationship of the *Klebsiella* capsule to virulence, however, has not been demonstrated.

Another similarity to the pneumococcus is the ability of *Klebsiella pneumoniae* to cause classic lobar pneumonia; this association is rare, however, and cases usually involve individuals severely compromised by age or disease. Most *Klebsiella* pneumonias are indistinguishable from those produced by other members of the Enterobacteriaceae. *Klebsiella pneumoniae* is by far the most common species and the most frequent cause of infection. *Klebsiellae* are usually resistant to ampicillin and carbenicillin. Plasmid-mediated resistance to other antimicrobics is common.

Enterobacter

Motile

Enterobacter species generally ferment lactose promptly and produce colonies similar to those of *Klebsiella,* although not as mucoid. A differential feature is motility by peritrichous flagella, which are generally present in *Enterobacter* species but uniformly absent in *Klebsiella.*

Resistance to ampicillin and first-generation cephalosporins

β-Lactamase-derepressed mutants

Enterobacter species and infections are less common than those of *Klebsiella*. They are usually found in mixed infections, in which their significance must be decided on clinical and epidemiologic grounds. Several hospital outbreaks traced to contaminated parenteral fluid solutions have implicated *Enterobacter* species. Most isolates are resistant to ampicillin and first-generation cephalosporins, but may be susceptible to second- or third-generation cephalosporins, although mutants derepressed for β-lactamase production occur at relatively high frequency and confer resistance to many cephalosporins.

Serratia

Some yield red colonies; DNAase positive

Isolates often highly resistant

Serratia strains ferment lactose slowly (3–4 days), if at all. Some produce distinctive brick-red colonies. Although the least commonly isolated of the group, the genus produces the same range of opportunistic infections seen with the rest of the Enterobacteriaceae. *Serratia* strains show consistent resistance to ampicillin and cephalothin, with the frequent addition of plasmid-determined resistance to many other antimicrobics, including the aminoglycosides. Sporadic infections and nosocomial outbreaks with multiresistant strains have often been difficult to control, and some *Serratia* isolates are resistant to essentially all available antimicrobics.

Salmonelleae

The Salmonelleae tribe includes a range of pathogens that can infect otherwise healthy individuals. Most are associated with disease in a wide range of vertebrates, although *S. typhi,* the cause of typhoid fever, is a strict human pathogen. The organisms are motile by peritrichous flagella. *Salmonella* species do not ferment lactose; some *Arizona* and *Citrobacter* strains, however, may ferment lactose. The ability to produce hydrogen sulfides from sulfur-containing amino acids is a group feature that is used to identify colonies on primary isolation media. As members of the group resemble each other closely, detailed biochemical testing is necessary for differentiation at the species level.

Usually lactose negative; motile; produce H_2S

Classification

The genus *Salmonella* is presently classified into three antigenically homogenous species (*Salmonella typhi, Salmonella paratyphi* A and *Salmonella choleraesuis*) and also into a very large group (1500 +) of organisms distinguished on the basis of differences in their O and H antigenic structure and referred to as *Salmonella* serotypes. Serotypes have been given names such as typhimurium (mouse typhoid), budapest, seminole, tamale, and oysterbeds, which reflect the condition or place from which they were first isolated and add color to the microbiological literature. These serotypes are often designated as though they are species, for example, *Salmonella typhimurium* rather than as *Salmonella* serotype typhimurium. This simplifies description and will be used in the chapter. More than 80 O antigens have been found and numbered. Several are represented in any given strain, and strains with similar combinations of O antigens are organized into nine broad serogroups. There are also multiple flagellar H antigens, more than one of which may be represented on a flagellum. In addition, most *Salmonella* strains show the phenomenon of phase variation of their H antigens; that is, they can synthesize two distinct sets of flagella, termed *phase 1* and *phase 2*. Population shifts between these two phases depend on various cultural and immunologic conditions. Phase 1 and 2 flagellins are coded by genes termed H1 and H2. Expression is controlled by an H2 promoter, which can invert. In one orientation it activates H2 and an H1 repressor. In the other, H2 is not transcribed and H1 is expressed (see Chapter 4).

S. typhi, S. paratyphi A, S. choleraesuis, and group of 1500 + named serotypes

Serotypes distinguished by H and O antigenic structure

Flagellar antigen phase variation

Examples of antigenic formulas for the three species and two of the *Salmonella* serotypes are shown in Table 20.4.

Diseases and Pathogenesis

Salmonella serotype infections usually result from ingestion of numerous organisms in food or occasionally water. Smaller numbers may infect under conditions that decrease gastric acidity or transit time through the stomach (achlorhydria, vagotomy, gastrectomy), presumably because more viable bacteria reach the small intestine. Once in the small intestine, the organisms may multiply and produce an acute enterocolitis with fever, diarrhea, and evidence of inflammation of the bowel; however, infection and colonization may be asymptomatic. These *Salmonella* species have been shown experimentally to penetrate the intestinal mucosa, but do not multiply in

High infecting dose for Salmonella serotype infections

Enterocolitis

Table 20.4 Antigenic Composition of Some *Salmonella* Species and Serotypes

Species (serotype)	Sero-group	O Antigens	Surface Antigens	Phase of H Antigens 1	Phase of H Antigens 2
S. paratyphi A	A	1, 2, 12	—	a	1, 5
S. serotype *typhimurium*	B	1, 4, 5, 12	—	i	1, 2
S. serotype *durban*	D	9, 12	—	a	e, n, z_{15}
S. typhi	D	9, 12	Vi	d	None
S. choleraesuis	C	6, 7	—	c	1, 5

Possible role of toxins

the enterocyte to the extent that *Shigella* does. The factors that determine this invasion and spread by *Salmonella* are not known. Recently toxins with both cytotoxic (shigalike) and enterotoxic (choleralike) properties have been described in *Salmonella*. Although these could explain both the fluid outpouring and inflammatory components of *Salmonella* diarrhea, the association remains speculative. Table 20.5 compares pathogenic features of *Salmonella* and *Shigella*.

Salmonella septicemia associated with *S. choleraesuis*

Salmonella choleraesuis and some *Salmonella* serotypes invade the mucosa and spread to the bloodstream without producing enteritis. Bacteremia is demonstrable, and secondary infections can occur at almost any anatomic site. It must be reemphasized, however, that the most common disease caused by *Salmonella* is enterocolitis.

Enteric fever usually caused by *S. typhi* (typhoid fever)

Enteric fever represents yet another type of disease. It is usually caused by *S. typhi* and occasionally by *S. paratyphi* A or one of the group of serotypes. The infecting dose is less than that required for *Salmonella* enterocolitis, and infection is usually transmitted by fecally contaminated

Table 20.5 Pathogenic Features of *Salmonella* and *Shigella* Species

Species	Toxins Cyto-toxin	Toxins Entero-toxin	Epithelial Cell Invasion	Intracellular Multiplication	Primary Site	Bacteremia	Mortality (Untreated)
Salmonella							
S. typhi	?	?	+ +	Macrophage type phagocytes	RES	>90%	5–15%
S. choleraesuis	?	?	+ +	?	Small bowel; tissues	20–50%	Low
Serotypes[a]	+	+	+	+	Small bowel	<10%	Very low
Shigella							
S. dysenteriae, 1	Shiga	—	+ + +	Enterocytes	Large bowel	Variable	10–20%
Other	Shigalike	—	+ + +	Enterocytes	Large bowel	<10%	Very low

Abbreviation: RES = reticuloendothelial system.

[a] Based on studies primarily with *S. typhimurium*.

food or water. The disease begins with multiplication of *S. typhi* in the small intestine. The organism penetrates the mucosa without producing enterocolitis, but does not immediately spread to the blood and distant organs. Instead, upon reaching regional lymph nodes, it multiplies within mononuclear cells, then spreads to reticuloendothelial sites in the liver, spleen, and bone marrow through the lymphatic system and blood during the incubation period (approximately 10 days). The intracellular survival of *S. typhi* is associated with inhibition of the oxidative metabolic burst of host phagocytes. Continued multiplication results in reseeding of the bloodstream with bacteria, necrosis of reticuloendothelial cells, and onset of clinical enteric fever. In the course of the bacteremia, other sites such as intestinal lymphoid follicles and the biliary tract become infected, leading to reinfection of the intestinal tract. The disease is thus primarily caused by the multiplication of *S. typhi* in the reticuloendothelial system.

Many of the clinical findings in enteric fever are similar to those caused by Gram-negative endotoxin. The prolonged fever and toxic symptoms in particular tempt one to attribute the disease to continuously circulating endotoxin. Efforts to verify this hypothesis experimentally have been unsuccessful, because endotoxin tolerance develops. Similarly, efforts to correlate symptoms with endotoxin detection in clinical cases have failed. The duration of fever may be attributable to prolonged and diffuse inflammation in the reticuloendothelial system with release of IL1 (endogenous pyrogen) and TNF (tumor necrosis factor).

Salmonella typhi usually possesses a polysaccharide Vi (virulence) surface antigen, which is associated with enhanced capacity to invade the host. The mechanism may involve interference with host phagocytic cells or with serum bactericidal activity. Its presence is not essential for virulence, but appears to lower the infecting dose necessary to produce disease.

Invasion without enterocolitis

Involvement of reticuloendothelial system

Bacteremia

Infection of intestinal lymphoid follicles and biliary tract

Role of endotoxin

S. typhi Vi antigen

Immunity

Experimental models of *Salmonella* infection have shown both humoral and cell-mediated immune mechanisms to be important in resistance to infection. The T cells of animals immunized with live *Salmonella* direct activation and expansion of the macrophage pool with enhanced phagocytosis and intracellular killing. Specific antibody production is also important in accelerating the rate of phagocytosis. It is not clear yet which antigens (surface polysaccharides, outer membrane proteins, lipopolysaccharides, etc) are the most important in eliciting protective immune responses, and this remains an important question for vaccine development.

Most of the experimental work on *Salmonella* immunity has been in a *S. typhimurium* mouse model that has similarities to human typhoid fever. The fact that *S. typhimurium* does not produce typhoid in humans and *S. typhi* does not produce typhoid in mice demands caution in extrapolating experimental findings to human enterocolitis, bacteremia, and enteric fever.

Both humoral and cell-mediated immunity involved

Epidemiology

Infections by *Salmonella* serotypes and *S. choleraesuis* are acquired usually through ingestion of contaminated food or, less often, of water. Direct fecal–oral spread is also possible, particularly in children; this mode of spread is not as efficient as with *Shigella*, however, because the infecting dose of *Salmonella* is much higher. Contamination of foodstuffs is usually

Salmonella serotype infection usually from food contamination with animal strains

Range of animal hosts

from the large reservoir in animals for which *Salmonella* is a primary pathogen. Virtually all species of poultry, mammals, reptiles, and amphibians may be infected, but *Salmonella* infection is particularly important in cattle and poultry kept under conditions of intensive husbandry. Some serotypes are more adapted to certain animal species, but all are potentially transmissible to humans.

Approximately 20,000–40,000 cases of human *Salmonella* enterocolitis are reported in the United States each year, making it one of the most common bacterial causes of diarrhea. The vehicles of transmission vary according to the animal reservoir; however, they usually involve animal products that are contaminated with *Salmonella* during processing, then handled in ways that allow the bacteria to multiply to levels that increase the probability of infection and disease. This situation usually results when incompletely cooked or uncooked food is allowed to remain warm for a few hours, during which time *Salmonella* can multiply to as many as 10^7–10^9 organisms per gram.

Organism multiplies in food to produce infecting dose

The classic example of *Salmonella* infection is the community picnic or bazaar, where volunteers prepare poultry, potato salad, and other potential culture media to be eaten later in the day. The source of contamination is often turkey or chicken or the surfaces on which they have been prepared for cooking. Because refrigerators are filled with iced tea, beer, and soda, the food is left out in covered pans. An appropriate incubation temperature is provided by the still-warm contents and the afternoon sun, and the organisms enter logarithmic growth during the softball game. The bacteria usually produce no noticeable change in the food, and those who eat it are stricken the following day in rough proportion to their degree of consumption. This series of events also occurs frequently with other types of bacterial food poisoning (Chapter 65).

Poultry, meat and dairy products common source of *Salmonella* serotype infection

Approximately one-half of *Salmonella* cases traced to specific vehicles involve poultry or poultry products in fresh, frozen, or dehydrated form. Meat and dairy products are also common vehicles. A recent increase in the popularity of raw milk has been associated with outbreaks of *Salmonella* (and *Campylobacter*) infection. Other sources include some dried egg products and exotic pets such as turtles. Like other enteric infections, *Salmonella* enterocolitis has a seasonal pattern with peaks in the summer months.

S. typhi an exclusively human pathogen

Infecting dose may be low

As there is no animal reservoir, cases of typhoid fever originate from other human cases or carriers of *S. typhi*. The vehicle of transmission may be water or food contaminated by a preparer carrying the organism. The infecting dose is much lower than that of the *Salmonella* serotypes, and multiplication outside the body before ingestion is usually unnecessary. Most of the 400–500 cases of typhoid fever reported yearly in the United States are now associated with travel to an endemic area or can be traced to a chronic carrier, who may have had the disease many years previously. Water-borne infection is very rare in areas with adequate sewage systems. A typhoid outbreak in 1973 among migrant workers in Florida was traced to leakage of sewage into the water supply, failure of chlorination, and a chronic carrier as the original source. Strains of *S. typhi* can be "fingerprinted" by bacteriophage typing to assist in tracing sources of infection.

Role of chronic carrier

Bacteriophage typing of *S. typhi*

Clinical Manifestations of Salmonellosis

Enterocolitis (Food Poisoning).   Illness begins with nausea, vomiting, and diarrhea of varying severity 6–48 hr after ingestion. Myalgia, headache, fever, and other constitutional symptoms may also develop. The diarrhea is usually intermediate in nature between the voluminous watery diarrhea

Incubation period 6–48 hr; constitutional signs of mucosal invasion; diarrhea

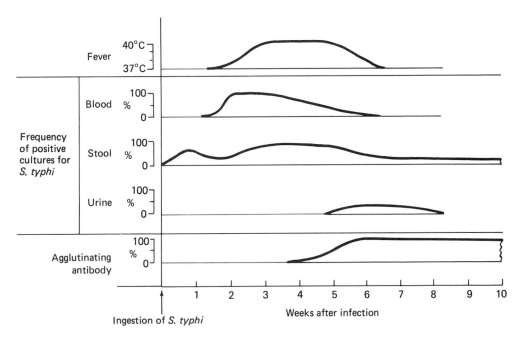

20.1 Natural history of enteric (typhoid) fever. The course of disease without antimicrobial therapy. Fever chart shows time course for typical patient. Culture and agglutinating antibody show timing and probability of positive results in a group of typhoid fever patients.

of cholera (Chapter 21) and the crampy diarrhea of shigellosis. Gross blood and pus are not common, but red and white cells may be seen on microscopic examination of the stool. The diarrhea usually reaches its peak within hours and typically lasts a few hours to a few days. There are considerable variations in severity and duration depending on host factors and inoculum size. For example, the infecting dose may be lower if the patient is on antibiotics to which the strain is resistant, presumably because of elimination of some competing flora. Infection tends to be more common, severe, and prolonged in infants, the aged, and the sick than in healthy adults. The usual case is self-limiting without extension beyond the gastrointestinal tract.

Enteric Fever. In contrast to *Salmonella* enterocolitis, diarrhea is not a prominent feature of enteric fever and is absent or mild in many cases (Figure 20.1). The illness has an insidious onset 10–14 days after ingestion of the organism, with fever, malaise, headache, and anorexia. Fever and constitutional signs increase over many days. Diarrhea may occur after 1 week, although the patient is often constipated. A maculopapular rash known as *rose spots* may appear on the abdomen in the second or third week, but rarely lasts more than a few days. Abdominal tenderness and distention are common as the disease progresses, and a palpable enlargement of the liver and spleen occurs in up to one-half of cases.

If the illness is not treated, the fever and other findings usually continue for 3–4 weeks, then decrease in a gradual stepwise fashion resembling the onset in reverse. The primary risk in enteric fever involves its com-

Disease usually self-limiting

Incubation period 10–14 days

Severe systemic disease lasting 3–4 weeks if untreated; diarrhea often absent

Complications of typhoid

Necrosis of intestinal lymphoid follicles with hemorrhage or rupture

infections in other organs (brain, bone, joints, heart valves), or local complications in the gastrointestinal tract. The latter involve infection, hyperplasia, and necrosis of the lymphoid aggregate follicles of the small intestine with ulceration of the intestinal mucosa. Intestinal hemorrhage from the necrotic patch or perforation into the peritoneal cavity is possible. Occasionally the enlarged, friable spleen ruptures. In the preantibiotic era, these complications were responsible for mortality as high as 15% in typhoid fever. With adequate antimicrobial therapy the infection, although still serious, is fatal in less than 1% of cases.

S. choleraesuis and S. enteritidis bacteremia

Osteomyelitis in sickle cell anemia and in the immunocompromised

Other Extraintestinal Infections. Bacteremia with signs of sepsis may be produced by *S. choleraesuis* or, sometimes, by *Salmonella* serotypes without associated diarrhea or even positive stool cultures, although the site of invasion is presumably the small intestine. Localization and abscess formation can occur in any anatomic site. Osteomyelitis is noteworthy, because it usually occurs in immunosuppressed patients and those with sickle cell anemia. *Salmonella* bacteremia may be potentiated by the presence of other infectious diseases. In parts of the world where typhus, malaria, and schistosomiasis are endemic, *Salmonella* bacteremia is an important complication of these and other systemic infections.

Carrier State

Typhoid carriage in the biliary tract

Excretion of *Salmonella* serotypes after enterocolitis may continue for a few weeks. Such cases are regarded as convalescent carriers; after 1 month, however, their frequency falls off sharply. Chronic carriage (more than 1 year), which often develops after *S. typhi* infection, is of great epidemiologic significance because carriers are the major reservoir for subsequent cases. The biliary tract is the primary site for chronic typhoid carriage, and eradication may be difficult in the presence of biliary tract disease. The presence of gallstones may require cholecystectomy to eliminate the carrier state.

Laboratory Diagnosis

Stool cultures for *Salmonella* serotype infection

Salmonella serotype enterocolitis is diagnosed by isolation of the causative organism from stool specimens using special indicator and selective media (for example, MacConkey, Hektoen, and xylose–lysine–deoxycholate). The media used most frequently are those appropriate for isolation of both *Salmonella* and *Shigella*. Enrichment broths such as selenite F are generally highly effective in detection of low concentrations of *Salmonella* from stools of cases and carriers. Serologic tests are not useful in the diagnosis or management of *Salmonella* serotype infection.

Blood cultures positive in early stages of enteric fever; stool cultures positive later

Serodiagnostic procedures of limited value

Enteric fever presents a special diagnostic problem because of its complex pathogenesis. As shown in Figure 20.1, the first specimens to yield the organism are blood cultures; stool and sometimes urine cultures become positive later in the clinical course. Most patients with typhoid fever develop agglutinating antibodies to the O and H antigens of *S. typhi* between the second and fourth weeks of illness. Tests for these antibodies may be used for diagnostic purposes; however, the timing of the antibody response (Figure 20.1), the effects of previous typhoid vaccination, and the occurrence of some false-positive and -negative results limits them to an adjunctive role. The diagnosis is best made by isolation of *S. typhi* from blood and/or stool as early in the illness as possible.

Treatment

Antimicrobics in *Salmonella* enterocolitis unhelpful

Uncomplicated enterocolitis rarely requires hospitalization or antimicrobial therapy. Fluid replacement by mouth is usually all that is necessary, unless there is evidence of spread beyond the intestinal tract. Treatment with antimicrobics does not significantly alter the clinical course, and it may cause prolonged excretion of *Salmonella*.

Antimicrobic treatment of enteric fever

Plasmid-mediated resistance

Treatment of chronic typhoid carriers

Enteric fever requires supportive fluid and nutritional therapy as well as an effective antimicrobial agent. *Salmonella typhi* is susceptible in vitro to many antimicrobics, but only chloramphenicol, ampicillin, trimethoprim-sulfamethoxazole and some quinolones and third generation cephalosporins have demonstrated clinical effectiveness. In recent years, therapy has been complicated by plasmid-mediated resistance including combined chloramphenicol-ampicillin resistance. Drug selection must be guided by susceptibility tests. Response to treatment is typically gradual, as with natural lysis of the disease. Treatment of the chronic carrier is difficult; for example, high-dose ampicillin therapy for 4–6 weeks is successful in only about 25% of cases without cholecystectomy. Trimethoprim-sulfamethoxazole may be more effective.

Prevention

Public health measures

Typhoid vaccines

Public health sanitary measures, good water and sewage treatment, and education on the proper means of cooking and storing food are the primary ways to prevent *Salmonella* infection. Typhoid vaccines consisting of whole, killed *S. typhi* are available for parenteral administration; the degree of protection is only relative, however, and the vaccines are associated with considerable reactions to their endotoxins. Recent studies with live, attenuated, and genetically engineered oral vaccines promise much more effective prophylaxis in the future.

Arizona

Reptiles major reservoir

Lactose fermentation common

The term *Arizona* refers to a group of closely related *Salmonella* serotypes originally isolated from lizards and gila monsters in Arizona. Their taxonomic status has varied over the years from that of a separate genus, to a species of *Salmonella,* and to a *Salmonella* serotype. Currently, they are referred to as *the Arizona group* of *Salmonella* serotypes. The most important practical difference from other salmonellas is fermentation of lactose by roughly one-half of strains. Many strains will therefore not be detected in routine stool culture procedures unless the laboratory is told of their possible presence. They are animal pathogens and isolation from humans has the same clinical significance as that of other *Salmonella* serotypes.

Citrobacter

Opportunists

The genus *Citrobacter,* although biochemically and serologically similar to *Salmonella,* does not cause typical *Salmonella* enterocolitis or enteric fever. These organisms, which may appear in the normal intestinal flora, are opportunistic pathogens like many other Enterobacteriaceae, such as *Enterobacter.* Despite reports of association of *Citrobacter* with diarrheal disease, present evidence does not indicate that the organism should be considered an enteric pathogen.

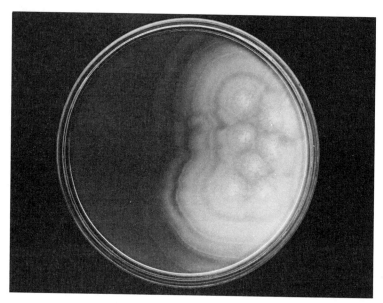

20.2 Swarming *Proteus*. This strain of *Proteus mirabilis* was inoculated at one spot on the blood agar plate. Note the waves of the spreading growth, which have covered the entire plate. On media containing bile salts (MacConkey agar) the swarming is inhibited and discrete colonies are formed.

Proteeae

Opportunists

The Proteeae, a group of organisms that includes the genera *Proteus, Morganella,* and *Providencia* (appendix), are also opportunistic pathogens found in varying frequencies in the normal intestinal flora. *Proteus mirabilis,* the most commonly isolated member of the group, is one of the most susceptible of the Enterobacteriaceae to the penicillins; this characteristic includes moderate susceptibility to penicillin G. Other Proteeae are regularly resistant to ampicillin and the cephalosporins. *Proteus mirabilis* and *Proteus vulgaris* share the ability to swarm over the surface of enriched media, rather than remaining confined to discrete colonies (Figure 20.2). This characteristic makes them readily recognizable in the laboratory—often with dismay, because the spreading growth covers other organisms in the culture and thus delays their isolation. *Proteus* and *Morganella* differ from other Enterobacteriaceae in the production of a very potent urease, which aids their rapid identification. It also leads to production of alkalinity and an ammoniac odor in urinary tract infections. *Providencia* species do not produce urease, are the least frequently isolated, and are generally the most resistant of the group to antimicrobics.

Swarming and nonswarming species

Proteus and *Morganella* elaborate potent urease

Yersinia

The genus *Yersinia* is now classified among the Enterobacteriaceae. Of the medically important species of the genus, *Yersinia pestis* and *Yersinia pseudotuberculosis* were previously included in the genus *Pasteurella* and are designated as such in the older literature. *Yersinia enterocolitica* was not described until the 1960s. Morphologically, *Yersinia* tend to be coccobacillary and to retain staining at the ends of the cells (bipolar staining); they otherwise resemble the rest of the Enterobacteriaceae. Their general growth and metabolic characteristics are the same as those of other Enterobacteriaceae, although some strains grow more slowly or have optimal growth temperatures below 37°C. *Yersinia* are primarily animal pathogens, with occasional transmission to humans through direct or indirect contact.

Primarily animal pathogens

Virulence mechanisms

Yersinia pestis is the cause of plague, one of the great pandemic infectious diseases in human history.

The virulence of *Yersinia* is related to its invasiveness, endotoxin, and in some instances, production of exotoxin. All three medically important species synthesize protein antigens, termed *V* and *W*, that are necessary for animal pathogenicity. In addition to the V and W proteins, *Y. pestis* also produces a capsular protein antigen termed *F1,* which has antiphagocytic properties. The expression of determinants of virulence of *Yersinia* differ with temperature and ionic environment and may reflect the need for *Y. pestis* to multiply in an insect vector (the flea), as well as in a warm-blooded host (see Chapter 31). Invasiveness is associated with a chromosomally determined protein. Spread and resistance to phagocytosis are mediated by the V and W proteins and in the case of *Y. pestis* by the F1 capsular protein. These are all encoded in plasmids and synthesized at body temperature under the ionic conditions that obtain within macrophages and other cells, but not in intercellular fluids. The sequence sites and significance of the synthesis of virulence factors in *Y. pestis* are described in Chapter 31.

Schemes for serotyping, biotyping, and bacteriophage typing have been developed for *Yersinia*. *Yersinia pestis* is antigenically homogenous, but *Y. pseudotuberculosis* and *Y. enterocolitica* have multiple O and H antigens (appendix). There are cross-reactions between *Y. pestis* and *Y. pseudotuberculosis.*

Yersinia pestis

Plague

Yersinia pestis causes plague in both man and animals. The pathogenesis, epidemiology, and clinical features of this important disease are covered in Chapter 31.

Yersinia pseudotuberculosis

Acute mesenteric lymphadenitis

In animals *Y. pseudotuberculosis* causes pseudotuberculosis, a disease characterized by lesions ranging from local necrosis to granulomatous inflammation in the lymph nodes, spleen, and liver. The organisms have been shown to survive and grow within mammalian cells. In humans the most common manifestation is an acute mesenteric lymphadenitis. The portal of entry is the gastrointestinal tract, and in most cases wild animals are a possible source of infection. The primary clinical manifestations are fever and abdominal pain, often mimicking acute appendicitis. Diagnosis is by isolation of *Y. pseudotuberculosis* from lymph nodes or from blood in the small proportion of cases that are bacteremic. The role of antimicrobial therapy in mesenteric lymphadenitis is uncertain, as the disease is usually self-limiting. The organism is usually susceptible to ampicillin, cephalosporins, aminoglycosides, tetracyclines, and chloramphenicol.

Yersinia enterocolitica

Invasive enterocolitis
Other syndromes

Yersinia enterocolitica, a more recently described pathogen, produces a wider variety of infections than other members of the genus. The most common infection is enterocolitis, usually occurring in children and characterized by fever, diarrhea, and abdominal pain. It also causes an acute mesenteric lymphadenitis similar to that produced by *Y. pseudotuberculosis,* terminal ileitis, septicemia, and a polyarthritic syndrome associated with its diarrheal manifestations. In addition to their ability to penetrate cells,

Y. enterocolitica strains have been shown to produce an enterotoxin with properties similar to *E. coli* ST toxin.

Geographic variation in the frequency of *Y. enterocolitica* infections is marked. The highest rates have been reported from some Scandinavian and other European countries, with much lower rates in the United Kingdom and the United States. Low isolation rates may be partially attributable to the difficulty of growing *Y. enterocolitica* from stool specimens. Few laboratories in the United States routinely screen stools for *Yersinia* because the yield has been low and good selective media are not available.

Yersinia enterocolitica enterocolitis is usually self-limiting, and the influence of antimicrobics on its course is not clear. The organism is susceptible to the same antimicrobics as *Y. pseudotuberculosis,* with the exception of penicillins and cephalosporins, to which it is usually resistant through production of β-lactamases.

Appendix 20.1 General Characteristics of Some Enterobacteriaceae

Organism	Serologic Type(s) (Antigens)	Bacteriologic Features						Major Disease(s)	Found in Normal Flora
		Lactose	Indole	Urease	Hydrogen Sulfide	Motility	Other		
Escherichieae									
Escherichia coli	150+ (O, K, H)	+	+	-	-	+		Urinary tract infections; diarrhea; opportunistic	Yes
Shigella dysenteriae	10 (O)	-	v	-	-	-		Dysentery (type 1, severe)	No
Shigella flexneri	6 (O)	-	-	-	-	-		Dysentery	No
Shigella boydii	15 (O)	-	v	-	-	-		Dysentery	No
Shigella sonnei	1 (O)	-	-	-	-	-		Dysentery	No
Klebsielleae									
Klebsiella pneumoniae	72 (K)	+	-	+[a]	-	-	Encapsulated	Pneumonia; opportunistic	Yes
Enterobacter sp.		+	-	-	-	+		Opportunistic	Yes
Serratia marcescens		-	-	v[a]	-	+	Red pigment	Opportunistic	Yes
Salmonelleae									
Salmonella serotypes	1500+ (O, H)	-	-	-	+	+		Diarrhea	No
Salmonella choleraesuis	1 (O, H)	-	-	-	v	+		Bacteremia	No
Salmonella typhi	1 (O, H, K)	-	-	-	+	+		Enteric (typhoid) fever	No
Salmonella paratyphi A.	(O, H)	-	-	-	+	+		Diarrhea; enteric fever	No
Citrobacter sp.		v	-	v[a]	+	+		Opportunistic	Yes

Appendix 20.1 General Characteristics of Some Enterobacteriaceae *(continued)*

Organism	Serologic Type(s) (Antigens)	Bacteriologic Features						Major Disease(s)	Found in Normal Flora
		Lactose	Indole	Urease	Hydrogen Sulfide	Motility	Other		
Proteeae									
Proteus mirabilis		–	–	+	+	+	Swarming[b]	Opportunistic	Yes
Proteus vulgaris		–	+	+	+	+	Swarming[b]	Opportunistic	Yes
Morganella morganii		–	+	+	–	+		Opportunistic	Yes
Providencia		–	+	v	–	+		Opportunistic	Yes
Yersinieae									
Yersinia pestis		–	–	–	–	–		Plague	No
Yersinia pseudotuberculosis	10 (O, H)	–	v	+[c]	–	+[c]		Mesenteric lymphadenitis	No
Yersinia enterocolitica	50+ (O, H)	–	–	+[c]	–	+[c]		Mesenteric lymphadenitis; enteric fever; diarrhea	No

Abbreviations: + = more than 90% of strains positive; – = less than 10% of strains positive; v = variable (some strains positive, others negative).

[a] Positive reactions weak or delayed compared to those of Proteeae.

[b] Growth swarms over surface of agar plates.

[c] Positive reactions seen at 25°C but not at 37°C.

Additional Reading

Cornelis, G., Larouche, T., Balligand, G., et al. 1987. *Yersinia Enterocolitica,* a primary model for bacterial invasiveness. *Rev. Infect. Dis.* 9:64–87. The complexities of virulence for the three major species are explained.

DuPont, H.L., Formal, S.B., Hornick, R.B., et al. 1971. Pathogenesis of *Escherichia coli* diarrhea. *N. Engl. J. Med.* 285:1–9. These in vitro and in vivo studies using human volunteers clearly differentiate the two mechanisms, invasion and enterotoxin production, by which *Escherichia coli* causes diarrhea.

Hornick, R.B., Greisman, S.E., Woodward, T.E., et al. 1970. Typhoid fever: Pathogenesis and immunologic control. *N. Engl. J. Med.* 283:686–691. All aspects of typhoid fever are reviewed in detail with emphasis on the relationships of pathogenesis and clinical features.

Levine, M.M. 1987. *Escherichia coli* that cause diarrhea: Enterotoxigenic, enteropathogenic, enteroinvasive, enterohemorrhagic, and enteroadherent. *J. Infect. Dis.* 155:377–389. This paper complements the Robins-Browne review with emphasis on experimental evidence for adherence as a mechanism of diarrhea.

O'Brien, A.D., and Holmes, R.K. 1987. Shiga and shiga-like toxins. *Microbiol. Rev.* 51:206–220. This scholarly review discusses both the toxins and their role in disease.

Reid, G., and Sobel, J.D. 1987. Bacterial adherence in the pathogenesis of urinary tract infections: A review. *Rev. Infect. Dis.* 9:470–487. This review covers all aspects of the pathogenesis of urinary tract infections with emphasis on adherence by *E. coli.*

Robins-Browne, R.M. 1987. Traditional enteropathogenic *Escherichia coli* of infantile diarrhea. *Rev. Infect. Dis.* 9:28–53. This is a comprehensive and readable review of pathogenic mechanisms and epidemiology with a good historical perspective.

Rowe, B., Taylor, J., and Bettelheim, K.A. 1970. An investigation of travellers diarrhea. *Lancet* 1:1–5. An outbreak of traveler's diarrhea among British soldiers is studied. This strain was later shown to produce enterotoxin.

21

Vibrio *and* Campylobacter

Kenneth J. Ryan

Vibrio

Vibrios are curved, Gram-negative rods commonly found in water. Cells may be linked end to end, forming S shapes and spirals. They are highly motile with a single polar flagellum, non-spore forming, oxidase positive, and can grow under aerobic or anaerobic conditions. The cell envelope structure is similar to that of other Gram-negative bacteria. Some species are pathogenic for humans, causing diarrheal illnesses. *Vibrio cholerae* is the cause of cholera.

Vibrio cholerae

Morphology.   Cholera vibrios are slim, short, curved rods, about 0.5 × 3 μm in size. Their motility is extremely rapid.

Growth.   The organism grows readily on the usual broth and solid media used in clinical laboratories. It has a low tolerance for acid, but grows under alkaline (pH 8.0–9.5) conditions that inhibit many other Gram-negative bacteria. It is facultatively anaerobic, but grows best under aerobic conditions.

Differential Features.   *Vibrio cholerae* is distinguished from other vibrios by its biochemical reactions, O antigenic structure, and production of a potent enterotoxin. From a medical standpoint, the nomenclature of the genus *Vibrio* is somewhat confusing because many strains with essentially the same biochemical reactions may or may not produce enterotoxin and cholera. The strains associated with epidemic cholera are limited to a single serogroup, 0:1, and are further divided into three serologic variants named *Ogawa, Inaba,* and *Hikojima.* A biochemical variant, *V. cholerae* biotype eltor, is sometimes called *Vibrio eltor.* Noncholera vibrios have

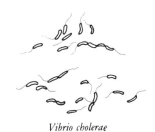

Vibrio cholerae

Rapid motility

Tolerance for alkaline conditions

Epidemic cholera limited to serotype 0:1 strains

Eltor biotype

385

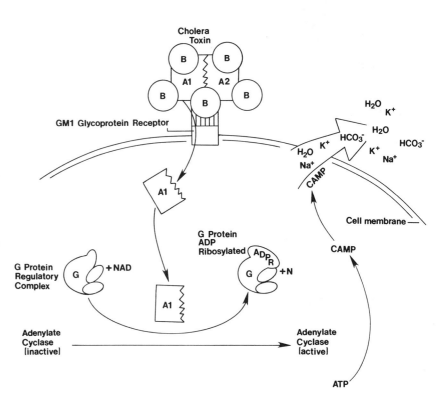

21.1 The action of cholera toxin. The complete toxin is shown binding to the GM1-ganglioside receptor on the cell membrane via the binding (B) subunits. The active portion (A₁) of the A subunit enters the cell and inactivates the G protein by ADP-ribosylation. Because the G protein acts to return adenylate cyclase from its active to inactive form, the net effect is persistent activation of adenylate cyclase. The increased adenylate cyclase activity results in accumulation of cyclic adenosine 3',5'-monophosphate (cAMP) along the cell membrane. The cAMP causes the active secretion of sodium (Na⁺), chloride (Cl⁻), potassium (K⁺), bicarbonate (HCO₃⁻), and water out of the cell into the intestinal lumen.

Environmental isolates

worldwide distribution and are frequently found in water, sewage, and various marine environments. Although they have occasionally been associated with diarrhea and with enterotoxin production, these organisms have not produced epidemic cholera.

Exotoxin with toxic unit and multiple binding units

Toxin. The outstanding feature of *V. cholerae* is the ability of virulent strains to produce and secrete a potent enterotoxic exotoxin responsible for the disease cholera. The structure and mechanism of action of cholera toxin has been studied extensively (Figure 21.1). Its molecule is an aggregate of multiple polypeptide chains organized into a toxic unit (A) and multiple binding units (B). The B units mediate tight binding to a ganglioside receptor on the cell membrane (the GM1-ganglioside). Once bound, the A unit enters the cytoplasm where it exerts its effect on the membrane-associated adenylate cyclase system. The target of the toxic component is a regulatory protein (G protein) that participates in converting adenylate cyclase from its active form to an inactive form. Cholera toxin catalyzes the ADP ribosylation and inactivation of the G protein, resulting in persistent activation of intracellular adenylate cyclase, which in turn stimulates the conversion of adenosine triphosphate to cyclic adenosine 3',5'-monophosphate (cAMP). The net effect is excessive accumulation of cAMP at the cell membrane, which causes hypersecretion of chloride, potassium, bicarbonate, and associated water molecules out of the cell with consequent diarrhea when the intestinal mucosa is involved. This reaction is not specific for intestinal cells, as adenylate cyclase is found in many other cell types. Understanding the mechanism of action of cholera toxin has acquired additional importance with the discovery that other enterotoxins, such as the heat-labile toxin (LT) of *Escherichia coli* (Chapter

Ganglioside receptor for toxin

Toxic subunit leads to ADP-ribosylation of regulatory protein and cAMP accumulation

Hypersecretion of water and electrolytes from increased cAMP causes diarrhea

Relation of cholera toxin to *E. coli* LT

20), utilize the same mechanism. Synthesis of cholera toxin is controlled by a chromosomal gene, whereas the *E. coli* LT gene is located on a plasmid.

Large infecting dose

Pathogenesis. To produce disease, *V. cholerae* must reach the small intestine in sufficient numbers to multiply and colonize. In healthy people, ingestion of large numbers of bacteria is required to offset the acid barrier of the stomach. Colonization is aided by the ability of the organism to penetrate the surface mucus covering of the intestinal mucosa and to adhere to the epithelial surface. The organism's motility, chemotaxis, and production of a mucinase contribute to the ability of *V. cholerae* to colonize, but the specific mechanisms of adherence have not been defined. The organism can colonize the entire intestinal tract from the jejunum to the colon and multiply to high numbers.

Penetration of mucus and adherence

Colonization of length of intestinal tract

The physiologic effects result from the intracellular action of toxin, which is produced at the epithelial surface. Their extent depends on the balance between the amount of bacterial growth, toxin production, fluid secretion, and fluid absorption in the entire gastrointestinal tract. In general, an alkaline environment ideal for continued growth of the organism is produced, and fluid loss in the form of voluminous, watery stools results. The outpouring of fluid and electrolytes is greatest in the small intestine, where the secretory capacity is high and absorptive capacity low. The diarrheal fluid can amount to many liters per day, with approximately the same sodium content as plasma but two to five times the potassium and bicarbonate concentrations. The result is dehydration (isotonic fluid loss), hypokalemia (potassium loss), and metabolic acidosis (bicarbonate loss). The diarrheal fluid also contains mucus flecks, giving it a gross appearance called *rice-water stools*. Surprisingly, the intestinal mucosa remains unaltered except for some hyperemia. *Vibrio cholerae* does not invade, and there are no inflammatory or destructive changes.

Extensive fluid, potassium, and bicarbonate loss

Intestinal mucosa structurally unaffected; no invasion

Lower infecting dose with achlorhydria

Immunity. Nonspecific defenses such as gastric acidity, gut motility, and intestinal mucus are important in preventing colonization with *V. cholerae*. For example, in persons who lack gastric acidity (gastrectomy or achlorhydria from malnutrition), the attack rate of clinical cholera is higher. Humoral antibodies against both the O antigens and the toxin appear after immunization and disease, but they are not long lasting and their association with immunity is not clear. Nevertheless, cholera patients demonstrate resistance to subsequent challenge with *V. cholerae;* and it is likely that this resistance is attributable to local rather than to systemic mechanisms. The immune state has been associated with production of IgA by lymphocytes in the subepithelial areas of the gastrointestinal tract, but the precise protective mechanism remains to be established. It includes the possibility of local action of antitoxin or of antibody blocking the attachment of the organism.

Immunity unassociated with circulating antibody; probably mediated by sIgA

Usual transmission of epidemic cholera through water

Epidemiology. Epidemic cholera is spread primarily by contaminated water under conditions of poor sanitation, although other vehicles are clearly important in some instances. During epidemics, numerous vibrios purged from the intestines of infected individuals reach the primary water supply and are transmitted to others via drinking, food preparation, or bathing. The maintenance of the organism in nature between epidemics is more obscure. It is fragile, surviving only a few days in the environment, but there is evidence that *V. cholerae* may be maintained in marine and fresh-water crustaceans. Convalescent human carriage is usually brief, and prolonged carriage very rare.

Interepidemic maintenance

The eltor biotype of *V. cholerae* has a longer survival in nature and is more likely to produce subclinical cases of cholera, both of which would aid its geographic spread and survival. This organism, first discovered in 1905 at El Tor quarantine camp for Mecca pilgrims, has been of increasing importance in the spread of epidemic cholera beyond its previous location in Africa and southern Asia. In the second half of the 20th century, cholera has slowly spread beyond its major endemic focus in the common delta of the Ganges and the Brahmaputra Rivers. This spread has involved Indonesia, south and central Asia, Africa, and western Europe. Since 1978, endemic cases of cholera caused by the eltor biotype have been recognized in the United States. Infection resulted from eating inadequately cooked crabs and shrimp caught off the Gulf Coast of Louisiana and Texas. *Vibro cholerae* has been shown to survive in crabs cooked less than 10 min.

Clinical Manifestations. Typical cholera has a rapid onset, beginning with abdominal fullness and discomfort, gurgling, rushes of peristalsis, and loose stools. Vomiting may also occur. The stools quickly become watery, voluminous, almost odorless, and contain mucus flecks. These characteristics account for their description as rice-water stools. There is no pus or blood in the stools, and the patient is afebrile. Clinical features of cholera result from the extensive fluid loss and electrolyte imbalance, which can lead to extreme dehydration, hypotension, and death within hours if untreated.

Diagnosis. The initial suspicion of cholera depends on recognition of the typical clinical features in an appropriate epidemiologic setting. *Vibrio cholerae* is not the only organism to cause watery diarrhea or rice-water stools, although it produces the most severe disease. A bacteriologic diagnosis is accomplished by isolation of *V. cholerae* from the stool. The organism grows on common clinical laboratory media such as blood agar and MacConkey agar, but its isolation is enhanced by the use of media and growth conditions that favor it selectively. These conditions include the use of an alkaline (pH 9.0) liquid medium and thiosulfate–citrate-bile salt–sucrose agar. Once isolated, the organism is readily identified by biochemical reactions; identification may be confirmed by agglutination with specific antisera, if available. In parts of the world where cholera is not endemic, these procedures are not routinely used in clinical laboratories and must be requested specifically.

Treatment. The outcome of cholera is dependent on balancing the diarrheal fluid and ionic losses with adequate fluid and electrolyte replacement. This balance is accomplished by oral and/or intravenous administration of solutions of glucose with near physiologic concentrations of sodium and chloride and higher than physiologic concentrations of potassium and bicarbonate. Exact formulas are available as packets to which a given volume of water is added. Oral replacement, particularly if begun early, is sufficient for all but the most severe cases and has substantially reduced mortality from the disease. Antimicrobial therapy shortens the duration of diarrhea and magnitude of fluid loss. Tetracyclines have been used most frequently, although ampicillin, chloramphenicol, and trimethoprim-sulfamethoxazole have also been effective.

Prevention. Epidemic cholera, a disease of poor sanitation, does not occur where treatment and disposal of human waste is adequate. As good sanitary conditions do not exist in much of the world, secondary local measures

---

Marginal notes (left column):

Spread of eltor biotype in recent years

Sporadic cases in United States associated with eating crabs and shrimp caught in Southeast

Extreme watery diarrhea with large fluid loss

Disease manifestations from dehydration and electrolyte imbalance

Stool culture using selective media

Fluid and electrolyte replacement

Antimicrobial therapy

Hygienic disposal of excreta

Water treatment

Vaccines

Development of nontoxigenic
live immunogens

Halophilic vibrios

V. parahemolyticus infections
from seafood

V. vulnificus sepsis and
wound infections

Similar morphology to
vibrios, but taxonomically
distinct

Slow growing microaerophiles

such as boiling or chemical treatment of water during epidemics are required. Vaccines prepared from whole cells, lipopolysaccharide, and cholera toxoid have all been evaluated with variable results. Some preparations
are protective, but do not yet confer the long-lasting immunity known to
result from natural infection. Currently there is considerable interest in
live avirulent vaccine strains because of their potential to stimulate the
local immune response that appears to be of primary importance in cholera. Through use of recombinant DNA technology, strains have been
constructed that have the toxin gene deleted or which produce only the
B subunit. The hope is that such nontoxigenic strains given orally could
multiply and stimulate mucosal sIgA immunity.

The occasional cases associated with crustaceans could be prevented by
adequate cooking and avoidance of recontamination from containers and
surfaces.

Other Vibrios

Several less common infections have been associated with *Vibrio* species
other than *V. cholerae*. Because of their salt requirement and normal habitat
in seawater, these species are sometimes called *halophilic vibrios*. Bacte-
riologically, they resemble *V. cholerae* in many respects, but are readily
distinguished on the basis of biochemical and serologic characteristics.

The most important of these species is *Vibrio parahemolyticus*, which
causes an acute illness characterized by severe cramping, abdominal pain,
and explosive watery diarrhea. Low-grade fever, chills, and headache are
occasionally present. The incubation period is short, typically 24–48 hr
after ingestion. *Vibrio parahemolyticus* is commonly present in coastal
waters throughout the world. Infection develops after ingestion of incompletely cooked seafood. In the United States, most cases have been detected in common source outbreaks involving shellfish. In countries such
as Japan, where raw fish is commonly eaten, *V. parahemolyticus* accounts
for a significant portion of all diarrheal illnesses. The disease is usually
self-limiting, and the course is not affected by antimicrobial therapy.

Other halophilic vibrio species may cause diarrhea or infections of cuts
and wounds contaminated with seawater. Such infections typically involve
seashore bathers or fishermen or follow after ingestion of raw shellfish.
The most virulent member of this group is *Vibrio vulnificus*, which in
addition to wound infections and gastroenteritis, can produce a life-threatening bacteremia. The bacteremic disease is most severe in persons with
liver disease, such as hepatic cirrhosis.

Campylobacter

Campylobacters are small, curved, oxidase-positive, Gram-negative rods
with polar flagella and motility similar to those of vibrios, although often
present in pairs to give a "seagull" appearance. For many years they were
classified as vibrios (*Vibrio fetus*), but differ from them in DNA base ratios
and in a variety of important bacteriological characteristics. Campylobacters grow well only on enriched media under microaerophilic conditions
(reduced oxygen tension but not strict anaerobiosis). Growth usually requires 2–4 days, sometimes as much as a week. In contrast to the vibrios
and members of the Enterobacteriaceae, campylobacters are biochemically
inactive. Campylobacter taxonomy is in a state of considerable flux with
species and subspecies designation changing as new information is gained.
From the standpoint of human disease, there are three species or "groups"

associated, respectively, with systemic illness, diarrhea, and gastritis and peptic ulcer disease. These will be referred to as *Campylobacter fetus, Campylobacter jejuni,* and *Campylobacter pylori.*

Probable zoonotic transmission

Campylobacters are commonly found in the normal gastrointestinal and genitourinary flora of animals, particularly sheep and cattle. Chickens, wild birds, and domestic animals such as dogs may also carry the organisms and probably play a significant role in transmission to humans.

Campylobacter fetus

Bacteremia in humans

Campylobacter fetus has long been recognized as a common cause of abortion in sheep and cattle and a rare cause of sepsis in humans. The most common human presentation is of intermittent fever without evidence of localized infection. Occasionally the meninges and heart valves may become infected, and thrombophlebitis is considered a typical feature although it occurs in only 10% of cases. The diagnosis is established by isolation of *C. fetus* from the blood.

Campylobacter jejuni

Before 1973, *C. jejuni* was not recognized as a cause of human disease. It was not until selective media for its isolation were developed in the late 1970s that its importance was appreciated. This organism is now recognized as one of the most common causes of infectious diarrhea.

Common cause of infectious diarrhea

Low infecting dose

Pathogenesis.   Infection is established by oral ingestion followed by colonization of the intestinal mucosa. The infecting dose is probably low, as volunteers have been infected with as few as 500 cells. Adherence of *C. jejuni* to a number of cell types has been demonstrated, but the binding ligand has not been identified.

Studies of the mechanisms by which *C. jejuni* produces diarrhea have been hampered by the lack of a practical small animal model that simulates human disease. A candidate enterotoxin and a cytotoxin have been described but not yet proved to play a role in human disease. Acquired immunity following natural infection with *C. jejuni* has been demonstrated in volunteer studies, but the mechanisms involved are unknown.

Epidemiology.   It is humbling to consider how a pathogen as common as *C. jejuni* could have been missed for so many years. Studies throughout the world show isolation of *C. jejuni* from 4 to 30% of all cases of infectious diarrhea with less than 1% of healthy persons carrying the organism. The primary reservoir is in animals. Usually the source is raw or partially cooked poultry, but outbreaks have been caused by contaminated rural water supplies and unpasteurized milk often consumed as a "natural" food. Sometimes a direct association can be made as with a sick household pet.

Commonest cause of zoonotic bacterial diarrheas

Clinical Manifestations.   The illness typically begins 1–7 days after ingestion with lower abdominal pain, which may be severe enough to mimic acute appendicitis. The abdominal pain is followed by diarrheal stools that usually contain blood and pus. Fever is commonly present.

Fever and evidence of mucosal invasion

The illness is typically self-limiting after 3–5 days, but may last 1–2 weeks. The diagnosis is confirmed by isolation of the organism from the stool using a special medium made selective for *Campylobacter* by inclusion of antimicrobics that inhibit the normal facultative flora of the bowel. Plates are incubated in a microaerophilic atmosphere.

Treatment. *Campylobacter jejuni* is generally susceptible to erythromycin, tetracycline, chloramphenicol, the aminoglycosides, and the quinolones, but not to penicillins and cephalosporins. Because the disease is usually self-limiting, the effects of antimicrobics on its course remain unclear. Erythromycin has been suggested for severe cases on the basis of in vitro data, and some clinical experience indicates that it may be effective if given early in the course of the illness.

Susceptibility to erythromycin

Helicobacter pylori (formerly Campylobacter pylori)

The association of "spiral bacteria," now known to be *H. pylori,* with the gastric mucosa was made many years ago, but their potential significance was not appreciated until very recently. It is now recognized that this organism has a very strong association with chronic inflammation of the mucus-secreting cells found in the antrum of the stomach. Antral gastritis is associated with the majority of gastric and duodenal ulcers. The etiologic significance of the organism is not entirely clear, because *H. pylori* is found in the stomach of many asymptomatic persons; however, epidemiologic studies indicate its presence is associated with a 10-fold increase in the risk of duodenal ulcer. Therapeutic trials have demonstrated reversal of antral gastritis with antimicrobics active against *H. pylori* and with bismuth preparations that also inhibit the organism.

Association with gastritis and gastric and duodenal ulcers

Etiologic role not yet proven

Helicobacter pylori itself is similar to campylobacters in its morphology and preference for microaerophilic growth conditions. One unique feature is the production of a potent urease. Urease activity can be detected directly in the gastric mucus of infected persons, an observation that in the past was attributed to activity of the mucosal cells themselves.

Additional Reading

Blake, P.A., Allegra, D.T., Snyder, J.D., Barrett, T.J., McFarland, L., Caraway, C.T., Feeley, J.C., Craig, J.P., Lee, J.V., Puhr, N.D., and Feldman, R.A. 1980. Cholera—A possible endemic focus in the United States. *N. Engl. J. Med.* 302:305–309. This study was the first to detail the epidemiologic features of cholera cases along the Gulf Coast of Louisiana.

Levine, M.M., Kaper, J.B., Black, R.E., and Clements, M.L. 1983. New knowledge on pathogenesis of bacterial enteric infections as applied to vaccine development. *Microbiol. Rev.* 47:510–550. The strategies proposed here for recombinant cholera vaccines are particularly interesting.

Marshall, B.J. 1986. *Campylobacter pyloridis* and gastritis. *J. Infect. Dis.* 153:650–657. This article provides an historic perspective on past and present views concerning the role of bacteria in one of the most common of all diseases.

Rettig, P.J. 1979. Campylobacter infections in human beings. *J. Pediatr.* 94:855–864. Both *Campylobacter fetus* and *Campylobacter jejuni* infections are reviewed in detail. The report nicely documents the importance of *C. jejuni* as an intestinal pathogen.

Walker, R.I., Caldwell, M.B., Lee, E.C., et al. 1986. Pathophysiology of *Campylobacter* enteritis. *Microbiol. Rev.* 50:81–94. Few conclusions can yet be made concerning the mechanisms by which this organism causes diarrhea, but leads that will be followed up in the coming years are contained here.

22

Pseudomonas *and Other Opportunistic Gram-Negative Bacilli*

Kenneth J. Ryan

A number of opportunistic Gram-negative rods of several genera not considered in other chapters are discussed herein. With the exception of *Pseudomonas aeruginosa* they rarely cause disease, and all are frequently encountered as contaminants and superficial colonizers. The significance of their isolation from clinical material thus depends on the circumstance and site of culture and on the clinical situation of the patient.

Pseudomonas aeruginosa

Gram-negative motile rod

Pseudomonas aeruginosa is an aerobic, motile, Gram-negative rod; its outstanding bacteriologic feature is the production of colorful water-soluble pigments. It is commonly found free living in moist environments, but is also a pathogen of plants, animals, and humans. As a cause of infection, it is particularly important in severely burned patients, in those with hematologic and other malignancies, and in the intubated urinary tract. It is also the most consistently resistant of all the medically important bacteria to antimicrobics.

Morphology and Structure

Polar flagella

Pseudomonas aeruginosa is generally slimmer and more pale staining than members of the Enterobacteriaceae, but its length is comparable ($0.5 \times 2.5 \mu m$). Its flagella are polar, but otherwise morphologic differences from other Gram-negative bacteria are not sufficiently consistent to be diagnostically useful. Ultrastructural features are similar to those of other Gram-negative bacteria. The lipopolysaccharide (LPS) present in the cell wall is structurally similar to that of the Enterobacteriaceae, but differs in some chemical groupings. The composition of the polysaccharide side chains extending from the outer membrane LPS is believed to determine serologic specificity and susceptibility to bacteriocins (pyocins) and bac-

LPS

Slime layer

teriophages. The slime layer has a mixed chemical composition but is primarily polysaccharide. Pili are present on the cell surface.

Growth and Metabolism

Aerobes with simple growth requirements

Pseudomonas aeruginosa is an aerobe sufficiently versatile in its growth and energy requirements to utilize simple molecules such as ammonia and carbon dioxide as sole nitrogen and carbon sources. Thus, it does not require enriched media for growth, and it can survive and multiply over a wide temperature range (20–42°C) in almost any environment, including those with a high salt content. The organism uses oxidative energy-producing mechanisms and synthesizes large amounts of cytochrome oxidase;

Oxidase positive

it is thus oxidase positive. Although an aerobic atmosphere is necessary for optimal growth and metabolism, most strains will multiply slowly in an anaerobic environment if nitrate is present as an electron acceptor.

Fringed, irregular colonies at 18 hr

Growth on all common isolation media is luxurious, although not as rapid as that of the Enterobacteriaceae. Colonies are well developed after overnight incubation, usually show green pigmentation, and have a delicate, fringed edge. Confluent growth often has a characteristic metallic sheen. Hemolysis may be produced on blood agar. In broth, a surface pellicle is formed, reflecting the organism's preference for aerobic conditions and chemotaxis toward oxygen.

Surface pellicle in liquid media

Classification

No lactose fermentation

Production of blue pyocyanin and yellow pyoverdin imparts green color to growth

Pseudomonas aeruginosa is one of several oxidase-positive, motile organisms to produce non–lactose-fermenting colonies on MacConkey agar. Its oxidase reaction differentiates it from the Enterobacteriaceae, and its production of blue, yellow, or rust-colored pigments from most other Gram-negative bacteria. The blue pigment, pyocyanin, is produced only by *P. aeruginosa;* its demonstration, however, requires a balance of magnesium, iron, and other ions not found in all media that support its growth. Pyoverdin, a yellow pigment that fluoresces under ultraviolet light, is produced; however, it is also produced by free-living nonpathogenic pseudomonads. Pyocyanin and pyoverdin combined produce a bright green color that diffuses throughout the medium. A rust-colored pigment, pyorubrin, is produced by a small proportion of strains. The combination of pyocyanin

Growth at 42°C

production and the ability to grow at 42°C is sufficient to distinguish *P. aeruginosa* from other pseudomonads.

Serologic, bacteriocin, and phage types

Several systems for subtyping *P. aeruginosa* have been developed; 7–29 serotypes have been defined depending on the particular scheme used. *Pseudomonas* bacteriocins (pyocins) and bacteriophages that lyse *P. aeruginosa* in up to 30 patterns have been isolated and organized into typing systems. Recently, DNA hybridization techniques have proved useful in distinguishing strains involved in outbreaks of infection.

Toxins and Extracellular Products

Extracellular enzymes

Most strains of *P. aeruginosa* produce extracellular products, including exotoxin A, proteolytic enzymes destructive to tissues, lecithinase, collagenase, and an elastase that digests the elastin found in the lung and arterial walls. Hemolysins (one of which is phospholipase C) and a leukocidin have also been described. An enterotoxin produces fluid accumulation in the intestinal tract of animals; it has not been clearly characterized, however, and its role in human disease is uncertain. *Pseudomonas*

LPS less toxic than that of Enterobacteriaceae

aeruginosa LPS endotoxin has biologic activities similar to other Gram-negative bacilli, but is roughly 10-fold less toxic than the endotoxin of Enterobacteriaceae.

Exotoxin A resembles diphtheria toxin

Exotoxin A, the most potent toxic factor, has been studied in greatest detail. It is 10,000 times more toxic to experimental animals than *Pseudomonas* endotoxin and is found in more than 90% of clinical isolates. Mutants that lack exotoxin A have much decreased virulence for experimental animals, and antitoxin protects animals against otherwise fatal challenge with exotoxin A-producing strains. The toxin acts to inhibit protein synthesis by a mechanism identical to that of diphtheria toxin (Chapter 17). It catalyzes the ADP-ribosylation and thus the inactivation of elongation factor 2, an essential component of the sequential elongation of proteins on the ribosome. This leads to cell death. Although its mechanism of action is the same, exotoxin A differs from diphtheria toxin in its amino acid structure and receptor-binding characteristics. It does not cross-react immunologically with diphtheria toxin.

Epidemiology

Primary habitat environmental

The primary habitat of *P. aeruginosa* and other pseudomonads is environmental. They are found in water, soil, and various types of vegetation throughout the world. *Pseudomonas aeruginosa* has been isolated from the throat and stool of 2–10% of healthy persons. Colonization rates may be higher in hospitalized patients.

Can produce invasive infections in immunocompromised hosts

Multiplication in humidifiers, solutions, and moist environments

Infection with *P. aeruginosa*, rare in previously healthy persons, is one of the most important causes of invasive infection in compromised patients with serious underlying disease, such as leukemia, cystic fibrosis, and extensive burns. The organism's ability to survive and proliferate in water with minimal nutrients can lead to heavy contamination of any unsterile water, such as that in the humidifiers of respirators. Inhalation of aerosols from such sources can bypass the normal respiratory defense mechanisms and initiate pulmonary infection. Infections have resulted from the growth of *Pseudomonas* in medications, contact lens solutions, and even in some disinfectants. Sinks and faucet aerators may be heavily contaminated and serve as the environmental source for contamination of other items. It is important to recognize, however, that the simple finding of a few *P. aeruginosa* in solutions or sites not normally sterile (for example, drinking water, food) is not in itself abnormal or a cause for alarm. The risk lies in the proximity between items susceptible to contamination and patients uniquely predisposed to infection.

Pathogenesis and Immunity

Need for break in first-line defenses

Although *P. aeruginosa* is an opportunistic pathogen, it is one of particular virulence. The organism usually requires a significant break in first-line defenses (such as a wound) or a route past them (such as a contaminated respirator or intratracheal tube) to initiate infection. Attachment to epithelial surfaces is the first step in infection and has been associated with pili and extracellular polysaccharide. The mucoid strains found in patients with cystic fibrosis (see "Clinical Manifestations") produce extensive extracellular polysaccharide, forming a matrix containing many bacteria. This arrangement promotes adherence to respiratory epithelium and resistance to phagocytosis. These features are similar to the adherence of streptococci to heart valves (Chapter 16) and of *Staphylococcus epidermidis* to plastics (Chapter 15). The *P. aeruginosa* extracellular polysaccharides has an un-

Pili and extracellular polysaccharide promote adhesion

usually complex structure with acetylation of disaccharide units. It resembles that found in some algae and is sometimes referred to as *alginate*. This structure may explain why immune responses are of little help in clearing chronic infections.

The relative roles of the cellular LPS and extracellular enzymes in virulence have been a source of some debate, but current opinion favors the latter as most important, particularly exotoxin A. The toxicity of *Pseudomonas* LPS is weak compared to that of the Enterobacteriaceae; it is a potent immunogen, however, and LPS-directed antibody may decrease the incidence of fatal burn infections. Exotoxin A production is associated with a fatal outcome in bacteremic patients, and antitoxin against it is associated with survival. No diphtherialike systemic effect of exotoxin has been demonstrated, but its cytotoxic action correlates with the primarily invasive and locally destructive lesions seen in *P. aeruginosa* infections.

Multifactorial nature of virulence

The virulence of *P. aeruginosa* is therefore probably multifactorial. After invasion, the protection from phagocytosis afforded by LPS and slime may provide sufficient time for production of collagenases, elastases, pyocyanin and other products, allowing spread and local tissue destruction. Exotoxin A may be an important contributor to local injury and the lethal effects of widespread infection. A recent group of in vitro studies has shown the pigment pyocyanin to inhibit mitogen-induced lymphocyte multiplication and also superoxide generation by polymorphonuclear leukocytes. Perhaps these factors are important in facilitating the establishment, spread, and persistence of infection.

Significance of humoral and cellular immune responses

Human immunity to *Pseudomonas* infection is not well understood, although some inferences can be drawn from animal studies and clinical observations. The importance of humoral immunity is supported by demonstration of a protective effect of various vaccines and passive transfer of immunity with immune globulin. The strong propensity of *P. aeruginosa* to infect the immune compromised host, particularly those with defective cell-mediated immunity, indicates that these responses are also important. Knowledge of the specific mechanisms involved is, however, lacking.

Clinical Manifestations

Range of opportunistic infections

Pseudomonas aeruginosa can produce any of the opportunistic extraintestinal infections caused by members of the Enterobacteriaceae, but *Pseudomonas* infections are generally less common. Burn, wound, urinary tract, skin, eye, ear, and respiratory infections all occur. Infection of severe burns is common; bacteremia may be a sequel to this or to other severe infection.

Burn infections

Bacteremia and ecthyma gangrenosum

In some cases of *P. aeruginosa* bacteremia, the cutaneous syndrome of ecthyma gangrenosum develops. It begins with a few painful maculopapular lesions of the skin. As they enlarge over 2–3 days a purple, then black, necrosis develops in the center of the lesion, as a result of direct invasion and destruction of blood vessel walls by the organism. *Pseudomonas aeruginosa* is also one of the most common causes of infection associated with injuries in which there is environmental contamination of the wound (for example, osteomyelitis after compound fractures, deep puncture wounds). Such injuries are the major route of deep-seated infection in immunologically normal persons.

Osteomyelitis after wounds

Pneumonia

Pseudomonas aeruginosa pneumonia is a severe infection. It may follow the use of respirators with contaminated humidifiers and occurs in hospitalized patients with granulocytopenia. It is particularly severe and associated with alveolar necrosis, vascular invasion, infarcts, and bacteremia. *Pseudomonas aeruginosa* is also a common cause of otitis externa, particu-

Otitis externa and folliculitis

larly the "swimmer's ear" seen in children who spend most of the summer in a pool, and of a rare but life-threatening "malignant" otitis externa in diabetics. Folliculitis of the skin may follow soaking in inadequately decontaminated hot tubs that can become heavily contaminated with the organism.

Eye infections

The organism can cause conjunctivitis, keratitis, or endophthalmitis when introduced into the eye by trauma or contaminated medication or contact lens solution. Keratitis can progress rapidly and destroy the cornea within 24–48 hr.

Cystic fibrosis infections

Pseudomonas aeruginosa is now the most common bacterial pathogen to complicate the management of patients with cystic fibrosis, an inherited disease of exocrine glands associated with excessive viscid mucus in the smaller respiratory passages. A high proportion of cases become colonized, and the organism may cause or contribute to tracheobronchitis or pneumonia. A striking feature of these infections is their association with the mucoid strains mentioned earlier. Most *P. aeruginosa* strains have genes for production of the alginate extracellular polysaccharide that are silent. The environment in the lung of cystic fibrosis patients apparently selects for their expression, but the mechanism is not understood. Strains often revert back to the nonmucoid phenotype on subculture.

Association with mucoid strains

Treatment and Prevention

Antimicrobic resistance

Of the pathogenic bacteria, *P. aeruginosa* is the organism most consistently resistant to antimicrobics. To a considerable extent this resistance is due to the structure of their outer membrane porins that restrict the entry of antimicrobics to the periplasmic space more than is the case with other Gram-negative bacteria. *P. aeruginosa* strains are regularly resistant to penicillin, ampicillin, cephalothin, tetracycline, chloramphenicol, sulfonamides, and the earlier aminoglycosides (streptomycin, kanamycin). Thus, it is fruitless to perform a susceptibility test with these agents. Much effort has been directed toward the development of antimicrobics with anti-*Pseudomonas* activity. The newer aminoglycosides, gentamicin, tobramycin, and amikacin are all active against most strains despite occasional mutational and plasmid-mediated resistance. Carbenicillin and ticarcillin are active and can be given in high doses, but plasmid-mediated resistance and permeability mutations occur more frequently than with the aminoglycosides. A primary feature of the third-generation cephalosporins (for example, cefotaxime, ceftazidime, and cefoperazone) is their activity against *Pseudomonas*. In general, urinary infections may be treated with a single drug; but more serious systemic *P. aeruginosa* infections are usually treated with a combination of an anti-*Pseudomonas* β-lactam antimicrobic and an aminoglycoside, particularly in neutropenic patients. Ciprofloxacin is also used in treatment of such cases. In all instances susceptibility must be confirmed in vitro.

Impermeability of outer membrane pores

Combined therapy

Vaccines

Vaccines incorporating somatic antigens from multiple *P. aeruginosa* serotypes have been developed and proved immunogenic in humans. The primary candidates for such preparations are patients with burn injuries, cystic fibrosis or immunosuppression. Although some protection has been demonstrated, these preparations are still experimental.

Other Pseudomonads

There are a large number of *Pseudomonas* species other than *P. aeruginosa;* however, the total number of infections produced by these species is far less than that produced by *P. aeruginosa* alone. They are most frequently

Table 22.1 Pseudomonads Associated with Human Infection

Group	Species	Bacteriologic Features				Disease
		Pyocyanin	Other Pigments	Growth at 42°C	Amino-glycoside Resistance[a]	
Fluorescent	*P. aeruginosa*	+	+	+	5–20%	Opportunistic
	P. fluorescens	−	+	−	Uncommon	Opportunistic
	P. putida	−	+	−	Uncommon	Opportunistic
Pseudomallei	*P. mallei*	−	−	−	—	Glanders
	P. pseudomallei	−	−	+	90%	Melioidosis
	P. cepacia	−	−	v	90%	Opportunistic
Other	*P. alcaligenes*	−	−	v	Uncommon	Opportunistic
	P. stutzeri	−	−	v	Uncommon	Opportunistic
	P. maltophilia	−	+	v	Uncommon	Opportunistic
	P. putrifaciens	−	−	v	Uncommon	Opportunistic
	P. acidovorans	−	−	v	Uncommon	Opportunistic

Abbreviations: v = variable; + = usually positive (more than 90%); − = usually negative (less than 10%).

[a] Aminoglycoside resistance refers to gentamicin, tobramycin, amikacin, etc.

seen as colonizers and contaminants. Those of medical importance are shown in Table 22.1. With the exception of the *Pseudomonas pseudomallei* group, they cause only opportunistic infections, and the assignment of species names has little clinical importance beyond differentiation from *P. aeruginosa*. Reports vary regarding the frequency of their isolation from cases of bacteremia, arthritis, abscesses, wounds, conjunctivitis, and urinary tract infections. In any individual case the significance of isolating one of these species must be decided on its own merits. In general, unless isolated in pure culture from a high-quality (direct) specimen, it is difficult to attach pathogenic significance to any of the miscellaneous *Pseudomonas* species.

Environmental habitat of *P. pseudomallei*

Pseudomonas pseudomallei can cause primary infections in otherwise healthy individuals. It is not found in temperate climates, but exists as a saprophyte in soil, ponds, rice paddies, and produce in Southeast Asia, the Philippines, Indonesia, and other tropical areas. Infection is acquired by direct inoculation or by inhalation of aerosols or dust containing the bacteria. The disease, melioidosis, is usually an acute pneumonia; however, it is sufficiently variable that subacute, chronic, and even relapsing infections may follow systemic spread. The clinical and radiologic features may resemble tuberculosis. In fulminant cases, rapid respiratory failure may ensue and metastatic abscesses develop in the skin or other sites. Tetracycline, chloramphenicol, sulfonamides, and trimethoprim–sulfamethoxazole have been effective in therapy.

Acute or chronic pulmonary infection

Metastatic abscesses

Glanders is a disease of horses and some other mammals caused by *Pseudomonas mallei*. Transmission to humans is extremely rare. The disease manifests as local suppurative or acute pulmonary infections.

Pseudomonas cepacia is an opportunistic organism that has been found to contaminate reagents, disinfectants, and medical devices in much the same manner as *P. aeruginosa*.

Acinetobacter

Coccoid forms common

The genus *Acinetobacter* comprises Gram-negative coccobacilli that occasionally appear sufficiently round on Gram smears to be confused with *Neisseria*. On primary isolation they closely resemble the Enterobacteriaceae in growth pattern and colonial morphology, but are distinguished by their failure to ferment carbohydrates or reduce nitrates. Although the two major species have well-defined characteristics, the taxonomy has been confused by the use of many names in the past, including *Mima* and *Herellea*. The organism previously classified as *Mima* is now termed *Acinetobacter calcoaceticus* var. *lwoffii* (*A. lwoffii*) and *Herellea vaginicola* as *Acinetobacter calcoaceticus* var. *anitratus* (*A. anitratus*).

Opportunistic pulmonary, urinary tract, and soft tissue infections

As with most of the organisms discussed in this chapter, the isolation of *Acinetobacter* from clinical material does not define infection, because they appear most frequently as colonizers and contaminants. Pneumonia is the most common infection, followed by urinary tract and soft tissue infections. Nosocomial respiratory infections have been traced to contaminated inhalation therapy equipment, and bacteremia to infected intravenous catheters. Treatment is complicated by frequent resistance to penicillins, cephalosporins, chloramphenicol, and occasionally aminoglycosides.

Moraxella

Moraxella is another genus of coccobacillary, Gram-negative rods that are usually paired end to end. Some species require enriched media, such as blood or chocolate agar. Their morphology, fastidious growth, and positive oxidase reaction can result in confusion with *Neisseria*. The organism now called *Moraxella lacunata*, originally described as a cause of angular conjunctivitis, is an uncommon isolate from any site. All species rarely cause disease. They are susceptible to penicillin.

Aeromonas and *Plesiomonas*

The genera *Aeromonas* and *Plesiomonas* have features similar to those of both the Enterobacteriaceae and *Pseudomonas*. They are aerobic and facultatively anaerobic, attack carbohydrates fermentatively, and demonstrate various other biochemical reactions. Their colonies and growth pattern resemble those of the Enterobacteriaceae. The major taxonomic resemblance to *Pseudomonas* is that both *Aeromonas* and *Plesiomonas* are oxidase positive with polar flagella. Their habitat is basically environmental (water and soil), but they can occasionally be found in the human intestinal tract. In addition to opportunistic infection, some evidence suggests an occasional role in gastroenteritis through production of an enterotoxin. This association is not yet strong enough to justify attempts to isolate them from diarrheal stools. Resistance to penicillins and cephalosporins is common. Most strains show susceptibility to chloramphenicol and tetracycline, with variable susceptibility to aminoglycosides, including gentamicin.

Other Gram-Negative Rods

Nonfermenters

The terms *miscellaneous* or *nonfermenter* are used loosely by bacteriologists to describe Gram-negative rods that do not ferment carbohydrates or that fail to react in many of the tests used to characterize other bacteria. Identification is frequently delayed as additional tests are tried or the organism is sent to a reference laboratory. As the clinical significance of all these organisms is essentially the same, the clinician will usually receive a report of a "nonfermenter" or another descriptive term and a susceptibility test result. The clinical significance of the isolate is then decided on other grounds. The major characteristics of some of these organisms are shown

Table 22.2   Characteristics of Miscellaneous Gram-Negative Bacilli

| Organism | Usual Habitat | Bacteriologic Features | | | | Infection |
		Growth on MacConkey Agar	Oxidase	Motility	Other	
Alkaligenes	Respiratory tract; intestinal tract	+	+	+		Blood; urine; wounds
Cardiobacterium	Respiratory tract; intestinal tract	−	+	−	CO_2 required	Endocarditis
Chromobacterium	Environmental (tropical)	+	+	v	Blue to yellow pigments	Blood; abscesses
Actinobacillus	Oral	−	+	+	CO_2 required	Endocarditis
Flavobacterium	Environmental	−	+	−	Yellow pigment	Meningitis; nosocomial
Eikenella	Respiratory tract	−	+	−	CO_2 required; pits agar	Abscesses; endocarditis

Abbreviations: + = usually positive (more than 90%); − = usually negative (less than 10%); v = variable.

in Table 22.2. All have little inherent virulence and rarely cause infection. The types of infection listed represent the most common among scattered case reports, and should not be interpreted as typical for each organism.

Some Gram-negative nonfermenters fail to conform to any of the species currently recognized, usually because of insufficient isolates or lack of interest in assigning any unifying bacteriologic or clinical significance. Such strains are usually referred by hospitals to reference centers, such as the Centers for Disease Control (CDC) in Atlanta. They are kept and assigned numbers to aid in comparison with similar past and future strains. Eventually, some are given designations such as "CDC group IIF," which may appear in clinical reports. Much later, a new genus and/or species name may be issued if agreement among taxonomists is sufficient.

Additional Reading

Döring, G., Holder, I.A., and Botzenhart, K., Eds. 1987. Basic research and clinical aspects of *Pseudomonas aeruginosa. Antibiot. Chemother.* 39:1–311. This monograph is a collection of papers from an international symposium and includes recent updates on virulence factors and prospects for immunotherapy. Some libraries index it as a book.

23

Haemophilus *and* Bordetella

Kenneth J. Ryan

Haemophilus and *Bordetella* are small, Gram-negative rods that tend to assume a coccobacillary shape. They are nonmotile, non-spore forming, and require complex media for growth. Members of both genera cause respiratory infections, and *Haemophilus influenzae* is responsible for a variety of systemic infections, including purulent meningitis.

HAEMOPHILUS

Haemophilus influenzae

Morphology and Structure

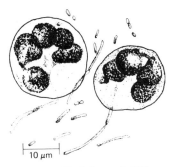

Haemophilus influenzae in CSF

Serotypes based on polysaccharide capsule

Organisms grown in broth or on agar plates usually show a highly regular shape. The rounded ends of short (1.0–1.5 μm) bacilli make many appear round, hence the term *coccobacilli*. The cells are so small that clear visualization requires optimal light microscopy. In clinical specimens such as sputum, the same morphology is generally seen; in cerebrospinal fluid (CSF), however, some of the cells may be elongated to several times their usual length.

The cell wall has a lipopolysaccharide–protein surface similar to that of other Gram-negative bacteria. *Haemophilus influenzae* may have a polysaccharide capsule, but other species of *Haemophilus* are not encapsulated. Capsulate *H. influenzae* are divided into six serotypes, a–f, based on the capsular polysaccharide antigen. Capsulate strains can be typed with specific antisera by use of slide agglutination, capsule swelling, or other serologic procedures for detecting surface antigens. The chemical nature of the capsular polysaccharides is known. For example, type b capsule is made up of a polymer of ribose, ribitol, and phosphate, called polyribitol phosphate (PRP). These surface polysaccharides are strongly associated with virulence, particularly in type b *H. influenzae*, which is responsible for

401

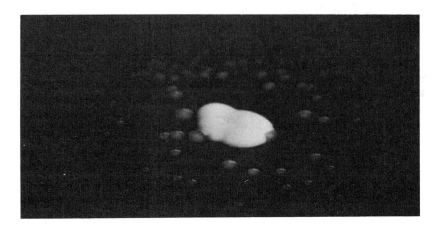

23.1 The satellite phenomenon. This blood agar plate has been evenly spread with *Haemophilus influenzae* and then touched with a wire containing *Staphylococcus aureus*. Note that the small colonies appear only around the *S. aureus*, which is producing V factor (NAD). Together with the X factor (hematin) from the blood, the requirement for both X and V factors are met only in this area.

most cases of serious systemic infection. Cell wall (somatic) antigens of capsulated and nonencapsulated *Haemophilus* have not been associated with virulence.

Growth

Growth factor requirements: hematin (X) and NAD (V)

In addition to the usual components of enriched culture media, *Haemophilus* species require added blood products for optimal growth (as indicated by the genus name, from the Greek *haema*, blood, and *philos*, loving). This requirement is attributable to the need for hematin and/or nicotinamide adenine dinucleotide (NAD) as growth factors. These growth factors, also termed *X factor* (hematin) and *V factor* (NAD), are both present in erythrocytes. In culture medium, optimal concentrations of X and, particularly, V factors are not available to *Haemophilus* from blood unless the red blood cells are lysed by gentle heat (chocolate agar) or some digestion process (Fildes agar). Although erythrocytes are the only convenient source of hematin, the V factor is present in a variety of biologic materials and is produced by some other bacteria and yeast. These conditions are responsible for the "satellite phenomenon," in which *H.*

Satellitism around colonies of *S. aureus*

influenzae grows on blood agar only in the vicinity of a colony of *Staphylococcus aureus* that is producing V factor (Figure 23.1).

Cultural characteristics

When their nutritional needs are met, most *Haemophilus* species grow rapidly, producing 1- to 2-mm translucent colonies after overnight incubation under aerobic or anaerobic conditions. Encapsulated strains may produce larger colonies with a glistening mucoid quality. Commonly used broth media lack sufficient X and V factors to support growth of *Haemophilus*, but when whole blood is added with the inoculum (as in blood cultures) the organisms will grow, but they require 2–3 days and usually do not become sufficiently numerous to produce turbidity. Rapid growth with large numbers of organisms is achieved if the pure growth factors or blood digest supplements are added.

Pathogenesis

Carrier rates in health

Various *Haemophilus* species are common inhabitants of the upper respiratory tract. Carrier rates for *H. influenzae* as high as 80% have been found in children and are commonly 20–50% in healthy adults. Most strains are nonencapsulated, but healthy carriers of encapsulated strains are not infrequent. The events that cause these organisms to initiate disease are poorly understood and differ for encapsulated and unencapsulated *Haemophilus* strains.

Invasive ability of *H. influenzae* type b

Type b *H. influenzae* strains are primary pathogens that can occasionally multiply and spread into the deeper tissues beyond the nasopharynx. This invasion may involve inflammation and edema of the epiglottis or facial and neck tissues. Bacteremia, which is common once the organisms spread beyond the nasopharynx, is probably the mechanism for entry into the central nervous system and for metastatic infections at distant sites such as bones and joints. Host factors probably determine whether meningitis, arthritis, or a more local infection results. Systemic spread is typical only for encapsulated *H. influenzae* strains, and over 90% of invasive strains are type b.

Localized infections with nonencapsulated strains

Nonencapsulated *H. influenzae* and other respiratory *Haemophilus* species can be regarded as opportunistic and produce disease when they gain access to usually protected areas connected to the respiratory tract often because local defenses are compromised, for example, by a viral infection. Invasion of the middle ear, respiratory sinuses, and bronchi are most common. The infections produced are more superficial than those with type b, and deep invasion and bacteremia are rare.

Antiphagocytic effects of capsules

Endotoxin action on ciliated cells

Absence of exotoxins

The pathogenic mechanism involved in *H. influenzae* infection remains to be fully understood. The capsule is antiphagocytic and probably the most significant determinant of virulence. Endotoxin is present in the cell wall. It is toxic to ciliated respiratory cells, but endotoxemia is not a feature of *Haemophilus* infection to the extent that it is with *Neisseria meningitidis*. *Haemophilus* influenzae produces no exotoxin, but has been reported to produce an IgA protease that may facilitate colonization.

Immunity

Anticapsular and bactericidal antibody

Immunity to *H. influenzae* infections, has been clearly associated with the presence of circulating antibodies, which are anticapsular, opsonic, and bactericidal in the presence of complement. The infant is usually protected by passively acquired maternal antibody for the first few months of life. Thereafter the presence of actively acquired antibody increases with age; it is present in the serum of most children by age 10. The peak incidence of *H. influenzae* type b infections is at 6–18 months of age, which corresponds to the nadir of the serum antibody curve (Figure 23.2). This inverse relationship between infection and serum antibody is analogous to that for *N. meningitidis* (Figure 19.2). The major difference is that prevention of infection requires antibody directed against several meningococcal serogroups but against only a single type of *H. influenzae* (type b). Thus, systemic *H. influenzae* infections (meningitis, epiglottitis, cellulitis) are rare in adults. When such infections develop, however, the immunologic deficit is probably the same as that with meningococci: lack of circulating antibody.

Type b infections most common at ages when antibody titer is lowest

Poor response to vaccine in early childhood

Studies using a vaccine of purified type b PRP have shown age-related differences in ability to respond to this antigen, probably because, like many polysaccharides, it fails to activate T helper cells or elicit a significant secondary response on reinjection. Infants respond poorly, whereas older children form high levels of antibody. Some infants fail to form anti-PRP antibody after systemic infection and have a second episode of invasive *H. influenzae* disease. A genetic basis for invasive *H. influenzae* type b disease is suggested by a statistical association of disease with a particular grouping of alloantigens of the major histocompatibility complex. There

Possible genetic predisposition

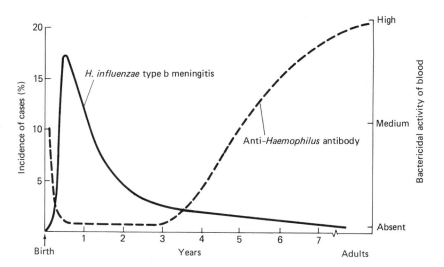

23.2 Relation of age incidence of *H. influenzae* meningitis to the bactericidal activity of blood against *H. influenzae*. (*Adapted from Fothergill and Wright.*)

is a high rate of disease among some ethnic groups such as Native Alaskans, but this may involve socioeconomic and environmental factors as well as genetic differences.

Epidemiology

Because it is not a public health requirement to report *H. influenzae* infections, accurate infection rates are not available; the frequency of *H. influenzae* meningitis, however, has been estimated at 8000 cases yearly in the United States. Virtually all of these cases occur in children under 6 and most under 2 years of age. Cases of epiglottitis and pneumonia tend to peak in the 2- to 5-year age range. Evidence indicates that the frequency of systemic type b disease has increased slowly over the past three to four decades and that adult infections are becoming more frequent. The reason for this trend is not known, but changes in the incidence of infection, virulence of the organism, and the impact of antimicrobic usage on development of immunity are possibilities.

> Age incidence of *H. influenzae* type b meningitis, epiglottitis, and pneumonia

In contrast to meningococcal meningitis, which has long been known to be communicable, *Haemophilus* meningitis was believed to be an isolated endogenous infection. Recent reports of outbreaks in closed populations, such as day-care centers, and careful epidemiologic studies of secondary spread in families have changed this view. The risk of serious infection for children under 4 years of age living with an index case is more than 500-fold that for nonexposed children. This risk indicates a need for prophylaxis for contacts in the susceptible age group. Although the effectiveness of various antimicrobics as chemoprophylactics has not been clearly established, rifampin is currently recommended for this purpose.

> Increased risk of infection in children who are close contacts

> Prophylaxis

Haemophilus influenzae Infections

Meningitis

This is almost invariably caused by type b strains. *Haemophilus* meningitis follows the same pattern as other causes of acute purulent bacterial meningitis (Chapter 67). Meningitis is often preceded by signs and symptoms

Morbidity and mortality

of an upper respiratory infection, such as nasopharyngitis, sinusitis, or otitis media. Whether these represent a predisposing viral infection or early invasion by the organism is not known. Just as often, meningitis is preceded only by vague malaise, lethargy, irritability, and fever. Mortality is currently 5–10% despite adequate therapy, and roughly one-third of all survivors have significant neurologic damage.

Acute Epiglottitis

Respiratory obstruction

Cherry-red swollen epiglottis

Need for maintaining airway

Acute epiglottitis is a dramatic infection caused by *H. influenzae* type b in which the epiglottis and surrounding tissues can obstruct the airway. Findings are those of a systemic infection with signs of increasing respiratory difficulty. The onset is sudden, with fever, sore throat, hoarseness, a barking cough, and rapid progression to severe prostration within 24 hr. The prostrated child has air hunger, inspiratory stridor, and retraction of the soft parts of the chest with each inspiration. The hallmark of the disease is an inflamed, swollen, cherry-red epiglottis that protrudes into the airway and can be visualized on lateral X-rays. As with meningitis, this infection is treated as a medical emergency with prime emphasis on maintenance of an airway (tracheostomy). Without an established airway, manipulations, including routine examination or attempting to take a throat swab, can be fatal by triggering acute obstruction.

Cellulitis

A tender, reddish-blue swelling in the cheek or periorbital areas is the usual presentation of *Haemophilus* cellulitis. This disease is also caused by type b strains. Fever and a moderately toxic state are usually present, and the infection may follow an upper respiratory infection or otitis media. A large proportion of cases are bacteremic, and some develop infections at other sites.

Arthritis

Most common cause of purulent arthritis in children under 2 years of age

Haemophilus influenzae type b is the leading cause of purulent arthritis in children in the susceptible age range, particularly those under 2 years of age. Infection may follow another manifestation of *H. influenzae* infection or appear as the primary illness. Local signs of inflammation in single, large, weight-bearing joints with fever and irritability are the usual features. *Haemophilus* arthritis is occasionally the cause of a more subtle set of findings, in which fever occurs without clear clinical evidence of joint involvement. Bacteremia is usually present.

Other Respiratory Infections

Role of noncapsulate strains in otitis media, sinusitis, and bronchitis

Haemophilus influenzae is one of several respiratory organisms that can cause otitis media, acute and chronic sinusitis, and exacerbation of chronic bronchitis. These infections usually result from displacement of the normal flora into normally sterile luminal structures. Thus, most *H. influenzae* infections are caused by nonencapsulated and thus nontypable strains found commonly in the respiratory flora. These infections usually remain localized without bacteremia. Disease may be acute or chronic, depending on the anatomic site and underlying pathology. For example, otitis media is acute and painful because of the small, closed space involved, but usually clears without sequelae after antimicrobic therapy and reopening of the eustachian tube. The association of *H. influenzae* with chronic bronchitis is more complex. There is evidence that *H. influenzae* and other bacteria play a role in inflammatory exacerbations, but a unique cause and effect relationship is difficult to prove. The underlying cause of the bronchitis is usually related to chronic damage resulting from smoking or other factors.

Haemophilus pneumonia may be caused by either encapsulated or non-encapsulated organisms. Encapsulated strains have been observed to produce a disease much like pneumococcal pneumonitis; however, unencapsulated strains may also produce pneumonia, particularly in patients with chronic bronchitis.

Diagnosis

Gram smear

Culture

Demonstration of growth factor requirement

Value of blood cultures in systemic infections

Detection of type b capsular antigen in body fluids

The combination of clinical findings and a typical Gram smear is usually sufficient to make a presumptive diagnosis of *Haemophilus* infection. This diagnosis must then be confirmed by isolation of the organism from the site of infection or from the blood, using appropriate media. Gram-negative rods that grow on chocolate agar but not blood agar (except around a staphylococcus colony) strongly suggest *Haemophilus*. Confirmation and speciation depends on demonstration of the requirement for X and V factors. Serotyping, which may be done by slide agglutination or capsular swelling (quellung) techniques, is usually unnecessary for clinical purposes.

Blood cultures are particularly useful in systemic *H. influenzae* infections. It is difficult, except with meningitis, to gain access to the site of infection (epiglottitis, pneumonia) or to obtain a purulent specimen (cellulitis); however, a large proportion of patients are bacteremic, and blood cultures will usually yield the organism.

Haemophilus influenzae type b PRP is released into body fluids and circulates during the course of infection. PRP may be detected in infected body fluid, blood, or urine by methods such as counterimmunoelectrophoresis and latex agglutination (Chapter 14). The procedures are not dependent on the presence of live organisms and can be helpful when cultures are negative because of antimicrobial therapy.

Treatment

Ampicillin-resistant strains

Plasmid-determined β-lactamase

Haemophilus influenzae is usually susceptible in vitro to ampicillin and amoxicillin, the newer cephalosporins, chloramphenicol, tetracycline, aminoglycosides, and sulfonamides. It is less susceptible to other penicillins and to erythromycin. *Haemophilus* meningitis has been treated effectively with ampicillin, chloramphenicol, and the newer cephalosporins. Since 1974, the therapy of systemic infections has been complicated by the emergence of ampicillin-resistant strains of *H. influenzae*. These strains produce a potent β-lactamase that is plasmid mediated and identical to that found in other Gram-negative bacteria, such as *Escherichia coli*. Infections with these strains do not respond to ampicillin therapy. The frequency of resistant strains varies between 5 and 50% in different geographic areas, but for therapeutic purposes all strains must be considered resistant until proved susceptible. Susceptibility is determined by direct testing for β-lactamase production from colonies and by modifications of standard susceptibility tests that satisfy the growth requirements of *Hae-*

Approaches to treatment

mophilus. Although ampicillin-resistant strains that do not produce β-lactamase have also been described, they are uncommon, as are chloramphenicol-resistant *H. influenzae.* Current practice is to start empiric therapy with chloramphenicol, ampicillin plus chloramphenicol, or with a third-generation cephalosporin (eg, ceftriaxone, cefuroxime). This can be changed when the results of susceptibility tests are known and administration of inappropriate antimicrobics is discontinued.

Nonencapsulated *Haemophilus* strains have demonstrated ampicillin resistance at about the same rate as the type b organisms. The therapeutic impact of this resistance is less clear, because other organisms may be involved in infections with which they are associated, and a specific etiologic diagnosis is often not established (for example, otitis media). The common use of ampicillin to treat such infections is now questioned, however, and may have been responsible in part for the increasing frequency of resistance. The use of sulfonamides, newer cephalosporins (eg, cefaclor), and various combinations (trimethoprim/sulfamethoxazole, penicillin/sulfonamide, erythromycin/sulfonamide) is under increasing consideration.

Prevention

Type b capsular vaccine

A purified PRP vaccine is now available for prevention of systemic disease produced by *H. influenzae* type b. It has been recommended for all children at 24 months of age and suggested at 18 months for children in known high-risk groups. This is far from ideal, because a large proportion of cases occur before 24 months, and, for reasons discussed above, the immunogenicity of the PRP cannot be guaranteed at 18 months. Furthermore, for unexplained reasons, occasional trials in limited geographic areas have failed to show efficacy, and for a week or so after immunization, susceptibility may actually be increased. Recent interest has focused on the long-known enhancement of the immune response to a weak carbohydrate immunogen when it is coupled to a protein carrier. A new class of poly-

Conjugate vaccines

saccharide–protein conjugate vaccines is being actively explored for prevention of *Haemophilus* disease. These include conjugates of PRP with diphtheria toxoid, tetanus toxoid, and an outer membrane protein from group B *Neisseria meningitidis.* The vaccines augment the antibody response to PRP. Results with the diphtheria toxoid-PRP conjugate vaccine are promising. Hopefully this line of investigation will lead to a vaccine that can be given early enough to prevent the majority of *H. influenzae* type b infections.

Other Species of *Haemophilus*

Several other *Haemophilus* species exist and are defined by their requirement for X and/or V factor, CO_2 dependence, and other cultural characteristics (Table 23.1). The respiratory species, of which *Haemophilus parainfluenzae* is the most common, have the same biology as the nonencapsulated strains of *H. influenzae.* An organism isolated from outbreaks of conjunctivitis, formerly assigned the name *Haemophilus aegyptius,* is now considered a variant of *H. influenzae.* Most of these species have been reported to cause systemic illness, including pneumonia, meningitis, arthritis, endocarditis, and soft tissue infections. Such cases are rare, as are those with nonencapsulated *H. influenzae.*

Table 23.1 Characteristics of *Haemophilus* Species

Haemophilus Species	Growth Factor Requirement		Hemolysis	Enhanced Growth with CO_2	Polysaccharide Capsular Antigen
	X	V			
H. influenzae (encapsulated)	+	+	−	−	Types a−f
H. influenzae (nonencapsulated)	+	+	−	−	−
H. parainfluenzae	−	+	−	−	−
H. haemolyticus	+	+	+	−	−
H. aphrophilus	−	−	−	+	−
H. paraaphrophilus	−	+	−	+	−
H. ducreyi	+	−	−	−	−

Abbreviations: X = hematin; V = nicotinamide adenine dinucleotide.

Haemophilus ducreyi

Rare sexually transmitted disease

Haemophilus ducreyi causes chancroid, a rare venereal disease in North America, although small outbreaks have occurred. The typical lesion is a tender papule on the genitalia that develops into a painful ulcer with sharp margins. Satellite lesions may develop by autoinfection, and regional lymphadenitis is common. The incubation period is usually short (2−5 days).

The diagnosis of chancroid is primarily clinical. It is considered in the differential diagnosis of genital ulcers along with more common causes such as syphilis and genital herpes. In this context, the lack of induration

Soft chancre

in chancroid has caused the primary lesion to be called *soft chancre* to distinguish it from the primary syphilitic chancre, which is typically indurated and painless. The presence of open genital sores due to *H. ducreyi* enhances the risk of transmission of human immunodeficiency virus, the etiologic agent of acquired immunodeficiency virus (AIDS), and this may contribute to the heterosexual spread of AIDS on the African continent.

Laboratory diagnosis

Isolation of *H. ducreyi* is difficult. This difficulty has led to reliance on relatively nonspecific diagnostic techniques, such as Gram staining from specimens inoculated into tubes of clotted rabbit blood. Recent studies show that the organism can be isolated directly from the lesion using chocolate agar, particularly if vancomycin is added to inhibit interfering flora. The bacteria are present in small numbers and may take up to 10 days to grow. Clinical laboratories should be specifically instructed to search for the organism when the disease is suspected.

Gardnerella vaginalis

Gardnerella vaginalis is a small Gram-variable coccobacillus discussed here because it is frequently encountered in the literature and was once called *Haemophilus vaginalis*. It resembles *Haemophilus* species in morphology and preference for chocolate agar for growth, but in little else. The species name relates to the long-held association of *G. vaginalis* with the clinical syndrome of bacterial vaginosis (Chapter 70). It is now thought to be only one of many secondary invaders and not a primary pathogen.

BORDETELLA

Bordetella pertussis

Bordetella pertussis is a coccobacillus with Gram stain morphology similar to that of *Haemophilus*. The organisms are strict aerobes and nonmotile. Infection of the human tracheobronchial epithelium produces pertussis (whooping cough), a prolonged disease marked by paroxysmal coughing.

Morphology and Structure

Small piliated Gram-negative coccobacilli

Bordetella pertussis is a tiny (0.5–1.0 μm), Gram-negative coccobacillus with highly regular staining characteristics. The cell wall has the structure typical of Gram-negative bacteria. Fresh isolates have capsules, pili, and a rodlike protein called *filamentous hemagglutinin* due to its ability to mediate agglutination of a variety of erythrocytes.

Growth

Bordetella pertussis is a slow-growing organism that requires specialized conditions for growth. Primary media require the addition of fresh blood, albumin, charcoal, starch, or ion exchange resins to an enriched base medium.

Bordet-Gengou medium

A widely used medium continues to be Bordet–Gengou agar containing fresh blood in a complex agar base. The function of the additives is not for nutrition, but for adsorption of substances toxic to *B. pertussis* that are normally found in culture media. The organism is also very susceptible to environmental changes and survives only briefly outside the human respiratory tract. Isolation requires direct plating onto a specially prepared medium. Aerobic incubation for 3–7 days is required for initial growth, which appears as tiny, glistening, compact colonies with the ap-

Small "drops of mercury" colonies

pearance of bisected pearls or drops of mercury. On media containing blood, a narrow zone of hemolysis is present around the colony. Growth may also be obtained in a suitable enriched broth. Several surface antigens have been identified that tend to change on subculture, a feature of importance in vaccine production, but of unknown significance in disease.

Toxins

In addition to cell wall endotoxin, *B. pertussis* produces at least three exotoxins. The best studied of these is *pertussis toxin,* also known as *lymphocytosis promoting factor.* The toxin is not directly cytotoxic, but stimu-

Pertussis toxin stimulates adenylate cyclase system

lates the adenylate cyclase system in a wide variety of cell types by ADP-ribosylating and inactivating a regulatory protein. Its action thus resembles diphtheria, cholera, and *Escherichia coli* heat-labile toxins, and *Pseudomonas* exotoxin A.

A wide variety of biologic effects are attributable to pertussis toxin, the net results depending on the cell type involved. These include histamine sensitization, lymphocytosis promotion, insulin secretion, and a variety of actions involving immune effector cells.

Extracellular adenylate cyclase toxin

Another recently discovered toxin is itself an adenylate cyclase. This extracellular enzyme has been shown to interfere with chemotaxis and superoxide production by polymorphonuclear leukocytes. The toxin is activated within the cell by calmodulin, a eukaryotic regulatory protein. This activation of a bacterial enzyme by an intracellular mammalian protein is unusual, but also seen with anthrax toxin (Chapter 17). A third toxin

23.3 A tracheal organ culture 72 hr after infection with *B. pertussis.* The organisms have attached to the cilia of some cells and killed them. These balloonlike cells with attached bacteria are extruded from the epithelium. The large arrow shows the *Bordetella* and the small arrow the cilia. Note the background of uninfected ciliated cells and denuded epithelium where nonciliated cells remain. (*Reproduced with permission from Muse, K. E., Collier, A. M., and Baseman, J. B. 1977. J. Infect Dis. 136:768–777. Figure 3, copyright 1977 by University of Chicago, publisher.*)

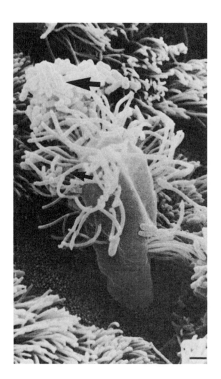

produced by *B. pertussis* is currently called *tracheal cytotoxin* because of its action on ciliated tracheal epithelium. It is closely associated with cell wall peptidoglycan.

Pathogenesis

Bordetella pertussis is a strict pathogen of humans. It has not been isolated from animals or as a member of the normal flora of healthy persons. When introduced into the respiratory tract, the organism has a remarkable tropism for ciliated bronchial epithelium. The bacteria first attach to and immobilize the cilia. This action begins a sequence in which the ciliated epithelial cells are progressively destroyed and extruded from the epithelial border (Figure 23.3). The nonciliated cells are not involved and maintain the integrity of the epithelial lining. All of these events occur without tissue invasion by *B. pertussis,* although considerable local inflammation and exudate are produced in the bronchi.

The mediator of the initial attachment to tracheal cilia is not known for certain, but the filamentous hemagglutinin and pertussis toxin appear to be involved. Following attachment, the subsequent injury to the respiratory epithelium is by the tracheal cytotoxin. Pertussis toxin is clearly responsible for many of the systemic manifestations of pertussis, such as lymphocytosis, but its role in local injury, cough, or the prolonged course of the disease is unclear. The adenylate cyclase probably plays an antiphagocytic role by virtue of its direct action on phagocytes.

Tropism for bronchial epithelium

Immobilization and destruction of ciliated epithelial cells; organisms noninvasive

Immunity

Although antibodies are produced during the course of pertussis and by immunization, their role in immunity is not well understood. Naturally acquired immunity is not lifelong, although second attacks, when recognized, tend to be mild. The high susceptibility of newborns and infants before immunization may reflect a low level of antibody in adults and thus lack of passive transfer to the infant at birth.

Epidemiology

High infectivity

Atypical or subclinical disease in adults

Effectiveness of immunization

Pertussis is spread by airborne droplet nuclei to those in close contact with a patient in the early stages of illness. It is highly infectious. Secondary spread in families is common; it is not always recognized, however, because of the mildness of symptoms in immunized patients. Such cases, particularly in adults, may serve as a significant reservoir of the organism. Outbreaks in highly susceptible populations, such as hospitalized newborns, have been traced to hospital employees with pertussis symptoms resembling those of the common cold.

The incidence of pertussis has been decreasing since the introduction of immunization in the 1940s. Sporadic epidemics occur, and there is no strong seasonal pattern to the disease. Rates of pertussis have increased when immunization rates have decreased, because of concern of vaccine potency and side effects. For example, when immunization rates in England fell below 50% in 1981, there were 47,000 cases in the first 9 months of 1982. Mortality has dropped in accordance with the decreased incidence of disease, but remains highest in infants. Over 70% of fatal cases are in children under 1 year of age, whereas less than 5% are in children over 5 years of age.

Clinical Manifestations

After an incubation period of 7–10 days, pertussis follows a prolonged course consisting of three overlapping stages: 1) catarrhal; 2) paroxysmal coughing; and 3) convalescent.

Catarrhal phase, highly communicable

In the catarrhal stage, the primary feature is a profuse and mucoid rhinorrhea that persists for 1–2 weeks. Nonspecific findings such as malaise, fever, sneezing, and anorexia may also be present. The disease is most communicable at this stage, as large numbers of organisms are present in the nasopharynx and the mucoid secretions.

Paroxysmal phase

Inspiratory whoop

The appearance of a persistent cough marks the transition from the catarrhal to the paroxysmal coughing stage. At this time, episodes of paroxysmal coughing occur up to 50 times a day for 2–4 weeks. The characteristic inspiratory whoop follows a series of coughs as air is rapidly drawn through the narrowed glottis. Vomiting frequently follows the whoop. The combination of mucoid secretions, whooping cough, and vomiting causes the child to be miserable, exhausted, and barely able to breathe. Fever is not present unless a complication such as bacterial superinfection or atelectasis develops. Marked leukocytosis, primarily a result of increased levels of circulating lymphocytes, reaches its peak in the paroxysmal stage. Absolute lymphocyte counts of $40,000/mm^3$ are typical, and much higher counts have been recorded.

High lymphocytosis

Convalescent phase

During the convalescent stage, which lasts 3–4 weeks, the frequency and severity of paroxysmal coughing episodes gradually diminish. Other features of the disease gradually fade as well.

Partially immune persons and infants under 6 months of age may not show all the typical features of pertussis. Some evolution through the three stages is usually seen, but paroxysmal coughing and lymphocytosis may be absent.

Pulmonary complications

The most common complications of pertussis involve the lung. Pneumonia, usually caused by a superinfecting organism such as *Streptococcus pneumoniae,* is the most serious complication and accounts for the majority of deaths caused by pertussis. Pneumonia typically appears at the height of the paroxysmal coughing stage and, in addition to the usual signs and symptoms, is associated with disappearance of the paroxysms. Atelectasis is also common but may be recognized only by radiologic examination. Other complications, including convulsions, hemorrhage, and hernias, are related to the pressure effects of the paroxysmal coughing and the anoxia produced by inadequate ventilation and apneic spells. Nutritional disturbances and dehydration may also be a problem over the prolonged course of the illness.

Diagnosis

Nasopharyngeal swab

A clinical diagnosis of pertussis is confirmed by isolation of *B. pertussis* from a nasopharyngeal swab. The organism is not found at distant sites, and bacteremia does not occur. Specimens collected early in the course of disease (during the catarrhal or early paroxysmal stage) provide the greatest chance of successful isolation. Unfortunately, the diagnosis is frequently not considered until paroxysmal coughing has been present for

Organisms often not present by paroxysmal phase

some time, and the number of organisms has decreased significantly. The nasopharyngeal swab is best collected by the pernasal route and plated directly onto either Bordet-Gengou or a special charcoal agar medium. Low concentrations of a penicillin or cephalosporin are usually added to these plates to inhibit members of the normal flora and to allow *B. pertussis* to grow. Characteristic colonies appear after 3–5 days of incubation and the organisms are identified serologically, because *B. pertussis* shows few specific metabolic activities.

Direct immunofluorescence

A direct immunofluorescent technique has been successfully applied to nasopharyngeal smears for rapid diagnosis of pertussis. Smears are stable on transport to the laboratory, whereas the organisms themselves may not survive without special precautions. Positive smears should always be confirmed by culture, if possible.

Treatment

No specific therapy by paroxysmal phase

Once the paroxysmal coughing stage has been reached, the treatment of pertussis is primarily supportive. By this stage the bronchial epithelium has already been damaged, and antimicrobial therapy will not reverse it. Antimicrobial therapy is useful at earlier stages and for limiting spread to other susceptible individuals. Some antimicrobics, including ampicillin,

Erythromycin treatment in catarrhal phase

tetracycline, erythromycin, and chloramphenicol are active in vitro against *B. pertussis.* Of these, erythromycin is preferred because of its clinical effectiveness and relative lack of toxicity. Penicillins, including ampicillin, have not been effective in clearing the organisms from the respiratory tract.

Prevention

Inactivated bacillary vaccine

Active immunization is the primary method of preventing pertussis. Vaccines are produced from inactivated whole cell suspensions or from partially purified preparations derived from whole cells. In the United States, the vaccine is combined with diphtheria and tetanus toxoids to produce

DPT

a triple vaccine, DPT. Three doses given at monthly intervals are begun as early in life as possible (6–8 weeks) because of the high susceptibility

Effectiveness and side effects
of vaccine

and mortality in infants. Booster doses later in childhood are recommended. Recent immunization reduces the attack rate upon exposure and the severity of disease upon infection. Side effects and vaccine-related complications have been a problem with some pertussis vaccine preparations. Local inflammation and febrile reactions have been common, and occasionally convulsions and brain damage have occurred.

Pertussis immunization has become a controversial, even emotional, issue in many countries, and small but vocal groups argue that the risk of neurologic sequelae outweigh those of the disease. Epidemiologic data do not support these claims, but it must be recognized that the whole-cell vaccine is among the crudest preparation routinely injected into humans. A more purified acellular vaccine containing primarily pertussis toxin and filamentous hemagglutinin has been produced but it has not yet been clearly shown to be as effective as the whole-cell preparation. Until more is known about the relative roles played by the *B. pertussis* virulence factors, it will be difficult to decide which component(s) to include in a "purified" vaccine.

Additional Reading

Fothergill, L.D., and Wright, J. 1933. Influenzal meningitis: The relation of age incidence to the bactericidal power of blood against the causal organism. *J. Immunol.* 24:273–284. A classic study, the first to advance the currently accepted concepts of humoral immunity in *Haemophilus influenzae* disease.

Friedman, R.L. 1988. Pertussis: The disease and new diagnostic methods. *Clin. Microbiol. Rev.* 1:365–376. In addition to an update on pathogenesis, this review discusses current and potential diagnostic methods.

Granoff, D.M., and Munson, R.S. 1986. Prospects for prevention of *Haemophilus influenzae* type b disease. *J. Infect. Dis.* 153:448–461. This article discusses the problem with immunogenicity of polysaccharide vaccines and the prospects for the polysaccharide–protein conjugate vaccines.

Muse, K.E., Collier, A.M., and Baseman, J.B. 1977. Scanning electron microscopic study of hamster tracheal organ cultures infected with *Bordetella pertussis*. *J. Infect. Dis.* 136:768–777. The unique tropism of *Bordetella pertussis* for ciliated cells and the subsequent destruction of those cells are shown experimentally and visually.

Ward, J.I., Fraser, D.W., Baraff, L.J., and Plikaytis, B.D. 1979. *Haemophilus influenzae* meningitis: A national study of secondary spread in household contacts. *N. Engl. J. Med.* 301:122–126. This study changed our thinking about the epidemiology of *Haemophilus influenzae* type b infections by elucidating the extent to which they are contagious.

Weiss, A.A., and Hewlett, E.L. 1986. Virulence factors of *Bordetella pertussis*. *Annu. Rev. Microbiol.* 40:661–686. A review of the action of all the virulence factors and what is known, or unknown, about their role in clinical pertussis.

24

Mycoplasma *and* Ureaplasma

Lawrence Corey

Smallest free-living organisms

Mycoplasma and *Ureaplasma* (formerly called *T-strain Mycoplasma*) are the smallest free-living microorganisms. They comprise the two genera of the family Mycoplasmataceae, members of which resemble other bacteria except in their lack of a cell wall. Species are ubiquitous in nature, and some are pathogens of animals, plants, and humans. DNA base ratio studies indicate that most species are unrelated and have different origins. Numerous *Mycoplasma* species that are associated with humans have been identified (Table 24.1), but only three species of the two genera have been associated with disease. *Mycoplasma pneumoniae* is a lower respiratory tract pathogen. *Mycoplasma hominis* and *Ureaplasma urealyticum* cause some genitourinary tract infections.

Absence of cell walls

These organisms have diameters of about 0.2–0.3 μm, but they are highly plastic and pleomorphic and may appear as coccoid bodies, filaments, and large multinucleoid forms. They have no cell wall, but are bounded by a single triple-layered membrane (Figure 24.1) that, unlike those of other bacteria, contains sterols. The sterols are not synthesized by the organism, but are acquired as essential components from the media or tissues in which it is growing. *Mycoplasma* stain poorly or not at all with the usual bacterial stains. Because of their lack of cell walls, they are completely insensitive to the penicillins and cephalosporins. Their genome is small probably because of lack of genes encoding a complex cell wall. It consists of double-stranded DNA with a molecular weight of about 5×10^8 that replicates like that of other bacteria. *Mycoplasma pneumoniae* is an aerobe, but most other species are facultatively anaerobic. All grow slowly in enriched liquid culture media and on special *Mycoplasma* agar to produce minute colonies only after several days of incubation. The center of the colony grows into the agar and appears denser to give an inverted "fried egg" appearance. Growth in culture is inhibited by specific antisera directed at the particular species.

Not stained by Gram's method

Slow growth in specialized artificial media

Inhibition of growth by antisera

Differential features

Different metabolic properties are characteristic of the various species

415

Table 24.1   Some Mycoplasma and Ureaplasma Species of Humans

Organism	Site	Prevalence	Disease
M. salivarium	Periodontal sulci	Very common	None
M. orale	Upper respiratory tract	Very common	None
M. pneumoniae	Upper and lower respiratory tract	Common	Primary atypical pneumonia
M. fermentans	Genitourinary tract	Rare	None
M. hominis	Genitourinary tract	Common	Postpartum fever; pelvic inflammatory disease
U. urealyticum	Genitourinary tract	Very common	Nongonococcal urethritis
M. genitalium	Genitourinary tract	Undetermined	Unknown

Hemadsorption by *M. pneumoniae*

of *Mycoplasma* and *Ureaplasma* and allow easy differentiation between those of importance in human medicine. Colonies of *M. pneumoniae* bind red blood cells that are washed onto the surface of agar plate cultures (hemadsorption). This is due to the affinity of a surface adhesin (protein P1) on the mycoplasma for neuraminic acid groups on red cell glycoproteins. This phenomenon also accounts for attachment of *M. pneumoniae* to respiratory epithelial cells. The species that infect the respiratory and genital tracts will be considered separately in this chapter because of their different epidemiologic characteristics.

Mycoplasma pneumoniae

Disease Syndromes

Range of infections and allergic reactions

Mycoplasma pneumoniae is an important respiratory tract pathogen of humans. Several syndromes have been associated with the infection, including pharyngitis, tracheobronchitis, inflammation of the tympanic membrane presenting as bullous myringitis, and pneumonitis. Occasionally, infection caused by *M. pneumoniae* is associated with arthritis, menin-

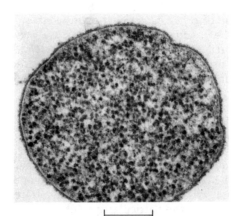

24.1 Electron micrograph of *Mycoplasma*. Note cytoplasmic membrane ribosomes and surface amorphous material with absence of cell wall. (*Kindly provided by the late Dr. E. S. Boatman.*)

├─────── 0.2 μm ───────┤

goencephalitis, hemolytic anemia, and rash. Allergic reactions (Stevens–Johnson syndrome and erythema multiforme) may develop.

Primary atypical (walking) pneumonia

Insidious onset

Frequent lobar distribution

In most populations, *M. pneumoniae* accounts for approximately 20% of all cases of pneumonia. Classically, it causes a disease less severe than common bacterial pneumonia that has been described as *primary atypical pneumonia* or *walking pneumonia.* Most cases do not require hospitalization. The disease is of insidious onset, with fever, headache, and malaise for 2–4 days before the onset of respiratory symptoms. Pulmonary symptoms generally comprise a nonproductive cough. X-rays reveal a lobar pneumonia, usually in the lower lobes, although multiple lobes are sometimes involved. Small pleural effusions are seen in 25% of cases. Any expectorated sputum is mucoid, and Gram staining of sputum usually shows some polymorphonuclear cells but a paucity of bacteria, because *M. pneumoniae* are not detectable by this stain.

Tracheobronchitis and pharyngitis

A milder tracheobronchitis with fever, cough, headache, and malaise is the most common syndrome associated with acute *M. pneumoniae* infection, although there is usually X-ray evidence of pulmonary involvement. Pharyngitis with fever and sore throat may also occur. The clinical signs and symptoms of *M. pneumoniae* pharyngitis are indistinguishable from those caused by viruses such as Epstein–Barr virus and by the group A streptococcus.

Bullous myringitis and otitis media

Acute hemorrhagic bullous myringitis is an uncommon but well-described syndrome associated with infection caused by *M. pneumoniae.* Nonpurulent otitis media or myringitis occurs concomitantly in approximately 15% of patients with *M. pneumoniae* pneumonitis. The presence of nonpurulent otitis media and lower respiratory illness in a teenager suggests *M. pneumoniae* infection.

Infection and Pathogenesis

Very low infecting dose

Infection with *M. pneumoniae* is acquired by droplet spread. In experimental challenge, the human infectious ID_{50} (the dose of organisms required to cause infection in 50% of volunteers) is only one colony-forming unit when inhaled in an aerosol and about 100 colony-forming units by intranasal inoculation.

Specific adherence to respiratory epithelium

Damage to epithelium; inflammatory response

Initially, the organism attaches to surface neuraminic acid receptors on the respiratory epithelium. It interferes with ciliary action and leads to desquamation of the involved mucosa and a subsequent inflammatory reaction and exudate. The inflammatory response is at first most pronounced in the bronchial and peribronchial tissue, although the alveoli may also be involved. Lymphocytes, plasma cells, and macrophages then infiltrate and thicken the walls of the alveoli and bronchioles.

Prolonged shedding of organisms

Organisms are shed in upper respiratory secretions for 2–8 days before the onset of symptoms, and shedding continues for as long as 14 weeks after infection.

Immune Responses

Complement fixing antibody titers

Cold hemagglutinins

Both local and systemic specific immune responses occur. Local immunoglobulin A(IgA) antibody is produced, but disappears 2–4 weeks after the onset of the infection. Complement fixing serum antibody titers reach a peak 2–4 weeks after infection and gradually disappear over 6–12 months. Nonspecific immune responses to the glycolipids of the outer membrane of the organism may develop. The most common of these responses involves the production of cold hemagglutinins, which are IgM antibodies that react with the I antigen of human red blood cells and cause agglutination at temperatures of 0–4°C. They are seen in about two-thirds of symptomatic patients infected with *M. pneumoniae*. Antibodies to the glycolipids of the outer membrane of the organism, which occasionally result in false-positive reagin tests for syphilis, may include antibody that reacts with a nonhemolytic streptococcus (*Streptococcus MG*).

Immunity incomplete and reinfection common

Immunity is not complete, and reinfection with *M. pneumoniae* is common. Clinical disease appears to be more severe in older than in younger children, which has led to the suggestion that many of the clinical manifestations of disease are the result of cellular immune responses rather than response to invasion by the organism.

Epidemiology

Worldwide endemic infection with intermittent epidemics

Most common age incidence 5–15 years

Outbreaks in families and closed communities

Endemic infections with *M. pneumoniae* occur throughout the year and are worldwide, but they are especially prominent in temperate climates. Epidemics at 4- to 6-year intervals have been noted in both civilian and military populations. The most common age for symptomatic *M. pneumoniae* infection is between 5 and 15 years, and the disease accounts for more than one-third of all cases of pneumonia in teenagers. Infections in children less than 6 months old are uncommon. The disease often appears as a sporadic, endemic illness in families or closed communities because of its relatively long incubation period (2–15 days) and because prolonged shedding in nasal secretions may cause infections to be spread over time. Attack rates in susceptible individuals within families approach 60%. Asymptomatic infections occur, but most studies have suggested that more than two-thirds of infected cases develop some evidence of respiratory tract illness.

Laboratory Diagnosis

Diagnosis usually serologic because of slow growth

Significance of single high complement fixing titers

Clinical diagnosis of *M. pneumoniae* infection may be difficult because of the overlap of manifestations with those of other bacterial and viral infections. Direct staining of clinical material is not useful. The organism can be isolated from throat swabs or sputum of infected patients on special enriched culture media; however, because of its relatively slow growth, more than 1 week of incubation is generally required. Thus, serologic tests rather than cultures are usually used for specific diagnosis. A fourfold rise in serum complement fixing antibody during the disease indicates active *M. pneumoniae* infection. A single high titer, such as greater than 1:128, indicates recent or concurrent infection, because complement fixing antibody is of short duration. With the relatively long incubation period and insidious onset of the disease, many patients will have high antibody titers at the time of presentation to the physician.

Significance of cold agglutinin titers

In many clinical situations, the demonstration of nonspecific anti-I antibody can be helpful, because more than two-thirds of patients with symptomatic lower respiratory *M. pneumoniae* infection develop high titers of cold hemagglutinins. It must be remembered that cold agglutinins are nonspecific and have been observed in adenovirus infections, infectious mononucleosis, and some other illnesses. The cold agglutinin test is simple, however, and can be performed rapidly in any clinical laboratory or even at the bedside.

Treatment

Erythromycin and tetracycline

Erythromycin and tetracycline are the agents used for treatment of *M. pneumoniae* infections. They will shorten the course of infection, although eradication from the nasopharynx may take much longer.

Infection by Genitourinary Tract *Ureaplasmas* and *Mycoplasmas*

Ureaplasma urealyticum

Urease production

The genus *Ureaplasma* contains a single species, *U. urealyticum,* of which some 14 serotypes have been described. *Ureaplasma* is distinguished from all other members of the order Mycoplasmatales by its production of urease. On special *Ureaplasma* agar media, colonies are small and circular and grow downward into the agar. In liquid media containing urea and phenol red, growth of *Ureaplasma* results in production of ammonia from the urea, with a resultant increase of pH and a change of color in the indicator.

Sexual transmission

Epidemiology. The main reservoir of human strains of *U. urealyticum* is the genital tract of sexually active men and women; it is rarely found before puberty. Colonization, which probably results primarily from sexual contact, occurs in more than 80% of individuals who have had three or more sexual partners.

Association with nongonococcal urethritis

Clinical Outline of Disease. Because of the high colonization rate, it has been difficult to associate specific illness with *Ureaplasma.* However, recent studies suggest that approximately one-half of cases of nongonococcal, nonchlamydial urethritis in men may be caused by *U. urealyticum.* In women, *Ureaplasma* has been shown to cause chorioamnionitis, and postpartum fever has been associated with it.

Responsiveness to tetracycline and spectinomycin

Diagnosis and Treatment. In the appropriate clinical situation, men with nongonococcal urethritis should be treated on the assumption that *Ureaplasma* infection may be involved. Tetracycline is the treatment of choice because it is also active against chlamydiae. Recently, tetracycline-resistant strains of *Ureaplasma* have been reported that have been associated with recurrences of nongonococcal urethritis in men. In such cases, spectinomycin treatment, or treatment with quinolone antimicrobics is also effective.

Mycoplasma hominis

Arginine breakdown

Mycoplasma hominis is another inhabitant of the genitourinary tract. Although some strains grow on ordinary blood agar as nonhemolytic pinpoint colonies, the organism is best detected on *Mycoplasma* agar, on which it grows rapidly. *Mycoplasma hominis* and *Ureaplasma* can be differentiated by demonstrating arginine breakdown by the former and urease activity by the latter. At least seven antigenic variants of *M. hominis* have been described. To date, the major clinical condition associated with *M. hominis*

Association with postpartum fever and pelvic inflammatory disease

infection is postabortal or postpartum fever. *Mycoplasma hominis* is isolated from the blood of about 10% of women with this condition, and *U. urealyticum* from another 10%. The diseases appears to be self-limiting, although antibiotic therapy may decrease the duration of fever and hospitalization. Recently, serologic studies and animal experiments have indicated that pelvic inflammatory disease syndromes in women may be associated with *M. hominis* infection of the Fallopian tubes. The organism

Susceptible to tetracycline; resistant to erythromycin

is sensitive to tetracycline. In contrast to *U. urealyticum* and *M. pneumoniae,* *M. hominis* is resistant to erythromycin.

Additional Reading

Broughton, R.A. 1986. Infections due to *Mycoplasma pneumoniae* in childhood. *Ped. Infect. Dis.* 5:71–85.

Cassell, G.H., and Cole, B.C. 1981. Mycoplasmas as agents of human disease. *N. Engl. J. Med.* 304:80–89.

Taylor-Robinson, D., and McCormack, W.M. 1980. The genital mycoplasmas. *N. Engl. J. Med.* 302:1003–1010, 1063–1067.

These are three excellent reviews of this chapter's topic.

25
Legionella

Kenneth J. Ryan

The widely publicized outbreak of pneumonia among attendees of the 1976 American Legion convention in Philadelphia led to the isolation of a new infectious agent, *Legionella pneumophila*. The event was unique in medical history; for months the American public had entertained theories of its cause that ranged from sabotage to viroids, only to find that a previously undescribed Gram-negative rod was responsible. It was an outstanding example of the benefits of pursuing sound epidemiologic evidence until it is explained by equally sound microbiologic findings. We now know the disease had occurred for many years: specific antibodies and organisms have been detected in material preserved from the 1950s, and a mysterious outbreak in 1965 has been solved retrospectively. The primary reasons the organism escaped detection for so long are that it stains poorly or not at all with common methods and will not grow on the usual bacteriologic media. *Legionella pneumophila* is only one of a growing list of over 20 *Legionella* species found in the environment and, in some cases, in human infections.

Legionella

Morphology

Legionella pneumophila is a thin, pleomorphic, Gram-negative rod 0.5–0.7 μm in width and 2–20 μm or more in length. Elongated, filamentous forms are common. In clinical specimens, the organism stains poorly or not at all by Gram stain or the usual histologic stains; it can be demonstrated, however, by certain silver impregnation methods (Dieterle stain) and by some simple stains that omit decolorization steps. It should be emphasized that these staining methods are nonspecific, but suggest *Legionella* when the organism is clearly demonstrable only by such manipulations. Ultrastructurally, *L. pneumophila* has features similar to those of Gram-negative

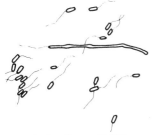

Legionella pneumophila

Stains with difficulty; Gram-negative cell wall structure

421

bacteria with a typical outer membrane, thin peptidoglycan layer, and cytoplasmic membrane. Polar, subpolar, and lateral flagella may be present. Most species of *Legionella* are motile. Spores are not found.

Growth

Legionella species will not grow on common enriched bacteriologic media such as blood agar, but require a medium containing a range of amino acids that is supplemented with L-cysteine and a source of ferric ions. The latter may be provided by hemoglobin or soluble ferric pyrophosphate. *Legionella pneumophila* grows optimally at a pH of 6.9, and it is sensitive to major variations from this value. Optimal growth occurs on properly supplemented agar media under aerobic conditions at 35°C. Colonies develop in 2–5 days and have a surface resembling ground glass. Although growth in fluid media is generally poor, it is interesting to note that good growth has been obtained in broth containing macrophages and in water containing photosynthetic bacteria, algae, and amebas.

Special media needed for growth

Classification

Legionella species are not closely related to any other groups of bacteria. They possess catalase, oxidase (weak), gelatinase, and β-lactamase activity, but do not grow or react positively in most other taxonomic tests used to classify other bacteria. Their identification and classification depends largely on antigenic features, chromatographic analysis of cellular fatty acid content, and on DNA homology tests. Antisera have been prepared that react specifically with *Legionella,* and the chromatographic profile of cellular branched and unbranched fatty acids is unique. Twelve serotypes of *L. pneumophila* have been defined by immunofluorescent procedures using whole organisms, but the nature of the responsible antigens is not known. In addition to *L. pneumophila,* over 20 related organisms have now been assigned species names within the *Legionella* genus (*L. bozemanii, L. dumoffii, L. micdadei,* etc.). These organisms share the poor staining characteristics and growth requirements for primary isolation of *L. pneumophila,* but differ in some cultural and other features, such as fluorescence of colonies under ultraviolet light. The most commonly encountered *Legionella* other than *L. pneumophila* is *L. micdadei. L. micdadei* is distinctive in demonstrating acid-fastness in sputum and tissue—a characteristic that is lost in culture. DNA homology has become the primary taxonomic tool in assigning new isolates to a species or in creating a new species. This approach is used when an isolate with the cultural characteristic of *Legionella* does not react with any of the typing sera available for *L. pneumophila* or the more common other legionellas.

Identification by antigenic structure and gas chromatographic patterns

Serotypes of L. pneumophila

Other Legionella species

Role of DNA homology tests in defining new species

Epidemiology

Two clinically and epidemiologically distinct syndromes are associated with *L. pneumophila.* The first, a severe pneumonia with an incubation period of 2–10 days, is called *Legionnaires' disease* and has mortality as high as 60%. The other, *Pontiac fever* (named for a 1968 Michigan outbreak), is a nonpneumonic febrile illness with an incubation period of 20–48 hr. Pontiac fever is a self-limiting illness that is not life threatening. The attack rate for Legionnaires' disease has been estimated at less than 5% of those exposed, whereas over 90% have had clinical illness in outbreaks of Pontiac fever.

Pneumonic and nonpneumonic diseases

Both syndromes can appear in sporadic or epidemic form. Most outbreaks have occurred in or around large buildings such as hotels, factories, and hospitals. Those outbreaks traced to a source have involved a cooling tower, evaporative condenser, or some other part of the building's air-conditioning system. Organisms contaminating the water are aerosolized and spread either directly or through the air ducts of the system. Some recent hospital outbreaks have implicated potable water found in sites such as faucets and shower heads, although the mechanisms of transmission from these sources is unclear. Person-to-person transmission has not been documented, and the organisms have not been isolated from healthy individuals. It is difficult to ascertain the overall incidence of *Legionella* infections, as most information has been from outbreaks. Serologic surveys indicate that outbreaks constitute only a small part of the total cases, many of which currently go undetected. Estimates based on seroconversions suggest approximately 25,000 cases in the United States each year and that the frequency of pneumonic disease is probably less than that of Pontiac fever. Both serologic and environmental studies indicate that *Legionella* has low virulence for humans.

Legionella pneumophila has been isolated not only from air-conditioning systems but from freshwater sites such as lakes and ponds, and the organism is known to survive as long as a year in unchlorinated tap water. It does not grow in sterile tap water, but will multiply if other environmental microorganisms are added. These include certain bacteria, algae, and free-living protozoa, which can provide necessary growth factors. Of particular interest are environmental amebas. *Legionella pneumophila* has been shown to penetrate them and multiply intracellularly in a manner entirely analogous to that observed in human macrophages (see "Pathogenesis and Pathology"). Although a direct link with transmission to humans has not been proven, such amebas have been found growing in cooling towers that have been the source of *Legionella* outbreaks. This suggests that amebas could act as the environmental reservoir for virulent legionellas.

Pathogenesis and Pathology

Legionella pneumophila is striking in its propensity to attack the lung and associated structures with minimal spread to other organs. The pneumonia is necrotizing and multifocal with a tendency for coalescence of the lesions. Microscopically, the process involves the alveoli and terminal bronchioles with relative sparing of the larger bronchioles and bronchi. Microabscess formation is common. The inflammatory exudate contains abundant fibrin and a mixture of both polymorphonuclear leukocytes and macrophages. Much less is known about the pathology, pathogenesis, and immunity of nonpneumophila infections because of their lower frequency, but it appears to resemble that seen with *L. pneumophila*.

Legionella pneumophila is a facultative intracellular pathogen. Its pathogenicity is strongly related to its ability to survive and multiply within cells of the monocyte–macrophage series. This process involves some characteristic steps which are illustrated in Figure 25.1. The organisms are taken into macrophages by a process called *coiling phagocytosis*. Once in the phagocyte, the *Legionella*-containing phagosome becomes lined with ribosomes and clusters of mitochondria. At this stage instead of being killed by the bactericidal mechanisms of the macrophage, the bacteria multiply extensively in the cell. These features have been demonstrated in experimental systems, in human infections, and in some free-living

Marginal notes:

Association with humidifying and cooling systems

No person-to-person transmission

Most infections subclinical

Water habitats

Necrotizing multifocal pneumonia

Facultative intracellular pathogen

Ability to multiply in macrophages

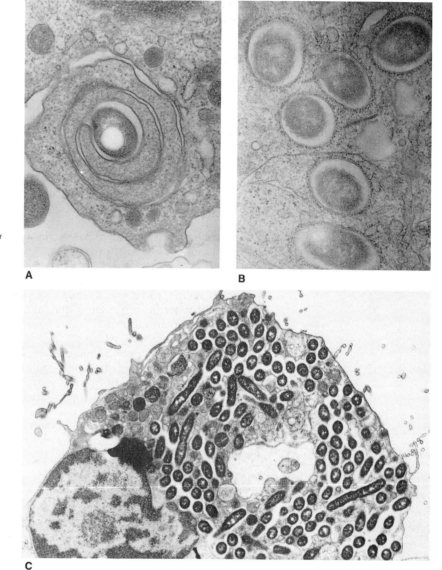

25.1 Multiplication of *Legionella pneumophila* in human macrophages. *Legionella pneumophila* enters the cell by coiling phagocytosis (**A**), and the phagosome created is lined by ribosomes and mitochondria (**B**). The bacteria multiply within the macrophages to reach very high numbers (**C**). (*Kindly provided by Dr. Marcus Horwitz.*)

Inhibits lysosome–phagosome fusion

amebas. The ability to escape intraphagocytic killing is related to inhibition of lysosomal fusion and thus of acidification of the phagosome. *Legionella pneumophila* also produce a toxin that inhibits the oxidative burst of phagocytosis. The relative contribution of these and other factors remains to be determined, but it is clear that once *L. pneumophila* reaches the lower airways, the alveolar macrophage becomes a haven rather than a death trap.

Immunity

Just as intracellular multiplication is the key to *L. pneumophila* virulence, its inhibition by cell-mediated mechanisms appears to be the most important aspect of immunity. Activated macrophages are able to inhibit

Roles of cell-mediated and humoral immunity

intracellular multiplication by both oxygen-dependent and -independent mechanisms. Gamma interferon appears to be one of the mediators of this activation. The role of antibody in immunity appears to be less. Antibody alone has no effect on the multiplication of *Legionella,* but in the presence of activated cellular immune responses it may play an ancillary role through enhancement of phagocytosis. These observations are based on in vitro and animal experiments. It is unknown whether humans who have had Legionnaires' disease have increased immunity to reinfection and disease.

Clinical Features

Severe toxic pneumonia

Legionnaires' disease is a severe toxic pneumonia that begins with myalgia and headache, followed by a rapidly rising fever. A dry cough may develop and later become productive, but sputum production is not a prominent feature. Chills, pleuritic chest pain, vomiting, diarrhea, confusion, and delirium may all be seen. Radiologically, patchy or interstitial infiltrates with a tendency to progress toward a nodular consolidation are present unilaterally or bilaterally. Liver function tests often indicate some hepatic dysfunction. In the more serious cases the patient becomes progressively ill and toxic over the first 3–6 days, and the disease terminates in shock and/or respiratory failure. The overall mortality is about 15%, but is particularly high in patients with serious underlying disease or immunosuppression. Mortality has been over 50% in some hospital outbreaks.

High mortality

Non-progressive, self-limiting disease

Pontiac fever begins similarly with fever and myalgia, and one-half of all patients have a dry cough. The disease does not progress, however, and recovery usually begins after 2–5 days. It would be considered a mild form of Legionnaires' disease were it not for the rather uniform clinical and epidemiologic features in documented outbreaks. In the Pontiac outbreak there were 144 cases with no deaths.

Diagnosis

The possibility of Legionnaires' disease should be considered in any patient with severe progressive pneumonia not shown to be caused by another organism. The best means of diagnosis for clinical purposes is direct microscopic examination and culture of infected tissues. For this purpose, a high-quality specimen such as that from a transtracheal aspirate, lung aspirate, or lung biopsy is usually necessary, because the organism is rarely found in sputum. Typically the Gram smear shows no bacteria; the organisms are demonstrated by direct immunofluorescent examination of the same material using *Legionella*-specific conjugates. This method is the most rapid means of diagnosis, but it is positive in only 25–50% of culture-proved cases.

High-quality specimens needed

Direct examination by fluorescence microscopy

Cultures on special media

Cultures should be made on routine media as well as on special agar media that meet the growth requirements of *Legionella.* Currently, the best agar medium is buffered charcoal yeast extract. This contains yeast extract as a source of amino acids and vitamins, the necessary L-cysteine and iron supplements, charcoal to adsorb toxic fatty acids or surfactants, and buffer to give the optimum pH for *Legionella* growth. The isolation of morphologically characteristic Gram-negative rods on this medium after 2–5 days, but not on routine culture plates (blood agar, chocolate agar), is presumptive evidence of *Legionella.* These findings are confirmed by direct immunofluorescent staining of smears prepared from the colonies. The medium also allows isolation of most other *Legionella* species. Occasional cases with positive direct immunofluorescent smears but negative cultures are still seen. These results are probably caused by strains for which growth conditions remain unmet.

Serodiagnosis by rising titer

The diagnosis can also be established by demonstrating a significant rise in specific serum antibody titer with an indirect immunofluorescent technique. As with most other serodiagnostic tests, this method requires paired (acute and convalescent) sera to demonstrate a rising titer; it is used primarily for retrospective diagnosis and in epidemiologic studies. In some communities elevated titers in single serum samples have been detected in as much as 25% of the population.

Diagnostic procedures for legionellosis should not be considered routine at present and may not be available in some hospital laboratories. This is particularly true for the direct immunofluorescence test. Therefore, the clinician should always advise the laboratory of the suspicion of Legionnaires' disease before submitting material. Specimens and smears can then, if necessary, be sent to a reference laboratory for processing.

Treatment and Prevention

The best information on antimicrobial therapy is still provided by the original Philadelphia outbreak. Because the etiology was completely obscure at the time, the cases were treated with many different regimens.

Erythromycin treatment

β-Lactamase producers

Patients treated with erythromycin clearly did better than those given the penicillins, cephalosporins, or aminoglycosides; subsequently, it was shown that *Legionella* are producers of β-lactamase, which explains the poor results with β-lactam antimicrobics. In vitro susceptibility tests and animal studies confirmed the activity of erythromycin and showed that tetracycline is also active, but less so than erythromycin. The organism is also susceptible to rifampin, but this agent is not used alone because of the frequency of resistant mutants. The organisms are susceptible to the newer quinolones, which show promise as therapeutic agents.

Preventive measures

The prevention of legionellosis involves preventing or minimizing contamination of aerosol sources in cooling towers and in water supplies of buildings. This is complicated by the fact that, compared to the Enterobacteriaceae, legionellas are relatively resistant to chlorine and heat. They have been isolated from hot water tanks held at over 50°C. Methods for decontaminating water systems are still under evaluation, although some outbreaks appear to have been aborted by disinfectants, by correcting malfunctions in air-conditioning systems, or by temporarily elevating water temperature above 70°C.

Additional Reading

Fraser, D.W., Tsai, T.R., Orenstein, W., Parkin, W.E., Beecham, H.J., Sharrar, R.G., Harris, J., Mallison, G.F., Martin, S.M., McDade, J.E., Shepard, C.C., Brachman, P.S., and the Field Investigation Team. 1977. Legionnaires' disease: Descriptions of an epidemic of pneumonia. *N. Engl. J. Med.* 297:1189–1197.

McDade, J.E., Shepard, C.C., Fraser, D.W., Tsai, T.R., Redus, M.A., Dowdle, W.R., and the Laboratory Investigation Team. 1977. Legionnaires' disease: Isolation of a bacterium and demonstration of its role in other respiratory disease. *N. Engl. J. Med.* 297:1197–1203. This study and the report by Fraser et al. describe the 1976 outbreak at the Philadelphia American Legion convention and the methods that led to the discovery of the cause of this "new" disease.

Winn, W.C., Jr. 1988. Legionnaires disease: Historical perspective. *Clin. Microbiol. Rev.* 1:60–81. This review delivers much more than indicated by the title. It is a comprehensive update on all aspects of this "new" disease.

26

Spirochetes

John C. Sherris and
James J. Plorde

The spirochetes are helical organisms; their morphology differs from that of other bacteria in that they have a flexible cell wall around which several fibrils are wound. These fibrils have the structure of flagella and are referred to as *endoflagella* (Figure 26.1). The cell wall and endoflagella are completely covered by an outer bilayered membrane similar to the outer membrane of other Gram-negative bacteria. Spirochetes are motile, exhibiting rotation and flexion; this motility is believed to result from movement of the endoflagellar filaments, although the mechanism is not clear. Like other bacteria, spirochetes divide by transverse fission.

Outer membrane is external to endoflagella wound around cell wall

Many spirochetes are very slim (0.15 μm or less) and can only be visualized by dark-field microscopy, electron microscopy, or special staining techniques that effectively increase their diameter to bring them within the resolving power of the light microscope. Others (*Borrelia*) are larger and visible in stained preparations. They are Gram negative, although they are more easily detected by other staining methods.

Many are too slim to be seen by light microscopy

Some spirochetes are free living, some are members of the normal flora of humans and animals, and three genera, *Treponema, Leptospira,* and *Borrelia,* include the causative agents of important human and zoonotic diseases.

Treponema, Leptospira, and *Borrelia*

Some spirochetes fail to grow in culture

Parasitic spirochetes grow more slowly in vitro than most disease-causing bacteria, and some, including the causative agent of syphilis, have not been grown beyond one or two generations in cell culture. Some are strict anaerobes, others require low concentrations of oxygen, and still others are aerobic.

Variable oxygen requirements

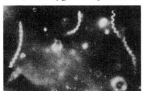

Treponema pallidum. Dark-field microscopy

Treponema pallidum and Syphilis

Treponema pallidum is the causative agent of syphilis, a venereal disease first recognized in the 16th century as an acute and often fatal disease that rapidly spread through Europe as a concomitant of the extensive military

427

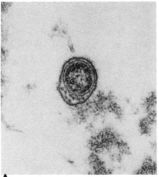

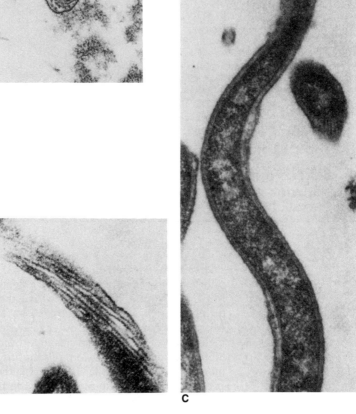

26.1 Spirochete of Lyme disease. Original magnification ×40,000. (A) and (B) Note endoflagella. (C) Note outer membrane. *(Reprinted with permission from Dr. A. C. Steere and of the N. Engl. J. Med. 1983, 308:736.)*

campaigns of the century. Over the intervening years, a state of more balanced parasitism developed; the disease is now a more chronic illness, but it can nonetheless have devastating effects.

Morphology

Treponema pallidum is a slim (0.15μm) spirochete 5–15 μm long with regular spirals of a wavelength of 1 μm and an amplitude of about 0.3 μm. It is not visible by transmitted light under the microscope, because its width is below the resolving power of the instrument and its refractive index is similar to that of the usual suspending media. It is readily seen by immunofluorescence techniques and by dark-field microscopy, which depends on reflection of light from the surface of particles (Chapter 14). It cannot be visualized with the usual bacteriologic stains; however, its width can be effectively increased by the use of techniques that deposit silver on its surface, and silver impregnation techniques are used to demonstrate it in histologic preparations. Viable *T. pallidum* shows characteristic rotational motility and flexion.

Failure to stain by routine methods

Flexional and rotational motility

Cultivation

Brief growth in some primary cell cultures only

Probably microaerophilic

Until recently, *T. pallidum* had not been shown to multiply in vitro. Using special tissue culture techniques and careful control of oxygen tension and pH, the organism has now been shown to multiply through several generations in primary cell culture, but has not been passed in subculture. It was previously thought that *T. pallidum* was an anaerobe, but it is now known to be capable of carrying out oxidative dissimilation of glucose and to incorporate radiolabeled amino acids in the presence of low concentrations of oxygen. The organism retains viability for considerable periods in liquid medium in the absence of oxygen. Other information about its metabolic properties is limited because of the extreme difficulty in obtaining sufficient organisms for study.

Resistance

Rapid death in environment

High susceptibility to penicillin

Treponema pallidum dies rapidly on drying and is readily killed by a wide range of disinfectant agents. These properties account for its almost exclusive transmission by direct contact. It is exquisitely sensitive to penicillin and is inhibited by low concentrations of tetracyclines, erythromycin, and many other antimicrobics. No resistance to chemotherapeutically useful agents appears to have developed.

Antigenic Structure

Treponemal antibodies

Nontreponemal antibodies

The outer membrane of the spirochete contains few proteins and is only weakly antigenic. However, during the course of a syphilitic infection, antibodies are produced that react with it and, in the presence of complement, immobilize the spirochete. These are referred to as *antitreponemal antibodies*. A number of somatic proteins have been detected and purified by recombinant DNA techniques and antibodies to them demonstrated in the sera of infected patients, but their role in immunity and diagnosis remains to be established. During infection, antibodies also develop that react with a phospholipid component, cardiolipin (diphosphatidyl glycerol), of normal human and animal tissues that is found in mitochondrial membranes. It remains unclear whether the antigen that stimulates production of this antibody is a product of the spirochete itself or a modified component of host cells. The difficulty in answering this question is compounded, because *T. pallidum* adsorbs lipids from the tissues in which it is multiplying.

Pathogenicity

Exclusively human pathogen under natural conditions

Experimental rabbit infection

Treponema pallidum is an exclusively human pathogen under natural conditions. In the laboratory, it can produce lesions when inoculated into the skin, cornea, or testicle of the rabbit. The latter yields large numbers of *T. pallidum,* which are a source of antigen for serologic tests. Infection in rabbits is nonprogressive and does not mimic the disease in humans. Some degree of passive protection is provided by sera from recovered animals.

Syphilis in Humans: Manifestations, Pathogenesis, and Immunity

Syphilis is considered is some detail in Chapter 70; thus, only salient clinical features will be considered here.

In most cases, *T. pallidum* infection is acquired from direct sexual con-

Infection from contact with primary or secondary lesions

Transplacental transmission

Penetration of epithelia

Spirochetes disseminate rapidly

Primary chancre is highly infectious with numerous spirochetes

Primary lesion may be inapparent

Numerous spirochetes and high infectivity in secondary syphilis

Secondary stage involves generalized superficial lesions and systemic disease

Immune complex component in secondary syphilis

Infection progresses to latency, tertiary disease, or cure

Tertiary gummatous lesions have protean manifestations

Absence of readily detectable spirochetes, except in most tertiary lesions

Possible autoimmune components of tertiary lesions

tact with an individual who has an active primary or secondary syphilitic lesion. Less commonly, the disease may be spread by nongenital contact with a lesion (for example, of the lip) or transplacental transmission to the fetus may occur within approximately the first 3 years of infection (Chapters 69 and 70). Occasional cases result from accidental inoculation of infected material. Modern precautions have essentially eliminated blood transfusion as a source of the disease. The spirochete reaches the subepithelial tissues through inapparent breaks in the skin or possibly by passing between the epithelial cells of a mucous membrane. It multiplies locally with a generation time of about 30 hr; although the primary lesion is local, the organism also disseminates rapidly to local lymph nodes, then to other organs by way of the bloodstream.

Initially, there is little tissue reaction to multiplication of *T. pallidum,* which appears to produce neither endotoxins nor exotoxins, but the primary lesion develops 2–10 weeks after infection as an indurated swelling at the site of infection. The surface necroses to yield a hard-based ulcerated lesion, termed the *chancre,* which is teeming with spirochetes and is highly infectious. The lesion is densely infiltrated with lymphocytes and plasma cells, and the small arterioles show swelling and proliferation of their endothelial cells, which reduces local blood supply and probably accounts for the necrotic ulceration. During this time, antibodies and cell-mediated immunity to spirochetal antigens develop. Untreated, the lesion heals within 3–8 weeks. The primary lesion is not always apparent, especially when it involves the female genital tract.

For reasons that are not understood, the disease is then silent for 2–10 weeks, during which a disseminated secondary stage develops with varying degrees of severity. Lesions are heavily infected with *T. pallidum,* which do not appear to differ antigenically from those causing the primary lesions. Secondary lesions present as a skin rash, as erosions of mucous membranes, and as wartlike condylomata lata in moist areas, such as the external female genitalia and perianal areas. The patient often shows systemic manifestations of infection with fever, malaise, enlarged lymph nodes, and patchy loss of hair. Immune complexes of antibody, spirochetal components, and complement are present in arteriolar walls and account for some of the clinical manifestations. This stage may last for several weeks and may relapse. It may be mild, however, and go unnoticed by the patient. Secondary lesions are highly infectious. The factors that control the secondary stage are unclear: humoral antibody has not been shown to play a role, and high titers of both treponemal and nontreponemal antibodies are present throughout.

After the secondary stage, nontreponemal antibody test results of one-fourth of patients revert to negative, possibly the result of spontaneous cure. In another 45%, serologic tests remain positive, but no further clinical manifestations appear. The remaining untreated cases develop tertiary manifestations several months to 30 years later. Most late syphilitic manifestations are destructive granulomatous lesions (gummatous lesions), again associated with the characteristic endarteritis of syphilis. They can affect skin, bone, joints, oral and nasal cavities, parenchymatous organs, the cardiovascular system, and the meninges and nervous system. Too few spirochetes are in the lesions to be demonstrated by microscopic techniques, except in general paresis, when large numbers are found in the cerebral cortex. Late disease is not infectious to others. It appears probable that late manifestations involve delayed-type hypersensitivity responses to the spirochete or its products or an autoimmune reaction to host tissues

Congenital syphilis

Immunity to reinfection
develops

Failure to control established
infection

Dark-field and fluorescent
antibody demonstration of
spirochetes

Nontreponemal cardiolipin
serodiagnostic tests

False-positive cardiolipin test
results

Cardiolipin tests are used for
screening and as tests of cure

Treponemal serodiagnostic
tests include FTA-ABS and
MHA-TP procedures

FTA-ABS is an indirect
immunofluorescent test

in areas in which spirochetes persist. Once again, however, the processes
are unclear.

Congenital syphilis may present with the major manifestations of secondary and tertiary syphilis. This illness is considered in Chapters 69 and
70.

In the early stages of syphilis, the patient rapidly becomes immune to
reinfection, but immunity is short-lived if the patient is successfully
treated. In the later stages, immunity to reinfection is more solid and
continues after treatment. From experiments in rabbits, it appears that
both antibody and cell-mediated immunity are significant, but as in humans
they are not sufficiently effective to eradicate established disease in most
instances. Syphilis in immunocompromised patients such as those suffering from the acquired immunodeficiency syndrome may present with unusually aggressive or atypical manifestations.

Laboratory Diagnosis

Treponema pallidum can be detected in primary and secondary lesions by
dark-field microscopy or by treating smears from lesions with polyclonal
fluorescent antitreponemal antibody preparations derived from sera of
infected rabbits. The recent introduction of monoclonal antibodies specific
for *T. pallidum* has improved both sensitivity and specificity of the direct
immunofluorescent test. Dark-field microscopy requires considerable skill
and experience and is prone to misinterpretation in the examination of
oral and rectal lesions, in which other spirochetes from the normal flora
may be numerous.

Most cases of syphilis are diagnosed serologically. Nontreponemal tests
such as the VDRL and RPR (rapid plasma reagin), which depend on immune flocculation of cardiolipin in the presence of lecithin and cholesterol,
become positive in the early stages of the primary lesion and are uniformly
positive during the secondary stage. They slowly wane in the later stages
of the disease (Chapter 70). In neurosyphilis, VDRL tests on cerebrospinal
fluid may be positive when the serum VDRL has reverted to negative.
Cardiolipin tests are nonspecific: they may become positive in a variety
of autoimmune diseases or in those involving substantial tissue destruction
or liver involvement, such as lupus erythematosus, viral hepatitis, infectious mononucleosis, and malaria. False-positive results can also occur
occasionally in pregnancy. Nontreponemal tests are thus used as screening
procedures for diagnosis and are confirmed by one of the treponemal tests
to be described below. They are, however, of substantial value as tests of
cure after treatment, because they slowly revert to negative or their titer
of reactivity decreases substantially after successful therapy. In contrast,
treponemal tests remain positive.

Treponemal tests involve direct detection of antibody to *T. pallidum.*
The spirochetes used in the tests are derived from rabbit testicular lesions.
Two procedures are now used most frequently, the fluorescent treponemal
antibody absorption test (FTA-ABS) and, increasingly, the microhemagglutination test for *T. pallidum* antibody (MHA-TP). The FTA-ABS procedure is an indirect immunofluorescent serodiagnostic test (Chapter 14).
It involves treatment of the patient's serum with extracts of a cultivated
treponema that is not *T. pallidum.* This treatment blocks potential nonspecific cross-reacting antibodies. The treated (absorbed) serum is then
applied to a slide to which *T. pallidum* has been fixed. After allowing any
specific antibody to react, nonbound constituents of serum are removed
by washing, and the presence of antibody on *T. pallidum* is detected by

application of a fluorescein-labeled antihuman globulin serum prepared by immunizing rabbits with human immunoglobulin. Positive results are indicated by the bright fluorescence of *T. pallidum* under the ultraviolet microscope.

MHA-TP involves adsorption of treponemal antigens to erythrocytes

The MHA-TP is simpler than the FTA-ABS procedure, and only slightly less sensitive. It is a hemagglutination test employing *T. pallidum* antigens adsorbed to erythrocytes that have been stabilized by tannic acid and formaldehyde. Appropriate blocking antigens are added to avoid nonspecific reactions.

Treponemal tests results are specific, but unaffected by treatment

Treponemal tests are considerably more specific than those using cardiolipin, but the titers of positive tests do not decrease significantly with cure. Thus, they are valuable confirmatory tests, but they are not helpful in monitoring therapy.

For consideration of other aspects of syphilis, including its epidemiology, prevention, and treatment, the reader should consult Chapter 70.

Nonvenereal Treponemal Diseases

Etiologic agents indistinguishable from *T. pallidum*

Three nonvenereal treponematoses, bejel (endemic syphilis), yaws, and pinta, occur in different geographic locations. In each case, the etiologic spirochete is indistinguishable morphologically and antigenically from *T. pallidum,* and the same difficulties have been encountered in attempting to grow them. Patients exhibit serologic responses in nontreponemal and treponemal tests similar to those of patients with syphilis, and it seems probable that each disease, and venereal syphilis itself, is caused by organisms that have diverged in evolution under particular local conditions. It has not been possible to determine which, if any, was the first human disease.

Occur under poor hygienic conditions

Major clinical manifestations involve the skin or oral cavity

The nonvenereal trematoses all occur in developing countries in which hygiene has been poor, little clothing is worn, and direct skin contact is common, often because of overcrowding. They frequently develop in childhood. The major manifestations of pinta and yaws involve the skin, and infection is transmitted by direct contact. In bejel, primary and secondary lesions usually involve the oral cavity, and spread may occur during suckling, by oral contact, or through fomites. All three diseases have primary and secondary stages, and tertiary manifestations may develop. Their features are summarized in Table 26.1. These infections are rarely transmitted venereally, and congenital infections do not occur. All are susceptible to penicillin. Their manifestations are well recognized by affected populations, and all have been greatly reduced in incidence by public health procedures designed to eradicate them.

Penicillin treatment and possibilities for eradication

Leptospira and Leptospirosis

Zoonotic disease transmitted through animal urine

Leptospirosis is a worldwide disease of a variety of animal species. It can be transmitted to humans, usually through water contaminated with animal urine. It is caused by *Leptospira interrogans,* the pathogenic member of the genus *Leptospira.* In the past, multiple species of pathogenic leptospires were recognized (for example, *L. icterohaemorrhagiae, L. canicola, L. pomona,* and *L. autumnalis*) based on geographic occurrence, differences in host species, and associated clinical syndromes, as well as antigenic differences. Now, however, 18 serogroups are recognized, many of which bear the names of the previously described species (for example, *L. interrogans,* serogroup pomona), and more than 170 serotypes are recognized within these groups. The clinical syndromes caused by the different se-

L. interrogans serogroups and serotypes

Table 26.1 Nonvenereal Treponemata

Disease	Cause	Major Geographic Location	Primary Lesion	Secondary Lesions	Tertiary Lesions
Bejel	*T. pallidum,* subspecies *endenicum*[a]	Middle East; arid, hot areas	Oral cavity[b]	Oral mucosa	Rare; gummatous lesions of skin, periosteum, bone, and joint
Yaws	*T. pallidum,* subspecies *pertenue*	Humid, tropical belt	Skin; papillomatous	Systemic; resemble syphilis	Rare; gummatous lesions of skin, periosteum, bone, and joint[c]
Pinta	*T. carateum*	Central and South America	Skin; erythematous papule	Skin; merge into primary lesion; altered pigmentation	Areas of altered skin pigmentation and hyperkeratoses

[a] Probably a variant of that causing venereal syphilis.
[b] Often inapparent.
[c] Neurologic manifestations usually absent.

rogroups have special features, but they show considerable overlap. The distinction between serogroups and serotypes is of epidemiologic and epizoologic importance rather than clinical significance.

Morphology and Cultivation

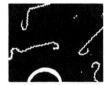

Leptospira. Dark-field microscopy
Grows in artificial culture

Leptospira interrogans is a slim (approximately 0.15 μm) spirochete 5–15 μm in length, with fine, closely wound spirals and hooked ends. As it is not visualized with the usual bacteriologic staining procedures, detection is most easily accomplished by dark-field or immunofluorescent microscopy. The organism's fine structure and motility conform to that described for the spirochetes as a group. It is an aerobe and can be grown in certain special enriched semisolid media.

Resistance

Survives in water under alkaline conditions

Sensitive to penicillin

Leptospira interrogans can survive for days or weeks in some waters in the environment at a pH of more than 7.0. Acidic conditions, such as those that may be found in urine, rapidly kill the organism. It is highly sensitive to drying and to a wide range of disinfectants. The organism is also susceptible to a number of antimicrobics, including penicillin and tetracycline.

Antigenic Structure

As indicated previously, *L. interrogans* can be divided into multiple serogroups and serovars (serotypes), although some antigens are common to all members of the species. Seroidentification is accomplished in reference laboratories by agglutination tests using highly specific absorbed antisera against the various antigenic components.

Animal Pathogenicity

Chronic renal infections in rodents, cattle, and household pets

The various serogroups of *L. interrogans* are pathogenic to a wide range of wild and domestic animal species, particularly rats, cattle, and dogs. These animals constitute the zoonotic reservoirs of the diseases. Infection is often subclinical, with organisms persisting in the renal tubules and being excreted in the urine for many weeks. Guinea pigs and some other small laboratory animals susceptible to intraperitoneal infection have been used to isolate the organism from clinical and environmental sources.

Leptospirosis in Humans

Transmitted by occupational or recreational exposure to contaminated water

Infection usually results from contact with water contaminated with the urine of infected animals or, in the case of the serogroup canicola, by direct contact with canine urine. Sewer workers, miners, farm workers, veterinarians, and slaughterhouse employees are all subject to exposure, although most clinical cases in North America are now associated with recreational exposure to contaminated water (for example, children playing in irrigation ditches).

Infection occurs through upper alimentary tract or skin

The organism gains entrance to the tissues through small skin lesions, the conjunctiva, or, most commonly, through ingestion and the upper alimentary tract mucosa. Most infections are subclinical and only detectable serologically, but after an incubation period of 7–13 days an influenzalike febrile illness with fever, chills, headache, and muscle pain may develop. This disease is associated with bacteremia. Leptospiras are also found in the cerebrospinal fluid at this stage, but without clinical or cytologic evidence of meningitis. The fever often subsides after about a week coincident with the disappearance of the organisms from the blood, but may recur with a variety of clinical manifestations depending partly on the serogroup involved. This second phase of the disease usually lasts 3 or more weeks and may present as an aseptic meningitis resembling viral meningitis (Chapter 67), or as a more generalized illness with muscle aches, headache, rash, pretibial erythematous lesions, and/or biochemical evidence of hepatic and renal involvement. In its most severe form (Weil's disease, usually caused by the icterohaemorrhagiae group), there is extensive vasculitis, jaundice, renal damage, and sometimes a hemorrhagic rash. The mortality in such cases is up to 10%.

Bacteremic phase

Disease sometimes biphasic

May present as aseptic meningitis

Weil's disease with hemorrhage, hepatitis, and renal involvement

Probable immunologic component to pathogenesis

Blind-ended infection in humans

The onset of the second phase of the disease correlates with the appearance of circulating IgM antibodies, and it appears probable that there is a major immunologic component to its pathogenesis. This is supported by absence of response to antimicrobics when given at this stage and failure usually to recover the organism from the cerebrospinal fluid in cases of leptospiral meningitis. Leptospirosis is essentially blind ended in humans with transmission to others being virtually unknown.

Laboratory Diagnosis

Blood culture in first week

Urine cultures may be successful in later stages

Serodiagnosis by agglutination tests

Leptospiras can be isolated from the blood or cerebrospinal fluid during the first week of the disease. Thereafter it can often be isolated from the urine if precautions are taken to initiate cultures immediately after the specimen is collected. Antibodies begin to appear within the first week of clinical disease, and the diagnosis is usually made by agglutination tests using serotypes common in particular regions as antigens. A titer of 1:100 or greater is suggestive of infection in the presence of a compatible clinical picture. A fourfold increase in titer is diagnostic.

Treatment

Antimicrobic treatment only effective in first few days

Penicillin and tetracycline treatment appear to modify the course of the disease if given within the first 4 days of the bacteremic phase. Later treatment is ineffective.

Prevention

Animal immunization

Rodent control and drainage

Vaccines are used extensively in cattle and household pets to prevent the disease, and this has reduced its occurrence in humans. Other measures include rodent control, drainage of waters known to be contaminated, and care on the part of those subject to occupational exposure to avoid contamination of food or skin lesions. Clinical disease is now unusual in the United States, and fewer than 100 cases are reported annually; however, many cases are probably unreported. It is impossible to eliminate the disease because of its reservoir in rodents. The infection is much more common in developing countries in which exposure to irrigated crops is extensive.

Disease is most common in developing countries

Borrelia recurrentis and Relapsing Fever

Endemic and epidemic diseases

Taxonomic complexities of relapsing fever borrelias

Relapsing fever is a disease transmitted to humans by ticks in the case of endemic relapsing fever or by body lice in the case of epidemic relapsing fever. The causative spirochetes have remarkable antigenic variability. In the past, various specific names have been given to strains associated with different species of ticks; similarities outweigh differences, however, and it has been shown experimentally that strains are not restricted to single vectors and that some tick-borne strains can infect lice and vice versa. Pending definitive DNA base composition and homology studies of different strains, it is reasonable to regard them all as members of a single species *Borrelia recurrentis,* and they will be so considered here. The disease is characterized by two or more relapses associated with selection of antigenic variants.

Morphology, Staining, and Culture

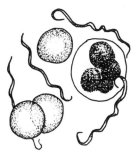

Borrelia recurrentis in blood smear

Borrelia recurrentis is a large spirochete 10–30 μm long and approximately 0.3 μm wide. In contrast to those of *Treponema* and *Leptospira,* spirals are irregular, with a wavelength of 2–4 μm. The basic organizational structure of the cell and its motility conform to that of other spirochetes, but unlike most, it is readily stained by aniline dyes. The organism is Gram negative, but it is seen most easily with Giemsa or Wright staining of smears of blood sampled during the bacteremic phase of the disease.

Borrelia recurrentis is an aerobe and has been successfully grown in artificial cultures.

Antigenic Structure and Variation

High-frequency variation of major protein antigens

Silent genes for each variable antigen are transposed sequentially to an expression site

The most characteristic antigenic property of *Borrelia* is its variability. Major surface protein antigens that are partly responsible for virulence and determine immunity vary dramatically at a frequency of about 10^{-4} per generation—a much higher rate than is usual for expressed mutations. It is now known that genes responsible for the different proteins exist in all cells of the *Borrelia,* but are transposed intermittently from a silent storage locus to an active expression site at which they displace the previously active gene. In some cases, it appears that genes encoding such proteins are carried extrachromosomally on linear plasmids. The characteristic relapses of the disease are due to selection of variants with major surface protein antigens that do not react with the antibodies produced in response to the original infection or a previous relapse. Antigenic switching by *Borrelia* is, thus, an important mechanism for avoiding host defenses resembling that used by gonococci (Chapter 19) and trypanosomes (Chapter 54).

Immunity to the disease is largely humoral and appears to involve lysis of the organism in the presence of complement. The disease is controlled when variants from the antigenic repertoire are no longer able to avoid the immune response. For further information on this antigenic variability, the reader should consult the references to the work of Barbour that are cited at the end of this chapter.

Antigenic switching allows Borrelia to avoid immune defenses; accounts for relapses

Pathogenicity

Tick-borne strains of *Borrelia recurrentis* infect a range of small rodents and other mammals and are pathogenic to humans. Soft-bodied ticks of the genus *Ornithodorus* can be infected from the animal reservoir; infected ticks are found in mountainous areas of North America and in other parts of the world in which the endemic disease occurs. The survival of the tick is not influenced by the infection, and the organism can be passed transovarially to subsequent generations. In louse-borne relapsing fever, the human body louse is infected by ingesting *Borrelia* from a case of the disease, but the infection is not transmitted transovarially. The relapsing nature of the disease in humans is reproduced in susceptible laboratory animals.

Rodent reservoir of tick-borne strains

Tick infection

Human body louse infection

Epidemiology

Endemic relapsing fever occurs in most areas of the world. It is contracted from the bite of an infected tick and is ultimately derived from the rodent reservoir. In addition to their ability to pass the infection to their progeny, ticks may remain infectious for several years when deprived of hosts. Human cases of endemic relapsing fever are usually sporadic, and in the United States they often develop after exposure to ticks during recreational activities.

Epidemic relapsing fever involves human-to-human spread by the body louse. In this case there is no transovarial spread, and the life span of the infected louse is not longer than 2 months. Infection results from scratching and crushing the infected louse into its bite or other superficial wounds. The disease is associated with overcrowding, war, poverty, and social breakdown, and without treatment the mortality may approach 30%. Currently, this variety of relapsing fever appears to be limited to east and central Africa, China, and the Peruvian Andes. As the life span of the infected louse is brief and human carriage is not documented, it is quite possible that epidemic relapsing fever can originate from cases of endemic tick-borne relapsing fever. This hypothesis remains to be proved, however, because outbreaks have occurred in areas where the endemic disease is not documented, and there are differences in some pathogenic characteristics of strains isolated from tick or louse borne disease.

Endemic infection is tick-borne

Transovarial transmission and longevity of ticks

Epidemic infection is louse-borne between humans

Association of epidemics with overcrowding, poverty, and war

Possible origin of epidemic from endemic disease

Disease in Humans

After a mean incubation period of 7 days, massive spirochetemia develops with high fever, rigors, severe headache, muscle pains, and weakness. The organism produces an endotoxinlike substance, which probably accounts

Spirochetemia and endotoxin-like effects

for some of the manifestations. The febrile period lasts about a week and terminates abruptly with the development of an adequate immune response. The disease relapses 2–4 days later, usually with less severity, but following the same general course. Epidemic relapsing fever is usually limited to two relapses, but with endemic disease three or four may occur.

Relapses

Epidemic relapsing fever is more severe than endemic disease, possibly because of the social conditions that predispose to it. Fatalities in endemic relapsing fever are rare. Most organs of the body are invaded by *Borrelia* during the disease, and mortality is usually associated with myocarditis.

Greater severity of epidemic disease

Laboratory Diagnosis

Diagnosis is readily made during the febrile period by Giemsa or Wright staining of blood smears. The appearance of the spirochete among the red cells is characteristic. Cultural and animal inoculation procedures are also used for recovery of the infecting organism. Specific serodiagnostic test are unhelpful; however, patients may develop antibodies to *Proteus* OXK, which can cause problems in differentiating the diagnosis from that of rickettsial disease (Chapter 30).

Spirochetes seen in direct blood smears during fever

Treatment

The disease responds well to tetracycline therapy, and single-dose treatment with this agent can be effective. As in the case of syphilis and leptospirosis, treatment often produces a Jarisch–Herxheimer reaction, which, at times, may even be fatal.

Tetracycline treatment

Prevention

Prevention of endemic relapsing fever involves attention to deticking and insecticide treatment and rodent control around habitations, such as mountain cabins, shown to be associated with infection.

Louse, tick, and rodent control

Epidemic relapsing fever is controlled by delousing, particularly dusting of clothing with appropriate insecticides. Ultimately, improved hygiene will stop an outbreak and prevent further occurrences.

Borrelia burgdorferi and Lyme disease

Lyme disease is a recently defined zoonotic disease that is transmitted to humans by *Ixodes* ticks. Human cases have been reported from the United States, Europe, Australia, the USSR, China and Japan. The disease is named for the town in Connecticut in which a cluster of cases was first recognized. It is initially characterized by a chronic migratory erythematous skin rash, fever, muscle and joint pains, and often some evidence of meningeal irritation. Later, the patient may develop meningoencephalitis, evidence of myocarditis, and a recurrent arthritis which can be severely disabling and develop over several years.

Zoonotic disease transmitted by *Ixodes* deer ticks

Morphology and Staining

Borrelia burgdorferi is a large spirochete measuring 10–30 μm in length and 0.2 μm in width with loose and irregular spirals. Its basic cell structure and motility conform to those of other spirochetes (Figure 26.1). Like other borrelias, *B. burgdorferi* is Gram negative, but is most easily visualized with Giemsa, Wright, or acridine orange stain. In histopathologic

Stains best with Giemsa or Wright stain

sections, the spirochete can sometimes be visualized with silver impregnation or immunofluorescence staining procedures.

Culture and Strain Identification

Microaerophil that can be grown in culture

Borrelia burgdorferi is microaerophilic and can be grown in artificial culture, a procedure that has been useful for both detection and antimicrobial susceptibility testing. Polyclonal antibodies prepared against purified cell components and monoclonal antibodies have indicated that there are probably several distinct strains of *B. burgdorferi*.

Epizoology and Epidemiology

I. dammini and *I. pacificus* are usual vectors in United States Adults feed on deer

In the United States, the disease is transmitted by *I. dammini* ticks in the eastern and central states and by *I. pacificus* in the west. Adult *Ixodes* ticks attach to, feed, and mate on deer in the late fall and winter. In the spring, fertile females, engorged from their blood meals, fall to the ground and deposit their eggs. During the summer, the tick larvae seek out and obtain a blood meal from the white-footed mouse, which is the main reservoir of *B. burgdorferi*. The spirochetes ingested by the larvae are maintained through the subsequent development stages of the tick. The following spring or summer, the small (1–2 mm) nymph stage feeds on a vertebrate host (including, again, white-footed mice) to obtain the blood required for maturation to adulthood; in the process they amplify the reservoir and may transmit the disease to humans among other mammals. The engorged, satiated nymphs fall off their host, mature into adult male and female ticks, and parasitize any available deer, thus completing a life cycle that has occupied a full 2 years. Deer are essential to the mating and survival of the tick and thus the disease does not occur in areas in which they are absent. Transovarial transmission of *B. burgdorferi* is rare, but its occurrence contributes to maintenance and spread of the organism in nature.

Larvae feed on murine reservoir of *B. burgdorferi*

Nymphs feed on vertebrate host (including humans); transmit disease if infected

Deer are essential to maintaining tick cycle

Vertebrates other than deer can be infected by both the adult and nymph stages of the tick, but human Lyme disease is acquired primarily from nymphs, because they are active when humans are most likely to invade their ecosystem. Many other mammals have been shown to develop infection with *B. burgdorferi*, including raccoons, opossums, voles, cattle, and the domestic dog.

Human infection usually follows bite of infected nymph

Lyme disease has been spreading rapidly in the United States and has now been reported from 43 states. It is prominent in the northeastern states, Wisconsin, Minnesota, and parts of California and Oregon. In 1988, 5000 cases were reported, and it is probable that very many more were unreported. The reasons for the extension of the habitat of infected ticks is not completely understood, but may involve carriage by birds and increasing deer populations. The increase in human cases partly reflects greater recreational use of infested areas and progression of suburbs into the habitats of the ticks and their primary hosts. The disease is usually acquired from infected nymphs between May and September and is commonest in children, probably because of greater skin exposure.

Rapid spread of Lyme disease in United States

Infection commonest in summer months

Lyme borreliosis in Humans

As with syphilis, Lyme borreliosis presents in stages. These comprise a primary lesion, a period of spirochetemia associated with fever and generalized manifestations of illness, and finally persistence of viable spirochetes in various organ systems leading to immunologically mediated damage. The disease is rarely fatal, but if untreated is often a source of chronic ill health.

Primary chronic migrating erythema at site of tick bite

The primary lesion occurs at the site of the tick bite, usually the thigh, groin, or axilla, 3 to 14 days after the feed. It begins as a macule or papule that expands to become an annular lesion with a raised, red border and central clearing. The lesion, known as *erythema chronicum migrans,* slowly expands. The center may become necrotic and new adjacent rings may form. Roughly half of untreated patients develop metastatic skin lesions that closely resemble the primary one. Skin biopsies show the presence of the spirochete and perivascular infiltrates of lymphocytes and histocytes. The patient frequently develops fever, muscle and joint pains, and some evidence of meningeal irritation. In the untreated patient, the skin lesions usually disappear over a period of weeks, but constitutional symptoms may persist for months.

Evidence of systemic spread

Some untreated patients develop neurologic or cardiac manifestations

The second stage of the disease usually begins weeks to months after the resolution of the primary lesion and generally involves the nervous system and/or heart. Approximately 15% of patients develop neurologic abnormalities. Typically, these present as a fluctuating meningitis accompanied by facial palsy and a peripheral neuropathy, which completely resolves within a period of several months. Heart disease occurs in about 10% of patients, usually as an atrioventricular block. In some cases, however, an acute myocarditis develops that can lead to cardiac enlargement. Cardiac abnormalities may also fluctuate in intensity but generally resolve completely in a matter of weeks.

Arthritis often develops months or years later

Arthritis marks the third stage of the disease and develops in almost two-thirds of patients weeks to years after the onset of infection. Typically, it too follows a fluctuating or intermittent course, generally infecting the large points, particularly the knees. In a small percentage of patients, the arthritis becomes chronic with erosion of the bone and cartilage. Synovial biopsies show vascular proliferations, perivascular infiltrates of lymphocytes and histiocytes, and fibrin deposits. The spirochetes are not demonstrable in the lesions by staining techniques. Occasionally, mild neurological dysfunctions or even frank encephalitis have been reported.

Pathogenesis of Lyme Disease

Pathogenetic mechanisms remain to be established clearly. It is known that the outer membrane of the spirochete contains a toxic lipopolysaccharide that differs, however, from the usual Gram-negative endotoxin. The spirochetal peptidoglycan has inflammatory properties, survives for considerable periods in tissues, and may contribute to arthritis when deposited in joint tissues.

Arthritis may involve inflammatory response to peptidoglycan deposition or autoimmunity

The rarity of spirochetes in affected tissues after the first stage of the disease indicates that autoimmune responses probably contribute to the chronic arthritis and other late clinical manifestations.

Laboratory Diagnosis

Antibodies develop slowly, but later stages are diagnosed serologically

In most cases, the laboratory diagnosis of the disease involves demonstration of circulating antibodies to the borrelia. These often take 4 weeks to develop, but IgG antibodies are almost uniformly present in symptomatic patients thereafter. Enzyme immunoassay tests for detecting IgM and IgG antibodies against *B. burgdorferi* are available commercially. Although the antibodies cross-react with many other spirochetes, patients with Lyme disease do not give positive VDRL or other cardiolipin antigen tests for syphilis.

Spirochetes usually not demonstrable in later lesions

Although *B. burgdorferi* certainly exists in later lesions, cultures and direct microscopic examinations are only occasionally positive. The organisms may sometimes be demonstrated in ticks that have been allowed to feed on infected patients under controlled conditions, but the procedure is impractical for routine diagnosis. The recent development of sensitive and specific DNA probes should facilitate detection of this organism in tissue by in situ hybridization techniques.

Treatment

Tetracycline and penicillin effective; later stages require prolonged parenteral penicillin

Tetracycline, penicillin, and erythromycin are all effective in the treatment of early Lyme disease. Approximately 15% of patients will experience a febrile (Jarisch–Herxheimer-like) reaction early in the course of therapy. In the second and third stages of the disease, prolonged administration of parenteral penicillin is usually necessary. In patients with chronic arthritis, antibiotic therapy is effective in only half the affected individuals, and nonresponders may require surgical intervention.

Prevention

Sensible clothing, tick removal, and insect repellents

Early treatment of first stage prevents complication

There is currently no vaccine available for Lyme borreliosis. In areas where the disease occurs, the most useful preventive measures are the use of clothes that reduce the likelihood of the infected nymph reaching the legs or arms, careful search for nymphs after potential exposure, and removal of the tick by its head using tweezers. Some insect repellents may provide added protection. Early diagnosis and treatment will prevent the more serious complications of later disease, and the public must be educated in the early manifestations of the infection.

Spirochetes of the Normal Oral Flora and Fusospirochetal Diseases

The oral cavity, particularly the dental crevice, harbors spirochetes of the genera *Treponema* and *Borrelia* as part of its normal flora. As described in Chapter 62, spirochetes from this source, together with fusobacteria (Chapter 18), can cause an anaerobic, synergistic, necrotizing, ulcerative infection of the gums, or similar ulcerations in the oral cavity or pharynx termed *Vincent's infection* or *trench mouth*. This opportunistic infection is usually seen with severe malnutrition, leukemia, or in the immunocompromised host, particularly with deficient phagocytic defenses. It may also follow trauma or complicate herpes simplex infections. The term *trench mouth* was derived from the common occurrence of infections of this type in troops under the appalling conditions that existed in the trenches during World War I, when reasonable oral hygiene could not be maintained.

Vincent's infection and ulcerative gingivitis
Disease associated with immunodeficiencies

Direct smear examination

Response to penicillin

The disease is readily diagnosed by examining specially stained smears of material taken directly from the ulcerated lesion. Its appearance is illustrated in Figure 26.2 in which the characteristic fusiform and spirochetal organisms are seen. Resolution is rapid with penicillin therapy supplemented with careful oral hygiene.

Additional Reading

Barbour, A.G. 1988. Antigenic variation of surface proteins of *Borrelia* species. *Rev. Infect. Dis.* 10 (suppl 2):S399–S402. A review of the molecular genetics of antigenic variation in relapsing fever borrelias by a major contributor to the field.

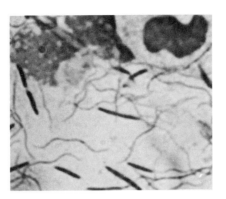

26.2 Fusospirochetal disease. Note the large number of fusiform organisms and spirochetes. *(Reproduced with kind permission from Leon J. Lebeau, Ph.D., Department of Pathology, University of Illinois Medical Center.)*

Barbour, A.G., and Hayes, S.F. 1986. Biology of *Borrelia* species. *Microbiol. Rev.* 50:381–400. A major and fully referenced review of the field, including a section on host–parasite interaction.

Baughn, R.E. 1987. Role of fibronectin in the pathogenesis of syphilis. *Rev. Infect. Dis.* 9(suppl 4):S372–S383. This paper reviews the factors mediating attachment of *T. pallidum* and the possible role of fibronectin–treponemal interactions in the immunology and pathogenesis of syphilitic lesions.

Burgdorfer, W. 1986. The enlarging spectrum of tick-borne spirochetoses. R.R. Parker Memorial Lecture. *Rev. Infect. Dis.* 8:932–940. An overview of *Borrelia* infections by the discoverer of *B. burgdorferi*.

Horton, J.M., and Blaser, M.J. 1985. The spectrum of relapsing fever in the Rocky Mountains. *Arch. Intern. Med.* 145:871–875. This paper analyzes the clinical manifestations, epidemiology, and treatment of 22 cases of tick-borne relapsing fever that occurred between 1944 and 1983 and describes in detail several of the later cases.

Lastavica, C.C., Wilson, M.L., Berardi, V.P., et al. 1989. Rapid emergence of a focal epidemic of Lyme disease in coastal Massachusetts. *N. Engl. J. Med.* 320:133–137. A fascinating account of an outbreak of the disease associated with an adjacent nature reserve. An excellent source of recent references.

Penn, C.W. 1987. Pathogenicity and immunology of *Treponema pallidum*. *J. Med. Microbiol.* 24:1–9. An up-to-date account of the subject that discusses both the limitations of present knowledge and the opportunities offered by biotechnology for future advances.

Stamm, L.V., Dallas, W.S., Ray, P.H., et al. 1988. Identification, cloning, and purification of protein antigens of *Treponema pallidum*. *Rev. Infect. Dis.* 10(suppl 2):S403–S407. A description of the application of recombinant DNA technology to obtaining purified protein antigens of an organism that has not been grown. These approaches are being used by several research groups and are beginning to clarify the immunology of syphilis and to produce improved diagnostic reagents.

Steere, A.C. 1989. Lyme Disease. *N. Engl. J. Med.* 321:586–596. An up-to-date review of the subject by Dr. Steere, whose work led to recognition of the disease and its importance.

27
Mycobacteria

John C. Sherris and
James J. Plorde

The mycobacteria are slim, rod-shaped organisms 0.2–0.4 × 2–10 μm in size. They are nonmotile and do not form spores. They have an unusual cell wall structure that contains N-glycolylmuramic acid in place of N-acetylmuramic acid and has a very high lipid content (60%), which renders the surface hydrophobic and makes mycobacteria difficult to stain with commonly used basic aniline dyes at room temperature. Mycobacteria can be stained with dyes by prolonged application or with heating; once they have taken up the stain, however, they resist decolorization with up to 3% hydrochloric acid. Some species also resist decolorization with 95% ethanol. These properties, which depend on the integrity of the cell wall, are described as *acid fastness* and *acid–alcohol fastness* and are exploited in selective stains that allow mycobacteria to be distinguished from other genera and species. For example, the Ziehl–Neelsen stain is commonly applied to slides from cultures or to clinical specimens such as sputum. The method involves flooding the slide with basic fuchsin (a red dye) in 5% phenol as a mordant. The slide is heated gently for several minutes before decolorization with 3% HCl in ethanol. After washing, the preparation is counterstained with methylene blue. Mycobacteria stain red, whereas other genera are decolorized and therefore take the blue color of the counterstain. There are various modifications of this procedure, including the use of fluorochromes as the primary stain. In this case, mycobacteria, but not other genera, fluoresce when examined microscopically at the excitor wavelength of the stain.

Mycobacteria are strictly aerobic, and the most important pathogen, *Mycobacterium tuberculosis*, shows enhanced growth in 10% carbon dioxide and at a pH of about 6.5–6.8. Nutritional requirements vary among species and range from the ability of some nonpathogens to multiply on the washers of water faucets to the strict intracellular parasitism of *Mycobacterium leprae*, which does not grow in artificial media or cell culture.

Mycobacteria grow more slowly than most human pathogenic bacteria

Acid and alcohol fastness

Ziehl–Neelsen stain

Fluorescence microscopic techniques

Aerobes

Slow growth of many species

because of their hydrophobic cell surface, which causes them to clump and inhibits permeability of nutrients into the cell. Addition of the surfactant Tween 80 to cultures of *M. tuberculosis* wets the surface and leads to dispersed and more rapid growth.

Distinguishing features

The major distinguishing features among different species of mycobacteria are nutritional and temperature requirements, growth rates, pigmentation of colonies grown in light or darkness, some key biochemical tests, and range of pathogenicity in experimental animals. Some of the more important characteristics are summarized in Appendix 27.1. The improved means of in vitro characterization have essentially eliminated the need for animal pathogenicity tests.

Pathogenicity

Mycobacteria include a wide range of species pathogenic for humans and animals. Some, such as *M. tuberculosis*, occur exclusively in humans under natural conditions. Others, such as *Mycobacterium intracellulare*, can infect various species, including humans, but also appear able to exist in the free-living state. Most nonpathogenic species are widely distributed in the environment.

Some mycobacteria are saprophytic

Diseases caused by mycobacteria tend to develop slowly, follow a chronic course, and elicit a granulomatous response. Infectivity of pathogenic species is quite high, but virulence for healthy humans is low; for example, disease following infection with *M. tuberculosis* is the exception rather than the rule.

Hypersensitivity to mycobacterial proteins

Mycobacteria do not produce classic exotoxins or endotoxins, and disease processes are largely a result of delayed-type hypersensitivity reactions to mycobacterial proteins. The hypersensitive state can be detected by intradermal injections of purified proteins from the mycobacteria. Cross-reaction of responses to proteins from different species is considerable.

Mycobacterium tuberculosis

Cause of most tuberculosis

Mycobacterium tuberculosis is the cause of almost all cases of human tuberculosis in developed countries. In the past a significant number of tuberculous infections were caused by the animal pathogen *Mycobacterium bovis*, usually from drinking milk from infected herds; now, however, the disease has been almost eliminated by eradication programs in cattle and by pasteurization of milk. A variant of *M. tuberculosis* designated *Mycobacterium africanum* causes many tuberculous infections in Africa, but its significance is the same as that of *M. tuberculosis* and it will not be considered separately here.

Tuberculosis due to *M. bovis* is rare in developed countries

Morphology, Staining, and Cultural Characteristics

Mycobacterium tuberculosis is a slim, strongly acid–alcohol-fast rod. It frequently shows irregular beading in its staining, appearing as connected series of acid-fast granules (Figure 27.1). It grows at 37°C, but not at room temperature, and requires enriched or complex media for primary growth from clinical specimens. Growth is enhanced by 5–10% CO_2, but is still very slow, with a mean generation time of 12–24 hr.

Growth on complex and semisynthetic media

Complex media are widely used for primary culture. One, Löwenstein–Jensen medium, is composed of 60% homogenized egg in nutrient base containing a low concentration of malachite green as an inhibitor of nonmycobacterial contaminants. The medium is solidified into slants by heating at 85°C until the egg protein coagulates. Colonies usually appear after 3–6 weeks of incubation. They become raised, warty, and adherent, with

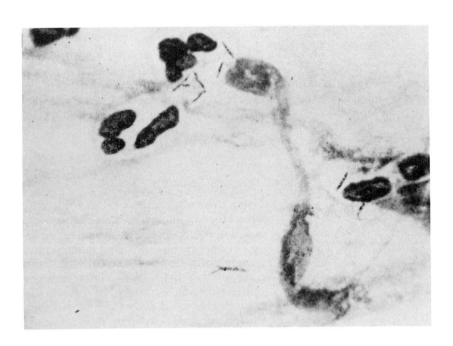

27.1 *Mycobacterium tuberculosis* in sputum stained by Ziehl–Neelsen technique. The mycobacteria retain the red carbol fuchsin through the decolorization step. The cells, background, and any other organisms stain with methylene blue counterstain.

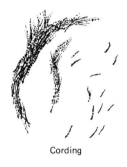

Cording

a buff pigmentation and are difficult to emulsify because of their high lipid content. Other commonly used media are oleic acid–albumin agar (7H-11), a semisynthetic plating medium that grows *M. tuberculosis* more rapidly, and oleic acid–albumin broth, which is used in some rapid radiometric detection systems. On oleic acid–albumin agar virulent strains show *cording* in which multiplying organisms remain attached in parallel bundles and form long intertwining cords or ropes. Cording is caused by a glycolipid termed *cord factor*. Its association with virulence is clear, but its role, if any, as a virulence factor is not. Although complex media are needed for primary isolation, a heavy inoculum of *M. tuberculosis* will grow well on the surface of a liquid medium containing only inorganic salts, asparagine, and glycerol. Under these conditions, the organism appears to produce a substance(s) needed for its own growth that is initially supplied by the heavy inoculum.

The major phenotypic tests for identification of *M. tuberculosis* are summarized in the appendix. Of particular importance is the ability of *M. tuberculosis* to produce large quantities of niacin, which is uncommon in other mycobacteria.

Range of Pathogenicity

Virulence for guinea pigs

Mycobacterium tuberculosis is highly virulent for guinea pigs, but much less so for other commonly used experimental animals; thus, much of our knowledge of the pathogenesis and immunity of tuberculosis has been derived from the guinea pig model. The minimal infecting dose for this animal is usually less than 10 cells, and after subcutaneous or intramuscular injection, a local and systemic infection develops with extensive involvement of lymph nodes, liver, and spleen. Untreated, the animal dies, usually after 6–12 weeks. Monkeys in captivity are also very susceptible to *M. tuberculosis* infection, which they contract from handlers or other infected monkeys. They can pose a serious source of infection to those working with them.

Resistance

Unusual resistance to
disinfectants but not to heat

Mycobacterium tuberculosis is unusually resistant to drying, to most disinfectants except formaldehyde and glutaraldehyde, and to acids and alkalis. This resistance, attributable to its hydrophobic lipid surface, is exploited in preparing contaminated clinical specimens for culture. Tubercle bacilli are quite heat sensitive; they are killed in milk by pasteurization for 30 min at 62°C. Individual organisms in droplet nuclei are susceptible to inactivation by ultraviolet light.

Antigenic Structure

Antibody responses occur but
are not involved in immunity

Mycobacterium tuberculosis has, as do all bacteria, a highly complex antigenic structure, and humoral immune responses are mounted to many of these antigens during the course of a tuberculous infection. Antibody responses do not appear to be involved in immunity to infection, however, and no commercially available serologic test has so far proved sufficiently sensitive and specific to be useful as a diagnostic procedure. A number of possibly specific antigens of *M. tuberculosis* have been described recently. If serological tests against cloned antigens prove to have sufficient sensitivity and specificity, they would have significant diagnostic value, particularly in patients with extrapulmonary forms of tuberculosis. Likewise, monoclonal antibodies against any specific antigens would be of value in seroidentification or even serotyping. At present, however, there are no practical tests for these purposes.

Cell-mediated immunity and
hypersensitivity to
tuberculoprotein

Tuberculin and PPD

Cellular immunity and cell-mediated hypersensitivity to tuberculoproteins develop during the course of tuberculous infection and contribute to both the pathology and the immunity of the disease. The most studied antigens are heat-stable proteins that are liberated into liquid culture media. The original preparation was a crude culture filtrate termed *Old Tuberculin*, but a purified protein derivative (PPD) of tuberculin is now used for skin testing for hypersensitivity and is standardized in tuberculin units according to skin test activity. Hypersensitivity does not result from repeated PPD injections in those who are skin test negative. However, the degree of hypersensitivity may be somewhat increased for a few weeks in those already allergic.

Virulence Mechanisms

Lack of toxins

Ability to multiply in
macrophages and in
developing lesions

Intracellular survival
associated with failure of
lysosome–phagosome fusion

The cells and cellular components of *M. tuberculosis* are remarkably nontoxic to humans and experimental animals not previously sensitized to tuberculin. Two of the cell wall lipids, Wax D and cord factor, will elicit granulomatous lesions, but the amounts required are considerably in excess of those to be expected in a natural lesion. No toxins have been found in the organism, and attempts to isolate single immunizing antigens have so far been unsuccessful, although modern procedures for detecting, separating, and producing protein antigens or synthetic peptides are only now being exploited. The organism owes its virulence to its ability to multiply within macrophages and in the physical and chemical conditions (low pH, high lactic acid, high CO_2) that obtain in developing lesions. It is essentially unaffected by the humoral antibody response that it elicits, and it can survive for long periods in macrophages that have been activated by the cellular immune response. Intracellular survival of *M. tuberculosis* appears attributable, at least in part, to inhibition of lysosome fusion to the phagocytic vacuole. This effect is caused by sulfatides in the mycobacterial cell

Table 27.1 Antimicrobics Commonly Used in Treatment of Tuberculosis

First-Line Drugs	Second-Line Drugs[a]
Isoniazid	*para*-Aminosalicylic acid
Ethambutol	Ethionamide
Rifampin	Cycloserine
Pyrazinamide	Fluoroquinolones
Streptomycin	Kanamycin, etc

[a] Second-line drugs added to combinations if resistance or toxicity contraindicate first-line agents.

wall. Disease manifestations result primarily from hypersensitivity to tuberculoprotein.

Antimicrobic Susceptibility

Mycobacterium tuberculosis is susceptible to several effective antimicrobics (Table 27.1). Isoniazid, ethambutol, rifampin, pyrazinamide, and streptomycin and combinations of these agents constitute the primary drugs of choice for treatment of tuberculosis. All of these, except for ethambutol, are bactericidal. Isoniazid and rifampin are active against both intra- and extracellular organisms, and pyrazinamide, a nicotinamide analog, acts at the acidic pH found within cells. Streptomycin does not penetrate into cells and is thus active only against extracellular organisms. The modes of action of these agents are considered in Chapter 13. *Mycobacterium tuberculosis* is also susceptible to other drugs that may be used to replace those of the primary group if they are inappropriate because of resistance or drug toxicity. The fluoroquinolones, such as ciprofloxacin and ofloxacin, are active against *M. tuberculosis* and penetrate well into infected cells. Their role in the treatment of tuberculosis is under evaluation.

Mutational resistance to antituberculous drugs occurs at frequencies of 10^{-7}–10^{-10}, and mutants often come to predominate and produce clinical relapse when a single drug is used to treat serious tuberculosis. This resistance develops because organisms in many tuberculous lesions are sufficiently numerous to include resistant mutants, which can grow under the conditions that exist in lesions during treatment and cause clinical relapse. Adequate, continuous treatment with two or three antituberculous drugs with different modes of action greatly reduces this problem, because the chance of a doubly resistant mutant being present among the number of organisms in a lesion is very low. Primary infections with drug-resistant strains continue to occur, and susceptibility tests are indicated for organisms from active cases of tuberculosis.

Tuberculosis

Tuberculosis is a disease of great antiquity that reached epidemic proportions during the major periods of urbanization in the 18th and 19th centuries: mortality reached 200–400 per 100,000 of the population per year, and morbidity was many times higher. The disease has major sociologic components, flourishing with ignorance, poverty, overcrowding, and poor hygiene and during the social disruptions of war and economic depression. Under these conditions, the poor are the major victims, but

Marginal notes:

Isoniazid, ethambutol, rifampin, pyrazinamide, and streptomycin

Role of second-line drugs; activity of fluoroquinolones

Combined therapy prevents selection of resistant mutants

History and prevalence

all sectors of society are at risk. Chopin, Paganini, Thoreau, Keats, Elizabeth Barrett Browning, and the Brontës, to name but a few, were all lost to the disease in their intellectual prime. With knowledge of its cause and transmission, the disease was increasingly brought under control in Western countries, but mortality and morbidity remain at 19th-century levels in many countries despite extensive national and international control programs. It is estimated that about 8 million new cases develop each year throughout the world and that the disease causes 2–3 million deaths annually. Particularly concerning for the future control of tuberculosis is the marked susceptibility of patients suffering from acquired immunodeficiency syndrome (AIDS).

Attack rates still high in many developing countries

Routes of Infection

The great majority of tuberculous infections are first contracted by inhalation of droplet nuclei carrying the causative organism; occasionally, infection occurs through the gastrointestinal tract or skin.

Most infections by respiratory route

It has been estimated that a single cough can generate as many as 3000 infected droplet nuclei and that less than 10 bacilli may initiate a pulmonary infection in a susceptible individual. The likelihood of acquiring infection thus relates to the numbers of organisms in the sputum of an open case of the disease, the frequency and efficiency of the coughs, the closeness of contact, and the adequacy of ventilation in the contact area. Epidemiologic data indicate that large doses or prolonged exposure to smaller infecting doses is usually needed to initiate infection in humans. In some closed environments, such as a submarine or a crowded nursing home, a single open case of pulmonary tuberculosis can infect the majority of PPD-negative individuals sharing sleeping accommodations.

Pathogenesis of Tuberculosis

Primary Infection. Primary tuberculosis is the response to initial infection in an individual not previously infected and sensitized to tuberculoprotein. The infection is usually pulmonary and develops at the periphery of the midzone of the lung. Tubercle bacilli that reach the small bronchi or alveoli with inhaled droplets are engulfed by macrophages. Those that survive continue to multiply within the macrophages and are carried to the hilar lymph nodes that drain the infected site. Multiplication of the organisms is relatively unimpeded, and the inflammatory reaction is minor and nonspecific. Dissemination of some bacilli through the lymphatic vessels and bloodstream is common at this time, and they may be deposited in many organs, including the liver, spleen, kidney, bone, brain, meninges, and the apices or other parts of the lung. Symptoms and signs of infection are absent or are manifested as a mild influenzalike disease; however, the primary site of infection and some enlarged hilar lymph nodes can often be detected radiologically.

Multiplication in aveolar macrophages

Low reactivity to the organism allows multiplication and dissemination

Cell-mediated immunity to *M. tuberculosis* and hypersensitivity to tuberculoprotein, both manifestations of the same process, develop 2–6 weeks after infection, with formation of classic histologic tubercles at the sites of bacillary multiplication. This process is initiated when immunologically competent lymphocytes encounter *M. tuberculosis*-containing macrophages. Lymphokines attract monocytes to the site and transform them into activated macrophages that surround the infected area and have increased activity against the bacteria that they ingest so that multiplication slows or stops. Morphologically, the tubercle is a microscopic granuloma

Hypersensitivity and cell-mediated immunity develop in 2–6 weeks

Development and morphology of the tubercle

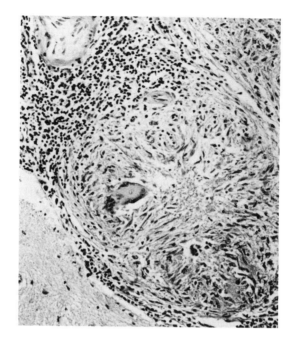

27.2 Microscopic tubercule of brain, showing giant cell and surrounding epithelioid cells and lymphocytes.

consisting of some multinucleated giant cells formed by the fusion of several macrophages (Langhans cells), many epithelioid cells (activated macrophages), and a surrounding collar of lymphocytes (Figure 27.2). When many bacteria are present and there is a high degree of hypersensitivity, enzymes and reactive oxygen intermediates are released by dying macrophages and lead to necrosis of the center of the granuloma, which is termed *caseous* because of its cheesy, semisolid character. Other macrophage secretions stimulate accumulation of fibroblasts and deposition of collagen.

Primary infections are usually handled well by the host. Bacterial multiplication ceases. Most organisms die, and the lesions in the lung and draining lymph nodes fibrose and sometimes calcify to produce the classic Ghon complex on X-ray. Most microscopic lesions in other areas of the body also heal by fibrosis, and the organisms in them slowly die. In others, the tubercle bacilli remain viable for long periods and serve as a potential source of reactivation many months or years later if host defenses weaken. Less commonly, the primary disease is not controlled and merges into the reactivation type of tuberculosis, or it disseminates to many organs to produce active miliary tuberculosis. The latter may result from a necrotic tubercle eroding into a small blood vessel.

Reactivation (Adult) Tuberculosis. In Western countries, reactivation of an old, quiescent lesion followed by clinical disease now occurs most often after the age of 50 and is more common in men. Frequently, reactivation is associated with malnutrition, alcoholism, diabetes, old age, and a dramatic change in the individual's life, such as loss of a spouse. When the disease was more common, reactivation tuberculosis was often seen in young adults of both sexes. Hospital house staff and nurses had a high attack rate, probably because of the long hours and inherent stresses of their jobs superimposed on the virtual inevitability of previous childhood

Caseation occurs with high levels of antigen and hypersensitivity

Most primary infections are controlled; lesions fibrose and sometimes calcify

The Ghon complex

Primary infection may progress to reactivation or miliary tuberculosis

Reactivation is most common in older men

Predisposing factors

infection at that time. Recently, reactivation and progressive primary tuberculosis among younger adults has increased as a complication of AIDS.

Commonest site is lung apex

Reactivation usually occurs in body areas of relatively high oxygen tension and low lymphatic drainage, most often in the apex of the lung. The lesions show spreading, coalescing tubercles with numerous tubercle bacilli and large areas of caseous necrosis. Necrosis often involves the wall

Discharge of caseous material forms pulmonary cavities

of a small bronchus from which the necrotic material is discharged, resulting in a pulmonary cavity and bronchial spread. Frequently, small blood vessels are also eroded. As a result, the sputum in these patients is often

Infectiousness of cavitary pulmonary tuberculosis

bloodstained and contains caseous material and numerous tubercle bacilli. Sputum droplets from such patients are the major source of infection to others. The disease is characterized by chronic fever and weight loss, probably mediated in part by macrophage-derived tumor necrosis factor (cachectin). Night sweats, productive coughing, and hemoptysis are frequent manifestations.

Extrapulmonary disease

Reactivation tuberculosis can also occur in other organs, such as the kidneys, bones, lymph nodes, brain, meninges, bone marrow, and bowel and, again, is an important complication in some AIDS patients.

Immunity to Tuberculosis

Innate immunity

As discussed previously, humans generally have a rather high innate immunity to development of disease. This immunity was dramatically illustrated in the Lübeck disaster of 1926: as a result of a laboratory error, 249 infants were fed a virulent culture of *M. tuberculosis* in place of the intended bacillus Calmette-Guérin (BCG) vaccine. Although the dose was very large, 173 of the children developed only minor lesions and survived; 76 children, however, died of acute disease. Among humans, there is

Racial differences in immunity reflect extent of exposure of forebears

excellent epidemiologic and historic evidence for differences in racial immunity. Races with a long history of urbanization and exposure to the epidemics of the 18th and 19th centuries have greater resistance than rural peoples or those whose exposure to infection was recent. Those of urbanized European stock appear to have a high degree of immunity, whereas native Americans and Eskimos, whose exposure was quite recent, are very susceptible and had high morbidity and mortality when the infection was introduced.

It is impossible to be precise about the extent of the influence of differences in innate immunity on morbidity and mortality, because cultural and environmental differences are also operative. Studies on attack rates in identical and nonidentical twins, however, have clearly shown genetic differences in susceptibility. When one twin is clinically infected, the attack rate in an identical twin is 75%; that in nonidentical twins is 25%.

Immunity is cell mediated, but incomplete; both T4 and T8 cells involved

Acquired immunity is cell mediated but incomplete. Both helper-inducer (T4) and cytotoxic (T8) cells are involved. Macrophages are activated at the site of infection by lymphokines from antigen-stimulated T4 cells and limit the multiplication and spread of *M. tuberculosis*. Cytotoxic T cells release bacilli from unactivated phagocytic cells and allow them to be ingested and handled by the activated macrophages. The concomitant de-

Delayed-type hypersensitivity enhances immunity to reinfection

layed-type hypersensitivity to tuberculoprotein plays an important part in immunity to reinfection by mobilizing immune cells and macrophages to the site of deposition of tubercle bacilli. In the past, it was believed that reinfection from external sources was extremely rare, but it is now clear that loss of hypersensitivity and cell-mediated immunity can occur over time and that reinfection developing into clinical tuberculosis can occur.

The role of delayed-type hypersensitivity in immunity of established

Hypersensitivity can precipitate caseation and spread in established disease

tuberculosis is more complex, because high degrees of sensitivity can precipitate caseous necrosis and lead to spread of the disease. Therapy by inoculation with large doses of tuberculin, as attempted at the turn of the century, leads to a systemic tuberculin reaction with hyperemia and even necrosis in tuberculous lesions, marked constitutional signs, and often spread of the disease. This treatment was abandoned rapidly when its effects were recognized.

The importance of cell-mediated immunity and hypersensitivity in modulating the course of tuberculosis is, perhaps, most dramatically illustrated in patients with AIDS. Those with minimal impairment of cellular immune responses develop typical tubercles containing relatively few bacilli. Those with advanced impairment demonstrate abundant acid-fast bacilli without epithelioid cell accumulation or associated tissue necrosis.

The Tuberculin Test

PPD test measures hypersensitivity to tuberculoprotein

The tuberculin skin test measures delayed-type hypersensitivity to tuberculoprotein. Purified protein derivative (PPD), derived from culture filtrates of *M. tuberculosis*, is standardized biologically against an international reference preparation and its activity expressed in tuberculin units (TUs). Most initial skin tests employ 5 TUs (intermediate strength). When an unusually high degree of hypersensitivity or eye or skin tuberculosis is suspected, then 1 TU (first strength) or less is used initially to avoid the risk of an excessive reaction locally or at the site of a mycobacterial lesion.

The test most commonly performed involves intradermal injection of 0.1 ml of PPD containing 5 TU. It is read 48–72 hr later. An area of measured induration of 10 mm or more accompanied by erythema constitutes a positive reaction, although smaller areas of induration and erythema indicate a lesser degree of sensitization to mycobacterial proteins. No induration indicates a negative reaction.

Interpretation of PPD test

A positive PPD test indicates that the individual has been infected at some time with *M. tuberculosis* or with a strongly cross-reacting mycobacterium of another species. It carries no implication about the activity of the infection, which may have been simply a primary complex contracted 20 years previously.

A negative PPD test in a healthy individual indicates that he or she has not been infected with *M. tuberculosis*, is in the prehypersensitive stage of a primary infection, or has finally lost tuberculin sensitivity along with disappearance of antigen from an old primary complex. Patients with severe disseminated disease, those on steroid or immunosuppressive drugs, or those with certain other diseases such as AIDS or measles may also become anergic, lose their tuberculin hypersensitivity, and become more susceptible to the disease.

Anergy may develop with therapy or disease affecting cell-mediated immunity

Induration below the 10-mm-diameter criterion for positivity indicates low-level sensitization, which may be attributable to *M. tuberculosis* infection or to a cross-reacting mycobacterial infection.

Clinical value depends on incidence of primary infections

The clinical value of the PPD test depends on the occurrence of primary infection in different age groups. In earlier years and in many underdeveloped countries, the test had little diagnostic value because primary infection, and thus a high positivity rate, was the rule by late childhood or early adult life. Now, in much of the Western world, primary infection is sufficiently uncommon that a negative test is frequently important in excluding tuberculosis, and a positive test in infancy or childhood has significance in diagnosis and can often be used to trace a household or

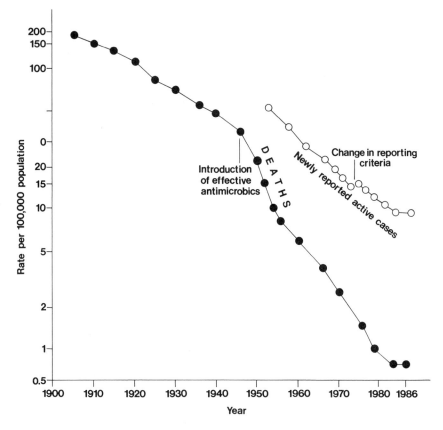

27.3 Morbidity and mortality of tuberculosis in the United States, 1900–1986.

Value in case finding

school source of infection. Epidemiologic surveys of tuberculin reactivity indicate trends in the incidence of infection and constitute the simplest way of monitoring the effectiveness of control measures.

Epidemiology of Tuberculosis

Decline in tuberculosis in developed countries

Reactivation tuberculosis commonest in older individuals

Explanations for cessation of decline in disease in the United States

AIDS patients are at special risk

The major factors determining the epidemiology of tuberculosis have already been mentioned. The change in mortality and occurrence of the disease in the United States over the last century is shown in Figure 27.3. As the incidence of infection in developed countries decreased, there was a major shift in the age of tuberculosis patients: most were over 50 and represented cases in which an old primary lesion, quiescent for decades, has become reactivated. The grandfather who has developed "chronic bronchitis" is a classic source of infection to children. Since 1984, the decline in reports of active cases and of deaths in the United States has ceased. This is partly attributable to infections developing in immigrants from countries in which primary infections are common, partly to social and economic changes that have left a subpopulation of impoverished and often homeless individuals living under conditions reminiscent of the 19th century, and partly because of the AIDS epidemic. It is estimated that patients with latent tuberculosis increase their risk of reactivation or acquisition of disease by factors of 200–300 with the acquisition of a human

Table 27.2 Some Indications for Isoniazid Prophylaxis of Tuberculosis

---

1. Radiologic evidence of active primary complex

2. PPD-positive close contact of infectious case

3. Child who is close contact of infectious case, whether or not PPD positive (retest after 12 weeks)

4. Known recent PPD converter (eg, laboratory worker who is regularly tested)

5. Patient with skin test, radiologic, or other evidence of primary infection who is immunosuppressed, undergoing corticosteroid treatment, or has a disease (eg, AIDS) predisposing to tuberculosis

---

Abbreviations: PPD = purified protein derivative; AIDS = acquired immunodeficiency syndrome.

immunodeficiency virus coinfection. Over 5% of AIDS patients develop active tuberculosis, usually within 3 years of diagnosis of AIDS.

Single-source epidemics still occur

A few single-source epidemics of tuberculosis occur each year, sometimes involving schoolchildren and a teacher with unrecognized cavitary pulmonary tuberculosis or tuberculous bronchopneumonia. Often the majority of such children exposed over time become PPD positive, and some develop clinical and radiologic evidence of primary infection. Such exposure in childhood is an indication for chemoprophylaxis. Recently, similar outbreaks have been described associated with shelters for the homeless and among medical personnel exposed during aerosol therapy to unusually large numbers of infected droplets from unrecognized cases of tuberculosis.

Treatment and Prophylaxis

Combined therapy to prevent resistance

Treatment of established tuberculosis always involves double or triple therapy to prevent the selection of resistant mutants. Such treatment with antimicrobics to which the organism is susceptible will usually render the patient noninfectious within a week or two, which has shifted the care of the tuberculous patient from isolation hospitals and sanatoriums to the home or the general hospital. After an initial intense phase of systemic chemotherapy, treatment is usually continued with oral antimicrobics and may need to be continued for a year or more, although successful therapy can often be completed in 6 to 9 months when isoniazid and rifampin are used concomitantly. The effectiveness of chemotherapy on most forms of tuberculosis has been dramatic and has greatly reduced the need for surgical procedures such as pulmonary lobectomy. Failure of chemotherapy is often associated with lack of adherence to the regimen by the patient.

Indications for chemoprophylaxis

Special role and limitations of isoniazid in chemoprophylaxis

Prophylactic chemotherapy, usually with isoniazid alone, is now used in situations in which known or suspected primary tuberculous infection poses the risk of clinical disease. Some indications for prophylaxis are summarized in Table 27.2. Isoniazid can be used alone in prophylaxis because the load of tubercle bacilli in a subclinical primary lesion is small in relation to that in reactivation tuberculosis, and experience has shown that the development of subsequent clinical disease from isoniazid-resistant strains selected by prophylaxis can be discounted. Unfortunately, isoniazid may cause a form of hepatitis, and the risk increases progressively after age 20. Its use in older subjects involves balancing risk against potential benefit and requires monitoring with liver function tests.

Immunoprophylaxis

BCG vaccine is a live attenuated derivative of *M. bovis*

At present the BCG vaccine (named for its originators, Calmette and Guérin) is the only available vaccine. It has been used for prophylaxis of tuberculosis in various countries since 1923; administration is usually intradermal. It is a live vaccine derived originally from a strain of *M. bovis* that was attenuated by repeated subculture in a bile-containing medium until it became of markedly reduced virulence, but would still induce tuberculin hypersensitivity. Since then, it has had a checkered history, with results in different controlled trials ranging from ineffectiveness to 80% protection. This disparity arose partly because cultures of BCG maintained in different countries varied in their immunizing ability, partly because of differences in the ages and low-level hypersensitivity status of the trial populations and partly because some populations already had a baseline immunity from infection with mycobacteria other than *M. tuberculosis*. On the basis of encouraging early trials, massive immunization campaigns sponsored by the World Health Organization were organized in underdeveloped countries.

Variable effectiveness of BCG in different studies

PPD conversion by BCG

BCG is used only in tuberculin-negative subjects. Successful vaccination leads to a minor local lesion, self-limiting multiplication of the organism locally and in draining lymphatic vessels, and development of tuberculin hypersensitivity. The latter results in loss of the PPD test as a diagnostic and epidemiologic tool, and when infection rates are low, as they are now in most Western countries, this loss may offset the possible immunity produced. In general, tuberculosis rates in the West have declined as rapidly in countries that have not used the BCG vaccine as in those that have adopted mass vaccination with its occasional complications. Its potential value in these countries is restricted to population groups at particular risk, but its role in developing countries remains a matter of some contention. The BCG vaccination is contraindicated for individuals in whom cell-mediated immune mechanisms are compromised, such as those infected with the human immunodeficiency virus.

Laboratory Diagnosis

Detection of mycobacteria in direct smears of clinical material

If present in sufficient numbers, acid–alcohol-fast bacilli can be detected microscopically in direct smears of clinical specimens or in smears of material concentrated for culture (see below). Smears are stained by the Ziehl–Neelsen procedure or one of its modifications, including the fluorescence staining method. About 65% of culture-positive sputum samples yield positive smears from concentrated specimens. These procedures are not specific for *M. tuberculosis* because other mycobacteria may have a similar morphology and may be etiologic agents of disease, members of the normal flora, or external contaminants. Their significance depends on the specimen. Acid-fast bacilli in sputum collected into a container not subject to contamination are highly significant for mycobacterial infection. A clean-voided male urine specimen, on the other hand, is often contaminated with *Mycobacterium smegmatis* from the prepuce, and the finding of acid-fast bacilli does not per se indicate infection. Bronchoscopy equipment and nasotracheal tubes or their lubricants are prone to contamination with free-living mycobacteria, and false conclusions have been drawn from smears of such preparations.

M. smegmatis and contaminating mycobacteria may yield "false" positives

Specimens used for culture

Cultural confirmation of a tentative diagnosis of tuberculosis is thus essential, and the organism must be isolated for identification and susceptibility testing. Specimens from protected sites, such as cerebrospinal fluid, bone marrow, pleural fluid, and ureteric urine can be seeded directly to culture media use for *M. tuberculosis* isolation. Those samples inevitably contaminated with normal flora, such as sputum, gastric aspirations (cultured when sputum is not available, for example, in young children), or voided urine, are treated with alkali, acid, or a detergent germicide under conditions that will kill the normal flora, but allow many mycobacteria to survive because of their resistance to these agents. The most commonly used treatment now employs *N*-acetylcysteine to dissolve mucus, combined with the antibacterial effect of a weak sodium hydroxide solution. The material is concentrated by centrifugation or filtration, neutralized or washed, and inoculated to culture media.

> Contaminated material must be treated to kill other organisms

Cultures on solid media usually take 3 or more weeks to show visible colonies. Growth may be detected radiometrically in about half the time by using liquid oleic acid–albumin broth containing ^{14}C-labeled palmitic acid, which is metabolized by mycobacteria to liberate $^{14}CO_2$. The labeled CO_2 is detected in the space above the medium using an automated sampling procedure. Incorporation of a specific inhibitor of *M. tuberculosis* in a parallel vial increases the specificity of the test.

> Traditional cultures take 3 + weeks; radiometric procedures are more rapid

Whichever procedure is used, specific identification of an isolated *Mycobacterium* is essential. It may be achieved with a number of cultural and biochemical tests, including those shown in the appendix, but the process usually takes several weeks. More rapid results can be obtained by high-resolution gas chromatographic analysis of fatty acids in mycobacterial colonies or by testing for homology between genetic probes of labeled mycobacterial DNA and ribosomal RNA extracted from the strain under test. Specific probes are now available commercially for detecting *M. tuberculosis* and the *M. avium–intracellulare* complex.

> All isolates must be speciated

> Hybridization tests with DNA probes speed identification

Susceptibility testing is important with newly diagnosed cases. When sufficient numbers of acid-fast bacilli are seen on direct smears, the treated clinical specimen can be seeded directly onto antimicrobic-containing media for susceptibility tests, thereby saving several weeks. If numbers are scanty, the initiation of tests must await primary isolation. More rapid test results can be obtained by incorporating antimicrobics in the medium used for radiometric detection of mycobacterial growth. These results show good concordance with conventional tests and are available 1–2 weeks earlier.

> Susceptibility testing by conventional and radiometric procedures

Because of the complexity of the laboratory diagnosis of mycobacterial diseases, the clinician and laboratory should cooperate closely in reviewing the progress of specimens and in the interpretation of smear, culture, and susceptibility test results.

> Interpretation of test results

Other Mycobacteria Causing Tuberculosislike Diseases

Mycobacteria causing diseases that often resemble tuberculosis are listed in the appendix. With the exception of *M. bovis*, they have become relatively more prominent as the incidence of tuberculosis has declined. All have known or suspected environmental reservoirs, and all the infections they cause appear to be acquired from these sources. Immunocompromised individuals or those with chronic pulmonary conditions or malignancies are more likely to develop disease with these organisms. There is no evidence of case-to-case transmission. The organisms grow on the same media as *M. tuberculosis*, but usually more rapidly. Colonies of some species produce yellow or orange pigment in the light (photochromogenic), some in the light and dark (scotochromogenic). Species are distinguished by these characteristics and by biochemical reactions. Envi-

> Acquired from the environment; no case-to-case transmission

> Some species are pigmented

ronmental mycobacteria that cause tuberculosislike infections are usually more resistant than *M. tuberculosis* to some of the antimicrobics used in the treatment of mycobacterial diseases, and susceptibility testing is often needed as a guide to therapy.

In the past, these organisms were referred to as *atypical* or *anonymous mycobacteria*. Both terms are now inappropriate, because these species are well characterized in their own right.

Mycobacterium kansasii

Photochromogen

Distribution

Mycobacterium kansasii is a photochromogenic mycobacterium that usually forms yellow-pigmented colonies after about 2 weeks of incubation in the presence of light. In the United States, infection is most common in Illinois, Oklahoma, and Texas and tends to affect urban residents; it is uncommon in the Southeast. There is no evidence of case-to-case transmission, but the reservoir has yet to be identified. It causes about 3% of mycobacterial disease in the United States.

Can cause progressive pulmonary disease

Cross-hypersensitivity to PPD from *M. tuberculosis*

Prolonged combined chemotherapy

Mycobacterium kansasii infections resemble tuberculosis and tend to be slowly progressive without treatment. Cavitary pulmonary disease, cervical lymphadenitis, and skin infections are most common, but disseminated infections also occur. Hypersensitivity to proteins of *M. kansasii* develops and cross-reacts almost completely with that caused by tuberculosis. Positive PPD tests may thus result from clinical or subclinical *M. kansasii* infection. Prolonged combined chemotherapy with antimycobacterial drugs, including rifampin, is usually effective.

Mycobacterium avium–Intracellulare Complex

Worldwide occurrence

Mycobacterium avium-intracellulare complex is a group of related acid-fast organisms that grow only slightly faster than *M. tuberculosis* and can be divided into a number of serotypes. Among them are organisms that cause tuberculosis in birds (and sometimes swine), but rarely cause disease in humans. Others may produce disease in mammals, including humans, but not in birds. They are found worldwide in soil and water and in infected animals. In the United States they are most common in the Southeast, Pacific Coast, and northcentral regions. They are second only to *M. tuberculosis* in significance and frequency of the diseases they cause.

Second only to *M. tuberculosis* as cause of disease in United States

Wide range of diseases; commonest are pulmonary

Relative resistance to antituberculous drugs

The most common infection in humans is cavitary pulmonary disease, often superimposed on chronic bronchitis and emphysema. Most of those infected are white men aged 50 or more. Cervical lymphadenitis, chronic osteomyelitis, and renal and skin infections also occur. The organisms in this group are substantially more resistant to antituberculous drugs than most other species, and treatment with the three or four agents found to be most active often requires supplementation with surgery. About 20% of cases relapse within 5 years of treatment.

Disseminated infection is a common complication of AIDS

Disseminated avium–intracellulare infections, once considered rare, are now the most common systemic bacterial infection in patients suffering from AIDS. They usually develop when the patient's general clinical condition and helper T4 (CD4+) lymphocyte concentrations are declining. Clinically, the patient experiences progressive weight loss and intermittent fever, chills, night sweats, and diarrhea. Histologically, granuloma formation is muted, and there are aggregates of foamy macrophages containing numerous intracellular acid-fast bacilli. The diagnosis is most readily made by blood culture, using a variety of specialized cultural techniques. Response to chemotherapeutic agents is marginal, and the prognosis is grave.

A PPD prepared from a strain of *M. intracellulare* (PPD-B) has been used to detect evidence of previous or present infection as well as in epidemiologic surveys. There is some cross-reaction with PPD from *M. tuberculosis*. Skin test surveys give evidence of a high level of subclinical infection in the population of the southeastern states. Currently, PPD-B is not available for routine use.

PPD-B

Mycobacterium scrofulaceum

Scotochromogen

Mycobacterium scrofulaceum is an acid-fast scotochromogen that occurs in the environment under moist conditions. It forms yellow colonies in the dark or light within 2 weeks, and it shares several features with the *Mycobacterium avium–intracellulare* complex.

Granulomatous cervical lymphadenitis in children

Mycobacterium scrofulaceum is now one of the more common causes of granulomatous cervical lymphadenitis in young children. It derives its name from *scrofula*, an old descriptive term for tuberculous cervical lymphadenitis. The infection is manifested by an indolent enlargement of one or more lymph nodes with little, if any, pain or constitutional signs. It may ulcerate or form a draining sinus to the surface. It does not cause PPD conversion. Treatment usually involves surgical excision.

Surgical excision usually needed

Mycobacterium leprae and Leprosy

Leprosy is a chronic granulomatous disease of the peripheral nerves and nasal mucosa. It is rare in the United States and other Western countries and for this reason is considered only briefly. It remains a major problem on a worldwide scale, however, with an estimated 10–12 million cases. Immigration into the Western countries from areas where the disease occurs has increased the numbers of cases seen.

Fails to grow in culture

Mycobacterium leprae is an acid-fast bacillus that has not been grown in artificial medium or tissue culture beyond, possibly, a few generations. It can, however, be grown in the footpads of normal mice, in thymectomized irradiated mice, and in the armadillo, which may also be infected naturally. The central reservoir of *M. leprae*, however, appears to be infected humans. Very rarely, cases develop in nonendemic areas without known case contacts. The infectivity of *M. leprae* is low. Most new cases have had prolonged close contact with an infected individual in the past. Transmission probably occurs most commonly by contamination of the nasal mucosa or minor skin lesions with infected nasal secretions from cases of lepromatous leprosy. Biting insects may also be involved. In vivo growth is very slow; as a consequence, the incubation period is measured in years or decades.

Growth in footpads of mice

Human reservoir

Low infectivity

Slow growth in vivo contributes to long incubation period

Two major forms of the disease are recognized, tuberculoid and lepromatous; intermediate forms occur, however, and the first form may merge into the second.

Tuberculoid Leprosy

Skin and nerve involvement

Tuberculoid leprosy involves the development of macules or large, flattened plaques on the face, trunk, and limbs with raised, erythematous edges and dry, pale, hairless centers. The organism may invade some peripheral sensory nerves, resulting in patchy anesthesia. Few *M. leprae* are seen in tuberculoid lesions, which are granulomatous with extensive ep-

Few *M. leprae* in lesions

ithelioid cell, giant cell, and lymphocytic infiltration. Patients show delayed hypersensitivity to lepromin, a tuberculin analog derived from leprous tissue. They mount an excellent cell-mediated immune response. The disease is indolent, with simultaneous evidence of slow progression and healing. Because of the small number of organisms present, this form of the disease is usually noncontagious.

Strong delayed hypersensitivity and cell-mediated immunity

Lepromatous Leprosy

Deficient cell-mediated immunity and anergy to lepromin

Many *M. leprae* in lesions

Extensive skin lesions produce "leonine fascies"

In lepromatous multibacillary leprosy, cell-mediated immunity is deficient, and patients are anergic to lepromin. Growth of *M. leprae* is, thus, relatively unimpeded. Histologically, lesions show dense infiltration with leprosy bacilli, and large numbers may reach the bloodstream. Skin lesions are extensive, symmetric, and diffuse, particularly on the face, with thickening of the looser skin of the lips, forehead, and ears, resulting in the classic leonine appearance. Damage may be severe, with loss of nasal bones and septum, sometimes of digits, and with testicular atrophy in men. The organism spreads systemically, with involvement of the reticuloendothelial system.

Laboratory Diagnosis

Stained smears and biopsies

Laboratory diagnosis of lepromatous leprosy involves preparation of Ziehl–Neelsen-stained scrapings of infected tissue, particularly nasal mucosa or earlobes. Large numbers of acid-fast bacilli are seen. Tuberculoid leprosy is diagnosed clinically and by histologic appearance of full-thickness skin biopsies.

Recently, glycolipid antigens unique to *M. leprae* have been identified, purified, and tested for their usefulness in serodiagnostic tests. The specificity has been excellent, but the sensitivity for tuberculoid leprosy is still unsatisfactory. It is likely that suitable serologic tests will be available for this disease in the near future.

Treatment and Prevention

Central role of sulfones

Combined therapy with rifampin

Treatment has been revolutionized by the development of sulfones, such as dapsone, which blocks *para*-aminobenzoic acid metabolism in *M. leprae*. When combined with rifampin, it will usually control or cure tuberculoid leprosy when given for 6 months. In lepromatous leprosy and multibacillary intermediate forms of the disease, a third agent (clofazimine) is added to help prevent the selection of resistant mutants, and treatment is continued for at least 2 years.

Prevention requires early diagnosis and treatment of cases

Prevention of leprosy involves recognition and treatment of infectious patients and early diagnosis of the disease in close contacts. Chemoprophylaxis with sulfones has been used for children in close contact with lepromatous cases. Immunization with BCG vaccine has been investigated, with varying results.

A possible diagnosis of leprosy elicits fear and distress in patients and contacts out of all proportion to its risks. Few clinicians in the United States have the experience to make such a diagnosis, and expert help should be sought from public health authorities before reaching this conclusion or indicating its possibility to the patient.

Other Mycobacterial Infections

Mycobacterium fortuitum Complex

Rapid growers

Abscesses and infections of prostheses

Mycobacterium fortuitum complex comprises free-living, rapidly growing, acid-fast bacilli that produce colonies within 3 days. Human infections are rare. Abscesses at injection sites in drug abusers are probably the most common lesions. Occasional secondary pulmonary infections develop. Some cases have been associated with implantation of foreign material, for example, breast prostheses and artificial heart valves. Except in the case of endocarditis, the infections usually resolve spontaneously with removal of the prosthetic device.

Mycobacterium marinum

Causes fish tuberculosis; fails to grow at 37°C

Human infections from swimming pools

Self-limiting skin granulomas

Mycobacterium marinum causes tuberculosis in fish, is widely present in fresh and salt waters, and grows at 30°C but not at 37°C. It occurs in considerable numbers in the slime that forms on rocks or on rough walls of swimming pools, and it can cause skin lesions in humans. Classically, a swimmer who abrades his elbows or forearms climbing out of a pool develops a superficial granulomatous lesion that finally ulcerates. It usually heals spontaneously after a few weeks, but is sometimes chronic. The organism may be sensitive to tetracycline as well as to some antituberculous drugs.

Mycobacterium ulcerans

Occurs in tropical areas

Severe, progressive ulcerations require surgical removal

Fails to grow at 37°C

Mycobacterium ulcerans is a much more serious cause of superficial infection. Cases usually occur in the tropics, most often in parts of Africa, New Guinea, and northern Australia, but have been seen elsewhere sporadically. Children are most often affected. The source and mode of transmission of the infection are unknown. Those infected develop severe ulceration involving the skin and subcutaneous tissue that is often progressive unless treated effectively. Surgical excision and grafting are usually needed. Antimicrobic treatment is often unsuccessful. Like *M. marinum, M. ulcerans* grows at 30°C, but not at 37°C.

Appendix 27.1 Mycobacteria of Major Clinical Importance[a]

Species	Reservoir	Virulence for Humans	Disease Caused	Case-to-Case Transmission	Growth Rate	Optimum Growth Temperature	Pigment Production[b]	Substantial Niacin Production[c]	Virulence for Guinea Pigs[a]
M. tuberculosis	Human	+++	Tuberculosis	Yes	S	37	-	+	+
M. bovis	Animals	+++	Tuberculosis	Rare	S	37	-	-	+
Bacillus Calmette-Guérin	Artificial culture	±	Local lesion	Very rare	S	37	-	-	-
M. kansasii	Environmental	+	Tuberculosislike	No	S	37	Photochromogen	-	-
M. scrofulaceum	Environmental	+	Usually lymphadenitis	No	S	37	Scotochromogen	-	-
M. avium-intracellulare	Environmental; birds	+	Tuberculosislike	No	S	37	±	-	-
M. fortuitum	Environmental	±	Local abscess	No	F	37	±	-	Local abscess
M. marinum	Water; fish	±	Skin granuloma	No	S	30	Photochromogen	-	-
M. ulcerans	Probably environmental; tropical	+	Severe skin ulceration	No	S	30	-	-	-
M. leprae	Human	+++	Leprosy	Yes	NG	NG	NG	NG	-
M. smegmatis	Human, external urethral area	-	None	-	F	37	-	-	-

Characteristics

Abbreviations: S = slow (colonies usually develop in 10 days or more); F = fast (colonies develop in 7 days or less); NG = not grown.
[a] Numerous nonpathogenic environmental mycobacteria exist and may contaminate human specimens.
[b] Yellow-orange pigment. Photochromogen = pigment produced in light; scotochromogen = pigment produced in dark or light.
[c] Many other differential biochemical tests used, eg, nitrate reduction, catalase production, Tween 80 hydrolysis.
[d] Disease following subcutaneous injection of light inoculum (eg, 10^2 cells).

Additional Reading

Chaisson, R.E., and Slutkin, G. 1989. Tuberculosis and human immunodeficiency virus infection. *J. Infect. Dis.* 159:96–100. A recent review of the impact of one of humankind's newest scourges on one of its oldest.

Daniel, T.M. 1982. Selective primary health care: Strategies for control of disease in the developing world. II. Tuberculosis. *Rev. Infect. Dis.* 4:1254–1265. A brief but excellent synopsis of the status of tuberculosis in the developing world, and potential strategies for its control in areas with limited financial and personnel resources.

Daniel, T.M. 1988. Antibody and antigen detection in the immunodiagnosis of tuberculosis. Why not? What more is needed? Where do we stand today? *J. Infect. Dis.* 158:678–680.

Dubos, R.J., and Dubos, J. 1952. *The White Plague. Tuberculosis, Man, and Society.* Boston: Little, Brown & Co. A scholarly and highly readable account of the history and impact of tuberculosis on western culture.

Gaylord, H., and Brennan, P.J. 1987. Leprosy and the leprosy bacillus. Recent developments in characterization of antigens and immunology of the disease. *Ann. Rev. Microbiol.* 41:645–675.

Hastings, R.C., Gillis, T.P., Krahenbuhl, J.L., et al. 1988. Leprosy. *Clin. Microbiol. Rev.* 1:330–348. The above two references are recent comprehensive reviews of this biblical disease, with an emphasis on its microbiology and immunology.

Snider, D., Jr., Bridbord, K., and Hui, F., Eds. 1989. Research towards global control and prevention of tuberculosis with an emphasis on vaccine development. *Rev. Infect. Dis.* 11(suppl 2):S335–S490. Proceedings of a Fogarty International Center Workshop with contributions by authorities covering the latest information on the topics considered in this chapter.

Woods, G.L., and Washington, J.A., II 1987. Mycobacteria other than *Mycobacterium tuberculosis*: Review of microbiologic and clinical aspects. *Rev. Infect. Dis.* 9:275–294. A recent highly readable and comprehensive summary of the mycobacteria that have been termed "atypical" and of the clinical diseases they produce.

28

Actinomyces *and* Nocardia

Kenneth J. Ryan

Actinomyces and *Nocardia* are bacteria with filamentous and branching growth, which caused them to be confused with fungi before the fundamental differences between eukaryotic and prokaryotic cells were recognized. They are Gram-positive rods related to the mycobacteria (some species are acid fast), but with a distinctive tendency to grow in a treelike branching network. They are opportunists that can sometimes produce indolent, slowly progressive diseases. A related genus, *Streptomyces*, is of medical importance as a producer of many antibiotics, but rarely causes infections. Important differential features of these groups and of the mycobacteria (Chapter 27) to which they are related are shown in Table 28.1.

Opportunists

Actinomyces and Actinomycosis

Microbiologic Characteristics

Members of normal flora

Actinomyces are normal inhabitants of some areas of the gastrointestinal tract of humans and animals from the oropharynx to the lower bowel. They grow only under microaerophilic or strictly anaerobic conditions both in vivo and in vitro, and prolonged incubation (4–10 days) is required before macroscopically visible growth appears in artificial culture. In culture and clinical lesions, the organisms typically appear as elongated Gram-positive rods that branch at acute angles and often show irregular staining. In young broth cultures, shorter forms appear as bent diphtheroids or in X and Y letterlike configurations; in pus, however, the most characteristic form is the *sulfur granule*. This yellow-orange granule, named for its gross resemblance to a grain of sulfur, is a small colony (usually less than 0.3 mm) of intertwined branching *Actinomyces* filaments solidified with elements of tissue exudate. The granule is so dense that the branching bacilli are visible only at the edges in a gram-stained preparation.

Species of *Actinomyces* are distinguished on the basis of biochemical

Slow-growing anaerobes

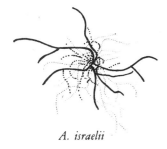

A. israelii

Table 28.1 Some Features of the Family Actinomycetales

Genus	True Branching	Acid Fast	Weakly Acid Fast[a]	Aerobic Growth	Penicillin Susceptible
Mycobacterium[b]	−	+[c]	+	+	−
Actinomyces	+	−	−	−	+
Nocardia	+	−	+[d]	+	−
Streptomyces	+	−	Rare	+	−

[a] Using weak decolorizer (1% H_2SO_4).
[b] See Chapter 27.
[c] Ziehl-Neelsen method for *M. tuberculosis*.
[d] Applies to *N. asteroides* and *N. brasiliensis* only.

Most infections due to *A. israelii*

reactions, cultural features, and cell wall composition. Most human actinomycosis is caused by *Actinomyces israelii*, but other species have been isolated from typical actinomycotic lesions. The related organism *Arachnia propionicus*, originally classified with the *Actinomyces*, can produce clinically similar disease. Other species of *Actinomyces* have been associated with dental and periodontal infections (see Chapter 62).

Pathogenesis and Pathology of Actinomycosis

Conditions for growth in tissues

Actinomyces are highly adapted to mucosal surfaces and do not produce disease unless they transgress the epithelial barrier under conditions that produce a sufficiently low oxygen tension for their multiplication. Such conditions usually involve mechanical disruption of the mucosa with necrosis of deeper, normally sterile tissues (for example, following tooth extraction). Once initiated, growth occurs as colonies in the tissues and extends locally through the tissues without regard to anatomic boundaries.

Sinus tracts

Pus and sulfur granules

The lesion is composed of sinus tracts filled with polymorphonuclear leukocytes surrounded by an indurated fibrous tissue reaction; the sinuses ultimately discharge to the surface. Sulfur granules are present within the pus, but are not numerous. Free *Actinomyces* or small branching units are rarely seen, although contaminating Gram-negative rods are common. As the lesion enlarges, it becomes firm and indurated. If near a cutaneous surface, sinus tracts usually open spontaneously and drain through the skin. Human cases provide little evidence of immunity to *Actinomyces*. Once established, infections typically become chronic and resolve only with the aid of antimicrobic therapy. Antibodies can be detected in the course of infection, but seem to reflect the antigenic stimulation of the ongoing infection rather than immunity.

Clinical Manifestations

Cervicofacial actinomycosis

Actinomycosis exists in several forms that differ according to the original site and circumstances of tissue invasion. Infection of the cervicofacial area, the most common site of actinomycosis, is usually related to poor dental hygiene, tooth extraction, or some other trauma to the mouth or jaw. Lesions in the submandibular region and the angle of the jaw give the face a swollen, indurated appearance.

Thoracic actinomycosis

Thoracic actinomycosis is very rare and may involve the lungs, pleura, mediastinal structures, or chest wall. It may follow aspiration of infected material, leading to an actinomycotic lung abscess that can erode through

Abdominal actinomycosis

the pleura and even the chest wall. It can also result from sinuses that initiated in actinomycotic lesions above or below the chest.

Abdominal actinomycosis is also rare. It can follow surgery or other trauma to the bowel, as well as perforations of ulcers or diverticula. Diagnosis is usually delayed, because only vague or nonspecific symptoms are produced until a vital organ is eroded or obstructed. The firm, fibrous masses are often initially mistaken for a malignancy.

Pelvic involvement as an extension from other sites also occurs occasionally. It is particularly difficult to distinguish from other inflammatory conditions or malignancies. A more localized chronic endometritis, apparently caused by *Actinomyces*, has been associated with the use of intrauterine contraceptive devices.

All are endogenous infections

Infections with *Actinomyces* are endogenous, and case-to-case transmission does not appear to occur.

Diagnosis

A clinical diagnosis of actinomycosis is based on the nature of the lesion, the slowly progressive course, and a history of trauma or of a condition predisposing to mucosal invasion by *Actinomyces*. The etiologic diagnosis

Paucity of *Actinomyces* in sinus drainage

can be difficult to establish with certainty: although the lesions may be extensive, the number of organisms in pus may be few and may remain concentrated in sulfur granule colonies deep in the indurated tissue. The diagnosis is further complicated by heavy colonization of the moist draining sinuses with other bacteria, usually small Gram-negative rods. This

Contamination of actinomycotic lesions with other species

contamination not only causes confusion regarding the etiology, but interferes with isolation of the slow-growing anaerobic *Actinomyces*.

Collection of pus for sulfur granules

Material for direct smear and culture should include as much pus as possible to increase the chance of collecting the diagnostic sulfur granules. Samples may be spread out in a petri dish lid to facilitate location of the granules, or they may be diluted with a large volume of saline; in the latter case, the granules tend to sediment to the bottom of the tube on standing.

Direct Gram stains

Granules crushed between two slides and stained show a dense, Gram-positive center with individual branching rods at the periphery. Granules should also be selected and macerated for culture, because culture of a simple swab from a draining sinus will usually grow only contaminants;

Anaerobic cultures

thus, detection of any *Actinomyces* is unlikely. Culture media and techniques are the same as those used for other anaerobes (Chapters 14 and 18). Incubation must be prolonged, because some strains require 7 days or more to appear. Identification requires a variety of biochemical tests to differentiate *Actinomyces* from propionibacteria (anaerobic diphtheroids), which may show a tendency to form short branches in fluid culture.

Biopsy

Biopsies for culture and histopathology are useful, but it may be necessary to examine many sections and pieces of tissue before sulfur granule colonies of *Actinomyces* are found. The morphology of the sulfur granule in tissue is quite characteristic with routine hematoxylin and eosin (H&E) or histologic Gram staining. With H&E, the edge of the granule shows amorphous eosinophilic "clubs" formed from the tissue elements and containing the branching actinomycotic filaments.

Treatment

Penicillin therapy

Penicillin G is the treatment of choice for actinomycosis, although a number of other antimicrobics (tetracycline, erythromycin, clindamycin) are active in vitro and have shown some clinical effectiveness. High doses of

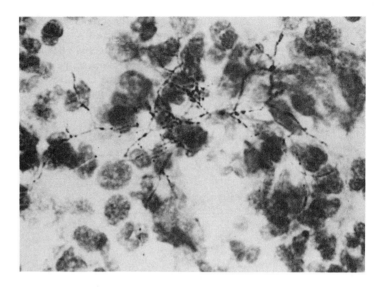

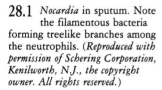

28.1 *Nocardia* in sputum. Note the filamentous bacteria forming treelike branches among the neutrophils. (*Reproduced with permission of Schering Corporation, Kenilworth, N.J., the copyright owner. All rights reserved.*)

penicillin must be used and therapy prolonged for 4–6 weeks or more before any response is seen. Although slow, response to therapy is often striking given the degree of fibrosis and deformity caused by the infection. Because detection of the causative organism is difficult, many patients are treated empirically as a therapeutic trial based on clinical findings alone.

Nocardia

Microbiologic Characteristics

Gram-positive aerobes

Nocardia species are Gram-positive, rod-shaped bacteria that show true branching both in culture and in clinical lesions. In contrast to *Actinomyces*, they are strict aerobes, and the species most common in human infection (*Nocardia asteroides* and *Nocardia brasiliensis*) are weakly acid fast. *Nocardia* species are commonly found in the environment, particularly in soil. They have been isolated in small numbers from the respiratory tract of healthy persons, but are not considered members of the normal human flora.

Environmental sources

Morphology similar to *Actinomyces*

The microscopic morphology is similar to that of *Actinomyces*, although *Nocardia* tend to fragment more readily and are found as shorter branched units throughout the lesion rather than concentrated in a few colonies or granules. Many strains take the Gram stain poorly, appearing "beaded" with alternating Gram-positive and Gram-negative sections of the same filament (Figure 28.1). Growth typically appears on ordinary laboratory medium (blood agar) after 2 days. Colonies initially have a dry, chalklike appearance and are usually adherent to the agar, sitting in a craterlike pit. With continued incubation, the colony becomes wrinkled and may develop white to orange pigment. Because of their need for aerobic conditions, colonies form a surface pellicle in broth culture.

Cultural characteristics

Classification

Speciation of *Nocardia* is a tedious process that involves tests for decomposition of substrates such as casein, tyrosine, and xanthine, as well as other tests not usually applied to most bacteria. Although the organism grows in a few days, these tests may require weeks to complete. The species of medical importance are *N. asteroides, N. brasiliensis*, and *Nocardia caviae.*

Pathogenesis and Pathology

Pulmonary Nocardiosis.   This begins with inhalation of *Nocardia* (usually

Usually due to *N. asteroides*

N. asteroides) that is present in dust or soil or contaminating mucosal surfaces. This event must be relatively common in comparison to the frequency of disease. Factors leading to disease are poorly understood, although roughly half of all patients with pulmonary nocardiosis have an underlying disease or have undergone treatment known to compromise

Predisposing factors; occurrence in the immunocompromised

immune defenses. These conditions include leukemia, lymphoma, chronic pulmonary disorders, and the use of immunosuppressive agents such as corticosteroids. There is evidence that effective cell-mediated immunity

Cell-mediated immunity

is important in host defense against *Nocardia* infection. Increased resistance to experimental *Nocardia* infection in animals has been linked to increased activity of activated macrophages. Neutrophils are prominent in nocardial lesions. Although they do not kill *Nocardia*, they slow its growth while an immune response is mounted. Activated macrophages kill *Nocardia* that they have engulfed. *Nocardia* are considered opportunists; their infectivity is low, and there is no case-to-case transmission.

The primary lesions in the lung show acute inflammation with suppuration and destruction of parenchyma. Multiple, confluent abscesses may occur. Unlike *Actinomyces* infections, there is little tendency toward

Pulmonary abscesses and dissemination to central nervous system

fibrosis and localization. Dissemination to distant organs, particularly the brain, may occur. In the central nervous system, multifocal abscesses are often produced. The great majority of *Nocardia* pulmonary and brain infections are produced by *N. asteroides.*

Skin and Subcutaneous Tissue Infections.   Infections can follow direct inoculation of *Nocardia.* This mechanism is usually associated with some kind of outdoor activity and with relatively minor trauma, such as a sliver

Usually due to *N. brasiliensis*

or thorn prick. Infection is usually with *N. brasiliensis*, which produces a superficial pustule at the site of inoculation. If *Nocardia* gain access to the subcutaneous tissues, lesions resembling actinomycosis may be produced, complete with draining sinuses and sulfur granules. This infection may occur with *Nocardia* species or related organisms such as *Actinomadura madurae* (formerly *Nocardia madurae*), a cause of the mycetoma syndrome (Chapter 49).

Clinical Manifestations

Bronchopneumonia

Pulmonary infection is usually a confluent bronchopneumonia that may be acute, chronic, or relapsing. Production of cavities and extension to the pleura are common. Symptoms are those of any bronchopneumonia,

Cerebral abscess

including cough, dyspnea, and fever. The clinical signs of brain abscess depend on its exact location and size: the neurologic picture can be particularly confusing when multiple lesions are present. The combination of current or recent pneumonia and focal central nervous system signs is suggestive of *Nocardia* infection. The cutaneous syndrome typically involves a pustule, fever, and tender lymphadenitis in the regional lymph nodes.

Diagnosis

The diagnosis of *Nocardia* infection is much easier than that of actinomycosis, because the organisms tend to appear throughout the lesions.

Direct Gram stain

Filaments of Gram-positive rods with primary and secondary branches can

Weak acid fastness of *N. asteroides*

usually be found in sputum and are readily demonstrated in direct aspirates from skin or other purulent sites. Demonstration of acid fastness, when combined with other observations, is diagnostic of *N. asteroides* or *N. brasiliensis*. The acid fastness of *Nocardia* species differs from that of mycobacteria (Chapter 27) in that they are less strongly acid fast. The staining method thus employs a weaker decolorizing agent than that used for mycobacteria. *Nocardia* do not show acid fastness with the regular Ziehl–Neelsen technique; mycobacteria, however, are acid fast by both methods (Table 28.1).

Culture on routine media

Culture of *Nocardia* is not difficult if the laboratory is alerted to the possibility of nocardiosis. The organisms grow on routine media used for Gram-positive bacteria (blood agar) or on those used for routine fungal cultures as long as they do not contain antibacterial agents.

Treatment

Sulfonamide therapy and drainage

Nocardia are usually highly sensitive to sulfonamides, but relatively resistant to penicillin. Combination of sulfonamides with drainage and surgery has been successful in treatment of this disease, which rarely enters spontaneous remission. Thus, pulmonary, cutaneous, and central nervous system nocardiosis remains one of the few indications for systemic sulfonamide therapy, although a significant proportion of patients do not respond. Technical difficulties in susceptibility testing have hampered the rational selection and study of other antimicrobics, but various reports support clinical activity of ampicillin, newer β-lactams (imipenem, ceftriaxone), minocycline, aminoglycosides, cycloserine, and trimethoprim–sulfamethoxazole. Antituberculous agents and antifungal agents such as amphotericin B have no activity against *Nocardia*.

Other antimicrobics

29

Chlamydia

Lawrence Corey

Chlamydia

Members of the genus *Chlamydia* are obligate, intracellular bacteria. They have nucleoids and ribosomes and a discrete cell envelope. They multiply in host cells by binary fission and are susceptible to several antibacterial antimicrobics. Two recognized species cause disease in humans, *Chlamydia psittaci* and *Chlamydia trachomatis*. A newly characterized species, *Chlamydia pneumoniae,* causes acute respiratory infections and differs from *C. psittaci* and *C. trachomatis*. It was previously termed *Chlamydia* strain TWAR.

Morphology and Structure

Obligate intracellular bacteria

Gram-negative type outer membrane; absence of peptidoglycan

Chlamydia species are small, generally rounded organisms that show morphologic variation during their replicative cycle. The cell envelope consists of inner and outer membranes, but differs from that of typical Gram-negative organisms in that there is no peptidoglycan layer between the membranes. *Chlamydia* possess ribosomes of the bacterial type and synthesize their own protein. Their DNA genome is one-fourth the size of that of *Escherichia coli* and one of the smallest among prokaryotes.

Metabolic Characteristics

Requires host-derived ATP

Chlamydia species are metabolically deficient compared to free-living bacteria, because they are dependent on the host cell for energy generation and cannot synthesize adenosine triphosphate (ATP) or reoxidize reduced nicotinamide adenine dinucleotide phosphate.

Replicative Cycle

The replicative cycle of *Chlamydia* is illustrated in Figure 29.1. It involves two forms of the organism, a small (0.3 μm) hardy infectious form termed the *elementary* body, and a larger (1+ μm) fragile intracellular reproductive

469

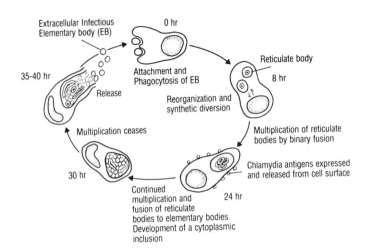

29.1 Reproduction cycle of *Chlamydia*.

Elementary body infects cell and transforms to reticulate body

form termed the *reticulate* body. The elementary body attaches to specific receptors on susceptible target cells (usually columnar or transitional epithelial cells) and enters by endocytosis within a vacuole derived from the host cell membrane. Metabolic changes that are incompletely understood lead the elementary body to reorganize within about 1–8 hr into the larger reticulate body. Using the ATP-generating capacity of the host cell, reticulate bodies divide by binary fission within the endocytic vacuole. The newly formed organisms finally occupy much of the infected host cell, producing a cytoplasmic inclusion body characteristic of *Chlamydia* infections. After 24–72 hr, the reticulate bodies reorganize and condense to yield multiple elementary bodies with the capacity to infect other host cells when the infected cell ruptures. Electron micrographs show that reticulate bodies have many more ribosomes than elementary bodies, as would be expected of growing and dividing cells.

Reticulate body divides by binary fission

Reticulate bodies produce multiple elementary bodies

Chlamydia trachomatis synthesizes large amounts of glycogen, which surrounds the reticulate bodies, and the inclusion bodies thus stain blue with iodine. *Chlamydia psittaci* and *C. pneumoniae* inclusions do not contain glycogen.

Inclusion bodies

Growth in the Laboratory

Growth in yolk sac of chick embryo and McCoy cells

Chlamydia can be grown in the yolk sac of the developing chick embryo, although it is sometimes difficult to grow certain strains of *C. trachomatis* in this way. They can also be grown in some cell cultures, such as those of the McCoy mouse heteroploid line. Treatment of the cells by irradiation or with antimetabolites (idoxuridine or cyclohexamide) before inoculation inhibits host cell replication and allows *C. trachomatis* to compete better for cell nutrients and, thus, to grow better. Chlamydiae may be detected in cell culture by the development of their characteristic intracytoplasmic inclusions, which are visualized with Giemsa stain or, in the case of *C. trachomatis* (Figure 29.2), with an iodine stain for glycogen. Staining for *Chlamydia* antigen in infected cells using immunofluorescence techniques is used in many laboratories and has greater sensitivity than iodine staining.

Antimetabolite treatment of McCoy cells for greater chlamydial growth

Antigenic Structure

Chlamydiae have common lipopolysaccharide antigens and specific cell envelope protein antigens by which they are divided into a number of serotypes. The antigenic difference between the various subtypes of *C.*

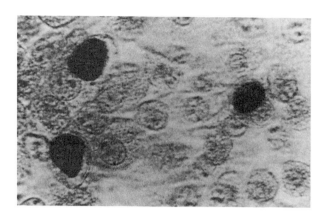

29.2 Iodine-stained inclusions of *C. trachomatis* in McCoy cell culture.

Association of specific serotypes with different disease syndromes

trachomatis appear to reside mainly in the major outer membrane protein, which comprises about 50% of the membrane. Each of the major disease syndromes caused by chlamydiae are associated with different serotypes (Table 29.1). The type-specific antigens elicit protective antibody in experimental animals, but the group antigens do not. Serotyping is performed by a fluorescence antibody procedure, but is not undertaken in routine diagnostic laboratories.

Pathogenesis of Chlamydial Diseases

Virulence of *C. psittaci* by respiratory route

Chlamydia psittaci and some strains of *C. trachomatis* are virulent to varying degrees to mice inoculated by the intravenous or intracerebral route or, in the case of the respiratory pathogen *C. psittaci,* by the intranasal route. *Chlamydia psittaci* is highly infectious to humans by the respiratory route and poses a significant risk to laboratory workers.

Prevention of lysosomal fusion

Competition with host cells for nutrients

The mechanisms of virulence of *Chlamydia* are incompletely understood. When ingested by phagocytic cells, they prevent lysosomal fusion with the phagocytic vacuole, and thus escape killing by lysosomal enzymes. All species produce heat-labile protein toxins that are lethal to mice on intravenous inoculation and specific to each serotype. Chlamydiae must compete with the host cell for essential nutrients, which may partially account for cell death and consequent tissue damage. There is some evidence that *C. trachomatis* may exist in a latent form and emerge to cause

Table 29.1 Association between Chlamydial Species, Serotypes, and Disease

Species	Subtype	Disease
C. psittaci	Many	Psittacosis
C. pneumoniae	One	Acute respiratory infection
C. trachomatis	A, B, C	Trachoma
	D, E, F, H, I, J, K	Nongonococcal urethritis; cervicitis; endometritis; salpingitis; proctitis; epididymitis; inclusion conjunctivitis in newborns; infant syndrome pneumonia
	L_1, L_2, L_3	Lymphogranuloma venereum

Table 29.2 Major Differential Features of *Chlamydia* Species That Cause Human Disease

Feature[a]	C. psittaci	C. trachomatis	C. pneumoniae
Natural habitat	Birds	Humans	Humans
Diseases	Pneumonitis	Conjunctivitis; genital tract infections; lymphogranuloma venereum	Upper and lower respiratory tract infections
Virulence in mouse	High	Variable (lymphogranuloma venereum strains only)	Less than *C. psittaci*
Glycogen containing discrete inclusion bodies	No	Yes	No
Sensitive to sulfonamides	No	Yes	No

[a] Information regarding serotypes is provided in Table 29.1.

relapses of infection in the immunosuppressed host. The mechanisms of latency are not understood.

Susceptibility

Failure to survive in environment

Susceptibility to tetracyclines

Chlamydiae are highly susceptible to environmental conditions and survive only briefly outside the body. Thus, transmission involves close contact or, in the case of *C. psittaci*, rapid spread by dust or droplet. They are susceptible to a considerable range of antimicrobics, of which the tetracyclines have been the most effective agents in clinical practice. In contrast to *C. psittaci* and *C. pneumoniae* many strains of *C. trachomatis* are sensitive to sulfonamides; this finding indicates that *C. trachomatis* synthesizes its own folic acid, whereas *C. psittaci* uses that provided by the host.

Species Differentiation

Little DNA homology is found between *C. psittaci*, *C. trachomatis*, and *C. pneumoniae* though they share a common group antigen. Their major differential features are shown in Table 29.2. Although data are incomplete, *C. pneumoniae* appears to have humans as a sole natural habitat.

Infections with *Chlamydia psittaci*

Zoonotic respiratory disease from birds

Human psittacosis (ornithosis) is a zoonosis contracted through inhalation of respiratory secretions, or dust from droppings, of infected birds. It was initially described in psittacines, such as parrots and parakeets, but was subsequently shown to occur in a wide range of avian species. The disease is usually latent in its natural host, but may become active, particularly with the stress of recent captivity or transport; *C. psittaci* is then excreted in large amounts.

Association with turkey processing and captive psittacine birds

Psittacosis in humans is seen mainly as an occupational hazard of poultry workers, especially those associated with processing turkey carcasses. It may also occur in owners of pet psittacine birds. There has been a marked reduction in cases of human psittacosis in the United States during the past 25 years. This decrease has been associated with the use of antimicrobics in poultry feeds and with quarantine regulations for imported psittacine birds.

C. *psittaci* pneumonitis

Diagnosis and treatment

Clinically, psittacosis in humans is an acute infection of the lower respiratory tract, usually presenting with acute onset of fever, headache, malaise, muscle aches, dry, hacking cough, and X-ray evidence of bilateral interstitial pneumonia. Occasionally, systemic complications such as myocarditis, encephalitis, and hepatitis may develop. The liver and spleen are often enlarged. The diagnosis of psittacosis should be suspected in a patient with acute onset of febrile lower respiratory illness with hepatosplenomegaly who gives a history of close exposure to birds. It must be remembered that spread can occur from both symptomatic and asymptomatic infections of birds. The specific diagnosis is usually made by demonstrating a fourfold rise in the titer of complement fixing antibody to chlamydial group antigen over several days of illness. *Chlamydia psittaci* can be isolated from the blood early in the disease and from sputum. Attempts to do so, however, must be made only in specialized laboratories because of the risk of laboratory infection and spread. Treatment with tetracycline or erythromycin is effective if given early in the course of illness.

Infections with *Chlamydia pneumoniae*

Respiratory infection of humans; droplet spread

Subclinical infections common

Recently, *C. pneumoniae* has been shown to be a cause of "walking pneumonia" in young adults in the United States. Epidemiologic evidence indicates that infection occurs throughout the year and is spread between humans by respiratory droplets. Most infections present as pharyngitis and/or lower respiratory tract disease, and the clinical spectrum is similar to that of *Mycoplama pneumoniae* infection. Serologic data show that infection is common, but, in most cases, subclinical. Tetracycline or erythromycin appear to be useful in ameliorating the signs and symptoms of *C. pneumoniae* infection.

Infections with *Chlamydia trachomatis*

Eye Infections

Trachoma and inclusion conjunctivitis due to different serotypes

There are two distinct distinct diseases, trachoma and inclusion conjunctivitis, which have some overlap in their clinical manifestations. Trachoma, a chronic infection caused by *C. trachomatis* immunotypes A, B, Ba, and C, is usually seen in less developed countries and often leads to blindness. Inclusion conjunctivitis is a worldwide disease of both adults and newborns. It is characterized as an acute inflammation of the conjunctiva, but is usually not associated with chronicity or permanent eye damage. It is caused by immunotypes D–K.

Leading cause of blindness in some developing countries

Chronicity of trachoma

Usually contracted in early life

Trachoma. Trachoma, a chronic follicular conjunctivitis, remains one of the leading causes of preventable blindness in the world. An estimated 20 million cases of blindness due to trachoma occur worldwide, and it is a major public health problem in North Africa, sub-Saharan Africa, and Central and Southeast Africa. In the United States, pockets of endemic trachoma exist, mainly among Native American populations in the Southwest. It is a complex disease that involves persistent infection and reinfection with *C. trachomatis,* hypersensitivity reactions to the organism, and superinfection with other bacterial species.

The disease is usually contracted in infancy or early childhood from the mother or other close contacts. First exposure results in acute conjunctivitis, which usually resolves. Persistence and reinfections and the

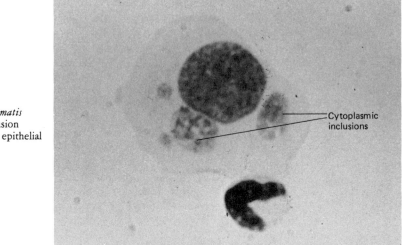

29.3 *Chlamydia trachomatis* cytoplasmic inclusion bodies in a conjunctival epithelial cell.

Cytoplasmic inclusions

Eyelid and corneal scarring

associated inflammatory responses provide the stimulus for the major pathologic effects of the disease in untreated cases. Chronic inflammation of the eyelids and increased vascularization of the corneal conjunctiva are followed by severe corneal scarring and conjunctival deformities. Visual loss often occurs 15–20 years after the initial infection.

Prevention of reinfection is most important

Antimicrobic therapy

Treatment of trachoma is difficult and generally directed toward prevention of continued reinfection during early childhood. From a public health point of view, improved hygiene appears to be the most effective approach and is aimed at decreasing transmission of infection within families. Treatment with systemic and topical antimicrobial agents such as sulfonamides, tetracycline, and erythromycin is often used to prevent reinfection or to treat persistent infection. Corrective surgery is required for severe corneal and blepharal conjunctival scarring.

Common form of neonatal conjunctivitis contracted from maternal genital infection

Inclusion Conjunctivitis.   Inclusion conjunctivitis is an acute infection of the conjunctiva seen in infants and adults among population groups in which the serotypes causing *C. trachomatis* genital infections are common. It is the most common form of neonatal conjunctivitis in the United States, occurring in 2–6% of newborn infants. The infection results from direct contact with infected cervical secretions of the mother at delivery.

Diagnosis and treatment

Inclusion conjunctivitis usually presents as an acute, copious, mucopurulent eye discharge 2–25 days after birth. The symptoms can resolve spontaneously and may not come to medical attention. Diagnosis can be made most easily by demonstrating characteristic cytoplasmic inclusions in smears of conjunctival scrapings (Figure 29.3). *Chlamydia trachomatis* can be isolated from conjunctival swabs. Topical antimicrobial treatment is usually effective for controlling eye disease, although it may fail in 10–30% of cases. Systemic therapy is preferred because the nasopharynx, rectum, and vagina may also be colonized and other forms of disease may develop, such as infant pneumonia syndrome. Inclusion conjunctivitis is less common in adults than in children and is usually associated with concomitant genital tract disease.

Genital Tract Infections

Clinical spectrum resembles that of *N. gonorrhoeae*

The clinical spectrum of sexually transmitted infections with *C. trachomatis* is similar to that of *Neisseria gonorrhoeae*. *Chlamydia trachomatis* can cause urethritis and epididymitis in men and cervicitis, salpingitis, and urethral syndrome in women. In addition, three serotypes of *C. trachomatis* cause the venereal disease lymphogranuloma venereum. *Chlamydia trachomatis* genital tract infections, like those caused by *N. gonorrhoeae*, are most prevalent in young adults, in those from lower socioeconomic groups, and in those with multiple sex partners.

Common cause of nongonococcal urethritis in men

Chlamydia trachomatis has been shown to cause about 40% of all cases of nongonococcal urethritis in men in industrialized societies. Approximately one-third to one-half of male sexual contacts of women with *C. trachomatis* cervicitis will develop nongonococcal urethritis after an incubation period of 2–6 weeks.

Cervicitis, salpingitis, and pelvic inflammatory disease in women

In women, *C. trachomatis* has been shown to cause both lower and upper genital tract infections. Infections of the uterine cervix are common and may be asymptomatic. Symptomatic infections present as mucopurulent cervicitis. Acute salpingitis and pelvic inflammatory disease can result from ascending infections. The organism has been isolated from 3 to 10% of women consulting private gynecologists for prenatal examinations.

Conjunctivitis in infants of infected mothers
Infant pneumonia syndrome

Approximately one-half of all infants born to mothers excreting *C. trachomatis* during labor will develop chlamydial diseases during the first year of life. Most will develop inclusion conjunctivitis, but 5–10% of them will develop infant pneumonia syndrome. *Chlamydia trachomatis* accounts for about one-third to one-half of all cases of interstitial pneumonia in infants. The illness usually develops between 6 weeks and 6 months of age and has a gradual onset. The child is usually afebrile, but develops difficulty in feeding, a characteristic staccato (pertussislike) cough, and shortness of breath. Radiography of the chest shows diffuse, bilateral interstitial infiltrates. Laboratory studies usually show a normal white blood cell count, but a slight increase in eosinophils. The disease is rarely fatal, but can be associated with prolonged illness and the need for hospitalization. Treatment with erythromycin or sulfonamides is currently recommended.

Three serotypes cause lymphogranuloma venereum

Lymphogranuloma venereum is a distinct venereal disease caused by three serotypes of *C. trachomatis* that are not associated with other chlamydial infections. It is one of the five "classic" sexually transmitted diseases (Chapter 70) and occurs principally in South America and Africa. The disease is uncommon in North America, but outbreaks have occurred. Lymphogranuloma venereum is one of the few diseases caused by *C. trachomatis* that produces both local and systemic manifestations.

More detailed consideration of all genital tract infections by *C. trachomatis* is given in Chapter 70.

Laboratory Diagnosis

Isolation of *Chlamydia*

Isolation of *C. trachomatis* is the best method of diagnosis. It is usually achieved by culture using idoxuridine- or cycloheximide-treated McCoy cells. Cell cultures are inoculated with samples obtained from potentially infectious areas such as the conjunctiva, sputum, urethra, or cervix. After incubation, the cells are treated with fluorescein-labeled monoclonal antibodies to detect the chlamydia. Staining with iodine demonstrates intracytoplasmic inclusions that contain glycogen, but is less sensitive than

Detection of *Chlamydia* by immunofluorescence

immunofluorescence. Procedures are now available for the direct detection of elementary body antigens in clinical specimens using monoclonal antibodies. These are nearly as sensitive as cell cultures in the case of symptomatic patients.

Serodiagnosis

Serodiagnostic methods are useful in diagnosis of acute infection. Detection of IgM antibodies against *C. trachomatis* is particularly helpful in cases of infant pneumonitis. Because of past infections, single high titers of IgG antibodies in sexually active persons cannot be considered indicative of recent *C. trachomatis* infection, and a rising antibody titer must be demonstrated.

Treatment

Effective antimicrobics

Strains of *C. trachomatis* are sensitive to many antimicrobics, of which those most commonly used are the tetracyclines, erythromycin, the sulfonamides, and rifampin. Erythromycin is the preferred systemic agent for pregnant women and infants because of the tooth staining that may result from tetracycline therapy (Chapter 13). Some of the quinolone antimicrobics are also effective, although their reliability is less than that of tetracycline.

Prevention

At present no effective vaccine is available for the prevention of *C. trachomatis* infection.

Use of eyedrops at birth to prevent chlamydial conjunctivitis

Instillation of tetracycline, erythromycin, or chloramphenicol eyedrops at birth decreases the subsequent development of chlamydial conjunctivitis. They are now used increasingly in routine conjunctival prophylaxis for newborns in areas of high prevalence, and they are also effective against most strains of *N. gonorrhoeae* for which prophylaxis is required by law. Silver nitrate eyedrops, which are effective in preventing gonococcal eye infections, are not active against *C. trachomatis*. No conjunctival prophylaxis will prevent colonization of the nasopharynx with *C. trachomatis* or the possible later development of infant pneumonia syndrome.

Additional Reading

Alexander, E.R., and Harrison, H.R. 1983. Role of *Chlamydia trachomatis* in perinatal infections. *Rev. Infect. Dis.* 5:713–719. A well-documented review of the role of *C. trachomatis* in perinatal morbidity.

Barron, A.L., Ed. 1989. *Microbiology of Chlamydia.* Boca Raton, Fla.: CRC Press. An up-to-date compendium on the microbiology of *Chlamydia* with excellent illustrations and fully referenced.

Cook, J.A., and Taylor, H.R., Eds. 1985. Infectious causes of blindness: trachoma and onchocerchiasis. *Rev. Infect. Dis.* 7:711–786. Papers in this review cover all aspects of *C. trachomatis* infection.

Grayston, J.T. 1989. *Chlamydia pneumoniae,* strain TWAR. *Chest* 95:664–669. A comprehensive review of the present status of knowledge about this organism by one of its discoverers.

Mardh, P-A., Holmes, K.K., Piot, P., et al. 1982. *Clamydia Infections.* New York: Elsevier Biomedical Press. An excellent monograph on *C. trachomatis* infections, with emphasis on sexually transmitted and neonatal diseases.

Reeve, R., Ed. 1989. *Chlamydial Infections.* Berlin/New York: Springer-Verlag.

A summary of up-to-date information by leaders in the field, with particular emphasis on *C. trachomatis.*

Thompson, S.E., and Washington, A.E. 1983. Epidemiology of sexually transmitted *C. trachomatis* infections. *Epidemiol. Rev.* 5:96–123. A useful detailed overview of the *Chlamydia* problem.

30
Rickettsia *and* Coxiella

Lawrence Corey

Obligate intracellular parasites

Rickettsia and *Coxiella* are members of the family Rickettsiaceae. They are obligate intracellular bacteria. They multiply by binary fission and possess nucleoids, ribosomes, and enzymes of the Krebs cycle. Most rickettsiae have animal reservoirs and are spread by insect vectors, which are prominent components of their life cycles. Pathogenic species are classified into two major groups based on their disease syndromes and vectors. One is the spotted fever group, which includes *Rickettsia rickettsii,* the etiologic agent of Rocky Mountain spotted fever; the other is the typhus group, which includes *Rickettsia prowazekii,* the cause of classic epidemic typhus. The only species of *Coxiella, C. burnetii,* causes a distinct systemic disease, Q fever. Its natural habitat is in wild animals and livestock. Spread to humans is usually by inhalation of dust from animal products.

Spotted fever and typhus groups of *Rickettsia*

RICKETTSIA

Morphology

Small, Gram-negative coccobacilli

Giemsa stain shows *Rickettsia* in infected cells

Richettsiae are small bacteria that appear as single coccobacilli or, more commonly, as diplobacilli with tapered ends. The latter usually show a transverse septum between the two bacilli, reflecting division by binary fission. They commonly measure no more than 0.3–0.5 μm. The Gram reaction is negative, but rickettsiae take the usual bacterial stains poorly or not at all. Tissue stains such as Giemsa demonstrate them more clearly, particularly in infected cells. The ultrastructural morphology, which is similar to that of other Gram-negative bacteria, includes a Gram-negative-type cell envelope, ribosomes, and a nuclear body. Chemically, the cell wall contains lipopolysaccharide in the outer membrane and peptidoglycan.

Growth and Metabolism

Growth in cytoplasm

Rickettsiae grow mainly in the cytoplasm of eukaryotic cells, an environment to which they are highly adapted. With one exception, they can be isolated and cultivated in the laboratory using living host cells such as cell

479

Slow growth compared to most bacteria

cultures or embryonated eggs. Their estimated generation time is much longer than that of bacteria such as *Escherichia coli,* but more rapid than that of *Mycobacterium tuberculosis.* Infection of the host cell begins by induction of an endocytic process analogous to phagocytosis, but which requires expenditure of energy by the rickettsiae. The organisms then escape the phagosome or endocytic vacuole to enter the cytoplasm, possibly by elaboration of a phospholipase. Intracytoplasmic growth eventually produces lysis of the cell and infection of another generation of host cells.

Induced phagocytosis

Exogenous cofactors and ATP required

The obligate intracellular parasitism of rickettsiae has several interesting features. Failure to survive outside the cell is apparently related to requirements for nucleotide cofactors (coenzyme A, nicotinamide adenine dinucleotide) and adenosine triphosphate (ATP). In the rickettsia-infected cytoplasm, host cell ATP is exchanged for rickettsial adenosine diphosphate by an exchange transport system similar to that found in mitochondria.

Rapidly loses infectivity outside host cell

Outside the host cell, rickettsiae not only cease metabolic activity, but leak protein, nucleic acids, and essential small molecules. This instability leads to rapid loss of infectivity, because the penetration of another cell requires energy. In summary, rickettsiae have the metabolic capabilities of other bacteria, but must borrow some essential elements from host cells for adequate growth, and thus do not survive well in the environment.

Pathogenesis of Infection

Infection of vascular endothelium

Most rickettsial infections of humans result in clinical illness. Rickettsiae infect the vascular endothelium, usually after the bite of an infected arthropod vector. The organisms multiply within these cells and become disseminated widely throughout the vascular system. Clinically the infection is manifested by fever and headache with widespread focal lesions, the most prominent of which is a rash. In the infected sites there is focal hyperplasia of the infected endothelial cells, inflammation, and thrombosis, leading to obstruction of small blood vessels and capillary leakage. An endotoxinlike shock has been demonstrated in animals on injection of whole rickettsial cells, but the nature and role of any toxin in human disease are unknown.

Vascular inflammation and obstruction

Possible role of endotoxin

Specific Diagnosis of Disease

Weil–Felix serodiagnostic test

In the early 1900s, it was observed that serum from patients with typhus caused agglutination of certain strains of *Proteus vulgaris.* This finding was developed into a serologic testing scheme called the *Weil-Felix test* in which three *Proteus* strains, OX-19, OX-2, and OX-K, have been used as antigens to detect rickettsial antibody (Table 30.1). Recently, more specific serologic tests such as complement fixation have been developed using type-specific rickettsial antigens. Isolation of rickettsiae in eggs or cell cultures is generally attempted only in reference centers, because the risk of laboratory infection requires special facilities and personnel experienced in handling the organisms.

Hazards of in vitro cultivation

Spotted Fever Group

Many tick-borne rickettsioses in different parts of world

A number of spotted fever rickettsioses are found in various parts of the world; the name often reveals the locale (for example, South African tick-bite fever and Queensland tick fever). They are caused by rickettsial species serologically related to, but distinct from, *R. rickettsii,* the cause of

Table 30.1 Examples of Pathogenic Rickettsiae

Disease	Organism	Commonest Geographic Distribution	Zoonotic Cycle		Weil–Felix Serology		
			Vector	Reservoir	OX-19	OX-2	OX-K
Spotted fever group							
Rocky Mountain spotted fever	*Rickettsia rickettsii*	North and South America	Tick	Rodents Dogs	+	+	−
Rickettsialpox	*Rickettsia akari*	United States, Soviet Union, Korea, Africa	Mite	Mouse	−	−	−
Typhus group							
Epidemic	*Rickettsia prowazekii*	Africa, Asia, South America	Body louse	Humans[a]	+	+/−	−
Brill's	*Rickettsia prowazekii*	Worldwide[b]	None[c]	Humans	+/−	−	−
Murine	*Rickettsia typhi*	Worldwide (pockets)	Flea	Rodents	+	+/−	−
Scrub	*Rickettsia tsutsugamushi*	South Pacific, Asia	Mite	Rodents	−	−	+
Trench fever	*Rickettsia quintana*[d] (*Rochalimaea quintana*)	Europe, Africa, Asia	Body louse	Humans	−	−	−

[a] An apparently identical organism has been isolated from flying squirrels in the United States.
[b] Related to immigration.
[c] Relapsing form of epidemic typhus.
[d] Closely related to *Rickettsia*, but has been grown in artificial culture.

the most important rickettsial disease in North America, Rocky Mountain spotted fever. This disease will be used to typify the spotted fevers; another less severe illness that occurs in North America, rickettsialpox, will also be discussed.

Rocky Mountain Spotted Fever

Rocky Mountain spotted fever is a common infection in the United States, with more than 1100 cases reported each year. In the past decade, the number of cases has been increasing, probably because of increased recreational exposure to areas where infected ticks exist. The disease has a significant mortality (7%), although most patients recover spontaneously.

Natural infection of ticks with *R. rickettsii*

Habitat. *Rickettsia rickettsii* is primarily a parasite of ticks. In the western United States, the wood tick (*Dermacentor andersoni*) is the primary vector. In the East the dog tick (*Dermacentor variabilis*) and in the Southwest the Lone Star tick (*Amblyomma americanum*) are the natural carriers and vectors of the disease. As *R. rickettsii* does not kill its arthropod host, the organism is passed through unending generations of ticks by transovarial spread. Rickettsiae acquired transovarially are thus present in the larval, nymph, and adult stages of development. The larval and nymph stages require a blood meal from a small mammal to proceed to the next stage. Adult females require a blood meal to lay eggs. Infected adult ticks have been shown to survive for as long as 4 years without feeding.

Transovarial spread

Infected ticks can survive for years without feeding

Epidemiology. The geographic distribution of Rocky Mountain spotted fever is illustrated in Figure 30.1. It has been found in all states except Maine, Alaska, and Hawaii. The highest attack rates are in the mid-Atlantic states, the Carolinas, and the Virginias. More than two-thirds of cases are in children less than 15 years of age. The illness is generally seen between April and September because of increased exposure to ticks. A history of tick bite can be elicited in approximately 70% of cases.

Most cases in children

Disease. The incubation period between the tick bite and the onset of illness is usually 2–6 days, but may be as long as 2 weeks. Fever, headache, rash, toxicity, mental confusion, and myalgia are the major clinical features. The rash is the most characteristic feature of the illness. It usually develops on the second or third day of illness as small erythematous macules that rapidly become petechial. The lesions appear initially on the wrists and ankles, then spread up the extremities to the trunk in a few hours. A diagnostic feature of Rocky Mountain spotted fever is the frequent appearance of the rash on the palms and soles, a finding not usually seen in the maculopapular eruptions associated with viral infections. Muscle tenderness, especially in the gastrocnemius, is characteristic and may be extreme. If untreated, or in occasional cases despite therapy, complications such as disseminated intravascular coagulation, thrombocytopenia, encephalitis, vascular collapse, and renal and/or heart failure may ensue.

Incubation period 2–6 days after tick bite

Fever, headache, and rash

Spread of rash from extremities to trunk

Complications

Rickettsial multiplication in endothelial cells causes vasculitis

The primary pathologic lesion is a vasculitis in which rickettsiae multiply in the endothelial cell lining of the small blood vessels. Focal areas of endothelial proliferation and perivascular infiltration lead to thrombosis and leakage of red blood cells into the surrounding tissues, accounting for the rash and petechial lesions; however, vascular lesions occur throughout the body, thus producing the systemic manifestations of the disease. They are obviously most apparent in skin, but most serious in the adrenal glands.

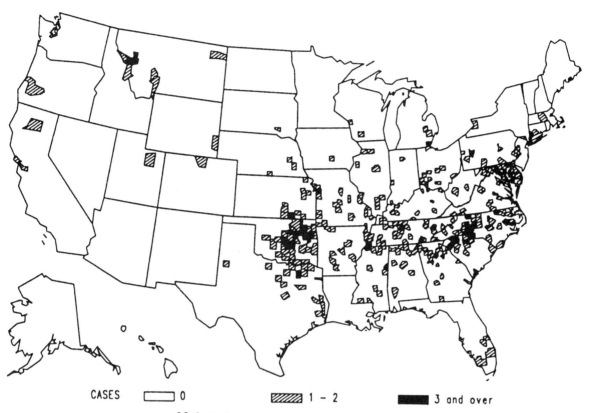

CASES [ ] 0   [////] 1 − 2   [████] 3 and over

30-1 Rocky Mountain spotted fever. Number of cases reported by county in the United States, 1987. (*Reproduced from Summary of notifiable diseases. United States 1987, Centers for Disease Control, U.S. Department of Health and Human Services.*)

Diagnosis and therapy based on clinical manifestations

Diagnosis. No laboratory test is generally available to establish the diagnosis of Rocky Mountain spotted fever early in the course of illness. Specific therapy must be started based solely on clinical signs, symptoms, and epidemiologic considerations. *Rickettsia rickettsii* may be identified by immunofluorescent staining of skin biopsy specimens, but this test is only undertaken in specialized laboratories. Complement fixation and immunofluorescent serologic tests are helpful in confirming the diagnosis, but the patient often does not develop high titers of antibody until late in the course of illness. A fourfold rise in antibody titer between acute and convalescent serum establishes the diagnosis. Rising titers to *Proteus* OX-19 or OX-2 or a single titer of 1:160 or greater in a patient with symptoms similar to Rocky Mountain spotted fever are presumptive evidence of infection. Low titers of antibody to these organisms (1:20 to 1:80) may be found in healthy individuals.

Serodiagnosis: rising titers against OX-19, OX-2, and rickettsial antigens

Importance of treatment during first week

Tetracycline or chloramphenicol

Therapy. Appropriate antibiotic therapy is highly effective if given during the first week of illness. If delayed into the second week or when pathologic processes such as diffuse intravascular coagulation are present, therapy becomes progressively less effective. The antibiotics of choice are tetracycline and chloramphenicol. Seriously ill patients and children less than 8 years of age are usually given chloramphenicol. Sulfonamides may enhance the disease process and are thus contraindicated. Before specific therapy became available, the mortality of Rocky Mountain spotted fever was approximately 25%. Treatment has reduced this figure to 5–7%. Death results primarily in patients in whom diagnosis and therapy are delayed into the second week of illness.

Prevention.   The major measure for prevention of Rocky Mountain spotted fever is the avoidance or reduction of tick contact. Frequent deticking in tick-infested areas is important, because ticks generally must feed for 4–6 hr before they can transmit the disease. Tick surveys in the Carolinas have shown infection in about 5% of samples. Killed vaccines prepared from infected ticks, embryonated eggs, and cell cultures have been developed, but, at present, none is licensed for clinical use.

Need for frequent deticking

Rickettsialpox

Benign disease transmitted by rodent mites

Rickettsialpox was first recognized in New York City in 1946. It is a benign rickettsial illness caused by *Rickettsia akari* and transmitted by a rodent mite. Distinguishing features of the disease include an eschar at the site of the bite, vesicular rash, and the absence of Weil–Felix agglutinins. The house mouse and other semidomestic rodents are the primary reservoir. Humans acquire infection when the mite seeks an alternative host.

Local eschar followed by fever and rash

Rickettsialpox is a biphasic illness. The first phase is the local lesion at the bite, which starts as a papulovesicle and develops into a black eschar over 3–5 days. Fever and constitutional symptoms appear as the organism disseminates. The second phase of the disease is a diffuse rash distributed randomly in the body, which, like the local lesion, becomes papulovesicular and develops into eschars. Rickettsialpox is self-limiting after 1 week, and no deaths have been reported. Tetracycline therapy shortens the course to 1–2 days.

Tetracycline therapy

Typhus Group

Primary Louse-Borne Typhus Fever

Severe louse-borne disease due to R. prowazekii

Primary louse-borne typhus fever is an acute, infectious disease caused by *R. prowazekii* that is transmitted to humans by the body louse. Historically, it has appeared during periods of war, famine, and social upheaval, which create conditions favorable to human body lice (crowding, infrequent bathing, and the like). The last North American epidemic was in Philadelphia in 1893; however, endemic typhus foci persist in Eastern Europe, Asia, Africa, and South America. During both world wars, louse-borne typhus infected millions and was particularly devastating in concentration camps. Although primarily a human disease, identical organisms have been recovered from flying squirrels and their ectoparasites in the southeastern United States, and a few human cases of sylvatic typhus have occurred in these areas.

Endemic foci

Cycle of infection: not passed transovarially in lice

The chain of epidemic typhus infection starts with *R. prowazekii* circulating in a patient's blood during an acute febrile infection. The human body louse becomes infected during one of its frequent blood meals, and, after 5–10 days of incubation, large numbers of rickettsiae appear in its feces. As the louse defecates while it feeds, the organisms can be rubbed into the louse-bite wounds when the host scratches the site. Dried louse feces are also infectious through the mucous membranes of the eye or respiratory tract. The louse dies of its infection in 1–3 weeks, and the rickettsiae are not transmitted transovarially.

Fever, headache, and rash

Fever, headache, and rash begin 1–2 weeks after the bite. A maculopapular rash appears first on the trunk, then spreads centripetally to the extremities, a pattern opposite to that of Rocky Mountain spotted fever. Headache, malaise, and myalgia are prominent components of the illness. Complications include myocarditis and central nervous system dysfunction. In untreated disease, the fatality rate increases with age from 10% to as high as 60%. The Weil–Felix reaction is positive with *Proteus* OX-19 and less commonly with OX-2 (both are positive in Rocky Mountain spotted fever). As with the spotted fever group, therapy with tetracycline or chloramphenicol is effective. Louse control is the best means of prevention and is particularly important in controlling epidemics. A killed vaccine grown in embryonated eggs is used only in persons at high occupational risk or risk of exposure during epidemics.

Complications; high mortality rate

Serodiagnosis; OX-19 positive

Treatment and prevention; louse control

Relapse of typhus after many years

Brill's Disease.   Brill's disease is a relapse or recrudescence of louse-borne typhus that occurs years after the primary attack. It is seen primarily in immigrants to other countries from Eastern Europe, whose initial infection often occurred during World War II. Factors triggering the relapse are unknown, but may involve fading immunity to rickettsiae that have remained dormant in reticuloendothelial cells. Because of partial immunity, the recrudescent infection is milder, shorter, and less debilitating than primary typhus. Titers to *Proteus* OX-19 are absent or low. Specific antibodies are of the immunoglobulin G class, in contrast to typhus, which shows a primary immune response predominantly with immunoglobulin M antibodies. Prolonged survival of *R. prowazekii* in the human host is important in the endemic maintenance of the disease.

Disease less severe than epidemic typhus

Importance in endemic maintenance of typhus

Murine Typhus

Transmitted by fleas from rat reservoir of *T. typhi*

Murine typhus is caused by *Rickettsia typhi* and transmitted to humans by the rat flea (*Xenopsylla cheopis*). Human illness is incidental to the natural transmission of the disease among urban rodents, which serve as the reservoir. Only 40–60 cases of murine typhus are reported in the United States each year. These occur predominantly in the southeastern and Gulf states, especially Texas.

The pathogenesis and transmission are similar to that of louse-borne typhus. The flea defecates when it takes a blood meal, and the infected feces gain access through the bite wound. After an incubation period of 1–2 weeks, illness begins with headache, myalgia, and fever. The rash is maculopapular, starting on the trunk and then spreading to the extremities in a manner similar to typhus. Serologically, the Weil–Felix reaction is similar in louse-borne and murine typhus. Because of antigens shared by *R. typhi* and *R. prowazekii,* even the complement fixation test may not separate the two diseases. In the untreated patient, fever may last 12–14 days. With tetracycline or chloramphenicol therapy, the course is reduced to 2–3 days. Mortality and complications are rare.

Resembles typhus, but less severe

R. typhi shares antigens with *R. prowazekii*

Scrub Typhus

R. tsutsugamushi transmitted from natural infection of mites

Scrub typhus is found in the Southwest Pacific, Southeast Asia, and Japan. The causative organism is *Rickettsia tsutsugamushi*. Mites that infest rodents are the reservoir and vectors, transmitting the rickettsiae to their own progeny via infected ova. Humans pick up the mites as they pass by low trees or brush. The mite larvae (chiggers) deposit rickettsiae as they feed.

Local eschar

Fever, headache, and rash

Hepatosplenomegaly

OX-K agglutinins

The typical initial lesion, a necrotic eschar at the site of the bite on the extremities, develops in only 50–80% of cases. Fever increases slowly over the first week, sometimes reaching 40.5°C. Later, headache, rash, and generalized lymphadenopathy follow. The maculopapular rash, which appears after about 5 days, is more evanescent than that seen with louse-borne or murine typhus. Hepatosplenomegaly and conjunctivitis may also appear. The diagnosis is primarily clinical, because the only responses by the Weil–Felix test are to OX-K, and titers are elevated in only one-half of cases. Differentiation from dengue, leptospirosis, malaria, or typhoid fever may be difficult. Both chloramphenicol and tetracycline constitute effective therapy.

COXIELLA

C. burnetii infection

Multiplies in phagolysosome

Resistant to drying

Coxiella burnetii is the cause of Q fever. It is a strict intracellular parasite, has similar morphological features to rickettsiae, but differs in G + C content and in many other regards from rickettsiae. *Coxiella burnetii* is taken into host cells by a phagocytic process that does not involve expenditure of energy by the parasite. It remains in the phagosome and multiplies extensively after lysosomal fusion, because its metabolism is optimal at low pH and it resists lysosomal enzymes. Vesicles containing *Coxiella* can occupy a large part of the cell before it ruptures and releases them. *Coxiella burnetii* is much more resistant to drying and other conditions outside the host cell than are rickettsiae, which partially accounts for the differences in modes of transmission. *Coxiella* infection does not lead to production of any of the Weil–Felix antibodies.

Q Fever

Zoonosis transmitted to humans by inhalation
Infected livestock

Infection of placental tissue

Prolonged viability in dust

Occupational exposure

Infection can result from ingestion

Systemic infection without rash

Lung involvement and hepatosplenomegaly

Q fever is transmitted from animals to humans by inhalation rather than by arthropod bite.

It is primarily a zoonosis, affecting cattle, sheep, goats, rodents, and marsupials. Distribution is worldwide. In domestic livestock, the infection is usually inapparent, but as many as 50–75% of animals in a herd may be infected in some areas. *Coxiella burnetii* grows particularly well in placental tissue, where it often attains levels of 10^9 organisms per gram of tissue. At the time of birth, the infected tissues contaminate the ground, where the organisms survive within dry dust particles for months. At 40°C, viability is retained for 1 or more years in dried fomites. This remarkable viability has suggested a sporogenic cycle in the organism, but this remains to be proved. The disease occurs sporadically among those who work with infected animals or their products. Epidemics of Q fever have occurred among workers in abattoirs in which infected animals are slaughtered, producing aerosols with massive contamination of employees. In textile plants, infection may occur among employees who break open bales of wool and do the preliminary washing and sorting. Infection in all of these circumstances is believed to result from inhalation. Infection can also occur from ingestion of contaminated milk or animal products. Temperatures now used for pasteurization are sufficient to kill *Coxiella*.

Q fever is a systemic infection that can occur with or without pneumonitis. The organism has a particular affinity for the reticuloendothelial tem. Little is known of the pathology, as fatal cases are rare. The disease usually begins 9–20 days after inhalation, with abrupt onset of fever, chills, and headache. There may be a mild, dry, hacking cough, and a patchy interstitial pneumonia. There is no typical rash. Hepatosplenomegaly is

Diagnosis and treatment

frequent, and abnormal results of tests of liver function are usual. Complications such as myocarditis, pericarditis, and endocarditis have been reported. The diagnosis is usually made by demonstrating high or rising titers of antibody to Q fever antigen by complement fixation, immunofluorescence methods, or enzyme-linked immunosorbent assay procedures. The organism can be grown in cell culture systems and experimental animals, but this is not normally used for routine diagnosis because of the considerable risk of laboratory infection with the organism. The disease responds to tetracyclines, and, when treated, death is uncommon. Experimental vaccines have been shown to be effective in those who are heavily exposed, but vaccines are not yet available commercially.

Additional Reading

Baca, O.G., and Paretsky, D. 1983. Q fever and *Coxiella burnetii:* A model for host-parasite interactions. *Microbiol. Rev.* 47:127–149. A comprehensive review of this organism and of the epidemiology, pathogenesis, and immunology of the disease that it causes.

Bernard, K.W., Helmick, C.G., and Kaplan, J.E., et al. 1982. Surveillance of Rocky Mountain spotted fever in the United States. 1978–1980. *J. Infect. Dis.* 146:297–299. The epidemiology of Rocky Mountain spotted fever is reviewed.

Hattwick, MA.W., Retailliau, H., and O'Brien, R.J., et al. 1978. Fatal Rocky Mountain spotted fever. *J. Am. Med. Assoc.* 240:1499–1503. Fatal results of delay in diagnosis and the rapid clinical course are reviewed.

McDade, J.E., and Newhouse, V.F. 1986. Natural history of *Rickettsia rickettsii. Annu. Rev. Microbiol.* 40:287–309. A review of the basic biology, distribution, and transmission of *R. rickettsii.*

Sawyer, L.A., Fishbein, D.B., and McDade, J.E. 1987. Q fever: Current concepts. *Rev. Infect. Dis.* 9:935–945. This paper reviews the clinical presentation, epidemiology, diagnosis, and treatment of the disease. An excellent source of references.

Weiss, E. 1982. The biology of rickettsiae. *Annu. Rev. Microbiol.* 36:345–370. A very valuable review of the basic microbiology, pathogenesis, and immunity of these organisms.

31

Some Bacteria Causing Zoonotic Diseases

Kenneth J. Ryan

Many bacterial, rickettsial, and viral diseases are classified as *zoonoses*, because they are acquired by humans either directly or indirectly from animals. This chapter considers bacteria causing four zoonotic infections that are not discussed in other chapters. All four, *Brucella*, *Yersinia pestis*, *Francisella tularensis*, and *Pasteurella multocida*, are Gram-negative bacilli that are primarily animal pathogens. The diseases that they cause, brucellosis, plague, tularemia, and pasteurellosis, are now rare in humans and develop only after unique animal contact. The full range of zoonoses considered in this and other chapters is shown in the appendix to this chapter.

Brucella and Brucellosis

Brucellosis (sometimes known as *undulant fever* or *Malta fever*) is a genitourinary infection of sheep, cattle, pigs, and other animals caused by several species of *Brucella*. Three are of importance in human medicine: *Brucella abortus*, *Brucella melitensis*, and *Brucella suis*. Humans become infected directly by occupational contact with these animals (farmers, slaughterhouse workers, veterinarians) or indirectly by consumption of contaminated animal products such as milk. In humans, the reticuloendothelial system is the primary target of infection, producing a prolonged febrile systemic illness.

Three species important in human disease

Microbiology

Gram-negative coccobacilli

Growth requirements

Slow growth

Brucella species are small, coccobacillary, Gram-negative rods that resemble *Haemophilus* and *Bordetella* morphologically (Chapter 23). They are non-motile, non-acid fast, and non-spore forming. Growth requires an aerobic environment and enriched media such as blood agar. One species, *B. abortus*, requires enrichment of the atmosphere to 5–10% carbon dioxide. Colonies are only visible on solid media after 2–3 days of incubation,

489

Table 31.1 Characteristic Features of *Brucella* Species

Characteristic	B. abortis	B. melitensis	B. suis
Carbon dioxide requirement	+	−	−
Hydrogen sulfide production	+	−	±
Growth in presence of			
Thionin[a]	−	+	+
Basic fuchsin[a]	+	+	−

[a] Concentration of 1:50,000 in nutrient medium.

and broth cultures may require more time depending on the size of the inoculum.

S to R variation

The antigenic structure of *Brucella* is complex. A smooth (S) even colony form, generally present on primary isolation, is associated with the presence of a small capsule and virulence. Rough (R) colonies have an uneven surface and tend to replace the S form on repeated subculture. They are composed of mutants that have lost their capsules and most of their virulence. Surface protein-lipopolysaccharide surface antigens designated *A* (abortus) and *M* (melitensis) are present in different amounts in all three species; A predominates in *B. abortus* and M in *B. melitensis*.

Protein-lipopolysaccharide A and M surface antigens

Species differentiation

Taxonomically, *Brucella* species are not closely related to any other genus, but are homogeneous as judged by analysis of nucleic acid base ratios and DNA homology. All species produce catalase, oxidase, and urease, but do not ferment carbohydrates. They are differentiated by the relative predominance of A and M antigens, CO_2 requirements for growth, hydrogen sulfide production, and the ability of particular concentrations of the dyes thionin and basic fuchsin to inhibit their growth (Table 31.1).

Epidemiology

Abortion in cattle, goats, and hogs

Brucellosis is an important cause of abortion, sterility, and decreased milk production in cattle, goats, and hogs. It is spread among animals by direct contact with infected tissues and ingestion of contaminated feed and causes chronic infection of the mammary glands, uterus, placenta, seminal vesicles, and epididymis. Although the associations are not absolute, each species is linked to a different animal: *B. abortus* tends to infect cattle, *B. melitensis*, goats, and *B. suis*, hogs.

Infection occupational and through unpasteurized dairy products

Humans acquire the infection by occupational exposure or consumption of unpasteurized dairy products. The organisms may gain access through cuts in the skin, contact with mucous membranes, inhalation, or ingestion. In the United States, the number of cases has dropped steadily from a maximum of more than 6000 per year in the 1940s to the current level of 150–200 per year. Of these cases, 50–60% are in abattoir employees, government meat inspectors, veterinarians, and others who handle livestock or meat products. Consumption of unpasteurized dairy products, which accounts for 8–10% of infections, is the leading source in persons who have no connection with the meat processing or livestock industries. Some recent cases of this type have been associated with "health" foods. In the United States, the distribution of human cases of brucellosis includes virtually every state, but is concentrated in those with large livestock industries (Iowa, Virginia, and Texas) or proximity to Mexico. A recent outbreak of *B. melitensis* in Texas was traced to unpasteurized goat cheese brought in from Mexico.

Pathogenesis and Immunity

Multiplication in macrophages

Spread to reticuloendothelial system

Activated macrophages inhibit growth

Immunity exclusively cell mediated

Erythritol in animal placentas stimulates growth

After penetration of the skin or mucous membranes, the organisms are carried within polymorphonuclear leukocytes through the lymph to the systemic circulation by way of the regional lymph nodes and the thoracic duct. Virulent *Brucella* can enter and multiply in macrophages in the liver sinusoids, spleen, bone marrow, and other components of the reticuloendothelial system. Smooth (virulent) *Brucella* strains possess a currently unknown virulence factor that allows some growth despite local macrophage activation and proliferation. The factors that ultimately control infection are complex, although it appears that activated macrophages from infected animals kill virulent organisms more readily than those activated by other stimuli. Thus, intracellular events in the monocyte determine the outcome of a *Brucella* infection, and control is dependent on active T-cell response. Antibodies to *Brucella* antigens can be detected in the sera of patients by a variety of methods, but there is no evidence that they alter the natural history of disease or confer immunity. Exotoxins, capsules, or antiphagocytic components are apparently not involved in virulence. In cows, sheep, pigs, and goats, erythritol, a four-carbon alcohol present in chorionic tissue, markedly stimulates growth of *Brucella*. This stimulation probably accounts for the tendency of the organism to locate in these sites. The human placenta does not contain erythritol.

Granulomas

Recurrent bacteremia

If not controlled locally, infection progresses with the formation of small granulomas in the reticuloendothelial sites of bacterial multiplication and with release of bacteria back into the systemic circulation. These recurrent bacteremic episodes are largely responsible for the recurrent chills and fever of the clinical illness. The entire cycle resembles that of another intracellular pathogen, *Salmonella typhi*, and its disease, typhoid fever (Chapter 20).

Clinical Illness

Night sweats

Periodic fever

Chronic illness and weight loss

Splenomegaly

Localized infection

Brucellosis starts with malaise, chills, and fever 7–21 days after infection. Drenching sweats in the late afternoon or evening are common, as well as temperatures in the range of 39.4–40°C. The pattern of periodic nocturnal fever (undulant fever) typically continues for weeks, months, or even 1–2 years, and the patient becomes chronically ill with associated body aches, headache, and anorexia. Weight loss of up to 20 kg may occur during prolonged illness. Despite these dramatic effects, physical findings and localizing signs are few. Less than 25% of patients show detectable enlargement of the reticuloendothelial organs, the primary site of infection. Of such findings, splenomegaly is most common, followed by lymphadenopathy and hepatomegaly. Occasionally, localized infection develops in the lung, bone, brain, heart, or genitourinary system. These cases usually lack the pronounced systemic symptoms of the typical illness.

Diagnosis

Cultural diagnosis

Definitive diagnosis requires isolation of *Brucella* from the blood or from biopsy specimens of the liver, bone marrow, or lymph nodes. Supplementation with CO_2 is needed for growth of *B. abortus*. The slow growth of some strains requires prolonged incubation of culture media to achieve isolation. Blood cultures in particular may require 2–4 weeks for growth, although most are positive in 2–5 days.

The diagnosis is often made serologically, but is subject to the same

Agglutinins ≥ 1:640

interpretive constraints as all serologic tests. Antibodies that agglutinate suspensions of heat-killed organisms typically reach titers of 1:640 or more in acute disease. Lower titers may reflect previous disease or cross-reacting antibodies. Titers return to the normal range within a year after successful therapy.

Treatment and Prevention

Tetracycline; aminoglycoside

Tetracycline is the primary antimicrobic for the treatment of brucellosis. In seriously ill patients, streptomycin or gentamicin may be added. The therapeutic response is not rapid; 2–7 days may pass before patients become afebrile. Up to 10% of cases have relapses in the first 3 months after therapy. Prevention is primarily by measures to minimize occupational exposure and by the pasteurization of dairy products. Control of brucellosis in animals involves using a combination of immunization with an attenuated strain of *B. abortus* and eradication of infected stock. No human vaccine is in use.

Pasteurization
Control in cattle

Yersinia pestis and Plague

Plague is an infection of rodents and small mammals caused by *Y. pestis*. It is transmitted to humans by the bite of infected fleas. The disease has two major cycles, urban and sylvatic, and two major clinical forms, bubonic and pneumonic. The combined pathogenic and epidemiologic potential of *Y. pestis* makes it one of the most potent and feared pathogens known.

Microbiology

Yersinia pestis is a nonmotile, non–spore-forming, Gram-negative bacillus with a tendency toward pleomorphism and bipolar staining. It has recently been reclassified as a member of the Enterobacteriaceae. Its biology is discussed in Chapter 20 with that of the other members of the genus *Yersinia*.

Epidemiology

Black Death

The term plague is often used generically to describe any explosive pandemic disease with high mortality. Medically it refers only to infection caused by *Y. pestis*, and this application was justly earned, because *Y. pestis* was the cause of the most virulent epidemic plague of recorded human history, the Black Death of the Middle Ages. In the 14th century, the estimated population of Europe was 105 million; between 1346 and 1350, 25 million died of plague. Pandemics continued through the end of the 19th and the early 20th century despite elaborate quarantine measures developed in response to the obvious communicability of the disease. Yersin isolated the etiologic agent in China in 1894 and named it after his mentor, Pasteur. Until recently, *Y. pestis* was known as *Pasteurella pestis*.

The plagues of the Middle Ages are examples of the urban cycle involving rats and humans. The first step probably involves infection of rats from a sylvatic source. Under poor hygienic conditions and when food sources elsewhere are scarce, rat populations in cities increase, which facilitates rat-to-rat transmission of *Y. pestis* by the rat flea (*Xenopsylla cheopis*). These conditions also bring the primary rat reservoir into closer contact with humans. When the number of nonimmune rats is sufficient, epizootic plague develops among them with bacteremia and high mortality.

Urban plague

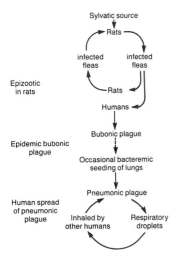

Sylvatic plague

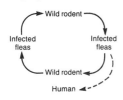

Most U.S. cases in California, Arizona, Utah, New Mexico, and Colorado

Increasing incidence in United States

Fleas feeding on the rat become infected, and the bacteria multiply in the intestinal tract of the flea to numbers that eventually block the proventriculus. As the infected rat dies, its hungry fleas seek a new host, which is usually another rat, but may be a human. The infected flea regurgitates *Y. pestis* from the proventriculus into the new bite wound. The probability of transmission to humans is thus greatest when both the rat population and rat mortality are high. The bite of the flea is the first event in the development of a case of bubonic plague, which, even if serious enough to kill the patient, is not normally contagious to other humans. Some patients with bubonic plague, however, develop a secondary pneumonia by bacteremia spread to the lungs. They can then transmit pneumonic plague directly to others by droplet spread. It is not hard to understand how rapid spread proceeds in conjunction with crowded unsanitary conditions and continued flea-to-human transmission. An urban plague epidemic is vividly described in Albert Camus' novel *The Plague*.

Although urban plague epidemics have been essentially eliminated by rat control and other public health measures, a sylvatic transmission cycle persists in many parts of the world, including North America. This cycle involves nonurban mammals such as prairie dogs, deer mice, rabbits, and wood rats. Transmission between them is accomplished by fleas. Coyotes or wolves may be infected by the same fleas or by ingestion of infected rodents. By their nature, these animals rarely come in contact with humans; when they do, however, the infected fleas they carry can transmit *Y. pestis*. The most common circumstance is a child exploring the outdoors who comes across a dead or dying prairie dog and pokes, carries, or touches it long enough to be bitten by the fleas leaving the animal. The result is a sporadic case of bubonic plague, which occasionally becomes pneumonic.

Sylvatic plague exists in most continents, is common in Southeast Asia, but is not found in Western Europe or Australasia. In the United States, the primary enzootic areas are the semiarid plains of the western states. Infected animals and fleas have been detected from the Mexican border to the eastern half of Washington.

Before 1965, human plague was a sporadic disease in the United States with zero to five cases per year. Since then, the incidence has steadily risen to a high of 30 to 40 cases in the mid-1980s. The geographic focus of plague in the United States is in the "four corners" area where Arizona, New Mexico, Colorado, and Utah meet, but cases have occurred in California, West Texas, Idaho, and Montana.

Pathogenesis and Immunity

Multiplication in flea

Mechanism of virulence

Yersinia pestis multiplies in the infected flea and blocks the foregut. The flea then regurgitates organisms into the next bite wound it produces. The organisms reach the regional lymph nodes of the newly infected individual through the lymphatic vessels. At the temperature of the flea (about 20–25°C), the F1 capsular antigen and the VW antigenic complex responsible for resistance to phagocytosis (Chapter 20), are not synthesized, and plague bacilli engulfed by polymorphonuclear leukocytes are killed. However, those ingested by macrophages survive, produce these virulence determinants within the cell, and emerge fully armed and resistant to subsequent phagocytic killing. The virulence factors of *Yersinia* are considered in more detail in Chapter 20.

Bubo

In the regional nodes, *Y. pestis* multiplies rapidly and produces a hemorrhagic suppurative necrosis that results in a painful swelling known as a *bubo*. The components of the organism responsible for the necrosis and

Bacteremia

Necrotizing pneumonia

Cyanosis (Black Death)

extreme systemic toxicity remain unclear, although both endotoxin and exotoxins are produced. Further spread leads to bacteremia and seeding of the lungs, liver, spleen, and occasionally the meninges. Pulmonary spread produces a fatal necrotizing hemorrhagic pneumonia known as *pneumonic plague*. Progression of plague pneumonia is rapid and so extensive that a terminal cyanosis is typical. Recovery from bubonic plague appears to confer lasting immunity, but for obvious reasons the mechanisms have not been extensively studied by modern immunologic methods. Animal studies suggest that antibody against the F1 capsular antigen is protective by enhancing phagocytosis, but cell-mediated mechanisms are required for intracellular killing. Because *Y. pestis* is a facultative intracellular parasite, the latter mechanisms must be at least as important as antibody in determining plague immunity.

Clinical Illness

Bubonic plague mortality 50–75% in untreated cases

The incubation period for bubonic plague is 2–7 days after the flea bite. Onset is marked by fever and the painful bubo, usually in the groin (bubo, from the Greek *boubon*, groin) or, less often, in the axilla. Without treatment, 50–75% of patients progress to bacteremia and die in Gram-negative septic shock within hours or days after development of the bubo. About 5% of victims develop pneumonic plague with mucoid, then bloody sputum. Primary pneumonic plague has a shorter incubation period (2–3 days) and begins with only fever, malaise, and a feeling of tightness in the chest. Cough, production of sputum, dyspnea, and cyanosis develop later in the course. Death on the second or third day of illness is common, and survival is rare without specific therapy. The course of the plague is identical whether it is acquired from urban or sylvatic sources.

Pneumonic plague fatal if untreated

Diagnosis

Direct Gram and immunofluorescent staining

Culture

Gram smears of aspirates from the bubo typically reveal bipolar-staining Gram-negative bacilli. An immunofluorescence technique is available in reference laboratories for immediate precise identification. *Yersinia pestis* is readily isolated on the media used for other members of the Enterobacteriaceae (blood agar, MacConkey agar), although growth may require more than 24 hr of incubation. The appropriate specimens are bubo aspirate, blood, and sputum. Laboratories must be notified of the suspicion of plague to avoid delay in the bacteriologic diagnosis and to guard against laboratory infection.

Treatment and Prevention

Streptomycin and tetracycline

Rat and flea control

Avoidance of sick or dead wild rodents

Streptomycin and tetracycline continue to be preferred antibiotics for treatment of both bubonic and pneumonic plague, because their effectiveness has been proven. Timely treatment reduces the mortality of bubonic plague from more than 50% to 10–15%. Of the 31 human cases of plague reported in the United States in 1984, 6 (19%) died.

Urban plague has been prevented by rat control and general public health measures such as use of insecticides. Sylvatic plague is virtually impossible to eliminate because of the size and dispersion of the multiple rodent reservoirs. Disease can be prevented by avoidance of sick or dead rodents and rabbits. Eradication of fleas on domestic pets, which have been known to transport infected fleas from wild rodents to humans, is recommended in endemic areas. The continued presence of fully virulent plague in its sylvatic cycle poses a risk of extension to the urban cycle and epidemic disease in the event of major disaster or social breakdown.

Chemoprophylaxis

Chemoprophylaxis with tetracycline is recommended for those who have had close contact with a case of pneumonic plague. It is also used for the household contacts of a case of bubonic plague, because they may have had the same flea contact. A formalin-killed plague vaccine is used only for those in high-risk occupations.

Francisella and Tularemia

Tularemia is a disease of wild mammals caused by *F. tularensis*. Humans become infected by contact with infected animals either directly or through the bite of a vector (tick or deer fly). The illness is characterized by high fever and severe constitutional symptoms. Many features of the clinical infection and its epidemiology are similar to those of plague.

Microbiology

Gram-negative coccobacilli

Special requirement for –SH compounds

Francisella tularensis is a small, facultative, coccobacillary, Gram-negative organism with much the same morphology as *Brucella*. It is one of the few bacterial species of medical importance that will not grow on the usual enriched media. This characteristic is due to a special requirement for sulfhydryl compounds, and growth occurs best on a cysteine-glucose blood agar medium incubated aerobically. On primary isolation, 2–10 days of incubation are required for appearance of the tiny transparent colonies. The species is antigenically homogeneous and not closely related to any other genus.

Epidemiology

Usually acquired from infected rabbit carcass or ticks

Transovarial transmission in ticks

Distribution throughout Northern Hemisphere

Humans most often acquire *F. tularensis* by contact with an infected rabbit or tick. Many other wild mammals can also be infected, including squirrels, muskrats, beavers, and deer. The most common history is of skinning wild rabbits on a hunting trip. The bite or scratch of a domestic dog or cat, probably after the animal ingested or mouthed an infected rodent or rabbit, has been implicated occasionally. Infected animals may not show signs of infection, because the organism is well adapted to its natural host. Ticks and deer flies are the usual vectors in animals. The tick may also serve as a reservoir of the organism by transovarial transmission to its offspring.

Tularemia is distributed throughout the Northern Hemisphere, although there are wide variations in specific regions. The highly virulent tick/rabbit-associated strains are common only in North America. It is not found in the British Isles. The number of human cases in the United States has decreased from as many as 10–20 per million in the 1940s to less than 1 per million at the present time.

Pathogenesis and Immunity

Low infecting dose

If directly injected or inhaled, the infecting dose of *F. tularensis* is very low (less than 100 organisms). Infection can follow virtually any kind of contact with the skin or mucous membranes, and the organism probably gains access to the tissues through unnoticed breaks in the epithelium.

Relatively little is known of the events that occur during the 2- to 5-day incubation period. The organism infects the reticuloendothelial organs, often forming granulomas, and the disease may sometimes follow a

Survival in monocytes

chronic relapsing course. These properties suggest multiplication within macrophages, and *F. tularensis* has been shown to survive in monocytes for long periods. A lesion often develops at the site of infection, which becomes ulcerated. Early bacteremic spread probably occurs although it is rarely detected. Other areas of multiplication are characterized by necrosis or granuloma production, and a mixture of abscesses and caseating granulomas may be seen in the same organ.

Focal necrosis and granulomas

Cell-mediated immunity

Naturally acquired infection appears to confer long-lasting immunity. Agglutinating antibody titers remain elevated for many years, but cellular immunity probably plays the major role in resistance to reinfection.

Clinical Illness

After an incubation period of 2–5 days, tularemia may follow a number of courses, depending on the site of inoculation and extent of spread. All begin with the acute onset of fever, chills, and malaise. In the ulceroglandular form, a local papule at the inoculation site becomes necrotic and ulcerative. Regional lymph nodes become swollen and painful. The oculoglandular form which follows conjunctival inoculation is similar except that the local lesion is a painful purulent conjunctivitis. Ingestion of large numbers of *F. tularensis* (more than 10^8) leads to typhoidal tularemia, with abdominal manifestations and a prolonged febrile course similar to that of typhoid fever. Inhalation of the organisms can result in pneumonic tularemia or a more generalized infection similar to the typhoidal form. Like plague pneumonia, tularemic pneumonia may also develop through seeding of the lungs by bacteremic spread of one of the other forms. Any form of tularemia may progress to a systemic infection with lesions in multiple organs. Without treatment, mortality ranges from 5 to 30%, depending on the type of infection. Ulceroglandular tularemia, the most common form, generally carries the lowest risk of a fatal outcome.

Ulceroglandular tularemia

Oculoglandular

Typhoidal

Pneumonic

Diagnosis

Special media needed
for culture

Immunofluorescent tests

Because tularemia is rare and *F. tularensis* has unique growth requirements, the diagnosis is easily overlooked. Laboratories must be alerted to the suspicion of tularemia so that specialized media can be prepared and precautions taken against the considerable risk of laboratory infection. An immunofluorescent reagent is available in reference laboratories for use directly on smears from clinical material.

Serodiagnosis

Because of the difficulty and risk of cultural techniques, many cases are diagnosed by serologic tests. Agglutinating antibodies are usually present in titers of 1:40 by the second week of illness, rising to 1:320 or greater after 3–4 weeks. Unless previous exposure is known, single high antibody titers are considered diagnostic.

Treatment and Prevention

Aminoglycosides

Streptomycin is the drug of choice in all forms of tularemia, although recent experience indicates that gentamicin may be just as effective. Tetracycline and chloramphenicol have also been effective, but relapses are more common than with streptomycin. Prevention is mainly by the use of rubber gloves and eye protection when handling potentially infected wild mammals. Prompt removal of ticks is also important. A vaccine exists, but is used only in laboratory workers and others who cannot avoid contact with infected animals.

Pasteurella multocida

Penicillin-sensitive, Gram-negative rods

Animal bites or scratches followed by cellulitis
Cellulitis

Involvement in bronchiectasis

Pasteurella multocida is one of many species of *Pasteurella* included in the normal respiratory flora of some animals. It is a small, coccobacilliary, Gram-negative organism that grows readily on blood agar but not on MacConkey agar. In addition, it is oxidase positive and ferments a variety of carbohydrates. Unlike most Gram-negative rods, *P. multocida* is highly susceptible to penicillin. Humans are usually infected by the bite or scratch of a domestic dog or cat. Infection develops at the site of the lesion, often within 24 hr. The typical infection is a diffuse cellulitis with a well-defined erythematous border. The diagnosis is made by culture of an aspirate of pus expressed from the lesion. Frequently, too few organisms are present to be seen on a direct Gram smear. *Pasteurella multocida* is by far the most common cause of an infected dog or cat bite. Twenty-one cases were seen in a 30-month period at the Arizona Health Sciences Center. For unknown reasons, *P. multocida* is occasionally isolated from the sputum of patients with bronchiectasis. Infections are treated with penicillin.

Additional Reading

Hubbert, W.T., McCulloch, W.F., and Schnurrenberger, P.R., Eds. 1975. *Diseases Transmitted from Animals to Man.* 6th ed. Springfield, Ill.: Charles C Thomas. An excellent multiauthored standard reference text on the subject.

McNeill, W.H. 1976. *Plagues and Peoples.* New York: Anchor Press/Doubleday. An account of the impact of infectious diseases, including zoonoses, on the course of human history.

World Health Organization. 1982. Technical Report Series 682. Bacterial and viral zoonoses. Geneva: World Health Organization. A report of an international committee on the health impact and control of zoonotic diseases.

Appendix 31.1 Some Important Bacterial and Rickettsial Zoonotic Infections

Disease	Etiologic Agent	Usual Reservoir	Usual Mode of Transmission to Humans	Transmission between Humans	Mode of Transmission between Humans	Special Characteristics
Anthrax	*Bacillus anthracis*	Cattle, sheep, goats	Infected animals or products	No[a]		Resistant spores
Bovine tuberculosis	*Mycobacterium bovis*	Cattle	Milk	No[a]		
Brucellosis	*Brucella* sp.	Cattle, swine, goats	Milk, infected carcasses	No[a]		
Campylobacter infection	*C. fetus, C. jejuni*	Wild mammals, cattle, sheep, pets	Contaminated food and water	Yes	Fecal-oral	
Leptospirosis	*Leptospira* sp.	Cattle, rodents	Water contaminated with urine	No[a]		
Lyme disease	*Borrelia bergdorferi*	Deer, rodents	Ticks; transplacentally	No[a]		Spreading relapsing disease

Appendix 31.1 Some Important Bacterial and Rickettsial Zoonotic Infections (*continued*)

Disease	Etiologic Agent	Usual Reservoir	Usual Mode of Transmission to Humans	Transmission between Humans	Mode of Transmission between Humans	Special Characteristics
Pasteurellosis	*Pasteurella multocida*	Animal oral cavities	Bites, scratches	No[a]		
Plague	*Yersinia pestis*	Rodents	Fleas	Yes	Droplet (pneumonic) spread	Great epidemic potential
Other *Yersinia* infections	*Y. enterocolitica, Y. pseudotuberculosis*	Wild mammals, pigs, cattle, pets	Fecal–oral	Yes	Fecal–oral	
Relapsing fever	*Borrelia* species	Rodents, ticks	Ticks	Yes	Body louse[b]	Epidemic potential
Salmonellosis	*Salmonella serotypes*	Poultry, livestock	Contaminated food	Yes	Fecal contamination of food	
Rickettsial spotted fevers	*R. rickettsii* (eg)	Rodents, ticks, mites	Ticks, mites	No[a]		
Murine typhus	*Rickettsia typhi*	Rodents	Fleas	No[a]		
Q fever	*Coxiella burnetii*	Cattle, sheep, goats	Contaminated dust and aerosols	No[a]		

[a] What never? No never. What *never*? Well, hardly ever! (W. S. Gilbert, "H.M.S. Pinafore").
[b] The relationship between tick-borne relapsing fever and epidemic relapsing fever by the body louse remains uncertain.

32
Respiratory Viruses

C. George Ray

Respiratory disease accounts for an estimated 75–80% of all acute morbidity in the U.S. population. Most of these illnesses (approximately 80%) are viral. Including episodes not requiring medical attention, the overall average is three to four illnesses per year per person, although incidence varies inversely with age (the frequency is greater among young children). Seasonality is also a feature; incidence is lowest in the summer months and highest in the winter.

Range of respiratory viruses

The viruses that are major causes of acute respiratory disease (ARD) include influenza, parainfluenza, rhinoviruses, adenoviruses, respiratory syncytial, and respiratory coronaviruses. Reoviruses are of questionable importance, but will also be considered. Others, such as enteroviruses and measles virus, can also cause respiratory symptoms, but are discussed in other chapters.

Short incubation period
Droplet or manual spread
Risk of bacterial superinfection

In addition to the ability to cause a variety of ARD syndromes, this somewhat heterogeneous group of viruses shares a relatively short incubation period (1–4 days) and a mode of spread from person to person. Transmission is direct, by infective droplet nuclei, or indirect, by hand contact with contaminated secretions and transfer to nasal or conjunctival epithelium. All of these agents are associated with an increased risk of bacterial superinfection originating in the damaged tissue of the respiratory tract, and all have a worldwide distribution.

Influenza Viruses

Habitat and History

Human, animal, and avian strains

Humans are the major hosts of the influenza viruses, and severe respiratory disease is the primary manifestation of infection. Influenza A viruses closely related to those prevalent in humans, however, circulate among many mammalian and avian species. Some of these may undergo antigenic

499

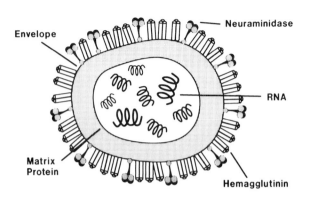

32.1 A diagrammatic view of influenza A or B virus, containing eight distinctive segments of single-stranded RNA.

mutation or genetic recombination and emerge as new human epidemic strains.

Characteristic influenza outbreaks have been described since the early 16th century; since then, outbreaks of varying severity have occurred nearly every year. Severe pandemics occurred in 1743, 1889–1890, 1918–1919 (the Spanish flu), and 1957 (the Asian flu). These episodes were associated with particularly high mortality; for example, the Spanish flu was thought to have caused at least 20 million deaths. Usually, the elderly and those persons of any age group with cardiac or pulmonary disease have the highest death rate.

Pandemic influenza

Age- and disease-associated mortality

Group Characteristics

Orthomyxoviruses

Types A, B, and C

Influenza viruses are members of the orthomyxovirus group, which are enveloped, pleomorphic, single-stranded RNA viruses. They are classified into three major serotypes, A, B, and C, each based on different ribonucleoprotein antigens. Influenza A is the most extensively studied of the three, and much of the following discussion is based upon knowledge of this type. It usually causes more severe disease and more extensive epidemics than the other types and has a greater tendency to undergo significant antigenic changes. Influenza B is somewhat more antigenically stable and usually occurs in more localized outbreaks; influenza C appears to be a minor cause of disease, in contrast to the other types.

Relative virulence and epidemic spread of different types

Enveloped RNA virus with segmented genome

Virus-specified hemagglutinin and neuramidase spikes

Influenza A and B viruses consist of a nucleocapsid containing segments of negative-sense, single-stranded RNA, which is enveloped in a glycolipid membrane derived from the host cell plasma membrane. The inner side of the envelope contains a layer of virus-specified protein. Two virus-specified glycoproteins, hemagglutinin and neuramidase, are embedded in the outer surface of the envelope and appear as "spikes" over the surface of the virion (Fig. 32.1). Influenza C differs considerably from the others in that it possesses only seven RNA segments and has no neuramidase, although it does possess other receptor-destroying capability (see below). In addition, the hemagglutinin of influenza C binds to a different cell receptor than that for types A and B.

Hemagglutinin and viral attachment

The virus-specified glycoproteins are antigenic and have special functional importance to the virus. Hemagglutinin is so named because of its ability to agglutinate red blood cells from certain species (for example, chickens, guinea pigs) in vitro. Its major biologic function is to serve as a point of attachment to mucoprotein receptor sites on human respiratory cell surfaces, which is a critical first step in initiating infection of the cell.

Neuraminidase and viral
invasion and release
from cell

Neuraminidase is an antigenic hydrolytic enzyme that acts on the mucoprotein hemagglutinin receptors by splitting off the terminal neuraminic acid. The result is destruction of receptor activity. Neuraminidase probably serves several functions. It may inactivate a free mucoprotein receptor substance in respiratory secretions that could otherwise bind to viral hemagglutinin and prevent access of the virus to the cell surface. It may be important in fusion of the viral envelope with the host cell membrane as a prerequisite to viral entry. It also aids in the release of newly formed virus particles from infected cells, thus making them available to infect other cells. Type-specific antibodies to neuraminidase appear to inhibit the spread of virus in the infected host and to limit the amount of virus released from host cells.

Viral replication, assembly,
and release

Nucleocapsid assembly takes place in the cell nucleus, but final virus assembly takes place at the plasma membrane. The ribonucleoproteins are enveloped by the plasma membrane, which by then contains hemagglutinin and neuraminidase. Virus "buds" are formed, and intact virions are released from the cell surface (See Chapter 6, Fig. 6.11).

Viral isolation

Culture in embryonated eggs

Cell culture

Influenza A viruses were initially isolated in 1933 by intranasal inoculation of ferrets, which developed febrile respiratory illnesses. At present, the viruses are often grown in the amniotic sac of embryonated hen's eggs, where their presence can be detected by the hemagglutination test. Most strains can also be readily isolated in cell culture systems, such as primary monkey kidney cells. Some will cause cytopathic effects in culture; however, the most efficient method of detection is by demonstrating hemadsorption on the infected cell surfaces.

Hemadsorption

Hemagglutination

Hemadsorption and
hemagglutination inhibition

Detection of
antihemagglutinin antibodies
in serum

Influenza virus can be detected in infected cell cultures by adherence of erythrocytes to infected cells containing hemagglutinin (hemadsorption) or by agglutination of erythrocytes by virus already released into the extracellular fluid (hemagglutination). The virus can then be identified specifically by neutralization or inhibition of these properties by addition of antibody directed specifically at the hemagglutinin. This method is called *hemadsorption inhibition* or *hemagglutination inhibition*, depending upon whether the test is performed on infected cells or extracellular virus, respectively. Also, because the hemagglutinin is antigenic, hemagglutination inhibition tests can be used to detect antibodies in infected subjects. It has been shown that antibody directed against specific hemagglutinin is highly effective in neutralizing the infectivity of the virus.

Influenza A

Influenza A will be considered in detail because of its great clinical and epidemiologic importance.

Influenza A genome

The influenza A virion contains at least eight segments of single-stranded RNA with defined genetic responsibilities. These functions include coding for virus-specified proteins and antigens. A unique aspect of influenza A viruses is their ability to develop a wide variety of subtypes

Mutability of virus

through the processes of mutation and recombination. These processes result in antigenic changes called *drifts* and *shifts*, which will be discussed shortly.

Subtypes based on H and N
antigens

A number of subtypes of hemagglutinin and neuraminidase antigens are known to exist among influenza A viruses. Of these, three hemagglutinins (H_1, H_2, and H_3) and two neuraminidases (N_1 and N_2) appear to be of greatest importance in human infections. These subtypes are designated according to the H and N antigens on their surface, for example, H_1N_1, H_3N_2. Within each subtype there may also be more subtle, but

Antigenic drifts

sometimes important, antigenic differences (drifts). These differences are designated according to the major representative virus to which they are most closely related antigenically, using the place of initial isolation, number of the isolate, and year of detection. For example, two H_3N_2 strains of influenza A viruses that differ antigenically only slightly are called A/Texas/1/77 (H_3N_2) and A/Bangkok/1/79 (H_3N_2).

Antigenic drifts within major subtypes can involve either the H or N antigens, as well as the genes coding for nonstructural proteins, and can result from as little as a single mutation in the viral RNA. The mutant may come to predominate under the selective immunologic pressures in the host population. Such drifts are frequent among influenza A viruses, occurring at least every few years and sometimes even during the course of a single epidemic. Drifts can also develop in influenza B viruses, but at a considerably lower frequency.

Major antigenic shifts

In contrast to the frequently occurring mutations that cause antigenic drift among influenza A strains, major antigenic changes in the H, N, or both subtypes can occur suddenly and unpredictably. These are referred to as *antigenic shifts*. They almost certainly result from recombinational events that can be readily reproduced in the laboratory. Simultaneously infecting a cell with two different influenza A subtypes yields progeny that contain antigens derived from either of the original viruses. For example, a cell infected simultaneously with influenza A (H_3N_2) and A (H_1N_1) may produce a mixture of influenza viruses of the following subtypes: H_3N_2, H_1N_1, H_1N_2, and H_3N_1. Alternative possibilities are that antigenic subtypes become latent in human host tissues, then become reactivated and spread to nonimmune contacts,* or that certain subtypes circulate into animal or avian reservoirs, only to reemerge and adapt to human hosts when a sufficient proportion of the population has little or no immunity to the "new" subtypes.

Epidemiology of major antigenic shifts

Major antigenic shifts, which have occurred approximately every 8–10 years in this century, have often resulted in serious epidemics or pandemics among populations with little or no preexisting antibody to the new subtypes. Examples include the appearance of an H_1N_1 subtype in 1947, followed by an abrupt shift to an H_2N_2 strain in 1957, which caused the pandemic of Asian flu. A subsequent major shift in 1968 to an H_3N_2 subtype (the Hong Kong flu) led to another, but somewhat less severe epidemic. The Russian flu, which appeared in late 1977, was caused by an H_1N_1 subtype very similar to that which dominated between 1947 and 1957 (Table 32.1).

Role of minor antigenic drifts in maintaining the virus

The concepts of antigenic shift and drift in human influenza A virus infections can be roughly summarized as follows: Periodic shifts in the major antigenic components appear, usually resulting in major epidemics in populations with little or no immunologic experience with the subtype. As the population of susceptible individuals is exhausted (that is, subtype-specific immunity is acquired by increasing numbers of people) the subtype continues to circulate for a time, undergoing mutation with subtle antigenic drift from season to season. This allows some degree of infection to continue to occur. Infectivity persists because subtype-specific immunity is not entirely protective against drifting strains; for example, an individual may have antibodies reasonably protective against influenza A/Texas/77 (H_3N_2), yet be susceptible in succeeding years to reinfection

---

* R.E. Hope-Simpson (*J. Hyg.* 86:35, 1981) suggests that seasonal reactivation in human carrier–hosts may result from seasonal stimuli related to solar radiation.

Table 32.1 Major Antigenic Shifts Associated with Influenza A Pandemics, 1947–1986

Year	Subtype	Prototype Strain
1947	H_1N_1	$A/FM_1/47$
1957	H_2N_2	A/Singapore/57
1968	H_3N_2	A/Hong Kong/68
1977	H_1N_1	A/USSR/77
1987	H_3N_2	No shift detected; strains circulating worldwide

by influenza A/Bangkok/79 (H_3N_2). Eventually, however, the overall immunity of the population becomes sufficient to minimize the epidemic potential of the major subtype and its drifting strains. Unfortunately, the battle is never entirely won, as the scene is set for the sudden and usually unpredictable appearance of an entirely new subtype that may not have circulated among humans for 20 years or more.

Doctrine of original antigenic sin

Continued anamnestic responses to first infecting subtype's antigens

Another concept helpful in understanding the behavior of influenza A virus in humans is the *doctrine of original antigenic sin*, which states that the immune response to all subsequent influenza A infection is dominated by a persistence of antibody to the first virus with which a person has contact through constant anamnestic response. This doctrine primarily describes the antibody response to the hemagglutinin antigen, but there is evidence that it also applies to neuraminidase antigen responses. To clarify the concept, the antibody response to the hemagglutinins is illustrated in the following example. An infant or young child never infected by any influenza A virus is immunologically "virgin" in this respect. The first infection may be with an H_1N_1 subtype, and the patient develops an antibody response to the H_1 antigen. Years later, the patient becomes infected with an H_2N_2 subtype and develops antibodies to the H_2 antigen; in addition, even though the H antigen is different in the second episode, an anamnestic antibody response to the initial (H_1) antigen develops. Throughout life, anamnestic "recall" will remain enhanced with regard to the first subtype encountered and, to a lesser extent, to subsequent subtypes, regardless of which influenza A virus later infects the patient. This phenomenon supports the presence of one or more shared (conserved) epitopes among all strains.

Explanation of age-specific attack rates

This immunologic recall response probably accounts for the variability in age-specific attack rates when newer subtypes are introduced into a population. For example, the appearance of the Russian flu (H_1N_1) in 1977–1978 was noteworthy in that a similar subtype had been prevalent during 1947–1956, but then disappeared. Individuals born after 1956 would not have experienced prior infection with the subtype, and the prediction that the highest attack rates would be among those less than 35 years of age was correct.

Unfortunately, none of these generalizations can be applied with great confidence to the individual patient. People vary in their immune responses to viruses, and other host factors, such as the aging process, can modify susceptibility to infection. Therefore, even though the H_1N_1 influenza A subtype is expected primarily to affect younger individuals, it is still considered prudent to attempt to protect high-risk groups such as the elderly, who might acquire severe, potentially life-threatening infections.

Infections Caused by Influenza Viruses

Clinical Disease and Outcome

As stated previously, influenza A and B viruses tend to cause the most severe illnesses, whereas influenza C seems to occur infrequently and generally causes milder disease. The typical acute influenzal syndrome will be described here.

Short incubation period

Acute disease

The incubation period is brief, lasting an average of 2 days. Onset is usually abrupt, with symptoms developing over a few hours. These include fever, myalgia, headache, and occasionally shaking chills. Within 6–12 hr, the patient is usually at the peak of illness severity, and a dry, nonproductive cough develops. The illness remains severe, sometimes with worsening cough, for 2–5 days, followed by gradual improvement. By a week after onset, the patient feels significantly better. Fatigue, nonspecific weakness, and cough, however, can remain frustrating lingering problems for an additional 2–3 weeks or longer.

Progressive respiratory infection

Other complications

Reye's syndrome

Occasional patients develop a progressive infection that involves the tracheobronchial tree and lungs to a greater extent. In these situations pneumonia, which can be lethal, is the result. Other unusual acute manifestations of influenza include central nervous system dysfunction, myositis, and myocarditis. In infants and children, a serious complication known as *Reye's syndrome* may develop 2–12 days after onset of the infection; it is characterized by severe fatty infiltration of the liver and cerebral edema (encephalopathy with fatty infiltration of the viscera). This syndrome is associated not only with influenza viruses, but with a wide variety of systemic viral illnesses; the risk may be enhanced by exposure to salicylates, such as aspirin.

Bacterial superinfection

The most common and important complication of influenza virus infection is bacterial superinfection. Such infections usually involve the lung, but bacteremia with secondary seeding of distant sites can also occur. The superinfection, which can develop at any time in the acute or convalescent phase of the disease, is often heralded by an abrupt worsening of the patient's condition after initial stabilization. The bacteria most commonly involved in such superinfections include *Streptococcus pneumoniae*, *Haemophilus influenzae*, and *Staphylococcus aureus*.

In summary, there are essentially three ways in which influenza may cause patient death:

Underlying disease with decompensation. People with limited cardiovascular or pulmonary reserves can be further compromised by any respiratory infection. Thus, the elderly and those of any age with underlying chronic cardiac or pulmonary disease are at particular risk.

Superinfection. Superinfection can lead to bacterial pneumonia and occasionally disseminated bacterial infection.

Direct rapid progression. Less commonly, direct rapid progression of the viral infection can lead to severe viral pneumonia with asphyxia.

Pathogenesis

Cilial damage and cell desquamation

Influenza viruses primarily infect the respiratory tract, and viremia is rarely detected. They multiply in ciliated respiratory epithelial cells, leading to functional and structural ciliary abnormalities. This is accompanied by a switch-off of protein and nucleic acid synthesis in the affected cells, the release of lysosomal hydrolytic enzymes, and desquamation of both ciliated and mucus-producing epithelial cells. There is, thus, substantial interference with the mechanical clearance mechanism of the respiratory tract. The process of cell death results in the cleavage of complement

Inflammatory response components, leading to localized inflammation. Early in infection, the primary chemotactic stimulus is directed toward mononuclear leukocytes, which comprise the major cellular inflammatory component. The respiratory epithelium may not be restored to normal for 2 to 10 weeks after the initial insult.

Viral toxicity The virus particles are also toxic to tissues. This toxicity can be demonstrated by inoculating high concentrations of inactivated virions into mice, which produces acute inflammatory changes in the absence of viral penetration or replication within cells.

Impairment of host defenses Other host cell functions are also severely impaired, particularly during the acute phase of infection. They include chemotactic, phagocytic, and intracellular killing functions of polymorphonuclear leukocytes and perhaps of alveolar macrophage activity.

The net result of these effects is that, on entry into the respiratory tract, the viruses cause cell damage, primarily to the respiratory epithelium, which elicits an acute inflammatory response and impairs mechanical and cellular host responses. This damage renders the host highly susceptible to invasive bacterial superinfection. In vitro studies also suggest that bacterial pathogens such as staphylococci are enhanced in their adherence to the surfaces of influenza virus-infected cells. Recovery from infection be-

Interferon and immune response gins with interferon production, which limits further virus replication, and with a rapid generation of natural killer cells. Shortly thereafter, cytotoxic T cells appear in large numbers to participate in the lysis of virus-infected cells and, thus, in initial control of the infection. This is followed by the appearance of local and humoral antibody along with an evolving, more durable, cellular immunity. Finally, there is repair of tissue damage.

Antibody Responses

Antibody responses Although cell-mediated immune responses are undoubtedly important in influenza virus infections, humoral immunity has been investigated more extensively. Typically, the patient responds to infection within a few days by the production of antibodies directed toward the group ribonucleoprotein antigen, the hemagglutinin, and the neuraminidase. Peak antibody titer levels are usually reached within 2 weeks of onset, then gradually wane over the following months to varying low levels. Antibody to the ribonucleoprotein appears to confer little or no protection against rein-

Protective effect of antihemagglutinin fection. Hemagglutination inhibition antibody is considered the most protective, as it has the ability to neutralize virus on reexposure; such immunity is relative, however, and quantitative differences in responsiveness exist between individuals. Furthermore, antigenic shifts and drifts often allow the virus to subvert the antibody response on subsequent exposures.

Antineuraminidase may limit viral spread Antibody to neuraminidase antigen is not as protective as hemagglutination inhibition antibody, but may play a role in limiting virus spread within the host.

Epidemiology

Seasonality Direct droplet spread is the most common mode of transmission. Influenza infections in temperate climates tend to occur most frequently during midwinter months. Major outbreaks of influenza A usually occur at 2- to 3-

Epidemic intervals

Increased absenteeism as indicator of epidemic

Excess mortality

year intervals; influenza B epidemics appear irregularly, usually every 4–5 years. The typical epidemic develops over a period of 3–6 weeks and may involve 10% of the population. Illness rates may exceed 30% among school-aged children, residents of closed institutions, and industrial groups. One major indicator of influenza virus activity is an abrupt rise in school or industrial absenteeism. In severe influenza A epidemics, the number of deaths reported in a given area of the country often exceeds the number expected for that period. This significant increase, referred to as *excess mortality*, is another indicator of severe, widespread illness. Influenza B rarely causes such severe epidemics.

Laboratory Diagnosis

Virus isolation and detection

Direct immunofluorescence

Serodiagnosis

During the acute phase of illness, influenza viruses can be readily isolated from respiratory tract specimens, such as nasopharyngeal and throat swabs. Most strains grow in primary monkey kidney cell cultures or in the amniotic cavity of embryonated hen's eggs, and they can be detected by hemadsorption. The presence of viral hemagglutinin in the amniotic fluid can be demonstrated after 2–3 days of incubation. More recently, diagnosis of infection within 2 hr was made possible by direct immunofluorescent detection of viral antigen in epithelial cells from the upper respiratory tract.

Serologic diagnosis is of considerable help epidemiologically and is usually made by demonstrating a fourfold or greater increase in complement-fixing or hemagglutination inhibition antibody titers in acute and convalescent specimens collected 10–14 days apart.

Prevention

Whole virus and "split" vaccines

Short duration of vaccine immunity

Indications for vaccination

Amantadine prophylaxis for influenza A

The best available method of control is by use of killed viral vaccine prepared from those strains related most closely to the antigenic subtypes currently causing infections. These inactivated vaccines may contain whole virions or "split" subunits composed primarily of hemagglutinin antigens. They are commonly used, in two doses given 1 month apart, for immunizing children who may not have been immunized previously; otherwise, single annual doses are recommended just prior to influenza season. Vaccine efficacy is variable, and annual revaccination is necessary to ensure maximal protection. Used in this way, the virus vaccines may be 70–85% effective.

It is recommended that vaccination be directed primarily toward the elderly, individuals of all ages who are at high risk (for example, those with chronic lung or heart disease), and perhaps those in essential jobs, such as medical personnel, police, and the like.

Amantadine hydrochloride, a symmetric amine, has been shown to be effective in short-term (several weeks) oral prophylaxis of influenza A infections. It appears to act by inhibiting viral uncoating or primary transcription of viral RNA. Amantadine can produce side effects, however, and is recommended only for high-risk patients until vaccine-induced immunity can be achieved. A typical example of its use would be during an epidemic in which an elderly, potentially susceptible patient may become exposed to infection within a short period. Oral amantadine prophylaxis may be initiated concurrently with administration of a vaccine containing the most current antigens and continued for 2 weeks. The immunogenic effect of the vaccine should ensure continued protection. It must be emphasized that amantadine has been proved effective for influenza A virus

Rimantadine equally effective

infections only; it is useless in the management and prevention of infections caused by other influenza types or by any other respiratory virus. A newer related drug, rimantadine, seems to be as efficacious as amantadine and may cause fewer adverse effects.

Treatment

Nonspecific therapy

The two basic approaches to management of influenzal disease are symptomatic care and anticipation of potential complications, particularly bacterial superinfection. Once the diagnosis has been made, rest, adequate fluid intake, conservative use of analgesics such as aspirin for myalgia and headache, and antitussives for severe cough are commonly prescribed. It must be emphasized that even nonprescription drugs must be used with caution. This applies particularly to those drugs containing salicylates and to children because the risk of Reye's syndrome must be considered.

Bacterial superinfection

Bacterial superinfection is often suggested by a rapid worsening of clinical symptoms after the patient has initially stabilized. Antibiotic prophylaxis has not been shown to enhance or diminish the likelihood of superinfection, but can increase the risk of acquisition of more resistant bacterial flora in the respiratory tract and make the superinfection more difficult to treat. Ideally, the physician should instruct the patient regarding the natural history of the influenza virus infection and be prepared to respond to bacterial complications, if they occur, with a specific diagnosis and therapy.

Amantadine therapy

When influenza A infection is proved or strongly suspected, 4–5 days of amantadine hydrochloride therapy may also be considered. It has been shown to benefit some patients to a modest degree, as measured by reduction of number of days of confinement to bed, of fever, and of functional respiratory impairment. These beneficial effects, however, have been observed only when the drug is administered early in the illness (within 12–24 hr of onset).

Parainfluenza Viruses

Paramyxoviruses

Structure like influenza viruses, but with unsegmented genome

Antigenic stability

There are four serotypes of parainfluenza viruses: parainfluenza 1, 2, 3, and 4. These enveloped viruses belong to the paramyxovirus group, contain nonsegmented, negative-sense, single-stranded RNA, and, like the influenza viruses, possess a neuraminidase and hemagglutinin. Their mode of spread and pathogenesis is similar to that of the influenza viruses. They differ from the influenza viruses in that nucleocapsid assembly occurs in the cytoplasm rather than the plasma membrane; in addition the antigenic makeup of each parainfluenza serotype is relatively stable, and significant antigenic shift or drift does not occur. Each serotype will be considered separately.

Parainfluenza 1

Association with croup

Parainfluenza 1 is the major cause of acute croup (laryngotracheitis) in infants and young children, but also causes less severe diseases such as mild upper respiratory illness (URI), pharyngitis, and tracheobronchitis in all age groups. Outbreaks of infection tend to occur most frequently during the fall months.

Parainfluenza 2

Parainfluenza 2 is of slightly less significance than parainfluenza 1 or 3. It has been associated with croup, primarily in children, with mild URI, and occasionally with acute lower respiratory disease. As with parainfluenza 1, outbreaks usually occur during the fall months.

Parainfluenza 3

Severe lower respiratory disease in infants

Parainfluenza 3 is a major cause of severe lower respiratory disease in infants and young children. It often causes bronchitis, pneumonia, and croup in children less than 1 year old. In older children and adults, it may cause URI or tracheobronchitis. Infections are common and can occur in any season; it is estimated that nearly one-half of all children have been exposed to this virus by 1 year of age.

Parainfluenza 4

Parainfluenza 4 is the least common of the group and is generally associated with mild upper respiratory illness only.

Frequency of disease in infants and children

The parainfluenza viruses are important because of the serious diseases they can cause in infants and young children. Parainfluenza 1 and 3 are particularly common in this regard. Overall, the group is thought to be responsible for 15–20% of all nonbacterial respiratory diseases requiring hospitalization in infancy and childhood. The onset of illness may be abrupt, as in acute spasmodic croup, but usually begins as a mild URI with variable progression over 1–3 days to involvement of the middle or lower respiratory tract. Duration of acute illness can vary from 4 to 21 days but is usually 7–10 days.

Course and duration

Transient immunity

Immunity to reinfection is transient; although repeated infections can occur in older children and adults, they are usually milder than the illnesses of infancy and early childhood.

Laboratory diagnosis

Specific diagnosis is based on virus isolation, usually in monkey kidney cell cultures, or on serology using the hemagglutination inhibition, complement fixation, or neutralization methods on paired sera. Direct immunofluorescence can also be used for rapid detection of antigen in respiratory epithelial cells.

There is currently no method of control or specific therapy for these infections.

Respiratory Syncytial Virus

Pneumovirus

Respiratory syncytial virus (RSV) is now classified as a pneumovirus within the paramyxovirus family. Its name is derived from its ability to produce cell fusion in tissue culture (syncytium formation). Unlike influenza or parainfluenza viruses, it possesses no hemagglutinin or neuraminidase. The RNA genome is nonsegmented, negative sense, single stranded, and codes for at least 10 different proteins. Among these are two matrix (M) proteins in the viral envelope. One forms the inner lining of the viral envelope; the function of the other is uncertain.

Syncytium formation

Enveloped RNA virus with unsegmented genome

G glycoprotein mediates attachment

Other notable antigens on the surface of the viral envelope include the G glycoprotein, which probably serves as an attachment site to host cell receptors, and the fusion (F) glycoprotein, which induces fusion of the viral envelope with the host cell surface. It is also responsible for fusion

F glycoprotein responsible for syncytium formation

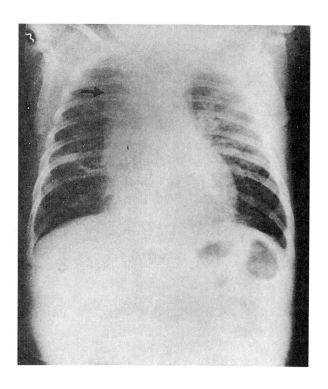

32.2 Chest radiograph of an infant with a severe case of respiratory syncytial virus pneumonia and bronchiolitis. Bilateral interstitial infiltrates, hyperexpansion of the lung, and right upper lobe atelectasis (arrow) are all present.

of infected cells in cell cultures, leading to the appearance of multinucleated giant cells (syncytium formation). Antibodies directed at the F glycoprotein neutralize the virus in vitro.

Antigenic variants

At least two antigenic subgroups (A and B) of RSV are known to exist. The epidemiologic and biological significance of these variants is not yet certain.

Respiratory syncytial virus is the single most important etiologic agent in respiratory diseases of infancy, and it is the major cause of bronchiolitis and pneumonia among infants under 1 year of age.

Clinical Outline of Disease and Outcome

Serious bronchiolitis and pneumonitis in infants

Duration and fatality

The usual incubation period is 1–4 days, followed by the onset of rhinitis; severity of illness progresses to a peak within 1–3 days. In infants, this peak usually takes the form of bronchiolitis and pneumonitis, with cough, wheezing, and respiratory distress. Clinical findings include hyperexpansion of the lungs, hypoxemia (low oxygenation of blood), and hypercapnea (carbon dioxide retention). Interstitial infiltrates, often with areas of pulmonary collapse, may be seen on chest radiography (Figure 32.2). Fever is variable. The duration of acute illness is often 10–14 days. The fatality rate among hospitalized infected infants is estimated to be 0.5–1%. Causes of death include respiratory failure, right-sided heart failure (cor pulmonale), and bacterial superinfection. Death has sometimes resulted from unnecessary procedures in patients in whom RSV infection was not considered. Bronchoscopy, lung biopsy, or overly aggressive therapy with corticosteroids and bronchodilators for presumed asthma can all pose a danger to such patients.

Older infants, children, and adults are also readily infected. The clinical illnesses in these groups are usually milder and include croup, tracheo-bronchitis, and URI. Respiratory syncytial virus can also cause acute fla-reups of chronic bronchitis and trigger acute wheezing episodes in asth-matic children.

Pathogenesis

The virus is spread to the upper respiratory tract by contact with infective secretions. Infection appears to be confined primarily to the respiratory epithelium, with progressive involvement of the middle and lower airways. Viremia occurs rarely. The direct effect of virus on respiratory tract ep-ithelial cells is similar to that previously described for influenza viruses, and cytotoxic T cells appear to play a similar role in early control of the acute infection.

The apparent enhanced severity of disease, particularly in very young infants, is not yet clearly understood, but may have an immunological basis. Factors that have been proposed to play a role include 1) qualitative or quantitative deficits in humoral or secretory antibody responses to critical virus-specified proteins; 2) excessive damage from antibody-dependent, cell-mediated cytotoxicity; 3) formation of antigen–antibody complexes within the respiratory tract resulting in complement activation; and 4) IgE-mediated histamine release.

Possible immunological basis for enhanced disease in infants

The usual mortality among infants hospitalized with RSV infections is 0.5 to 1%; however, this rises to 15% in children receiving cancer che-motherapy, 37% in infants with congenital heart disease, and 40% or greater among those with severe immunodeficiency. Infants with under-lying chronic lung disease are also considered to be at high risk for a lethal outcome.

Pathology

Bronchiolar and alveolar involvement

The major findings are in the bronchi, bronchioles, and alveoli. These findings include necrosis of epithelial cells, interstitial mononuclear cell inflammatory infiltrates, which sometimes also involve the alveoli and alveolar ducts, and plugging of smaller airways with material containing mucus, necrotic cells, and fibrin (Figure 32.3). Multinucleated syncytial cells with intracytoplasmic inclusions are occasionally seen in the affected tracheobronchial epithelium.

Immune Response

Brief immunity to reinfection

Infection results in IgG and IgA humoral and secretory antibody re-sponses. Immunity to reinfection is quite tenuous, however, as demon-strated by patients who have recovered from a primary acute episode and have become reinfected with disease of similar severity in the same or succeeding year. Illness severity appears to diminish with increasing age and successive reinfection.

Epidemiology

High attack rate

Community outbreaks of RSV infection occur annually and can commence at any time from late fall to early spring. The usual outbreak lasts 8–12 weeks and can involve nearly one-half of all families with children. In the family setting, it appears that older siblings often introduce the virus into the home, and secondary infection rates can be almost 50%. The usual

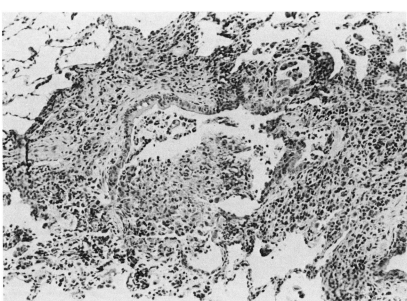

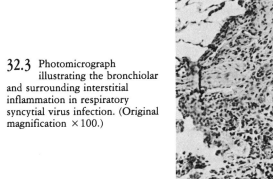

32.3 Photomicrograph illustrating the bronchiolar and surrounding interstitial inflammation in respiratory syncytial virus infection. (Original magnification × 100.)

duration of virus shedding is 5–7 days; young infants, however, may shed virus for 9–20 days or longer.

Nosocomial infection

Spread of RSV in the hospital setting is also a major problem. Control is difficult, but includes careful attention to hand washing between contacts with patients, isolation, and exclusion of personnel and visitors to the ward who have any form of respiratory illness. The effectiveness of masks in controlling nosocomial spread is questionable.

Laboratory Diagnosis

Direct immunofluorescent antibody detection

Cell culture

Serodiagnosis

Rapid diagnosis of RSV infection can be made by immunofluorescent antibody detection of viral antigen in the cytoplasm of nasopharyngeal epithelial cells. The virus can also be isolated from the respiratory tract by prompt inoculation of specimens into cell cultures without prior freezing. Syncytial cytopathic effects develop over 2–7 days. The cell cultures of choice are heteroploid cell lines. Serodiagnosis may also be employed, but requires acute and convalescent sera and is less sensitive than antigen detection methods or culture.

Prevention and Treatment

Ribavirin

No vaccine is available; however recent studies suggest that ribavirin aerosol treatment might be effective. Attenuated live virus vaccines are under investigation, but it is uncertain whether they will be of value.

Supportive treatment

Treatment is primarily directed at the underlying pathophysiology and includes adequate oxygenation, ventilatory support when necessary, and close observation of complications such as bacterial superinfection or right-sided heart failure.

Adenoviruses

Multiple serotypes of naked, double-stranded DNA viruses

Of the almost 100 different serotypes of adenoviruses, 41 are known to affect humans. These viruses are naked, icosahedral, and possess double-stranded DNA. Replication and assembly occur in the nucleus, and virions

Table 32.2 Clinical Syndromes Associated with Adenovirus Infection

Syndrome	Common Serotypes Found[a]
Childhood febrile illness; pharyngoconjunctival fever	1, 2, *3*, 5, 7, *7a*
Pneumonia and other acute respiratory illnesses	1, 2, *3*, 5, 7, *7a*, *7b* (4 in military recruits)
Pertussislike illness	1, *2*, *3*, 5, *19*, 21
Conjunctivitis	2, 5, 7, *8*, *19*, 21
Keratoconjunctivitis	*3, 8, 9, 19*
Acute hemorrhagic cystitis	11
Acute gastroenteritis	40, 41

[a] Italicized serotypes are those commonly associated with outbreaks.

Potential for prolonged infection without disease

are released by cell destruction. All adenoviruses share a common group-specific, complement-fixing antigen associated with the hexon component of the viral capsid. Adenoviruses are characterized by their ubiquity and their ability to reside in the host for periods ranging from a few days to several years. Their ability to produce infection without disease is illustrated by the frequent recovery of virus from tonsils or adenoids removed from healthy children (the group name is derived from its discovery in 1953 as a latent agent in many adenoid tissue specimens) and by prolonged intermittent shedding of virus from the pharynx and intestinal tract after initial infection.

Spread by respiratory or fecal–oral route

Types 1 and 2 are highly endemic; type 5 is the next most common. Most primary infections with these viruses occur early in life. The spread of the virus can be either respiratory or by fecal-oral contamination.

Most infections are subclinical

Overall, only about 45% of adenovirus infections result in disease. Their most significant contribution to acute illness is in children, particularly those under 2 years of age (10.6% of acute febrile illness). They are also major causes of acute respiratory disease in military recruits, usually by types 4 and 7.

Clinical Outline of Disease and Outcome

Upper respiratory infections

The diversity of major syndromes and commonly associated serotypes are summarized in Table 32.2. The acute respiratory syndromes vary in both clinical manifestation and severity. Symptoms include fever, rhinitis, pharyngitis, cough, and conjunctivitis. Adenoviruses are also common causes of nonstreptococcal exudative pharyngitis, particularly among children less than 3 years of age. Acute, and occasionally chronic, conjunctivitis and keratoconjunctivitis have been associated with several serotypes. More severe disease, such as laryngitis, croup, bronchiolitis, or severe pneumonia, may also occur. Occasionally, the illness may be prolonged for several weeks and can clinically resemble pertussis. A syndrome of pharyngitis and conjunctivitis (pharyngoconjunctival fever) is classically associated with adenovirus infection. Adenoviruses can also cause acute hemorrhagic cystitis, in which hematuria and dysuria are prominent findings. More recently, some serotypes that are difficult to cultivate in the laboratory have been recognized as significant causes of gastroenteritis (Chapter 38).

Conjunctivitis

More severe disease

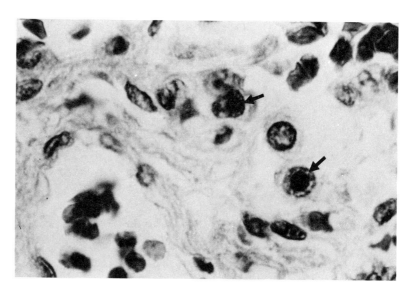

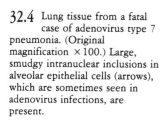

32.4 Lung tissue from a fatal case of adenovirus type 7 pneumonia. (Original magnification × 100.) Large, smudgy intranuclear inclusions in alveolar epithelial cells (arrows), which are sometimes seen in adenovirus infections, are present.

Pathogenesis

Routes of infection

The adenoviruses usually enter the host by inhalation of droplet nuclei or by the oral route. Direct inoculation onto nasal or conjunctival mucosa by hands or by contaminated towels and ophthalmic medications may also occur. The virus replicates in epithelial cells, producing cell necrosis and inflammation. Viremia sometimes occurs and can result in spread to distant sites, such as the kidney, bladder, liver, lymphoid tissue (including mesenteric nodes), and occasionally the central nervous system. In the acute phase of infection, the distant sites may also show inflammation; for example, abdominal pain is occasionally seen with severe illnesses and is believed to result from mesenteric lymphadenitis caused by the viruses.

Viremic spread and remote disease

Latency and reactivation

After the acute phase of illness, the viruses may remain in tissues, particularly lymphoid structures such as tonsils, adenoids, and intestinal Peyer's patches, and become reactivated and shed without producing illness for 6–18 months thereafter. This reactivation is enhanced by stressful events (stress reactivation), such as infection by other agents.

Toxic pentons

A potentially important pathogenic feature of the virion is the presence of pentons, which are located at each of the 12 corners of the icosahedron. They are fiberlike projections with knoblike terminal structures and appear to be responsible for a toxic effect on cells, which is manifested by clumping and detachment in vitro.

Pathology

Like that of the viruses described previously, the primary pathology is epithelial cell necrosis with a predominantly mononuclear inflammatory response. In some instances, smudgy intranuclear inclusions may be seen in infected cells (Figure 32.4).

Immune Responses

Type-specific immunity

Immunity after infection is serotype specific and usually long lasting. In addition to type-specific immunity, group-specific complement-fixing antibodies appear in response to infection. These antibodies are useful indicators of infection, but do not specify the infecting serotype.

Epidemiology

Infections caused by serotypes 1, 2, and 5 are generally most frequent during the first few years of life. All serotypes can occur during any season of the year, but are encountered most frequently during late winter or early spring. Sharp outbreaks of disease caused by serotypes 3 and 7 have been traced to inadequately chlorinated swimming pools. Conjunctivitis is the illness most commonly associated with these episodes. Other outbreaks of conjunctivitis have been traced to physicians' offices and appear to have been spread by contaminated ophthalmic medications or diagnostic equipment.

Swimming pool conjunctivitis

Iatrogenic infections

Laboratory Diagnosis

Viral isolation

Problems of associating isolates with disease

The viruses can be readily isolated in heteroploid cell cultures. There is little difficulty in relating the virus isolate to the illness in question when the isolate has been obtained from a site other than the upper respiratory or gastrointestinal tract (for example, lung biopsy, conjunctival swabs, urine); because of the known tendency for intermittent asymptomatic shedding into the oropharynx and feces, however, isolates from these sites must be interpreted more cautiously. If their significance is questionable, serologic testing of acute and convalescent sera may be necessary to confirm the relationship between the virus and the illness in question.

Prevention and Treatment

In the past, killed virus vaccines produced from serotypes 3, 4, and 7 were found effective in reducing illness in military recruits. The vaccine was discontinued, however, when it was found that types 3 and 7 were capable of inducing tumors in newborn hamsters. More recently, a live virus vaccine containing serotypes 4 and 7, enclosed in enteric coated capsules and administered orally, has been used in military recruit groups. The viruses are released into the small intestine, where they produce an asymptomatic, nontransmissible infection. This vaccine has been found effective, but is neither available nor recommended for civilian groups. There is no specific therapy for infection.

Rhinoviruses

Multiple serotypes of small, naked RNA viruses

Optimum temperature 33°C

The rhinovirus group comprises 89 accepted serotypes and many more that are not yet classified. They are picornaviruses—small (20–30 nm), naked particles containing single-stranded, positive-sense RNA—and are distinguished from enteroviruses by their acid lability and an optimum temperature of 33°C for in vitro replication. This temperature approximates that of the nasopharynx in the human host and may be a factor in the localization of pathological findings at that site. These viruses are most consistently isolated in cultures of human diploid fibroblasts.

Clinical Disease

Common cold viruses

Rhinoviruses are known as the *common cold viruses*. They represent the major causes of mild URI syndromes in all age groups, especially older children and adults. Lower respiratory tract disease caused by rhinoviruses is uncommon. The usual incubation period is 2–3 days, and acute symptoms usually last 3–7 days.

Epidemiology

Rhinovirus infections may be seen at any time of the year. Epidemic peaks tend to occur in the early fall or spring months.

Prevention and Treatment

No effective method of prevention

Barriers to effective vaccines

There are no current methods of prevention with vaccines and no specific therapy. Prospects for the development of an appropriate vaccine appear dim. The multiplicity of serotypes and their tendency to be type specific in the production of antibodies would seem to demand the development of a multivalent vaccine, which would be extremely difficult to accomplish. However, recent studies have shown that a monoclonal antibody directed at a single cellular receptor might block attachment of the majority of rhinovirus serotypes, or even displace previously bound virions. It remains to be seen whether this observation can be translated into effective preventive or therapeutic applications. At present, the attitude toward these viruses is best summed up by Sir Christopher Andrewes, who suggested that we should perhaps accept these infections as "one of the stimulating risks of being mortal".*

Coronaviruses

Common cold virus

Coronaviruses contain a single-stranded, positive-sense RNA genome. This is surrounded by an envelope that includes a lipid bilayer derived from intracellular rough endoplasmic reticulum and Golgi membranes of infected cells. Petal- or club-shaped spikes (peplomers) measuring approximately 13 nm project from the surface of the envelope, giving the appearance of a crown of thorns or a solar corona. The peplomers play an important role in inducing neutralizing and cellular immune responses. Like the rhinoviruses, coronaviruses are considered primary causes of the common cold. Based on serologic studies, it is estimated that they may cause as many as 5–10% of common colds in adults and a similar proportion of lower respiratory illnesses in children.

The number of serotypes is unknown. Two strains (229E and OC43) have been studied to some extent; it is clear that they can cause outbreaks similar to those of the rhinoviruses, and that reinfection with the same serotype can occur.

Reoviruses

Uncertain association with human disease

The reoviruses (*r*espiratory *e*nteric *o*rphans) are naked virions that contain segmented, double-stranded RNA and replicate in the cytoplasm of infected cells. They are extremely ubiquitous and have been found in humans, simians, rodents, cattle, and a variety of other hosts. They have been studied in great detail as experimental models, revealing much basic knowledge about viral genetics and pathogenesis at the molecular level. Three serotypes are known to infect humans; however, their role and importance in human disease remains uncertain. Sporadic cases of febrile URI, exanthems, pneumonia, hepatitis, encephalitis, and gastroenteritis have all been reported to be associated with these viruses. Asymptomatic

---

* Andrewes, C.H. 1964. The complex epidemiology of respiratory virus infections. *Science* 146:1274.

shedding of reoviruses also occurs, which makes it difficult to prove association with disease.

Reoviruses can be isolated in cell cultures, particularly primary monkey kidney or human kidney monolayers.

Additional Reading

Influenza Viruses

Abramson, J.S., and Mills, E.L. 1988. Depression of neutrophil function induced by viruses and its role in secondary microbial infections. *Rev. Infect. Dis.* 10:326–341. This article reviews the functional neutrophil defects induced by influenza viruses, as well as what is known with respect to other viral agents.

Webster, R.G., Laver, W.G., Air, G.M., et al. 1982. Molecular mechanisms of variation in influenza viruses. *Nature* 296:115–121. An excellent review of "drifts," "shifts," and virulence.

Respiratory Syncytial Virus

Hall, C.B., Powell, K.R., MacDonald, N.E., et al. 1986. Respiratory syncytial viral infection in children with compromised immune function. *N. Engl. J. Med.* 315:77–81. An update on the impact of infection on normal children and those with underlying disorders.

Henderson, F.W., Collier, A.M., Clyde, W.A., et al. 1979. Respiratory-syncytial-virus infections, reinfections, and immunity in young children. *N. Engl. J. Med.* 300:530–534. Examination of the effect of prior exposure on subsequent infection with the same virus suggests that illness upon second infection may be no less severe than that with the first; however, the next reinfection may be modified.

Parainfluenza Viruses

Glezen, W.P., Frank, A.L., Taber, L.H., et al. 1984. Parainfluenza virus type 3: Seasonality and risk of infection and re-infection in young children. *J. Infect. Dis.* 150:851–857. The epidemiology and impact of infection caused by the most common parainfluenza serotype is discussed.

Adenoviruses

Fox, J.P., Hall, C.E., Cooney, M.K., et al. 1977. The Seattle virus watch VII. Observations of adenovirus infections. *Am. J. Epidemiol.* 105:362–386. The epidemiology and problems involved in associating adenoviruses with illnesses are analyzed.

Rhinoviruses

Collono, R.J., Callahan, P.L., and Long, W.J. 1986. Isolation of a monoclonal antibody that blocks attachment of the major group of human rhinoviruses. *J. Virol.* 57:7–12. The possibility of a novel immunologic approach to prevention, and even treatment, of picornavirus infections is raised.

Fox, J.P. 1976. Is a rhinovirus vaccine possible? *Am. J. Epidemiol.* 103:345–354. A good review of the immunologic relationships among the many rhinovirus serotypes.

Gwaltney, J.M., Jr., Moskalski, P.B., Hendly, J.O., et al. 1978. Hand-to-hand transmission of rhinovirus colds. *Ann. Intern. Med.* 88:463–467. An interesting study of the efficiency of spread of rhinoviruses by various routes.

Reoviruses

Sharpe, A.H., and Fields, B.N. 1985. Pathogenesis of viral infections: basic concepts derived from the reovirus model. *N. Engl. J. Med.* 312:486–497. A clearly presented review of the molecular basis of reovirus pathogenesis, drawing interesting comparisons with other viruses.

33

Viruses of Mumps and Childhood Exanthems

C. George Ray

The major viruses to be described in this chapter (mumps, measles, rubella, and the human parvovirus B19) represent totally different virus families; however, they share several common epidemiologic characteristics: 1) distribution is worldwide, with a high incidence of infection in nonimmune individuals; 2) humans appear to be the sole reservoir of infection; and 3) person-to-person spread is primarily via the respiratory (aerosol) route.

The other disease discussed in this chapter is roseola infantum, a common infection of which little is known concerning pathogenesis.

Mumps

Paramyxovirus

Enveloped single-stranded RNA virus; hemagglutinating and neuraminidase activity

Mumps virus is a paramyxovirus, and only one antigenic type is known. Like fellow members of its genus, it contains single-stranded, negative-sense RNA surrounded by an envelope. There are two glycoproteins on the surface of the envelope; one mediates neuraminidase and hemagglutinating activity, and the other is responsible for lipid membrane fusion to the host cell. It shares the morphologic and cultural features of parainfluenza virus type 2; however, there is no apparent cross-immunity between the two viruses.

Clinical Outline of Disease and Outcome

Incubation period

Parotitis

Complications involving other organs

After an incubation period of 12–29 days (average, 16–18 days), the typical case is characterized by fever and swelling with tenderness of the salivary glands, especially the parotid glands. Swelling may be unilateral or bilateral and persists for 7–10 days. Several complications can occur, usually within 1–3 weeks after onset of illness. All appear to be a direct result of virus spread to other sites and illustrate the extensive tissue

517

tropism of mumps. Complications, which can occur without parotitis, include infection of the following:

1. *Meninges.* Approximately 10% of all infected patients develop meningitis. It is usually mild, but can be confused with bacterial meningitis. In about one-third of these cases, associated or preceding evidence of parotitis is absent.

2. *Brain.* Encephalitis is occasionally severe.

3. *Spinal cord and peripheral nerves.* Transverse myelitis or polyneuritis are rare.

4. *Pancreas.* Pancreatitis is suggested by abdominal pain and vomiting.

5. *Testes.* Orchitis is estimated to occur in 10–20% of infected men. Although there is concern regarding subsequent sterility, it appears that such a sequel is quite rare.

6. *Ovaries.* Oophoritis is an unusual, usually benign inflammation of the ovarian glands.

7. Other rare and transient complications occur, including myocarditis, nephritis, arthritis, thyroiditis, thrombocytopenic purpura, mastitis, and pneumonia.

The complications are acute and usually resolve without sequelae within 2–3 weeks; occasional permanent effects have been noted, however, particularly in cases of severe central nervous system infection, where sensorineural hearing loss and other impairment can occur.

Pathogenesis and Immunity

Viremic phases

After initial entry into the respiratory tract, the virus replicates locally. Replication is followed by viremic dissemination to target tissues such as the salivary glands or central nervous system. It is also possible that before development of immune responses, a secondary phase of viremia may result from virus replication in target tissues, for example, initial parotid involvement with later spread to other organs. Viruria is common, probably as a result of direct spread from the blood into the urine as well as active viral replication in the kidney. Virtually all infections are associated with discernible impairment of renal function.

Spread to target tissues

Viruria

Possible roles of cellular immune responses in pathogenesis and immunity

Immunity is associated with the presence of neutralizing antibody. The role of cellular immune responses is not clear, but they may contribute both to the pathogenesis of the acute disease and to recovery from infection. It is known that acute infection can cause a transient diminution of delayed-type hypersensitivity to previously recognized antigens, such as tuberculin protein.

Pathology

The tissue response is that of cell necrosis and inflammation with predominantly mononuclear cell infiltration. In the salivary glands swelling and desquamation of necrotic epithelial lining cells, accompanied by interstitial inflammation and edema, may be seen within dilated ducts.

Antibody Responses

Lifelong IgG response

As in most viral infections, the early antibody response is predominantly with IgM, which is replaced gradually over several weeks by specific IgG antibody. The latter persists for a lifetime, but can often be detected only by specific neutralization assays. After primary infection, immunity to reinfection is virtually always permanent.

Epidemiology

High infectivity

The highest frequency of infection is observed in the 5- to 15-year age group. Infection is rarely seen in the first year of life. Although about 85% of susceptible household contacts will acquire infection, approximately 30–40% of these contacts will not develop clinical disease. The disease is communicable from approximately 7 days before until 9 days after onset of illness; however, virus has been recovered in urine for up to 14 days following onset. The highest incidence of infection is usually during the late winter and spring months, but can occur during any season.

Laboratory Diagnosis

Specimens

Cell culture

Mumps virus can be readily isolated early in the illness from the saliva, pharynx, and other affected sites, such as the cerebrospinal fluid. The urine is also an excellent source for virus isolation. Mumps virus grows well in primary monolayer cell culture derived from monkey kidney, producing syncytial giant cells and viral hemagglutinin, and can be isolated in other cell systems as well as in the allantoic cavity of embryonated hen's eggs.

Detection of viral antigen

Rapid diagnosis can be made by direct detection of viral antigen in pharyngeal cells or urine sediment by direct immunofluorescence.

Serodiagnosis by complement fixation

V and S antigens

Serologic diagnosis is usually accomplished with the complement fixation test. Two virion antigens can be employed: the S (soluble) nucleocapsid antigen and the V (viral) antigen, which is a component of the viral envelope. Antibody to the S antigen rises as quickly as 3 days after onset of symptoms, then usually disappears in 6–8 months. Antibody to the V antigen rises more slowly; it peaks 2–4 weeks after onset, then remains detectable for years afterward. Other serologic tests may also be used, such as hemagglutination inhibition and neutralization. Of these, the neutralization test is the most sensitive for detection of immunity to infection.

Prevention

Live vaccine

Since 1968, a live, attenuated vaccine has been available that is safe and highly effective. It is produced by serial propagation of virus in chick embryo cell tissue cultures. A single dose causes seroconversion in more than 95% of recipients. Duration of immunity, although not yet established, appears to be greater than 10 years and may be lifelong. This vaccine is currently recommended for infants after the first year of life and for adults (particularly men) who may be susceptible and at high risk of exposure.

Treatment

Immune serum globulin or mumps hyperimmune globulin are no longer recommended for the prevention or treatment of mumps. No specific therapy is available.

Measles

Paramyxovirus

Common synonyms for measles include *rubeola*, *5-day measles*, or *hard measles*. The virus is classified in the paramyxovirus family, genus *Morbillivirus*. It contains linear, negative-sense, single-stranded RNA, which

Enveloped single-stranded RNA virus with hemagglutinating and fusion glycoproteins

codes for at least six virion structural proteins. Of these, three are in the envelope, comprising a matrix (M) protein that plays a key role in viral assembly and two glycoprotein projections (peplomers). One of the projections is a hemagglutinin (H), which mediates adsorption to cell surfaces; the other (F) mediates cell fusion, hemolysis, and viral entry into the cell. No neuraminidase activity is present. Only a single serotype restricted to human infection is recognized. Two antigenically similar viruses, rinderpest of cattle and canine distemper virus, have not been shown to cause human infection.

Clinical Outline of Disease and Outcome

Incubation period

Prodromal signs

Koplik's spots

Rash

Systemic signs

The incubation period ranges from 7 to 18 days. A typical illness usually begins 9–11 days after exposure, with cough, coryza, conjunctivitis, and fever. One to three days after onset, pinpoint gray-white spots surrounded by erythema (grains-of-salt appearance) appear on mucous membranes. This sign, called *Koplik's spots*, is usually most noticeable over the buccal mucosa opposite the molars and persists for 1–2 days. Within a day of the appearance of Koplik's spots, the typical measles rash begins, first on the head, then on the trunk and extremities. The rash is maculopapular and semiconfluent; it persists for 3–5 days before fading. Fever and severe systemic symptoms gradually diminish as the rash progresses to the extremities. Lymphadenopathy is also common with particularly noticeable involvement of the cervical nodes.

Disease can be severe

The disease can be very severe, especially in immunocompromised or malnourished patients. Death may result from overwhelming viral infection of the host, with extensive involvement of the respiratory tract and other viscera, or from other related causes. In some developing countries, mortality of 15–25% has been recorded.

Bacterial superinfection

Bacterial superinfection, the most common complication, occurs in 5–15% of all cases. Such infections include acute otitis media, mastoiditis, sinusitis, pneumonia, and sepsis.

Central nervous system effects

Clinical signs of encephalitis will develop in 1 of 500–1000 cases. This complication, which usually occurs 3–14 days after onset of illness, can be extremely severe. The mortality in measles encephalitis is approximately 15%, and permanent neurologic damage among survivors is estimated at 25%.

Thrombocytopenic purpura

Acute thrombocytopenic purpura may also develop during the acute phase of illness, leading to bleeding episodes. Abdominal pain and acute appendicitis can occur secondary to inflammation and swelling of lymphoid tissue.

Depressed cell-mediated immunity

Subacute sclerosing panencephalitis

Both wild and attenuated (vaccine) measles viruses have been shown to depress delayed hypersensitivity and cell-mediated immunity significantly for as long as several weeks. Exacerbation of chronic granulomatous infections such as tuberculosis can result. Measles has also been implicated in a rare, smoldering, usually fatal encephalitis known as *subacute sclerosing panencephalitis*, which will be discussed later in this section.

Pathogenesis and Immunity

Local multiplication

Effect of virus on the cell

After implantation in the upper respiratory tract, viral replication proceeds in the respiratory mucosal epithelium. The effect within individual respiratory cells is profound. Even though measles does not directly restrict host cell metabolism, susceptible cells are damaged or destroyed by virtue of the intense viral replicative activity and the promotion of cell fusion

Viremic dissemination

with formation of syncytia. This results in disruption of the cellular cytoskeleton, chromosomal disorganization, and the appearance of inclusion bodies within the nucleus and cytoplasm. Replication is followed by viremic and lymphatic dissemination throughout the host to distant sites, including lymphoid tissues, bone marrow, abdominal viscera, and skin. Virus can be demonstrated in the blood, in the prodromal phase of illness, and viruria persists for up to 4 days after the onset of rash. During the viremic phase, measles infects T and B lymphocytes, circulating monocytes, and polymorphonuclear leukocytes without producing cytolysis.

Effects on immune mechanisms

The effect on B lymphocytes has been shown to suppress immunoglobulin synthesis; in addition, generation of natural killer cell activity appears to be impaired. There is also evidence that the capability of polymorphonuclear leukocytes to generate oxygen radicals is diminished, perhaps directly by the virus or by activated T suppressor cells. This may further explain the observed enhanced susceptibility to bacterial superinfections. In addition, virion components can be detected in biopsy specimens of Koplik's spots and vascular endothelial cells in the areas of skin rash.

Role of CMI in disease and immunity

Although cell-mediated immune responses to other antigens may be acutely depressed during measles infection, there is evidence that measles virus-specific cell-mediated immunity developing early in infection plays a role in mediating some of the features of disease, such as the rash, and is necessary to promote recovery from the illness. Antibodies to the virus appear in the first few days of illness, peak in 2–3 weeks, then persist at

Lifelong immunity

low levels. Immunity to reinfection is lifelong and is associated with the presence of neutralizing antibody. In patients with defects in cell-mediated immunity, including those with severe protein–calorie malnutrition, the infection is prolonged, tissue involvement is more severe, and complications such as progressive viral pneumonia are common.

Pathology

In addition to necrosis and inflammatory changes in the respiratory tract epithelium, several other features of measles virus infection are noteworthy. The skin lesions show vasculitis characterized by vascular dilatation, edema, and perivascular mononuclear cell infiltrates. The lymphoid tissues show hyperplastic changes, and large multinucleated giant cells are often observed (Warthin-Finkeldey cells). Some of the giant cells contain intracytoplasmic and intranuclear inclusions. Similar giant cells can be found in the respiratory tract epithelium and urinary sediment.

Vasculitis

Giant cells

Inclusions

Lesions in encephalitis

The major findings in measles encephalitis include areas of edema, scattered petechial hemorrhages, perivascular mononuclear cell infiltrates, and necrosis of neurons. In some cases, perivenous demyelination in the CNS is also observed, suggesting an autoimmune pathogenesis.

Epidemiology

Childhood disease

The highest attack rates have been in childhood, usually sparing infants less than 6 months of age because of passively acquired antibody; however, a shift in age-specific attack rates to greater involvement of adolescents and young adults has been observed recently in the United States. This

Recent increase in infection in young adults

shift is believed to be attributable to the influence of immunization: younger children may be better immunized to limit spread of the virus, whereas older age groups may have missed effective immunization or earlier infection by the wild virus.

Epidemic cycles

Epidemics tend to occur during the winter and spring in 1- to 3-year cycles. The infection rate among exposed susceptible subjects in a classroom or household setting is estimated at 85%, and over 95% of those infected will become ill. The period of communicability is estimated to be 3–5 days before appearance of the rash to 4 days afterward.

High infectivity

Laboratory Diagnosis

Virus isolation

Giant cells in cell culture

Rapid diagnosis by fluorescent antibody

Serodiagnosis

The typical measles infection can usually be diagnosed on the basis of clinical findings. When the disease is atypical, laboratory confirmation may be necessary. Virus isolation from the oropharynx or urine is usually most productive in the first 5 days of illness. Measles grows on a variety of cell cultures, producing multinucleated giant cells similar to those observed in infected host tissues. If rapid diagnosis is desired, measles antigen may be identified in urinary sediment or pharyngeal cells by direct fluorescent antibody methods. Serologic diagnosis using complement fixation, hemagglutination inhibition, or indirect fluorescent antibody methods is also commonly used and requires acute and convalescent serum samples.

Prevention

Live, attenuated vaccine

Vaccination after 1 year of age

Long duration of immunity after vaccination

Contraindications to vaccination

Passive protection

Dangers of killed vaccines

Live, attenuated measles vaccine is available and highly immunogenic. To ensure effective immunization, the vaccine should be administered to infants after the first year of life (preferred routine immunization is at 13–15 months of age). In children less than 1 year old vaccine efficacy is occasionally impaired, probably because of the persistence of maternal antibody and the relatively lower immunologic responsiveness to some antigens early in life. Immunity induced by the vaccine may be lifelong. Reactions to vaccination, usually in the form of fever and occasional rash, are rarely severe. This is no clear evidence of vaccine-caused encephalitis to date. Because the vaccine contains live virus, it should not be administered to immunocompromised patients, and it is not recommended for pregnant women, except in exceptional situations.

Exposed susceptible patients who are immunologically compromised (including small infants) may be given immune serum globulin intramuscularly. This treatment can modify or prevent disease if given within 6 days of exposure, but protection is transient.

Killed measles virus vaccines, commonly used before 1965, are no longer available. It has been shown that vaccine virus killed or inadvertently inactivated by improper storage methods is not only a poor immunogen, but may also cause other difficulties: 1) It can sensitize some individuals, who will then develop severe local inflammatory reactions upon subsequent inoculation with live vaccine; and 2) the sensitization may result in severe atypical illness (atypical measles syndrome) when the patient is exposed to the wild virus later in life. This syndrome is characterized by abrupt onset of high fever, often with abdominal pain and pneumonia, and the appearance of a rash, predominantly over the extremities. The rash may be papular, vesicular, or hemorrhagic.

Treatment

No specific therapy is available other than supportive measures and close observation for the development of complications such as bacterial superinfection.

Subacute Sclerosing Panencephalitis

Progressive neurologic disease of children

Subacute sclerosing panencephalitis is a progressive neurologic disease of children, which usually begins 2–10 years after a measles infection. It is characterized by insidious onset of personality change, poor school performance, progressive intellectual deterioration, development of myoclonic jerks (periodic muscle spasms), and motor dysfunctions such as spasticity, tremors, loss of coordination, and ocular abnormalities, including cortical blindness. Neurologic and intellectual deterioration generally progresses over 6–12 months, with the child eventually becoming bedridden and stuporous. Dysfunctions of the autonomic nervous system, such as difficulty with temperature regulation, may develop. Progressive inanition, superinfection, and metabolic imbalances eventually lead to death.

Pathologic features

Most of the pathologic features of the disease are localized to the central nervous system and retina. Both the gray and the white matter of the brain are involved, the most noteworthy feature being the presence of intranuclear and intracytoplasmic inclusions in oligodendroglial and neuronal cells.

Chronic measles virus infection

The disease is a result of chronic measles virus infection of the central nervous system. Evidence for this conclusion includes 1) elevated measles antibody titers in the cerebrospinal fluid (CSF); 2) intranuclear and intracytoplasmic inclusions characteristic of a paramyxovirus in brain cells; 3) demonstration of measles-specific antigen by immunofluorescent testing in brain cells; and 4) isolation of measles virus from brain tissue and lymph nodes by cocultivation rescue techniques. Patients with subacute sclerosing panencephalitis have been shown to fail to respond immunologically to the M (matrix) protein of the measles virus, which plays a key role in virus assembly, probably in nucleocapsid alignment beneath the cytoplasmic membrane before budding. Further studies have shown that patients have a variety of patterns of missing measles virus structural proteins in brain tissue. Thus, any of several defects in viral gene expression may prevent normal viral assembly, allowing persistence of defective virus at an intracellular site with failure of immune eradication.

Incomplete measles virus in brain tissue

Rarely, a similar progressive, degenerative neurologic disorder may be related to persistent rubella virus infection of the central nervous system. This condition is seen most often in adolescents who have had congenital rubella syndrome. Rubella virus has been isolated from brain tissue in these patients, again using cocultivation techniques.

Epidemiology

The mean annual incidence of subacute sclerosing panencephalitis in the United States is 3.5 cases per 10 million persons less than 20 years of age. The disease appears to be twice as frequent in male as in female subjects. Its occurrence in the United States has decreased markedly over the past 15 years with the widespread use of live measles vaccine.

Reduced incidence after introduction of measles vaccine

At present, there is no accepted effective therapy of subacute sclerosing panencephalitis.

Rubella

Enveloped, single-stranded RNA togavirus

Rubella, commonly known as *German measles* or *3-day measles*, is classified as a member of the togavirus family. It is enveloped and contains single-stranded RNA. There is only one serotype, and no extrahuman reservoirs are known to exist. The virus can agglutinate some types of red blood cells, such as those obtained from 1-day-old chicks and trypsin-treated human type O cells.

Hemagglutinin

Teratogenicity

Rubella was considered a mild, benign exanthem of childhood until 1941, when the Australian ophthalmologist Sir Norman Gregg described the profound defects that could be induced in the fetus as a result of maternal infection. Since 1962, when the virus was first isolated, knowledge regarding its extreme medical importance and biologic characteristics has increased rapidly.

Clinical Outline of Disease and Outcome

Mild illness with lymphadenopathy

Rash

Arthralgia

The incubation period for acquired infection is 14–21 days (average, 16 days). Illness is generally very mild, consisting primarily of low-grade fever, upper respiratory symptoms, and lymphadenopathy, which is most prominent in the posterior cervical and postauricular areas. A macular rash often follows within a day of onset and lasts for 1–3 days. This rash is usually most prominent over the head, neck, and trunk, and may be quite faint. Petechial lesions may also be seen over the soft palate during the acute phase. The most common complication is arthralgia or overt arthritis, which may affect joints of the fingers, wrists, elbows, knees, and ankles. The joint problems, which occur most frequently in women, rarely last longer than a few days to 3 weeks. Other, rarer complications include thrombocytopenic purpura and encephalitis.

Mimicry of other viral infections

Because of the rather nonspecific nature of the illness, a diagnosis of rubella cannot be made on clinical grounds alone. More than 30 other viral agents, which will be discussed later in this chapter, can produce a similar illness. Confirmation of the diagnosis requires laboratory studies.

Fetal damage

High risk in first trimester

Major lesions of congenital rubella

The major significance of rubella is not the acute illness, but the risk of fetal damage in pregnant women, particularly when they contract primary infection during the first trimester. The risk of fetal malformation and chronic fetal infection, which is estimated to be as high as 80% if infection occurs in the first 2 weeks of gestation, decreases to 6–10% by the 14th week. The overall risk during the first trimester is estimated at 20–30%. Clinical manifestations of congenital rubella syndrome vary, but may include any combination of the following major findings: 1) cardiac defects, commonly patent ductus arteriosus and pulmonary valvular stenosis; 2) eye defects such as cataracts, chorioretinitis, glaucoma, coloboma, cloudy cornea, and microphthalmia; 3) nerve deafness; 4) enlargement of liver and spleen; 5) thrombocytopenia; and 6) intrauterine growth retardation. Other findings include 1) central nervous system defects such as microcephaly, mental retardation, and encephalitis; 2) anemia; 3) transient immunodeficiency; 4) interstitial pneumonia, sometimes chronic; and 5) intravascular coagulation, hepatitis, rash, and other congenital malformations. Late complications of congenital rubella syndrome have also been described, including an apparent increased risk of diabetes mellitus, chronic thyroiditis, and occasionally the development of a progressive, subacute panencephalitis in the second decade of life.

Late complications of congenital rubella

Some congenitally infected infants may appear entirely normal at birth, and sequelae such as hearing or learning deficits may not become apparent until months later. The spectrum of defects thus varies from subtle to severe.

Pathogenesis and Immunity

Upper respiratory infection and viremic spread

In acquired infection, the virus enters the host via the upper respiratory tract, replicates, then spreads via the bloodstream to distant sites, including lymphoid tissues, skin, and organs. Viremia in these infections has been

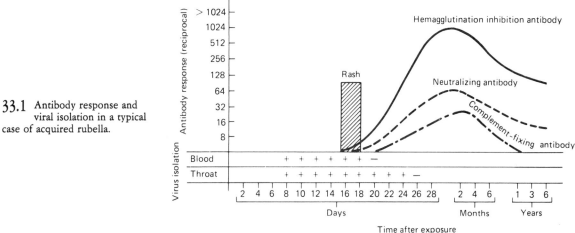

33.1   Antibody response and viral isolation in a typical case of acquired rubella.

Role of cell-mediated immunity and immune complexes

detected for as long as 8 days before to 2 days after onset of the rash, and virus shedding from the oropharynx can be detected up to 8 days after onset (Figure 33.1). Cellular immune responses and circulating virus–antibody immune complexes are thought to play a role in mediating the inflammatory responses to infection, such as rash and arthritis. After infection the serum antibody titer rises, with a peak within 2–3 weeks after onset. Natural infection also results in the production of specific secretory IgA antibodies in the respiratory tract. Immunity to disease is nearly always lifelong; however, reexposure can lead to transient respiratory tract acquisition, with an anamnestic rise in IgG and secretory IgA antibodies, but without resultant viremia or illness.

Transmission to fetus

Persistent fetal infection

Reasons for fetal defects

Congenital infection occurs as a result of maternal viremia, placental infection, and transplacental spread to the fetus. Once fetal infection occurs, it persists chronically. Such persistence is probably related to an inability to eliminate the virus by immune or interferon-mediated mechanisms. There is too little inflammatory change in the fetal tissues to explain the pathogenesis of the congenital defects. Possibilities include placental and fetal vasculitis with compromise of fetal oxygenation, chronic viral infection of cells leading to impaired mitosis, cellular necrosis, and induction of chromosomal breakage. Any or all of these factors may operate at a critical stage of organogenesis to induce permanent defects. Viral persistence with circulating virus–antibody immune complexes may evoke inflammatory changes postnatally and produce continuing tissue damage.

Continuing infection and dissemination after birth

After birth, affected infants continue to excrete the virus in the throat, urine, and intestinal tract (Fig. 33.2). Virus may be isolated from virtually all tissues in the first few weeks of life. Shedding of virus in the throat and urine, which persists for at least 6 months in most cases, has been known to continue for as long as 30 months. Virus has also been isolated from lens tissue removed 3–4 years later. These observations underscore the fact that such infants are an important reservoir in perpetuating virus transmission.

The prolonged virus shedding is somewhat puzzling, as it does not represent a typical example of immunologic tolerance. The affected infants

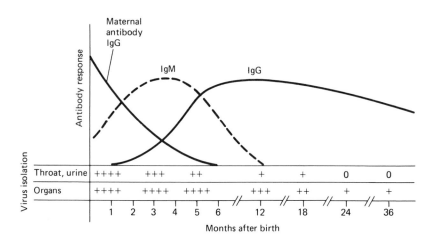

33.2 Persistence of rubella virus and antibody in congenitally infected infants.

are usually able to produce circulating IgM and IgG antibodies to the virus (Figure 33.2), although antibodies may decrease to undetectable levels after 3–4 years. Many infants show evidence of depressed rubella virus-specific cell-mediated immunity during the first year of life.

Pathology

Postnatal disease

Because postnatally acquired disease is usually mild, little is known about its pathology. Mononuclear cell inflammatory changes can be observed in tissues, and viral antigen can be detected in the same sites (for example, skin and synovial fluid).

Fetal disease

Congenital infections are characterized primarily by the various malformations. Necrosis of tissues such as myocardium and vascular endothelium may also be seen, and quantitative studies suggest a decrease in cell quantity in affected organs. In severe cases, normal calcium deposition in the metaphyses of long bones is delayed, which creates a "celery-stalk" appearance on a radiograph.

Epidemiology

Seasonality

Infections are usually observed during the winter and spring months. In contrast to measles, which has a high clinical attack rate among exposed susceptible individuals, only 30–60% of rubella-infected susceptible persons will develop clinically apparent disease. Although rubella is highly contagious, an estimated 15% of young adults escape natural infection during childhood. A major focus of concern is the susceptible woman of childbearing age, who carries a risk of exposure during pregnancy. Disease in patients with primary acquired infections is contagious from 7 days before to 7 days after the onset of rash; as mentioned previously, congenitally infected infants may spread the virus to others for 6 months or more after birth.

Low virulence, high infectivity

Duration of infectivity

Laboratory Diagnosis

Cell cultures: rarely used in routine diagnosis

The virus may be isolated from respiratory secretions in the acute phase (and from urine, tissues, and feces in congenitally infected infants) by inoculation into a variety of cell cultures. The cell cultures required are not usually employed routinely in the laboratory, however, and isolation can be expensive, tedious, and time consuming, requiring as long as 2 weeks for the development of interfering or cytopathic effects.

Serodiagnosis

Serologic diagnosis is usually employed in acquired infections; paired acute and convalescent samples collected 10–21 days apart are used. The

Hemagglutination inhibition test

hemagglutination inhibition test is used most often, but complement fixation, indirect fluorescent antibody, enzyme-linked immunosorbent assay, and other tests are available.

Determination of IgM-specific antibody is sometimes useful to ascertain whether an infection occurred in the past several months; it has also been used in the diagnosis of congenital infections. Unfortunately, there are

Value and pitfalls of IgM tests

certain pitfalls in interpreting this test: Some individuals (less than 5%) with acquired infections may have persistent elevations of IgM-specific antibodies for 200 days or more afterward, and some congenitally infected infants will not produce detectable IgM-specific antibodies.

Serologic tests to detect susceptibility

Serologic testing is also used to determine potential susceptibility or immunity to infection. The presence of antibodies at or above the threshold level (for example, 1:8 or 1:10 with the hemagglutination inhibition test) indicates a very high probability of immunity (titers of 1:16 or greater are particularly reassuring), whereas titers below the threshold (undetectable) suggest lack of immunity. Such testing is often done to determine which individuals are susceptible, such as female adolescents, who require closer surveillance and consideration for immunization when such a pro-

Role in preventing or detecting fetal exposure

cedure can be safely performed. It is particularly important to determine the immune status of women who are pregnant or contemplating pregnancy, in case exposure should occur subsequently. If the woman has serologic proof of prior immunity, the risk to the fetus if she is accidentally exposed is nil; if not, and exposure occurs during pregnancy, careful serologic monitoring is necessary. Termination of the pregnancy may be considered if there is serologic evidence of primary infection.

Prevention

Live, attenuated rubella vaccine

Since 1969, live attenuated rubella vaccines have been available for routine immunization. The current vaccine virus, grown in human diploid fibroblast cell cultures (RA 27/3), has been shown to be highly effective: it causes seroconversion in approximately 95% of recipients. Interestingly, significant seroconversion is often associated with excretion of the vaccine virus in the pharynx; however, it does not appear to be communicable. Routine immunization is now recommended for infants after the first year of life

Indications for immunization

and for other individuals with no history of immunization and lack of immunity by serologic testing. Target groups include female adolescents

Complications and contraindications

and hospital personnel in a high-risk setting. Complications of the vaccine, although similar to those of the acquired, wild virus disease, are far less frequent and usually milder. They include occasional rash, fever, and joint complaints; the latter are more common in women. The vaccine is contraindicated in immunocompromised patients and in pregnancy. To date, over 200 instances of accidental vaccination of susceptible pregnant women have been reported, with no clinically apparent adverse effects on the fetus; however, it is strongly recommended that immunization be avoided in this setting, and that nonpregnant women avoid conception for at least 3 months after receiving the vaccine.

Duration of artificial immunity

Vaccine-induced immunity may be lifelong. Further follow-up is necessary, however, before any conclusions can be made. Studies to date indicate that the duration of protection is at least 16 years.

Immune serum globulin has not been shown of significant value in post-exposure prophylaxis, and it is not routinely recommended.

Treatment

Other than supportive measures, there is no specific therapy for either the acquired or the congenital infection.

Parvovirus B19 Infections

Small naked, single-stranded DNA viruses

Parvoviruses are very small (18–26 nm), naked virions containing a linear single-stranded DNA molecule that codes for as few as three proteins. Diseases due to parvoviruses have been recognized among nonhuman hosts for a number of years. Notable among these are canine parvovirus and feline panleukopenia virus, which produce particularly severe infections among puppies and kittens, respectively. These do not appear to cross species barriers. Recently, a human parvovirus, B19, has been discovered and described, but our understanding of it is far from complete. At least two clinical syndromes are now associated with this virus: aplastic crisis and erythema infectiosum.

Human parvovirus associated with aplastic crisis and erythema infectiosum

Replicates in erythroid precursor nuclei

Inhibits erythropoiesis

Little is currently known regarding the pathogenesis of parvovirus B19. It can be grown in cultures of human bone marrow cells from some patients with hemolytic anemias, and the site of replication appears to be the nucleus of an immature cell in the erythrocyte lineage. Such infected cells then cease to proliferate, resulting in an impairment of normal erythrocyte development. The clinical consequences of this effect are generally trivial, unless the patient is already compromised by a chronic hemolytic process, such as sickle-cell disease or thalassemia, in which maximal erythropoiesis is continually needed to counterbalance increased destruction of circulating erythrocytes. Primary infection by parvovirus B19 in such patients often produces an acute, severe, sometimes fatal anemia manifested as a rapid fall in red blood cell counts and hemoglobin. This may present initially with no clinical symptoms other than fever.

Aplastic crisis

Erythema infectiosum

Another more common disease that is now clearly attributable to parvovirus B19 is erythema infectiosum (also referred to as *fifth disease* or *academy rash*). After an incubation period of 4–12 days, a mild illness appears, characterized by fever, malaise, headache, myalgia, and itching in varying degrees. A confluent, indurated rash appears on the face, giving a "slapped-cheek" appearance. The rash spreads in a day or two to other areas, particularly exposed surfaces such as the arms and legs, where it is usually macular and reticular (lacelike). During the acute phase, generalized lymphadenopathy or splenomegaly may be seen, along with a mild leukopenia and anemia. The illness lasts 1 to 2 weeks, but rash may recur for periods of 2 to 4 weeks thereafter, exacerbated by heat, sunlight, exercise, or emotional stress. Arthralgia sometimes persists or recurs for weeks to months, particularly in adolescent or adult females. Overt arthritis has also been reported in some. Serious complications are extremely rare; however, like rubella, active transplacental transmission of parvovirus B19 can occur during primary infections in pregnancy, sometimes resulting in stillbirth of fetuses that are profoundly anemic. The progress can be so severe that hypoxic damage to the heart, liver, and other tissues leads to extensive edema (hydrops fetalis). The frequency of such adverse outcomes is as yet undetermined.

Occasional severe fetal infection

Epidemiology

Epidemiologic evidence suggests that spread of the virus is primarily via the respiratory route, and high transmission rates occur in households.

Laboratory diagnosis

Outbreaks tend to be small and localized, particularly during the spring months, with the highest rates among children and young adults. Sero-epidemiologic studies have demonstrated evidence of past infection in 30–60% of adults. Laboratory confirmation of infection is presently difficult to obtain. Viremia, which usually lasts 7–12 days, may be detected by specific DNA probe or immunoprecipitation methods. Alternatively, the presence of IgM-specific antibody late in the acute phase or during convalescence strongly supports the diagnosis. It is important to be aware that erythema infectiosum is extremely variable in its clinical manifestations, and even the "classic" presentation can be mimicked by other agents, such as rubella or echoviruses. Before a firm diagnosis is made on clinical grounds, especially during outbreaks, it is wise to exclude the possibility of atypical rubella infection.

Roseola Infantum (Exanthem Subitum)

Association with human herpesvirus Type 6 and other viruses

Roseola infantum is a common, presumably viral, disease of infants and children 6 months to 4 years of age. Its alternative name, exanthem subitum, means "sudden rash." The apparent etiologic agent has been transmitted to human volunteers and monkeys and is now thought to be human herpesvirus type 6 (HHV-6) or a similar virus. The illness is characterized by abrupt onset of high fever, sometimes accompanied by brief, generalized convulsions and leukopenia. After 3 to 5 days, the fever diminishes rapidly, followed in a few hours by a faint, transient, macular rash.

Several other agents, including adenoviruses, Coxsackie viruses, and echoviruses, have been occasionally noted to cause this syndrome.

Other Causes of Rubella-like Rashes

In addition to erythema infectiosum, diseases due to numerous other agents can mimic rubella clinically. These agents include at least 17 echoviruses, nine Coxsackie viruses, several adenoviral serotypes, arboviruses such as dengue, Epstein–Barr virus, scarlet fever, and toxic drug eruptions, among others. Because of the wide variety of diagnostic possibilities, it is not possible to diagnose or rule out rubella confidently on clinical grounds alone. Therefore, a specific diagnosis requires specific laboratory studies. Because rubella is an infection with such significant impact on the fetus, serologic study to rule out this possibility is mandatory if the diagnosis is suspected during early pregnancy.

Additional Reading

Mumps

Beard, C.M., et al. 1977. The incidence and outcome of mumps orchitis in Rochester, Minnesota, 1935–1974. *Mayo Clin. Proc.* 52:3–7. Long-term follow-up and incidence and sequelae of mumps orchitis are discussed.

Hayden, G.F., et al. 1978. Current status of mumps and mumps vaccine in the United States. *Pediatrics* 62:965–969. The vaccine and its effectiveness and safety are reviewed.

Measles

Baczko, K., et al. 1986. Expression of defective measles virus genes in brain tissues of patients with subacute sclerosing panencephalitis. *J. Virol.* 59:472–478. A molecular study that helps clarify our current concepts of measles virus persistence.

Frank, J.A., Jr., et al. 1985. Major impediments to measles elimination. *Am. J. Dis. Child.* 139:881–888. Reviews the modern epidemiology of measles and future strategies for elimination.

Johnson, R.T., et al. 1984. Measles encephalomyelitis—Clinical and immunologic studies. *N. Engl. J. Med.* 310:137–141. Well-presented studies of patients, showing that measles encephalomyelitis probably has a pathogenesis similar to experimental allergic encephalomyelitis.

McChesney, M.B., et al. 1986. Viruses disrupt functions of lymphocytes. II. Measles virus suppresses antibody production by acting on B lymphocytes. *J. Exp. Med.* 163:1331–1336. This report reveals insight into the immunopathogenesis of measles.

Rubella

Miller, E., et al. 1982. Consequences of confirmed maternal rubella at successive stages of pregnancy. *Lancet* 2:781–784. A precise analysis of the risks of infection at various times during gestation.

Polk, B.F., et al. 1980. An outbreak of rubella among hospital personnel. *N. Engl. J. Med.* 303:541–545. The contagiousness of the virus and its impact in high-risk settings are illustrated.

Preblud, S.R. 1985. Some current issues relating to rubella vaccine. *J. Am. Med. Assoc.* 254:253–256. This article summarizes the key information concerning rubella vaccine over the previous 15 years.

Parvovirus B19

Anderson, L.J. 1987. Role of parvovirus B19 in human disease. *Pediatr. Infect. Dis. J.* 6:711–718. A review of the biology of the agent and its current relevance in humans.

Chorba, T., et al. 1986. The role of parvovirus B19 in aplastic crisis and erythema infectiosum (fifth disease). *J. Infect. Dis.* 154:383–393. Description of the epidemiology and laboratory diagnosis of a 1984 outbreak.

Ozawa, K., et al. 1986. Replication of the B19 parvovirus in human bone marrow cell cultures. *Science* 233:883–886. This study provides information on pathogenesis of the virus at cellular level.

Roseola Infantum (Exanthem Subitum)

Asano, Y., et al. 1989. Viremia and neutralizing antibody response in infants with exanthem subitum. *J. Pediatr.* 114:535–539. Virologic and serologic studies of 38 children with acute illness showed a high frequency of early human herpesvirus type 6 viremia with subsequent antibody responses.

34

Poxviruses

C. George Ray

The poxvirus family includes viruses that infect birds, mammals, and even insects. They are large, brick-shaped or ovoid, DNA-carrying virions (Figure 34.1) measuring approximately $100 \times 200 \times 300$ nm; their structure is complex, and replication occurs in the cytoplasm of infected cells. They possess an envelope, which is not acquired by budding and not essential for infectivity. The agents most important in human disease are variola, vaccinia, molluscum contagiosum, orf, cowpox, and pseudocowpox.

Variola (Smallpox)

Until very recently, smallpox played a significant role in world history with regard to both the serious epidemics recorded since antiquity and the sometimes dangerous measures taken to prevent infection.

Variola major and minor

Two types are known: variola major and variola minor (alastrim). Although the viruses are indistinguishable antigenically, their fatality rates differ considerably (less than 1% for variola minor, 3–35% for variola major). They are also difficult to distinguish in the laboratory; variola major, however, has slightly greater virulence in embryonated hen's eggs.

It is remarkable that, although these viruses are exceedingly infectious, they have been eradicated worldwide. Thus, any discussion of smallpox is now of more historic than practical interest.

Jenner's vaccination experiments

The first major step toward modern prevention and subsequent eradication of smallpox can be credited to Edward Jenner, who noted that milkmaids who develop mild cowpox lesions on their hands appeared immune to smallpox. He published evidence in 1798 indicating that purposeful inoculation of individuals with cowpox material could protect them against subsequent infection by smallpox. The concept of vaccination gradually evolved, with the modern use of live vaccinia virus, a poxvirus of uncertain origin, to produce specific immunity.

In 1967, the World Health Organization launched an ambitious pro-

531

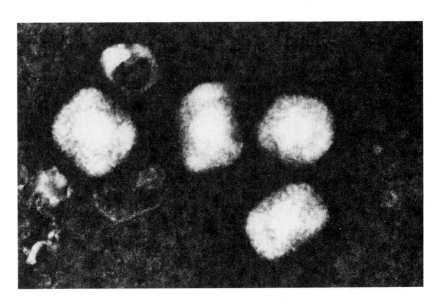

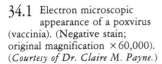
34.1 Electron microscopic appearance of a poxvirus (vaccinia). (Negative stain; original magnification ×60,000). (*Courtesy of Dr. Claire M. Payne.*)

Human reservoir only

No healthy carriers

Eradication by case finding, quarantine, and immunization

gram aimed at eradication of smallpox. This goal was considered realistic for two major reasons: 1) no extrahuman reservoir of the virus was known to exist; and 2) asymptomatic carriage apparently did not occur. The basic approach included intensive surveillance for clinical cases of smallpox, prompt quarantine of such patients and their contacts, and vaccination of contacts to prevent further spread. A tremendous amount of effort was involved, but the results were astonishing—the last recorded case of naturally acquired smallpox occurred in Somalia in 1977. After 2 more years of surveillance with discovery of no further infections, global eradication of smallpox was confirmed in 1979 and accepted by the World Health Organization in May 1980. Global eradication was followed up by destruction of virus kept by laboratories (one tragic episode of laboratory-transmitted smallpox occurred in 1978), with the exception of virus retained by two reference laboratories, one in Atlanta, Georgia, and one in Moscow, USSR. Vaccination is therefore no longer deemed necessary, except for the very few laboratory workers who may handle the virus.

Surveillance continues, including studies of poxviruses of animals (for example, whitepox, monkeypox) that are antigenically somewhat similar to smallpox. Some virologists remain legitimately concerned that an animal poxvirus could undergo mutation and become highly virulent to humans, although the probability of such an occurrence seems very low. Also, the possibility of escape of virus from a laboratory source, although highly unlikely, must be considered. Stockpiles of vaccine are maintained by several countries to block spread from any such event.

Clinical Outline of Disease and Outcome

The incubation period of smallpox was usually 12–14 days, although in occasional fulminating cases it could be as short as 4–5 days. The typical onset was abrupt, with fever, chills, and myalgia, followed by a rash 3–4 days later. The rash evolved to firm papulovesicles that became pustular over 10–12 days, then slowly healed. In contrast to varicella, only a single crop of lesions (all in the same stage of evolution) developed; these lesions were most prominent over the head and extremities (Figure 34.2). Some

Rash and clinical course

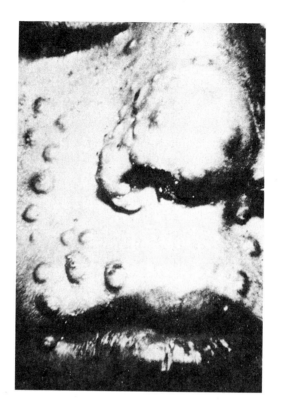

34.2 Close-up of facial lesions of smallpox during the first week of the illness.

Modifying effects of previous vaccination

cases of variola major were fulminant, with a hemorrhagic rash ("sledgehammer" smallpox). Death could result from the overwhelming primary viral infection or from bacterial superinfection. Previous vaccination, usually more than 3 years before the onset of infection, could shorten the evolution of the disease or modify it to a degree that sometimes made diagnosis difficult. The disease was highly contagious, and the virus could survive well in the extracellular environment. Acquisition of infection by respiratory spread or by exposure to dried crusts from skin lesions, contaminated articles, and fomites has been well documented.

Respiratory and fomite spread

Laboratory Diagnosis

Variola produces lesions (pocks) on the chorioallantoic membranes of embryonated hen's eggs; it will also infect a variety of cell cultures in vitro. Cytology of lesions shows cytoplasmic inclusions, but neither intranuclear inclusions nor giant cells. Direct electron microscopy and immunoprecipitin tests have also been applied to lesion specimens for rapid diagnosis.

Vaccinia

Origin

Vaccinia virus is serologically related to smallpox, although its exact origin is unknown. Some virologists believe it is a recombinant virus derived from smallpox and cowpox; others suggest it originated from a poxvirus of horses. The virus is usually propagated by dermal inoculation of calves, and the resultant vesicle fluid ("lymph") is lyophilized and used as a live virus vaccine in humans. The vaccine is inoculated into the epidermis and produces a localized lesion, which indicates successful immunization. The

Vaccination

Local reactions

Duration of immunity

Severe reactions

lesion becomes vesicular, then pustular, followed by crusting and healing over 10–14 days. The local reaction is sometimes severe and accompanied by systemic symptoms such as fever, rash, and lymphadenopathy.

Vaccinia-produced immunity to smallpox wanes rapidly after 3 years, becoming virtually absent after 20 years.

In addition to the local reactions, several other potentially serious and lethal complications can occur with vaccinia infection. These complications include encephalitis, progressive vaccinia (vaccinia gangrenosum, usually seen in immunocompromised patients), disseminated vaccinia, autoinoculation into the eye or mucous membranes, allergic reactions, and bacterial superinfection.

Recombinants as immunogens against unrelated agents

There has been a recent resurgence of scientific interest in vaccinia as a possible vector for active immunization against other diseases, such as hepatitis B, herpes simplex, or even human immunodeficiency virus. It has been shown that gene sequences coding for specific immunogenic proteins of other viruses can be inserted into the vaccinia virus genome, with subsequent expression as the virus replicates. For example, a recombinant vaccinia strain carrying the gene sequence for hepatitis B surface antigen (HbsAg) can infect cells, lead to production of HbsAg, and stimulate an antibody response to it. Theoretically, gene sequences coding for a variety of antigens could be packaged in a single viable vaccinia virus vector, thus allowing simultaneous active immunization against multiple agents. Whether such an approach will become safely applicable in clinical medicine remains to be seen.

Molluscum Contagiosum

Molluscum contagiosum is a benign, cutaneous poxvirus disease of humans, spread by direct contact with infected cells. It is usually acquired

Infection routes

by inoculation into minute skin abrasions; events that commonly lead to transmission include roughhousing in shower rooms and swimming pools, sharing of towels, and sexual contact.

Local lesions

After an incubation period of 2–8 weeks, nodular, pale, firm (pearl-like) lesions usually 2–10 mm in diameter develop in the epidermis. These lesions are painless and umbilicated in appearance. A cheesy material may be expressed from the pore at the center of each lesion. Local trauma may cause spread of lesions in the involved skin area. The lesions are not associated with systemic symptoms, and they disappear in 2–12 months without treatment. Specific treatment, if desired, is usually by curettage or careful removal of the central core by expression with forceps.

Histology

The pathologic findings, which are limited to the epidermis, include hyperplasia, ballooning degeneration, and acanthosis. The diagnosis, made on clinical grounds, can be confirmed by demonstration of large, eosinophilic cytoplasmic inclusions (molluscum bodies) in the affected superficial epithelial cells.

Orf

Orf is an old Saxon term for a human infection caused by a parapoxvirus of sheep and goats. Synonyms for the infection in animals include contagious pustular dermatitis, ecthyma contagiosum, pustular ecthyma, and "scabby mouth." Humans usually acquire the infection by close contact with young infected animals and accidental inoculation through cuts or abrasions on the hand or wrist. The typical skin lesion is solitary; it begins as a vesicle, then evolves into a nodular mass that later develops central necrosis. Regional lymphadenopathy sometimes develops; dissemination is rare. The average duration of the lesion is 35 days, followed by complete resolution. The diagnosis is usually made on the basis of clinical appearance and occupational history. Serologic confirmation or electron microscopy of the lesion can be done, but are rarely necessary.

Milker's Nodules and Cowpox

Milker's nodules (pseudocowpox) is a cutaneous poxvirus disease of cattle, distinct from cowpox, that can cause local skin infections similar to orf in exposed humans. Healing of the skin lesions may take 4–8 weeks. There is no cross-immunity to cowpox.

Cowpox is now very rare in the United States. It produces a vesicular eruption on the udders of cows and similar, usually localized, vesicular lesions in humans who are accidently exposed.

Additional Reading

Smith, G.L., et al. 1983. Infectious vaccinia virus recombinants that express hepatitis B virus surface antigen. *Nature* 302:490–495. This paper details the potential novel use of vaccinia virus recombinants as immunogens against totally unrelated infectious agents.

White, P.J., and Shackelford, P.G. 1983. Edward Jenner, M.D. and the scourge that was. *Am. J. Dis. Child.* 137:864–869. An informative review of the history of smallpox and its eradication.

35

Enteroviruses

C. George Ray

Enteroviruses comprise a major subgroup of small RNA viruses (picornaviruses) that readily infect and are shed from the intestinal tract. They include the polioviruses, Coxsackie viruses, echoviruses, and more recently discovered agents that are simply designated enteroviruses. The number of serotypes that can infect humans has grown to a total of 68, and more are likely to be found in the future.

Enteroviruses cause paralytic disease, mild acute aseptic meningitis syndromes, pleurodynia, exanthems, pericarditis, nonspecific febrile illness, and occasional fulminant encephalomyocarditis of the newborn. As more has been learned, it is apparent that the spectrum of disease is even broader. Some infections can lead to permanent damage, and others may trigger chronic, active disease processes.

These viruses, which have many features in common, will first be considered as a group. Some of the special features of important serotypes will be discussed in more detail later in this chapter.

Group Characteristics

Habitat

Worldwide occurrence

The enteroviruses of humans and animals are ubiquitous and have been found worldwide. Their name is derived from their ability to infect intestinal tract epithelial and lymphoid tissues and to be shed into the feces.

Morphologic and Biologic Features

Small, single-stranded RNA viruses

As a group, the enteroviruses are extremely small (22–30 nm in diameter), naked virions with icosahedral symmetry. They possess single-stranded, positive-sense RNA and four major polypeptides. Following replication and assembly in the cellular cytoplasm, new virus is released by cell destruction.

537

Table 35.1   Human Enteroviruses

Class	Number of Serotypes
Poliovirus	3
Coxsackie virus	
Group A	23
Group B	6
Echovirus	31
Enterovirus	5[a]

[a] More recently discovered enteroviruses, which have overlapping biologic characteristics, are identified numerically (types 68–72).

Enteroviruses are distinguished from rhinoviruses, which are also members of the picornavirus family, by their resistance to acid (pH 3.0), capability to replicate efficiently at 37°C, and a higher buoyant density. Another feature is cationic stability; in the presence of molar magnesium chloride, the viruses become more resistant to thermal inactivation. They are also resistant to many common disinfectants such as 70% alcohol, substituted phenolics, ether, and various detergents that readily inactivate most enveloped viruses. Chemical agents, such as 0.3% formaldehyde or free residual chlorine at 0.3–0.5 ppm, are effective; however, if there is sufficient extraneous organic debris present, the virus can be protected and survive for long periods.

Although some of the enterovirus serotypes share common antigens detectable by complement fixation, there are no significant serologic relationships between the major classes listed on Table 35.1. There are, thus, conserved and variable regions of enteroviral genomes within and between classes. Genetic variation within specific strains occurs, and mutants that exhibit antigenic drift and altered tropism for specific cell types are now recognized.

Polioviruses, which have been most extensively studied as enterovirus prototypes, are known to have epitopes on three surface structural proteins (VP1, VP2, and VP3) that induce type-specific neutralizing antibodies. This appears to be generally the case for all enteroviruses; definitive identification of isolates usually requires neutralization tests.

Growth in the Laboratory

Most of these agents can be isolated in primate (human or simian) cell cultures and show characteristic cytopathic effects; some strains, however, particularly several Coxsackie A serotypes, are grown with difficulty in cell cultures, and inoculation of newborn mice may be necessary for detection of virus. The newborn mouse, in fact, is one basis for originally classifying Coxsackie A and B viruses. After inoculation of mice at 24 hr of age or less and observing for 2–12 days, Coxsackie A viruses primarily cause a widespread, inflammatory, necrotic effect on skeletal muscle, leading to flaccid paralysis and death; similar inoculation of Coxsackie B viruses causes encephalitis, resulting in spasticity and occasionally convulsions. Other organs are variably affected, and histopathologic examination is sometimes helpful in distinguishing the two. Echoviruses and polioviruses rarely have an adverse effect on mice, unless special adaptation procedures are first employed. The higher-numbered enteroviruses (types 68–72),

(Margin notes: Resistance to chemical inactivation; Effectiveness of formaldehyde and hypochlorite; Mutations and drifts; Identification by neutralization tests; Growth in primate cell cultures; Effects of Coxsackie A and B viruses on newborn mice)

which have overlapping, variable growth and host characteristics, have been classified separately. Hepatitis A virus has been classified as enterovirus 72 or as a heparnavirus and is discussed in Chapter 36.

Host Range

Humans are the major natural host for the polioviruses, Coxsackie viruses, and echoviruses. There are enteroviruses of other animals with limited host ranges that do not appear to extend to humans. Conversely, viruses thought to be identical or related to human enteroviruses have been isolated from dogs and cats. Whether these agents cause disease in such animals is debatable, and there is no evidence of spread from animals to humans.

Epidemiology

Asymptomatic infections common

The enteroviruses have a worldwide distribution, and asymptomatic infection is common. The proportion of infected individuals who will develop illness varies from 2 to 100%, depending upon the serotype or strain involved and the age of the patient. Secondary infections in households are common and range as high as 40–70%, depending upon factors such as family size, crowding, and sanitary conditions.

Variation in dominant epidemic strains

In some years, certain serotypes emerge as dominant epidemic strains; they then may wane, only to reappear in epidemic fashion years later. For example, echovirus 16 was a major cause of outbreaks in the eastern United States in 1951 and 1974. Coxsackie B_1 virus was common in 1963, echovirus 9 in 1962, 1965, 1968, and 1969, and echovirus 30 in 1968 and 1969. The emergence of dominant serotypes is quite unpredictable from year to year.

Prevalence in summer and fall

All enteroviruses show a seasonal predilection; epidemics are usually observed during the summer and fall months. In subtropical and tropical climates, the duration of greatest transmission sometimes extends into the winter months.

Fecal–oral transmission

Direct or indirect fecal–oral transmission is considered the most common mode of spread. After infection, the virus will persist in the oropharynx for 1–4 weeks, and it can be shed in the feces for 1–18 weeks. Thus, sewage-contaminated water, fecally contaminated foods, or passive transmission by insect vectors (flies, cockroaches) may occasionally be the source of infection. More commonly, however, spread is directly from person to person. This mode of transmission is suggested by the high infection rates seen among young children, whose hygienic practices tend to be less than optimal, and in crowded households. Approximately two-thirds of all isolates are from children 9 years of age or younger.

Spread usually person to person

Most infections in children

Short incubation periods

Incubation periods vary, but relatively short intervals (2–10 days) are frequent. Often, illness will be seen concurrently in more than one family member, and the clinical features will vary within the household.

Pathogenesis and Pathology

Replication in upper respiratory and gastrointestinal tracts

After primary replication in the epithelial cells and lymphoid tissues in the upper respiratory and gastrointestinal tracts, viremic spread to other sites can occur. Potential target organs vary according to the virus strain and its tropism, but may include the central nervous system, heart, vascular endothelium, liver, pancreas, lungs, gonads, skeletal muscles, synovial tissues, skin, and mucous membranes. Histopathologic findings include cell

Viremic spread

Histopathology

Antibody response terminates replication

Clinical manifestations from lytic effects of virus

Probable immunopathologic manifestations include Coxsackie B myocarditis

Virus-induced autoimmune response

Serotype specificity of immunity

necrosis and mononuclear cell inflammatory infiltrates; in the central nervous system, the inflammatory cells are localized most prominently in perivascular sites. The initial tissue damage is thought to result from the lytic cycle of virus replication; secondary spread to other sites may ensue. Viremia is usually undetectable by the time symptoms appear, and termination of virus replication appears to correlate with the appearance of circulating neutralizing antibody, interferon, and mononuclear cell infiltration of infected tissue. The early antibody response is with immunoglobulin M(IgM), which usually wanes 6–12 weeks after onset to be progressively replaced by IgG-specific antibodies. The important role of antibodies in termination of infection, demonstrated in mouse models of Coxsackie B virus infections, is supported by the observation of persistent echovirus and poliovirus replication in patients with antibody deficiency diseases.

Although initial acute tissue damage may be caused by the lytic effects of the virus on the cell, the secondary sequelae may be immunologically mediated. Enterovirus-caused poliomyelitis, disseminated disease of the newborn, aseptic meningitis, encephalitis, and acute respiratory illnesses, thought to represent primary lytic infections, can usually be identified through routine methods of virus isolation and determination of specific antibody titer changes. On the other hand, syndromes such as myopericarditis, nephritis, and myositis have been associated with enteroviruses primarily because of serologic and epidemiologic evidence. In many of these cases, viral isolation is the exception rather than the rule. The pathogenesis of these latter infections is not clear; however, observations suggest that the acute infectious phase of the virus may be mild or subclinical and often subsides by the time clinical illness becomes evident. Illness may represent a host immunologic response to tissue injury by the virus or to viral or virus-induced antigens that persist in the affected tissues. In experimental Coxsackie B virus myocarditis, mononuclear inflammatory cells (monocytes, natural killer lymphocytes) seemed to play a greater role than antibody in termination of infection, and the persistence of inflammation after disappearance of detectable virus or viral antigen appeared to be mediated by cytotoxic T lymphocytes. Experimental findings have led to another hypothesis regarding pathogenic mechanisms that is called *molecular mimicry*. This is best conceptualized as a form of virus-induced autoimmune response. It is known that small peptide sequences on viral epitopes can sometimes be shared by host tissues. Thus, an immune response produced by the virus may also generate antibodies or cytotoxic cross-reactive effector lymphocytes that recognize shared determinants located on host cells. For example, a monoclonal antibody directed against a neutralizing site of a Coxsackie B virus has also been shown to strongly react with normal myocardial cells.

Immune Responses

Infection by a specific serotype in an immunologically normal host is followed by a humoral antibody response, which can often be detected by neutralization methods for many years thereafter (Figure 35.1). There is relative immunity to reinfection by the same serotype; however, reinfection has been reported, usually resulting in subclinical infection or mild illness. Although there is some antigenic sharing between serotypes in some of the enterovirus classes (for example, Coxsackie B viruses), there

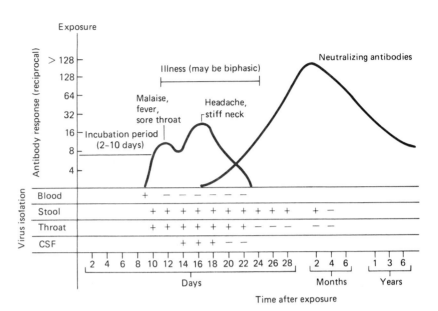

35.1 Antibody response and viral isolation in a typical case of enteroviral infection.

is no evidence of significant heterotypic immunity to infection by different serotypes.

Laboratory Diagnosis

Viral isolation in acute phase of disease

In acute enterovirus-caused syndromes, diagnosis is most readily established by virus isolation from throat swabs, stool or rectal swabs, body fluids, and occasionally tissues. Viremia is usually undetectable by the time symptoms appear. When there is central nervous system involvement, cerebrospinal fluid cultures taken during the acute phase of the disease may be positive in 10–85% of cases (except in poliovirus infections, in which virus recovery from this site is rare), depending upon the stage of illness and the viral serotype involved. Direct isolation of virus from affected tissues or body fluids in enclosed spaces (for example, pleural, joint, pericardial, or cerebrospinal fluid) usually confirms the diagnosis. Isolation

Significance of isolates from pharynx and stool

of an enterovirus from the throat is highly suggestive of an etiologic association, as the virus is usually detectable at this site for only 2 days to 2 weeks after infection; isolation of virus from fecal specimens only must be interpreted more cautiously, as asymptomatic shedding from the bowel may persist for as long as 4 months (Figure 35.1).

The diagnosis may be further supported by fourfold or greater neutralizing antibody titer changes between paired acute and convalescent serum samples. This method is often expensive and cumbersome, however, requiring careful selection of serotypes for use an antigens. Sero-

Limited value of serodiagnosis

diagnosis is generally reserved for critical situations in which the etiology is questioned, such as isolation of a virus only from a peripheral source such as the feces, or in illnesses such as myopericarditis, in which the yield on routine culture is low and number of serotypes that might be expected to be involved is limited. Quantitative interpretations of antibody titers on single serum samples are rarely helpful, because of the wide range of titers to different serotypes that can be found in groups of healthy individuals. In acute poliovirus infections, antibody titer determinations on acute and convalescent sera can aid in diagnosis.

Prevention

Vaccines, which are available only for the prevention of poliovirus infections, will be discussed in detail later in this chapter. Although proper disposal of feces and careful personal hygiene are recommended, the usual quarantine or isolation measures are relatively ineffective in controlling the spread of enteroviruses in the family or community.

Treatment

No specific therapy

None of the currently available antiviral agents has been shown effective in treatment or prophylaxis of enterovirus infections. Treatment is entirely symptomatic and supportive.

Infections Caused by Major Pathogenic Enteroviruses

Polioviruses

Three serotypes

Worldwide, the most important enteroviruses are the three poliovirus serotypes (types 1, 2, and 3). They first emerged as important causes of disease in developed temperate-zone countries during the latter part of the 19th century, and they have become increasingly important elsewhere as living conditions improve in developing countries. This somewhat paradoxical situation is related to the fact that the risk of paralytic disease resulting from infection increases with age. Improvement of sanitary conditions tends to impede spread of the viruses; thus, individuals may become infected not in early infancy but later in life, when paralysis is more likely to occur.

Risk of paralysis from infection increases with age

CNS tropism

The particular tropism of polioviruses for the central nervous system (CNS), which they usually reach by passage across the blood–CNS barrier, is perhaps favored by reflex dilatation of capillaries supplying the affected motor centers of the anterior horn of the brainstem or spinal cord. An alternate pathway is via the axons or perineural sheaths of peripheral nerves. Motor neurons are particularly vulnerable to infection and variable degrees of neuronal destruction. The histopathologic findings in the brainstem and spinal cord include necrosis of neuronal cells and perivascular "cuffing" by infiltration with mononuclear cells, primarily lymphocytes (Figure 35.2).

Motor neuron necrosis

Subclinical infections

Clinical Outline of Disease and Outcome. Most infections (perhaps 90%) are either completely subclinical or so mild that they do not come to attention. When disease does result, the incubation period can be from 4 to 35 days, but is usually between 7 and 14 days. The disease falls into three classes: The first, *abortive poliomyelitis*, is a nonspecific febrile illness of 2- to 3-day duration with no signs of CNS localization. In addition to these signs, *aseptic meningitis* (nonparalytic poliomyelitis) is characterized by signs of meningeal irritation (stiff neck, pain, and stiffness in the back). Recovery is rapid and complete, usually within a few days. The third class, *paralytic poliomyelitis*, is the major possible outcome of infection and is often preceded by a period of minor illness, sometimes with 2 or 3 symptom-free days intervening. There are signs of meningeal irritation, but the hallmark of paralytic poliomyelitis is *asymmetric flaccid paralysis*, with no

Abortive poliomyelitis

Aseptic meningitis

Paralytic poliomyelitis

Flaccid paralysis

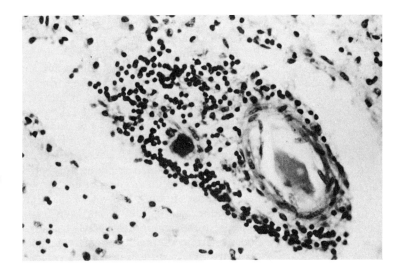

35.2 Section of spinal cord from a fatal case of poliomyelitis, demonstrating perivenous mononuclear cell inflammatory reaction. (*Kindly provided by Dr. Peter C. Johnson.*)

significant sensory loss. The extent of involvement varies greatly from case to case; in its most serious forms, however, all four limbs may be completely paralyzed or the brainstem may be attacked, with paralysis of the cranial nerves and muscles of respiration (bulbar polio). The maximum extent of involvement is evident within a few days after first paralysis. Thereafter, as temporarily damaged neurons regain their function, recovery begins and may continue for as long as 6 months; paralysis persisting after this time is permanent.

Recovery phase

Prevention. Two types of poliovirus vaccines are currently licensed in the United States: inactivated polio vaccine and live oral attenuated virus vaccine. Each contains the three serotypes of poliomyelitis virus.

Inactivated vaccine

Inactivated polio vaccine (IPV; also known as *killed polio vaccine* or *Salk vaccine*) was introduced in 1955; its use was associated with a dramatic decline in paralytic cases (Figure 35.3). It remains the only vaccine used

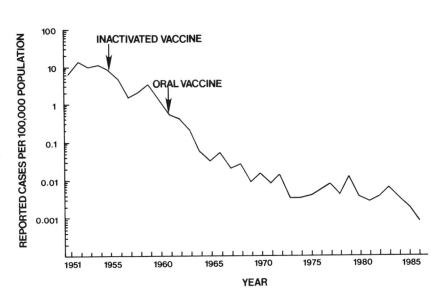

35.3 Reported paralytic poliomyelitis attack rates in the United States, 1951–1986. (*From the Centers for Disease Control, Summary of Notifiable Diseases United States, issued September 1987.*)

in some countries, notably Sweden and the Netherlands, and its efficacy has been generally excellent. Vaccination is by subcutaneous injection. Primary vaccination with four doses (three doses 4–8 weeks apart and the fourth 6–12 months later) produces antibody responses in more than 95% of recipients. The current product is considered quite safe, with no significant deleterious side effects. A newer, high-potency IPV is now available and may significantly reduce the number of doses required.

Live vaccine

Oral polio vaccine [OPV; also known as *poliovirus vaccine, live vaccine, oral trivalent vaccine* (TOPV), or *Sabin vaccine*] is composed of live, attenuated viruses that have undergone serial passage in cell cultures from humans and subhuman primates. It was first licensed in the United States in 1963. The vaccine is given orally as a primary series of three doses (the first two doses usually 6–8 weeks apart, and the third 8–12 months later) and produces antibodies to all three serotypes in more than 95% of recipients; these antibodies persist for several years. As with IPV, recall boosters are recommended to maintain adequate antibody levels. Like wild poliovirus, OPV viruses infect and replicate in the oropharynx and intestinal tract and can be spread to other persons.

Vaccine-associated poliomyelitis

One disadvantage of OPV is the remote risk of vaccine-associated paralytic disease in some recipients or their household contacts, including immunocompromised persons. Adults also have a slightly higher risk. There is speculation that some instances of vaccine-associated paralytic disease may be related to reversion of attenuated virus to more virulent characteristics in vivo after serial passage from person to person. The incidence of vaccine-associated paralytic poliomyelitis is estimated at approximately 1 per 3.7 million doses distributed.

Although there are no currently recognized areas of wild poliovirus prevalence in the United States, it must be kept in mind that importation of these strains can readily occur from endemic areas in contiguous countries such as Mexico, as well as from developing nations abroad. Once introduced into a community, the virus can spread rapidly among susceptible individuals. Thus, continuing immunization programs are of utmost importance in preventing spread of this disease.

Coxsackie Viruses and Echoviruses

The Coxsackie viruses and echoviruses are widespread throughout the world. The basic features of their epidemiology and pathogenesis appear to be the same as those of the polioviruses. Unlike polioviruses, they have a greater tendency to affect the meninges and occasionally the cerebrum, and only rarely affect anterior horn cells.

Most infections subclinical

The consequences of infection with these agents are highly variable and related only in part to virus subgroup and serotype. Up to 60% of infections are subclinical. The main interest in these agents stems from their ability to cause more serious illness, which becomes most evident during epidemics of infection with a particular agent.

Wide range of clinical manifestations

Inapparent infection is common, but varies with the infecting strain and the host involved. The range of illness manifestations varies from mild to lethal and from acute to chronic. Table 35.2 lists the major syndromes and serotypes commonly associated with each. Considerable overlap occurs, however, and one should not be surprised if an enteroviral serotype found in connection with a specific syndrome differs from that most often encountered. The one generalization that can be made is that the Coxsackie B group appears to have the greatest latitude with regard to tissue tropism.

Table 35.2 Clinical Syndromes and Commonly Associated Enterovirus Serotypes[a]

| Syndrome | Coxsackie Virus | | Echovirus and Enterovirus (E) |
	Group A	Group B	
Aseptic meningitis, encephalitis	2, 4, 7, 9, 10	1, 2, 3, 4, 5	*4, 6, 9, 11, 16, 30*; E70, E71
Muscle weakness and paralysis (poliomyelitislike disease)	7, 9	2, 3, 4, 5,	2, 4, 6, 9, 11, 30; *E71*
Cerebellar ataxia	2, 4, 9,	3, 4	4, 6, 9
Exanthems and enanthems	*4, 5, 6, 9, 10, 16*	2, 3, 4, 5	*2, 4, 5, 6, 9, 11, 16, 18, 25*
Pericarditis, myocarditis	4, 16	*2, 3, 4, 5*	1, 6, 8, 9, 19
Epidemic myalgia (pleurodynia), orchitis	9	*1, 2, 3, 4, 5*	1, 6, 9
Respiratory	9, 16, *21, 24*	1, 3, 4, 5	*4, 9, 11*, 20, 25
Conjunctivitis	*24*	1, 5	*7; E70*
Generalized disease (infants)	—	1, *2, 3, 4, 5*	3, 6, 9, 11, 14 17, 19

[a] Serotypes most commonly associated with syndrome are italicized.

In terms of relative frequency and significance, aseptic meningitis is the most important clinical illness associated with enterovirus infections. This syndrome can be mild and self-limiting, lasting 5–14 days; however, it is occasionally accompanied by encephalitis, which can lead to permanent neurologic sequelae, particularly in infants. Overall, enteroviruses cause the majority of all nonbacterial CNS infections now observed in the United States.

Acute inflammation of the heart muscle (myocarditis) and/or its covering membranes (pericarditis) can be caused by a variety of viral agents; however, it is estimated that as many as 50% of cases are associated with infection by Coxsackie B viruses. Such infections are usually self-limiting, but can lead to a fatal outcome (arrhythmia or heart failure) or cause chronic heart disease.

The exanthems may or may not be associated with CNS inflammation. The observed rashes usually resemble rubella, roseola infantum, or adenoviral macular or maculopapular exanthems, but may also appear as vesicular or hemangiomalike lesions. One interesting syndrome is hand-foot-and-mouth disease, which usually affects children and is characterized by a vesicular eruption over the extremities and the oral cavity. Coxsackie A16 virus is the specific enterovirus most frequently implicated, but others, such as enterovirus 71, can cause a similar illness. Herpangina is an enanthematous (mucous membrane) disease characterized by the acute onset of fever and sore throat. Characteristic small vesicles or white papules (lymphonodules) surrounded by a red halo are seen over the posterior half of the palate, pharynx, and tonsillar areas. This mild, self-limiting (1–2 weeks) illness has usually been associated with infection by several different Coxsackie A serotypes.

Epidemic myalgia

Generalized disease of newborn

Other diseases

Epidemic myalgia (pleurodynia or Bornholm disease) is characterized by fever and sudden onset of intense upper abdominal or lower thoracic pain, often accompanied by a frontal headache. The pain may be aggravated by movement, such as breathing or coughing, and usually persists for 3–14 days. Coxsackie B viruses are most frequently implicated.

Generalized disease of the newborn is a highly lethal expression of enteroviral infection, in which the infant may be overwhelmed by simultaneous virus infection of the heart, brain, liver, and other organs.

It is apparent from Table 35.2 that the spectrum of disease produced by these viruses is enormous, and recent observations suggest that many other illnesses may also result from infections by this subgroup. Recently, epidemics of acute hemorrhagic keratoconjunctivitis associated with enterovirus 70 have been reported in Asia, and localized outbreaks of disease resembling paralytic poliomyelitis caused by enterovirus 71 infection have occurred in Bulgaria and the United States. In addition, there is some recent evidence that certain enteroviruses, particularly Coxsackie B serotypes, may somehow participate in the pathogenesis of at least some cases of insulin-dependent diabetes mellitus, acute arthritis, polymyositis, and idiopathic acute nephritis. At the moment, however, such associations between these viruses and the diseases mentioned have not been elucidated; further investigation will be required to establish whether or not they are significant.

Additional Reading

Diamond, D.C., Kohara, M., Abe, S., et al. 1985. Antigenic variation and resistance to neutralization in poliovirus type 1. *Science* 229:1090–1093. This article illustrates how a single point mutation can cause significant changes in an enteroviral phenotype.

Horstmann, D.M. 1982. Control of poliomyelitis: A continuing paradox. *J. Infect. Dis.* 146:540–551. A good discussion of pathogenesis and problems in prevention.

Ray, C.G., Fulginiti, V.A. 1989. Coxsackievirus and echovirus infections. In *Infectious Diseases.* 4th ed. P.D. Hoeprich, M.C. Jordan, Eds. Philadelphia: J.B. Lippincott Co., pp. 1142–1149, 1360–1369. Reviews of the clinical and epidemiological features of enteroviral infections.

36
Hepatitis Viruses

Lawrence Corey

Hepatitis means inflammation of the liver, and as a disease entity, it has been recognized since the days of Hippocrates. The causes of hepatitis are varied and include viruses, bacteria, and protozoa, as well as drugs and toxins (for example, isoniazid, carbon tetrachloride, and ethanol). The clinical symptoms and course of acute hepatitis can be similar, regardless of etiology, and determination of a specific cause depends primarily on 1) epidemiologic and clinical history; 2) use of laboratory tests for the detection of viruses or other causes; 3) microscopic findings of liver biopsy; and 4) long-term clinical course. The nomenclature *viral hepatitis* has become synonymous with hepatitis A, hepatitis B, Delta hepatitis (due to hepatitis D virus), and non-A, non-B hepatitis (including that due to the recently described hepatitis C virus). Other viruses, such as Epstein-Barr virus, cytomegalovirus, varicella–zoster virus, and yellow fever viruses, can also cause inflammation of the liver. The major characteristics of the four principal causes of viral hepatitis are summarized in Table 36.1.

Multiple causes of hepatitis

Hepatitis A

Biology of the Agent

Hepatitis A virus is the cause of what was formerly termed *infectious hepatitis* or *short-incubation hepatitis*. It was first detected in the early 1970s in stools of patients incubating the disease. Subsequently, the virus has been successfully cultivated in primary marmoset liver cell cultures and in fetal rhesus monkey kidney cell cultures.

Hepatitis A virus is an unenveloped, single-stranded RNA virus with cubic symmetry and a diameter of 27 nm (Figure 36.1). It is not inactivated by ether and is stable at $-20°C$ and low pH. These properties are similar to those of enteroviruses, and hepatitis A virus has now been formally classified as enterovirus type 72. At present, only one major serotype of hepatitis A virus has been demonstrated.

Unenveloped, single-stranded, small RNA virus; grows in specialized cell cultures

547

Table 36.1 Comparison of A, B, D (Delta) and Non-A, Non-B Hepatitis

Feature	A	B	D	Non-A, Non-B
Virus type	Single-stranded RNA	Double-stranded DNA	Single-stranded RNA	Unknown
Cultured in vitro	Yes	No	No	No
Incubation period (days)	15–45 (mean, 25)	7–160 (mean, 60–90)	28–45	15–160 (mean, 50)
Onset	Usually sudden	Usually slow	Variable	Insidious
Age preference	Children, young adults	All ages	All ages	All ages
Transmission				
Fecal-oral	+ + +	+/−	+/−	Maybe
Sexual	+	+ +	+ +	Maybe
Transfusion	−	+ +	+ + +	+ + +
Severity	Usually mild	Moderate	Often severe	Usually mild
Chronicity	None	10%	50–70%	30% after transfusion
Carrier state	None	Yes	Yes	Yes
Immune serum globulin protective[a]	Yes	Yes	Yes[b]	Equivocal
Serologic detection methods	Yes	Yes	Yes	Yes (one type)

Abbreviation: Plus signs indicate relative frequencies.   [a] Hyperimmune globulin more protective.
[b] Prevention of hepatitis B will prevent hepatitis D.

Humans are natural hosts

Humans appear to be the major natural hosts of hepatitis A virus. Several other primates (including chimpanzees and marmosets) are susceptible to experimental infection, and natural infections of these animals may occur.

Clinical Disease

Mean incubation period of 25 days

The most commonly recognized manifestation of hepatitis A virus infection is acute hepatitis. The incubation period of 14–40 days (mean, 25 days) is usually followed by acute onset of fever, anorexia (poor appetite),

36.1 Diagram of the proposed structure of the hepatitis A virus. The protein capsid is made up of four viral polypeptides (VP_1 to VP_4). Inside the capsid is a single-stranded molecule of RNA (molecular weight 2.5×10^6), which has a genomic viral protein (VPG) on the 5' end. (*Reproduced by kind permission of Dr. J.A. Hoffnagle and of Abbott Laboratories, Diagnostic Division, North Chicago, Illinois.*)

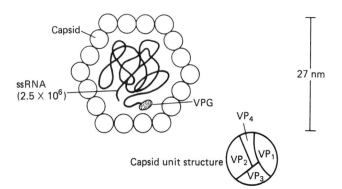

Signs and symptoms of acute hepatitis

nausea, pain in the right upper abdominal quadrant, and, within several days, jaundice. Dark urine and clay-colored stools may be noticed by the patient 1–5 days before the onset of clinical jaundice. The liver is enlarged and tender, and serum transaminase and bilirubin levels are elevated as a result of hepatic inflammation and damage.

Most infections are subclinical

Does not lead to chronic viral hepatitis

Many persons who have serologic evidence of acute hepatitis A infection are asymptomatic or only mildly ill, without jaundice (anicteric hepatitis A). The infection-to-disease ratio for hepatitis virus is dependent on age; it may be as high as 20:1 in children and approximately 7:1 in older adults. The vast majority of cases of hepatitis A are self-limiting. Chronic hepatitis such as that seen with hepatitis B or non-A, non-B hepatitis is very rare. In rare cases, fulminant fatal hepatitis associated with extensive liver necrosis may occur.

Pathogenesis of Infection

Virus replicates in intestinal mucosa during incubation period

Viremic spread to liver; hepatic response to infection

The virus is believed to replicate initially in the enteric mucosa. It can be demonstrated in feces by electron microscopy for 10–14 days before onset of disease. In most patients with symptoms of the disease, complete virus is no longer found in fecal specimens; viral antigen, however, has been demonstrated in feces for up to 14 days thereafter. Multiplication in the intestines is followed by a period of viremia with spread to the liver. The response to replication in the liver consists of lymphoid cell infiltration, necrosis of liver parenchymal cells, and proliferation of Kupffer cells. The extent of necrosis often coincides with the severity of disease. A variable degree of biliary stasis may be present.

Immune Response

Antibody to hepatitis A virus can be detected during early illness when the virus is still found in feces, and most patients with symptoms or signs of acute hepatitis A already have detectable antibody in serum. Early antibody responses are predominantly IgM, which can be detected by radioimmunoassay for several weeks or months. During convalescence, antibody of the IgG class predominates.

IgM antibody response develops before symptoms

Later IgG response gives long-term immunity

Detectable levels of IgG antibody to hepatitis A virus persist indefinitely in serum, and patients with anti-hepatitis A virus antibodies are immune to reinfection.

Epidemiology

Fecal–oral spread

Association with crowding and poor hygiene

No chronic carriers

The major mode of spread of hepatitis A is fecal–oral. Inoculation of infectious material intramuscularly can produce disease; transmission through blood transfusion, while possible, is not an important means of spread. Most cases of hepatitis A are not linked to a single contaminated source, but occur sporadically. The disease is common under conditions of crowding, and it occurs at high frequency in mental hospitals, schools for the retarded, and day-care centers. As a chronic carrier state has not been observed with hepatitis A, perpetuation of the virus in nature presumably depends on sporadic subclinical infections and person-to-person transmission. Outbreaks of hepatitis A have been linked to the ingestion of uncooked seafood, usually shellfish. In most instances, the water in which the shellfish lived was found to be contaminated with human feces.

Variations in attack rates for different populations

The disease is widespread but seroepidemiologic studies have shown marked variation in infection rates among various population groups. For example, rates are higher among those of lower socioeconomic status and among male homosexuals. Less than one-half of the general population of the United States now has serologic evidence of prior hepatitis A virus infection, however, and age-specific prevalence rates are decreasing, apparently because of better sanitation and less crowding. In contrast, in many underdeveloped countries, more than 90% of the adult population shows evidence of previous hepatitis A infection; in most cases, however, the evidence is of asymptomatic infection during childhood. The risk of overt disease is much higher in nonimmune infected adults than in children; travelers from developed countries who enter endemic areas are particularly susceptible.

High incidence in developing countries

Risk of disease greatest in nonimmune adults

Laboratory Diagnosis

Serodiagnosis

The most common method of laboratory diagnosis of hepatitis A virus is to demonstrate high titers of specific IgM antibody to the virus in serum drawn during the acute phase of illness. Because IgG antibody persists indefinitely, its demonstration in a single serum sample is not indicative of recent infection; a rise in titer between acute and convalescent sera must be documented. Immune electron microscopic identification of the viral antigen in fecal specimens, or isolation of the virus in cell cultures remain research tools.

Prevention

Passive immunization is protective

Immune serum globulin (ISG), manufactured from pools of plasma from large segments of the general population, is protective if given before or during the incubation period of the disease. It has been shown to be about 80–90% effective in preventing clinically apparent type A hepatitis. In some cases, infection occurs, but disease is ameliorated; that is, the patient develops anicteric, usually asymptomatic, hepatitis A. At present, ISG should be administered to household contacts of hepatitis A patients and those known to have eaten uncooked foods prepared or handled by an infected individual. Once clinical symptoms have appeared, the host is already producing antibody, and adminstration of ISG is not indicated. Persons from areas of low endemicity traveling to areas with high infection rates should receive ISG before departure and at 3- to 4-month intervals as long as potential heavy exposure continues.

Treatment

There is no specific treatment for patients with acute episodes of hepatitis A infection. Supportive measures include adequate nutrition and rest.

Hepatitis B

Structure

Enveloped, double-stranded DNA virus

Hepatitis B virus is a double-stranded enveloped DNA virus belonging to the family Hepadnaviridae. It is unrelated to any other human virus; however, related hepatotropic agents have been identified in woodchucks, ground squirrels, and kangaroos. A schematic of the hepatitis B virus is illustrated in Figure 36.2. The complete virion (the Dane particle, named for the worker who first saw it by electron microscopy) is a 42-nm, spher-

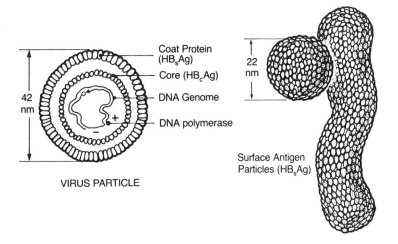

36.2 Schematic diagram of hepatitis B virion. The 42-nm particle is the "Dane particle" or the hepatitis B virus. The 22-nm particles are the filamentous and circular forms of hepatitis B surface antigen or protein coat.

Coat Protein (HB$_s$Ag)
Core (HB$_c$Ag)
DNA Genome
DNA polymerase

22 nm

VIRUS PARTICLE

Surface Antigen Particles (HB$_s$Ag)

42 nm

ical particle that consists of an envelope around a 27-nm core. The core comprises a nucleocapsid that contains the DNA genome.

Core comprises DNA genome, DNA polymerase, c and e antigens

The viral genome consists of partially double-stranded DNA with a short, single-stranded piece. It comprises approximately 3000 nucleotides. Closely associated with the viral DNA is a DNA polymerase. Other components of the core are a hepatitis B core antigen (HBcAg) and the hepatitis B e antigen (HBeAg), which is a low-molecular-weight glycoprotein. The major genes of hepatitis B virus and their products are shown in Table 36.2.

Envelope antigen, HBsAg

The envelope of the virus contains the hepatitis B surface antigen (HBsAg), formerly called *hepatitis-associated antigen* or *Australia antigen*. This was the first antigen of the hepatitis B virus to be detected. The antigen has been shown to possess a group-specific determinant, termed *a*, and two sets of mutually exclusive subtype determinants, *d* and *y* and *w* and *r*. Thus, there are four major subtypes of hepatitis B surface antigen, and adw, ayw, adr, and ayr denote the phenotypes of the virion. These subtypes are important in epidemiologic typing, but not in immunity, because there is antigenic cross-reactivity and cross-protection between subtypes. Aggregates of HBsAg are often found in great abundance in

Aggregates of HBsAg in serum

serum during infection. They may assume spherical or filamentous shapes with a mean diameter of 22 nm and may contain portions of the nucleocapsid (Figure 36.2). Hepatitis B DNA can also be detected in serum and is an indication that infectious virions are present there. In infected liver

Table 36.2 Major Genes of the Hepatitis B Virus and Their Products

Gene	Product (molecular weight)	Function of Product
S	25,000 and 30,000	Major envelope protein, HBsAg
C	17,000–22,000	Internal core proteins HBcAg and HBeAg
P	65,000	Virus-associated DNA polymerase
X	17,000–28,000	5′ protein linking to negative strand of viral DNA

tissue, evidence of HBcAg, HBeAg, and hepatitis B DNA are found in the nuclei of infected hepatocytes, whereas BHsAg is found in cytoplasm.

Despite extensive attempts, hepatitis B virus has not been propagated in the laboratory. Humans appear to be the major host; as with hepatitis A, however, infection of subhuman primates has been accomplished experimentally.

Virus not yet propagated in tissue culture

Replication Cycle

The replication of hepatitis B virus involves a reverse transcription step and as such is unique among DNA viruses. The double-stranded DNA is organized as two strands. One, a short strand, is associated with the viral DNA polymerase and is of positive polarity. The complete, or long strand, is complementary and thus of negative polarity. In viral replication, full-length "positive" viral RNA transcripts are inserted into maturing core particles late in the replicative cycle. These mRNA strands form a template for a reverse transcription step in which negatively stranded DNA is synthesized. The RNA template strands are then degraded by ribonuclease activity. A positive-stranded DNA is then initiated, although this is not completed prior to virus maturation and release and thus results in the variable-length short positive DNA strands found in the virions.

DNA organized as short-positive strand and complete negative strand

Replication involves a reverse transcription step

One positive DNA strand is not completed before viral release

Clinical Disease

The clinical picture of hepatitis B is highly variable. The incubation period may be as brief as 7 days or as long as 160 days (mean, approximately 10 weeks). Acute hepatitis B is usually manifested by the gradual onset of fatigue, loss of appetite, nausea, pain, and fullness in the right upper abdominal quadrant. Early in the course of disease, pain and swelling of the joints and occasionally frank arthritis may occur. Some patients develop a rash. With increasing involvement of the liver, there is increasing cholestasis and, hence, clay-colored stools, darkening of the urine, and jaundice. Symptoms may persist for several months before finally resolving.

In general, the symptoms associated with hepatitis B are more severe and more prolonged than those of hepatitis A; however, anicteric disease and asymptomatic infection occur. The infection-to-disease ratio, which varies according to age and method of acquisition, has been estimated to be approximately 6 or 7:1. One important difference between hepatitis A and hepatitis B is the development of chronic hepatitis in approximately 10% of patients with hepatitis B infection. This development is associated with ongoing replication of virus in the liver and usually with the presence of HBsAg in serum. Fulminant hepatitis, leading to extensive liver necrosis and death, develops in less than 1% of cases.

Variable incubation period (mean, 10 weeks)

Symptoms and signs, gradual onset

Course sometimes prolonged

Anicteric cases common

Can cause chronic hepatitis with HBsAg in serum

Pathogenesis and Pathology of Infection

In the past, hepatitis B was best known as a form of posttransfusion hepatitis or as hepatitis associated with the use of illicit parenteral drugs (serum hepatitis). Over the past few years, however, it has become clear that the major mode of acquisition is through close contact with infected secretions or blood of acute cases of disease or of chronic carriers of the virus. Hepatitis B surface antigen has been found in most body fluids, including saliva, semen, and cervical secretions. Transmission by person-to-person contact has been documented, as has vertical mother-to-child transmission, usually at the time of birth. Under experimental conditions, as little as

HBsAg can appear in most body fluids and secretions

Transmission by contact with infected blood or secretions

Vertical transmission to infants

Table 36.3 Nomenclature for Hepatitis B Virus Antigens and Antibodies

Abbreviation	Description
HBV	Hepatitis B virus; 42-nm double-shelled virus; Dane particle
HBsAg	Hepatitis B surface antigen; found on surface of virus; formed in excess and seen in serum as 22-nm spherical and tubular particles; four subdeterminants (adw, ayw, adr, and ayr) identified
HBcAg	Core antigen (nucleocapsid core); found in nucleus of infected hepatocytes by immunofluorescence
HBeAg	Glycoprotein; associated with the core antigen; utilized epidemiologically as marker of serious potential infectivity; seen only when HBsAg is also present
Anti-HBs	Antibody to HBsAg; correlated with protection against and/or resolution of disease
Anti-HBc	Antibody to HBcAg; seen in acute infection and chronic carriers; utilized as marker of past infection; apparently not important in disease resolution
Anti-HBe	Antibody to HBeAg

0.0001 ml of infectious blood has produced infection. Transmission is therefore possible by vehicles such as inadequately sterilized hypodermic needles or instruments used in tattooing and ear piercing.

The factors determining the different clinical manifestations of acute hepatitis B are largely unknown; however, some appear to involve the immunologic responses of the host. The serum sickness-like rash and arthritis that may precede the development of symptoms and jaundice appear related to circulating immune complexes that activate the complement system. Antibody to the HBsAg is protective and associated with resolution of the disease. Cellular immunity also may be important in the host response, because patients with depressed T-lymphocyte function have a high frequency of chronic infection with the hepatitis B virus. Antibody to the HBcAg, which appears during infection, is present in chronic carriers with persistent hepatitis B virion production. It does not appear to be protective.

The morphologic lesions of acute hepatitis B resemble those of hepatitis A and non-A, non-B hepatitis. In chronic active hepatitis B, the continued presence of inflammatory foci of infection results in necrosis of hepatocytes, collapse of the reticular framework of the liver, and progressive fibrosis. The increasing fibrosis can result in the syndrome of postnecrotic hepatic cirrhosis.

Rash and arthritis early in disease from immune complexes

Anti-HBsAg protective

Role of cell-mediated immunity

Hepatic damage and postnecrotic cirrhosis

Antigenemia and Immune Response

The nomenclature of hepatitis B antigens and antibodies is shown in Table 36.3. During the acute episode of disease, when there is active viral replication, large amounts of HBsAg and HBV DNA can be detected in the serum, as can fully developed virions (Dane particles) and high levels of DNA polymerase and HBeAg. Although HBcAg is also present, antibody against it invariably occurs and prevents its detection. With resolution of acute hepatitis B, HBsAg and HBeAg disappear from serum with the

Serum HBsAg associated with acute disease and chronic carriage

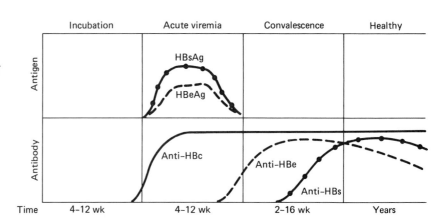

36.3 Sequence of appearance of viral antigens and antibodies in acute self-limiting cases of hepatitis B. HBsAg = hepatitis B surface antigen; HBeAg = hepatitis B e antigen; anti-HBc = antibody to hepatitis B core antigen; anti-HBe = antibody to HBeAg; anti-HBs = antibody to HBsAg.

Anti-HBs associated with elimination of infection and immunity

development of antibodies (anti-HBs and anti-HBe) against them. The development of anti-HBs is associated with elimination of infection and protection against reinfection. Anti-HBc is detected early in the course of disease and persists in serum for years. It is an excellent epidemiologic marker of infection, but is not protective. A schematic diagram of these responses is shown in Figure 36.3.

In patients with chronic hepatitis B, evidence of viral persistence can be found in serum. HBsAg can be detected throughout the active disease process and anti-HBs does not develop, which probably accounts for the chronicity of the disease. Anti-HBc is, however, detected. Two types of chronic hepatitis can be distinguished. In one, HBsAg is detected, but not HBeAg; these patients usually show minimal evidence of liver dysfunction. In the other, both antigens are found; the processs is more active, with continued hepatic damage that may result in cirrhosis. The occurrence of serum antigen and antibody is shown in Figure 36.4.

Presence of both HBeAg and HBsAg in chronic carriage suggests continued hepatic damage

Epidemiology

Hepatitis B infection is found worldwide, with prevalence rates varying markedly between countries. Chronic carriers of hepatitis B surface antigen (which indicates that intact virus is also present) constitute the main reservoir of infection: in some tropical countries as many as 5–15% of all persons are chronic carriers, although most are asymptomatic.

HBsAg-positive carriers main reservoir

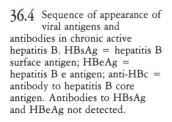

36.4 Sequence of appearance of viral antigens and antibodies in chronic active hepatitis B. HBsAg = hepatitis B surface antigen; HBeAg = hepatitis B e antigen; anti-HBc = antibody to hepatitis B core antigen. Antibodies to HBsAg and HBeAg not detected.

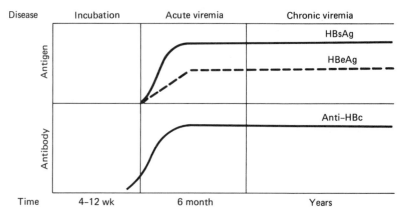

In the United States, it is estimated that 0.1–0.5% of the population comprises chronic carriers of hepatitis B. The occurrence of HBsAg is higher in certain populations, such as male homosexuals, patients on hemodialysis or immunosuppressive therapy, patients with Down's syndrome, and drug addicts using injection methods. Routine screening of blood donors for HBsAg and the elimination of commercial blood banks has markedly decreased the incidence of posttransfusion hepatitis B; 90% of cases developing after transfusion are now caused by non-A, non-B or delta hepatitis viruses. Some multiple-pool blood products, however, are still significant vehicles of transmission, as are inadequately sterilized, blood-contaminated needles. Exposure to hepatitis viruses from direct contact with blood or other bodily fluids, probably through small lesions, has resulted in sporadic outbreaks of acute viral hepatitis B in medical personnel. Attack rates are also high in spouses and sexual partners of affected patients.

Most hepatitis B infection of infants does not appear to be transplacentally transmitted to the fetus in utero, but is acquired during the birth process by swallowing infected blood or fluids or through abrasions. The rate of virus acquisition is high in infants born to mothers who are suffering from acute hepatitis B infection or carrying HBsAg and HBeAg. Most infants do not develop clinical disease; infection in the neonatal period is associated with failure of antibody production to HBsAg, however, and thus with chronic carriage and epidemiologic perpetuation by transmission in the family setting.

Hepatocellular carcinoma has been strongly associated with persistent carriage of hepatitis B virus by serologic tests and detection of viral nucleic acid sequences integrated in tumor cell genomes. In many parts of Africa and Asia, primary liver cancer accounts for 20–30% of all types of malignancies, but for only 1–2% in North and South America and Europe. The relative risk of developing the malignancy is increased over 200-fold in those patients with chronic hepatitis B. The mechanism of the association is unclear. Integration of hepatitis B viral DNA in hepatocellular cancer tissue occurs at variable sites for both viral and cellular DNA, but no activation of oncogenes has yet been identified. Chromosomal deletions have been shown in one hepatocellular cell line that is infected with hepatitis B virus.

Laboratory Diagnosis

The laboratory diagnosis of active acute and chronic hepatitis B is best made by demonstrating the HBsAg in serum. Almost all patients who develop jaundice will be HBsAg positive at the time of clinical presentation. In patients with self-limiting anicteric disease, the period of HBsAg detection in serum may be short; other serologic markers, such as antibodies to the core antigen (anti-HBc), may thus help to indicate that the disease was hepatitis B. Past infection with hepatitis B is best determined by detecting anti-HBc, anti-HBs, or both.

Prevention

Both active and passive prophylaxis of hepatitis B infection can be accomplished. Most preparations of ISG contain only moderate levels of anti-HBs; however, hyperimmune globulin (HBIG) with significant protective activity is now available. Hyperimmune globulin is prepared from sera of subjects who have high titers of antibody to HBsAg, but are free

---

Population groups with higher carrier rates in United States

Sources of infection

Infection at birth associated with development of chronic carriage

Association with hepatic carcinoma

Acute infection and carriage diagnosed by demonstrating serum HBsAg

Passive immunization with HBIG for exposed subjects

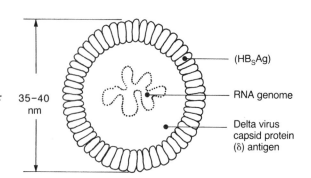

36.5 Schematic of delta hepatitis virus. Note outer layer derived from hepatitis B surface antigen.

35–40 nm

(HB$_S$Ag)

RNA genome

Delta virus capsid protein (δ) antigen

Active immunization with blood derived and recombinant HBsAg vaccines

of the antigen itself. Administration of HBIG soon after exposure to the virus greatly reduces acquisition of symptomatic disease. Two types of inactivated subunit hepatitis B vaccine are available. One has been developed by purification and inactivation of HBsAg from the blood of chronic carriers. The other is a recombinant surface antigen made in yeast. Excellent protection has been shown with both in studies on homosexual men and medical personnel. These groups and others, such as laboratory workers, who come into contact with blood or other potentially infected materials should receive hepatitis B vaccine.

Combined active and passive immunization gives excellent protection to exposed infants and other subjects

A combination of active and passive immunization is the most effective approach to prevent neonatal transmission and, thus, the development of chronic carriage in the neonate. Most hospitals recommend routine screening of pregnant women for the presence of HBsAg. Infants born to those who are positive should receive hepatitis B immune globulin in the delivery room followed by hepatitis B vaccine at 24 hr, 1 month, and 6 months after birth.

A similar combination of passive and active immunization should also be used for medical personnel who have been exposed to the disease by needle stick or similar injuries involving cases of hepatitis B disease or carriage.

Treatment

Risks of corticosteroid therapy

There is no specific treatment for typical acute hepatitis B. A high-calorie diet is desirable. Corticosteroid therapy has no value in uncomplicated typical acute viral hepatitis, and recent studies suggest that it may increase the severity of chronic hepatitis caused by hepatitis B virus.

Delta Hepatitis

Small, single-stranded RNA virus that requires coinfection with hepatitis B virus

Delta hepatitis is caused by the hepatitis D virus. This is a small single-stranded RNA virus that requires the presence of hepatitis B surface antigens for its transmission but not its replication. Delta hepatitis is thus found only in persons with acute or chronic hepatitis B infection. Strategies directed at preventing hepatitis B are also effective in preventing delta hepatitis.

Protein–RNA complex surrounded with HBsAg coat

The method of transcription of hepatitis D viral RNA is not clear. Associated with the RNA are proteins of 27 and 29 kilodaltons that comprise the delta antigen. This protein RNA complex is surrounded by hepatitis B surface antigen (Figure 36.5). Thus, while the delta virus produces its own antigens, it co-opts the hepatitis B surface antigen in assembling its coat. Methods are available to detect both delta antigen and IgM and

IgG antibodies directed against it. These are the means by which delta infection is diagnosed.

Clinical Manifestations

Two major types of delta infection have been noted: simultaneous delta and hepatitis B infection or delta superinfection in those with chronic hepatitis B. Simultaneous infection with both delta and hepatitis B results in clinical hepatitis that is indistinguishable from acute hepatitis A or B. However, fulminant hepatitis is much more common than with hepatitis B virus alone. The delta agent causes its greatest morbidity by increasing the severity and accelerating the pace of chronic hepatitis B infection.

Persons with chronic hepatitis B who acquire infection with hepatitis D suffer relapses of jaundice and have a high likelihood of developing chronic cirrhosis. Epidemics of delta infection in populations with a high incidence of chronic hepatitis B have occurred and have resulted in rapidly progressive liver disease resulting in death in up to 20% of infected persons.

Hepatitis D virus associated with greater disease severity

Epidemiology

Delta hepatitis is most prevalent in groups at high risk of hepatitis B. Drug addicts are those at greatest risk in the United States, and localized epidemics have occurred in this group. Because blood is not yet routinely screened for the delta agent, blood products and dialysis transmission are possible sources for those who have prior hepatitis B. Nonparenteral and vertical transmission can also occur.

Epidemics in intravenous drug abuses

Diagnosis

Diagnosis is made most commonly by demonstrating IgM and/or IgG antibodies to the delta antigen in serum. IgM antibodies appear within 3 weeks of infection and persist for several weeks. IgG antibodies persist for years.

Prevention

Because the capsid of delta hepatitis is HBsAg, measures aimed at limiting the transmission of hepatitis B will prevent the transmission of delta hepatitis.

Non-A, Non-B Hepatitis

The curious designation *non-A, non-B hepatitis* reflects that little is known about other hepatitis viruses, although 90% of cases of posttransfusion hepatitis are now associated with etiologic agents other than hepatitis A or B. In addition to transmission by blood transfusion, non-A, non-B hepatitis has occurred in patients undergoing hemodialysis and renal transplantation and accounts for approximately 20% of cases of sporadic hepatitis presenting for medical evaluation. Intensive investigations over the past 10 years have been directed at defining the etiology of this disease.

Posttransfusion hepatitis

Non-A, non-B hepatitis is usually insidious in onset, mild, and anicteric, but results in chronic liver disease in many patients. As most transmitters of the disease are asymptomatic, a chronic carrier state is presumed. Transmission to nonhuman primates with development of two distinct patho-

Disease usually mild, but may cause chronic liver damage

logic entities has been documented, and two suspected viral candidates have been described. No cross-immunity seems to occur between these two candidate viruses.

The occurrence of multiple bouts of non-A, non-B hepatitis among drug abusers also supports the probability of more than one transfusion-associated non-A, non-B hepatitis agent. In addition, another non-A, non-B type of hepatitis has been noted in India, especially in pregnant women. The causative agent appears to be waterborne and the epidemiology of the disease resembles more closely that of hepatitis A.

Recently, it has been shown that 70–75% of transfusion-associated non-A, non-B hepatitis cases worldwide, and many community-acquired infections, are due to an RNA virus, tentatively termed *hepatitis C virus*. This agent has not yet been isolated in cell culture; however, evidence for its existence and role in the etiology of transfusion-associated non-A, non-B hepatitis was accomplished by preparing numerous complementary DNA clones from the presumed RNA virus in infectious serum. Peptides encoded in these clones were then tested for reaction with antibody from cases of non-A, non-B hepatitis and one was found to be highly specific. The data derived from the nature of the viral genome suggest that it is most closely related to togaviruses or flaviviruses. This technical tour-de-force, which is referenced under "Additional Reading" at the end of the chapter, has provided a serological test for screening donated blood and will certainly help to clarify the epidemiology and natural history of this important disease.

Additional Reading

Choo, Q-L., Kuo, G., Weiner, J., et al. 1989. Isolation of a cDNA clone derived from a blood borne non-A, non-B viral hepatitis genome. *Science* 244:359–362.

Kuo, G., Choo, Q-L., Alter, H.J., et al. 1989. An assay for circulating antibodies to a major etiologic virus of human non-A, non-B hepatitis. *Science* 244:362–364. The Choo et al. and Kuo et al. papers describe how specific antigens have been prepared using cloned cDNA derived from an RNA hepatitis virus that has not been grown. The findings are of great significance to the safety of the blood supply and to unravelling the epidemiology of non-A, non-B hepatitis.

Hadler, S.C., De Monzan, M., Ponzetto, A., et al. 1984. Delta virus infection and severe hepatitis. *Ann. Intern. Med.* 100:339–344.

Krugman, S. 1982. The newly licensed hepatitis B vaccine. Characteristics and indications for use. *J. Am. Med. Assoc.* 247:2012–2015. A review of hepatitis B vaccine and its use.

Krugman, S., and Gocke, D.J. 1978. Viral hepatitis. In *Major Problems in Internal Medicine*. Smith, L.H., Ed. Vol. XV. pp. 1–147. Philadelphia: Saunders. A classic monograph by major contributors to knowledge of the disease.

Lemon, S.M. 1984. Hepatitis. New developments in an old disease. *N. Engl. J. Med.* 313:1059–1067.

37

Herpesviruses

Lawrence Corey

Large-enveloped, double-stranded DNA viruses

Molecular differences among herpesviruses

Host range differences

Wide spectrum of diseases

The group *Herpesvirus*, of the family Herpetoviridae, comprises large, enveloped, double-stranded DNA viruses found in both animals and humans. They are ubiquitous and are one of the most commonly acquired infectious agents. The major members of the group to infect humans are two herpes simplex viruses (HSV), cytomegalovirus (CMV), varicella–zoster virus (VZV), and Epstein-Barr virus (EBV), and the recently discovered human herpesvirus type 6. Occasionally, the simian herpesvirus, herpes B virus, has caused human disease.

All herpesviruses are morphologically similar. The nucleic acid core is about 30–45 nm in diameter, surrounded by an icosahedral capsid. The capsid is covered by a glycoprotein envelope. Despite the morphologic similarity between these agents, substantial differences in the molecular composition of the genome are reflected in the structural glycoproteins and polypeptides. Serologic tests can readily differentiate among herpesviruses despite some cross-reactions (for example, between HSV and VZV).

The host ranges of these agents under experimental conditions differ considerably. Herpes simplex virus has the widest range; it replicates in numerous animal and human host cells, although it only affects humans in nature. Varicella–zoster virus is much more restricted; it does not replicate in experimental animals, other than subhuman primates, and is best grown in cells of human origin, although some laboratory-adapted strains can grow in primate cell lines. Human CMV replicates well only in human fibroblast cell lines. Epstein-Barr virus does not replicate in most commonly used cell culture systems, but can be grown in continuous human or primate lymphoblastoid cell cultures. Human herpesvirus type 6 grows in lymphocyte cell cultures.

The clinical diseases caused by herpesviruses range from asymptomatic infections to diseases of high morbidity and mortality, such as herpes simplex encephalitis or CMV pneumonia in the immunocompromised pa-

Table 37.1   Major Clinical Syndromes of Herpesviruses in Humans

Virus	Major Clinical Syndrome	Site of Latent Infection
Herpes simplex virus Type 1	Gingivostomatitis in children and young adults; recurrent oral-labial infection (cold sores); infection of the cornea (keratitis); herpes encephalitis	Trigeminal nerve root ganglion and autonomic ganglia of superior cervical and vagus nerves
Type 2	Genital herpes; neonatal herpes	Sacral nerve root ganglia
Varicella-zoster	Chickenpox (primary infection); shingles (zoster)	Thoracic cervical or lumbar nerve root ganglia
Cytomegalovirus	Asymptomatic infection; heterophile-negative mononucleosis; fever hepatitis syndrome in neonates and transplant patients; interstitial pneumonia in immuno-compromised patients	Leukocytes (neutrophils and lymphocytes)
Epstein-Barr virus	Heterophile-positive mononucleosis	B lymphocytes
Human herpesvirus type 6	Roseola	B and T lymphocytes

Viral latency and disease reactivation

tient. Characteristically, all of these agents produce an initial overt infection followed by a period of latent infection in which the genome of the virus is present in the cell, but infectious virus is not recovered (Table 37.1). Reactivation of virus may then result in recurrent infection. Complex host-virus interactions determine the expression of disease. With all of these agents, immunocompromised patients, especially those with altered cellular immunity, have more frequent and severe episodes of disease.

Herpes Simplex

Biology of the Agent

HSV-1 and HSV-2

The term *herpes* (from the Greek *herpein*, to creep) and the clinical description of cold sores date back to Hippocrates. Two distinct epidemiologic and antigenic types of HSV exist (HSV-1 and HSV-2). The DNA genomes of both are linear, double-stranded molecules with molecular weights of approximately 10^8. Their nucleic acids demonstrate approximately 50% base-sequence homology, which is considerably greater than that shown between these viruses and other herpesviruses. HSV-1 and HSV-2 share antigens in almost all their surface glycoproteins and other structural polypeptides. Numerous strains of both HSV-1 and HSV-2 exist. In fact, by restriction endonuclease analysis of the viral genome,

Strain differentiation by restriction endonuclease techniques

most strains of HSV-1 or HSV-2 are found to differ somewhat, except in epidemiologically related cases such as mother-infant or sexual partner transfer.

Mechanisms of Acute and Latent Infection

HSV DNA replication and viral assembly occur in the nucleus

Herpes simplex virus produces both acute and latent infections, in which the virus–cell interaction and the manifestations of an infection differ. In acute infections, the initial stages entail attachment of the virus to the cell membrane and entry into the cytoplasm. Viral DNA released in the cytoplasm migrates to the nucleus. New viral DNA synthesis and transcription of mRNA occurs in the nucleus; mRNA then migrates to the cytoplasm. After translation of virus-specified protein in the cytoplasm, these proteins migrate back to the nucleus, where they encapsulate the viral DNA. The virus "buds" through the nuclear membrane; this process adds the envelope material to the virus particles, which are then released through the cytoplasm.

α-Polypeptides produced initially

Later β-polypeptides include virus-specified thymidine kinase

γ-Polypeptides are structural components of virus

The molecular events involving synthesis of virus-specific gene products are coordinated and regulated. Three classes of mRNA coding for three groups of virus polypeptides have been identified. The initial products, designated the α-polypeptides, are synthesized 2–4 hr after infection. The exact function of these α-polypeptides, five of which have been identified, is unknown; however, some authorities believe that they may be related to the development of latent infection. The β-polypeptides include virus-specified thymidine kinase and DNA polymerase. These virus-specified enzymes differ from host cell enzymes and are important in chemotherapy, as currently available antiviral drugs inhibit their activity. The synthesis of β-polypeptides shuts off the synthesis of α-polypeptides and induces the synthesis of a third group of polypeptides. The γ-polypeptides, synthesized 12–15 hr after infection, largely represent the structural components of the viral particle.

Latency not associated with detectable β- or γ-polypeptides or whole virions

Latent infection of nervous tissue by HSV does not result in the death of the cell; however, the exact mechanism of viral genome interaction with the cell is incompletely understood. Recent evidence has shown that the HSV genome exists in a circular form in latently infected neuronal cells. It appears that transcription of only a small portion of the viral genome occurs. As latent infection does not appear to be associated with detectable amounts of β- or γ-polypeptides, antiviral drugs directed at the viral DNA polymerase or thymidine kinase enzymes do not eradicate the virus in its latent state.

Diseases Caused by Herpes Simplex Virus, Type 1

Vesicular lesions become pustular and then ulcerate

Infection with HSV-1 is usually "above the waist." It consists characteristically of grouped or single vesicular lesions that become pustular and coalesce to form single or multiple ulcers. On dry surfaces, these ulcers scab before healing; on mucosal surfaces, they reepithelialize directly. Herpes simplex virus can be isolated from almost all lesions until the crusting stage, but the titer of virus decreases as the lesions progress. Infections generally involve embryonic ectoderm (skin, mouth, vagina, conjunctiva, nervous system). The major clinical manifestations of HSV-1 disease include mucocutaneous superficial infection of the pharynx, skin, and eye and infection of the brain.

Primary infections often asymptomatic

Primary infection with HSV-1 is often asymptomatic. When symptomatic, it appears most frequently as gingivostomatitis, usually in 3- to 5-year-old children. There can be fever, irritability, and vesicular or ulcer-

Primary gingivostomatitis in childhood

ative lesions involving the buccal mucosa, tongue, gums, and pharnyx. The lesions are quite painful, and the illness usually lasts 5–12 days. After this initial infection, HSV may become latent within sensory nerve root ganglia of the trigeminal nerve.

Recurrent cold sores usually unilateral

Lesions usually recur over the anterior buccal mucosa, lips, or perioral area of the face and, because reactivation is usually from a single latent source, are typically unilateral. These lesions are commonly called *cold sores* or *fever blisters*. Symptoms are milder than those with primary infections because of the development of partial immunity. Systemic complaints are unusual, and the episode generally lasts approximately 7 days. It should be noted that HSV may be reactivated and excreted into the saliva with no apparent mucosal lesions present. Herpes simplex virus has been isolated from saliva in 5–8% of children and 1–2% of adults who were asymptomatic at the time.

Virus in saliva with asymptomatic reactivation

Ulcerative pharyngitis

Herpes simplex virus may also cause pharyngitis, usually in young adults. The disease presents as a sore throat associated with an ulcerative lesion of the posterior pharynx. Pharyngitis is usually a manifestation of primary infection; the subsequent history of this infection involves latency in the trigeminal nerve root ganglion, with reactivation of disease manifested by cold sores.

Herpetic whitlow

Herpes simplex virus sometimes infects the finger and nail area. This infection, termed *herpetic whitlow*, is an occupational hazard of nurses, physicians, and laboratory technicians. It usually results from the inoculation of infected secretions through a small cut in the skin. Painful vesicular lesions of the finger develop and pustulate. These lesions are accompanied by "lymphatic streaking" and epitrochlear and axillary lymphadenopathy. The disease, which often recurs, is frequently misdiagnosed as staphylococcal or streptococcal infection. As with other HSV infections, reactivation and recurrence are possible.

Herpetic corneal and conjunctival infection: local antiviral treatment

Herpes simplex virus infection of the eye is one of the most common causes of corneal damage and blindness in industrialized nations. Infections usually involve the conjunctiva and cornea, and characteristic dendritic ulcerations are produced. With recurrence of disease, there may be deeper involvement with corneal scarring. Occasionally there may be extension into deeper structures of the eye, especially if topical steroids are used. Debridement of the cornea and topical antiviral therapy with idoxuridine, adenine arabinoside, trifluorothymidine, or acyclovir are effective in ameliorating the course of disease. None of these treatments, however, decreases the rate of recurrence.

Herpes encephalitis

Encephalitis may sometimes result from HSV-1 infection. Herpes encephalitis accounts for approximately 10% of all cases of viral encephalitis in the United States. Only about 1 in 100,000 persons infected with HSV-1, however, will actually develop HSV encephalitis. The pathogenesis of HSV encephalitis is not well understood. Most cases occur in adults with high levels of anti-HSV-1 antibody, suggesting reactivation of latent virus in the trigeminal nerve root ganglion and extension of productive (lytic) infection into the temporal–parietal area of the brain. Alternatively, reinfection with a different strain of HSV with neurotropic spread of the virus from peripheral sites up the olfactory bulb into the brain may also result in parenchymal brain infection. It is unknown why reactivation of disease may result in this devastating complication in a small proportion of latent infections.

Encephalitis is localized: high mortality if untreated

Classically, the disease affects one temporal lobe, leading to focal neurologic signs and cerebral edema. If untreated, mortality is 70%. Clinically, the disease can resemble brain abscess, tumor, or intracerebral hemor-

Value of antiviral therapy

rhage. The virus is easily isolated from brain tissue, and diagnostic brain biopsy remains the most definitive method of diagnosis. Intravenous acyclovir or vidarabine effectively reduces the mortality of the disease. Rapid diagnosis is very important.

Diseases Caused by Herpes Simplex Virus, Type 2

Association of HSV-2 with genital herpes

Primary and recurrent genital herpes

May cause self-limiting aseptic meningitis

Genital herpes is an important sexually transmitted disease. Both HSV-1 and HSV-2 can cause the disease; but 70% of first episodes of genital HSV infection in the United States are caused by HSV-2. Genital HSV-2 disease is also more likely to recur than genital HSV-1 infection.

Primary genital herpes is analogous to primary gingivostomatitis and symptoms such as fever, headache, malaise, and myalgia are commonly present. Characteristically, the patient has multiple (20–30) coalesced, bilaterally distributed, tender lesions of the genital area. Pain, irritation, dysuria, and vaginal or urethral discharge are the predominant local symptoms. In addition, 1–2% of patients develop herpetic aseptic meningitis (Chapter 67). Unlike HSV-1 encephalitis, HSV-2 aseptic meningitis is a self-limiting disease with no mortality. Like oral–labial disease, recurrent genital herpes is usually a localized skin infection and lasts for a shorter time than primary infections. Details of the clinical course are discussed in Chapter 70.

Neonatal herpes: severe disease with high mortality

Neonatal herpes usually results from transmission of disease during delivery by contact with infected genital secretions from the mother. In utero infection, although possible, is uncommon. The prevalence rate of neonatal herpes varies greatly among populations, but is estimated at approximately 1 per 7000 live births in the United States. Because a normal immune response is absent in the neonate, neonatal HSV infection is an extremely severe disease with an overall mortality of more than 60% in untreated subjects. Manifestations vary; some infants show disseminated vesicular lesions with a widespread internal organ involvement and necrosis of the liver and adrenal glands. The mortality of such disseminated disease is more than 90%. Some infants have involvement of the central nervous system only, with listlessness and seizures; the overall mortality of this syndrome is 50%. Vidarabine and acyclovir decrease the mortality of neonatal herpes, although the morbidity remains high.

Antiviral therapy reduces mortality

Relationship of HSV-2 to carcinoma of cervix is unknown

Some epidemiologic and molecular biologic studies have shown an association between HSV-2 and cervical carcinoma. Recent studies have linked another genitourinary pathogen, the human papilloma virus (HPV) of genital warts (Chapter 42), more closely to these tumors. The role of HSV or the interrelationship between HSV and HPV in genitourinary neoplasms is still unknown.

Pathogenesis of Infection

Transmission by contact

Initial lesions are inflammatory and necrotic

Neuronal spread and latent infection of sensory and autonomic nerve ganglia

Herpes simplex viruses are transmitted through contact with infected lesions or secretions. The incubation period is 2–14 days. Pathologic changes during acute infections consist of development of multinucleated giant cells, ballooning degeneration of epithelial cells, focal necrosis, eosinophilic intranuclear inclusion bodies (Figure 37.1), and an inflammatory response characterized by an initial polymorphonuclear neutrophil infiltrate and a subsequent mononuclear cell infiltrate. The virus can spread intra- or interneuronally or through supporting cellular networks of an axon or nerve, resulting in latent infection of sensory and autonomic nervous ganglia. In humans, latent infection by HSV-1 has been demonstrated

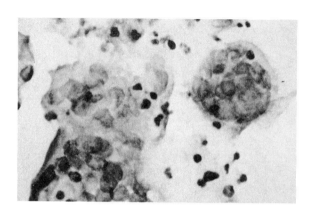

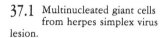
37.1 Multinucleated giant cells from herpes simplex virus lesion.

by cocultivation techniques in trigeminal, superior cervical, and vagal nerve ganglia, and occasionally in the S_2–S_3 dorsal sensory nerve root ganglia. Latent HSV-2 infection has been demonstrated in the sacral (S_2–S_3) region.

Reactivation of latent virus

Reactivation of virus from latently infected ganglionic cells with subsequent release of infectious virions appears to account for most recurrences of both genital and oral–labial infections. The mechanisms by which latent infection is maintained or reactivated are unknown. Two alternative theories have been postulated to explain how latent virus reaches peripheral sites. According to the ganglionic theory, metabolic changes in latently infected cells "switch on" the viral replicative cycle; the virus then travels down the peripheral nerves to the skin, where it replicates in epidermal cells and produces the lesions. An alternative explanation, the skin trigger theory, suggests chronic multiplication of virus in the ganglion with intermittent shedding of the virus through the nerve axon to the skin. Local alterations in host immune status then initiate replication in skin. Precipitating factors that initiate reactivation of herpes simplex are largely unknown; exposure to ultraviolet light appears to be important in some patients with recurrent oral–labial herpes. Experimentally, mucocutaneous herpes may be caused by exogenous reinfection with different strains of the same subtype; but this is uncommon in nature.

Ganglionic theory

Skin trigger theory

Precipitating factors

Immunity to Infection

Evidence for development of partial immunity

Host factors have a major effect on clinical manifestations of HSV infection. Many episodes of HSV infection are either asymptomatic or mildly symptomatic. Initial symptomatic clinical episodes of the disease are more severe than recurrent episodes, probably because of the presence of anti-HSV antibodies and immune lymphocytes in persons with recurrent infections. Prior infection with HSV-1 will shorten the duration of symptoms and lessen the severity of first infections with HSV-2.

Cell-to-cell transfer in presence of neutralizing antibody

Both cellular and humoral immune responses are important in immunity to herpes. Experimentally, neutralizing antibody to HSV can be shown to inactivate extracellular virus; however, the persistence of viral spread through cell-to-cell transfer helps to explain recurrence of HSV in the presence of high titers of neutralizing antibody. Cell-mediated immunity has also been shown to retard viral replication, and recurrences of HSV are clinically of shorter duration and more localized than primary infections. In immunosuppressed patients, especially those with depressed

Evidence for cell-mediated immunity

cell-mediated immunity, reactivation of HSV may be associated with prolonged viral excretion and persistence of lesions. Viremia and dissemination through visceral organs has been shown to occur occasionally, even in the presence of detectable neutralizing antibody to HSV.

Epidemiology

No animal reservoirs

Herpes simplex viruses have worldwide distribution. There are no known animal vectors, and humans appear to be the only natural reservoir. Direct contact with infected secretions is the principal mode of spread. Seroepidemiologic studies indicate that the prevalence of HSV antibody varies according to the age and socioeconomic status of the population studied. In most underdeveloped countries, 90% of the population have HSV-1 antibody by the age of 30. In the United States, HSV-1 antibody is currently found in approximately 50–60% of middle-class populations; among lower socioeconomic groups, however, the percentage approaches 90%.

Relationship of spread to socioeconomic status

Detection of HSV-2 antibody before puberty is unusual. The virus is associated with previous sexual activity, and sexual transmission is the major mode of spread. Approximately 20–35% of sexually active adults in Western industrialized countries have HSV-2 antibody. The virus can also be isolated from the cervix and urethra of approximately 5–12% of adults attending sexually transmitted disease clinics; many of these patients are asymptomatic.

Extent of infection with HSV-2

Laboratory Diagnosis

Grow in many cell culture systems

Herpes simplex viruses are best demonstrated by isolation from infected secretions or lesions. They grow in a wide variety of cell culture systems; most clinical laboratories, however, use diploid fibroblast lines and/or rabbit kidney cells for isolation. The cytopathic effects of HSV, which can usually be demonstrated 24–96 hr after inoculation, are similar for HSV-1 and HSV-2 in most cell systems. Isolates of HSV-1 and HSV-2 can be differentiated presumptively by a number of biologic or immunologic methods. The most commonly used procedures are to stain virus-infected cells with type-specific monoclonal antibodies to the two types or to analyze restriction enzyme digests of purified viral DNA. In this latter assay each type shows characteristic bands of DNA fragments on agar gel electrophoresis. This technique has also revealed numerous strains of HSV-1 and HSV-2 and can be used to recognize epidemiologically related strains, that is, strains acquired between sexual partners or through mother–infant transmission. Serologic studies can be used to document evidence of past infection. Because of cross-reaction, however, it may be difficult to demonstrate a convincing serologic response to HSV-2 in the presence of high titers of HSV-1 antibody.

HSV-1 and -2 distinguished by type-specific monoclonal antibodies

Typing and subtyping by analyses of restriction endonuclease digests of DNA

Prevention

No specific form of prevention is available. Avoiding contact with individuals with lesions reduces the risk of spread; however, virus may still be shed asymptomatically from the saliva, urethra, and cervix. Because of the high morbidity and mortality of neonatal infection, special attention must be paid to prevention of spread from infected mothers. In many cases abdominal delivery (cesarean section) may be used to minimize con-

Prevention of neonatal infection

tact of the infant with infected maternal genital secretions. Cesarean section may not be effective if rupture of the membranes precedes delivery.

Treatment

Several antiviral drugs directed at inhibiting virus-specified enzymes have been developed. The most effective and commonly used is the nucleoside analog acyclovir (see Chapter 13), which is phosphorylated first by viral and then by cellular enzymes to the triphosphate form, which is a potent inhibitor of the viral DNA polymerase. Acyclovir decreases the duration of primary infection and suppresses recurrences. Recent studies show that acyclovir decreases the duration of mucocutaneous HSV infections. If taken daily it can also suppress recurrences of genital and oral–labial HSV. In its intravenous form it is effective in reducing mortality of HSV encephalitis and neonatal herpes. Vidarabine has also been shown to decrease the mortality of HSV encephalitis and, when given systemically, of neonatal infection. No antiviral agents have been developed that decrease the risk of subsequent reactivation of disease.

Varicella–Zoster Virus

Morphologically, VZV is indistinguishable from HSV. In addition, lesions of VZV may sometimes be confused with those of HSV, and vice versa. As with HSV, pathologic changes in skin consisting of ballooning degeneration of cells, formation of giant cells, and nuclear eosinophilic inclusion bodies are characteristic of the disease. Varicella–zoster virus is more difficult to isolate in cell culture than HSV and grows best in diploid fibroblast cells. Compared with HSV, it has a narrower host range and a slower replicative cycle, and it appears to be less readily released from the cell.

Clinical Disease

Chickenpox virus

Latency and herpes zoster (shingles)

Manifestations of chickenpox

Varicella–zoster virus produces a primary infection in normal children characterized by a generalized vesicular rash termed *chickenpox*. After clinical infection resolves, the virus may persist for decades in the absence of clinical manifestation. Reactivation of latent virus results in a unilateral vesicular eruption, generally in a dermatomal distribution, that is clinically diagnosed as herpes zoster or "shingles."

Chickenpox lesions generally appear on the back of the head and ears, then spread centrifugally to the face, neck, trunk, and extremities. Involvement of mucous membranes is common, and fever may occur early in the course of disease. Lesions appear in different stages of evolution; this characteristic was one of the major features used to differentiate varicella from smallpox, in which lesions were concentrated on the extremities and appeared at the same stage of disease. Varicella lesions are pruritic (itchy), and the number of vesicles may vary from 10 to several hundred.

Severe disease in immunocompromised patients

Immunocompromised children may develop progressive varicella, which is associated with prolonged viremia, visceral dissemination, and the development of pneumonia, encephalitis, hepatitis, and/or nephritis. Progressive varicella has an estimated mortality of approximately 20%.

Reactivation to zoster commonest in elderly

Reactivation of VZV is associated with the disease herpes zoster. Although zoster is seen in patients of all ages, it increases in frequency with advancing age. Clinically, pain in a sensory nerve route distribution may herald the onset of the eruption, which occurs several days to a week or

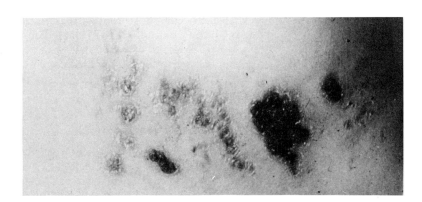

37.2 Herpes zoster lesion of the thorax. Note dermatomal distribution and presence of vesicles, pustules, ulcerated and crusted lesions.

Zoster lesions follow sensory nerve distribution

two later. The vesicular eruption is usually unilateral, involving one to three dermatomes (Figure 37.2). New lesions may appear over the first 5–7 days. Multiple attacks of VZV infection are uncommon; if recurrent attacks of a vesicular eruption occur in one area of the body, HSV infection should be considered.

The complications of varicella are varied and depend upon age and host immune factors. Postherpetic neuralgia is a common complication in elderly adults. It involves persistence of severe pain in the dermatome after resolution of the lesions of zoster and appears to result from damage to the involved nerve root. Immunosuppressed patients may develop disseminated zoster with visceral infection, which resembles progressive varicella. Bacterial superinfection is also possible.

Postherpetic neuralgia after zoster

Disseminated zoster and visceral spread in the immunocompromised

Pathogenesis and Immunity

The relationship between zoster and varicella was first described by Von Bokay in 1892, when he observed several instances of varicella in households after the introduction of a case of zoster. On the basis of these epidemiologic observations, he proposed that zoster and varicella were different clinical manifestations of a single agent. The cultivation of VZV in vitro by Weller in 1954 confirmed Von Bokay's hypothesis: the viruses isolated from chickenpox and from varicella–zoster were identical. Latency of varicella–zoster occurs in ganglia, and VZV genome has been demonstrated by in situ hybridization methods in dorsal root ganglia of adults many years after varicella infection.

Latency of varicella virus in ganglion cells and reactivation to produce zoster

Both humoral and cell-mediated immunity are important factors in determining the frequency of reactivation and severity of varicella–zoster. Circulating antibody prevents reinfection, and cell-mediated immunity appears to control reactivation. In patients with depressed cell-mediated immune responses, especially those with bone marrow transplants, Hodgkin's disease, acquired immunodeficiency syndrome (AIDS), or lymphoproliferative disorders, zoster infections are more frequent and more severe.

Circulating antibody prevents reinfection; cell-mediated immunity controls reactivation

Epidemiology

Varicella–zoster infection is ubiquitous. Nearly all persons contract the disease before adulthood, and 90% of cases occur before the age of 10. The virus is highly contagious, with attack rates among susceptible contacts of 75%.

Infection usually by respiratory route and before adulthood

Seasonality, incubation period, and infectivity

Varicella occurs most frequently during the winter and spring months. The incubation period is 11–21 days. The major mode of transmission is respiratory, although direct contact with vesicular or pustular lesions may result in disease. Infectivity is greatest 24–48 hr before the onset of rash and lasts 3–4 days into the rash. Virus is rarely isolated from crusted lesions.

Laboratory Diagnosis

Diagnosis usually clinical

Rapid confirmation by immunofluorescent staining

Varicella or herpes zoster infection can be readily diagnosed clinically. For confirmation, scrapings of lesions in which to look for multinucleated giant cells may be useful. The virus can be isolated from aspirated vesicular fluid inoculated onto human diploid fibroblasts; however, cytopathic effects are usually not seen for 5–9 days. For rapid viral diagnosis, varicella–zoster antigen may be demonstrated in exfoliated cells from lesions by immunofluorescent antibody staining.

Prevention

Passive immunization of exposed immunocompromised individuals

Need for isolation of cases in hospital

Live vaccine under evaluation

High-titer immune globulin administered within 72 hr after exposure is useful in decreasing infection and ameliorating disease in patients at risk of serious complications. Immunosuppressed children who are household or play contacts of patients with primary varicella are candidates for immunoprophylaxis. Once infection has occurred, high-titer immune globulin has not proved useful in ameliorating disease or preventing dissemination. In nonimmunosuppressed children varicella is a relatively mild disease, and passive immunization is not indicated. Varicella is a highly contagious disease, and rigid isolation precautions must be instituted in all hospitalized cases. A live vaccine, developed by a group of Japanese workers, is now under investigation. It appears to be effective in both immunosuppressed and immunocompetent persons. Recommendations regarding short- and long-term use of this vaccine are now under discussion.

Treatment

Antiviral chemotherapy in immunocompromised patients

Uncomplicated varicella in children requires no specific therapy. In immunosuppressed patients, controlled trials of acyclovir and interferon have shown efficacy in reducing dissemination. In addition, controlled trials of acyclovir, vidarabine, and interferon have demonstrated effectiveness in the treatment of herpes zoster in immunocompromised patients. These substances also speed healing. Acyclovir is the treatment of choice at present. In some instances, acyclovir may also be used to treat VZV infections in immunocompetent adults. Analgesics and sometimes prednisone are given to treat and prevent postherpetic neuralgia.

Cytomegalovirus

Nuclear and perinuclear cytoplasmic inclusions; latent infection of leukocytes

Human CMV possesses the largest genome of the herpes viruses. It produces cytopathic effects in tissue culture more slowly than varicella–zoster virus and HSV. In addition to the nuclear inclusions characteristic of HSV and varicella–zoster, CMV produces perinuclear cytoplasmic inclusions. It can cause latent infection of leukocytes. Clinical manifestations of CMV infection vary with the age, antibody status, and immune response of the patient.

Table 37.2   Diseases Associated with Cytomegalovirus Infections

Neonatal infection
   Congenital transplacental infection
     Symptomatic
     Asymptomatic at birth, subsequent neurologic impairment
  Infection acquired during or after birth (usually asymptomatic)

Infection of children and adults
   Heterophile-negative mononucleosis
   Interstitial pneumonia
   Postperfusion syndrome
   Granulomatous hepatitis
   Guillain-Barré syndrome
   Rare cases of encephalitis
   Genitourinary syndromes
     ? Cervicitis
     ? Urethral syndrome

Infections in immunosuppressed patients
   Interstitial pneumonia
   Posttransplant (fever, hepatitis) syndrome
   Alimentary tract infection
     Esophagitis
     Duodenitis
   Central nervous system infections
     Chlorioretinitis
     Encephalitis/myelitis

Biology of the Agent

Strains of CMV demonstrate considerable genomic and phenotypic heterogeneity. As with HSV, restriction endonuclease analysis of viral DNA has shown heterogeneity between strains isolated from different persons except for those epidemiologically related (eg, isolates from mothers and their infants and from sex partners).

CMV infects epithelial cells and lymphocytes. In epithelial cells it produces intranuclear inclusions and eccentrically placed intracytoplasmic inclusions surrounded by a clear halo, resulting in an "owls eye" appearance. In vitro, CMV DNA can be demonstrated in monocytes showing no cytopathology, indicating a restricted growth potential in these cells.

Clinical Syndromes Caused by Cytomegalovirus

Teratogenicity of some congenital CMV infections

Clinical syndromes associated with CMV are listed in Table 37.2. The most serious is congenital CMV disease. Worldwide, 1% of infants excrete CMV in urine or nasopharynx at delivery as a result of infection in utero. On physical examination, 90% of these infants appear normal; however, long-term follow-up has indicated that 20% will go on to develop sensory nerve hearing loss and/or psychomotor mental retardation. The infants with symptomatic illness (about 0.1% of all births) may have a variety of congenital defects or other disorders (hepatosplenomegaly, jaundice, anemia, thrombocytopenia, low birth weight, microcephaly, and chorioretinitis).

Perinatal infection asymptomatic or mild

In contrast to these devastating findings with some congenital infections, acquired neonatal infection appears to be associated with no adverse outcome. Most population-based studies have indicated that 10–15% of all mothers are excreting CMV from the cervix at delivery. Approximately one-third to one-half of all infants born to mothers excreting CMV at delivery will acquire disease. Almost all of these perinatally infected infants have no discernible illness. Infection is only determined if cultures for CMV from urine or nasopharynx are performed. Follow-up of these infants has also shown no incidence of neurologic abnormalities.

Most CMV infections are asymptomatic

As with intrapartum acquisition of disease, most CMV infections during childhood and adulthood are totally asymptomatic. In young adults, CMV may cause a mononucleosislike syndrome. In immunosuppressed patients, latent CMV may be reactivated, possibly resulting in diffuse involvement of the lung and severe hypoxia (CMV pneumonia). In patients receiving bone marrow transplants, interstitial pneumonia caused by CMV is the leading cause of death (90% mortality). In AIDS patients CMV often disseminates to visceral organs, causing hepatitis, cholecystitis, and chorioretinitis. This latter syndrome may lead to progressive blindness.

CMV pneumonia, visceral, and eye infections in immunosuppressed and AIDS patients

Epidemiology and Transmission

High infection rates in early childhood and early adulthood

Presence in saliva, urine, semen, and cervical secretions

Viral latency in leukocytes: transmission by transfusions

Cytomegalovirus is ubiquitous, and at least 80% of adults have antibody to it. Age-specific prevalence rates show very high rates of acquisition of infection during the first 5 years of life, after which they level off. The rate subsequently increases during young adulthood, probably through sexual transmission of disease. The virus has been isolated from saliva, cervical secretions, semen and urine, and white blood cells; it may be present and can be isolated from patients with circulating neutralizing antibody. Latent infection, which may reside primarily in leukocytes and their precursors, accounts for transfusion-associated disease. In a recent study, more than one-third of infants born to CMV-negative mothers who received blood from donors with CMV antibody subsequently developed infection. Although most infections from transfusions of CMV-contaminated blood may be asymptomatic, persistent fever, hepatitis, and/or pneumonitis may occur. Granulocyte transfusions may also lead to transmission of CMV. Excretion of virus is prolonged after congenital and perinatal infections, probably because of immunological tolerance. High titers of virus have been isolated for more than 5 years after birth. Transmission of infection in day-care centers has been shown to occur from asymptomatic excretors to other children and parents.

Prolonged excretion and infectivity with congenital or perinatal infections

Difficulty in establishing relationship of viral isolation to disease

Because of the high prevalence of asymptomatic carriers and the known tendency of CMV to persist for weeks or months in infected individuals, it is frequently difficult to associate a specific disease entity with the isolation of the virus from a peripheral site. Thus, the isolation of CMV from urine of immunosuppressed patients with interstitial pneumonia does not constitute evidence of CMV as the etiology of that illness. The virus must be isolated from the lung.

Immunology

Disease in immunocompetent individuals related only to primary infection

Both humoral and cellular immune responses are important in CMV infections. In immunocompetent persons, almost all clinical disease is related to primary infection, but subclinical reactivation with viral excretion in cervical excretions or semen can occur in spite of high circulating levels of antibody. During primary infections, CMV infection of monocytes results in dysfunction of these phagocytes. In immunocompromised patients this increases predisposition to fungal and bacterial superinfection.

Laboratory Diagnosis

Cell culture, serodiagnosis, and detection of inclusion-bearing cells

Laboratory diagnosis of CMV infection depends on isolating the virus, finding virus particles in body fluid by electron microscopy, or demonstrating a rise in antibody titer. Cytomegalovirus can be grown readily in serially propagated diploid fibroblast cell lines. Demonstration of cytopathic effect generally requires 3–14 days, depending on the concentration of virus in the specimen. The presence of large inclusion-bearing cells in urine sediment may be detected in widespread CMV infection. This technique is insensitive, however, and provides positive results only when large quantities of virus are present in the urine.

Prevention and Therapy

Measures to prevent infection of immunocompromised subjects

Ganciclovir

The use of blood from CMV seronegative donors or blood that is treated to remove white cells decreases transfusion-associated CMV. Similarly, the disease can be avoided in seronegative transplant recipients by using organs from CMV seronegative donors. Hyperimmune human anti-CMV globulin has been used to ameliorate CMV disease associated with renal transplants. A live attenuated CMV vaccine is now undergoing trials.

Recently, ganciclovir, a nucleoside analog of acyclovir, has been shown to inhibit CMV replication and reduce the severity of some CMV syndromes, such as retinitis and colitis. When given with hyperimmune globulin, gancyclovir reduces the very high mortality of CMV pneumonia in bone marrow transplant patients.

Epstein–Barr Virus

Biology

Etiologic agent of heterophile-positive infectious mononucleosis

Cultivation in lymphoblastoid cell lines

EBV-infected cultured cells are transformed

Replication in epithelial cells of mouth and cervix

Epstein–Barr virus was discovered in 1964 during the search for a suspected viral etiology of African Burkitt's lymphoma. Infection with EBV is common, worldwide, and usually occurs as a subclinical infection in early childhood. The virus has been established as the etiologic agent of "heterophile-positive" infectious mononucleosis. Although morphologically similar to the other herpesviruses, EBV is unique in that it can be cultured easily only in lymphoblastoid cell lines derived from B lymphocytes of humans and higher primates. The virus generally does not produce cytopathic effects or the characteristic intranuclear inclusions of other herpesvirus infections. After infection with EBV, lymphoblastoid cells containing viral genome can be cultivated continuously in vitro; they are thus transformed, or immortalized. Recent studies suggest that most of the viral DNA in transformed cells remains in circular, nonintegrated form as an episome. Some cell lines produce mature virions, which can be detected by demonstrating capsid antigen with immunofluorescence. Other cell lines, called *nonproducers*, contain no evidence of mature virions, although certain virus-associated antigens may still be detected. Epstein–Barr virus has been shown to replicate in vitro and in vivo in epithelial cells of both the mouth and cervix. This helps explain the observation that EBV can be cultured from saliva of some asymptomatic patients. Excretion may persist for weeks to months. At present there appears to be much less genomic strain difference among EBV isolates than other herpesviruses.

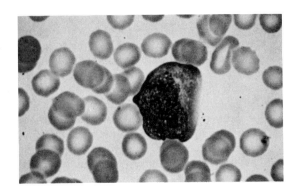

37.3 Atypical lymphocyte
(Downey cell) in blood
smear from a patient with
infectious mononucleosis. Note
indented cell membrane.

Pathogenesis

The pathogenesis of EBV infections is a result of viral replication and host
immune responses to viral antigens. The initial site of infection and replication is the epithelial cell. Shortly thereafter, productive infection of B
lymphocytes occurs. During the acute phase of infectious mononucleosis,
up to 20% of circulating B lymphocytes will demonstrate EBV antigens.
After infection subsides, EBV can be isolated from only about 1% of such
cells.

Productive infection of B lymphocytes

Epstein–Barr virus enters B lymphocytes by means of the CD3 receptor; 18 to 24 hr later EBV nuclear antigens are detectable within the
nucleus of infected cells. Expression of the viral genome, which encodes
at least two viral proteins, is associated with immortalization and proliferation of the cell. The EBV-infected B lymphocytes are polyclonally
activated to produce immunoglobulin and express a lymphocyte-deter-
mined membrane antigen that is the target of host cellular immune responses to virus-infected B lymphocytes. Only a minority of virus-infected
cells transcribe all the viral proteins; these cells are, thus, lytically infected
and succumb.

Immortalization and proliferation of infected B cells

T-Cell response against infected B cells

The host mounts a cellular immune response to control B-cell proliferation. T8 cytotoxic lymphocytes are activated for this function; later,
memory T cells maintain the capacity to limit proliferation of infected B
cells.

Clinical Disease

Widespread asymptomatic infection: disease most common in young adults

Infection is widespread. Antibodies to EBV occur in all population groups
studied and are usually found in 90–95% of adults. Most early infections
are asymptomatic; clinically apparent EBV infection occurs most frequently in populations in which primary EBV exposure has been delayed
until the second decade of life. The disease is thus seen most often in
young adults; it consists of a constellation of clinical findings, including
fever, lymphadenopathy (especially in the cervical area), sore throat, and
fatigue and malaise, which may last from days to several weeks. Laboratory
examination reveals a markedly raised lymphocyte and monocyte count
with more than 10% atypical lymphocytes, called *Downey cells* (Figure
37.3). Alterations in liver function tests may also occur, and enlargement
of the liver and spleen is a frequent finding. During acute disease, EBV
can be isolated from throat washings. Seroconversion and high titers of
immunoglobulin M antibody to EBV capsid antigen are usually present.

Infectious mononucleosis syndrome

Immune Response in Infectious Mononucleosis

Antiviral and heterophile antibodies

Virus-induced infectious mononucleosis results in the synthesis of circulating antibodies against viral antigens, as well as against unrelated antigens found in sheep, horse, and some beef red blood cells. These heterophile antibodies, a heterogeneous group of predominantly IgM antibodies long known to correlate with episodes of infectious mononucleosis, are commonly used as diagnostic tests for the disease. They do not cross-react with antibodies specific for EBV, and there is no good correlation between the heterophile antibody titer and the severity of illness. Some other immunologic functions are also effected by EBV infection. Cutaneous anergy and decreased cellular immune responses to mitogens and antigens are seen early in the course of mononucleosis.

Decreased cellular immune responses

Atypical lymphocytes in infectious mononucleosis are T cells

Viral carriage after recovery

The lymphocytosis associated with infectious mononucleosis is caused by an increase in the number of circulating T cells. It has been hypothesized that the atypical lymphocytes are activated cells developed in response to the virus-infected B lymphocytes. With recovery from illness, the atypical lymphocytosis gradually resolves and cell-mediated immune functions return to preinfection levels. The virus may be cultivated intermittently from oropharyngeal washings and blood for 12–18 months after recovery from infectious mononucleosis. Immunosuppressed patients have a higher frequency of EBV in saliva than immunocompetent patients; the virus can be cultured from throat washings from 10–20% of normal healthy adults and from 50% of renal transplant recipients.

Epidemiology of Infection

Low contagiousness of infectious mononucleosis: spread by repeated contact

Secondary attack rates low

Epstein–Barr virus is acquired by contact with infected secretions. The virus is of low contagiousness, and most cases of infectious mononucleosis are contracted after repeated contact between susceptible persons and those asymptomatically shedding the virus. Secondary attack rates of infectious mononucleosis are low (less than 10%), because most family or household contacts already have antibody to the agent. Infectious mononucleosis has also been transmitted by blood transfusion, and infections have developed after open heart surgery. Most transfusion-associated mononucleosis syndromes, however, are attributable to CMV virus.

Association with Burkitt's lymphoma and nasopharyngeal carcinoma

Epstein–Barr virus has been implicated in several malignancies including African Burkitt's lymphoma, anaplastic nasopharyngeal carcinoma (a common neoplasm in Southeast China), and certain B-cell lymphomas (Chapter 42). Epstein–Barr virus DNA is found in cells of nearly all Burkitt's lymphomas and nasopharyngeal carcinomas and in half of the cases of B-cell lymphomas that occur in immunosuppressed and AIDS patients. The precise etiologic relationship of EBV to these tumors still remains unclear. One theory is that polyclonal stimulation and proliferation of B cells increases the chance of a chromosomal translocation occurring with selective proliferation of the aberrant B-cell clone.

Laboratory Diagnosis

Heterophile antibody test

Tests for heterophile antibodies, recently modified as the *Monospot test*, are used most commonly for diagnosis of infectious mononucleosis. In the heterophile antibody test, the patient's serum is first absorbed with guinea pig kidney homogenate to remove cross-reacting antibodies that may develop in other situations, such as serum sickness. With infectious mononucleosis, heterophile antibody is still present and is usually detected

Table 37.3 EBV-Specific Antibodies

Antibody Specificity	Time of Appearance in Infectious Mononucleosis	Duration	Comments
Viral capsid antigen			
IgM	Early in illness	1–2 months	Indicator of primary infection
IgG	Early in illness	Lifelong	Standard EBV titer reported by most commercial and state labs; major utility is as a marker for prior or current infection in epidemiological studies
Early antigen			
EA diffuse protein	Peaks 3–4 weeks after onset	3–6 months	Presence in IM patients; IgA antibodies useful for prediction of NPC in high-risk populations
EA restricted	Several weeks after onset	Months to years	Present in higher titer in African Burkitt's lymphoma; may be useful as an indicator of reactivation of EBV
EBNA	3–6 weeks after onset	Lifelong	Late appearance of anti-EBNA antibodies in IM makes seroconversion a useful marker for primary infection; persists for life; indication of latency

Abbreviations: Ig = immunoglobulin; EA = early antigen; EBV = Epstein–Barr virus; IM = infectious mononucleosis; NPC = nasopharyngeal carcinoma; EBNA = EBV nuclear antigen.

Tests for antiviral antibodies

by agglutination of sheep red blood cells. The heterophile antibody titer is the highest dilution of the absorbed serum to agglutinate these erythrocytes.

Virus-specific antibodies to the EBV viral capsid antigen or nuclear antigen can also be determined. These antibodies are specific for the virus and can be utilized to document infection. The most commonly used test is for antibody to the viral capsid antigen. Titers to the EBV capsid antigen rise quickly in disease and persist for life. Antibodies to the nuclear antigen rise later in disease (after about 1 month) and also persist in low titers for life. Thus, a high titer to viral capsid antigen and no titer to nuclear antigen are indicative of recent EBV infection, whereas antibody titers to both antigens are indicative of past infection. In the last few years, virus specific serologic diagnosis of EBV infections has been used increasingly. This test is especially important in young children (less than 6 years of age), who do not produce heterophile antibodies with acute EBV infections. Table 37.3 summarizes these tests.

Treatment and Prevention

Treatment of infectious mononucleosis is largely supportive. More than 95% of patients recover uneventfully. In a small percentage of patients, splenic rupture may occur; thus, restriction of contact sports or heavy lifting during the acute illness is recommended. The DNA polymerase enzyme of EBV has been shown to be sensitive to acyclovir, and acyclovir can decrease the amount of replication of EBV in tissue culture. In selected patients, systemic acyclovir may offer temporary benefit. Viral replication increases once administration of the drug is discontinued. No vaccine is available.

Herpesvirus Type 6

Association with roseola infantum

Recently, a new human herpesvirus, now called *human herpesvirus type 6*, has been identified. The virus, which is genetically distinct but morphologically similar to other herpesviruses, replicates in lymphoid tissue and is cytopathic for T lymphocytes in cell culture. It appears to be the etiologic agent of roseola infantum (see Chapter 33) and may be a cofactor in human immunodeficiency virus infections. Its relationship to other human infections is presently unclear. Serologic studies indicate that almost all children acquire infection by the age of 5. It appears to be capable of reactivating in immunosuppressed patients, but its clinical significance in this situation is not understood.

Additional Reading

Herpes Simplex Virus

Corey, L.C., and Spear, P.G. 1986. Infections with herpes simplex viruses. *N. Engl. J. Med.* 314:686–691, 749–757. A two-part series reviewing the biology and pathogenesis of HSV infections.

Strauss, S.E., Moderator. 1985. Herpes simplex virus infection: Biology, treatment, prevention. An NIH conference. *Ann. Int. Med.* 103:404–419.

Cytomegalovirus

Adler, S.P. 1983. Transfusion-associated cytomegalovirus infections. *Rev. Infect. Dis.* 5:977–993. A review of an important aspect of CMV infections.

Ho, M. 1982. *Cytomegalovirus, Biology and Infection.* New York: Plenum. A valuable monograph on cytomegalovirus.

Varicella–Zoster

Strauss, S.E., Moderator. 1988. Varicella-zoster virus infections: Biology, natural history, treatment, prevention. An NIH conference. *Ann. Int. Med.* 108:221–237. A valuable up-to-date review of the subject.

Weller, T.H. 1983. Varicella and herpes zoster: Changing concepts of the natural history, control, and importance of a not-so-benign virus. *N. Engl. J. Med.* 309:1362–1368, 1434–1440. A review of the epidemiology and clinical complications of this infection by the person who first isolated this agent.

Epstein-Barr Virus

Kieff, E., Dambaugh, T., Heller, M., et al. 1982. The biology and chemistry of Epstein-Barr virus. *J Infect. Dis.* 146:506–517.

38

Viruses of Diarrhea

C. George Ray

Acute diarrheal disease is an illness, usually of rapid evolution (within several hours), that lasts less than 3 weeks. A variety of infectious agents can be responsible; overall, bacteria and protozoa have been implicated as etiologic agents in approximately 20–25% of cases. In many of the remaining cases, viruses have been considered as the cause. Unfortunately, investigations have been hampered because most of these viruses cannot be readily cultivated in the laboratory. Viruses that can be cultivated, such as enteroviruses and many adenoviruses, replicate in the intestinal tract; however, epidemiologic studies have failed to implicate them as primary, important causes of acute gastrointestinal disease.

Until the past decade or so, proof of viral causation of acute diarrhea was usually based on exclusion of known bacterial or protozoan causes and supported by feeding cell-free filtrates of diarrheal stools to human volunteers in an attempt to reproduce the disease. As might be expected, the results of such experiments were variable, and the methods were not applicable to routine laboratory diagnosis.

One aspect of such infections that proved of great help was that many were associated with abundant excretion of virus particles during the acute phase of illness. Particle numbers in excess of 10^8 per gram of diarrheal stool are relatively common; these particles can often be readily visualized with an electron microscope. In recent years, direct electron microscopy and immune electron microscopy have been employed to detect and identify the presumed causative viruses; the latter method can also be used to detect humoral antibody responses to infection.

Visualization of a specific virus in the stools of symptomatic patients is not sufficient to establish the role of the virus in causing disease. Other criteria to be fulfilled include the following: 1) establish that the virus is detected in ill patients significantly more frequently than in asymptomatic, appropriately matched controls and that virus shedding temporally correlates with symptoms; 2) demonstrate significant humoral and/or secre-

Most cultivated with difficulty or not at all

Many viral particles in stool

Visualization by electron microscopy

Criteria for establishing etiologic relationship

577

Table 38.1   Biologic and Epidemiologic Characteristics of Viruses Causing Diarrhea

Special Features	Rotavirus	Norwalk Virus
Biologic		
Nucleic acid	Double-stranded RNA	Unknown
Diameter, shape	70 nm, naked, double-shelled capsid	23–34 nm, naked, round
Replication in cell culture	Incomplete, poor	None
No. of serotypes	5 groups (A–E) 15 + serotypes	3, perhaps many more
Pathogenic		
Site of infection	Duodenum; jejunum	Jejunum
Mechanism of immunity	Local intestinal IgA	Unknown
Epidemiologic		
Epidemicity	Epidemic or sporadic	Family and community outbreaks
Seasonality	Usually winter	None known
Ages primarily affected	Infants, children <2 yr old	Older children and adults
Method of transmission	Fecal–oral	Fecal–oral; contaminated water and shellfish
Incubation period (days)	1–3	1–2
Major diagnostic tests	EM, ELISA	EM, IEM, RIA

tory antibody responses in patients shedding the virus; 3) reproduce the disease by experimental inoculation of nonimmune human or animal hosts (usually the most difficult criterion to fulfill); and 4) exclude other known causes of diarrhea, such as bacteria, bacterial toxins, and protozoa. Using these criteria, three groups of viruses have been clearly established as important causes of gastrointestinal disease: the rotaviruses, the Norwalk viruses, and some adenovirus serotypes. Other viruses have also been implicated; as all of the above criteria have not been fulfilled, however, they are currently regarded only as "candidate" causes of gastrointestinal disease.

Rotaviruses, Norwalk viruses, and adenoviruses

Other "candidate" viruses

The currently established and candidate viruses are listed in Table 38.1, in which it can be seen that much remains unknown about most of these viruses. All have several features in common, including a tendency toward brief incubation periods, fecal–oral spread by direct or indirect routes, and production of vomiting, which generally precedes or accompanies the diarrhea. The latter feature has influenced physicians to use the term *acute viral gastroenteritis* to describe the syndrome associated with these agents.

Rotaviruses

Habitat

Most common cause of winter gastroenteritis in children <2 years old

The human intestinal rotaviruses were first found in1973 by electron microscopic examination of duodenal biopsy specimens from infants with diarrhea. Since then, they have been found worldwide, and they are believed to account for 40–60% of cases of acute gastroenteritis occurring during the cooler months in infants and children less than 2 years of age. These viruses have been detected in intestinal contents and in tissues from the upper gastrointestinal tract.

Astrovirus	Calicivirus	Coronaviruslike	Adenovirus
?Single-stranded RNA	Single-stranded RNA	Unknown	Double-stranded DNA
28–38 nm, naked, star shaped	29–33 nm, naked, cuplike surfaces	80–300 nm, enveloped, pleomorphic	70–90 nm, naked, icosahedral
None	None	None	None or incomplete
5, perhaps more	2, perhaps more	Unknown	Unknown
?Small intestine	?Small intestine	?Small intestine	?Small intestine
Unknown	Unknown	Unknown	Unknown
Sporadic	Sporadic	Sporadic	Sporadic
None known	None known	None known	None known
Infants, children	Infants, children	Neonates, immunocompromised children and adults	Infants, children
?Fecal–oral	?Fecal–oral	?Fecal–oral; ?perinatal	Fecal–oral
?1–2	?1–2	?1–2	8–10
EM	EM	EM	EM

Abbreviations: IgA = immunoglobulin A; EM = electron microscopy; IEM = immune electron microscopy; RIA = radioimmunoassay; ELISA = enzyme-linked immunosorbent assay.

Group Characteristics

Double-stranded RNA viruses

Antigenic types based on capsid structure

Animal rotaviruses

Interspecies spread not demonstrated in nature

The rotaviruses belong to the family Reoviridae. They are naked, spherical particles 65–75 nm in diameter (smaller forms have also been described) with a genome containing 11 segments of double-stranded RNA and a double-shelled outer capsid. Their name is derived from the Latin *rota* (wheel) because of the outer capsid, which resembles a wheel attached by short spokes to the inner capsid and core (Figure 38.1). At least four serotypes, based on type-specific antigens on the outer capsid, are known to affect humans. Rotaviruses can replicate in the cytoplasm of infected cell cultures in the laboratory, but are difficult to propagate because the replicative cycle is usually incomplete; that is, mature, infectious virions are not produced. However, successful propagation of human strains in vitro has been achieved in some instances.

Rotaviruses of animal origin are also highly prevalent and produce acute gastrointestinal disease in a variety of species. The very young, such as calves, suckling mice, piglets, and foals, are particularly susceptible. The animal rotaviruses can often replicate in cell cultures, and infection across species lines has been accomplished experimentally; there is no evidence, however, that such interspecies spread occurs in nature (for example, animal rotaviruses are not known to affect humans and vice versa).

Human Rotavirus Infections

Short incubation period
Vomiting, diarrhea

Clinical Outline of Disease and Outcome. After an incubation period of 1–3 days, there is usually an abrupt onset of vomiting, followed within hours by watery, brown, copious, frequent stools. In severe cases, the stools may become clear; the Japanese refer to the disease as *hakuri*, the white stool diarrhea. Fever, usually low grade, is often present. Vomiting may persist for 1–3 days, and diarrhea for 5–8 days.

38.1 Viruses of diarrhea. (A) Rotavirus. (B) Norwalk virus. (C) Astrovirus. (D) Calicivirus. (E) Coronaviruslike particle. (*Kindly provided by Claire M. Payne.*)

Dehydration

The major complications result from severe dehydration, occasionally associated with hypernatremia. This complication can lead to death, particularly in very small or malnourished infants.

Upper intestinal involvement

Pathogenesis and Pathology. Rotaviruses appear to localize primarily in the duodenum and proximal jejunum, causing destruction of villous epithelial cells with blunting (shortening) of villi and variable, usually mild, infiltrates of mononuclear and a few polymorphonuclear inflammatory cells within the villi. The gastric and colonic mucosa are unaffected; however, for unknown reasons, gastric emptying time is markedly delayed.

Transient malabsorptive state

The primary pathophysiologic effects are 1) a decrease in absorptive surface in the small intestine and 2) decreased production of brush border enzymes, such as the disaccharidases. The net result is a transient malabsorptive state, with defective handling of fats and sugars. It may take as long as 3–8 weeks to restore the normal histologic and functional integrity of the damaged mucosa.

Duration of viral excretion

Viral excretion usually lasts 2–12 days but can be greatly prolonged, with persistent symptoms, in malnourished or immunodeficient patients.

Type-specific humoral and IgA antibodies

Protective role of breast-feeding

Immune Responses. Patients with rotavirus infection respond with production of type-specific humoral antibodies that appear to last for years, perhaps a lifetime. In addition, type-specific secretory IgA (sIgA) antibodies are produced in the intestinal tract, and their presence seems to correlate best with immunity to reinfection. Breast-feeding also seems to play a protective role against rotavirus disease in young infants, probably because of the presence of sIgA antibodies to rotaviruses in colostrum and their continued secretion in breast milk for several months postpartum.

Seasonality and age incidence

Epidemiology. Outbreaks of rotavirus infection are common, particularly during the cooler months, among infants and children 1–24 months of age. Older children and adults can also be affected, but attack rates are usually much lower. Recently, outbreaks among elderly, institutionalized patients have also been recognized.

Infection of infants without disease

Although newborn infants can be readily infected with the virus, such infections often result in little or no clinical illness. This finding is illustrated by reported infection rates of 32–49% in some neonatal nurseries, but mild illness in only 8–28% of the infants. It is unclear whether this transient resistance to disease is a result of host maturation factors or transplacentally conferred immunity.

Most older children and adults immune

Seroepidemiologic studies have been useful in demonstrating the ubiquity of these viruses, and perhaps help to explain the age-specific attack rates. By the age of 4 years, over 90% of individuals have humoral antibodies, suggesting a high rate of virus infection early in life.

Electron microscopic or serologic detection of virus

Laboratory Diagnosis. Diagnosis of acute rotavirus infection is usually by detection of virus particles in the stools during the acute phase of illness. Detection can be accomplished by direct examination of the specimen by electron microscopy or by immunologic detection of antigen with latex agglutination, enzyme-linked immunosorbent assay, or radioimmunoassay methods. In the latter two techniques, unlabeled specific antirotavirus antibody is used to "capture" the viral antigen on a solid surface. The antigen is then demonstrated by addition of enzyme- or radioisotope-labeled specific antibody, which attaches to the antigen and can be detected by the presence of a color change when an appropriate substrate for the enzyme is added, or by radioactivity.

Fluid and electrolyte replacement

Treatment and Prevention. There is no specific treatment. Vigorous replacement of fluids and electrolytes, often required in severe cases, can be life-saving.

Vaccines: live, attenuated, or recombinant

The rotaviruses are highly infectious and can spread quickly in family and institutional settings. Control consists of rigorous hygienic measures, including careful hand washing, and adequate disposal of enteric excretions. Live, attenuated vaccines derived from bovine or rhesus monkey rotaviruses have been developed and are being tested in humans. The findings to date suggest that such an approach to control or amelioration of the natural infection may be safe and feasible. In addition, live recombinant viruses containing genomic combinations of human and animal strains are being developed for clinical testing as vaccines.

Norwalk Viruses

Although the Norwalk viruses were the first to be clearly associated with outbreaks of gastroenteritis, considerably less is known about their biology than about that of the rotaviruses. They were first associated with an outbreak in Norwalk, Ohio, in 1968, and their role was confirmed by production of disease in human volunteers fed fecal filtrates. The original virus was thus called the *Norwalk agent*, and subsequent, similar viruses have been given names such as Hawaii agent, Montgomery County agent, Ditchling agent, and so on.

Group Characteristics

Small, round unenveloped viruses

Nucleic acid category unknown

Several serotypes

Not yet grown

Small, round viruses or parvo/ picornaviruses

The viruses are small, naked, round particles 23–34 nm in diameter; their appearance is similar to that of the DNA-containing parvoviruses and hepatitis A virus (Figure 38.1). At present, their nucleic acid content is unknown. The viruses appear to be extremely hardy; their infectivity persists after exposure to acid, ether, and heat (60°C for 30 min).

At least three different serotypes have been demonstrated by immune electron microscopy with convalescent sera from affected patients. Knowledge of the antigenic characteristics and biology of these viruses has been seriously hampered by the current inability to grow them in the laboratory and by their lack of known pathogenicity for animals. In addition to the Norwalk viruses, a number of other small (20–30 nm) featureless agents have been described in association with gastroenteritis. Even less is known concerning their nature or role in disease, and they are often referred to as small, round viruses (SRV) or *parvo/picornaviruses*. Whether some of these are biologically related to Norwalk viruses remains to be seen.

Infections Caused by Norwalk Viruses

Clinical picture similar to that of rotavirus infection

Clinical Outline of Disease and Outcome.   The incubation period is 1–2 days, followed by abrupt onset of vomiting and diarrhea—a syndrome clinically indistinguishable from that caused by rotaviruses. Respiratory symptoms rarely coexist, and the duration of illness is relatively brief (usually 1–2 days).

Pathogenesis and Pathology.   Both the pathogenesis and the pathology are similar to those described for rotaviruses. The mucosal changes usually revert to normal within 2 weeks after onset of illness. Virus shedding in the feces generally lasts no more than 3–4 days.

Reinfection can occur

Immune Responses.   Patients and experimentally infected volunteers respond to infection with the production of humoral antibodies, which persist indefinitely; their role in protection from reinfection, however, appears minimal. Reinfection and illness with the same serotype occurs, and the role of local antibody has not been well defined. It is possible that other nonimmune or genetic factors are essential for protection.

Sharp outbreaks

Older children and adults usually affected

Epidemiology.   Sharp family and community outbreaks are common and can occur in any season. Unlike rotaviruses, the Norwalk viruses are much more common causes of gastrointestinal illness in older children and adults. This difference in age-specific predilection is perhaps reflected in serosurveys, which have shown that the prevalence of antibodies rises slowly, reaching approximately 50% by the fifth decade of life—a striking contrast to the frequent acquisition of antibodies to rotaviruses early in life. Transmission is primarily fecal–oral; outbreaks have also been associated with consumption of contaminated water, uncooked shellfish, and other foods.

Diagnostic tests similar to
those for rotavirus infection

Laboratory Diagnosis.   These viruses can be detected by electron microscopy or immune electron microscopy in stools during the acute phase of illness. In addition, radioimmunoassay methods have been developed for detection of antigen as well as for measurement of humoral antibody responses to infection.

Prevention and Treatment.   As with rotavirus infection, there is no specific treatment other than fluid and electrolyte replacement. Prevention requires good hygienic measures.

Adenoviruses and Candidate Viruses

Some adenoviruses, most of which are exceedingly difficult to cultivate in vitro (in contrast to those associated with respiratory diseases), are now recognized as significant intestinal pathogens. They may account for an estimated 5–15% of all viral gastroenteritis in young children. These include serotypes 40, 41, and perhaps 38.

Other viruses associated with gastrointestinal diseases include astroviruses, caliciviruses, coronaviruslike agents, and some Coxsackie A viruses (the latter primarily cause gastrointestinal symptoms in severely immunocompromised patients). Characteristics of the major ones are listed in Table 38.1. This list may grow in the future, and some of the candidates are becoming accepted more widely as causes of such diseases; however, much remains to be learned about their biology and epidemiologic behavior.

Additional Reading

Christensen, M.L.. 1989. Human viral gastroenteritis. *Clin. Microbiol. Rev.* 2:51–89. A thorough review of the viruses involved, with extensive references.

Kapikian, A.Z., et al. 1986. Rotaviruses: The major etiologic agent of severe infantile diarrhea may be controllable by a "Jennerian" approach to vaccination. *J. Infect. Dis.* 153:815–822. An excellent review of the biology and immunology of rotaviruses and the rationale for live vaccine development.

Morse, D.L., et al. 1986. Widespread outbreaks of clam and oyster-associated gastroenteritis: role of Norwalk virus. *N. Engl. J. Med.* 314:678–681. This report illustrates the potential magnitude of Norwalk agent-caused outbreaks. The accompanying editorial on pp. 707–708 will provide the reader with further reason to avoid eating raw or slightly steamed shellfish.

39

Arthropod-Borne and Other Zoonotic Viruses

C. George Ray

The arboviruses (arthropod-borne viruses) comprise more than 400 agents with worldwide distribution. Their name is taken from their mode of transmission, which is primarily by infected bloodsucking insects such as mosquitoes, ticks, and phlebotomus flies (sandflies). Many of these viruses appear to be involved primarily in infections of lower vertebrates; others have not yet been associated with disease in any host. Members of this group are from diverse taxonomic families, including primarily the Togaviridae, Bunyaviridae, Flaviviridae, Rhabdoviridae, and Reoviridae.

Include members of several virus families

This chapter will describe the arboviruses of greatest importance in human disease; in addition, non–arthropod-borne viruses considered to be of zoonotic origin will be discussed.

Arboviruses

Range of diseases

On a worldwide basis the most important arboviruses (in terms of amount and seriousness of disease caused) include yellow fever, dengue, Japanese B encephalitis, St. Louis encephalitis, western equine encephalitis, eastern equine encephalitis, Russian spring–summer encephalitis, West Nile fever, and sandfly fever. In addition to dengue and yellow fever, other agents cause outbreaks of severe hemorrhagic disease; however, these latter agents are important only in very restricted areas. They include the viruses of Kyasanur forest disease in India and Omsk hemorrhagic fever in Russia.

Arboviral infections in United States

The western equine, eastern equine, St. Louis, and California encephalitis viruses are the most important arboviral agents in the United States. Dengue and yellow fever are present in many tropical areas, including the Caribbean, and Venezuelan equine encephalitis is endemic in Central America. As appropriate vectors still exist, these viruses can and occasionally have spread into nearby areas of the southern United States.

The arboviruses can produce disease ranging from simple, febrile, in-

585

Table 39.1   Selected Arboviruses of Major Importance to Humans

Genus and Member	Major Geographic Distribution	Primary Arthropod Vector	Usual Disease Expression
Togaviridae			
Alphavirus			
Western equine encephalitis	North America	Mosquito	Encephalitis
Eastern equine encephalitis	North America	Mosquito	Encephalitis
Venezuelan equine encephalitis	Central and South America	Mosquito	Encephalitis
Chikungunya	Africa and Asia	Mosquito	Febrile illness
Flaviviridae			
Flavivirus			
St. Louis encephalitis	North America	Mosquito	Encephalitis
Dengue	All tropical zones	Mosquito	Febrile illness or hemorrhagic fever
Yellow fever	Africa, South America, and Caribbean	Mosquito	Hemorrhagic fever
West Nile fever	Africa	Mosquito	Febrile illness
Murray Valley encephalitis	Australia	Mosquito	Encephalitis
Russian Spring–Summer encephalitis	Eastern Soviet Union and Central Europe	Tick	Encephalitis
Powassan	Canada	Tick	Encephalitis
Japanese B encephalitis	Japan, Korea, and Philippines	Mosquito	Encephalitis
Bunyaviridae			
Bunyavirus			
California	North America	Mosquito	Encephalitis
Bunyamwera	Africa	Mosquito	Febrile illness
Rift Valley fever	Africa	Mosquito	Febrile illness
Sandfly fever	Mediterranean	Phlebotomus	Febrile illness
Reoviridae			
Orbivirus			
Colorado tick fever	North America	Tick	Febrile illness

fluenzalike illness to hemorrhagic disease or encephalitis. Representative viruses, their classification, their vectors, and the primary diseases they cause are summarized in Table 39.1.

General Virology

Most arboviruses are members of the families Togaviridae, Flaviviridae, and Bunyaviridae. In general, the viruses are named according to location of initial isolation (for example, St. Louis encephalitis) or on the basis of disease produced (for example, yellow fever). It has been possible, how-

Taxonomy

ever, to assign most to one or another virus family on the basis of morphologic and biochemical features, and some to genera within the families on the basis of antigenic as well as molecular relationships. For example, the St. Louis encephalitis and dengue viruses are both members of the family Flaviviridae, and they share antigens common to the genus *Flavivirus*. These antigenic similarities can be detected by serologic tests such as complement fixation or hemagglutination inhibition. The following sections provide a general description of the families represented by major arboviruses of importance in human disease.

Single-stranded, positive-sense, RNA-enveloped virion

Togaviridae and Flaviviridae. These are enveloped virions containing single-stranded, positive-sense RNA and measuring 40–70 nm in external diameter. The envelope contains a hemagglutinin and lipoproteins. The lipid of the envelope is an essential component, and lipid solvents such as ether and deoxycholate can readily inactivate these viruses. They mature by budding from cellular membranes. Replication can occur in cells of infected arthropods and vertebrate hosts.

The genera in which most arthropod-borne viruses are classified are *Alphavirus* and *Flavivirus*; rubella virus (*Rubivirus*) is also a togavirus, but it is not arthropod borne. Each genus possesses its own unique primary structure of the RNA genome. Viruses within each of these genera are frequently serologically related to one another, but not to others. Representatives are listed in Table 39.1.

Single-stranded, negative-sense RNA-enveloped virion

Bunyaviridae. Bunyaviruses are enveloped and contain single-stranded, negative-sense RNA. They are spherical, measuring approximately 90–100 nm in external diameter. Unlike alphaviruses and flaviviruses, they mature by budding into smooth-surfaced vesicles in or near the Golgi region. The LaCrosse and snowshoe hare antigenic subtypes of California virus are the most important bunyaviruses in North America.

Double-stranded RNA nonenveloped virion

Reoviridae. The most important North American arbovirus of the family Reoviridae is Colorado tick fever. A member of the genus *Orbivirus*, it possesses 12 segments of double-stranded RNA in a nonenveloped virion of cubic symmetry that measures about 80 nm in diameter.

Growth in the Laboratory and Diagnosis

Intracerebral inoculation of newborn mice

The arboviruses may be isolated in various culture systems; for most agents, however, intracerebral inoculation of newborn mice is used, which often results in encephalitis and death.

Virus from blood and infected tissue

The viruses may be found in the blood (viremia) from a few days before onset of symptoms through the first 1–2 days of illness; attempts at isolation from blood, however, are generally useful only when viremia is more prolonged, as in dengue, Colorado tick fever, and some of the hemorrhagic fever viruses. Virus is not present in the stool and is rarely found in the throat; viral recovery from cerebrospinal fluid is also unusual. Virus can be isolated readily from affected tissue during the acute phase of illness, but this approach is seldom practical in diagnosis. Specific diagnosis

Serodiagnosis

is usually accomplished by serologic techniques, using acute and convalescent sera. Various tests have been utilized, including hemagglutination inhibition, complement fixation, and virus neutralization methods. Other serologic tests, such as precipitin and enzyme-linked immunosorbent assay techniques, have also been employed in selected instances. Early, rapid presumptive diagnosis can sometimes be made by the detection of IgM-specific antibodies that often appear within a few days of onset (except in Colorado tick fever, where they may be delayed by 1–2 weeks) and persist for 1–2 months.

Reservoirs and Transmission

Arthropod infection and transmission

As noted previously, the arboviruses can infect cells of arthropods, humans, and a variety of lower vertebrate hosts. Infection in the arthropod usually does not appear to harm the insect; a period of virus multiplication (extrinsic incubation period) is required, however, to enhance the capacity to transmit infection by bite. The consequences of infection transmitted from the arthropod to susceptible vertebrate hosts are variable; some will develop illness of varying severity, with transient viremia, whereas others will become viremic without clinical disease. Vertebrate hosts can be a

Virus amplification in vertebrate hosts

source of further spread of the virus by *amplification*, in which noninfected arthropods feeding on viremic hosts acquire the virus, thereby increasing the risk of transmission. Transient viremia is often insufficient, however, to sustain transmission of the viruses for an appreciable length of time;

Blind-ended infections

those affected, including humans and higher vertebrates (for example, horses and cattle), are often referred to as *blind-end hosts*.

In contrast, if viremia is sustained for longer periods (for example, a week or longer in dengue, yellow fever, and Colorado tick fever in humans; weeks to months in a variety of togavirus, flavivirus, and bunyavirus

Significance of vertebrate reservoir

infections in lower vertebrates), the vertebrate host becomes highly important as a reservoir for continuing transmission.

Obviously, the usual arthropod vectors are rarely present during all seasons. The question then arises of how the arboviruses survive between the time the vector disappears, then reappears in subsequent years. Several

Mechanisms of overwintering in arthropods

mechanisms can operate to sustain the virus between transmission periods (often referred to as *overwintering*): 1) sustained viremia in lower vertebrates such as small mammals, birds, and snakes, from which newly mature arthropods can be infected when taking a blood meal; 2) hibernation of infected adult arthropods that survive from one season to the next; and 3) transovarial transmission, whereby the infected female arthropod can transmit virus to its progeny.

Pathogenesis and Pathology

Viremia

Infection of the human by a biting arthropod is followed by viremia, which is apparently amplified by extensive virus replication in the reticuloen-

Localization in target organs

dothelial system and vascular endothelium. After replication the virus becomes localized in various target organs, depending upon its tropism, and illness results. The viruses produce cell necrosis with resultant inflammation, which leads to fever in nearly all infections.

CNS infection with aseptic meningitis or encephalitis

If the major viral tropism is for the central nervous system (CNS), virus reaching this site by crossing the blood–brain barrier or along neural pathways can cause meningeal inflammation (aseptic meningitis) or neuronal dysfunction (encephalitis). The CNS pathology consists of meningeal and perivascular mononuclear cell infiltrates, degeneration of neurons with neuronophagia, and occasionally destruction of the supporting structure of neurons.

Liver tropism and hemorrhage in yellow fever

In some infections, especially yellow fever, the liver is the primary target organ. Pathologic findings include hyaline necrosis of hepatocytes, which produces cytoplasmic eosinophilic masses called *councilman bodies*. Degenerative changes in the renal tubules and myocardium may also be

Hemorrhagic fevers

Effect of dengue virus on
vascular system

Increased vascular
permeability and DIC

Immune-complex
contribution to disease

Possible enhancing effect of
antibody on the infection

Possible contributions of
cytokines

seen, as well as microscopic hemorrhages throughout the brain. Hemorrhage is a major feature of yellow fever, largely because of the lack of liver-produced clotting factors as a result of liver necrosis.

Hemorrhagic fevers other than those related to primary hepatic destruction have a somewhat different pathogenesis which has been studied most extensively in dengue infections. In uncomplicated dengue fever, which is associated with a rash and influenzalike symptoms, there are changes in the small dermal blood vessels. These alterations include endothelial cell swelling and perivascular edema with mononuclear cell infiltration. More severe infection [dengue hemorrhagic fever (DHF), often complicated by shock] is characterized by widespread effusions into serous cavities such as the pleura, hemorrhage, and perivascular edema. The spleen and lymph nodes show hyperplasia of lymphoid and plasma cell elements, and there is focal necrosis in the liver. The pathophysiology seems related to increased vascular permeability and disseminated intravascular coagulation (DIC), which is further complicated by liver and bone marrow dysfunction (for example, decreased platelet production, decreased production of liver-dependent clotting factors). The major vascular abnormalities may be provoked by circulating virus–antibody complexes (immune complexes), which mediate activation of complement and subsequent release of vasoactive amines. The precise reason for this phenomenon is not clear; it may be related to the intrinsic virulence of the virus strain involved and to host susceptibility factors. Two hypotheses are based on the existence of four distinct but antigenically related serotypes of dengue virus, any of which can generate group-specific cross-reacting antibodies, which are not necessarily protective against other serotypes. One possibility is that preexisting group-specific antibody at a critical concentration serves as "enhancing" rather than neutralizing antibody. In the presence of enhancing antibody, virus–antibody complexes are more efficiently adsorbed to and engulfed by monocytes and macrophages. Subsequent replication leads to spread throughout the host. Alternatively, or in concert with this, activation of previously sensitized T cells by viral antigen present on the surfaces of macrophages may result in release of cytokines, which mediate the development of shock and hemorrhage.

Immune Responses

The usual humoral antibody responses (hemagglutination inhibition, complement fixation, neutralization, precipitation) in relation to onset of illness are illustrated in Figure 39.1. One exception to this general pattern is Colorado tick fever, in which increases in complement fixation antibody titer may be delayed by 3–6 weeks. The rise in antibody titer generally correlates with recovery from infection. Neutralizing antibodies, which are the most serotype specific, generally persist for many years after infection. Hemagglutination inhibition and complement fixation antibodies to togaviruses and bunyaviruses are group specific; that is, they do not always clearly distinguish between members of a specific genus, such as the flaviviruses. Hemagglutination inhibition antibodies may persist for several years after infection, whereas complement fixation antibodies are relatively short lived; the presence of the latter suggests relatively recent infection (within 1–2 years). If IgM-specific antibodies are found, these indicate that primary infection likely occurred within the preceding 2 months. Immunity to reinfection is serotype specific and appears to be permanent.

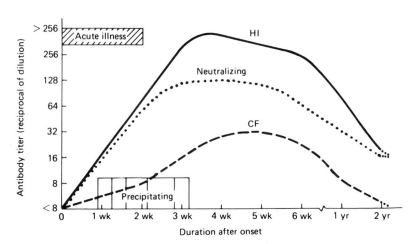

39.1 Typical patterns of antibody response after arbovirus infection. HI = hemagglutination inhibition antibodies; CF = complement fixation antibodies; precipitating = precipitating antibodies detected by immunodiffusion (sometimes used in diagnosis of California virus encephalitis).

Epidemiology

Most are zoonoses involving lower vertebrates and arthropods

With the possible exception of urban dengue and sandfly fever, all arbovirus diseases are zoonoses; that is, their basic reservoir mechanism involves both arthropods and lower vertebrates, which typically experience only subclinical infections. For most, human infection is a blind end in the chain of transmission.

Seasonal incidence

In temperate climates, such as the United States, arboviruses are major causes of disease during the summer and early fall months, the season of greatest activity of the arthropod vectors (usually mosquitoes or ticks). When climatic conditions and ecologic circumstances (for example, swamps and ponds) are optimal for arthropod breeding and egg hatching, arbovirus amplification may begin.

Amplification

An example of amplification is provided by western equine encephalitis. When the mosquito vectors become abundant, the level of transmission among the basic reservoir hosts (birds and small mammals) increases, and the mosquitoes also turn to other susceptible species such as domestic fowl. These hosts experience a rapidly developing asymptomatic viremia, which permits still more arthropods to become infected upon biting. At this point, spread to blind-end hosts such as humans or horses becomes likely, with the development of clinical disease. This occurrence depends upon the accessibility of the host to the infected mosquito and on mosquito feeding preferences, which for unknown reasons vary from one season to another.

The several basic cycles of arbovirus transmission are as follows.

Examples of cycles

Urban. As the term suggests, the urban cycle is favored by the presence of relatively large numbers of humans living in close proximity to arthropod (usually mosquito) species capable of virus transmission. The

Human reservoir

cycle is

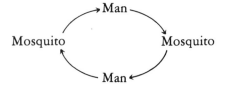

Examples of this cycle include urban dengue, urban yellow fever, and the occasional urban outbreaks of St. Louis encephalitis.

Sylvatic or jungle. In the sylvatic cycle, a single nonhuman vertebrate reservoir may be involved as follows:

Single nonhuman reservoir

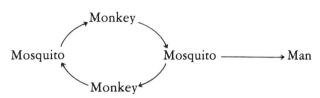

In this situation the human, who becomes a tangential host through accidental intrusion into a zoonotic transmission cycle, is not important in maintaining the infection cycle. An example of this cycle is jungle yellow fever.

Multiple reservoirs

In contrast, multiple vertebrate reservoirs may be involved in this cycle:

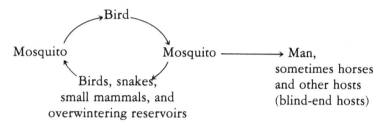

Examples of this cycle include the western equine encephalitis, eastern equine encephalitis, and California viruses. In some situations, such as St. Louis encephalitis and yellow fever, the urban and sylvatic cycles may operate concurrently.

Arthropod sustained. Arthropods, especially ticks, may sustain the reservoir by transovarial transmission of virus to their progeny, with abetment of the cycle by spread to and from small mammals:

Maintenance by transovarial transmission

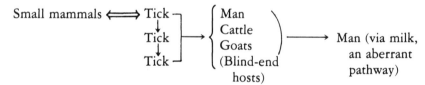

Tick-borne encephalitis in the Soviet Union is transmitted by this cycle.

Treatment and Prevention

Other than supportive care, there is no specific treatment for arboviral infections. Prevention is primarily by avoidance of contact with potentially infected arthropods, a task that can be extremely difficult, even with the use of adequate screening and insect repellents. In some settings, vector control can be accomplished by elimination of arthropod breeding sites (pools and the like) and sometimes by attempts to eradicate the arthropods with careful use of insecticides. Such measures have been highly effective in the control of urban yellow fever, in which elimination of urban breeding sites and attempts to eradicate the principal mosquito vector species (*Aëdes aegypti*) have been used. Those viruses maintained in complex sylvatic cycles, however, are considerably more difficult to control without risking major environmental disruption and inestimable expense.

Arthropod vector control

Equine encephalitis vaccines

Vaccines are available for immunization of horses against western, eastern and Venezuelan equine encephalitis virus infections; the latter vaccine has also been used for some laboratory personnel who work with the virus. The only other arbovirus vaccine in general use for humans is a live, attenuated yellow fever virus vaccine (17-D strain), which is used to protect rural populations exposed to the sylvatic cycle and for international

Live attenuated yellow fever vaccine

travelers to endemic areas. In fact, many countries in tropical Africa, Asia, and South America require proof of yellow fever vaccination before allowing travelers to enter. A single subcutaneous dose results in the appearance of antibodies that persist for at least 16–19 years, which correlates well with protective immunity. If booster doses are desired, they need not be given more than once every 10 years to maintain protection.

Specific Arboviruses of Major Importance

Western Equine Encephalitis. The agent that causes western equine encephalitis is prevalent in the western United States, particularly in the central valley of California, eastern Washington (Yakima Valley), Colorado, and Texas. It has also been responsible for outbreaks in midwestern states (Minnesota, Wisconsin, Illinois, Missouri, and Kansas) and as far east as New Jersey. Horses and humans represent blind-end hosts; both are susceptible to infection and illness, commonly manifested as encephalitis. Although human infection in endemic areas is commonplace, overall only 1 of 1000 infections results in clinical illness. In young infants (under 1 year of age), however, 1 of every 25 infections may produce severe illness. The attack rates are therefore far higher in young infants than in other groups.

The disease spectrum may range from mild, nonspecific febrile illness to aseptic meningitis or severe, overwhelming encephalitis. Mortality is estimated at 5% for cases of encephalitis. It is a very serious disease in infants less than 1 year of age: as many as 60% of survivors have permanent neurologic impairment.

Eastern Equine Encephalitis. The eastern equine encephalitis virus is largely confined to the Atlantic seaboard states from New England down the coast of Florida, although it may extend down the Atlantic coast of Central and South America. The mosquito vector (principally *Culiseta melanura*) generally restricts its feeding to horses and birds, although occasional outbreaks among humans have occurred. The virus can cause severe encephalitis in horses and also in wild pheasants. The attack rate in humans is highest in infants and children; the mortality in this group is estimated at 20% or greater, and the incidence of severe sequelae among survivors is high.

St. Louis Encephalitis. The St. Louis encephalitis virus is a major cause of arbovirus encephalitis in the United States. Although its geographic distribution and major mosquito vector (*Culex tarsalis*) are similar to that of western equine encephalitis, it has been much more active in eastern states, Texas, Mississippi, and Florida. It infects but causes no disease in horses. The disease spectrum is similar to that of western equine encephalitis, but the major morbidity and mortality as well as the highest attack rates are among adults over 40 years of age. Infants and young children are relatively spared.

California Virus. Although California virus was first isolated in that state, its major distribution in the United States has been in the Midwest; outbreaks are particularly prevalent in Wisconsin, Ohio, Minnesota, and Indiana. Studies elsewhere in North America and throughout the world, however, indicate that California virus or closely related agents are present nearly everywhere. In the upper midwestern states of Wisconsin and Minnesota, California virus is considered the most important cause of encephalitis. The primary mosquito vector (*Aëdes triseriatus*) is commonly

---

Marginal notes:

Western United States and Midwest

Infection in humans common: disease rare

Aseptic meningitis: encephalitis

Severity in infants

Atlantic seaboard of United States
Mosquito, bird, horse cycle

Major morbidity in children

Major morbidity and mortality in adults

Major occurrence in Midwest

Highest attack rates age 5–18

encountered in suburban or rural environments. Unlike western equine, eastern equine, and St. Louis encephalitis viruses, the highest attack rates are seen in those aged 5–18 years. Infection is often characterized by abrupt onset of encephalitis, often with seizures.

Central and South America and Africa

Yellow Fever.   Geographically, yellow fever is distributed throughout the Caribbean, Central America, the Amazon Valley in South America, and a broad central zone in Africa from the Atlantic coast to the Sudan and Ethiopia. It continues to be a potential threat to the southeastern United States because of the presence of an urban vector (*Aëdes aegypti*) in that area.

Nonencephalitic systemic disease involving liver

The clinical disease is characterized by abrupt onset of fever, chills, headache, and hemorrhage; it may progress to severe vomiting (sometimes with gastric hemorrhage), bradycardia, jaundice, and shock. If the patient recovers from the acute episode, there are no long-term sequelae.

Middle East, Africa, Far East, and Caribbean

Dengue.   There are four related serotypes of dengue, any of which may exist concurrently in a given endemic area. These agents are widespread throughout the world, particularly in the Middle East, Africa, the Far East, and the Caribbean Islands, and they have invaded the United States in the past. The vector (*Aëdes aegypti*) is the same as the domestic vector of yellow fever. The known transmission cycle is man–mosquito–man, although a sylvatic cycle involving monkeys may also exist.

Nonencephalitic systemic disease, sometimes hemorrhagic

The characteristic clinical illness usually results in fever, severe pain in the back, head, muscles, and joints, and erythematous rash. Especially in the Far East (the Philippines, Thailand, and India), the disease has periodically assumed a severe form characterized by shock, pleural effusion, and hemorrhage (DHF), often followed by death.

Japanese B Encephalitis.   The *Flavivirus* species that causes Japanese B encephalitis is prevalent on the eastern coast of Asia, on its offshore islands (Japan, Taiwan, and Indonesia), and in India. Its transmission cycle resembles that of the St. Louis encephalitis and western equine encephalitis viruses. A high proportion of human infections are subclinical, especially in children; when encephalitis does develop, however, it is severe and often fatal.

Powassan Virus.   Powassan virus is the only known tick-borne *Flavivirus* species of North America. First isolated in Ontario from a fatal case of encephalitis, it has been found in infected ticks in Ontario, British Columbia, and Colorado. Its significance to humans is not yet established, as only a few cases of encephalitis proved to be caused by this agent have been described. Serologic evidence, however, suggests that the virus is prevalent in many areas of North America.

Tick-borne encephalitis

Colorado Tick Fever.   The tick-borne *Orbivirus* species that causes Colorado tick fever has been found throughout the western United States, including Washington, Oregon, Colorado, and Idaho, and also on Long Island. It is frequently found in *Dermacentor andersoni,* which are also vectors for *Rickettsia rickettsii.* The typical illness, which occurs 3–6 days after the tick bite, is characterized by a sudden onset with headache, muscle pains, fever, and occasionally encephalitis. Leukopenia is a consistent feature of infection. It is estimated that no more than one clinical illness occurs for every 100 infections with this agent.

Arenaviruses

Enveloped, single-stranded RNA virions containing host ribosomes

The family Arenaviridae comprises enveloped spherical or pleomorphic viruses containing single-stranded, negative-sense RNA in several segments and measuring 50–300 nm in diameter. They mature by budding from host cell cytoplasmic membranes and contain host cell ribosomes in their interior. These ribosomes confer a granular appearance to the viruses, hence their name (from the Latin *arenosus*, sandy). They can be isolated by inoculation of clinical specimens (blood, cerebrospinal fluid, and the like) into mice, hamsters, guinea pigs, and a variety of tissue cultures.

Reservoir in small rodents

Vertical transmission

A common feature of the arenaviruses is their zoonotic reservoir, particularly small rodents, in which they may be sustained for long periods. Primary infection of mature rodents often results in disease and death, whereas intrauterine or perinatal infection (vertical transmission) usually leads to chronic lifelong viremia with persistent shedding of virus into the feces, urine, and respiratory secretions. Although chronically infected rodents are somewhat tolerant to the virus (that is, infection is persistent without causing illness), they do produce antibodies, and evidence of deleterious effects can be found in older hosts, usually in the form of immune-complex glomerulonephritis. The viruses are perpetuated by vertical transmission from infected mothers to their offspring. When environmental contact becomes close, spread from the rodent reservoir to humans (and, in some instances, subhuman primates) can occur via aerosols, through exposure to infective urine, feces, or tissues, or directly by rodent bites.

Spread to humans

Lymphocytic Choriomeningitis Virus

Human chronic meningitis or meningoencephalitis from contact with rodents

Infection with lymphocytic choriomeningitis virus is particularly common in hamsters and mice. In the United States, most human illnesses have been traced to contact with rodent breeding colonies in research or pet supply centers and to pet hamsters in the home. The illness usually consists of fever, headache, and myalgia, although meningitis or meningoencephalitis also occurs occasionally. Such CNS infections may persist for as long as 3 months.

The diagnosis is suggested by a history of rodent contact. The virus may be isolated in the early stages of disease by intracerebral inoculation of blood or cerebrospinal fluid into weanling mice or young guinea pigs. More commonly, the diagnosis is confirmed by serologic testing of acute and convalescent sera using complement fixation, indirect immunofluorescence, or neutralization tests. No person-to-person transmission of infection has been documented.

Arenaviruses Associated with Hemorrhagic Fevers

Transmission from rodent reservoir or by secretions and body fluids between humans

The agents of hemorrhagic fevers are transmitted from infected rodents to humans, although person-to-person spread via contact with secretions and body fluids can also occur readily. The viruses in this group include the South American hemorrhagic fever agents (Junin virus, the cause of Argentinian hemorrhagic fever, and Machupo virus, the cause of Bolivian hemorrhagic fever) and Lassa virus, the cause of Lassa fever in West Africa.

Systemic disease with high mortality

These viruses have pathogenic and pathologic features similar to those described for the arboviruses that cause hemorrhagic fevers; however, the mechanisms involved in the coagulation abnormalities are not understood. All are characterized by fever, usually accompanied by hemorrhage manifestations, shock, neurologic disturbances, and bradycardia. Lassa fever also frequently causes hepatitis, myocarditis, and exudative pharyngitis. Mortality is estimated to be 10–50% for Lassa fever and 5–30% for the others. All are considered highly dangerous in terms of infectivity. Importation of cases to nonepidemic areas has occurred, with significant risk of spread to medical and laboratory personnel.

Risk of nosocomial infection of medical and laboratory staff

The diagnosis is suggested primarily by the recent travel history of the patient and the clinical syndromes. Although virus isolation and serologic diagnosis can be done, *these procedures should not be attempted in a hospital diagnostic laboratory*. Any patient suspected of having such an infection should be immediately isolated and public health authorities notified. Because of the high risk of spread of infection from body fluids and excreta, even routine laboratory studies are best deferred until the diagnosis and proper disposition of specimens can be resolved. Viremia can persist for 1 month, and virus shedding in the urine may continue for more than 2 months after the onset of illness.

Treatment is primarily supportive; however, intravenous ribavirin, if begun within 6 days of illness onset, has been shown to be helpful in Lassa fever.

Other Viruses of Apparent Zoonotic Origin

Marburg and Ebola Viruses

Enveloped, single-stranded RNA filamentous viruses

These are enveloped, single-stranded, negative-sense RNA viruses. They are filamentous and highly pleomorphic, averaging 80 nm in diameter and 300–14,000 nm in length as they bud from the cell membranes. They have been classified as members of the family Filoviridae.

The association of the Marburg virus with serious disease did not become apparent until 1967, when 26 cases of hemorrhagic fever occurred among persons in Germany and Yugoslavia who were handling a group of African green monkeys imported from central Uganda. The agent was later identified as Marburg virus, apparently transmitted by the infected monkeys. In 1975 it was associated with a similar disease in three travelers in South Africa and in 1980 in Kenya.

Marburg virus transmitted from infected monkeys

In 1976, severe outbreaks of hemorrhagic fever occurred in northern Zaire and the southern Sudan. The illnesses were similar to those described for Marburg virus. They were later shown, however, to be caused by an antigenically different agent now known as *Ebola virus*, named after a small river in Zaire. Two distinct antigenic types are now recognized.

Ebola virus outbreaks in Zaire and Sudan

Ebola virus produces disease in humans and subhuman primates; onset is within 4–6 days of inoculation. The reservoir, although uncertain, is thought to be in small mammals, perhaps rodents.

High mortality during epidemics

Serosurveys of humans residing in the areas where outbreaks have occurred suggest that human infection may be relatively common; as much as 7% of the survey group had antibodies, indicating past infection. In symptomatic infections, the mortality for both Marburg and Ebola viruses is extremely high (30–80%).

Person-to-person spread of Ebola virus

As with the arenavirus-associated hemorrhagic fevers, the diagnosis of infection by these agents is suggested by a similar syndrome and recent travel history. Person-to-person transmission similar to that described for Lassa fever occurs in Ebola virus infections and may be possible with Marburg virus. Diagnosis can be confirmed by isolation of virus in Vero cells (a continuous line of African green monkey kidney), mice, and guinea pigs, as well as by serologic methods employing indirect immunofluorescence. As with the arenavirus-associated hemorrhagic fevers, however, utmost care in isolation precautions and *prompt* notification of public health authorities is mandatory for suspected cases *before* any diagnostic attempts are made. There is no specific therapy for the infections.

Vesicular Stomatitis Virus

A rhabdovirus, vesicular stomatitis virus, that causes outbreaks of disease in cattle, pigs, and horses can be transmitted by arthropods. Human infection acquired by contact with infected animals is unusual; it consists of a self-limited febrile illness and occasional herpeslike eruptions over the lips and oral mucosa.

Korean Hemorrhagic Fever and Related Agents

As its name implies, Korean hemorrhagic fever (KHF) is endemic to Korea and surrounding areas in the Far East. It is an important cause of hemorrhagic fever, often complicated by varying degrees of acute renal failure. The first reported isolation of KHF was in 1978, when the antigen was detected in the lung tissues of wild rodents (*Apodemus* species) by indirect immunofluorescence using convalescent sera from affected patients. No illness was apparent in the rodents, suggesting a reservoir mechanism and mode of transmission similar to those described for the arenaviruses. Additional work using the Hantaan virus (a prototype strain serially propagated in a continuous cell line from a human pulmonary carcinoma) indicates that the agent is a member of the family Bunyaviridae.

Evidence has accumulated indicating that other agents with close antigenic similarities to KHF virus are responsible for hemorrhagic-renal syndromes occurring throughout northern Eurasia, including the Soviet Union, eastern Europe, Finland, and Scandinavia. These syndromes have been given a variety of names, including nephropathia epidemica (NE). Methods similar to those used to detect KHF antigen have detected the NE antigen in the lungs of small rodents (bank voles) in Finland. Antigens and antibodies related to Hantaan virus have been detected in urban rat species in Maryland, Pennsylvania, and Louisiana. Thus there is a possibility that human infection with disease may occur in the United States. There is no evidence of human-to-human transmission, but some investigators believe that transmission by arthropod vectors is possible.

Additional Reading

Halstead, S.B. 1988. Pathogenesis of dengue: Challenges to molecular biology. *Science* 239:476–481. An excellent review of antibody-dependent enhancement in the pathogenesis of viral infection.

McCormick, J.B., et al. 1986. Lassa fever. Effective therapy with ribavirin. *N. Engl. J. Med.* 314:20–26. This paper demonstrates approaches and difficulties encountered in evaluating a new antiviral drug for a serious disease.

Pang, T. 1983. Delayed-type hypersensitivity: Probable role in the pathogenesis of dengue hemorrhagic fever/dengue shock syndrome. *Rev. Infect. Dis.* 5:346–352. An excellent discussion of dengue pathogenesis (including work of Dr. Scott Halstead), which may eventually apply to our knowledge of some other infectious disease processes.

Schmaljohn, C.S., et al. 1985. Antigenic and genetic properties of viruses linked to hemorrhagic fever with renal syndrome. *Science* 227:1041–1044. This is a good example of how to utilize basic studies for characterizing viruses and their habitat distribution.

Zweighaft, R.M., Fraser, D.W., Hattwick, M.A., et al. 1977. Lassa fever: Response to an imported case. *N. Engl. J. Med.* 297:803–807. The extreme concern regarding infectivity and diagnosis of hemorrhagic fever viruses is illustrated.

40

Rabies

Lawrence Corey

Single-stranded RNA virus

Rabies is an acute viral illness of the central nervous system. It can affect all mammals and is transmitted between them by infected secretions, usually saliva.

Agent

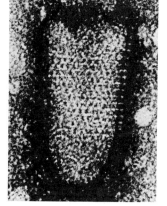

Rabies virus *

The rabies virus is a bullet-shaped, enveloped, single-stranded RNA virus of the rhabdovirus group. Other pathogens in this group include the vesicular stomatitis virus (Chapter 39). Rabies virus is large, with a diameter of about 180 × 70 nm. Knoblike glycoprotein excrescences, which elicit neutralizing and hemagglutination inhibiting antibodies, cover the surface of the virion.

The virus, which can be grown in tissue culture, produces rapid encephalitis when injected intracerebrally into laboratory rodents. In the past, a single antigenically homogeneous virus was believed responsible for all rabies. However, differences in cell culture growth characteristics of isolates from different animal sources, some differences in virulence for experimental animals, and antigenic differences in surface glycoproteins have indicated strain heterogeneity among rabies virus isolates. These studies may help to explain some of the biologic differences noted, as well as the occasional case of "vaccine failure."

Clinical Manifestations

Transmitted to humans from rabid animals

Rabies in humans usually results from a bite by a rabid animal or contamination of a wound by its saliva. It presents as an acute, fulminant, fatal encephalitis; human survivors have been reported only occasionally. The

*Rabies virus particle figure reproduced with permission of Dr. K. Hummuler. Hummuler, K., Koprowski, M., and Wiktor, T.J. 1967. *J. Virol.* 1:152–170.

disease begins as a nonspecific illness marked by fever, headache, malaise, nausea, and vomiting. Abnormal sensations at or around the site of viral inoculation occur frequently and probably reflect local nerve involvement. The onset of encephalitis is marked by periods of excess motor activity and agitation. Hallucinations, combativeness, muscle spasms, signs of meningeal irritation, seizures, and focal paralysis appear. Periods of mental dysfunction are interspersed with completely lucid periods; as the disease progresses, however, the patient lapses into coma. Autonomic nervous system involvement often results in increased salivation. Brain stem and cranial nerve dysfunction is characteristic, with double vision, facial palsies, and difficulty in swallowing. The combination of excess salivation and difficulty in swallowing produces the traditional picture of "foaming at the mouth." Hydrophobia, the painful, violent involuntary contractions of the diaphragm and accessory respiratory, pharyngeal, and laryngeal muscles initiated by swallowing liquids, is seen in about 50% of cases. Involvement of the respiratory center produces respiratory paralysis, the major cause of death. The median survival after onset of symptoms is 4 days, with a maximum of 20 days unless artificial supporting measures are instituted. Recovery is rare and has only been seen in partially immunized individuals.

Encephalitic manifestations; survival very rare

Hydrophobia from dysphagia

Brief course with development of respiratory paralysis

Occasionally rabies may appear as an ascending paralysis resembling Guillain-Barré syndrome.

Pathogenesis

The essential first event in human or animal rabies infection is the introduction of virus through the epidermis, usually as a result of an animal bite. Inhalation of heavily contaminated material, such as bat droppings, can also cause infection. Rabies virus first replicates in striated muscle tissue at the site of inoculation. It then enters the peripheral nervous system at the neuromuscular junctions and spreads up the nerves to the central nervous system, where it replicates exclusively within the gray matter. It then passes centrifugally along autonomic nerves to reach other tissues, including the salivary glands, adrenal medulla, kidneys, and lungs. Passage into the salivary glands in animals facilitates further transmission of the disease by infected saliva. The incubation period ranges from 10 days to a year, depending on the amount of virus introduced, the amount of tissue involved, the host immune mechanisms, and the distance the virus must travel from the site of inoculation to the central nervous system. Thus, the incubation period is generally shorter with face wounds than with leg wounds. Immunization early in the incubation period frequently aborts the infection.

Routes of infection

Initial replication in muscle followed by spread from nerves to brain

Centrifugal spread in autonomic nerves; salivary gland involvement

Factors influencing incubation period that varies from 10 days to 1 year

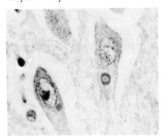

Negri body in cytoplasm of neuron.*

Pathology

The neuropathology of rabies resembles that of other viral diseases of the central nervous system, with infiltration of lymphocytes and plasma cells into central nervous system tissue and nerve cell destruction. The pathognomic lesion is the Negri body, an eosinophilic cytoplasmic inclusion distributed throughout the brain, particularly in the hippocampus, cerebral cortex, cerebellum, and dorsal spinal ganglia. As Negri bodies are not seen in at least 20% of rabies victims, their absence does not rule out the diagnosis.

---

*Negri bodies figure provided by Dr. Daniel P. Perl.

Laboratory Diagnosis

Immunofluorescent
examination of infected tissue

Intracerebral inoculation of
suckling mice

Demonstration of Negri
bodies

Laboratory diagnosis of rabies is accomplished by indirect or direct demonstration of virus. Viral antigen can be demonstrated rapidly in brain tissue by immunofluorescent procedures. Intracerebral inoculation of infected brain tissue or secretions into suckling mice results in death in 3–10 days. Histologic examination of their brain tissue shows Negri bodies; both Negri bodies and rhabdovirus particles may be demonstrated by electron microscopy. Specific antibodies to rabies virus can be detected, but generally only late in the disease.

Epidemiology and Epizoology

Urban and sylvatic animal
rabies

Infections of cattle and
humans are blind ended

Most human cases are derived
from infected dogs or cats

Rabies exists in two epizoologic forms: urban, which is associated with unimmunized dogs or cats; and sylvatic, which occurs in wild skunks, foxes, wolves, raccoons, mongooses, and bats. Human infection, or the much more common infection of cattle, is incidental, blind ended, and does not contribute to maintenance or transmission of the disease. In the United States, more than 75% of reported cases of rabies in animals occur among wildlife. Most human exposure, however, is from bites by unimmunized dogs or cats. Infection in domestic animals usually represents a spillover from infection in wildlife reservoirs. Human infection tends to occur where animal rabies is common and where there is a large population of unimmunized domestic animals. Worldwide, the occurrence of human rabies is estimated to be about 15,000 cases per year, with the highest attack rates in Southeast Asia, the Philippines, and the Indian subcontinent. In the United States, one to five cases of human rabies are reported yearly. A recent addition to the epidemiology of rabies in the United States has been the transmission of disease through transplantation of infected corneal tissue from a recently deceased but undiagnosed case.

Bat rabies in United States

In most areas of the world, the dog is the most important vector of the rabies virus to human. Other important sources of disease are the wolf in eastern Europe, the mongoose in Africa, the fox in western Europe, and the bat in Latin America and the United States.

Prevention and Treatment

Prevention is the mainstay of controlling human rabies. Intensive supportive care has resulted in two or three long-term survivals; despite the best modern medical care, however, the mortality still exceeds 90%. In addition, because of the infrequency of the disease, many cases die without definitive diagnosis.

Pasteur's vaccine

In the late 1800s Pasteur, noting the long incubation period of rabies, suggested that a vaccine to induce an immune response before the development of disease might be useful in prevention. He apparently successfully vaccinated Joseph Meister, a boy severely bitten and exposed to rabies, with multiple injections of a crude vaccine made from dried spinal cord of rabies-infected rabbits. This treatment emerged as one of the best known and noteworthy accomplishments in the annals of medicine.

Preexposure prophylaxis for
individuals at special risk

Human diploid cell culture
vaccine

Currently, the prevention of rabies is divided into preexposure and postexposure prophylaxis. Preexposure prophylaxis is recommended for individuals at high risk of contact with rabies virus, such as veterinarians, spelunkers, laboratory workers, and animal handlers. Two types of vaccine are currently licensed in the United States for preexposure prophylaxis; however, only one is commercially available. This employs an attenuated

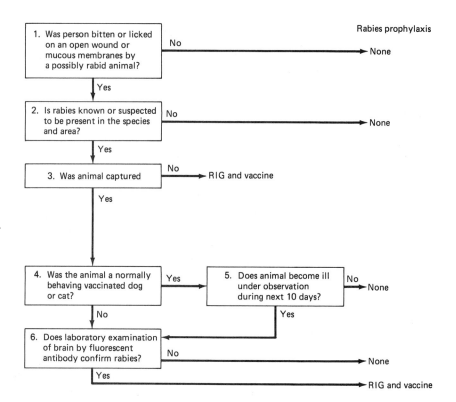

40.1 Postexposure rabies
     prophylaxis algorithm.
RIG = rabies immune globulin.

rabies virus grown in human diploid cell culture and inactivated with β-propiolactone. Preexposure prophylaxis consists of two subcutaneous injections of vaccine given 1 month apart, followed by a booster dose several months later.

Postexposure prophylaxis

Factors influencing decision to immunize after possible exposure

Postexposure prophylaxis requires careful evaluation and judgment. Every year more than one million Americans are bitten by animals, and in each instance a decision must be made whether to initiate postexposure rabies prophylaxis. In this decision the physician must consider 1) whether the individual came into physical contact with saliva or another substance likely to contain rabies virus; 2) whether there was significant wounding or abrasion; 3) whether rabies is known or suspected in the animal species and area associated with the exposure; 4) the circumstances surrounding the exposure (that is, whether the bite was provoked or unprovoked); and 5) whether the animal is available for laboratory examination. Any wild animal or ill, unvaccinated, or stray domestic animal involved in a possible rabies exposure, such as an unprovoked bite, should be captured and killed. The head should be sent immediately to an appropriate laboratory, usually at the state health department, for search for rabies antigen by immunofluorescence. If examination of the brain by this technique is negative for rabies virus, it can be assumed that the saliva contains no virus and that the exposed person requires no treatment. If the test is positive, the patient should be given postexposure prophylaxis. It should be noted that rodents and rabbits are not important vectors of rabies virus.

Concurrent active and passive immunization

Postexposure prophylaxis is based on 1) immediate thorough washing of the wound with soap and water; 2) passive immunization with hyperimmune globulin of which at least half the dose should be instilled around the wound site; and 3) active immunization with antirabies vaccine. With human diploid vaccine, six doses given on days 1, 3, 7, 14, and 90 are recommended. An algorithm illustrating the approach to postexposure prophylaxis is shown in Figure 40.1.

Critical need for consultation

The physician in private practice in the United States should always seek the advice of the local health department when the question of rabies prophylaxis arises.

Additional Reading

Anderson, L.J., Nicholson, K.G., Tauxe, R.V., et al. 1984. Human rabies in the United States, 1960–1979. Epidemiology, diagnosis, and prevention. *Ann. Int. Med.* 100:728–735. An excellent general review of this problem.

Baer, G.M., Bridbord, K., Hui, F.W., et al, Eds. 1988. Research towards rabies prevention. *Rev. Infect. Dis.* 10(suppl 4):S573–S815. A symposium dealing with a world-wide perspective. It includes consideration of control of rabies in wildlife.

Recommendation of the Immunization Practices Advisory Committee. 1984. Rabies prevention: United States. 1984. *MMWR* 33:393–402, 407–408. An authoritative guide to rabies prophylaxis in humans with a subsequent addition in MMWR, 1986, 35:767–768.

41

Retroviruses

James J. Champoux

Single-stranded RNA
enveloped viruses carrying
reverse transcriptase

Include oncoviruses and
lentiviruses

Rapidly inactivated outside
the body

Oncoviruses cause tumors in
many animals

HTLV-I and -II associated
with human leukemias

The retroviruses are enveloped, single-stranded RNA viruses. They encode reverse transcriptase (an RNA-dependent DNA polymerase) that copies their genome into proviral double-stranded DNA. Representatives of two major groups will be considered in this chapter, the oncoviruses (*onco-*: related to a tumor) and the lentiviruses (*lenti-*: slow). Like most enveloped viruses, all retroviruses are highly susceptible to factors that affect surface tension and are thus not transmissible through air, dust, or fomites under normal conditions, but require intimate contact with the infecting source.

Oncoviruses of this group have long been associated with a variety of cancers in animals, including leukemias, lymphomas, and sarcomas, but until recent years had not been found to infect humans. The first human retrovirus, human T-lymphotropic virus I (HTLV-I), was discovered in the late 1970s. It was shown to cause adult T-cell leukemia, a rare malignancy found only in Japan, Africa, and the Caribbean, although serological evidence shows that the virus also occurs in the United States and has raised the possibility of an association with some chronic neurological conditions. A relative of HTLV-I, HTLV-II, has been associated with some cases of human leukemias, including hairy cell leukemia, but its precise role in these diseases remains unclear.

HIV-1 and -2 are lentiviruses
that cause AIDS

The most important human retrovirus infection, the acquired immunodeficiency syndrome (AIDS) is caused by one of two lentiviruses termed the *human immunodeficiency viruses* (HIV-1 and HIV-2). This devastating disease, for which there is no present cure, has spurred unprecedented research efforts to determine the nature and pathogenic mechanisms of HIV and other retroviruses in the hopes of finding effective drugs and vaccines. Most of our present knowledge of HIV is derived from studies on HIV-1, which is the major cause of AIDS worldwide.

Oncoviruses usually not
cytolytic; transduce or
activate oncogenes

Oncoviruses do not kill the cell that they infect, but instead usually continue to produce new virus indefinitely. This property, combined with

41.1 Structure of HIV particle. The two RNA molecules enclosed within the capsid (CA) are coated with the nucleocapsid protein (NC). The matrix protein (MA) lies just inside the membrane envelope. The envelope contains the two membrane glycoproteins, gp41 and gp120, also called the *transmembrane protein* (TM) and *surface protein* (SU), respectively.

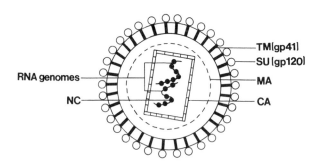

the fact that they can transduce growth-promoting genes called *oncogenes* into the recipient cell, accounts in part for their ability to cause malignancies (see below). With lentivirus infections, the cell–virus relationship is quite different. Lentiviruses can persist for years in a latent state without causing much cell killing, only to become highly cytolytic when the infected cells are subjected to certain stimuli. The prototype lentivirus is the visna virus, which causes a slow degenerative neurological disease in sheep. Like visna, HIV can persist for long periods of time without serious effects, but eventually is induced to replicate to high levels resulting in cell death. Although HIV can infect a variety of human cell types, its most drastic effects appear to result from destruction of the T4 subclass of lymphocytes, which play a central role in the capacity of the host to mount effective and protective immunological reponses to a wide range of infections.

> Lentiviruses become cytopathic after long latency

> HIV specifically attacks T4 lymphocytes

Structure of Retroviruses

All retroviruses are remarkably similar in their basic composition. The structure of HIV is depicted in Figure 41.1. The virion is about 100 nm in diameter. It contains two copies of a single-stranded RNA genome and is thus diploid. The RNA genome is coated with the nucleocapsid protein and the RNA–protein complexes are enclosed in a capsid composed of multiple subunits. Like all enveloped viruses, the membrane is acquired during budding from the host cell, but the surface (SU) and transmembrane (TM) glycoproteins found in the envelope are virally encoded. Between the capsid and the envelope is a matrix (MA) protein. In addition to structural proteins shown in Figure 41.1, the virion contains three virus-specific proteins that are essential for viral replication: reverse transcriptase, (RT), protease (PR), and an integrase (IN). The relationship between viral genes (*gag, pol,* and *env*) and the proteins they encode are presented in Table 41.1.

> Virion contains two single-stranded RNA molecules

> Envelope acquired during budding contains two viral glycoproteins

> Viral genome encodes structural and replicative proteins

Retroviral Life Cycle

The diagram shown in Figure 41.2 depicts the life cycle of a typical retrovirus and serves to illustrate the many unique aspects of retroviral replication that could be potential targets for therapeutic intervention.

Table 41.1 Retroviral Proteins

Gene[a]	Protein Products	Function
gag	Matrix	Structural
	Capsid	Structural
	Nucleocapsid	Structural
	p10–21	Unknown
	Protease[b]	Protein processing
pol	Protease[b]	Protein processing
	Reverse transcriptase	DNA synthesis
	Integrase	Integration
env	Surface glycoprotein	Adsorption
	Transmembrane protein	Anchor for surface glycoprotein

[a] Each gene encodes a polyprotein that is subsequently processed by proteolysis to yield the individual proteins.
[b] The protease is encoded in either the *gag* gene or the *pol* gene, depending on the virus.

41.2 Retroviral Life Cycle

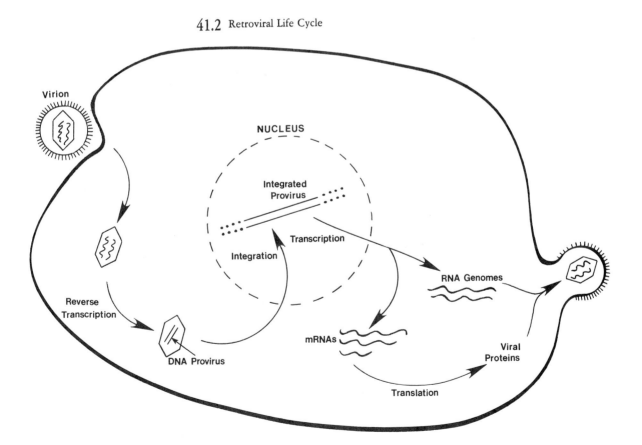

Viral Entry

Surface glycoprotein gp 120 attaches to CD4 cell receptor in case of HIV

The virions adsorb to cellular membrane receptors and either enter the cell by receptor-mediated endocytosis (see Chapter 6) or by direct fusion with the plasma membrane. For HIV, the virion attachment protein is the SU glycoprotein gp120, and the cell receptor is the CD4 molecule that occurs primarily on the plasma membrane of T4 lymphocytes and cells of the monocyte–macrophage series and some other target cells. The HIV transmembrane (TM) protein gp41 is responsible for fusion of viral and cell membranes, a process that apparently mediates entry of the virus into the host cell.

Transmembrane protein mediates fusion of viral and cell membranes

HIV can also infect cells such as fibroblasts and certain brain cells that lack the CD4 surface molecule, apparently because the fusion-inducing activity of the TM protein is sufficient in these cases to promote entry. Fusion activity may also play an important role in amplification of the effects of the virus infection, because infected cells expressing viral glycoproteins in their membranes readily fuse with uninfected T4 lymphocytes to form large syncytia. This process appears to provide a means for cell-to-cell transmission of the virus that bypasses the usual extracellular phase and also damages the membrane of uninfected cells and affects their viability.

Fusion of infected and uninfected cells allows viral transmission

Viral RNA Replication

Reverse transcriptase copies RNA to double stranded DNA

Among the RNA viruses, retroviral replication is unique. Soon after entry of the viral core into the cytoplasm of the infected cell, the RNA is copied into double-stranded DNA by reverse transcriptase, the virion-associated DNA polymerase. The overall process is referred to as *reverse transcription* and results in a linear *proviral* DNA that enters the nucleus and integrates at random into a host cell chromosome. Once the viral genetic information has been converted to DNA and integrated, it essentially becomes part of the cellular genome. The viral genes are therefore replicated and faithfully inherited as long as the infected cell continues to divide.

DNA provirus integrates into host chromosome and replicates with the cell

Provirus includes its own promoter and signals that control transcription

Special sequences contained within the RNA are duplicated during the reverse transcription process so that the integrated provirus contains identical long terminal repeats (LTRs) at its ends. The LTR sequences contain the appropriate promoter and other signals required for transcription of the viral genes by the host RNA polymerase II. Transcription produces both a full-length RNA genome and one or more spliced mRNAs. The predominant spliced mRNA is translated to produce the envelope glycoproteins, but in HIV a series of spliced mRNAs are produced that also encode a variety of viral regulatory proteins. Unlike most retroviruses, HIV apparently exerts considerable control over whether primary transcripts are allocated to full-length RNA or are spliced to produce mRNAs (see below). With the exception of these regulatory proteins, all retroviral proteins are initially translated as polyproteins that are subsequently processed by proteolysis into the individual protein molecules. The enzyme responsible for most of these protein cleavages is the virus-specific protease (PR) that is either encoded in the *gag* gene or the *pol* gene of the viruse (see Table 41.1).

Genomic RNA and spliced mRNA's are both produced: the latter encode surface glycoproteins and regulatory proteins

HIV can control extent of genomic or spliced mRNA production

A simplified view of retroviral RNA replication is presented in Figure 41.3. In addition to a DNA polymerase activity, the reverse transcriptase possesses an RNase H activity that is responsible for degrading the RNA

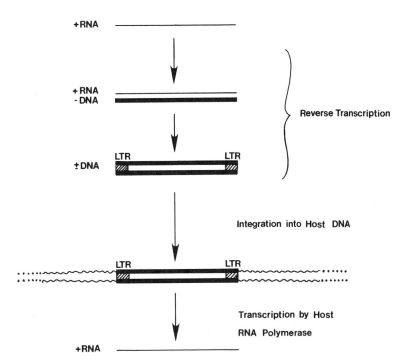

41.3 Retroviral RNA
Replication

RNase H activity degrades
original RNA genome, which
was reverse transcribed

portion of the DNA–RNA hybrid (+RNA/−DNA) produced in the first phase of reverse transcription. The immediate product of reverse transcription is a linear double-stranded DNA molecule that is flanked by the LTR sequences. The viral integrase (IN), in conjunction with at least one host factor, mediates the integration of the linear DNA into host DNA. The integration process is highly specific with respect to the viral DNA, and one or two base pairs (depending on the virus) are lost from each end of the DNA. However, the choice of a target site for integration into the

Integration is random in host
DNA

cellular DNA appears to be nearly random. A short sequence of base pairs in the target DNA (four to six depending on the virus) is duplicated during the integration process and the sequences immediately flank the integrated provirus. The replication process is completed by transcription of the

Integrated DNA is
transcribed by host RNA
polymerase

proviral DNA by the host RNA polymerase.

It should be noted that the scheme represented in Figure 41.3 also describes the replication cycle for hepatitis B virus (see Chapter 36). However, instead of packaging the RNA form of the genome as occurs with retroviruses, hepatitis B virus packages the double-stranded DNA that is the immediate product of reverse transcription.

Variation in HIV

Of all the known retroviruses, HIV possesses the most error-prone reverse transcriptase. This property accounts for the many nucleotide differences observed between different isolates (even from the same infected individual) and for the variability of the gp120 antigen. It may explain in part the failure of the immune system to control the infection and the increases in viral virulence that appear to occur during the course of the infection.

Marked error proneness of
HIV reverse transcriptase

Different isolates from the
same patient can differ in
virulence and antigenically

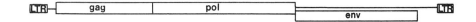

Retroviral Genomes

Typical retrovirus

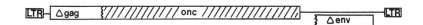

**Defective acute
transforming retrovirus**

HIV

41.4 Maps of the integrated forms of various retroviral genomes are drawn with the
genes and long terminal repeats (LTRs) shown as boxes. The vertical displacements
of the boxes above and below the lines depict the relative reading frames of the coding
segments.

Retroviral Genes

The organization of the genome of different types of retroviruses is shown
in Figure 41.4 (see also Table 41.1). The order of the genes for a typical
retrovirus is *gag–pol–env*. The *gag* (group-specific antigen) gene encodes
the structural proteins of the virus and in some cases the protease. The
pol (polymerase) gene encodes the reverse transcriptase, the integrase, and
sometimes the protease. The *env* (envelope) gene encodes the two membrane glycoproteins found in the viral envelope. Not surprisingly, the
surface protein (gp120 in HIV) is responsible for the host range of the
virus and its antigenicity. As indicated previously, the HIV *env* gene is
found to exhibit extensive variation from one isolate to another, resulting
in considerable polymorphism of gp120.

Roles of *gag, pol,* and *env*
genes

The genomes of acute transforming oncoviruses have a variety of structures, but the feature that is common to nearly all of them is that some
viral genes are replaced by genes derived from their hosts that render
them oncogenic (see below). In every case, the signals required for reverse
transcription and transcription of the integrated virus, which are located
near the ends of the RNA, are retained in the infecting virus. In the
example shown in Figure 41.4, the *pol* gene and parts of both the viral
gag and *env* genes are deleted, but other configurations are possible. Such
oncoviruses are defective and only replicate in the presence of a helper
virus that can supply the missing functions.

Some retroviruses carry host
genes rendering them
oncogenic

Most acute transforming
oncogenic viruses are
defective and require helper
virus for replication

A comparison of the genetic makeup of HIV with that of a typical
retrovirus (Figure 41.4) reveals a larger number of genes and a much more

Table 41.2 HIV and HTLV-I Regulatory Proteins

Gene	Protein	Function
HIV–*tat* HTLV–*tax*	TAT TAX	Transactivation of viral gene expression
HIV–*rev* HTLV–*rex*	REV REX	Promote synthesis of viral structure proteins at level of mRNA transport
HIV–*nef*	NEF	Negative regulator of transcription
HIV–*vif*	VIF	Facilitate virus maturation during budding

Abbreviations: HIV = human immunodeficiency virus; HTLV = human T-lymphotropic virus.

Complexity of HIV; multiple regulatory genes control latency and virulence

complex organization. HIV contains, in addition to the usual ensemble of genes, an array of other genes (*tat, rev, nef, vif, vpr,* and *vpu*). Expression of these genes requires mRNA splicing, and all apparently encode proteins that serve regulatory roles important in determining the long period of latency exhibited by the virus (see below). HTLV-I encodes a similar array of regulatory proteins. The names of the genes that have been best characterized and the proteins and functions that they determine are given in Table 41.2.

Transformation by Retroviruses

Oncogenic retroviruses appear to transform cells to an oncogenic state by three distinct mechanisms (see Chapter 7).

First, the acute transforming viruses (see Figure 41.4) have acquired a cellular gene (called an *oncogene*) that when expressed in the infected cell results in loss of normal growth control. Upon infection, the oncogene is expressed immediately from the viral LTR promoter, resulting in a rapid and acute onset of malignant disease. Persistent transformation by oncogene transduction is only possible for those retroviruses that are not cytocidal. More that 25 different oncogenes have been identified in a variety of animal retroviruses, but no human retroviruses are known that transform by this mechanism.

Noncytocidal viruses carrying cellular oncogenes can produce persistent transformation

The second mechanism is called *insertional mutagenesis*. Integration of a retrovirus in the vicinity of particular cellular genes can cause inappropriate expression of the gene resulting in uncontrolled cell growth. These cellular genes are called *protooncogenes*, and insertional activation by the virus is apparently due to the close proximity of the integrated viral promoter or enhancer to the gene. Cancers that are caused by this mechanism have very long latent periods, because integration is random and only rarely occurs near a cellular protooncogene. No human cancers are known to be caused by this mechanism.

Integration adjacent to cellular protooncogenes can activate them

HTLV-I, the causative agent of adult T-cell leukemia, exemplifies the third mechanism. In this case, the integrated provirus in the leukemic cells from any one patient is found at a unique location on a particular chromosome. Thus, the tumors are probably monoclonal. However, the cancer is not the result of insertional mutagenesis, because the chromosomal location of the provirus is never the same in any two patients. Instead, transformation results from the continual expression of the viral *tax* gene (the HTLV-I homolog of the HIV *tat* gene, see Table 41.2). Apparently, the TAX protein can not only activate viral transcription in the same manner as TAT, but can also activate the expression of one or more cellular genes (possibly protooncogenes) resulting in malignant transformation.

HTLV-1 transforms by production of TAX, which activates cellular transforming genes

Human Immunodeficiency Virus Latency

A unique feature of HIV and other members of the lentivirus subfamily is the ability to produce a complex array of regulatory proteins that appear to be responsible for latent periods that can extend for months or years. In some cases, virus-specific DNA has even been detected in individuals who show no immunological response, suggesting that the viral genome can exist for prolonged periods of time in a quiescent state without expressing viral proteins.

Although much remains to be determined about the regulatory circuits that modulate HIV gene expression, the following features of the process have been established. Regulation appears to occur at three levels: mRNA production, transport of unspliced versus spliced mRNAs from the nucleus to the cytoplasm, and the maturation of viral proteins during budding. It may also occur at the level of mRNA translation. The HIV regulatory proteins and their functions are listed in Table 41.2. In the absence of the viral regulatory proteins, two features of the expression of the HIV proviral DNA are significant. First, the viral promoter in the LTR is intrinsically weak. Second, transport of the full-length, unspliced mRNA to the cytoplasm is so inefficient that the only mRNAs produced are spliced. Extensive splicing precludes production of the virion structural proteins and the enzymes required for virus production. Thus, shortly after integration, viral gene expression is restricted to the viral envelope glycoproteins and the regulatory proteins. One of these regulatory proteins is the NEF protein, which is apparently responsible for maintaining the latent state. NEF acts on a DNA sequence (NRE) in the viral LTR near the promoter to further suppress the transcription of the integrated proviral DNA.

Two of the regulatory proteins, TAT and REV, play a positive role in promoting viral gene expression. The TAT protein increases the rate of viral mRNA synthesis, and REV facilitates the transport of full-length mRNA to the cytoplasm before it can be spliced. The combined action of these two regulatory proteins is to promote the production of virus particles. Therefore, TAT acts to counter the activity of NEF, whereas REV promotes the production of virion structural proteins at the expense of its own production and that of other regulatory proteins. The VIF protein promotes virus production at the level of maturation.

Superimposed on this complex regulatory network is the fact that the viral promoter contains elements that are sensitive to specific cellular transcription factors. This observation may help explain why virus production in T4 lymphocytes is greatly increased when the cells are activated. Clearly the outcome of an HIV infection is determined by a complex interplay between a very large number of different factors.

Pathogenesis of HIV Infection

The pathogenesis of HIV infection is incompletely understood and very complex, but the following factors are likely to be important in the disease-causing process.

1. HIV can infect a large number of different cell types, primarily those with the CD4 surface antigen, including monocytes, macrophages, glial brain cells, and, of central importance, the T4 lymphocytes. The virus replicates slowly in macrophages, which may well be the first cells infected and a reservoir for continued expansion of the infection, including migration and spread across the blood–brain barrier.

Latency may be terminated
by proviral mutational
changes or activation of the
host cell

2. Several factors can terminate the long latent period of HIV. Mutations occur in the proviral genome that appear to enhance induction of virulent virus forms of increased cytopathic capacity and altered cell tropisms. If this is the case, the more virulent mutants are unlikely to be the transmitted form of the virus, because the natural history of the disease does not appear to have changed. A second factor may be a requirement for activation of infected T cells to permit virus production and cell death, and this may involve a variety of mitogenic and antigenic stimuli occurring after infection.

Cell fusion allows viral spread
and damages uninfected cells

3. Fusion between susceptible cells, most carrying the CD4 marker, allows virus to spread without being exposed to any neutralizing antibody and can also lead to damage to the membrane of uninfected cells, thus indirectly causing their death.

Primary defect is viral or
immunological destruction of
T4 cells or their functional
impairment

AIDS involves generalized
failure of cell-mediated
immune responses and of
specific antibody responses

4. The primary defect in AIDS results from the reduction in numbers and effectiveness of T4 helper-inducer lymphocytes both in absolute numbers and relative to T8 suppressor cells. This is due to direct killing of T4 cells by virus; to secondary killing of uninfected cells during cell fusion; to autoimmune processes that lead to the elimination of T4 cells by opsonophagocytosis; and possibly to antibody-dependent, cell-mediated cytotoxicity directed at gp120 expressed on the T4 surface. There are also functional defects in T4 cells affecting lymphokine production and leading to inhibition of some macrophage functions including low levels of interleukin 1 and interferon alpha. Effects on T4 cells thus lead to a generalized failure of cell-mediated immune responses, but there is also an effect on antibody production due to polyclonal activation of B cells, possibly associated with other viral infections of these cells. This overwhelms the capacity of infected individuals to respond to specific antigens. The end result of these processes is the susceptibility of AIDS patients to a range of viral, fungal, and bacterial infections to which, at present, they ultimately succumb. Acquired immunodeficiency syndrome as a disease is considered in more detail in Chapter 73.

Additional Reading

Levy, J.A. 1989. Human immunodeficiency viruses and the pathogenesis of AIDS. *JAMA* 261:2997–3006. An excellent up-to-date review of the pathogenesis of HIV infections.

Scientific American. 1988. Vol. 259, No. 4. This entire issue is devoted to the subject of AIDS. Even though some details may soon be out of date, this remains one of the most readable, informative, and well-written reviews of the subject.

42

DNA *Tumor* *Viruses*

Lawrence Corey and
John C. Sherris

Epstein–Barr, hepatitis B, and
human papillomaviruses are
associated with human tumors

Among DNA viruses, only three groups have thus far been unequivocally associated with the occurrence of tumors in humans. These are the Epstein–Barr virus (EBV), the hepatitis B virus, and the human papillomavirus (HPV).

Several other DNA viruses have been considered candidates for causing human tumors, but have not so far been shown to do so. The polyomaviruses, which fall with the papillomaviruses in the papovavirus family, produce tumors in experimental animals, but not in their natural hosts, and have not been associated with benign or malignant tumors in humans. They are considered in more detail later in the chapter because of the light that they have cast on mechanisms of oncogenesis. Some serotypes of adenoviruses can transform a number of cells lines in vitro and can cause tumors in newborn rodents, but, again, they have not been shown to be oncogenic in humans. During the past two decades, suspicion fell on herpes simplex virus type 2 as a cause of carcinoma of the uterine cervix in humans, but recent studies support the concept that certain types of HPV are the agents involved.

Only a small proportion of
infected individuals develop
tumors

The mechanisms by which DNA viruses predispose to tumors are not well understood. It is apparent from the ubiquity of these agents that only a small proportion of infected individuals develop tumors and usually after many years. Cofactors are almost certainly involved, and there is no clear evidence that DNA virus infections, in and of themselves, are the direct cause of cancers in humans.

Epstein–Barr Virus-Associated Tumors

EBV is associated with
Burkitt's lymphoma and
nasopharyngeal carcinoma

The EBV virus has been considered in Chapter 37 in some detail. It is the cause of infectious mononucleosis and has been associated with two types of tumors, African Burkitt's lymphoma and nasopharyngeal carcinoma. The factors that render the EBV infections oncogenic in these two cases are obscure. The distribution of EBV infections in Africa has suggested an infectious cofactor, such as human immunodeficiency virus or malaria infections, which may cause immunosuppression and predispose to EBV-related malignancy. Parts of the EBV genome are found in Burkitt's lymphoma cells.

EBV transforms B lymphocytes in vitro

In vitro, EBV virus infects human B lymphocytes and certain epithelial cells, including nasopharyngeal cells. The virus transforms B lymphocytes into lymphoblastlike cells that are able to multiply indefinitely. The DNA genome of the virus is present in the nucleus of transformed cells either integrated into the genome or more often as an extrachromosomal plasmid in multiple copies. Only partial transcription of viral proteins occurs (about 10 of the 60–70 genes). Two of these have been shown to be transforming genes, but the precise mechanisms by which transformation occurs is unclear.

Transformed cells possess integrated or extrachromosomal circularized viral genome

In the in vivo situation, EBV-associated lymphomas have been shown to be of both monoclonal or polyclonal origin. Chromosomal translocations in B cells are characteristic of Burkitt's lymphoma and involve specific breaks in chromosomes at sites of genes encoding immunoglobulins. These translocations lead to expression of oncogenes that may contribute to clonal activation and ultimately to malignancy. Some breakdown in immune surveillance also appears to play a role in the development of malignancy because immunosuppressed patients are more prone to develop B-cell lymphomas.

Chromosomal translocations in immunoglobulin genes occur in Burkitt's lymphoma and activate oncogenes

Breakdown in immune surveillance probably contributes to oncogenesis

The two classes of cancer associated with EBV are commonest in restricted geographic areas, which offers the possibility of prevention by immunization with virus specific antigen(s). This approach is under exploration at the present time. A subunit vaccine has proved effective in preventing the development of tumors in tamarin monkeys, which are highly susceptible to the oncogenic effects of the virus under experimental conditions.

Geographic limitation of tumor occurrence offers prospect of artificial immunization

Hepatitis B-Associated Tumors

The association of chronic hepatitis B infection (see Chapter 36) with hepatocellular carcinoma of the liver is well documented. The malignancy develops several decades after the initial infection, and prospective studies in Taiwan have shown that men in the age range of 40 to 60 who have hepatitis B surface antigen (HBsAg) detectable in their blood are more than 200 times as likely to develop hepatocellular carcinoma as those who are HBsAg negative.

Chronic hepatitis B may result in hepatocellular carcinoma long after infection

Integrated hepatitis B viral DNA can be found in nearly all hepatocellular carcinomas. The virus has not been shown to possess a transforming gene, but may well activate a cellular oncogene. It is also possible that the virus does not play such a direct molecular role in oncogenicity, because the natural history of chronic hepatitis B infection involves cycles of damage or death of liver cells interspersed with periods of intense regenerative hyperplasia. This significantly increases the opportunity for spontaneous mutational changes that may activate cellular oncogenes. Whatever the mechanism, the association of chronic viral infection and hepatocellular carcinoma is clear, and liver cancer is a major cause of disease and death in countries in which chronic hepatitis B infection is common. The proven success of combined active and passive immunization in aborting hepatitis B infection in infancy or childhood makes hepatocellular carcinoma of the liver a potentially preventable disease.

Integrated viral genome in tumor cells may activate cellular oncogenes

Tumors could also result from mutations in regenerating liver cells

Hepatocellular carcinoma is potentially preventable by immunization

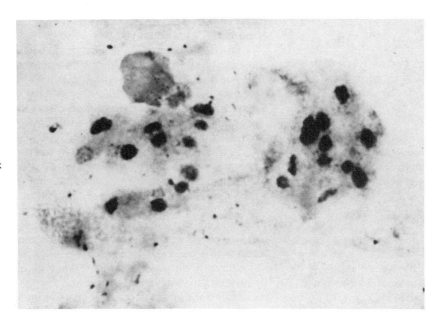

42.1 Human papillomavirus (HPV) type 16 DNA demonstrated in a cervical smear by in situ hybridization. The dark circles represent detection of HPV DNA sequences by the DNA probe.

Papillomaviruses and Associated Tumors

Members of papovavirus group; naked double-stranded DNA viruses

The papillomaviruses share membership of the papovavirus group with the polyomaviruses. Papillomaviruses are small, unenveloped, double-stranded DNA viruses exhibiting cubic symmetry (Figure 42.1). They are about 55 nm in diameter. They cause epidermal papillomas and warts in a wide range of higher vertebrates. Different members of the group are generally species specific. For example, bovine and human papillomaviruses only infect the hosts reflected in their names. In some cases, tumors caused by these agents can become malignant.

Cause of species specific papillomas and warts in higher vertebrates

Shope rabbit papillomas can become malignant; cofactors hasten the progress

Papillomaviruses were the first DNA viruses linked to malignant changes. In the mid-1930s it was demonstrated by Shope that benign rabbit papillomas were due to filterable agents and could advance to become malignant squamous cell carcinomas. External cofactors, such as coal tar, could hasten this process. However, work on the biology and mechanism by which these agents foster malignant transformation has been impeded by the inability to cultivate papillomaviruses in vitro. Molecular probes to detect viral products in vivo indicate that replication and assembly of these viruses takes place only in the differentiating layers of squamous epithelia—a situation that has not been reproduced in vitro.

Papillomaviruses have not been grown in cell culture

Genomes of papillomaviruses have been cloned and compared: many genotypes infect humans and are associated with specific diseases

The genomes of many of the papillomaviruses have now been cloned from infected lesions into bacterial plasmids and compared by restriction endonuclease and DNA homology procedures (Chapters 4 and 14). These studies have shown a wide genomic diversity among papillomaviruses that infect different species, and also among those infecting humans. They have led to the allocation of numbers for the different genotypes.

Viral components detectable in infected cells

Range of lesions caused by human papillomaviruses

Over 50 genotypes of HPV have been identified in human papillomas and warts. Some of the genotypes are serologically (phenotypically) different and groups of genotypes are associated with specific lesions. Viral components can be detected in infected cells by labeled specific antibody or by in situ hybridization with cloned viral DNA. Human papillomaviruses have been identified in plantar warts, flat and papillomatous warts of other skin areas, juvenile laryngeal papillomas, and in a variety of genital hyperplastic epithelial lesions, including cervical, vulvar, and penile warts and papillomas.

The first evidence that HPVs could be associated with human malignant disease came from observations on epidermodysplasia verruciformis. This disease has a genetic basis that results in unusual susceptibility to HPV types 5 and 8, which produce multiple flat warts. About a third of affected patients develop squamous-celled carcinoma from the lesions. The HPV genomic material is detectable in the nuclei of both the benign and malignant tumors.

Twelve genotypes found in human genital lesions; silent infections are common

Twelve genotypes of HPV have been identified in genital lesions of humans, and there are many apparently silent infections with these viruses. The incidence of HPV infections has almost certainly been increasing, and they now constitute perhaps the commonest sexually transmitted disease. From 20 to 60% of adult women in the United States are infected with one or other of the genotypes. Human papillomavirus types 6 and 11 are associated most commonly with benign genital warts in males and females, and with some cellular dyplasias of the cervical epithelium, but these lesions rarely become malignant. They can be perinatally transmitted and cause infantile laryngeal papillomas. Types 16, 18, and 31 may also cause warty lesions of the vulva, cervix, and penis, but infections with viral types more often progress to malignancy. Viral genomes of these types are found in a large proportion of markedly dysplastic uterine cervical cells, carcinomas in situ, and in cells of frankly malignant lesions. Human papillomavirus infection is now considered to be a prerequisite for the majority of carcinomas of the cervix.

HPV types 6 and 11 associated with benign genital warts

Types 16, 18, and 31 infections may progress to malignancy; associated with most carcinomas of the cervix

The mechanisms of oncogenicity of HPV is less clear, and much of what follows has been extrapolated from studies on a bovine papilloma virus that can be grown in mouse cell lines. Cells infected with this virus are transformed and produce tumors when injected into nude (T cell-deficient) mice. The viral genome exists as multiple copies of a circular episome within the nucleus of transformed cells, but is not integrated into the cellular genome. This appears also to be the case with benign human lesions. In malignant tumors, part of the viral genome is found integrated in the cellular genome, but integration is not site specific. Both the integrated viral genome and the extrachromosomal form carry their own transforming genes. Host cells normally produce a protein that inhibits expression of papillomavirus-transforming genes, but this can be inactivated by products of the virus and possibly by other infecting viruses, thus allowing malignant transformation to occur.

Both integrated and extrachromosomal viral genomes occur

Viral genome carries transforming genes

The role of HPV in genital lesions and in the etiology of carcinoma of the cervix is considered in additional detail in Chapter 70.

Polyomaviruses

The polyomaviruses include polyomavirus, the J.C. and B.K. viruses of humans, and the simian SV 40 virus. Polyomaviruses, like the papillomaviruses, are members of the papovavirus family. They are also double-stranded, naked capsid DNA viruses and are widely distributed among various animal species, usually without causing apparent disease. They are, however, able to transform cells of a variety of heterologous cell lines in culture.

Polyomaviruses usually cause no disease in natural hosts; transform cells in culture

Polyomaviruses can produce malignant tumors in certain experimental animals, but, interestingly, do not do so in their natural hosts. For example, SV 40 can produce lymphocytic leukemia and a variety of reticuloendothelial cell sarcomas in baby hamsters, but is not oncogenic in its natural

May produce tumors in experimental animals, but not in their natural hosts

monkey host. Fortunately, even though it can transform some human cells in vitro, it fails to produce disease in humans, a fact that became apparent on follow-up of recipients of early batches of poliomyelitis vaccine that were contaminated with live SV 40 virus. The J.C. virus (Chapter 43), which is a polyomavirus of humans, also produces cerebral tumors in baby hamsters. The majority of humans show serological evidence of having been infected with it at one time or another, usually without any clinical manifestations. It does not produce tumors in humans, but has been associated occasionally with a neurodegenerative disease in humans (see Chapter 43).

J.C. virus infects humans but does not cause human tumors

The reason why polyomaviruses fail to produce tumors in their natural hosts is uncertain, but may be because they are usually cytocidal under these conditions. From a biological point of view, the polyomaviruses are particularly useful models of oncogenicity because they can be readily studied in vitro and interact with cells in different ways. In some, they can produce lytic infections and cell death with production of complete virions. In others, they integrate randomly into cell genome and cause transformation by the expression of one or more of the viral genes. In no case has a human tumor been shown to have been caused by polyomaviruses.

Valuable experimental models of oncogenicity

It merits stressing that DNA viruses have not yet been proven to be the *immediate* cause of malignant as opposed to benign tumors in humans. In most cases there is a period of years between infection and the development of malignancy. Other factors such as benign cellular hyperplasia or immunologically mediated damage to infected cells may increase the chances of somatic mutations leading to malignancy. As in the case of retroviruses (Chapter 41), the field is one of very active research and is helping to clarify the processes by which cancers develop and extend.

DNA virus-associated tumors may result from mutations in hyperplastic or immunologically damaged host cells

Further Reading

Ciba Foundation Symposium 120. 1986. *The Papillomaviruses*. New York: John Wiley & Sons, pp. 1–246. An excellent monograph on the molecular biology and epidemiology of HPV.

43

Persistent Viral Infections of the Central Nervous System

Lawrence Corey

Progressive neurologic diseases

Evidence has accumulated during the past 30 years that a variety of progressive neurologic diseases in both animals and humans are caused by viral or other filtrable agents that share some of the properties of viruses (Table 43.1). These illnesses have been termed *slow viral diseases* because of the protracted period between infection and the prolonged course of the illness, but a better term is *persistent viral infection*.

Involve well-differentiated cells

It is of interest that most persistent viral infections involve well-differentiated cells, such as lymphocytes and neuronal cells. They can be classified as 1) diseases associated with "conventional" viral agents that possess nucleic acid genomes and protein capsids, induce immune responses, and can be grown in cell culture systems and 2) diseases associated with "unconventional" viruses, which are small, filterable infectious agents transmissible to certain experimental animals, but that do not appear to be associated with immune or inflammatory responses by the host and have not been cultivated in cell culture.

Unconventional agents do not produce immune or inflammatory responses

Contributors to viral persistence

Viral persistence can result from integration of viral nucleic acid into the host genome, mutations that interfere with viral replication or antigenicity, failure of host immune systems to recognize virus or infected cells, or perhaps because the causative "virus" is itself encoded in the normal host cell genome.

Diseases Associated with Conventional Agents

The following are the major persistent infections due to conventional viral agents. They are summarized in Table 43.1.

Subacute Sclerosing Panencephalitis

Subacute sclerosing panencephalitis has been considered in detail in Chapter 33. It is a rare chronic measles virus infection of children that produces progressive neurologic disease characterized by an insidious onset of per-

Chronic measles infection of children

619

Table 43.1   Slow Virus Infections

Disease	Agent
Conventional Viruses	
Subacute sclerosing panencephalitis	Measles virus
Progressive panencephalitis after congenital rubella	Rubella virus
Progressive multifocal leukoencephalopathy	Papovaviruses, J.C. virus, SV40-like agent
AIDS dementia complex	Human immunodeficiency virus
Persistent enterovirus infection of the immunodeficient	Picornaviruses
Unconventional Viruses[a]	
Kuru	
Creutzfeld–Jakob disease	
Scrapie (sheep and goats)	
Transmissible mink encephalopathy	

[a] Subacute spongiform encephalopathies.

sonality change, progressive intellectual deterioration, and both motor and autonomic nervous system dysfunctions.

Progressive Post Rubella Panencephalitis

Rarely, a degenerative neurologic disorder similar to measles subacute sclerosing panencephalitis may be related to persistent rubella virus infection of the central nervous system. This condition is seen most often in adolescents who have had congenital rubella syndrome. Rubella virus has been isolated from brain tissue in these patients using cocultivation techniques.

Progressive Multifocal Leukoencephalopathy

Progressive neurologic disease of immunocompromised adults

Progressive multifocal leukoencephalopathy (PML) is a rare, subacute, degenerative disease of the brain found primarily in adults with other chronic diseases, especially the acquired immunodeficiency syndrome (AIDS), reticuloendothelial malignancies, or those receiving immunosuppressives. The disease is characterized by the development of impaired memory, confusion, and disorientation, followed by a multiplicity of neurologic symptoms and signs that includes hemiparesis, visual disturbances, incoordination, seizures, and visual abnormalities. The disease is progressive, with death usually occurring 3–6 months after onset of symptoms. The cerebrospinal fluid (CSF) findings are often normal, although some patients show a slight increase in lymphocytes, and elevated protein levels may be present.

Pathologic features

Pathologically, foci of demyelination are found, surrounded by giant, bizarre astrocytes containing intranuclear inclusions. The demyelination is due to viral damage to oligodendroglial cells, which synthesize and maintain myelin.

Viral damage to myelin-synthesizing cells

Although the clinical diagnosis may be difficult to make, the pathologic

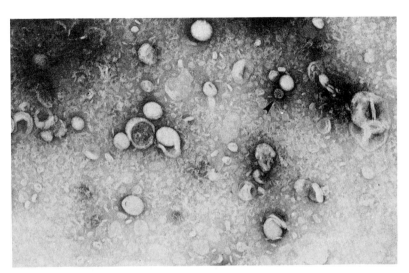

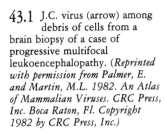

43.1 J.C. virus (arrow) among debris of cells from a brain biopsy of a case of progressive multifocal leukoencephalopathy. (*Reprinted with permission from Palmer, E. and Martin, M.L. 1982. An Atlas of Mammalian Viruses. CRC Press, Inc. Boca Raton, Fl. Copyright 1982 by CRC Press, Inc.*)

Association with papovaviruses, including J.C. virus

features of the disease are relatively pathognomonic. Electron microscopic studies have demonstrated papovaviruslike particles within the nuclei of oligodendrocytes. In addition, papovavirus antigen has been demonstrated by immunofluorescence, and two types of papovaviruses have been isolated from brain tissue of patients with the disease. One of these agents is related to the SV 40 virus of primates. The other virus has been called the *J.C. virus* (the initials are those of the patient from whom it was first isolated) (Figure 43.1). The J.C. virus has been grown in primary human fetal glial culture cells and isolated from the urine of some immunosuppressed patients. Seroepidemiologic studies have indicated that antibody to J.C. virus can be found in about 70% of adults in the United States, although no defined clinical symptoms have been associated with the infection that occurred. It appears that progressive multifocal leukoencephalopathy is a rare manifestation of infection with these agents, although the high frequency of PML in AIDS patients appears related in part to induction of latent J.C. virus by the human immunodeficiency virus (HIV).

Persistent Enterovirus Infection in Immunodeficient Patients

Association with immunodeficiency

Persons with congenital or severe acquired immunodeficiency, especially those with agammaglobulinemia, may develop a chronic central nervous system infection due to an echovirus or other enterovirus. Headache, confusion, lethargy, seizures, and CSF pleocytosis are the common manifestations. The virus can be isolated from the CSF. Clinical improvement

Temporary improvement with hyperimmune globulin

is often achieved by the administration of human hyperimmune globulin to the infecting virus type. However, relapse occurs if therapy is discontinued, indicating persistence of virus despite the therapy.

AIDS Dementia Complex

The HIV causes a persistent infection of the central nervous system in as many as half those with symptomatic CDC class III or IV (see Chapter 73) infection. The clinical course may vary from a mild subacute illness to severe progressive dementia. Loss of complex cognitive function is

Severe loss of mental acuity

usually the first sign of illness. Progression to severe memory loss, depression, seizures, and coma may ensue. Cerebral atrophy involving primarily cortical white matter is characteristic. Histologically, focal vacuolation of the affected brain tissue with perivascular infiltration of macrophages are noted. Multinucleated giant cells with syncytia formation surround the perivascular infiltrates. Some neuronal cells appear to have CD-4 receptors, and these cells may be bound to HIV-infected macrophages. HIV can be isolated from the CSF and high titers of antibodies to HIV can be demonstrated in the CSF.

Neuronal cells have CD4 receptors

HIV may also cause other neurologic syndromes, such as peripheral neuropathies and aseptic meningitis. These are discussed in Chapter 67.

Diseases Caused by Unconventional Viral Agents: Subacute Spongiform Encephalopathies

These are a group of progressive degenerative diseases of the central nervous system that have been shown to be caused by infectious agents with unusual physical and chemical properties (see Table 43.1). Two of the illnesses, kuru and Creutzfeldt–Jakob disease, occur in humans; two others, scrapie in sheep and goats and progressive encephalopathy in mink, occur in animals. Although the pathogenesis of these four illnesses is not well understood, they have similar features. There are varying degrees of neuronal loss, spongiform neurologic changes, and astrocyte proliferation. The incubation periods are months to years. The diseases have a protracted and inevitably fatal course. All four have been transmitted to experimental animals by inoculation of infected tissues.

Kuru and Creutzfeldt–Jakob disease

Transmissible to experimental animals

The nature of these unconventional agents is still obscure. They are small and filterable to diameters of 5 nm or less, have wide host ranges, multiply to high titers in the reticuloendothelial system and brain, produce characteristic infections, and can remain viable even in formalinized brain tissue for many years. They are resistant to ionizing radiation, boiling, and many common disinfectants. Recognizable virions have not been found in tissues, and the agents have not been grown in cell culture. Treatment of infectious material with proteases and nucleases does not decrease infectivity. The characteristics of the agents are summarized in Table 43.2.

Unusual characteristics of infectious agents

Absence of immune response

Concentrated and purified proteinaceous extracts of brain tissue have been shown to transmit disease in very high dilutions. Brain extracts from scrapie-infected animals contain a glycoprotein of 27,000 to 30,000 molecular weight, which is not found in the brains of normal animals and is associated with transmission of the disease. This protein has been termed a *prion* (proteinaceous infectious particle), and considerable evidence has been produced that it is responsible for transmission and infection. Repeated attempts to find associated nucleic acids have been generally unrewarding. It is now clear that the prion protein is encoded in a host gene, and specific prion mRNA has been found in both normal and infected tissue. Why the mRNA is translated in the disease, and how prion production is apparently initiated by an external source of infectious prion protein remains to be determined. During scrapie infection, prion protein may aggregate into birefringent rods and form filamentous structures termed *scrapie-associated fibrils*, which are found in membranes of scrapie-infected brain tissues.

Prion protein associated with infectivity

Absence of nucleic acids in prions

Prion protein encoded in host cell genome

Scrapie-associated fibrils

Kuru was a subacute, progressive neurologic disease of the Fore people of the Eastern Highlands of New Guinea. Although the illness was localized

Occurrence in women and children of the Fore people of New Guinea

Table 43.2   Biologic and Physical Properties of Unconventional Viruses

Chronic progressive pathology without remission or recovery

No pathologic evidence of an inflammatory response

Filterable to estimated diameter of ≤ 5 nm

No virionlike structures visible by electron microscopy

Replication to high titers in susceptible tissue

Transmissible to experimental animals

No alteration in pathogenesis by immunosuppression or immunopotentiation

No interferon production or interference by other viruses

Unusual resistance to ultraviolet radiation

Resistance to inactivation by alcohol, 10% formalin, β-propiolactone, boiling water, proteases, and nucleases

Can be inactivated by 5% sodium hypochlorite, 1N sodium hydroxide, and autoclaving; partially inactivated by acetone and ether

Clinical and pathologic features of Kuru

and decreasing in incidence, its study has thrown light on the transmissibility and infectious nature of similar transmissible encephalopathies. In the local Fore dialect, *kuru* means "to tremble with fear or to be afraid." The disease was brought to the attention of the Western world by Drs. Carleton Gadjusek and Vincent Zigas in the mid-1950s. Epidemiologic studies indicated that kuru usually afflicted adult women or children of either sex. The disease was rarely observed outside of the Fore region, and outsiders in the region did not contract the disease. The symptoms and signs were ataxia, hyperreflexia, and spasticity, which led to progressive starvation and death. Mental alertness was unaffected until the late stages of illness. Pathologic examination revealed changes only in the central nervous system, with diffuse neuronal degeneration and spongiform changes of the cerebral cortex and basal ganglia. No inflammatory response was noted. Inoculation of infectious brain tissue into primates produced a disease that caused similar neurologic symptoms and pathologic manifestations after an incubation period of approximately 40 months. Epidemiologic studies indicated that transmission of the disease in humans was associated with ritual cannibalism, practiced mainly by women and young children and occasionally by men. This ritual involved the handling and ingestion of organs of deceased relatives. Inoculation through lesions in the skin and mucous membranes was shown to be the most likely mode of transmission, with clinical disease developing 4–20 years after exposure. Since the elimination of cannibalism from the Fore culture, kuru has disappeared.

Transmissibility to primates

Association of Kuru with cannibalism

Progressive disease of the elderly

Creutzfeldt–Jakob disease is a progressive, fatal illness of the central nervous system that is seen most frequently in the sixth and seventh decades of life. The initial clinical manifestations are a change in cerebral function, usually diagnosed initially as a psychiatric disorder. Forgetfulness and disorientation progress to overt dementia, with the development of changes in gait, increased tone in the limbs, involuntary movement and seizures. These manifestations resemble those of Kuru. The disorder runs a course of 12 months to 4–5 years, eventually leading to death.

Pathologic features and transmission to animals

The pathology of Creutzfeldt–Jakob disease is identical to that of kuru.

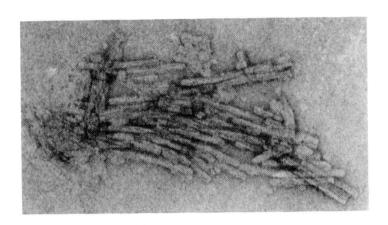

43.2 Amyloidlike fibrils (scrapie-associated fibrils) observed in brain extract of a patient with Creutzfeldt–Jakob disease. (*Reprinted from Bockman, J.M., Kingsbury, D.T., McKinley, M.P., et al. 1985. Creutzfeldt–Jakob disease prion proteins in human brains. N. Engl. J. Med. 312:73–82. With permission.*)

It has been transmitted to chimpanzees, mice, and guinea pigs by inoculation of infected brain tissue, leukocytes, and certain organs. High levels of infectious agent have been found, especially in the brain, where they may reach 10^{-7} infectious doses per gram of brain. Nonpercutaneous transmission of disease has not been observed, and there is no evidence of transmission by direct contact or airborne spread.

Scrapielike structures seen in brain

Brains from patients with Creutzfeldt–Jakob disease have the birefringent rods and fibrillar structures noted in scrapie (Figure 43.2). Antibodies to their component 27,000-molecular-weight proteins are found in CSF and may be a useful diagnostic adjunct to neuropathological examination of brain tissue.

Very low incidence of disease; natural mode of acquisition unknown

Creutzfeldt–Jakob disease is found worldwide, with an incidence of disease of one case per million per year. Most cases are sporadic, although 20% develop in family members. The mode of acquisition is unknown, but a higher incidence of the disease among Israelis of Libyan origin who eat sheep eyeballs has led to speculation that the disease may be transmitted by the ingestion of scrapie-infected tissue. Infection has been transmitted by corneal transplants, contact with infected electrodes used in a neurosurgical procedure, and by pituitary-derived human growth hormone. In these cases, the incubation period of the disease was approximately 15–20 months. Other evidence suggests that a longer latency may follow natural infection.

Nosocomial infections

Prevention of nosocomial infections from transplants or instruments

There is no effective therapy of Creutzfeldt–Jakob disease, and all cases have been fatal. The risk of nosocomial infection can be greatly reduced. Stereotactic neurosurgical equipment, especially that used in patients with undiagnosed dementia, should not be reused. In addition, organs from patients with undiagnosed neurologic disease should not be used for transplants. Growth hormone from human tissue has now been replaced by a recombinant genetically engineered product. The agent of Creutzfeldt–Jakob disease has not been transmitted to animals by inoculation of body secretions, and no increased risk of disease has been noted in family members or medical personnel caring for patients. Disinfection of potentially infectious material can be accomplished by treatment for 1 hr with 0.5% sodium hypochlorite solution or by autoclaving at 121°C for 1 hr.

Gerstmann-Straussler-Schwinker disease (GSS) is a rare fatal illness characterized by ataxia and dementia. The onset of disease is usually in the fifth decade of life, and it progresses slowly over 2–10 years. Amyloid deposits in brain, scrapie-associated fibrils, and antibodies to scrapie prion proteins are found in the brain of these patients.

Additional Reading

Bockman, J.M., Kingsbury, D.T., McKinley, M.P., et al. 1985. Creutzfeldt–Jakob disease prion proteins in human brains. *N. Engl. J. Med.* 312:73–82.

Gajdusek, D.C. 1985. Unconventional viruses causing subacute spongiform encephalopathies. In *Virology*, Fields, B.N., Ed. New York: Raven Press, Chapter 63, pp. 1519–1557. A superb review of this field by the discoverer of the epidemiology of Kuru and the nature of its agent.

Prusiner, S.B. 1987. Prions and neurodegenerative diseases. *N. Engl. J. Med.* 317:1571–1581. An excellent consideration of this fascinating topic.

Southern, P., and Oldstone, M.B.A. 1986. Medical consequences of persistent viral infection. *N. Engl. J. Med.* 314:359–367. Excellent review of the pathogenesis and virus–host interactions of persistent viral infections.

44

Characteristics of Fungi

Kenneth J. Ryan

Fungi are a distinct class of microorganisms, a few of which can produce diseases in humans. These diseases, the *mycoses*, have some unique clinical and microbiologic features. Fungi are eukaryotes with a higher level of biologic complexity than bacteria. They represent a degree of differentiation toward multicellular organization resembling that of plants. The mycoses vary greatly in their manifestations, but tend to be subacute to chronic diseases with indolent, relapsing features. Acute disease such as that produced by many viruses and bacteria is uncommon in fungal infections.

The Nature of Fungi

Eukaryotic cell structure

The fungal cell has typical eukaryotic features, including a nucleus with chromosomes, a nuclear membrane, and cytoplasmic organelles, such as mitochondria and an endoplasmic reticulum. Fungi are usually in the haploid state, although diploid nuclei are formed through nuclear fusion in the process of sexual reproduction. The cell structure includes a rigid cell wall and a cytoplasmic membrane in which ergosterol predominates; in contrast, cholesterol is the dominant sterol in mammalian membranes. The chemical and antigenic structure of the cell wall is markedly different from that of bacterial cells in that it does not contain peptidoglycan, glycerol or ribitol teichoic acids, or lipopolysaccharide. In their place are *peptidomannan, glucan*, and *chitin* in close association with each other and with structural proteins. Peptidomannans are mannose-based polymers (mannan) found on the surface and in the structural matrix of the cell wall where they are linked to protein. They are major determinants of serologic specificity because of variations in the composition and linkages of the polymer side chains. *Glucans* are glucosyl polymers, some of which form fibrils that increase the strength of the fungal cell wall, often in close association with chitin. Chitin is composed of long unbranched chains of

Rigid cell wall; ergosterol in cell membrane

Cell wall mannan linked to structural proteins

Chitin and glucans add rigidity to cell wall

627

poly-N-acetylglucosamine. It is inert, insoluble, and rigid and provides structural support in a manner analogous to the chitin in crab shells or cellulose in plants. It is a major component of the cell wall of filamentous fungi. In yeasts, chitin appears to be of most importance in forming cross-septa and the channels through which nuclei pass from mother to daughter cells during cell division.

Heterotrophic metabolism

Fungal metabolism is heterotrophic, requiring exogenous organic energy sources. Metabolic diversity is great, but most fungi will grow with only an organic carbon source and ammonium or nitrate ions as a nitrogen source. In nature, nutrients for free-living fungi are derived from decaying organic matter. A major difference between fungi and plants is that fungi lack photosynthetic energy-producing mechanisms. Most are strict aerobes, although some can grow under anaerobic conditions. None are strict anaerobes.

Lack of photosynthetic mechanisms

Asexual and sexual reproductive elements are termed conidia and spores respectively

Fungi may reproduce by either asexual or sexual processes. Reproductive elements produced asexually are termed *conidia*. Those produced sexually are termed *spores*. Asexual reproduction involves mitotic division of the haploid nucleus and is associated with production by budding spore-like conidia or separation of hyphal elements. In sexual reproduction, the haploid nuclei of donor and recipient cells fuse to form a diploid nucleus, which then divides by classic meiosis. Some of the four resulting haploid nuclei may be genetic recombinants, and all may undergo further division by mitosis. Highly complex specialized structures may be involved. Detailed study of this process in fungal species such as *Neurospora crassa* has been important in understanding basic cellular genetic mechanisms.

Fungal Growth and Morphology

Variations in size and complexity

The size of fungi varies immensely. A single cell without transverse septa may range from bacterial size (2–4 μm) to a macroscopically visible structure. The morphologic forms of growth vary from colonies superficially resembling those of bacteria to the formation of some of the most complex, multicellular, colorful, and beautiful structures seen in nature. Mushrooms are an example and can be regarded as complex colonies of fungi showing structural differentiation.

Some show multicellular differentiation

Mycology, the science devoted to the study of fungi, has many terms to describe the morphologic components that make up these structures. Fortunately, the terms and concepts that must be mastered can be limited by considering only the fungi of medical importance and accepting some simplification.

Yeasts multiply by budding

Initial growth from a single cell may follow either of two courses, yeast or mold (Figure 44.1). The first and simplest is the formation of a bud, which extends out from a round or oblong parent, constricts, and forms a new cell. These buds are called *blastoconidia* (Figure 44.1) and fungi that reproduce in this manner are called *yeasts*. On plates, yeasts form colonies that resemble and can be mistaken for those of bacteria. In broth, yeasts produce diffuse turbidity or grow as sediments in unshaken cultures.

Blastoconidia

Molds produce septate or nonseptate hyphae

Fungi may also grow through the development of *hyphae* (sing. *hypha*), which are tubelike extensions of the cell with thick, parallel walls. As the hyphae extend, they form an intertwined mass called a *mycelium*. Most fungi form hyphal *septa* (sing. *septum*), which are cross-walls perpendicular to the cell walls that divide the hypha into subunits (Figure 44.2). Some species are nonseptate; they form hyphae and mycelia as a single, continuous cell. In both septate and nonseptate hyphae, multiple nuclei are present with free flow of cytoplasm along the hyphae or through pores

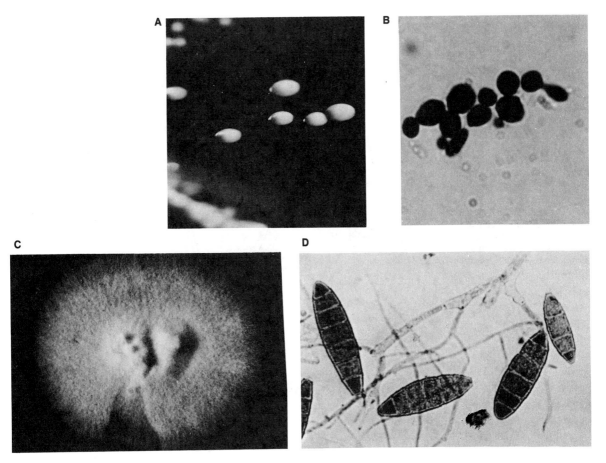

44.1 The yeast and mold forms of fungal growth. (**A**) Yeasts form colonies similar to those of bacteria. (**B**) Microscopically, they are large oval cells with occasional buds (blastoconidia). (**C**) Molds form fuzzy often pigmented colonies. (**D**) Microscopically, molds are a complex of hyphae and associated conidia. (*Parts C and D reproduced with permission from Dr. E. S. Beneke and the Upjohn Company: Scope Publications. Human Mycoses.*)

Vegetative mycelium

Aerial mycelium bears reproductive structures

Pseudohyphae

Morphology of reproductive conidia and spores

in any septa. A portion of the mycelium (*vegetative* mycelium) usually grows into the medium or organic substrate (for example, soil) and functions, like the roots of plants, as a collector of nutrients and moisture. The more visible surface growth assumes a fluffy character as the mycelium becomes *aerial*. The hyphal walls are rigid enough to support this extensive, intertwining network, commonly called a *mold*. The aerial hyphae bear the reproductive structures of this class of fungi. Some fungi form structures called *pseudohyphae* (Figure 44.3), which differ from true hyphae in having recurring budlike constrictions and less rigid cell walls.

The reproductive conidia and spores of the molds and the structures that bear them assume a great variety of sizes, shapes, and relations to the parent hyphae, and the morphology of these structures is the primary basis of identification of medically important molds. The mycelial structure plays some role in identification, depending on whether the hyphae are septate or nonseptate, but differences are not sufficiently distinctive to identify or even suggest a fungal species.

Exogenously formed asexual conidia may arise directly from the hy-

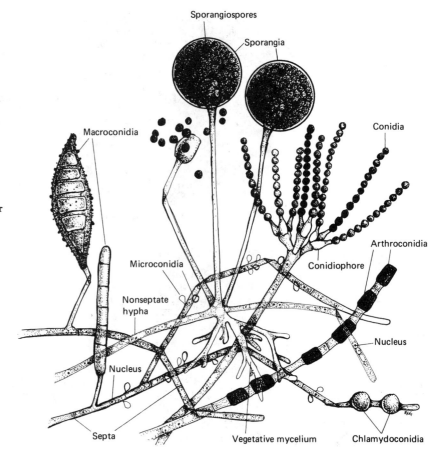

44.2 Forms of molds. The tubelike hyphae form their basic structure. Examples of spores and conidia and of the structures that bear them are shown. They develop from the hyphal wall.

Conidiophores

Macroconidia, microconidia, chlamydoconidia, and arthroconidia

Ascospores

Dimorphism

phae, or on a special stalklike structure, the *conidiophore*. Occasionally, terms such as *macroconidia* or *microconidia* are used to indicate the size and/or complexity of these conidia. Conidia that develop within the hyphae are called either *chlamydoconidia* or *arthroconidia*. Chlamydoconidia become larger than the hypha itself; they are round, thick-walled structures that may be borne on the terminal end of the hypha or along its course. Arthroconidia conform more to the shape and size of the hyphal units, forming a series of delicately attached conidia that break off and disseminate when disturbed. The most common sexual spore is termed an *ascospore*. Four or eight ascospores may be found in a saclike structure, the *ascus*. The structures are illustrated in Figures 44.2 and 44.3.

In general, fungi grow either as yeasts or as molds; mold forms show the greatest diversity. Some species can grow in either a yeast or a mold phase, depending on environmental conditions. These species are known as *dimorphic* fungi. Several human pathogens demonstrate dimorphism: they grow in the yeast phase in infected tissue, but in the mold phase in their environmental reservoir and in culture at ambient temperatures. For most, it is possible to manipulate the cultural conditions to demonstrate both yeast and mold phase in vitro. Yeast phase growth requires conditions similar to those of the parasitic in vivo environment, such as 35–37°C incubation and enriched media. Mold growth requires minimal nutrients and ambient temperatures. The asexual spores produced in the mold phase may be infectious and serve to disseminate the fungus.

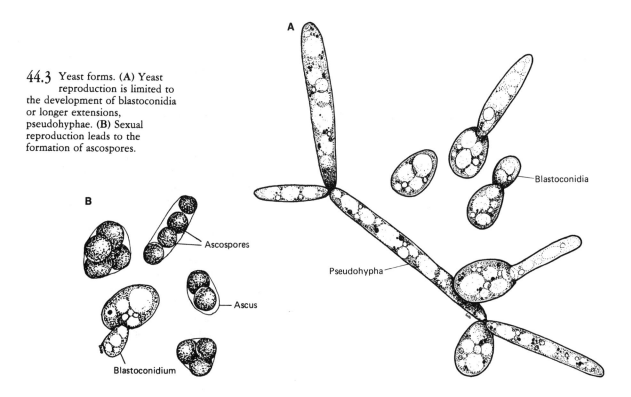

44.3 Yeast forms. (A) Yeast reproduction is limited to the development of blastoconidia or longer extensions, pseudohyphae. (B) Sexual reproduction leads to the formation of ascospores.

Classification

Taxonomy

Although asexual conidia are more readily observed, the taxonomy of fungi depends on the nature of sexual spores and septation of hyphae as its fundamental characteristics. On this basis, four classes—Zygomycetes, Ascomycetes, Basidiomycetes, and Deuteromycetes—are defined as shown in Table 44.1. Some medically important species appear in the Zygomycetes and Ascomycetes, but none in the Basidiomycetes. Most pathogenic species, because they lack a sexual reproductive cycle, have been allocated to the class Deuteromycetes. The mycologist's dislike for

Fungi imperfecti

this lack of symmetry is indicated by the term *fungi imperfecti*, which is synonymous with Deuteromycetes. It suggests that the sexual spores have been lost during evolution or are so rarely produced that they have not been detected. Indeed, some fungi originally classified in the Deutero-

Table 44.1   Taxonomic Classes of Fungi

| Class | Hyphae | Reproductive Elements | | Biology |
		Sexual	Asexual	
Zygomycetes	Nonseptate	Various types	Sporangioconidia	Saprophytes; rare pathogens[a]
Ascomycetes	Septate	Ascospores	Conidia	Saprophytes; rare pathogens
Basidiomycetes	Septate	Basidiospores	Conidia	Mushrooms, smuts; nonpathogenic
Deuteromycetes (fungi imperfecti)	Septate	None	Conidia	Common pathogens; saprophytes

[a] Pathogenicity for humans. Many fungi are plant pathogens.

Some pathogenic fungi have sexual phases

mycetes have been transferred to the Ascomycetes on isolation of a sexual (perfect) form. These discoveries do not necessarily simplify classification; for instance, when the sexual stage of *Trichophyton mentagrophytes* was demonstrated, it was found to be identical to that of an already named ascomycete (*Arthroderma benhamiae*). This type of finding and the morphologic similarity of the asexual forms suggest a close relationship between the classes Ascomycetes and Deuteromycetes.

Classification by disease states

Superficial fungi

Subcutaneous fungi

Opportunistic fungi

Systemic pathogens

The grouping of medically important fungi used in the following chapters is based on the type of tissues they parasitize and the diseases they produce, rather than on the principles of basic mycologic toxonomy, because the disease state is how they appear to the clinician. The *superficial* fungi, such as the dermatophytes, cause indolent lesions of the skin and its appendages commonly known as *ringworm* and *athlete's foot*. The *subcutaneous* pathogens characteristically cause infection through the skin, followed by subcutaneous and/or lymphatic spread. The *opportunistic* fungi are those found in the environment or in the normal flora that occasionally produce disease, usually in the compromised host. They may sometimes appear as contaminants on culture media. The *systemic* pathogens are the most virulent fungi and may cause serious progressive systemic disease in previously healthy persons. They are not members of the normal human flora and are rarely, if ever, encountered as contaminants of culture media. Although their major potential is to produce deep-seated visceral infections and systemic spread (systemic mycoses), they may also produce superficial infections as part of their disease spectrum or as the initiating event. The superficial mycoses do not spread to deeper tissues. As with all clinical classifications, overlaps and exceptions occur. In the end, the organism defines the disease, and it must be isolated or otherwise demonstrated.

Epidemiology

Origin of infection

Only dermatophyte infections are communicable

Most fungal infections arise from contact with an environmental reservoir or from the patient's own fungal flora. Some superficial mycoses can be transmitted from person to person by very close contact, such as sharing a comb with an individual who has scalp ringworm; others can be acquired from ringworm infections of animals. Other fungal infections are not communicable between humans or animals, and infected patients need not be isolated.

Laboratory Diagnosis of Fungal Infections

Direct examination in KOH preparations

Because of their large size, fungi often demonstrate distinctive morphologic features on direct microscopic examination of infected pus, fluids, or tissues. The simplest method is to mix the specimen with a 10% solution of potassium hydroxide (KOH preparation) and place it under a coverslip. The strong alkali digests or clears the tissue elements (epithelial cells, leukocytes, debris), but not the rigid cell walls of both yeasts and molds. After digestion of the material, the fungi can be observed under the light microscope with or without staining (Figure 46.1B). Some yeasts will stain with common stains such as the Gram stain, to which they are usually Gram positive. Histopathologic examination of tissue biopsy specimens is widely used and shows the relationship of the organism to tissue elements and responses (blood vessels, phagocytes, granulomatous reactions). Most fungi can be seen in sections stained with the hematoxylin and eosin (H&E) method routinely used in histology laboratories (Figure

Gram reaction of yeasts

Visualization in histologic preparations

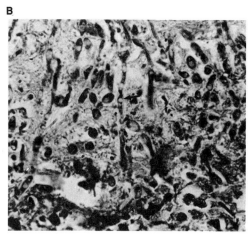

44.4 Direct examinations for fungi. (A) Fungi such as *Candida albicans* are large enough to be demonstrated microscopically at low magnification. (B) In histologic sections the invasive pseudomycelia (arrow) may be seen. (*Part A reproduced with permission from Dr. E. S. Beneke and from the Upjohn Company: Scope publications. Human Mycoses.*)

Periodic acid-Schiff and methenamine silver stains

Growth in culture

Importance of selective media

Sabouraud's agar

Other selective media

Yeast identification

44.4B). Specialized staining procedures such as the periodic acid-Schiff and methenamine silver methods are frequently used because they stain almost all fungi. The pathologist should be alerted to the suspicion of fungal infection when tissues are submitted, because special stains and searches for fungi are not made routinely.

Fungi can be grown by methods similar to those used to isolate bacteria. Growth occurs readily on enriched bacteriologic media commonly used in clinical laboratories (for example, blood agar and chocolate agar). Many fungal cultures, however, require days to weeks of incubation for initial growth; bacteria present in the specimen will grow more rapidly and may interfere with isolation of a slow-growing fungus. Therefore, the culture procedures of diagnostic mycology are designed to favor the growth of fungi over bacteria and to allow incubation to continue for a sufficient time to isolate slow-growing strains.

The most commonly used medium for cultivating fungi is *Sabouraud's agar,* which contains only glucose and peptones as nutrients. Its pH is 5.6, which is optimal for growth of dermatophytes and satisfactory for that of other fungi. Most bacteria associated with humans fail to grow or grow poorly on Sabouraud's medium.

Blood agar or another enriched bacteriologic agar medium is used when pure cultures would be expected. It is made selective for fungi by the addition of antibacterial antibiotics such as chloramphenicol and gentamicin. Cyclohexamide, an antimicrobic that inhibits some saprophytic fungi, is sometimes added to Sabouraud's agar to prevent overgrowth of contaminating molds from the environment, particularly for skin cultures. Media containing these selective agents cannot be relied on exclusively because they can interfere with growth of some pathogenic fungi or because the "contaminant" may be producing an opportunistic infection. For example, cyclohexamide inhibits *Cryptococcus neoformans*, and chloramphenicol may inhibit the yeast forms of some dimorphic fungi. Selective media are not needed for growing fungi from sterile sites such as cerebrospinal fluid or tissue biopsy specimens. In contrast to most parasitic bacteria, many fungi grow best at 25–30°C, and temperatures in this range are used for primary isolation. Paired cultures incubated at 35–37°C may be used to demonstrate dimorphism.

Once a fungus is isolated, identification procedures depend on whether it is a yeast or mold. Yeasts are identified by biochemical tests analogous to those used for bacteria, including some that are identical (for example,

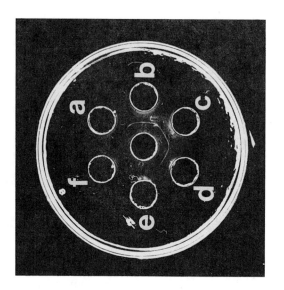

44.5 Exoantigen test. In this immunodiffusion plate the center well contains an antiserum known to react with mycelial antigens of *Coccidioides immitis* and the outer wells contain extracts from the mycelia of known and unknown molds. **A** and **D** are positive controls, and **B** and **C** are molds isolated from patients. Note the precipitin lines between the center well, the positive controls, and isoalte **B**, which is thus identified as *C. immitis*.

Pseudohyphal formation in yeasts

urease production). Some fungi that ordinarily grow as yeast can be induced to form elongated buds called *pseudohyphae*. These differ from true hyphae in their lack of rigid parallel cell walls; they also have a budlike constriction at their origin. The ability to form pseudohyphae is taxonomically useful among the yeasts.

Mold identifcation

Molds are most often identified by the morphology of their asexual conidia and conidiophores. Other features such as the size, texture, and color of the colonies help to characterize molds, but without demonstrating conidiation they are not sufficient for identification. The ease and speed with which various fungi produce conidia vary greatly. Minimal nutrition, moisture, good aeration, and ambient temperature favor conidia development.

Microscopic fungal morphology is usually demonstrated by methods that allow in situ microscopic observation of the fragile asexual conidia and their shape and arrangement. Morphology may also be examined in fragments of growth teased free of a mold and examined moist in preparations containing a dye called *lactophenol cotton blue*. The dye stains the

Lactophenol cotton blue preparations

mycelia and spores. Conidia production may not occur for days or weeks after the initial growth of the mold. It is somewhat like waiting for flowers to bloom, and it can be frustrating when the result has immediate clinical application.

Demonstration of dimorphism

It is desirable, but not always possible, to demonstrate both the yeast and mold phases with dimorphic fungi. In some cases, this result can be achieved with parallel cultures at 22°C and 37°C. The tissue form of *Coccidiodes immitis* is not readily produced in vitro.

Exoantigen test

An alternate approach has been developed for identification of some of the dimorphic systemic fungi, based on soluble antigens prepared from mycelial growth (exoantigens), called the *exoantigen test*. When these react with specific antibody in an immunodiffusion procedure, precipitin lines are formed between the unknown antigen and its homologous antibody (Figure 44.5). Results are usually available much more rapidly than those of cultural tests.

Serologic tests

Serum antibodies directed against a variety of fungal antigens can be detected in patients infected with those agents. Except for some of the systemic pathogens, the sensitivity and/or specificity of these tests has not been sufficient to recommend them for use in diagnosis or therapeutic monitoring of fungal infections. The tests of value will be discussed in sections on specific agents.

Additional Reading

A number of good texts on medical mycology are available. All give more in-depth coverage of the mycologic, epidemiologic, and clinical aspects of mycoses than this book. Several are listed below.

Conant, N.F., Smith, D.T., Baker, R.D., and Calloway, J.L. 1971. *Manual of Clinical Mycology*. 3rd ed. Philadelphia: Saunders. Concise but complete coverage of epidemiologic, diagnostic, and clinical features is provided.

Emmons, C.W., Binford, C.H., Utz, J.P., and Kwon-Chung, K.J. 1977. *Medical Mycology*. 3rd ed. Philadelphia: Lea & Febiger. Coverage of pathologic features is particularly good.

Rippon, J.W. 1988. *Medical Mycology: the Pathogenic Fungi and Pathogenic Actinomycetes*. 3rd ed. Philadelphia: Saunders. Detailed, comprehensive coverage, including historic aspects, is given.

45

Pathogenesis, Immunity, and Chemotherapy of Fungal Infections

Kenneth J. Ryan

We all have regular contact with fungi. They are so widely distributed in our environment that thousands of fungal spores are inhaled or ingested every day. Other species are so well adapted to humans that they are common members of the normal flora. Despite this ubiquity, clinically apparent systemic fungal infections are quite uncommon even among persons living within the geographic habitat of the more pathogenic species. However, when systemic infections need treatment they often pose some of the most difficult therapeutic problems in infectious disease. The purpose of this chapter is to give an overview of the pathogenesis and immunology of fungal infections, and of the activity of antifungal agents. Details relating to specific fungi are given in Chapters 46–49.

Pathogenesis

Compared with bacterial, viral, and even parasitic disease, less is known about the pathogenic mechanisms and virulence factors involved in fungal infections. Analogies with bacterial diseases come the closest because of the apparent importance of adherence to mucosal surfaces, invasiveness, extracellular products, and interaction with phagocytes. Most fungi are opportunists producing serious disease only in individuals with impaired host defense systems. Only a few fungi are able to cause disease in previously healthy persons.

Most fungi are opportunists

Adherence

A number of fungal species, particularly the yeasts, are able to colonize the mucosal surfaces of the gastrointestinal and female genital tract. It has been shown experimentally that the ability to adhere to buccal or vaginal epithelial cells is associated with colonization and virulence. Within the genus *Candida* (Chapter 47), the species that adhere best to epithelial cells

Adherence mediated by fungal adhesins and host cell receptors

Peptidomannan is the adhesin of *C. albicans* and fibronectin, the receptor

are those most frequently isolated from clinical infections. Adherence usually requires a surface adhesin on the microbe and a receptor on the epithelial cell. In the case of *Candida albicans*, peptidomannan components extending from the cell wall have been implicated as the adhesin and fibronectin, a glycoprotein commonly found on epithelial cell surfaces, as the receptor. Specific binding mediators have not been identified for other fungi.

Invasion

Traumatic and respiratory infections with environmental fungi

Passing an initial surface barrier, whether skin, mucous membrane, or respiratory epithelium, is an important step for most successful pathogens. Some fungi are introduced through mechanical breaks. For example, *Sporothrix schenckii* infection (Chapter 49) typically follows a thorn prick or some other obvious trauma.

Most fungi that initially infect the lung grow as molds in the soil, and fungal spores or conidia are disturbed into the air and carried in the airstream past the upper airway defenses. For example, arthroconidia of *Coccidioides immitis* can remain suspended in air for a considerable time, are small enough ($2 \times 3-6 \mu m$) to reach the alveoli, and can initiate pulmonary coccidioidomycosis.

C. albicans invasion across mucosal barriers

Invasion directly across mucosal barriers by the yeast *C. albicans* is associated with the formation of hyphae and pseudohyphae, but the mechanisms that allow them to penetrate and spread are not known. Extracellular enzymes (proteases, elastases, etc) have also been associated with virulent species of *Candida* and with some of the dimorphic systemic fungi. Although it is tempting to attribute some aspect of invasion or spread to these enzymes, their role, if any, remains to be proven.

Phagocyte Interactions

There is considerable evidence that normal persons have a high level of natural resistance to most fungal infections. This is particularly true of opportunistic molds. An important component of this resistance is the ability of healthy neutrophils to kill hyphae of most fungi if they reach the tissues. A small number of species, all of which are dimorphic (Chapters 48 and 49), are sometimes able to produce mild to severe disease in otherwise healthy individuals. In vitro studies have shown these fungi to be more resistant to killing by neutrophils than the opportunists. *Coccidioides immitis*, one of the best-studied species, has been shown to contain a component in the wall of its hyphal (infective) phase that is antiphagocytic. As the hyphae convert to the spherule (tissue) phase they also become resistant to phagocytic killing because of their size and surface characteristics. The tissue yeast form of *Histoplasma capsulatum* is resistant to phagocytic killing after ingestion and, in fact, multiplies within macrophages. These mechanisms of avoiding phagocytic killing appear to allow many dimorphic fungi to multiply sufficiently to produce an infection that can only be controlled by the immune response.

Resistance of tissue phases of dimorphic fungi to phagocytic killing

H. capsulatum multiplies with macrophages

Tissue Injury

No classical exotoxins known to be produced in vivo

None of the extracellular products of opportunistic fungi or dimorphic pathogens have been shown to directly injure the host during infection in a manner analogous to bacterial toxins. The presence of necrosis and infarction in the tissues of patients with invasion of fungi such as *Aspergillus* suggest a toxic effect, but direct evidence is lacking. A number of fungi do produce exotoxins, called *mycotoxins*, in the environment but not in vivo. The structural components of the cell do not cause effects similar to the endotoxin of Gram-negative bacteria, although mannan is known to circulate widely in the body. The injury caused by fungal infections seems to be primarily due to the inflammatory and immune responses that are stimulated by the prolonged presence of the fungus.

Injury primarily due to inflammatory and immunological responses

Immunity

A recurrent theme with fungal infections is the importance of an intact immune response in preventing infection and progression of disease. Most fungi are incapable of producing even a mild infection in an immunocompetent individual.

A small number of species (see Chapters 46, 48, and 49) are able to cause clinically apparent infection that usually resolves once there is time for activation of normal responses. In instances in which it has been adequately investigated the action of neutrophils and T-cell-mediated immune responses have been found to be of primary importance in this resolution. Progressive, debilitating, or life-threatening disease with these agents is commonly associated with depressed or absent cell-mediated immune responses, and the course of any fungal disease is worse in immunocompromised than previously healthy persons.

Importance of T-cell-mediated responses

Progressive fungal diseases in immunocompromised patients

Humoral Immunity

Antibodies can be detected at some time during the course of almost all fungal infections, but for most there is little evidence that they contribute to immunity. *Cryptococcus neoformans* (Chapter 48) is the best example of a fungus against which antibody is probably important in controlling infection.

Experimentally, opsonizing antibody enhances killing of *C. neoformans* by phagocytes, and recovery from clinical illness is associated with rising titers of antibody against the capsule of the organism. The capsule of *C. neoformans* is unique among the pathogenic fungi and has similar antiphagocytic properties to those of encapsulated bacterial pathogens (*Streptococcus pneumoniae, Haemophilus influenzae*, etc) against which humoral immunity is the primary defense mechanism. Antibody also plays a role in control of *C. albicans* infections by enhancing fungus–phagocyte interactions, and this is probably true for other yeasts. In some other fungal infections, the lack of protective effect of antibody is striking. In coccidioidomycosis, for example, high titers of *C. immitis*-specific antibodies are associated with dissemination and a worsening clinical course.

Opsonizing antibody effective in some yeast infections

Cellular Immunity

There is considerable clinical and experimental evidence pointing toward the importance of cellular immunity in fungal infections. Most patients with severe systemic disease have obvious defects in neutrophil function, neutropenia, or in T-cell-mediated immune reactions. These can result from factors such as steroid treatment, leukemia, Hodgkin's disease, and, more recently, acquired immunodeficiency syndrome. In other cases, an immunological deficit can usually be demonstrated by absence of delayed type hypersensitivity responses or by direct in vitro assays of T-cell responsiveness to the fungus in question. In the latter case, it is possible

Association of systemic disease with deficiencies in neutrophils and cell-mediated immunity

that hyporesponsiveness is due at least in part to activation of suppressor cells or continued circulation of fungal antigen.

Although not all fungi have been studied to the same degree, a unified picture is emerging from clinical and experimental animal studies. When hyphae or yeast cells of the fungus reach deep tissue sites, they are either killed by neutrophils or resist destruction by the antiphagocytic mechanisms described above. When the dimorphic fungi convert to yeast or spherule phases in the tissue, their growth may be slowed by macrophages, but they are not killed. The turning point comes when the macrophages are activated by mediators produced by T cells that have interacted with the fungal antigen. Where they have been identified, these mediators are interleukin 2 or gamma interferon, which can directly activate macrophages. The activated macrophages are then able to restrict the growth of the fungus, and the infection is controlled. Defects that disturb this cycle lead to progressive disease. To the extent that they are known, the specifics of these reactions will be discussed in the following chapters.

Dimorphic fungi normally controlled by cytokine-activated macrophages

Chemotherapy

Compared to antibacterial agents, relatively few antimicrobics are available for treatment of fungal infections. Many substances with antifungal activity have proved to be either unstable, toxic to humans, or have undesirable pharmacologic characteristics, such as poor diffusion into tissues. Of the agents in current clinical use, none approach the degree of selective toxicity of most antibacterial antimicrobics.

Antifungals generally show less selective toxicity than antibacterials

Fortunately, most fungal infections are self-limiting and require no chemotherapy. Superficial mycoses are the most commonly treated, but topical therapy can be used, thus limiting toxicity to the host. The remaining small group of deep mycoses that are uncontrolled by the host's immune system require the prolonged use of relatively toxic antifungals. This, combined with the fact that most of these patients have underlying immunosuppression, makes them the most difficult of all infectious diseases to treat successfully.

The characteristics of currently used antifungal chemotherapeutics are discussed below and summarized in Table 45.1. Their primary targets are the nucleic acid synthesis mechanisms and the ergosterol-rich fungal cytoplasmic membrane of fungi. No clinically useful antifungal acts on the cell wall in a manner analogous to the penicillins, although inhibitors of both glucan and chitin synthesis have been discovered and are under evaluation.

Most act on fungal nucleic acid synthesis or cytoplasmic membrane

Antifungal Antibiotics

Polyenes. The polyenes are produced by *Streptomyces* and have essentially the same modes of action and antifungal spectra. They are lipophilic and bind to sterols, particularly to ergosterol, which predominates in the fungal cytoplasmic membrane. Following binding to the membrane, pore formation occurs, the function of the membrane is disrupted, and leakage of the cell contents results.

Bind to ergosterol in fungal cell membranes; cause membrane disruption

The only polyenes in clinical use in the United States are *nystatin*, which is limited to topical use, and *amphotericin B*, which has been the most reliable antifungal for systemic use for many years. Amphotericin B is insoluble in water and must be administered intravenously as a colloidal suspension. It is not absorbed from the gastrointestinal tract.

Ampherotericin B in treatment of systemic life-threatening mycoses

Almost all fungi are susceptible to amphotericin B, and the development of resistance is too rare to be a consideration in its use. The major

Table 45.1   Characteristics of Antifungal Agents

Antifungal	Action	Route of Administration[a]			Spectrum
		Topical	Oral	Parenteral	
Amphotericin B	Membrane disruption	−	−	+	All fungi
Nystatin	Membrane disruption	+	−	−	All fungi
Griseofulvin	Microtubule function	−	+	−	Dermatophytes
Flucytosine	Nucleic acid synthesis	−	+	−	*Candida, Torulopsis, Cryptococcus,* other yeasts
Potassium iodide	?	−	+	−	*Sporothrix schenckii*
Clotrimazole	Ergosterol synthesis	+	−	−	Most fungi[b]
Miconazole	Ergosterol synthesis	+	−	−	Most fungi[b]
Ketoconazole	Ergosterol synthesis	−	+	−	Most fungi[b]
Tolnaftate	?	+	−	−	Dermatophytes

[a] Indicates predominant current usage.
[b] Generally not active against *Aspergillus*.

Toxicity results from some affinity for host cell membranes

Nephrotoxicity

limitation to amphotericin B therapy is toxicity of the agent, because its affinity for fungal and mammalian membranes is relatively close. Infusion is commonly followed by chills, fever, headache, and dyspnea, but the most serious toxicity is renal and is seen in virtually every patient receiving a therapeutic course. Experienced clinicians learn to titrate the dosage for each patient to minimize the nephrotoxic effects. For obvious reasons, use of amphotericin B is limited to progressive life-threatening fungal infections. In these cases, despite its toxicity, it often remains the antifungal agent of choice.

Active only against superficial mycoses

Acts on microtubules and nuclear division

Concentrates in keratinized skin layers

Griseofulvin.   Griseofulvin is a product of a species of the mold penicillium. It is active only against the agents of superficial mycoses. Griseofulvin is actively taken up by susceptible fungi and acts on the microtubules and associated proteins that make up the mitotic spindle. It interferes with cell division and possibly other cell functions associated with microtubules. It is absorbed from the gastrointestinal tract after oral administration and concentrates in the keratinized layers of the skin. Clinical effectiveness has been demonstrated for all causes of dermatophyte infection, but the response is slow. Difficult cases may require 6 months of therapy to effect a cure.

Synthetic Antifungals

Potassium Iodide.   Potassium iodide is the oldest-known oral chemotherapeutic for a fungal infection. It is effective for only one mycosis, sporotrichosis. Its activity is somewhat paradoxical, because the mold phase of the etiologic agent, *Sporothrix schenckii*, can grow on media containing 10% potassium iodide. It appears that molecular iodine is active against the pathogenic yeast form of this dimorphic fungus that develops in vivo.

Flucytosine. Flucytosine was originally developed as an anticancer drug. It is an antimetabolite analog of cytosine, which is well absorbed after oral administration. In the cell, flucytosine is converted by cytosine deaminase to 5-flurouracil, which disrupts protein synthesis when incorporated into RNA by uridine phosphorylase.

Flucytosine is well absorbed after oral administration. It is active against most clinically important yeasts, including *C. albicans* and *C. neoformans*, but has little activity against molds or dimorphic fungi. A significant limitation is the development of resistance that can occur by single-step mutation during therapy. In addition to the involvement of cytosine deaminase and uridine phosphorylase, a permease is required for entry of flucytosine into the cell, and flucytosine resistance has been shown to result from mutation in any one of these enzymes.

Potential resistance limits flucytosine use to mild yeast infections or treatment in combination with amphotericin B for life-threatening systemic infections. Use in combination reduces the chance of flucytosine resistance and allows a lower dose of amphotericin B to be used. In some instances, the combination is synergistic. The primary toxicity of flucytosine is a reversible bone marrow suppression that can lead to neutropenia and thrombocytopenia. This effect is dose related and can be controlled by drug monitoring.

Imidazoles. The imidazoles are a large family of synthetic organic compounds containing the imidazole ring. They include members with antibacterial, antifungal, and antiparasitic properties. The important antifungals are *clotrimazole, miconazole*, and *ketoconazole*. Others are under development or evaluation. The antifungal activity of the imidazoles is based on interference with the incorporation of ergosterol and possibly other lipids into the cytoplasmic membrane. The effect is primarily fungistatic rather than fungicidal. Clotrimazole and miconazole are now used only in topical preparations having been eclipsed by ketoconazole as the imidazole with the greatest promise for systemic therapy.

Ketoconazole may be given orally. Although nausea, vomiting, and elevation of hepatic enzymes complicate the treatment of some patients, it is much less toxic than amphotericin B. Clinical experience has been favorable with most systemic fungal infections except aspergillosis, and there are a few reports of succcess with systemic candidosis. Central nervous system penetration of ketoconazole is poor, which limits its effectiveness in systemic coccidioidomycosis and cryptococcosis, which characteristically spread to the meninges. Currently, ketoconazole is used for treatment of some systemic fungal infections and as an alternative for superficial mycoses in which the standard therapy either fails or is not tolerated by the patient. Other imidazoles and related compounds are under evaluation for both topical and systemic antifungal treatment. Of these, itraconazole is the most promising because of desirable pharmacological properties (long half-life) and potential activity against *Aspergillus*.

Tolnaftate. Tolnaftate is a derivative of naphthiomate. It has activity against dermatophytes (Chapter 46), but not against yeasts. It has been

---

Marginal notes:

Product of flucytosine incorporated in RNA; disrupts protein synthesis

Specifically active against yeasts
Single-step mutations to resistance

Use in combined therapy to prevent resistance

Reversible bone marrow suppression

Interfere with sterol incorporation in cytoplasmic membrane

Fungistatic activity

Hepatotoxicity of ketoconazole

Ketoconazole used for some systemic mycoses

effective in topical treatment of dermatophytoses and is available in over-the-counter preparations.

Selection of Antifungals

As with all chemotherapy, the selection of antifungal agents for treatment of superficial, subcutaneous, and systemic mycoses involves balancing probable efficacy against toxicity. The factors to be considered are 1) the threat of morbidity or mortality posed by the specific infection; 2) the immune status of the patient; 3) the toxicity of the antifungal; and 4) the probable activity of the antifungal agent against the fungus. In vitro susceptibility testing has proved less helpful in individual cases of fungal infection than has been the case with bacterial infections (Chapter 13). Broth and agar dilution methods have been applied to fungal susceptibility tests, but there are no agreed standard methods, and the results are markedly influenced by different media and by whether a dimorphic fungus is in the yeast or mold phase. Molds are particularly difficult to test. Antifungal susceptibility tests done in reference laboratories can sometimes be helpful, but the clinician must usually rely on knowledge of the etiologic agent and of the expected spectrum of each agent (Table 45.1).

> Decisions on antifungal therapy balance dangers of disease against toxicity of treatment

In the case of superficial mycoses, the risks of appropriate therapy are small, and a number of agents may be tried. At the other extreme, an immunocompromised patient will most likely be treated with amphotericin B for proven or even suspected systemic fungal infection, because it has been shown to be most effective, and the risk of a fatal outcome outweighs the toxicity of the drug.

Additional Reading

Drouhet, E., and Dupont, B. 1987. Evolution of antifungal agents: past, present, and future. *Rev. Infect. Dis.* 9:S4–S14. A readable summary of the current status of antifungal therapy including mechanisms of action and clinical usage.

Fromtling, R.A., and Shadomy, H.J. 1986. An overview of macrophage-fungal interactions. *Mycopathologia* 93:77–93. This review focuses on the experimental evidence for immune mechanisms in the major fungal infections.

Reiss, E. 1986. *Molecular Immunology of Mycotic and Actinomycotic Infections.* New York/Amsterdam: Elsevier. This monograph gives a detailed account of the antigenic structure of all medically important fungi and how it relates to their pathogenesis.

46

Superficial Fungal Pathogens

Kenneth J. Ryan

Dermatophytoses are superficial infections of the skin and its appendages, commonly known as *ringworm, athlete's foot*, and *jock itch*. They are caused by species of the genera *Microsporum*, *Trichophyton*, and *Epidermophyton*, which are collectively known as *dermatophytes*. These fungi are highly adapted to the nonliving, keratinized tissues of nails, hair, and the stratum corneum of the skin.

Dermatophytes

Microbiology

Molds

Identification based on characteristics of conidia

Best growth at 25°C

Septate hyphae

Dermatophytes are molds that have been classified among the Deuteromycetes (fungi imperfecti). More recently, sexual spores corresponding to two ascomycete genera have been discovered in many of the *Microsporum* and *Trichophyton* species. Dermatophytes are still called by their previous names in the medical literature for reasons of familiarity and because identification procedures continue to be based on the characteristics of asexual conidia. Many species cause dermatophyte infections, the most common of which are shown in Table 46.1. They require a few days to a week or more to initiate growth. Most grow best at 25°C on Sabouraud's medium, which is usually used for culture. The hyphae are septate, and the conidia may be borne directly on the hyphae or on conidiophores. Small microconidia may or may not be formed; however, the larger and more distinctive macroconidia (Figure 46.1C) are usually the basis for identification.

Pathogenesis

Infection through minor lesions

Dermatophytoses begin when minor traumatic lesions come in contact with the fungi. Once the stratum corneum is penetrated the organism can proliferate, but does not invade deeper structures. The course of the in-

Table 46.1 Agents of Superficial Mycoses

Fungus	Infection Site(s)	Fungal Growth In Lesion	In Culture (25°C)
Dermatophytes			
Microsporum canis	Hair,[a] skin	Mycelia	Mold
Microsporum audouini	Hair[a]	Mycelia	Mold
Microsporum gypseum	Hair, skin	Mycelia	Mold
Trichophyton tonsurans	Hair, skin, nails	Mycelia	Mold
Trichophyton rubrum	Hair, skin, nails	Mycelia	Mold
Trichophyton mentagrophytes	Hair, skin	Mycelia	Mold
Trichophyton violaceum	Hair, skin, nails	Mycelia	Mold
Epidermophyton floccosum	Skin	Mycelia	Mold
Other mycoses			
Pityrosporum orbiculare	Skin (pink to brown)[b]	Yeast (mycelia)[c]	Yeast
Cladosporium werneckii	Skin (brown-black)[b]	Mycelia	Yeast (mold)
Trichosporon cutaneum	Hair (white)[b]	Mycelia	Mold
Piedraia hortae	Hair (black)[b]	Mycelia	Mold

[a] Specimens fluoresce under ultraviolet light.
[b] Color of clinical lesions.
[c] Denotes less frequent findings.

Balance between growth and desquamation

fection is then dependent on the anatomic location, the dynamics of skin growth and desquamation, the speed and extent of the inflammatory response, and the infecting species. For example, if the organisms grow very slowly in the stratum corneum, and turnover by desquamation of this layer is not retarded, the infection will probably be short lived and cause minimal signs and symptoms. Inflammation tends to increase skin growth and desquamation rates and help to limit infection, whereas immunosuppressive agents such as corticosteroids decrease shedding of the keratinized layers and tend to prolong infection. Most infections are self-limiting, but those in which fungal growth rates and desquamation are balanced and in which the inflammatory response is poor tend to become chronic. The lateral spread of infection and its associated inflammation produce the characteristic sharp advancing margins that were once believed to be the burrows of worms. This characteristic is the origin of the common name *ringworm* and the Latin term *tinea* (worm) that is often applied to the clinical forms of the disease (Figure 46.1A).

Most infections self-limiting

Ringworm and tinea

Infection may spread from skin to other keratinized structures, such as hair or nails, or may invade them primarily. The hair shaft is penetrated by hyphae, which extend as arthroconidia either exclusively within the shaft (endothrix) or both within and without the shaft (ectothrix). The end result is damage to the hair shaft structure, which often breaks off. Loss of hair at the root and plugging of the hair follicle with fungal elements may result. Invasion of the nail bed causes a hyperkeratotic reaction, which dislodges or distorts the nail.

Involvement of hair and nails

Endothrix and ectothrix infections

Nail bed infection

Immunity

The great majority of dermatophyte infections pass through an inflammatory stage to spontaneous healing. Little is known about the factors that mediate the host response in these self-limiting infections or whether

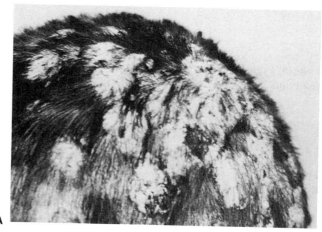

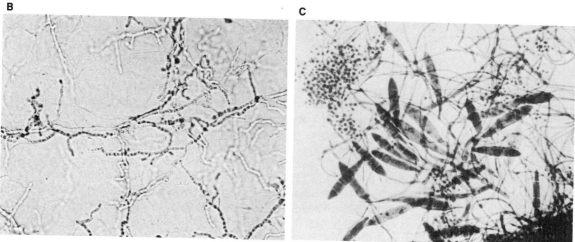

46.1 Dermatophyte infection of scalp (ringworm). **(A)** Scalp lesions. Note the annular margination. **(B)** Scrapings taken from the edge of the scalp lesion in KOH. Only the hyphal elements are visible. **(C)** Culture. Both hyphae, macroconidia, and microconidia are present. The macroconidia are characteristic for *Trichophyton*. (*Reproduced with permission from Dr. E. S. Beneke and the Upjohn Company: Scope monograph. Human Mycoses.*)

they confer immunity to subsequent exposures. Antibodies may be formed during infection, but they play no known role in immunity. Most clinical and experimental evidence points to the importance of cell-mediated immunity as with other fungal infections. Enhanced desquamation with the inflammatory response helps remove infected skin.

Occasional dermatophyte infections become chronic and widespread. This progression has been related to both host and organism factors. Approximately half of these patients have underlying diseases affecting their immune responses or are receiving treatments which compromise T-cell function. These chronic infections are particularly associated with *Trichophyton rubrum* to which both normal and immunocompromised persons appear to be hyporesponsive. Although a number of mechanisms have been proposed, how this organism is able to grow without stimulating much inflammation is unexplained.

Epidemiology

Human, animal, or soil reservoirs

There are both ecologic and geographic differences in the occurrence of the various dermatophyte species. Some are primarily adapted to the skin of humans, others to animals. Many wild and domestic animals, including dogs and cats, are infected with certain dermatophyte species and represent a large reservoir for infection of humans. Other pathogenic dermatophytes are found primarily in the soil. There are large differences between temperate and tropical climates in the frequency of cases and isolations from nonhuman sources of the different species. Many of these differences are changing with shifts in population.

Human-to-human transmission

Human-to-human transmission usually requires very close contact with an infected subject or infected materials, because dermatophytes are of low infectivity and virulence. Transmission usually takes place within families or in situations involving contact with detached skin or hair, such as barber shops and locker rooms. No special precautions beyond hand washing need be taken by the medical attendant after contact with an infected patient.

Clinical Manifestations

Variations in clinical severity

Dermatophyte infections range from inapparent colonization to chronic progressive eruptions that last for months or years, causing considerable discomfort and disfiguration.

Clinical syndromes

Dermatologists often give each infection its own "disease" name, for example, *tinea capitis* (scalp), *tinea pedis* (feet, athlete's foot), *tinea manuum* (hands), *tinea cruris* (groin), *tinea barbae* (beard, hair), and *tinea unguium* (nail beds). Skin infections not included in this anatomic list are called *tinea corporis* (body). There are some general clinical, etiologic, and epidemiologic differences between these syndromes, but there is also considerable overlap. The primary differences between etiologic agents that infect different sites are shown in Table 46.1.

Hair infections

Infection of hair begins with an erythematous papule around the hair shaft, which progresses to scaling of the scalp, discoloration, and eventually fracture of the shaft. Spread to adjacent hair follicles progresses in a ring-like fashion, leaving behind broken, discolored hairs and sometimes black dots filled with fungal debris. The degree of inflammatory response markedly affects the clinical appearance and in some cases can cause constitutional symptoms. In most cases symptoms beyond itching are minimal.

Skin infections

Skin lesions begin in a similar pattern and enlarge to form sharply delineated erythematous borders with skin of nearly normal appearance in the center. Multiple lesions can fuse to form unusual geometric patterns on the skin. Lesions may appear in any location, but are particularly common in moist, sweaty skin folds. Obesity and the wearing of tight apparel increase susceptibility to infection in the groin and beneath the breasts. Another form of infection, which involves scaling and splitting of the skin between the toes, is commonly known as *athlete's foot*. Moisture and maceration of the skin provide the mode of entry.

Nail bed infections

Nail bed infections first cause discoloration of the subungual tissue, then hyperkeratosis and apparent discoloration of the nail plate by the underlying infection. Direct infection of the nail plate is uncommon. Progression of hyperkeratosis and associated inflammation cause disfigurement of the nail but few symptoms until the nail plate is so dislodged or distorted that it exposes or compresses adjacent soft tissue.

Diagnosis

Diagnostic value of KOH mounts of skin scrapings and infected hairs

The goal of diagnostic procedures is to distinguish dermatophytoses from other skin diseases, such as mimicking infections caused by bacteria and other fungi, and from noninfectious inflammatory skin disorders, such as psoriasis and contact dermatitis. The most important step is microscopic examination of material from lesions to detect the fungus. Potassium hydroxide preparations of scales scraped from the advancing edge of a dermatophyte lesion demonstrate septate hyphae (Figure 46.1B). Examination of infected hairs reveals hyphae and arthrospores penetrating the hair shaft. Broken hairs give the best yield. Some species of dermatophyte fluoresce, and selection of hairs for examination can be aided by the use of an ultraviolet lamp (Wood's lamp).

Importance of culture in typical infections with negative KOH preparations

The same material used for direct examination can be cultured for isolation of the offending dermatophyte. Mild infections with typical clinical findings and positive KOH preparations are often not cultured, because clinical management is not influenced significantly by the identity of the etiologic species. Clinically typical infections with negative KOH preparations require culture. The major reason for false-negative KOH results, however, is failure to collect the scrapings or hairs properly.

Treatment and Prevention

Local tolnaftate, miconazole, or clotrimazole

Griseofulvin treatment in more refractory cases

Many local skin infections resolve spontaneously without chemotherapy. Those that do not may be treated with topical tolnaftate, miconazole, or clotrimazole. Scalp, nail bed, and more extensive skin infections require systemic therapy with griseofulvin often combined with topical therapy. Therapy must be continued over weeks to months, and relapses are common.

Dermatophyte infections can usually be prevented simply by observing general hygienic measures. No specific preventive measures such as vaccines exist.

Other Superficial Mycoses

Tinea (pityriasis) versicolor occurs primarily in the tropics; it is characterized by discrete areas of hypopigmentation associated with induration and scaling. Lesions are found on the trunk and arms; some assume pigments ranging from pink to yellow-brown, hence the term *versicolor*. The cause (*Pityrosporum orbiculare*) can be seen in skin scrapings as clusters of budding yeast cells mixed with hyphae. It grows primarily in the yeast form in culture.

Tinea versicolor and tinea nigra occur primarily in tropics

Tinea nigra, another tropical infection, is characterized by brown to black macular lesions, usually on the hands or feet. There is little inflammation or scaling. The cause (*Cladosporium werneckii*) is a black-pigmented fungus found in soil and other environmental sites. Scrapings of the lesion show brown-black-pigmented septate hyphae. In culture initial growth is in the yeast form, with slow development of hyphal elements.

Piedra

Piedra is an infection of the hair characterized by black or white nodules attached to the hair shaft. White piedra (caused by *Trichosporon cutaneum*) infects the shaft in hyphal forms, which fragment with occasional buds. Black piedra (caused by *Piedraia hortae*) shows branched hyphae and ascospores in sections of the hair.

Additional Reading

Wilson, J.W., and Plunkett, O.A. 1965. *The Fungous Diseases of Man*. Berkeley: University of California Press. This general mycology text can still be found on the shelves of most medical libraries. Its outstanding characteristic is the photographic presentation of dermatophytoses and other cutaneous manifestations of fungal disease.

Candida *and* Other Opportunistic Fungi

Kenneth J. Ryan

The fungi considered in this chapter are usually found as members of the normal flora or as saprophytes in the environment. With breakdown of host defenses they can produce disease ranging from superficial skin or mucous membrane infections to systemic involvement of multiple organs. The most common opportunistic infections are caused by *Candida albicans*, a common member of the skin, gastrointestinal, and genital floras. The diseases caused by *Candida* and other species are summarized in Table 47.1.

Candida

Candida species are usually regarded as yeasts, because they grow as typical 4- to 6-μm, budding, round or oval yeast cells (Figure 44.1) under most conditions and at most temperatures. Under specialized conditions, they can form pseudohyphae or hyphae. Some species form chlamydoconidia. Many *Candida* species have been defined; those most commonly associated with disease in humans are shown in Table 47.2. Species identification is based on a combination of biochemical and morphologic characteristics, such as carbohydrate assimilation and fermentation and the ability to produce hyphae, pseudohyphae, and chlamydoconidia. Particular attention is given to the differentiation of *C. albicans* from other species, because it is the most frequent cause of disease. *Candida albicans* forms sproutlike hyphae directly from yeast cells that are incubated in serum at 37°C. These structures are called *germ tubes* (Figure 47.1A) and are produced within 2–3 hr. The organism also forms terminal thick-walled chlamydoconidia under certain conditions (Figure 47.1B). Other *Candida* species do not have this combination of properties.

Most *Candida* species, including *C. albicans*, grow rapidly on Sabouraud's medium and on enriched bacteriologic media. Smooth, white, 2- to 4-mm colonies resembling those of staphylococci are produced on blood

Margin notes:

Budding yeasts

Hyphae and pseudohyphae may develop

C. albicans

Germ tube development

Chlamydoconidia formation

Bacterialike colonies

651

Table 47.1 Agents of Opportunistic Mycoses

Organism	Infection	Growth		
		Tissue	Culture (25°C)	Culture (37°C)
Candida	Skin, mucous membranes, urinary, disseminated	Yeast (pseudomycelia)[a]	Yeast (mycelia)[a]	Yeast
Aspergillus	Lung, disseminated	Mycelia (septate)	Mold	Mold
Absidia	Rhinocerebral, lung	Mycelia (nonseptate)	Mold	Mold
Mucor	Rhinocerebral, lung	Mycelia (nonseptate)	Mold	Mold
Rhizopus	Rhinocerebral, lung	Mycelia (nonseptate)	Mold	Mold

[a] Less common feature.

agar after overnight incubation. Fluid cultures typically show a deposit at the bottom but diffuse growth may occur if the broth is well aerated.

Candida albicans *Infections*

Normal floral organism

Pathogenesis. *Candida albicans* is normally present in small numbers in the oral cavity, lower gastrointestinal tract, and female genital tract. This colonization is aided by the ability of *C. albicans* to adhere to mucosal cells, a feature that distinguishes it from most other *Candida* species. Numerous studies implicate fibrillar peptidomannan components on the yeast surface as the adhesin. The receptor appears to be fibronectin on the host cell surface. Under certain conditions *C. albicans* may become locally invasive, sending pseudohyphae down into the tissue and producing acute inflammation and tissue destruction (Figure 44.4). The factors that trigger this invasion, beyond some disruption of anatomic barriers or other compromise of host defenses, are not clear. For example, dry, normal skin is more resistant to infection than wet, macerated skin.

C. albicans has adhesin for some epithelial cells

Local tissue invasion and acute inflammatory response

Factors that allow *C. albicans* to increase its relative proportion of the

Table 47.2 Medically Important *Candida* and *Torulopsis* Species

Species	Germ Tubes[a]	Pseudohyphae	Chlamydoconidia
C. albicans	+	+	+
C. krusei	−	+	−
C. parapsilosis	−	+	−
C. tropicalis	−	+	−[b]
C. guilliermondii	−	+	−
Torulopsis glabrata	−	−	−

[a] Rapid production (4 hr or less).
[b] Occasional strains produce chlamydoconidia morphologically different from those of *C. albicans*.

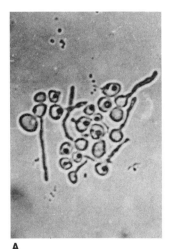
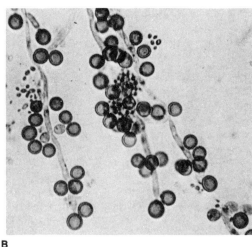

47.1 *Candida albicans.* (A) When incubated at 37°C, *C. albicans* rapidly forms elongated hyphae called germ tubes. (B) On specialized media, *C. albicans* forms thick-walled chlamydoconidia, which differentiate it from other *Candida* species. (*Reproduced with permission from Dr. E. S. Beneke and from the Upjohn Company: Scope Publications, Human Mycoses.*)

A   **B**

Predisposing effects of antibacterial therapy, neutrophil dysfunction, and T-cell dysfunction

Invasion associated with production of hyphae and pseudohyphae

Dissemination

flora (antibacterial therapy), that compromise the general immune capacity of the host (leukopenia or corticosteroid therapy), or that interfere with T-cell function (eg, AIDS) are often associated with local and invasive infection. Diabetes mellitus creates a general predisposition toward *C. albicans* infection, as well as many other infections. The invasive process itself is associated with a shift from formation of blastoconidia to formation of pseudohyphae and hyphae (Figure 47.2A). These differ from blastoconidia in morphology and also possess antigens not present in the parent cell. Invasion may be aided by the digestive action of an acid proteinase (Figure 47.2B).

Disseminated *C. albicans* infections are associated with parenchymal

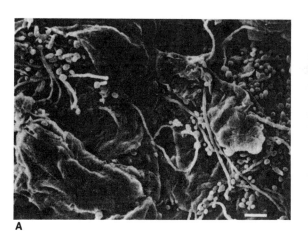
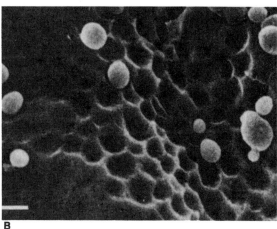

A   **B**

47.2 Invasiveness of *Candida albicans.* Two features of invasiveness are seen in these scanning electron micrographs taken from experiments with murine corneocytes. In **A**, both blastoconidia and mycelial elements are present. The mycelial elements spread over the surface and invade the cell cuticle. In **B**, a *C. albicans* strain that produces a protease is seen producing cavitylike depressions in the cell surface. This action could play a role in invasion of the cell. (*Reproduced with permission of Thomas L. Ray and Candia D. Payne. 1988. Infect Immun. 56:1945–1947, Figures 4,6B. Copyright. American Society for Microbiology.*)

invasion, microabscesses, and, occasionally, chronic granulomatous inflammatory responses. Cases of disseminated disease may begin with superficial infection, but usually involve a major breach of the host's local defenses or general immune responses. Many of the newer technologic devices used in medicine, such as indwelling catheters, monitoring devices, prostheses, and particularly hyperalimentation procedures, can provide a convenient route for *Candida* (and other organisms) to gain access to deeper organs. The organism's resistance to antibacterial drugs and its invasive capacity facilitate production of disease in these circumstances.

Immunity.   Both humoral and cell-mediated immunity are important in defense against *Candida* infections. *Candida albicans* yeast forms are readily phagocytosed and killed when opsonized by antibody and complement. In the absence of antibody, the process is less efficient. Mycelial forms are too large to be ingested by neutrophils, but there is evidence these cells can still kill the fungi by attaching to the hyphae and discharging oxidative metabolites generated by the respiratory burst and lysosomal enzymes. There is recent evidence that *C. albicans* possesses surface receptors for the iC3b component of complement similar to those on human neutrophils: iC3b bound to the candidal surface by these receptors is, thus, oriented in a fashion that makes it unavailable for opsonization. Enhanced production of such receptors under various conditions, for example, elevated glucose concentration, could explain some of the circumstances associated with *Candida* infection. The association of chronic mucocutaneous candidiasis (see below) with a number of T-cell immunodeficiencies emphasizes the importance of this arm of the immune system in fungal infections.

Epidemiology.   Most *C. albicans* infections are caused by endogenous flora, except in cases of direct mucosal contact with lesions in others (for example, through sexual intercourse). Nosocomial *C. albicans* infections are also derived more frequently from the patient's own flora than from cross-infection; they are often associated with the invasive procedures mentioned previously.

Clinical Manifestations.   Superficial invasion of the mucous membranes by *C. albicans* produces a white, cheesy plaque that is loosely adherent to the mucosal surface. The lesion is usually painless, unless the plaque is torn away and the raw, weeping, invaded surface is exposed. Oral lesions, called *thrush*, occur on the tongue, palate, and other mucosal surfaces as single or multiple ragged white patches. A similar infection in the vagina, vaginal *candidiasis*, produces a thick, curdlike discharge and itching of the vulva.

Candida albicans skin infections have an appearance similar to that of intertriginous dermatophyte infections and occur in similar circumstances. Crural folds and other areas in which wet, macerated skin surfaces are opposed are the sites most commonly affected. For example, one type of diaper rash is caused by *C. albicans*. Other infections of the skin folds and appendages occur an association with recurrent immersion in water. For example, *Candida* infections of the nail beds (paronychia) is an occupational disease of dishwashers and laundry workers. The initial lesions are erythematous papules or confluent areas associated with tenderness, erythema, and fissures of the skin. Infection usually remains confined to the chronically irritated area, but may spread beyond it, particularly in infants. In rare persons with specific T-cell defects in cell-mediated immune de-

---

Marginal notes (left column):

Infection through medical devices

Opsonized yeast forms are phagocytosed and killed

Neutrophil products may kill extracellular hyphal forms

Antiopsonic activity of *C. albicans* complement receptors

Significance of cell-mediated immunity

Superficial infections

Thrush

Vaginal candidiasis

Skin infections of moist areas

Diaper rash and paronychia

Chronic mucocutaneous candidiasis associated with defect in CMI

fense against *Candida* antigens, a chronic, relapsing form of candidiasis called *chronic mucocutaneous candidiasis* develops. Infections of the skin, hair, or mucous membranes are initially similar to those seen in other patients, but fail to resolve with adequate therapy and management. The mucocutaneous junctions are often involved, with considerable disfigurement and discomfort, particularly when the disease is accompanied by a granulomatous inflammatory response. Although lesions may become extensive, they usually do not disseminate. To some degree this disease may represent a clinical example of immunologic tolerance. The cutaneous anergy to *C. albicans* antigens commonly seen in these patients is often reversed during antifungal chemotherapy suggesting that it is due to chronic antigen excess.

Esophagitis

Inflammatory patches similar to those in thrush may develop in the esophagus with or without associated oral candidiasis. Painful swallowing and substernal chest pain are the most common symptoms. Extensive ulcerations, deformity, and occasionally perforation of the esophagus may ensue. Although similar lesions may develop in the stomach, they are less frequent than those of the esophagus. Superficial and deep ulcerative lesions of the small and large intestine, which may also occur in immunosuppressed patients, are rare in immunologically normal persons. *Candida* proctitis is often a complication of broad-spectrum antibacterial therapy.

Intestinal candidiasis

Urinary candidiasis

The presence of *C. albicans* in the genital flora and anterior urethra allows these organisms to enter the urinary bladder under the same conditions as the more common bacterial causes of urinary infection (Chapter 66). *Candida* cystitis is particularly associated with diabetes mellitus. Infection of the kidneys via the hematogenous or ascending routes may produce acute pyelonephritis, abscesses, perinephric abscess, or expanding fungus ball lesions in the renal pelvis.

Disseminated infection

Association with immunocompromise

Candida infections of visceral organs with or without further dissemination to multiple organs have a particularly strong association with immunologic compromise or some other violation of normal defense mechanisms. The organs most commonly involved are the kidneys, brain, heart, and eye. Involvement of many other sites, including the lung, is possible, but less frequent. As discussed previously, dissemination may occur from a superficial infection; more commonly, however, the primary mechanism for access to deep tissues involves a medical device, such as an infected intravenous catheter. Multiple organ involvement is typical, particularly if the mechanism of entry causes a continuous fungemia.

Central nervous system candidiasis

Endophthalmitis

Cardiac infections

The clinical findings in disseminated infections are generally not sufficiently characteristic to suggest *C. albicans* rather than bacterial pathogens, which more commonly produce infection of deep organs. Central nervous system infection may appear as meningitis, with a predominantly lymphocytic cell count in the cerebrospinal fluid (CSF) or as multifocal microabscesses. A contaminated ventricular shunt can be a direct route for CSF infection. *Candida* endophthalmitis has the characteristic funduscopic appearance of a white cotton ball expanding on the retina or floating free in the vitreous humor. Endophthalmitis and infections of other eye structures can lead to blindness. A full range of *Candida* cardiac infections may be produced, including pericarditis, myocarditis with microabscesses, and endocarditis. *Candida* endocarditis is particularly associated with cardiac surgery, but is otherwise similar in clinical findings to bacterial endocarditis.

Laboratory Diagnosis.   Superficial *C. albicans* infections are among the easiest to diagnose, but deep organ involvement is very difficult to estab-

KOH and Gram smears of superficial lesions

lish. In addition to their characteristic clinical appearances, superficial infections such as thrush or vaginitis provide ready access to diagnostic material. Exudate or epithelial scrapings are examined by potassium hydroxide or Gram smear. In either case, abundant budding yeast cells are seen; if pseudohyphae are present, the infection can be assumed to be caused by *C. albicans*, and culture may not be needed.

Difficulties in diagnosing systemic candidiasis

Deep organ involvement is difficult to diagnose because the infected tissues are not accessible for sampling. For example, isolation of *C. albicans* from the sputum of a patient with suspected *Candida* pneumonia is not diagnostic, because the organism is part of the normal flora of the mouth or may come from a superficial oral mucous membrane lesion. Even positive blood cultures may not necessarily be conclusive; they may represent contamination of the intravenous catheters present in patients prone to systemic candidiasis. An invasive sampling procedure, such as a direct aspirate or surgical biopsy, is often required to establish the diagnosis.

Culture and identification

Culture of *Candida* species is not difficult. On isolation, the organisms grow rapidly as yeasts on blood or Sabouraud's agar. The primary identification procedure involves presumptive differentiation of *C. albicans* from other *Candida* species with the germ tube test. Germ-tube-negative strains may be further identified or reported as "yeast not *C. albicans*," depending on their apparent clinical significance. Other *Candida* species are much less virulent than *C. albicans*; a possible exception is *Candida tropicalis*, which can be invasive.

Blood culture

Candida albicans is readily isolated from the blood in media used for bacteriologic culture, but cultures must be well aerated. The atmospheric conditions present in most commercial blood culture bottles are not satisfactory unless they are vented (aerated) in the laboratory. The newer lysis–centrifugation blood culture procedures that place the blood concentrate on the surface of plates provide good conditions for growth of *Candida* and other fungi. Growth usually appears in 1–4 days. *Candida* endocarditis represents a special diagnostic problem, because blood cultures have often been negative in established cases. It is likely that the relatively large yeasts are filtered out in the capillary beds and thus prevented from reaching the venous circulation, from which blood samples are collected. Arterial blood cultures, although sometimes successful in this situation, are not a routine procedure.

Serodiagnostic procedures

Many serologic tests have been developed for *C. albicans* infection; none has the sensitivity or specificity needed for clinical diagnosis, although *Candida* antibodies can be demonstrated. Chromatographic or immunologic techniques show promise in detection of *Candida* metabolites or cell components such as mannan, but none are yet sensitive enough for clinical use.

Detection of *C. albicans* products

Local treatment

Treatment. *Candida albicans* is usually susceptible to amphotericin B, nystatin, flucytosine, and the imidazoles. Superficial infections are generally treated with topical nystatin. Measures to decrease moisture and chronic trauma are important adjuncts in treating *Candida* skin infections. Deeper *C. albicans* infections may resolve spontaneously with elimination or control of predisposing conditions. Removal of an infected catheter, control of diabetes, or rise in peripheral leukocyte counts are often associated with recovery without antifungal therapy. Persistent relapsing or disseminated candidiasis is treated with amphotericin B, flucytosine, ketoconozole, or a combination of amphotericin B and flucytosine. Ketoconazole is the primary treatment for chronic mucocutaneous candidiasis.

Recovery without specific therapy

Amphotericin B, flucytosine, and ketoconazole therapy

Infection with Other Opportunistic Yeasts

Species of *Candida* other than *C. albicans* (Table 47.2) produce infections in circumstances similar to those described previously, but less frequently. When contamination of an indwelling device is the portal of entry, the probability of infection by these other species increases. The adherence and invasive properties for *C. albicans* are also seen with *Candida tropicalis*. Both experimental and clinical evidence indicate that *C. tropicalis* has virulence equal to or greater than *C. albicans*. Infections with this organism, although uncommon, may be particularly serious. Another distinctive organism is *Torulopsis glabrata*. This species is a small (2–4 μm) yeast with characteristics similar to those of *Candida*, with the exception of failure to produce hyphae or pseudohyphae in culture. It is a member of the normal gastrointestinal and genital flora. The most common infections are in the urinary tract, but occasionally other deep tissue involvement and fungemia occur. The organism may appear in the same nosocomial settings as *C. albicans*, including intravenous catheters. In deep tissue infections, the organisms are small enough to be confused with *Histoplasma capsulatum* in histologic preparations. Therapy is similar to that for *C. albicans* infections, although *T. glabrata* is more likely to be resistant to flucytosine on primary isolation.

Aspergillus

Microbiology

Molds

Differentiation on basis of conidiophores and conidia

Aspergillus species are rapidly growing molds with septate hyphae and characteristic asexual conidia (Figure 47.3A). Fluffy colonies appear in 1–2 days and by 5 days may cover an entire plate with pigmented growth. Many species in this genus are defined on the basis of differences in the structure of the conidiophore and the arrangement of the conidia. The most important species in human infections are *Aspergillus fumigatus* and *Aspergillus flavus*, but others, such as *Aspergillus niger*, can be involved.

Epidemiology

Environmental organisms

Aspergillus species are widely distributed in nature and found throughout the world. They seem to adapt to a wide range of environmental conditions, and the heat-resistant conidia provide a good mechanism for dispersal. Hospital air and air ducts have received attention as sources of nosocomial *Aspergillus* isolates. Occasionally, building remodeling or other kinds of major environmental disruption have been associated with increased frequency of *Aspergillus* contamination, colonization, or infection.

Aspergillosis

Allergic responses to aspergilli

Aspergillus can cause clinical allergies or occasional invasive infection. In both cases, the lung is the organ primarily involved. Allergic aspergillosis, which can be a mechanism of exacerbation in patients with asthma, is characterized by transient pulmonary infiltrates, eosinophilia, and a rise in *Aspergillus*-specific immunoglobulin G. These conditions follow direct inhalation of fungal elements or, more commonly, colonization of the respiratory tract. Areas of the bronchopulmonary tree with poor drainage because of underlying disease or anatomic abnormalities may serve as a site for growth of organisms and continuous seeding with antigen. A par-

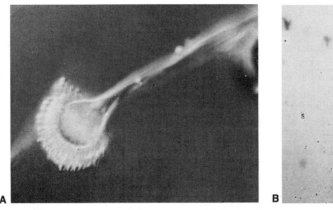

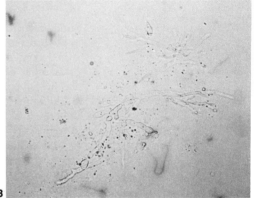

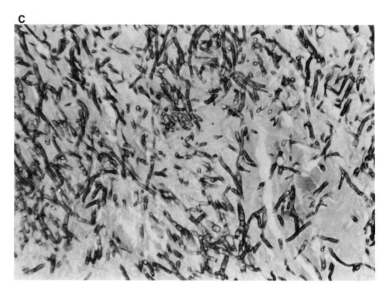

47.3 *Aspergillus.* (A) This asexual conidia forming structure is characteristic of
Aspergillus species. The conidia are borne at the end of the fingerlike extensions at
the end of the conidiophore. These structures are rarely produced in vivo. (B) This tissue
aspirate mixed with KOH shows branching, septate hyphae. (C) Histologic sections also
show branching, septate hyphae, but because the conidia shown in **A** are not seen the
findings are not diagnostic of *Aspergillus.* (*Reproduced with permission from Dr. E. S. Beneke
and from the Upjohn Company: Scope Publications, Human Mycoses.*)

Farmer's lung

Localized and invasive
pulmonary aspergillosis

Fungus ball

ticular form of allergic bronchopulmonary disease known as *farmer's lung*
is associated with inhalation of large numbers of *Aspergillus* conidia as well
as those of other fungi. Acute, recurrent, and chronic pulmonary symptoms are associated with dispersion from haystacks, silos, and similar environments.

Invasive aspergillosis occurs in a similar setting of preexisting pulmonary disease (bronchiectasis, chronic bronchitis, asthma, tuberculosis), particularly when dilated bronchi or cavities are present. Colonization with
Aspergillus can lead to extensive growth, with eventual invasion into the
tissue by branching septate hyphae. Mycelial masses can grow to such an
extent that they form a radiologically visible *fungus ball* within a cavity.

Tissue invasion may involve blood vessels, causing hemoptysis, or erosion into other structures with development of fistulas.

A more acute form of pneumonia may occur in severely immunosuppressed patients. Multifocal infiltrates expanding to consolidation with high fever are present; this finding, however, is no more characteristic of *Aspergillus* than of many other causes of opportunistic pneumonia in these patients. In contrast to that of the more chronic illness, the prognosis is grave. Dissemination to other organs is common. Invasive aspergillosis outside the lung in nonimmunosuppressed patients is very rare. A few cases of endocarditis have been described, and *Aspergillus* is isolated occasionally from otitis externa and other superficial skin lesions.

Diagnosis

Aspergillus is relatively easy to isolate and identify. Its rapidly spreading mold growth and all too frequent contamination of cultures cause it to be regarded by microbiologists as a kind of weed. The diagnostic problem in aspergillosis is not in isolating the organism, but in distinguishing contamination and colonization with *Aspergillus* from invasive disease. This differentiation cannot be certain without the use of invasive procedures such as lung aspiration or open biopsy. With tissue directly from the lesion, the combination of KOH preparation or histologic findings (large, branching, septate hyphae; Figures 47.3B and C) and culture is diagnostic. The histologic picture alone is suggestive but not diagnostic, because other fungi can have similar appearances. Occasionally the complete fruiting bodies are produced in vivo, creating a striking and diagnostic histologic picture. Serologic methods have been developed to demonstrate *Aspergillus* antibodies. Although these tests may be helpful in suggesting allergic aspergillosis, their value in invasive disease is unclear, because antibody is common in healthy persons.

Treatment

Amphotericin B is the treatment of choice for invasive or disseminated aspergillosis. Ketoconazole and other imidazoles are not effective. It is not clear whether flucytosine is active either alone or in combination with amphotericin B. In cases with pulmonary structural abnormalities and fungus balls, chemotherapy has little effect. Surgical intervention is sometimes needed.

Zygomycosis

Zygomycosis (Mucormycosis) is a term applied to infection with any of a group of zygomycetes, the most common of which are *Absidia, Rhizopus,* and *Mucor*. These fungi are ubiquitous saprophytes in soil and are commonly found on bread and many other foodstuffs. They occasionally cause disease in persons with diabetes mellitus and in immunosuppressed patients receiving corticosteroid therapy. Diabetic acidosis has a particularly strong association with mucormycosis.

Pulmonary or rhinocerebral disease is acquired by inhalation of conidia. The pulmonary form has clinical findings similar to those of other fungal pneumonias; the rhinocerebral form, however, produces a dramatic clinical syndrome in which agents of mucormycosis show striking invasive capacity. They penetrate the mucosa of the nose, paranasal sinuses, or

Severe rhinocerebral infections

palate, often resulting in ulcerative lesions. Once beyond the mucosa, they progress through tissue, nerves, blood vessels, fascial planes, and often the vital structures at the base of the brain. The clinical syndrome begins with headache and may progress in less than 2 weeks through orbital cellulitis and hemorrhage, cranial nerve palsy, vascular thrombosis, coma, and death.

Nonseptate and non-spore forming in tissues

The pathologic cerebral and pulmonary findings are distinctive: the zygomycetes involved all show large, nonseptate hyphae in tissue, although conidia are not seen. As with *Aspergillus*, tissue biopsies are necessary to demonstrate the invasive hyphae, unless they can be seen on scrapings from palatal or nasal ulcers. For reasons that are obscure, biopsy cultures are frequently negative even from tissue containing characteristic hyphae. Therapy involves control of underlying disease, amphotericin B, and occasionally surgery.

Additional Reading

Bennett, J.E. 1987. Rapid diagnosis of candidiasis and aspergillosis. *Rev. Infect. Dis.* 9:398–402. This review critically examines the current status of diagnostic tests for the two most opportunistic fungi and the possibilities for improvement in the future.

Calderone, R.A., and Scheld, W.M., 1987. Role of fibronectin in the pathogenesis of candidal infections. *Rev. Infect. Dis.* 9(suppl 4):S400–403. In addition to the evidence for fibronectin as a receptor, this short review covers the general topic of *Candida* adherence.

48

Systemic Fungal Pathogens

Kenneth J. Ryan

The fungi discussed in this chapter cause a variety of deep-seated infections, all of which can range in severity from mild to progressive and fatal. Growth in environmental sites is an important part of their biology, but they rarely, if ever, contaminate laboratory cultures or colonize healthy humans. Their isolation from clinical material is considered diagnostic of the mycoses that they cause.

Cryptococcus neoformans

Microbiology

Yeast with large capsule

Cryptococcus neoformans is a yeast 4–6 μm in diameter that produces a characteristic capsule (Figure 48.1) that extends the overall diameter to 25 μm or more. It is the only pathogenic fungus to form such a capsule that is composed of a complex polysaccharide with a mannose backbone. There are some differences between serogroups based on acetylation and substitution of carbohydrates. Cross-reactions with some serotypes of *Streptococcus pneumoniae* have been demonstrated. *C. neoformans* gives a positive test for urease, in contrast to *Candida* and most other yeasts. It grows in 2–5 days at 35–37°C on a variety of media, including blood agar, chocolate agar, and Sabouraud's agar, to produce mucoid, bacterialike colonies. Some strains are inhibited by cyclohexamide, and media containing this selective agent should not be relied on for isolation. A sexual phase has been demonstrated for *C. neoformans*. Under the conditions used in clinical laboratories, however, it grows only in the yeast phase.

Urease production
Growth characteristics

Pathogenesis and Immunity

Infection by inhalation

Cryptococcal infection is usually acquired by inhalation of fungal conidia, followed by pulmonary infection or disease. In most instances symptoms and signs must be minimal, because cryptococcal pulmonary infections are

661

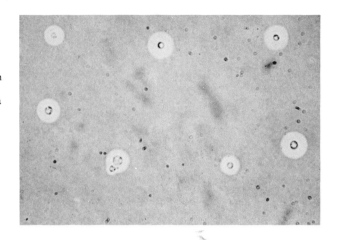

48.1 *Cryptococcus neoformans.*
This India ink preparation was made by mixing CSF containing cryptococci with India ink. The yeast cells can be seen within the clear space caused by the large polysaccharide capsule. (*Reproduced with permission from Dr. E. S. Beneke and the Upjohn Company: Scope Monograph, Human Mycoses.*)

Most infections are unrecognized and self-limiting

rarely seen, or at least rarely diagnosed. In most cases, the inhaled cryptococci are phagocytosed and killed by polymorphonuclear leukocytes or macrophages despite the antiphagocytic effect of the capsule. Occasionally the infection progresses in the lungs or spreads to the central nervous system. Roughly half of all such patients have received chemotherapy or have underlying disorders that compromise immunity. The capsule is the primary determinant of virulence, and noncapsulated variants are avirulent.

Association with other diseases and defects in acquired immunity

Tissue reaction to *C. neoformans* may vary from little or none to purulent or granulomatous. Many cases of pulmonary, cutaneous, and even meningeal cryptococcal infection show a remarkable paucity of inflammatory response. Anticryptococcal antibodies are formed in the course of infection, and there is evidence that they play a role in control of infection.

Immunity to cryptococcal infection in health is substantial and appears to involve both the humoral and cellular immune responses. The capsule interferes with phagocytosis by neutrophils and macrophages, but the organism is opsonized when specific antibody to the capsule develops and is then ingested by phagocytes. Intracellular killing is enhanced by factors that activate phagocytes. In patients with cryptococcal infection the appearance of circulating antibody is often associated with improvement or recovery. The presence and extent of antigenemia with capsular antigen also has prognostic significance. A declining antigen level and rising antibody titer are favorable signs. Cryptococcosis in immunocompromised patients occurs primarily in those with defects in T-cell function caused by underlying disease (eg. acquired immunodeficiency syndrome, AIDS) or in those treated with immunosuppressives (eg. steroids). There is also evidence that patients with cryptococcosis who have no known immune defects often have subnormal cellular immune functions as measured by lymphocyte blastogenesis or absent or reduced delayed hypersensitivity responses to cryptococcal and other antigens. Clinical recovery in such cases is associated with return of cellular immune functions.

Opsonizing effect of anticapsular antibodies

Significance also of cell-mediated immunity

Most clinically infected patients have immunological defects

Epidemiology

Reservoir in birds and soil

Cryptococcus neoformans is found throughout the world in pigeon or other bird droppings and in soil contaminated with them. The birds themselves do not appear to be infected. Little is known about the mechanism of human infection. Cases appear sporadically, with no particular occupa-

Lack of occupational association

tional predisposition. Surprisingly, no increased risk of disease has been found in pigeon fanciers or in those who work with the organism in the laboratory. Case-to-case transmission in humans has not been documented. It is possible that an infectious form, not yet identified, is produced in the environment, but not in vitro.

Clinical Manifestations

Cryptococcal meningitis: chronic course

Central Nervous System. Meningitis is the most commonly recognized form of cryptococcal disease; it usually has a slow, insidious onset with relatively nonspecific findings until late in the course. Intermittent headache, irritability, dizziness, and difficulty with complex cerebral functions appear over weeks or months with no consistent pattern. Behavioral changes have been mistaken for psychoses. Fever is usually, but not invariably, present. Seizures, cranial nerve signs, and papilledema may appear later in the clinical course, as may dementia and decreased levels of consciousness. A more rapid course may be seen in immunosuppressed patients, particularly those receiving steroids.

Cryptococcal pneumonia usually asymptomatic
Other sites of infection

Other Infections. Cryptococcal pneumonia is often asymptomatic or mild. Sputum production is minimal, and no findings are sufficiently specific to suggest the etiology. Skin and bone are the sites most frequently involved in disseminated disease; skin lesions are sometimes the presenting sign and are often remarkable for their lack of inflammation. The diagnosis is sometimes made when lesions are biopsied as suspected neoplasms.

Laboratory Diagnosis

Cryptococcus neoformans may be demonstrated by direct examination or by cultural isolation. It is important to remember that the number of organisms present may be quite small. Thus, perseverance and attention to detail are important in establishing the diagnosis.

The typical cerebrospinal fluid (CSF) findings in cryptococcal meningitis are increased pressure, CSF pleocytosis (usually 100 cells or more) with predominance of lymphocytes, and depression of CSF glucose levels. In some cases, one or all of these findings may be absent, yet cryptococci are isolated on culture. *Cryptococcus neoformans* are often demonstrable in

Direct India ink preparation

CSF by mixing centrifuged sediment with India ink and examining it under the microscope. The yeast and its capsule, which excludes the India ink (Figure 48.1), can often be seen. Some experience is necessary to avoid confusion of lymphocytes with cryptococci. Although this examination is positive in roughly 50% of cases, only a few cryptococci may be present in any single preparation.

Culture

Cryptococcus neoformans may be cultured from CSF or other infected sites. The more material cultured, the less the chance of missing cases with small numbers of organisms. In cases with negative cultures, the

Antigen detection methods

polysaccharide capsular antigen may be present in the CSF and can be demonstrated immunologically. Test kits containing latex particles coated with antibody to cryptococcal polysaccharide are available for this purpose. The particles agglutinate in the presence of cryptococcal antigens. This method has been the only means of attaining a specific diagnosis in some cases.

Histology

Cryptococcus neoformans stains poorly or not at all with routine histologic stains; thus, it is easily missed unless special fungal stains are used. Once stained, the cells themselves are not distinctive; however, histochemical

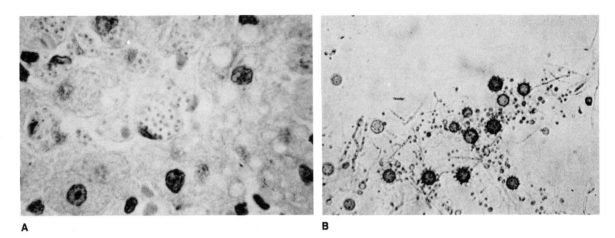

48.2 *Histoplasma capsulatum.* (**A**) Multiple organisms are present within macrophages in the liver. (**B**) The mold is shown with characteristic tuberculate macroconidia. (*Reproduced with permission from Dr. E. S. Beneke and the Upjohn Company: Scope Monograph, Human Mycoses.*)

methods for demonstrating the capsule can differentiate *C. neoformans* from other yeasts.

Treatment

Amphotericin and flucytosine

Amphotericin B, flucytosine, or a combination of both drugs is the usual treatment for systemic cryptococcal disease. Flucytosine alone is effective, but its use is limited by development of resistance during therapy. Although three-fourths of cases of meningitis respond to treatment, a significant portion suffer relapses after antifungal therapy is stopped; many become chronic and require repeated courses of therapy. One-half of those cured have some kind of residual neurologic damage.

Histoplasma capsulatum

Microbiology

Dimorphic fungus

Histoplasma capsulatum is a dimorphic fungus that grows in the yeast phase both in tissue (Figure 48.2A) and in cultures incubated at 37°C. The mold phase grows in cultures incubated at 22–25°C and as a saprophyte in soil.

Small yeast cells

The yeast forms are small for fungi (2–4 μm) and reproduce by budding (blastoconidia). The mycelia are septate and produce microconidia and macroconidia. The diagnostic structure is termed the *tuberculate macroconidium* because of its thick wall and radial, fingerlike projections (Figure 48.2B). Growth is obtained on blood agar, chocolate agar, and Sabouraud's agar, but may take many weeks to develop. As with *C. neoformans*, a sexual stage has now been discovered (*Ajelomyces capsulatus*), but the asexual name continues to be used in the medical literature. The designation *H. capsulatum* is actually a misnomer, because no capsules are formed: the unstained areas seen around the yeasts in tissue sections (Figure 48.2A) are artifacts of the staining and fixation procedures.

Tuberculate macroconidium
Growth

Absence of capsules

Pathogenesis and Immunity

Reticuloendothelial system
infection

Intracellular habitat

The hallmark of histoplasmosis is infection of the reticuloendothelial system with intracellular growth in phagocytic macrophages. The initial infection is pulmonary, through inhalation of infectious conidia, which convert to the yeast form in the host. This conversion is stimulated by the temperature (37°C) of the host and associated with changes in energy-generating pathways of the fungus. How this relates to the organism's ability to multiply within macrophages is unknown.

Primary pulmonary lesion

A primary lesion with lymphatic spread very similar to that seen in tuberculosis (Chapter 27) develops. The vast majority of cases never advance beyond this stage, leaving only a calcified node and a positive histoplasmin skin test as evidence of infection. The extent of spread to the reticuloendothelial system within macrophages during primary infection is unknown, but such spread is presumed to occur and account for the distribution of lesions in disseminated disease. Old lesions may reactivate in a small proportion of cases.

Granulomatous response

Pathologically, granulomatous inflammation with necrosis is prominent in pulmonary lesions. *Histoplasma capsulatum* may be difficult to find even with specific fungal stains. Extrapulmonary spread involves the reticuloendothelial system with enlargement of the liver and spleen. Numerous organisms within macrophages may be found in these organs, in lymph nodes, or in bone marrow (Figure 48.2A).

Cell-mediated immunity and
hypersensitivity
Histoplasmin skin test

Long-lasting immunity

Infection with *H. capsulatum* is associated with the development of cell-mediated immunity as demonstrated by a positive delayed hypersensitivity skin test to histoplasmin. Histoplasmin is a filtrate prepared from mycelial-phase cultures of the fungus. Infection is believed to confer long-lasting immunity, the most important component of which is T-cell mediated. In experimental infections, macrophages activated by T-cell-derived lymphokines (IL1 and gamma interferon) have been shown to inhibit intracellular growth of *H. capsulatum*. Although relapses have been documented, their overall frequency and their relationship to disseminated disease are not well defined. Infected immunosuppressed persons tend to develop disseminated disease.

Epidemiology

Environmental sources

High incidence of infection in
central United States

Point source outbreaks from
bird roosts and bat caves

Histoplasma capsulatum grows in soil containing bird or bat droppings under certain climatic conditions, and disease is acquired from the environment. Although evidence of worldwide distribution is increasing, the greatest concentration by far is in the areas of the United States drained by the Ohio and Mississippi Rivers. Over 50% of residents of states in this area show skin test evidence of previous infection. An African variant with larger yeast-phase cells infects skin and lymph nodes, but rarely produces lung lesions. Disturbances of bird roosts, bat caves, and soil have been associated with point source outbreaks of infection by airborne conidia. The disease is not transmitted from person to person.

Clinical Manifestations

Primary infection of
respiratory tract

Most cases of *H. capsulatum* infection are asymptomatic or show only fever and cough for a few days or weeks. Mediastinal lymphadenopathy and slight pulmonary infiltrates may be seen if X-rays are taken. The histoplasmin skin test becomes positive after about 3 weeks. More severe cases

Chronic infection

Progressive pulmonary
disease

may have chills, malaise, chest pain, and more extensive infiltrates, which usually resolve nonetheless. A residual nodule may continue to enlarge over a period of years, causing a differential diagnostic problem with pulmonary neoplasms. Progressive pulmonary disease occurs in a form similar to that of pulmonary tuberculosis, including the development of cavities, with sputum production, night sweats, and weight loss. The course is chronic and relapsing, lasting many months to years.

Disseminated histoplasmosis

Disseminated histoplasmosis generally appears as a febrile illness with enlargement of reticuloendothelial organs. The central nervous system, skin, gastrointestinal tract, and adrenal glands may also be involved. Painless ulcers on mucous membranes are a common finding. The course is typically chronic with manifestations that depend on the organs involved. For example, chronic bilateral adrenal failure (Addison's disease) may develop when the adrenal glands are involved.

Diagnosis

Direct examination of sputum
rarely helpful

In most forms of histoplasmosis, the organisms are not readily accessible for demonstration by direct examination or culture. They are rarely present in sputum in primary pulmonary infections, and repeated cultures are necessary to ensure positive findings in chronic cavitary disease. In disseminated disease, smears of a superficial mucous membrane lesion or biopsy samples of a reticuloendothelial organ are the specimens most likely to contain *Histoplasma*. Because of their small size, the yeast cells are difficult to see in potassium hydroxide preparations, and their morphology is not sufficiently distinctive to be diagnostic. Selective fungal stains such as methenamine silver demonstrate the organism, but may not differentiate it from other yeasts. Hematoxylin-eosin (H&E)-stained tissue

Histological examination of
bone marrow or other
affected organs

or Wright-stained bone marrow will often demonstrate the organisms and their intracellular location in macrophages (Figure 48.2A). Specimens must be examined carefully under high magnification ($100 \times$, oil immersion).

Culture and identification

The organism may be grown from tissue, bone marrow, or sputum. The latter poses special problems, as *H. capsulatum* grows slowly in comparison to other bacteria and fungi. Identification requires demonstration of dimorphism and of the typical conidia. Prolonged incubation may be necessary.

Serologic diagnosis

Serologic tests have been developed using histoplasmin or yeast cell antigens. Antibodies can be detected by immunodiffusion or complement fixation (CF). In histoplasmosis, CF titers typically rise to 1:32 or greater, but false-negative results are common in all clinical forms of the disease.

False negatives and cross-
reactions with *Blastomyces*
occur
Histoplasmin skin tests

False-positive findings also occur, and definite cross-reactions are found in cases of blastomycosis. The histoplasmin skin test is useful for epidemiologic studies but is often difficult to interpret in clinical situations. Skin testing may stimulate antibodies and thus confuse serologic diagnosis. Neither serologic nor skin test positivity alone is sufficient evidence of disease to initiate therapy. Cultural isolation or clear histologic demonstration is necessary for a firm diagnosis. Specific mycelial antigens can be demonstrated by immunodiffusion once the mold form is isolated (exoantigen test, Chapter 44).

Treatment

Amphotericin B and
ketoconazole

Amphotericin B has long been the treatment of choice for histoplasmosis. Its toxicity, however, limits its use to cases of extensive disease, such as progressive pulmonary disease and disseminated histoplasmosis. Keto-

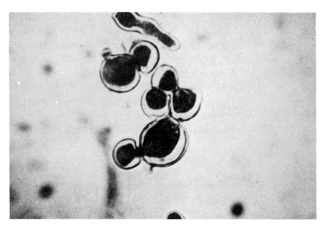

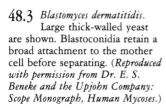

48.3 *Blastomyces dermatitidis.*
Large thick-walled yeast
are shown. Blastoconidia retain a
broad attachment to the mother
cell before separating. (*Reproduced
with permission from Dr. E. S.
Beneke and the Upjohn Company:
Scope Monograph, Human Mycoses.*)

conazole is active against *H. capsulatum*, and clinical experience to date
suggests that it or one of the newer imidazoles may replace amphotericin
B as the treatment of choice for all forms of progressive disease. Primary
infections and localized lung lesions usually require no treatment.

Blastomyces dermatidis

Microbiology

Dimorphic fungus

Large, thick-walled yeasts

Blastomyces dermatitidis is a dimorphic fungus with characteristics similar
to those of *Histoplasma*. Growth develops in the yeast phase in tissues and
in cultures incubated at 37°C. The yeast cells are typically larger (8–15
μm) than those of *H. capsulatum*, with broad-based buds and a thick wall
(Figure 48.3). A smaller variant with morphologic characteristics identical
to those of *Histoplasma* is occasionally seen. The mold phase appears in
culture at 25°C. Hyphae are septate and produce round to oval conidia
sufficiently similar to those produced by *H. capsulatum* to cause confusion
between the two in young mold cultures. Although older cultures may
produce chlamydoconidia, *B. dermatitidis* produces no structure as distinctive as the tuberculate macroconidium of *Histoplasma*.

Pathogenesis and Immunity

Much less is known about blastomycosis than about the more common
systemic mycoses, such as histoplasmosis and coccidioidomycosis. The
lower frequency of disseminated infections and the less specific performance of skin and serologic tests are partly responsible for this lack of
information. Much of what is believed to be true of blastomycosis is based
on analogy with histoplasmosis.

Primary pulmonary infection

The primary infection is pulmonary after inhalation of conidia, which
are believed to develop in soil. A mixed inflammatory response results,
which ranges from neutrophil infiltration to well-organized granulomas
with giant cells. The organisms appear as large yeast cells, most of which
still have blastospores attached. They appear to have a double wall in H&E
sections because of shrinkage of the cytoplasm and dense staining of its
periphery. A significant difference from *Histoplasma* is that the yeast cells
are primarily extracellular rather than within macrophages. This may be
due to their relatively large size, but there is little to suggest that *B.*

Yeasts are extracellular

dermatitidis shares the propensity for intracellular parasitism that is characteristic of *H. capsulatum*. The organism can spread to the skin and less often to bone and viscera. Considerable necrosis and fibrosis can lead to large, expanding lesions at infected sites.

Considerable antigenic cross-reactivity with other fungi has greatly hampered the study of immunity to this organism. A number of clinical and experimental observations indicate that T-cell-mediated responses are important, as with other fungi, but the relative contribution of humoral and cellular immunity to recovery from blastomyces infection is unknown.

Epidemiology

Geography

Cases of blastomycosis follow a geographic distribution similar to that of histoplasmosis. Most infections occur in the middle and eastern portions of North America, but cases have been reported in South America and Africa. Again the lack of a specific skin test limits study of the endemic area.

Clinical Manifestations

As mild cases are difficult to diagnose, most infections are recognized at advanced or disseminated stages of the disease. This problem was also posed by the other systemic mycoses before the development of sensitive and specific diagnostic procedures.

Pulmonary blastomycosis

Pulmonary infection is evidenced by cough, sputum production, chest pain, and fever. Hilar lymphadenopathy may be present, as well as nodular pulmonary infiltrates with alveolar consolidation. The total picture may mimic a pulmonary tumor, tuberculosis, or some other mycosis. Skin lesions are common and were once considered a primary form of the disease. In contrast to those in histoplasmosis, lesions develop on exposed skin; mucous membrane infection is uncommon. Extensive necrosis and fibrosis may produce considerable disfigurement. Bone infection has features similar to those of other causes of chronic osteomyelitis. The urinary and genital tracts are the most common visceral sites; the prostate is especially prone to infection. Prostatitis is an occasional initial complaint.

Skin lesions

Bone, urinary, and genital tract lesions

Diagnosis

Direct examination and biopsy diagnosis

Direct demonstration of typical large yeasts with broad-based buds (blastoconidia) in KOH preparations is the most rapid means of diagnosis. Biopsy specimens also have a high yield, and the organisms are visible with either H&E or special fungal stains. *Blastomyces dermatitidis* will grow on routine mycologic media, but culture may take as long as 4 weeks. Some strains may be inhibited by cyclohexamide in selective media. Conidia are not particularly distinctive, and demonstration of dimorphism and typical yeast morphology is essential to avoid confusion with other fungi, including *Histoplasma*. The exoantigen test (Chapter 44) from mycelial-phase cultures is particularly useful in differentiation from strains of *Histoplasma*, which are slow to produce characteristic conidia.

Culture

Exoantigen test

Antigens for CF tests are available, but CF antibodies are absent in up to 50% of cases. Skin tests have no value.

Treatment

Although amphotericin B is the preferred therapy, it is only used for progressive or disseminated disease. As with other systemic mycoses, response to treatment is slow, and relapse is common. Ketoconazole shows

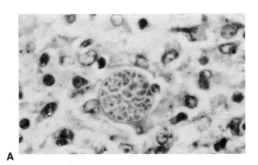

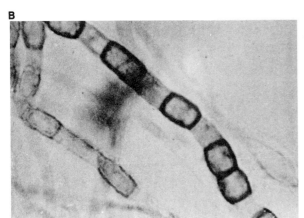

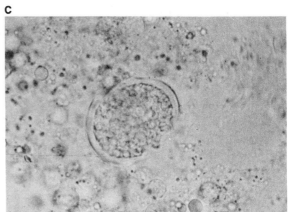

48.4 *Coccidioides immitis.* (A) Tissue with thick-walled spherule containing multiple endospores. (B) Mold phase with septate hyphae and arthroconidia. (C) KOH preparation of sputum showing thick-walled spherule, which has just burst. (*Reproduced with permission from Dr. E. S. Beneke and the Upjohn Company: Scope Monograph, Human Mycoses.*)

promise as an alternative agent, but relapses have occurred in some clinical series.

Coccidioides immitis

Microbiology

Dimorphic fungus

Coccidioides immitis is also a dimorphic fungus, but instead of a yeast phase, a large (12–100 μm), distinctive, round-walled spherule (Figure 48.4A) is produced in the invasive tissue form. Multiple endospores develop

Spherules form in tissues and release endospores

within the spherule and are released when the spherule ruptures. They serve as the reproductive unit in vivo. On routine culture, *C. immitis* grows only as a mold at room temperature and 37°C. Growth becomes visible

Arthroconidia form in mold hyphae at ambient temperature

in 2–5 days. The hyphae are septate and produce thick-walled, barrel-shaped arthroconidia (Figure 48.4B), which are the infectious unit in nature and highly infectious when they develop in the laboratory. Spherules have been produced in vitro under specialized conditions.

Pathogenesis

Respiratory infection

Inhaled arthroconidia are small enough (2–6 μm) to bypass the defenses of the upper tracheobronchial tree and lodge in the alveoli. There, the arthroconidia convert to the spherule stage, which begins its slow growth,

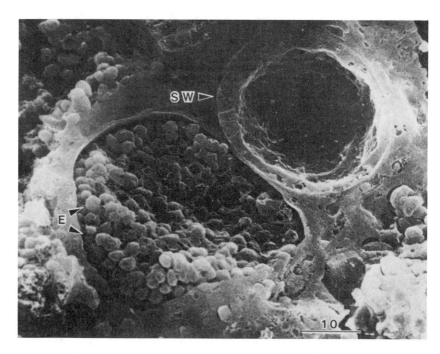

48.5 *Coccidioides immitis.* This electron micrograph of infected mouse lung shows a spherule filled with endospores (E) and one that has discharged its endospores into the surrounding tissue. Note the thickness of the spherule wall (SW). (*Reproduced with permission from Drutz, D.J., and Huppert, M. 1983. J. Infect Dis. 147:379. Figure 7. Copyright University of Chicago Publisher.*)

Inflammatory responses

stimulating a macrophage and neutrophil cellular response. The outer portion of the wall of the arthroconidium has antiphagocytic properties, which persist in the early stages of spherule development. As the spherule grows, its size makes effective phagocytosis difficult, although neutrophils are able to digest the wall. Later, as the spherules enlarge and multiply, the overall inflammatory response is granulomatous with some giant cells. Rupture of spherules with release of hundreds of endospores (Figure 48.5) stimulates an acute inflammatory response, which has an uncertain effect. The young endospores are released in packets with a surrounding matrix derived from the spherule, which may further protect them from destruction by the host. They then develop into new spherules.

Development of immunity and hypersensitivity

Occasional progressive and disseminated disease

In most cases, this mixed inflammatory response is associated with early resolution of the infection and development of a positive delayed hypersensitivity skin test. In a few cases, the infection is not controlled. These infections may progress to a chronic pulmonary form of the disease or become disseminated to other organs. The mechanism for dissemination is not precisely known, although an elastase and a protease have been identified in spherule/endospore lysates, which could aid in spherule rupture, and endospore escape to distant sites. In animals, suppression of cellular immunity is associated with more progressive disease, and dissemination in humans is accompanied by skin test anergy.

Immunity

Cell-mediated immunity

Immunity to coccidioidomycosis is associated with strong T-cell-mediated responses to coccidioidal antigens, and progressive disease is associated with weak or absent cellular immunity. The central events appear to be the reaction to arthroconidia or to endospores released from ruptured spherules. When phagocytosed before an immune response is mounted, they appear to be able to impair phagosome—lysome fusion. This does not

Endospores destroyed by activated macrophages

occur when macrophages are activated. In most infected persons the disease is, thus, controlled following mild or inapparent illness. The disease progresses if cell-mediated immunity and consequent macrophage activation do not develop. Such immune deficits may be a result of disease (eg, leukemia, AIDS) or immunosuppressive therapy or occur in patients with no other known cellular immune compromise.

Progressive disease with defects in cell-mediated immunity

Antibody production inversely related to disease progress

Antibody is not known to play any role in immunity. In fact, the presence and level of complement-fixing antibody is inversely related to the progress of disease. Persons with strong T-lymphocyte responses to *C. immitis* have little if any detectable antibody to the organisms. Those with disseminated disease and absent cellular immunity have high titers of antibody.

Epidemiology

Geography

Coccidioidomycosis is the most geographically restricted of the systemic mycoses, because *C. immitis* grows only in the semiarid climates known as the Lower Sonoran life zone. These areas are characterized by hot, dry summers, mild winters with few freezes, and annual rainfall of about 10 inches during brief rainy seasons. Areas with these conditions are found scattered throughout the Americas; some are ecologic "islands." The primary endemic zones in the United States are in the southwestern states of Arizona, Nevada, New Mexico, and western Texas and the arid parts of central and southern California. Infection does not normally occur outside the endemic areas, although visits of only a few hours to an endemic zone have resulted in infection. One such anecdote involves a gas station attendant with coccidioidomycosis, whose only contact with an endemic area was changing a flat tire on a truck from California. In another instance, a recent storm that blew inland dust into the San Francisco Bay area, which is outside the endemic zone, was associated with many cases of coccidioidomycosis. Earth-moving operations and archeologic digs have also been associated with outbreaks.

Dust-borne spread

High infection but low disease rates in affected regions

Persons living in the endemic areas are at high risk of infection, although disease is much less common. Positive skin test rates of 50–90% occur in longtime residents of highly endemic areas. Coccidioidomycosis is not transmissible from person to person.

Clinical Manifestations

Primary infection is usually asymptomatic and self-limiting

More than one-half of those infected with *C. immitis* suffer no symptoms, or the disease is so mild that it cannot be recalled when skin test conversion is discovered. Others develop malaise, cough, chest pain, fever, and arthralgia 1–3 weeks after infection. This disease, which lasts 2–6 weeks, is known as *valley fever* by the local populations in the United States. Objective findings are few. The chest X-ray is usually clear or shows only hilar adenopathy. Erythema nodosum may develop midway through the course, particularly in women. In most cases, resolution is spontaneous, but only after considerable discomfort and loss of productivity. In over 90% of cases, there are no pulmonary residua. A small number of cases progress to a chronic pulmonary form characterized by cavity formation and a slow relapsing course that extends over years. Less than 1% of all primary infections disseminate to foci outside the lung.

Valley fever

Erythema nodosum

Chronic and disseminated disease

Racial incidence

Disseminated disease is more common in men, in dark-skinned races, particularly Filipinos, and in immunosuppressed persons. Evidence of extrapulmonary infection almost always appears in the first year after primary

Sites of disseminated disease

infection. The most common sites are bones, joints, skin, and meninges. Coccidioidal meningitis develops slowly with gradually increasing headache, fever, neck stiffness, and other signs of meningeal irritation. The CSF findings are similar to those in tuberculosis and other fungal causes of meningitis, such as *C. neoformans*. Mononuclear cells predominate in the cell count, but substantial numbers of neutrophils are often present. If untreated, the disease is slowly progressive and fatal.

Meningitis

Diagnosis

Direct examination for spherules

With enough persistence, direct examinations are usually rewarding. The thick-walled spherules are so large and characteristic (Figures 48.4A and C) that they are difficult to miss in a KOH preparation. Skin and visceral lesions are most likely to be positive, CSF least. The spherules released into expectorated sputum are often small (10–15 μm) and immature without well-developed endospores. Some experience is necessary to differentiate them from artifacts. Spherules stain well in histologic sections by either H&E or the special fungal stains.

Culture

Risk of laboratory infection with arthrospores

Detection of exoantigen

Culture of *C. immitis* from sputum, visceral lesions, or skin lesions is not difficult, but must only be undertaken by those with experience and proper biohazard protection. Cultures from CSF are rarely positive. Laboratories must be warned of the possibility of coccidioidomycosis to ensure diagnosis and avoid inadvertent laboratory infection. The latter is particularly significant outside the endemic areas, where routine precautions may not be enforced. Identification requires growth of typical arthroconidia and demonstration of conversion to spherules either in vitro or in animals. The exoantigen immunodiffusion test (Figure 44.5) is also useful for differentiation of *C. immitis* from other fungi that produce arthroconidia, and it is more rapid than methods for demonstration of spherules.

Skin and serologic tests

Skin and serologic tests are very useful in diagnosis and management of coccidioidomycosis. The coccidioidin skin test usually becomes positive 1–4 weeks after the onset of symptoms of primary infection, and remains so for life. Disseminated disease is frequently associated with anergy, particularly when it is severe. The skin test does not interfere with serologic tests, as it does in histoplasmosis.

IgG levels reflect presence and severity of infection

One-half to three-quarters of patients with primary infection will develop serum IgM precipitating antibody in the first 3 weeks of illness. These conditions persist for 2–4 months. Immunoglobulin G antibodies detected by complement fixation (CF) tests appear somewhat later in symptomatic infections. The amount and duration depend on the extent of disease. Antibodies disappear with resolution and persist with continuing infection. The height of the CF titer is a measure of the magnitude of antigenic stimulation, and thus of the extent of disease. The presence of CF antibody in the CSF is also important in the diagnosis of coccidioidal meningitis, because cultures are usually negative. The precipitating and CF antibodies may be detected by classic methods or by more recently developed immunodiffusion procedures.

Treatment

Amphotericin B
in progressive disease

Primary coccidioidomycosis is self-limiting, and no antifungal therapy is indicated. Progressive pulmonary disease and disseminated disease require the use of antifungal agents, usually amphotericin B. The newer imidazoles, particularly ketoconazole, show some promise; and they are less toxic than amphotericin B, but have not yet been proved effective.

Paracoccidioides brasiliensis

Paracoccidioides brasiliensis is the cause of paracoccidioidomycosis (South American blastomycosis), a disease limited to tropical and subtropical areas of Central and South America. The organism is a dimorphic fungus, the most noteworthy feature of which is the production of multiple blastoconidia from the same cell. Characteristic 5- to 40-μm cells covered with budding blastoconidia may be seen in tissue or in yeast-phase growth at 37°C. The disease is primarily manifested by chronic mucocutaneous or cutaneous ulcers. The ulcers spread slowly and develop a granulomatous mulberrylike base. Regional lymph nodes, reticuloendothelial organs, and the lungs may also be involved. Little is known of the pathogenesis of the disease, although the route of infection is believed to be inhalation. Progression in experimental animals is associated with depressed T-cell-mediated immune responses. The disease has a striking predilection for men. Treatment is with sulfonamides, amphotericin B, and, more recently, the imidazole compounds.

Additional Reading

Drutz, D.J., and Huppert, M. 1983. Coccidioidomycosis: factors affecting the host-parasite interaction. *J. Infect. Dis.* 147:372–390. This review of pathogenesis is beautifully illustrated with electron micrographs.

Smith, C.E., Saito, M.T., and Simons, S.A. 1956. Pattern of 39,500 serologic tests in coccidioidomycosis. *J. Am. Med. Assoc.* 160:546–552. This study is the basis for the unique application of serologic tests to the diagnosis and prognosis of coccidioidomycosis.

49

Subcutaneous Fungal Pathogens

Kenneth J. Ryan

Assignment of fungal organisms to the category of subcutaneous fungi is somewhat arbitrary, because fungal pathogens can produce many subcutaneous manifestations as part of their disease spectrum. Those considered here are introduced traumatically through the skin and mainly involve subcutaneous tissues, lymphatic vessels, and contiguous tissues. They rarely spread to distant organs. The diseases they cause include sporotrichosis, chromoblastomycosis, and mycetoma. Only sporotrichosis has a single specific etiologic agent, *Sporothrix schenckii*. Chromoblastomycosis and mycetoma are clinical syndromes with multiple fungal etiologies (Table 49.1).

Sporotrichosis

Microbiology

Dimorphic fungus
Cigar-shaped yeast at 37°C

Sporothrix schenckii is a dimorphic fungus that grows as a cigar-shaped, 3- to 5-μm yeast (Figure 49.1A) in tissues and in culture at 37°C. The mold, which grows in culture at 25°C, is presumably the infectious form in nature. The hyphae are thin and septate, producing clusters of conidia at the end of delicate conidiophores (Figure 49.1B).

Epidemiology

Saprophyte

Traumatic infection

Occupational incidence

Sporothrix schenckii is a ubiquitous saprophyte found in soil, in decaying organic matter, and on the surfaces of various plants. Infection is acquired by traumatic inoculation through the skin of material containing the organism. Exposure is largely occupational or related to hobbies. The skin of gardeners, farmers, and rural laborers is frequently traumatized by thorns or other material that may be contaminated with spores of *S. schenckii*. An unusual outbreak of sporotrichosis involving nearly 3000 miners

675

Table 49.1   Agents of Subcutaneous Mycoses

Organism	Disease	Growth		
		Tissue	Culture (25°C)	Culture (37°)
Sporothrix schenkii	Sporotrichosis	Yeast (rare)	Mold	Yeast
Phialophora	Chromoblastomycosis; mycetoma	Mycelia[a]	Mold	Mold
Cladosporium	Chromoblastomycosis	Mycelia[a]	Mold	Mold
Petriellidium	Mycetoma	Mycelia	Mold	Mold

[a] Pigmented, often blunted to form round to oval bodies.

was traced to *S. schenckii* in the timbers used to support mine shafts. Infection is occasionally acquired by direct contact with infected pus or through the respiratory tract; these modes of infection, however, are much less common than the cutaneous route.

Pathologic Features

Pyogenic and granulomatous lesions

Local multiplication of the organism stimulates both acute pyogenic and granulomatous inflammatory reactions. The infection spreads along lymphatic drainage routes and reproduces the original inflammatory lesions at intervals. The organisms are scanty in human lesions.

Clinical Features

Skin infection ulcerates

A skin lesion begins as a painless papule that develops a few weeks to a few months after inoculation. Its location can usually be explained by occupational exposure; the hand is most often involved. The papule enlarges slowly and eventually ulcerates, leaving an open sore. Draining lymph channels are usually thickened, and pustular or firm nodular lesions

Lymphatic involvement and spread

A

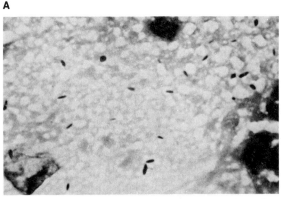

B

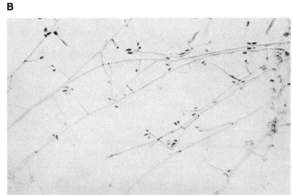

49.1   *Sporothrix schenckii.* (**A**) The yeast form of *S. schenckii* is typically cigar-shaped but is rarely seen in human lesions. This smear is from infected mouse testis. (**B**) Mold phase cultures develop delicate hyphae and conidiophores bearing fingerlike clusters of conidia. (*Reproduced with permission from the Scope monograph, Human Mycoses and from Dr. E. S. Beneke and from the Upjohn Company.*)

may appear around the primary site of infection or at other sites along the lymphatic drainage route. Once ulcerated, lesions usually become chronic. Multiple ulcers often develop if the disease is untreated. Symptoms are those directly related to the local areas of infection. Constitutional signs and symptoms are unusual.

Rare infections in other sites

Occasionally, spread occurs by other routes. The bones, eyes, lungs, and central nervous system are susceptible to progressive infection if the organisms reach them; such spread, however, occurs in less than 1% of all cases. Primary pulmonary sporotrichosis occurs but is also rare.

Diagnosis

Frequent failure of direct examination for fungi

Direct microscopic examination for *S. schenckii* is usually unrewarding because there are too few organisms to detect readily with potassium hydroxide preparations. Even specially stained biopsy samples and serial sections are usually negative, although the presence of a histopathologic structure, the asteroid body, is considered diagnostic. This structure is composed of *S. schenckii* yeast cells surrounded by amorphous eosinophilic "rays."

Grows readily in culture

Definitive diagnosis depends on culture of infected pus or tissue. The organism grows within 2–5 days on all media commonly used in medical mycology. Identification requires demonstration of the typical asexual spores and of dimorphism (Figures 49.1A and B).

Treatment and Prevention

Potassium iodide treatment

Cutaneous sporotrichosis is effectively treated with potassium iodide administered orally. Systemic infections require the use of amphotericin B. There is little therapeutic experience with the newer antifungal agents. Eradication of the environmental reservoir of *S. schenckii* is not usually practical, although the mine outbreak mentioned previously was stopped by applying antifungal agents to the mine shaft timbers.

Chromoblastomycosis

Tropical disease
Multiple etiologies

Wartlike, pigmented lesions

Chromoblastomycosis is primarily a tropical disease caused by multiple species of two genera of fungi, *Phialophora* and *Cladosporium*. The disease occurs typically on the foot or leg. It appears as papules that develop into scaly, wartlike structures, usually under the feet. Fully developed lesions have been likened to the tips of a cauliflower. Extension is by satellite lesions; it is slow and painless and does not involve the lymphatic vessels. The organisms are found in the soil of endemic areas, and most infections occur in those who work barefoot.

The outstanding mycologic feature is the presence of brown-pigmented hyphae on direct examination or in culture. Branching septate hyphae, which are often blunted, can be demonstrated in KOH preparations of scrapings or in histologic sections. Cultures grow as molds, but may take weeks to appear and longer for demonstration of characteristic conidia.

Difficulties in treatment

Surgery and antifungal therapy have been used in chromoblastomycosis, but results in advanced disease are disappointing. Flucytosine has been the antifungal agent most frequently used.

Mycetoma

Multiple etiologies

Mycetoma is another unusual infection associated with trauma to the foot and inoculation of any of several fungal species. The most common species in nontropical areas is *Petriellidium boydii*. The usual clinical appearance

Induration and sinuses on
feet

is of massive induration with draining sinuses. Some of the fungi that cause mycetoma are geographically widespread; most cases, however, occur in the tropics, probably because the chronically damp, macerated skin of the feet that causes predisposition toward mycetoma occurs most often in the tropical environment. This finding is illustrated by the case of a college rower in Seattle who developed mycetoma: he was the only member of his shell who insisted on rowing barefoot. Once established, the treatment of mycetoma is difficult. No antimicrobic stands out as particularly helpful.

Microcolonial granules

The precise microbiologic features depend on the agent involved. Hyphae are usually present in tissue, but may be difficult to demonstrate because of a tendency to form microcolonial granules, as in actinomycosis. *Petriellidium* grows relatively rapidly, but some of the other causes may take weeks for initial growth. Identification is by morphology of the asexual conidia.

Actinomycotic mycetoma

Essentially the same disease can be caused by some branching bacteria of the genus *Nocardia* (Chapter 28).

50

Pneumocystis carinii

James J. Plorde

Pneumocystosis is a highly lethal pneumonitis of immunocompromised patients and premature infants caused by *Pneumocystis carinii*, an organism of uncertain classification. It is now seen most frequently in patients undergoing cancer chemotherapy, organ transplant recipients receiving suppressive therapy, and in patients with acquired immunodeficiency syndrome (AIDS).

Organism

Probably a fungus

Cystic and noncystic forms

Microscopic demonstration of *P. carinii*

Although previously widely believed to be a protozoan, the taxonomic position of *P. carinii* remains unsettled. Recent data indicate that the ribosomal RNA sequence of *Pneumocystis* grown in rats corresponds to that of fungi rather than protozoa. These sequences are highly conserved in nature, and the evidence thus supports classifying the organism as a fungus despite morphologic studies suggesting that it is a protozoon. The organism exhibits cystic forms which are 5–8 μm in diameter and contain two to eight small bodies that are released with rupture of the cyst. These mature to pleomorphic organisms that have been termed *trophozoites*. They possess a single eccentric nucleus, a reticular cytoplasm, mitochondria, and a poorly developed cell membrane. These forms develop into the characteristic cysts. Both forms can be demonstrated in tissue with phase or fluorescent microscopy. Methenamine silver, Gram-Weigert, and toluidine blue stains preferentially stain the cyst wall (Figure 50.1), whereas Giemsa, Wright, and Gram stains stain the trophozoite form. In tissues, the cysts occur in clumps, and their walls are typically flattened at points of contact, presenting a characteristic honeycomb appearance. Organisms morphologically identical to the human parasite have been found in the lungs of several lower animals. Immunologic studies have revealed significant antigenic differences, suggesting the existence of separate strains or species.

679

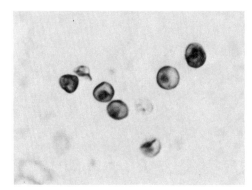

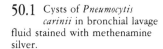 Cysts of *Pneumocytis carinii* in bronchial lavage fluid stained with methenamine silver.

Animal, but not human strains have been cultured

Limited in vitro cultivation, a necessary prerequisite to detailed study of any microbe, has been accomplished in a variety of cell culture lines for rodent strains of *P. carinii*. Human strains have not yet been grown.

Pneumocystosis

Epidemiology

Latent infection

Latent pulmonary infection occurs worldwide in a broad spectrum of animal life. Serologic and histologic evidence suggests a similar pattern in humans. Specific antibodies, detected by indirect immunofluorescence, are present in nearly all normal children by the age of 4, and autopsy studies have demonstrated organisms in the lung tissue of patients without clinical evidence of disease. Manifest illness, when it occurs, may appear in either an epidemic or a sporadic pattern.

Occasional epidemic infection in infants

Epidemics of pneumocystosis were first documented in Europe after World War II, when nursery outbreaks of interstitial pneumonia involving debilitated and premature infants were ultimately proved to be caused by *P. carinii*. Clinical and serologic data collected at that time suggested that the disease was contagious, possibly spreading from person to person via aerosols. With economic recovery and improvement in infant nutrition, the epidemic form of disease disappeared from Europe; however, it continues to be reported occasionally from other parts of the world, most recently in orphanages in Southeast Asia. In contrast, cases in the United States have occurred sporadically among immunocompromised patients.

Sporadic cases in immunocompromised hosts

In infants the disease is associated with congenital immunodeficiencies; in older children and adults, it has generally occurred as a complication of immunosuppressive therapy, particularly corticosteroid administration to patients with lymphoreticular malignancy, collagen vascular disease, or organ transplants.

Frequent occurrence of serious *Pneumocystis* infection in AIDS

In the last decade, AIDS has become the most common predisposing condition in the United States. Pneumocystosis is often the presenting manifestation of AIDS, being present in approximately half of all patients at the time of initial diagnosis. Eventually, at least 80% of AIDS patients develop one or more bouts of *P. carinii* pneumonitis, often in conjunction with another opportunistic infection, such as cytomegaloviral pneumonia. With a mortality rate of 30–50%, pneumocystosis is the leading cause of death in this patient population.

Origin of sporadic cases

It is generally believed that the sporadic cases in immunocompromised patients represent activation of latent infection. However, secondary cases

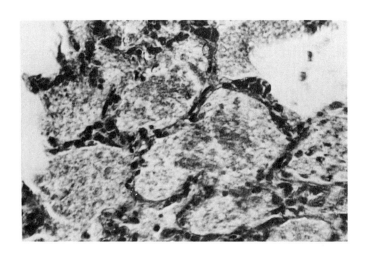

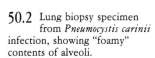
50.2 Lung biopsy specimen from *Pneumocystis carinii* infection, showing "foamy" contents of alveoli.

in the families of some patients and the occasional clustering of cases in cancer wards suggest that this form of the disease may also be contagious.

Pathogenesis and Pathology

Opportunistic pathogen

Pneumocystis carinii is evidently an organism of low virulence that seldom produces disease in a host with normal T-cell function. In experimental animals, progressive infection can be initiated with starvation or corticosteroid administration, presumably by suppressing T-cell function and allowing the activation of a latent infection. Concurrent viral, bacterial, fungal, and protozoan infections are found frequently in human cases, suggesting that *P. carinii* may also require the presence of another microbial agent for its multiplication.

Predisposition with conditions suppressing T-cell function

Latency and development of pulmonary lesions

Histologically, latent infections are characterized by the presence of scattered, isolated cysts found in contact with one class of alveolar cell (type I pneumocytes). In clinically manifest disease, the alveoli are filled with desquamated alveolar cells, monocytes, organisms, and fluid, producing a distinctive foamy appearance (Figure 50.2); hyaline membranes may be present. Proliferation of type II pneumocytes is common and round cell infiltrates may be visible in the septa. Fibrosis, when present, is usually minimal. These changes are generally reversible with therapy, although calcification and persistent fibrosis have been documented occasionally. Lesions outside the lung have been noted, but are extremely rare.

Clinical Manifestations

Progressive, diffuse pneumonitis

In the immunocompromised host, the disease presents as a progressive, diffuse pneumonitis. Illness may begin after discontinuation or a sudden decrease in the dose of corticosteroids or, in the case of acute lymphatic leukemia, during a period of remission. In infants and AIDS patients the onset is typically insidious, and the clinical course is 3–4 weeks in duration. Fever is mild or absent. In older individuals and patients who have previously been on high doses of corticosteroids, the onset is more abrupt, and the course is both febrile (38–40°C) and abbreviated. In both populations, the cardinal manifestation is progressive dyspnea and tachypnea; cyanosis and hypoxia eventually supervene. A nonproductive cough is

Progressive difficulty in breathing and hypoxia

present in one-half of all patients. Clinical signs of pneumonia are usually absent, despite the presence of infiltrates on X-ray. These infiltrates are alveolar in character and spread out symmetrically from the hili, eventually affecting most of the lung. Pleural effusions are uncommon. Clinical and radiographic abnormalities are generally accompanied by a decrease in arterial oxygen saturation, diffusion capacity of the lung, and vital capacity. Death occurs by progressive asphyxia.

Diagnosis

Definite diagnosis depends upon finding organisms of typical morphology in appropriate specimens. Although the organism has been found in sputum, tracheal aspirates, and gastric contents, the yield from such specimens is generally low. In AIDS patients, presumably because of the larger number of organisms present, sputum induced with hypertonic saline has been reported to be positive in roughly half of all patients subsequently shown to have pneumocystosis. Bronchial lavage and endobronchial brush biopsies have been found more helpful, being positive in 90% of AIDS patients and 50% of those with other predisposing conditions. Percutaneous needle aspiration of the lung, needle biopsy, and open lung biopsy, although somewhat more sensitive techniques, are accompanied by more complications, including pneumothorax and hemothorax.

Several tests have been developed to detect circulating antibodies, but none to date has been sufficiently sensitive and specific to warrant routine application.

Sputum positive in some AIDS cases

Bronchial lavage and endobronchial biopsy

Lung biopsy

Treatment and Prevention

Patients with acquired immunodeficiency syndrome excepted, appropriate management of this disease can reduce mortality from 100 to 30%. Oxygen therapy must be administered to maintain adequate oxygenation. In some patients, mechanical ventilatory assistance may be required. The organism is inhibited by trimethoprim-sulfamethoxazole, which should be given orally or intravenously for 14 days. It has been shown recently that long-term, low-dose administration of trimethoprim-sulfamethoxazole will significantly decrease the incidence of *P. carinii* pneumonia in high-risk patients and prevent relapse in AIDS patients.

AIDS patients respond more slowly to treatment, continue to excrete organisms after standard doses of trimethoprim–sulfamethoxazole, and suffer relapse more often. This necessitates administration for a minimum of 21 days. Unfortunately, those patients also have a high incidence of adverse effects to trimethoprim–sulfamethoxazole frequently requiring its discontinuation and the completion of therapy with the equally effective but more toxic pentamidine. A number of newer therapeutic agents are currently undergoing trial.

Trimethoprim-sulfamethoxazole treatment

Additional Reading

Burke, B.A., and Good, R.A. 1973. *Pneumocystis carinii* infection. *Medicine (Baltimore)* 52:23–51. A classic review.

Kovacs, J.A., Hiemenz, J.W., Macher, A.M., et al. 1984. *Pneumocystis carinii* pneumonia: a comparison between patients with acquired immunodeficiency syndrome and patients with other immunodeficiencies. *Ann. Intern. Med.* 100: 663–671.

Mills, J. 1986. *Pneumocystis carinii* and *Toxoplasma gondii* infections in patients with AIDS. *Rev. Infect. Dis.* 8:1001–1011. A recent review.

51

Introduction to Pathogenic Parasites: Pathogenesis and Chemotherapy of Parasitic Diseases

James J. Plorde

This chapter provides an overview of parasitic diseases and of antiparasitic therapy. The student may find it valuable to reread it after studying the subsequent chapters in this section.

Definition. Within the context of this section, the term *parasite* will refer to organisms belonging to one or two major taxonomic groups: *protozoa* and *helminths*. The former are microscopic, single-celled eukaryotes superficially resembling yeasts in both size and simplicity. The helminths, in contrast, are macroscopic, multicellular worms possessing differentiated tissues and complex organ systems; they vary in length from a meter to less than a millimeter. The majority of both protozoa and helminths are free living, play a significant role in the ecology of the planet, and seldom inconvenience the human race. The less common disease-producing species are typically obligate parasites, dependent on vertebrate and/or arthropod hosts for their survival. When their level of adaptation to a host is high, their presence typically produces little or no injury. Less complete adaptation leads to a more serious disturbance of the host and, occasionally, to death of both host and parasite.

Significance of Human Parasitic Infections

The relative infrequency of parasitic infections in the temperate, highly sanitated societies of the industrialized world has sometimes led to the parochial view that knowledge of parasitology has little relevance for physicians practicing in these areas. However, the continuing presence of parasitic disease among the impoverished, immunocompromised, sexually active, and peripatetic segments of industrialized populations means that most physicians will regularly encounter those pathogens.

Parasitic diseases remain among the major causes of human misery and death in the world today and, as such, are important obstacles to the

Eukaryotic single-celled protozoa and multicellular macroscopic helminths

Most are free living
Disease-producing species usually obligate parasites

Major causes of disease and death

683

Table 51.1 Prevalence of Parasitic Infections in 1982

Disease	Estimated Population Involved
Amebiasis	10% of world population
Malaria	
Population at risk	>1 billion
Population infected	177 million
Annual deaths	1 million
African trypanosomiasis	
Population at risk	35 million
New cases/year	≥ 10,000
American trypanosomiasis	
Population at risk	35 million
New cases/year	≥ 10,000
Schistosomiasis	>200 million
Opisthorciasis	19 million
Paragonimiasis	3.2 million
Fasciolopsiasis	10 million
Filariasis	250 million
Onchocerciasis	>20 million
Dracunculiasis	50–80 million
Ascariasis	650 million
Hookworm	450 million
Trichuriasis	350 million
Strongyloidiasis	35 million
Cestodiasis	65 million

development of the economically less favored nations (Table 51.1). Moreover, a number of recent medical, socioeconomic, and political phenomena have combined to produce a dramatic recrudescence of several parasitic diseases with important consequences to both the United States and the developing world.

Currently, over a billion people live in malarious areas, and of these, approximately 200 million are infected at any given time. At least a million children die of malaria each year. *Plasmodium falciparum*, the most deadly of the malarial organisms, has developed resistance to a major category of antimalarial agents, and resistant strains are now found throughout Southeast Asia, parts of the Indian subcontinent, large areas of tropical America, and, most recently, several areas of Africa. Growing resistance of the mosquito vector of malaria to the less toxic and less expensive insecticides has resulted in a cutback of many malaria control programs. In countries such as India, Pakistan, and Sri Lanka, where eradication efforts had previously interrupted parasite transmission, the disease incidence has increased 100-fold in recent years. In tropical Africa, the intensity of transmission defies current control measures. Of direct interest to American physicians is the spillover of this phenomenon to the United States. Presently, approximately 1000 cases of imported malaria are reported annually.

Malaria

Resistance of malarial parasites to chemotherapeutics

Resistance of insect vectors to insecticides

Recent increases in incidence of malaria

Amebic dysentery

Entamoeba histolytica, an intestinal protozoan, infects 10% of the world's population, including 2–3% in the United States. Invasive strains produce amebiasis, a disease characterized by intestinal ulcers and liver abscesses. It is more commonly seen in the poorly sanitated areas of the world, but occurs in the United States as well, particularly in institutions for the mentally retarded and among migrant workers and male homosexuals.

Trypanosomiasis

In Latin America, *Trypanosoma cruzi* infects an estimated 10 million individuals annually, leaving many with the characteristic heart and gastrointestinal lesions of Chagas' disease. In Africa, from the Sahara Desert in the north to the Kalahari in the south, a related organism, *Trypanosoma brucei*, causes one of the most lethal of human infections, sleeping sickness. Animal strains of this same organism limit food supplies by making the raising of cattle economically infeasible.

Leishmaniasis

Leishmaniasis, a disease produced by another intracellular protozoan, is found in parts of Europe, Asia, Africa, and Latin America. Clinical manifestations range from a self-limiting skin ulcer, known as *oriental sore*, through the mutilating mucocutaneous infection of espundia, to a highly lethal infection of the reticuloendothelial system (kala azar).

Parasitic worm infections

In 1947 Stall, in an article entitled "This Wormy World," estimated that between the tropics of Cancer and Capricorn there were many more intestinal worm infections than people. The prevalence was judged to be far lower in temperate climates. Warren, however, recently estimated that 27% of the American population harbored worms. The most serious of

Schistosomiasis

the helminthic diseases, schistosomiasis, affects an estimated 200 million individuals in Africa, Asia, and the Americas. Individuals with heavy worm levels develop bladder, intestinal, and liver disease, which may ultimately result in death. Unfortunately, the disease is frequently spread as a consequence of rural development schemes. Irrigation projects in Egypt, the Sudan, Ghana, and Nigeria have significantly increased the incidence of the disease in these areas, often mitigating the economic gains of the development program itself.

Filariasis

Two closely related filarial worms, *Wucheria bancrofti* and *Brugia malayi*, which are endemic in Asia and Africa, interfere with the flow of lymph and can produce grotesque swellings of the legs, arms, and genitals. Another filaria produces onchocerciasis (river blindness) in millions of Africans and Americans, leaving thousands blind.

Common parasitic diseases in the United States

Toxoplasmosis, giardiasis, trichomoniasis, and pinworm infections are four cosmopolitan parasitic infections well known to American physicians. The first, a protozoan infection of cats, infects possibly one-third of the world's human population. Although it is usually asymptomatic, infection acquired in utero may result in abortion, stillbirth, prematurity, or severe neurologic defects in the newborn. Asymptomatic infection acquired either before or after birth may subsequently produce visual impairment. Immunosuppressive therapy may reactivate latent infections, producing severe encephalitis.

Biology, Morphology, and Classification

Protozoa

Morphology.   Protozoa range in size from 2 to more than 100 μm. Their protoplasm consists of a true membrane-bound nucleus and cytoplasm. The former contains clumped or dispersed chromatin and a central nucleolus or karyosome. The shape, size, and distribution of these structures are useful in distinguishing protozoan species from one another.

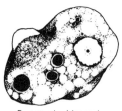

Prototypic rhizopod

(ameba)

10 μm

Table 51.2   Classes of Protozoa

Class	Organelles of Locomotion	Method of Reproduction
Rhizopods (amebas)	Pseudopods	Binary fission
Ciliates	Cilia	Binary fission
Flagellates	Flagella	Binary fission
Sporozoa	None	Schizogony/sporogony

The cytoplasm is frequently divided into an inner endoplasm and a thin outer ectoplasm. The granular endoplasm is concerned with nutrition and often contains food reserves, contractile vacuoles, and undigested particulate matter. The ectoplasm is organized into specialized organelles of locomotion. In some species, these organelles appear as blunt, dynamic extrusions known as *pseudopods*. In others, highly structured threadlike cilia or flagella arise from intracytoplasmic basal granules. Flagella are longer and less numerous than cilia and possess a structure and a mode of action distinct from those seen in prokaryotic organisms.

Classification.   Mode of reproduction and type of locomotive organelle are used to divide the protozoa into four major classes (Table 51.2). Although most rhizopods (amebas) are free living, several are found as commensal inhabitants of the intestinal tract in humans. One of these organisms, *E. histolytica*, may invade tissue and produce disease. Occasionally, free-living amebas may gain access to the body and initiate illness. The majority of ciliates are free living and seldom parasitize humans. Flagellates of the genera *Trypanosoma* and *Leishmania* are capable of invading the blood and tissues of humans, where they produce severe chronic illness. Others, such as *Trichomonas vaginalis* and *Giardia lamblia*, inhabit the urogenital and gastrointestinal tracts and initiate disease characterized by mild to moderate morbidity but no mortality. Sporozoan organisms, in contrast, produce two of the most potentially lethal diseases of humankind, malaria and toxoplasmosis.

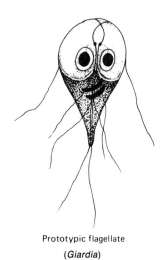

Prototypic flagellate

(*Giardia*)

10 μm

Facultative anaerobes

Nutrients engulfed by phagocytosis or pinocytosis

Extrusion of wastes

Many protozoa form resistant cysts

Reproduction

Physiology.   Most parasitic protozoa are facultative anaerobes. They are heterotrophic and must assimilate organic nutrients. This assimilation is accomplished by engulfing soluble or particulate matter in digestive vacuoles, processes termed *pinocytosis* and *phagocytosis*, respectively. In some species, food is ingested at a definite site, the peristome or cytostome. Food may be retained in special intracellular reserves, or *vacuoles*. Undigested particles and wastes are extruded at the cell surface by mechanisms that are the reverse of those used in ingestion.

Survival is ensured by highly developed protective and reproductive techniques. Many protozoa, when exposed to an unfavorable milieu, become less active metabolically and secrete a cyst wall capable of protecting the organism from physical and chemical conditions that would otherwise be lethal. In this form, the parasite is better equipped to survive passage from host to host in the external environment. Immunoevasive mechanisms described under "Immunity" contribute to survival within the host. Reproduction is accomplished primarily by simple *binary fission*. In one class of protozoa, the *Sporozoa*, a cycle of *multiple fission* (schizogony) alternates with a period of sexual reproduction (sporogony).

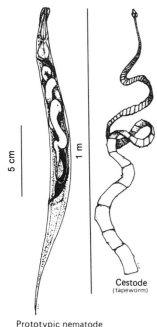

Prototypic nematode
(roundworm)

Great variation in size

Differentiated organs: no
circulatory system

Table 51.3 Classification of Helminthic Parasites of Humans

Characteristic	Roundworm (Nematode)	Tapeworm (Cestode)	Fluke (Trematode)
Morphology	Spindle shaped	Head with segmented body (proglottids)	Leaf shaped with oral and ventral suckers
Sex	Separate sexes	Hermaphroditic	Hermaphroditic[a]
Alimentary tract	Tubular	None	Blind
Intermediate host	Variable[b]	One[c]	Two[d]

[a] *Schistosoma* group has separate sexes.
[b] Tissue nematodes have intermediate hosts; intestinal nematodes do not.
[c] *Diphyllobothrium* group has two.
[d] *Schistosoma* group has one.

Helminths

Morphology and Classification.   Worms are elongated, bilaterally symmetric animals that vary in length from less than a millimeter to a meter or more. The body wall is covered with a tough acellular cuticle, which may be smooth or possess ridges, spines, and tubercles. At the anterior end there are often suckers, hooks, teeth, or plates used for the purpose of attachment. All helminths have differentiated organs. Primitive nervous and excretory systems and a highly developed reproductive system are characteristic of the entire group. Some have alimentary tracts; none possess a circulatory system.

The common helminthic parasites of humans can be placed in one of three classes on the basis of body and alimentary tract, configuration, nature of the reproductive system, and need for more than a single host species for the completion of the life cycle (Table 51.3).

Roundworms, or nematodes, have a cylindric fusiform body and a tubular alimentary tract that extends from the mouth at the anterior end to the anus at the posterior end. The sexes are separate, and the male worm is typically smaller than the female. These worms can be divided into those that dwell within the gastrointestinal tract and those that parasitize the blood and tissues of humans. Unlike the latter, those in the gastrointestinal tract generally do not require intermediate hosts.

Tapeworms, or cestodes, have flattened, ribbon-shaped bodies. The anterior end, or scolex, is armed with suckers and frequently with hooklets, which are used for attachment. Immediately behind the head is a neck that generates a chain of reproductive segments, or proglottids. Each segment contains both male and female gonads. The worm lacks a digestive tract and presumably absorbs nutrients across its cuticle. One or sometimes two intermediate hosts are required for the completion of the life cycle.

Flukes, or trematodes, are leaf-shaped organisms with blind, branched alimentary tracts. Particulate waste is regurgitated through the mouth. Two suckers, one surrounding the mouth and the second located more distally on the ventral aspect of the body, serve as organs of attachment and locomotion. Most are hermaphroditic and require two intermediate hosts. The blood-dwelling schistosomes, however, are unisexual and require but a single intermediate.

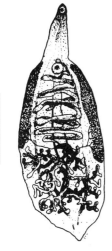

Prototypic trematode
(flukes)

Table 51.4 Transmission and Distribution of Four Representative Parasites

Organism	Infective Form	Mechanism of Spread	Distribution
Trichomonas vaginalis	Trophozoite	Direct (venereal)	Worldwide
Entamoeba histolytica	Cyst/trophozoite Cyst	Direct (venereal) Indirect (fecal-oral)	Worldwide Areas of poor sanitation
Ascaris lumbricoides	Egg	Indirect (fecal-oral)	Areas of poor sanitation
Plasmodium falciparum	Sporozoite	*Anopheles* mosquito	Tropical and subtropical areas

Physiology. Helminthic parasites are nourished by ingestion or absorption of the body fluids, lysed tissue, or intestinal contents of their hosts. Carbohydrates are rapidly metabolized, and the glycogen concentration of the worms is high. Respiration is primarily anaerobic, although larval offspring frequently require oxygen. A large part of the energy requirement is devoted to reproductive needs. The daily output of offspring can be as high as 200,000 for some worms. Typically, helminths are oviparous (excrete eggs), but a few species are viviparous (give birth to living young). The egg shells of many parasites with an aquatic intermediate host possess a lidded opening, or *operculum*, through which the embryo escapes once the egg reaches water. Whether hatched or free borne, the resulting *larva* is morphologically distinct from the mature worm and undergoes a series of changes or *molts* before it achieves adulthood.

Protection from the host's digestive and body fluids is afforded by the tough cuticle and the secretion of enzymes. Some worms, such as the schistosomes, can protect themselves from immunologic attack by the incorporation of host antigens into their cuticles. The life span of the adult helminth is often measured in weeks or months, but some, such as the hookworms, filaria, and flukes, can survive within their hosts for decades.

Life Cycles, Transmission, and Distribution

Single-Host Parasites

As is evident from the previous discussion, many parasites require but a single host species for the completion of their life cycles. The method by which the parasite is transmitted from individual to individual within that species is determined in large part by its viability in the external environment and, in the case of helminths, by the conditions required for the maturation of offspring. The mode of transmission, in turn, determines the social, economic, and geographic distribution of the parasite. A few illustrative examples are summarized in Table 51.4.

The protozoan *T. vaginalis* does not produce protective cyst forms. Although its active, or trophozoite, form is relatively hardy, it can survive only a few hours outside of its normal habitat, the human genital tract. Thus, for all practical purposes, transmission requires the direct genital contact of sexual intercourse. As a result, trichomoniasis is cosmopolitan,

Margin notes:

Anaerobic respiration of adult worm

High fertility

Protection from environment and immunological attack

Longevity

Direct contact transmission

Fecal-oral transmission

occurring wherever human hosts engage in sexual activity with multiple partners.

Another protozoan, *E. histolytica*, inhabits the human gut and produces hardy cysts that are passed in the stool. Transmission occurs when another individual ingests these cysts. Like *T. vaginalis*, the organism can be passed by direct physical contact, in this case by oral-anal sexual activity. This mode of transmission, in fact, accounts for the high incidence of amebic infections in male homosexuals. Unlike *T. vaginalis*, however, the cysts can survive for prolonged periods of time in the external environment, where they may eventually contaminate food or drinking water. Thus, in environments such as mental institutions, where the level of personal hygiene is low, or in populations in which methods for the sanitary disposal of human wastes are not available, amebiasis is common.

Fecal-oral transmission with infectivity developing in soil

The intestinal helminth *Ascaris lumbricoides* illustrates still another transmission pattern. In this infection, highly resistant eggs are passed in the human stool. Unlike the situation with *E. histolytica* described previously, the eggs are not immediately infective, but must incubate in soil under certain conditions of temperature and humidity before they are fully embryonated and infectious. As a result, this parasite cannot be transmitted directly from host to host. The organism spreads only when indiscriminate human defecation results in deposition of eggs on soil and subsequent exposure of that soil to the climatic conditions required for embryonation of the eggs. For this reason, *Ascaris* infections are most prevalent in poorly sanitated areas of the tropics and subtropics.

Multiple-Host Parasites

A few protozoa and many helminths require two or more host species in their life cycle. To avoid confusion, it is customary to refer to the species in which the parasite reproduces sexually as the *definitive host;* that in which asexual reproduction or larval development takes place is the *intermediate host.* When there is more than one intermediate, they are known simply as the first or second intermediate hosts. In some cases, such as that of *Taenia saginata*, the beef tapeworm, both host species are vertebrates; humans serve as the definitive host and cattle as the intermediate. Among parasites that inhabit the blood and tissues of humans, it is more common for a blood-feeding arthropod to serve as a second host and as the transmitting vector. An example is malaria, in which the causative plasmodium is transmitted from person to person by the bite of an infected female mosquito of the genus *Anopheles*. In this particular instance, sexual reproduction occurs in the mosquito, making it the definitive host and relegating the human host to the role of a mere intermediate.

Definitive and intermediate hosts

Influence of distribution of nonhuman hosts on disease occurrence

The distribution of parasites requiring a nonhuman host is limited to the ecologic niche occupied by this second host. Thus, the areas in which malaria is endemic are restricted by the distribution of *Anopheles*. The area of disease distribution is, in fact, generally smaller than that of the nonhuman host, because conditions favoring parasite transmission may also differ. For example, both the abundance of *Anopheles* and the speed with which the malarial parasite completes its development within them are directly related to the ambient temperature and humidity. Among temperate-zone *Anopheles*, the number of infected mosquitoes may be insufficient to sustain parasite transmission. In tropical areas, transmission is more likely to be constant and intense. In another more obvious example, infections with *T. saginata* are found only in areas where cattle are raised for human consumption and, within those areas, only where indiscriminate human defecation and the ingestion of raw or undercooked beef are common.

Immunity

The large size, complex structure, varied metabolic activity, and synthetic prowess of most parasites provide their human host with an intense antigenic challenge. The resulting immunologic response is, generally, vigorous, but its role in modulating the parasitic invasion differs significantly from that in viral and bacterial infections. It is apparent from the chronic course and frequent recurrences typical of many parasitic diseases that acquired resistance is often absent. When present, it is generally incomplete, serving to moderate the intensity of the infection and its associated clinical manifestations rather than to destroy or expel the causative pathogen. In fact, clinical recovery and resistance to reinfection in some parasitoses requires the persistence of viable organisms at low concentration within the body of the host (premunition). Complete sterilizing immunity with prolonged resistance to reinfection is exceptional.

This pusillanimous response does not result from any dearth of immunologic mechanisms available to the host. All those generally exercised against the more primitive microorganisms, including antibodies, cytotoxic T cells, activated macrophages, natural killer cells, antibody-dependent cell-mediated toxicity, lymphokines, and complement activation have been shown to play a part in moderating parasitic infection. In worm infections, some of these mechanisms find unique implementation. On invasion of tissue, helminths stimulate the production of IgE, the Fc portion of which binds to mast cells and basophils. Interaction of the antibody with parasitic antigen triggers the release of histamine and other mediators from the attached cells. These may injure the worm directly, or, by increasing vascular permeability and stimulating the release of chemotactic factors, they may lead to the accumulation of other cells and IgG antibodies capable of initiating antibody-dependent, cell-mediated destruction of the parasite. The specific killer cell involved is often the eosinophil. These cells attach by their Fc receptor site to IgG antibody-coated parasites and degranulate, releasing a major basic protein that is directly toxic to the worm.

The techniques by which parasites have been shown to evade the consequences of the host's specific acquired immunity are numerous. Included among them are seclusion within immunologically protected areas of the body, continual alteration of surface antigens, and active suppression of the host's effector mechanisms. A number of protozoa are shielded from humoral defenses by virtue of their intracellular location. Some have even found ways to avoid or survive the normally lethal environment of the phagolysosome of the macrophage. *T. cruzi*, for example, lyses the phagosomal membrane, providing escape into the cytoplasm, whereas *Toxoplasma gondii* inhibits fusion of the phagosome with lysosomes. *Leishmania*, capable of neither of these feats, are resistant to the action of lysosomal enzymes and survive in the phagolysosomes.

Toxoplasma, cestode larvae, and *Trichinella spiralis* armor themselves against immunologic attack by encysting within the tissue of the host. The gut lumen is, perhaps, the largest immunologic sanctuary within the body, because, unless the integrity of the intestinal mucosa is breached by injury or inflammation, this barrier protects lumen-dwelling parasites from most of the effective humoral and cellular immune mechanisms of the host, allowing almost unfettered growth and multiplication.

Most immune effector mechanisms are directed against the surface an-

Response to parasites vigorous but often relatively infective

IgE response to worm infections attracts eosinophils

Eosinophils bind to IgG-coated parasite and release toxic protein

Some intracellular protozoa avoid phagolysosome destruction

Encysted and intestinal parasites relatively inaccessible to host defenses

Antigenic shifts with
developmental change

tigens of the parasite, and alteration of these antigens may blunt the immunologic attack. Many parasites undergo developmental changes within their hosts that are generally accompanied by alterations in surface antigens. Immune responses directed at an early developmental stage may be totally ineffective against a later stage of the same parasite. Such stage-specific immunity has been demonstrated in malaria, schistosomiasis, and trichinosis, accounting for the seeming paradox of parasite survival in a host resistant to reinfection with the same strain of organism. Even more

Trypanosomal antigenic
variation outpaces
immunologic response

Antigenic glycoprotein
variants of trypanosomes
selected from preexisting
genetic repertoire

intriguing is the ability of some parasites to vary the antigenic characteristics of a single developmental stage. The trypanosomes causing African sleeping sickness circulate in the bloodstream coated with a thick layer of glycoprotein. The development of humoral antibody to this coating results in the elimination of the parasite from the blood. This is followed with successive waves of parasitemia, each associated with a new glycoprotein antigen on the parasite against which the previously produced antibody is ineffective. The parasite is capable of producing over 100 glycoprotein variants, each encoded by a different structural gene. The expression of individual genes from this large genetic repertoire is controlled by the sequential transfer of a duplicate copy of each gene to an area of the parasite responsible for gene expression.

Antigenic shedding and
masking

A number of protozoan and helminthic pathogens are thought to be capable of neutralizing antibody-mediated attack by shedding and, later, regenerating specific surface antigens. Adult schistosomes, in addition, may immunologically hide from the host by masking themselves with a host blood-group antigens and immunoglobulins.

Destruction by parasites of
immunologic mediators

Immunologic suppression by
some parasites

A number of parasites can destroy or inactivate immunologic mediators. Tapeworm larvae produce anticomplementary chemicals, and *T. cruzi* splits the Fc component of attached antibodies, rendering it incapable of activating complement. Several protozoa, most notably *T. brucei*, the etiologic agent of African sleeping sickness, induce polyclonal B-cell activation leading to the production of nonspecific immunoglobulins and eventual exhaustion of the antibody-producing capacity of the host. This and other protozoa can produce nonspecific suppression of both cellular and humoral effector mechanisms, enhancing the host's susceptibility also to a variety of unrelated secondary infections. Patients with disseminated leishmaniasis display a specific inability to mount a cellular immune response to parasitic antigens in the absence of evidence of generalized immunosuppression.

Finally, the thick, tough cuticle of many adult helminths renders them impervious to immune effector mechanisms designed to deal with the less robust microbes.

Pathogenesis

Humans as definitive and
intermediate hosts

In helminthic infections, humans may serve as the definitive host to the sexually mature adult worms (for example, *T. saginata*) or as the intermediate host to the larval stages (for example, *Echinococcus granulosus*). Occasionally, they serve as both the definitive and the intermediate host to the same worm (for example, *Trichinella spiralis, Taenia solium*). Unlike protozoan parasites, most adult helminths are incapable of increasing their numbers within their definitive host. As a result, the severity of clinical illness is related to the total number of worms acquired by the host over time. Most small worm loads are, in fact, asymptomatic and may not require therapy. Many worms are long lived, however, and repeated infections can result in very high worm loads with subsequent disability.

Most adult helminths do not
multiply within host

Significance of reinfection
and worm loads

The pathogenesis of both protozoan and helminthic disease is highly variable. The fish tapeworm *Diphyllobothrium latum* competes with the host for nutrients. The protozoan *G. lamblia* and the helminth *Strongyloides stercoralis* interfere with the absorption of food across the intestinal mucosa. Hookworm infections cause loss of iron, an essential mineral. Other helminths, such as *Clonorchis sinensis* and *Schistosoma haematobium*, compromise the function of important organs by obstruction, secondary bacterial infection, and induction of carcinomatous changes. Occasionally, as in the case of echinococcosis, disease results from pressure and displacement of normal tissue by the slow growth of the parasitic cyst. In malaria, the primary pathogenic mechanism appears to be the invasion and subsequent alteration and/or destruction of human erythrocytes. Similarly, many helminthic larvae are capable of tissue invasion and destruction. *Entamoeba histolytica* can destroy host cells without actual cellular invasion. Finally, immunologic mechanisms are responsible for tissue damage and clinical manifestations in many diseases. Allergic or anaphylactic reactions play a major role in the cutaneous reactions to invading hookworm, strongyloides, and schistosome larvae (ground itch, swimmer's itch) and in the fever, rash, and lymphadenopathy that accompanies the therapeutic destruction of onchocercal microfilariae (Mazzotti reaction) Transient pneumonias induced by the pulmonary migration of *Ascaris* and other nematode larvae (Loeffler's syndrome); nocturnal paroxysms of asthma in some patients with filariasis (tropical pulmonary eosinophilia); and the shock, asthma, and urticaria that follows rupture of a hydatid cyst are all immunologically mediated. Hemolysis in malaria and cardiac damage in Chagas' disease is thought, at least in part, to reflect antibody-mediated cytotoxicity. Immune complex diseases are seen in schistosomiasis (Katayama syndrome) and malaria (nephrosis). The granulomatous reaction to schistosomal eggs, the muscle damage in trichinosis, and the entire clinicopathologic spectrum of the leishmanial infections appear to be due to cell-mediated immune responses.

Diagnosis

Although parasitic diseases are not as common in the United States as elsewhere, they do occur and may, at times, be life threatening. In addition, the continuous arrival of travelers and immigrants from endemic areas necessitates consideration of these diseases in differential diagnoses. Unfortunately, the clinical manifestations of parasitic infections are seldom sufficiently characteristic to raise this possibility in the clinician's mind. Moreover, routine laboratory tests are seldom of aid. Although eosinophilia has been recognized as an important clue to the diagnosis of parasitic disease, this phenomenon is characteristic only of helminthic infection, and even in these cases it is frequently absent. Eosinophilia, which presumably reflects an immunologic response to the complex foreign proteins possessed by worms, is most marked during tissue migration. Once migration ceases, the eosinophilia may decrease or disappear entirely. Thus, the clinician must usually rely on a detailed travel, food intake, transfusion, and socioeconomic history to raise the possibility of parasitic disease.

Once considered, diagnosis is usually straightforward. Typically, it rests upon the demonstration and morphologic identification of the parasite or its progeny in the stool, urine, sputum, blood, or tissues of the human host.

In intestinal infections, a simple wet mount and/or stained smear of the stool is often adequate. Some parasites, however, are passed in the feces

Wide range of direct
pathogenetic mechanisms

Immunopathological
contribution to parasitic
diseases

Need to consider indigenous
and imported infections

Variable eosinophilia in
helminthic infections

Demonstration and
identification of intestinal
parasites

Stool concentration
techniques for intestinal
parasites

intermittently or in fluctuating numbers, and repeated specimens are needed. Ova of worms and cysts of protozoa may be concentrated by sedimentation or flotation techniques to increase their numbers for diagnosis. Occasionally, specimens other than stool must be examined. In the case of small-bowel infections such as giardiasis and strongyloidiasis, aspirates of the duodenum or a small-bowel biopsy may be required to establish the diagnosis. Similarly, the recovery of large-bowel parasites such as *E. histolytica* and *Schistosoma mansoni* may require proctoscopy or sigmoidoscopy with aspiration or biopsy of suspect lesions. Eggs of pinworms (*Enterobius*) and tapeworms (*Taenia*) may be found on the perineal skin when they are absent from the stool.

Demonstration and
identification of blood and
tissue parasites

Parasites dwelling within the tissue and blood of the host are more difficult to identify. Direct examination of the blood is useful for the detection of malarial parasites, leishmania, trypanosomes, and filarial progeny (microfilariae). The concentration of organisms in the bloodstream often fluctuates, however, requiring the collection of multiple specimens over several days. Both wet mount and stained preparations of thin and thick blood smears (Chapter 52) are used. Lung flukes and occasionally other helminths discharge their offspring in the sputum and may be found there with appropriate concentration techniques. In others, larvae can be recovered with skin (onchocerciasis) or muscle (trichinosis) biopsy.

Serologic tests

In some infections, parasite recovery is uncommon. Reliable serologic tests have been developed for several, including toxoplasmosis, amebiasis, South American trypanosomiasis, trichinosis, echinococcosis, and *Toxocara* infections. The recent introduction of purified homologous antigens and the adaptation of enzyme-linked immunosorbent assays to detection of parasitic infections will undoubtedly increase the number of useful tests in the near future.

Chemotherapy

The study and management of parasitic disease was seminal to the initiation of the chemotherapeutic era. Amazonian Indians first employed quinine-containing extracts of cinchona tree bark to treat malarious patients over 300 years ago. It was in the attempt to synthesize this same antimalarial compound that 19th-century German chemists discovered aniline dyes. The circle closed in the early years of this century when Ehrlich, while investigating the suitability of these dyes as protozoan stains, developed the concept that chemicals might be found that had the capacity to selectively destroy microbial pathogens without damage to the tissues of the human host. Although the most dramatic confirmation of that concept came with the introduction of arsenical compounds for the treatment of syphilis, his first successful chemotherapeutics were directed against protozoan agents. By 1930, chemically synthesized drugs had been marketed for the treatment of malaria, trypanosomiasis, and schistosomiasis.

History of antiparasitic
chemotherapy

The introduction and explosive increase in the number and variety of antimicrobic agents introduced in the second and third quarters of this century forever changed the face of medicine. Unfortunately, however, few were effective against parasites because they share the eukaryotic characteristics of their hosts. With the resources of the pharmaceutical companies directed to the development and introduction of antibacterial agents, work on antiparasitics lagged. Safer alternatives lacking, chemotherapeutics synthesized in the preantibiotic era remained critical elements of the parasitologist's therapeutic armamentarium until very recently. Most required prolonged or parenteral administration, the effectiveness of many was restricted to particular disease stages, and the toxicity of a few mandated that use be limited to very severe or life-threatening conditions. With time, and at a pace much slower than that seen for the antibacterials, newer antiparasitic agents were developed that overcame many of these problems. Their numbers are still limited, and only recently has their safety and efficacy begun to match that of their antibacterial equivalents.

Therapeutic Goals

The process of antiparasitic drug development and utilization has been shaped to a significant degree by the concentration of these diseases in the impoverished areas of the world. Community-based public health measures aimed at interrupting pathogen transmission, such as provision of sanitary facilities and clean water supplies, are still often beyond the capacity of tightly constrained budgets, and the major burden of mitigating the impact of parasitic illnesses in endemic areas often falls on medical auxiliaries or village health workers who, operating in remote and relatively primitive conditions, must examine, diagnose, and treat sick patients with whom they have only fleeting contact. Given these limitations and the large numbers of the afflicted, optimal therapy requires drugs that are effective in a single dose, easily administered, safe enough to be dispensed with limited medical supervision, and sufficiently inexpensive to be widely used.

Few such agents exist. Pharmaceutical companies, faced with the enormous costs of drug development and approval, have been reluctant to expend resources they are unlikely to recover. Until the international community provides the resources needed for the development of more suitable agents, the full potential of antiparasitic chemotherapy will not be realized.

The practical aspects of antiparasitic therapy are illustrated in the principles governing the treatment of worm infections, which differ significantly from those applied to prokaryotic or protozoan infections. Helminths, with few exceptions, do not multiply within the human host, and severe infections thus require the repeated acquisition of infectious stage parasites. Interestingly, the intensity of infection or worm burden does not follow a normal distribution in human populations. Most infected individuals harbor fewer than a dozen adult worms; a small minority harbor very large worm numbers. As there is a direct correlation between worm burden and clinical disease, it is only this minority that suffers significant morbidity. Concentrating treatment on those few clinically ill patients moderates the medical impact of a helminthic disease on a community at a cost dramatically lower than that required for mass treatment. Moreover, it is usually unnecessary to eradicate all worms from treated patients; a significant decrease in the worm burden is adequate to alleviate clinical symptoms. This can often be accomplished with short, subcurative doses that further reduce cost and minimize the likelihood of drug toxicity. Because this approach can dramatically decrease the total community worm burden, the number of worm progeny shed into the environment is similarly reduced and the transmission of the disease slowed or, at times, eliminated.

Structure and Action

With few exceptions, antiparasitic agents have been synthesized de novo rather than developed from naturally occurring substances. Most are relatively simple and often contain benzene or other ring structures.

Budgetary and practical factors influencing therapy in developing countries

Ideal agents would be cheap, of low toxicity, and effective in single doses

Concentration of effort on those most heavily parasitized

Most antiparasitics are synthetic

Modes of action and
differential toxicity

It is believed that the majority of antiprotozoan drugs interfere with nucleic acid synthesis or, less commonly, with carbohydrate metabolism. Antihelminthics, on the other hand, apparently act by compromising the worm's glycolytic pathways or neuromuscular function. In most cases, the parasite and host cells have functionally equivalent target sites. Differential toxicity is achieved by preferential uptake, metabolic alteration of the drug by the parasite, or differences in the susceptibility of functionally equivalent sites in parasite and host.

Acquired mutational resistance usually involves reduced uptake of drug

As has been the case for antibacterial agents, the impact of many antiparasitics has been compromised by the development of resistance in the parasite. This seems to have resulted from mutation and selection in the face of intensive, often prophylactic, drug use. The mechanisms responsible have been studied for only a few parasites, but appear to be related to reduced uptake of drug.

Drugs

Heavy Metals.   Arsenic and antimonial compounds have been used since ancient times. They form stable complexes with sulfur compounds and probably exert their biologic effects by binding to sulfhydryl groups. They are toxic to the host as well as to the parasite and have their greatest impact on cells that are most metabolically active such as neuronal, renal tubular, intestinal epithelial, and bone marrow stem cells. Their differential toxicity and therapeutic value is due to enhanced uptake by the parasite and its intense metabolic activity. Only one trivalent arsenical, Melarsoprol (Mel B), is now widely used. It is capable of penetrating the blood–brain barrier and is effective in all stages of trypanosomiasis. Because of its toxicity, it is employed only when less toxic agents have failed or the central nervous system is involved. The recently introduced less toxic trypanocides that penetrate the blood–brain barrier may soon replace this drug.

Arsenic and antimonial compounds inactivate –SH groups

Poor differential toxicity

Melarsoprol is active against all stages of trypanosomiasis

Antimonials used only for leishmanial infections

Antimonial agents are now restricted to the management of leishmanial infections. Two pentavalent compounds, sodium stibogluconate (Pentostam) and meglumine antimoniate (Glucantime), are used for all forms of leishmaniasis. In disseminated disease, prolonged therapy is usually required and relapses often occur. In localized cutaneous leishmaniasis, cure is usually achieved with a relatively brief course. Toxic side effects are similar to those of the arsenicals.

Quinine and quinoline analogs active against malaria

Antimalarial Quinolines.   Cinchona bark was employed in Europe for the treatment of fever as early as 1640. It was only after Pelletier and Caventou isolated quinine from cinchona in 1820 that this alkaloid gained widespread acceptance as an antimalarial. Synthesis of new quinolines was stimulated by the interruption of quinine supplies during two world wars and, after 1961, by the growing impact of drug-resistant falciparum malaria in several areas of the world. Among the most effective are those that share the double-ring structure of quinine.

Quinoline ring

Accumulate in parasitized cells, block DNA synthesis

Current analogs fall into three major groups, the 4-aminoquinolines, 8-aminoquinolines, and 4-quinolinemethanols. Most appear to block nucleic acid synthesis by intercalation into double-stranded DNA, but failure of the 4-quinolinemethanols to intercalate indicates that other mechanisms, perhaps interference with hemoglobin digestion by the malarial parasite, are involved. Selective destruction of intracellular parasites results from accumulation of drug by parasitized host cells. Quinine, 4-aminoquinolines, and 4-quinolinemethanols concentrate in parasitized

Quinine, 4-aminoquinolines (eg, chloroquine), and 4-quinolinemethanols suppress malarial infection

erythrocytes and rapidly destroy the erythrocytic stage of the parasite that is responsible for the clinical manifestations of malaria. These agents can thus be used prophylactically to suppress clinical illness should infection occur or therapeutically to terminate an acute attack. They do not concentrate in tissue cells, and thus organisms sequestered in exoerythrocytic sites, particularly the liver, survive and may later reestablish erythrocytic infection and produce a clinical relapse. The 8-aminoquinolines accumulate in tissue cells, destroy hepatic parasites and effect a radical cure.

8-Aminoquinolines (eg, primaquine) effect radical cure

Chloroquine phosphate, a 4-aminoquinoline, is the most widely used of the blood schizonticidal drugs. In the doses used for long-term malarial prophylaxis, it has proven remarkably free of untoward effects. Primaquine phosphate, the 8-aminoquinoline used to eradicate persistent hepatic parasites, has toxic effects related to its oxidant activity. Methemoglobinemia and hemolytic anemia are particularly frequent in patients with glucose-6-phosphate dehydrogenase deficiency, because they are unable to generate sufficient quantities of the reduced form of nicotinamide adenine dinucleotide to respond to this oxidant stress. Typically the anemia is severe in patients of Mediterranean and Oriental ancestry and mild in blacks.

Toxic effects of Primaquine

Quinine is the most toxic of the quinolines and is currently used primarily to treat the strains of *Plasmodium falciparum* resistant to several blood schizonticidal agents that are spreading rapidly through Asia, Latin America, and Africa. Chloroquine resistance is the most frequent and worrisome, because suitable alternatives to this safe and highly effective agent are few. The mechanism of resistance is not clearly understood, but resistant organisms fail to accumulate chloroquine. Experimental reversal of resistance with calcium channel blockers suggests the failure to accumulate this agent results from a rapid release mechanism. Mefloquine, a newly developed oral 4-quinolinemethanol, presently displays a high level of activity against most chloroquine-resistant parasites. However, its structural similarity to choloroquine, and ready in vitro development of mefloquine resistance in *P. falciparum* raises the specter that cross-resistance to this agent may develop quickly.

Quinine is active against many chloroquine resistant malarial strains

Folate Antagonists. Folic acid serves as a critical coenzyme for the synthesis of purines and ultimately DNA. In protozoa, as in bacteria, the active form of folic acid is produced in vivo by a simple two-step process. The first, the conversion of *para*-aminobenzoic acid to dihydrofolic acid, is blocked by sulfonamides. The second, the transformation of dihydro- to tetrahydrofolic acid, is inhibited by folic acid analogs (folate antagonists), which competitively inhibit dihydrofolate reductase. Used together with sulfonamides, folate antagonists are very effective inhibitors of protozoan growth.

Sulfonamide and folate antagonists inhibit protozoa

Trimethroprim, an inhibitor of dihydrofolate reductase, is used in combination with sulfamethoxazole to treat toxoplasmosis and *Pneumocystis* infection. Another folate antagonist, pyrimethamine, has a high affinity for sporozoan dihydrofolate reductase and has been particularly effective when used with a sulfonamide in the management of malaria and toxoplasmosis. Acquired protozoal resistance is mutational and has been generally limited to species of malarial parasite.

Trimethoprim effective in *Toxoplasma* and *Pneumocystis* infections

Folate antagonists may result in folate deficiency in individuals with limited folate reserves, such as newborns, pregnant women, and the malnourished. This is of great concern when large doses are used for prolonged periods of time, as in the treatment of acute toxoplasmosis. When used with sulfonamides, the entire range of sulfonamide toxicities may be

Side effects of folate antagonists and sulfonamides

seen. Patients with acquired immunodeficiency syndrome appear to suffer an unusually high incidence of toxic side effects to trimethoprim–sulfamethoxazole.

Nitroimidazoles. Metronidazole, a nitroimidazole, was introduced in 1959 for the treatment of trichomoniasis. Subsequently, it was found to be effective in the management of giardiasis, amebiasis, and a variety of infections produced by obligate anaerobic bacteria. Energy metabolism in all of them depends on the presence of low redox potential compounds, such as ferredoxin, to serve as electron carriers. These compounds reduce the 5-nitro group of the imidazoles to produce intermediate products responsible for the death of the protozoal and bacterial cells, possibly by alkylation of DNA. Resistance, although uncommon, has been noted in strains of *T. vaginalis* lacking nitroreductase activity. Of greater concern is in vitro evidence of mutagenicity. Metronidazole is the drug of choice for trichomoniasis and invasive amebiasis. It is effective in giardiasis although not yet approved by Food and Drug Administration for use in this infection. Tinidazole, a newer nitroimidazole not yet available in the United States, appears to be both a more effective and less mutagenic antiprotozoan agent.

Benzimidazoles. As the name implies, the basic structure of these antiparasitic agents consists of linked imidazole and benzene rings. Unlike their antiprotozoal cousins discussed above, the benzimidazoles are broad-spectrum antihelminthic agents. The prototype drug, thiabendazole, acts against both adult and larval nematodes and was shown to be useful in the management of cutaneous larva migrans, trichinosis, and most intestinal nematode infections soon after its introduction in the early 1960s. The mechanism by which it exerts its antihelminthic action is uncertain; it is known to inhibit fumarate reductase, an important mitochondrial enzyme of helminths. Most side effects are mild, related to the gastrointestinal tract or liver, and rapidly disappear with the discontinuation of the drug. Hypersensitivity reactions, induced either by the drug or by antigens released from the damaged parasite, may occur.

Mebendazole, a carbamate benzimidazole introduced in 1972, has a spectrum similar to that of thiabendazole, but also has been found to be effective against a number of cestodes including *Taenia, Hymenolepsis,* and *Echinococcus.* It irreversibly blocks glucose uptake of both adult and larval worms resulting in glycogen depletion, cessation of ATP formation, and paralysis or death. It does not appear to affect glucose metabolism in humans and is thought to exert its effect in worms by binding to tubulin, thus interfering with the assembly of cytoplasmic microtubules, structures essential to glucose uptake. Unlike thiabendazole, the drug is not well absorbed from the gastrointestinal tract and may owe part of its effectiveness against intestinal dwelling adult worms to its high concentrations in the gut. Toxicity is uncommon. Teratogenic effects have been observed in experimental animals; its use in infants and pregnant women is contraindicated.

Albendazole, a new benzimidazole carbamate not yet approved for use in the United States, has a spectrum similar to that of its close relative, mebendazole. It may be more effective than mebendazole in the management of echinococciasis. It is effective in the management of many intestinal nematode infections when administered as a single-dose treatment.

Active against extracellular protozoa

Metronidazole

Mutagenicity of metronidazole

Broad-spectrum antihelminthics

Benzimidazole nucleus

Mebendazole blocks glucose uptake by adult and larval worms

Teratogenic effects

Antibiotics that influence
nematode's neurotransmitter

Activity against filariae

Praziquantel

Causes loss of intracellular
calcium in cestodes and
trematodes

Avermectins. These macrocyclic lactones are produced as fermentation products of *Streptomyces avermitilis.* Structurally similar to the macrolide antibiotics, they are effective at extremely low concentration against a wide variety of nematodes and arthropods. The avermectins appear to induce neuromuscular paralysis by acting on a receptor of the parasites' peripheral neurotransmitter, γ-aminobutyric acid (GABA). In mammals, GABA is confined to the central nervous system and as the avermectins do not cross the blood–brain barrier in significant concentration, they do not appear to produce significant untoward effects in the mammalian host. Ivermectin, a derivative of avermectin B_1, is currently undergoing evaluation for the treatment of human filariasis. It appears to be effective in the treatment of onchocerciasis when given as a single oral dose. Its usefulness in other parasitic infections of humans remains to be established.

Praziquantel. This heterocyclic pyrazino-isoquinoline is an important new antihelminthic effective against a broad range of cestodes and trematodes, many of which had been poorly responsive to previously available agents. It is rapidly taken up by susceptible helminths in which it appears to induce the loss of intracellular calcium, tetanic muscular contraction, and destruction of the tegument. Its differential toxicity may be related to the inability of susceptible worms to metabolize the drug. Aside from transient, mild gastrointestinal symptoms, praziquantel appears remarkably free of side effects in humans. It is currently the drug of choice for the treatment of schistosomiasis, clonorchiasis, opisthorchiasis, and neurocysticercosis. Good activity has been demonstrated against other common trematode and cestode infections. Its effectiveness is in a single dose. Its high level of safety suggests this agent may well play a significant role in worldwide mass therapy campaigns.

Other Antiparasitics. A number of those used in therapy, their properties and clinical use are listed in Appendix 51.1.

Control

The control of diseases spread by the fecal-oral route depends upon the improvements in personal hygiene and sanitation that accompany general economic development. In contrast, efforts at preventing the spread of multihost parasites is usually focused on the simultaneous treatment of infected humans and the control or elimination of the nonhuman host.

Problems of epidemiological
control in developing
countries

Approaches to vaccine
development

To be effective, such measures must be applied in a comprehensive and coordinated manner over large areas. Administrative problems, political imbroglios, development of resistance in parasites and intermediate hosts, technical difficulties, and funding shortages have, individually and together, limited the success of such efforts. A case in point was the failure of the worldwide malaria eradication effort launched by the World Health Organization in 1955. This has refocused attention on alternative control measures, including immunization. Until recently, the development of effective parasitic vaccines has been constrained by the complexities of their immunologic interactions with the human host. Monoclonal antibodies have helped to identify antigens responsible for the induction of immunity to a number of parasitic infections, including malaria, leishmaniasis, and schistosomiasis. The subsequent cloning of the structural genes encoding such antigens has made a large-scale production of vaccine antigen feasible. It is further possible that the entire step of antigen production and purification could be bypassed by the use of synthetic peptide or anti-idiotype vaccines. All these approaches are currently being developed. Malaria vaccines are undergoing clinical trials.

Appendix 51.1 Miscellaneous Antiparasitic Medications

Compound	Drug Class	Route	Mechanism of Action	Clinical Use	Comments
Bithionol	Phenol	Oral	Uncouples phosphorylation	Paragonimiasis	Not commercially available in U.S.
Diethylcarbamazine	Piperazine	Oral	Neuromuscular paralysis	Filiarial infections	Allergic reactions to filarial antigens
Difluoromethylornithine (DFMO)	Ornithine analogue	Oral	Inhibits ornithine decarboxylase	African trypanosomiasis	Effective in CNS disease
Diloxanide furoate	Acetanilide	Oral	Unknown	Intestinal amebiasis	Used only for asymptomatic carriers
Iodoquinol (Diiodohydroxyquin)	Halogenated quinoline	Oral	Unknown	Intestinal amebiasis; dientamoeba infections	Related drug has caused optic atrophy
Niclosamide	Phenol	Oral	Uncouples phosphorylation	Intestinal tapeworms	Does not kill eggs
Nifurtimox	Nitrofuran	Oral	Alkylates DNA	Acute Chagas' disease	Toxic, therapy prolonged, effectiveness marginal
Pentamidine	Diamidine	IV	Binds DNA	Pneumocystosis, leishmaniasis; trypanosomiasis	Toxic
Pyrantel pamoate	Tetrahydro-pyrimidine	Oral	Neuromuscular blockade; inhibits fumarate reductase	Pinworm infection; hookworm infection; ascariasis	Single dose therapy
Suramin	Sulfated naphthylamine	IV	Inhibits a glycerophosphate oxidase & dehydrogenase	African trypanosomiasis Onchocerciasis	Not effective in CNS disease; renal toxic

Abbreviations: CNS = central nervous system; IV = intravenous.

Additional Reading

Campbell, W.C., and Rew, R.S., Eds. 1986. *Chemotherapy of Parasitic Diseases*. New York: Plenum. This is the most recent comprehensive publication on this subject.

Cohen, S., and Warren, K.S., Eds. 1982. *Immunology of Parasitic Infections*. 2nd ed. Oxford: Blackwell Scientific Productions. This relatively comprehensive monograph discusses general immune responses to parasitic infections as well as the immunity, immunopathology, and immunodiagnosis of specific parasitic diseases.

Desowitz, R.S. 1981. *New Guinea Tapeworms and Jewish Grandmothers: Tales of Parasites and Peoples*. New York: Norton. A delightful look at the host–parasite relationship.

Dorozynski, A. 1976. The attack on tropical disease. *Nature* 262:85–88 A brief look at the World Health Organization's efforts to relieve mankind of one of its major burdens.

Gutteridge, W.E. 1982. Chemotherapy. In *Modern Parasitology:* a textbook of parasitology. Cox, F.E.G. Ed. Oxford: Blackwell Scientific Publications. Chap. 9. Brief, but informative chapter with most data presented in tabular form.

Handbook of Antimicrobial Therapy. 1986. New Rochelle, NY: The Medical Letter. Includes a synoptic review of antiparasitic therapy.

Stoll, N.R. 1947. This wormy world. *J. Parasitol.* 33:1–18.

Warren, K.S. 1974. Helminthic disease endemic in the United States. *Am. J. Trop. Med. Hyg.* 23:723–730.

52

Sporozoa

James J. Plorde

Intracellular protozoa with alternating sexual and asexual cycles

Sporozoa are a unique class of intracellular protozoa distinguished by their alternating cycles of sexual and asexual reproduction. Asexual multiplication occurs by a process of multiple fission termed *schizogony*. In it, the nucleus of a trophozoite divides into several parts, forming a multinucleated *schizont*. Cytoplasm then condenses around each nuclear portion to form new daughter cells, or *merozoites*, which burst from their intracellular location to invade new host cells. After the completion of one or more of these asexual cycles, some merozoites differentiate into male and female gametocytes, initiating the cycle of sexual reproduction known as *sporogony*. The gametocytes mature and effect fertilization, forming a *zygote*. Upon encysting, the zygote is known as an *oocyst. Sporozoites* formed within the oocyst are released, penetrate host tissue cells, and begin another asexual cycle as trophozoites.

Malaria, toxoplasmosis, and cryptosporidiosis

Two sporozoan infections, malaria and toxoplasmosis, are common diseases of humans; together, they affect more than one-third of the world's population and kill or deform perhaps a million neonates and children each year. A third infection, cryptosporidiosis has only recently been found to be an important cause of diarrhea, particularly in immunocompromised hosts.

MALARIA

Plasmodia: The Malarial Parasites

Of all infectious diseases there is no doubt that malaria has caused the greatest harm to the greatest number. . . .

Laderman, 1975

Definition. The plasmodia are sporozoa in which the sexual and asexual cycles of reproduction are completed in different host species. The sexual

701

Sexual phase in mosquito

Asexual phase in humans

Species of malarial parasites

phase occurs within the gut of mosquitoes. These arthropods subsequently transmit the parasite while feeding upon a vertebrate host. Within the red cells of the vertebrate, the plasmodia reproduce asexually; they eventually burst from the erythrocyte and invade other uninvolved red cells. This event produces periodic fever and anemia in the host, a disease process known as *malaria*. Of the many species of plasmodia, four are known to infect humans and will be considered here: *Plasmodium vivax, Plasmodium ovale, Plasmodium malariae,* and *Plasmodium falciparum.*

Life Cycle of Malarial Parasites

Female *Anopheles* mosquito ingests gametocytes

Sporozoites from oocyst reach mosquito salivary glands

Sporogony, or the sexual cycle, begins when a female mosquito of the genus *Anopheles* ingests circulating male and female gametocytes while feeding upon a malarious human. In the gut of the mosquito, the gametocytes mature and effect fertilization. The resulting zygote penetrates the gut wall, lodges beneath the basement membrane, and vacuolates to form an oocyst. Within this structure thousands of sporozoites are formed. The enlarging cyst eventually ruptures, releasing the sporozoites into the body cavity. Some penetrate the salivary glands, rendering the mosquito infectious for humans. The time required for the completion of the cycle in mosquitoes varies from 1 to 3 weeks, depending upon the species of insect and parasite as well as on the ambient temperature and humidity.

Humans infected by mosquito bite

Hepatic asexual cycle in humans

Schizogony, the asexual cycle, occurs in the human and begins when the infected *Anopheles* takes a blood meal from another individual. Sporozoites from the mosquito's salivary glands are injected into the human's subcutaneous capillaries and circulate in the peripheral blood. Within 1 hr they invade liver cells (hepatocytes). In *P. vivax* and *P. ovale* infections, some of the sporozoites enter a dormant state immediately after cell invasion. The remaining sporozoites initiate *exoerythrocytic* schizogony, each producing about 2000 to 40,000 daughter cells, or merozoites. One to two weeks later, the infected hepatocytes rupture, releasing merozoites into the general circulation.

Erythrocytic asexual cycle in humans

Cyclical rupture and reinfection of erythrocytes

Some gametocytes formed; mosquito ingests gametocytes with blood meal

Intrahepatic dormancy causes relapses with *P. vivax* and *P. ovale*

The erythrocytic phase of malaria starts with the attachment of a released hepatic merozoite to a specific receptor on the red cell surface. After attachment, the merozoite invaginates the cell membrane and is slowly endocytosed. The intracellular parasite initially appears as a ring-shaped trophozoite, which enlarges and becomes more active and irregular in outline. Within a few hours, nuclear division occurs, producing the multinucleated schizont. Cytoplasm eventually condenses around each nucleus of the schizont to form an intraerythrocytic cluster of 6–24 merozoite daughter cells. About 48 (*P. vivax, P. ovale,* and *P. falciparum*) to 72 (*P. malariae*) hr after initial invasion, infected erythrocytes rupture, releasing the merozoites and producing the first clinical manifestations of disease. The newly released daughter cells invade other red cells, where most repeat the asexual cycle. Other daughter cells are transformed into sexual forms or gametocytes. These latter forms do not produce red cell lysis and continue to circulate in the peripheral vasculature until ingested by an appropriate mosquito. The recurring asexual cycles continue, involving an ever-increasing number of erythrocytes until finally the development of host immunity brings the erythrocytic cycle to a close. The dormant hepatic sporozoites of *P. vivax* and *P. ovale* survive the host's immunologic attack and may, after a latent period of months to years, resume intrahepatic multiplication. This leads to a second release of hepatic merozoites

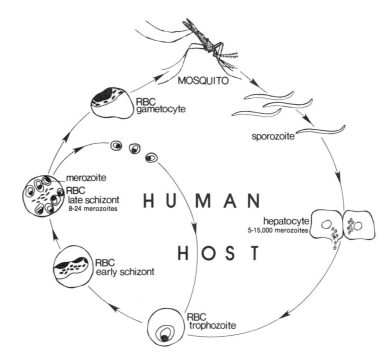

52.1 Life cycle of the malarial parasite.

and the initiation of another erythrocytic cycle, a phenomenon known as *relapse*. The life cycle of malarial parasites is summarized in Figure 52.1.

Morphology

The morphology of the stained intraerythrocytic parasites is shown in Figure 52.2. In stained smears, three characteristic features aid in the identification of plasmodia, red nuclear chromatin; blue cytoplasm; and brownish-black malarial pigment, or hemozoin, consisting largely of a hemoglobin degradation product, ferriprotoporphyrin IX. The change in the shape of the cytoplasm and the division of the chromatin at different stages of parasite development are obvious. Gametocytes can be differentiated from the asexual forms by their large size and lack of nuclear division. Some of the infected erythrocytes develop membrane invaginations, which appear in the stained cell as pink cytoplasmic granules.

52.2 Examples of erythrocytic stages of malarial parasites. *Note:* Trophozoite and schizont forms of *Plasmodium falciparum* occur in visceral capillaries rather than in blood. Male and female gametocytes show distinctive morphological differences.

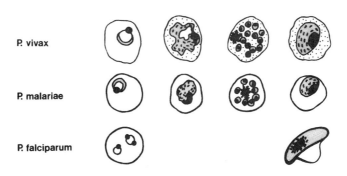

Table 52.1 Differential Characteristics of *Plasmodium* Species

Characteristics	*P. vivax*	*P. ovale*	*P. malariae*	*P. falciparum*
Erythrocyte				
Enlarged, pale	+	+	−	−
Oval, fimbriated	−	+	−	−
Schüffner's dots	+	+	−	−
Maurer's dots	−	−	−	+
Parasite				
All asexual stages seen	+	+	+	−
Band forms	−	−	+	−
Double infections	−	−	−	+
Double chromatin dots	−	−	−	+
Banana-shaped gametocytes	−	−	−	+

Morphologic differences between intraerythrocytic parasites

The appearance of each of the four species of plasmodia that infect humans is sufficiently different to allow their differentiation in stained smears. The parasitized erythrocyte in *P. vivax* and *P. ovale* infections is pale, enlarged, and contains numerous small granules known as *Schüffner's dots*. All asexual stages (trophozoite, schizont, merozoite) may be seen simultaneously. Cells infected by *P. ovale* are elongated and frequently irregular or fimbriated in appearance. In *P. malariae* infections, the red cells are not enlarged and contain no granules. The trophozoites often present as "band" forms, and the merozoites are arranged in rosettes around a clump of central pigment. In *P. falciparum* infections, the rings are very small and may contain two rather than a single chromatin dot. There is often more than a single parasite per cell, and parasites are frequently seen lying against the margin of the cell. Intracytoplasmic granules known as *Maurer's dots* may be present, but are often cleft shaped and fewer in number than Schüffner's dots. Schizonts and merozoites are not present in the peripheral blood. Gametocytes are large and banana shaped. These characteristics are summarized in Table 52.1.

Physiology

Parasites vary in ability to attack subpopulations of erythrocytes

Species of plasmodia differ significantly in their ability to invade subpopulations of erythrocytes; *P. vivax* and *P. ovale* attack only immature cells (reticulocytes), whereas *P. malariae* attacks only senescent cells. During infection with these species, therefore, no more than 1–2% of the cell population is involved. *Plasmodium falciparum*, in contrast, invades red cells *regardless of age* and may produce very high levels of parasitemia and particularly serious disease. In part, these differences may be related to the known differences in the red cell receptor sites available to the individual *Plasmodium* species. In the case of *P. vivax*, the site is closely related to the Duffy blood group antigens (Fy[a] and Fy[b]). Duffy-negative individuals, who constitute the majority of people of West African ancestry, are therefore resistant to vivax malaria. Red cell sialoglycoprotein, particularly glycoprotein A, has been implicated as the *P. falciparum* receptor site.

Relation of Duffy antigen to *P. vivax* receptor

Effect of sickle cell trait on intensity of *P. falciparum* infection

Certain red cell abnormalities may also effect parasitism. The altered hemoglobin (hemoglobin S) associated with the sickle cell trait limits the intensity of the parasitemia caused by *P. falciparum* and thereby provides a selective advantage to individuals who are heterozygous for the sickle cell gene. As a result, the sickle cell gene, which would otherwise be disadvantageous, is found at high frequency in populations living in malarious areas. The mechanism of the increased resistance is uncertain. Parasite growth appears to be retarded in red cells heterozygous for hemoglobins S (SA) when they are exposed to conditions of reduced oxygen tension such as might be present in the visceral capillaries. Sickling may also render the erythrocyte more susceptible to phagocytosis or directly damage the parasite. A similar protective effect may be exerted by hemoglobins C, D, and E; thalassemia; and glucose-6-phosphate dehydrogenase (G6PD) or pyridoxal kinase deficiencies, as these abnormalities have also been found more frequently in malarious areas. The protection in these conditions may be related to the increased susceptibility of such red cells to oxidant stress. In thalassemia, the protection may also be related in part to the production of fetal hemoglobin, which retards maturation of *P. falciparum.*

Changes in erythrocytes

Once invasion has occurred, malarial parasites may induce changes in erythrocytic membranes. In addition to invaginations or clefts, elevated knobs or excrescences may form on the surface, particularly in *P. falciparum* infections. These outgrowths have been shown to fuse with endothelial cell membranes, suggesting that they may play a role in the known tendency of *P. falciparum*-infected cells to sequester in the capillaries of the deep organs, where they can produce obstruction and microinfarcts. Malarial parasites may also alter the lipid composition of the erythrocytic membrane, and proteins from the parasite may modify both its osmotic properties and its susceptibility to immunologic attack.

Association with microinfarcts

Metabolism of malarial parasites

Malarial parasites generate energy by the anaerobic metabolism of glucose. They appear to satisfy their protein requirements by the degradation of hemoglobin within their acidic food vacuoles, resulting in the formation of the malarial pigment (hemozoin) mentioned previously. It has been estimated that the average plasmodium destroys between 25 and 75% of the hemoglobin of its host erythrocyte. Unlike their vertebrate hosts, malarial parasites synthesize folates de novo. As a result, antifolate antimicrobics such as pyrimethamine are effective antimalarious agents.

Growth in the Laboratory

Continuous in vitro cultivation of plasmodia in human erythrocytes was first achieved in 1976. The technique, which employs dilute cultures with low initial parasite densities in a reduced oxygen atmosphere, provides new opportunities for studying the biology, immunology, and chemotherapy of human malaria. Its most immediate impact has been on the development of methods for testing the sensitivity of *P. falciparum* to chemotherapeutic agents.

Malaria Infections

Epidemiology

Distribution

Malaria has a worldwide distribution between 45°N and 40°S latitude, generally at altitudes below 1800 m. *Plasmodium vivax* is the most widely distributed of the four species and, together with the uncommon *P. malariae*, is found primarily in temperate and subtropical areas. *Plasmodium falciparum* is the dominant organism of the tropics. *Plasmodium ovale* is rare and found principally in Africa.

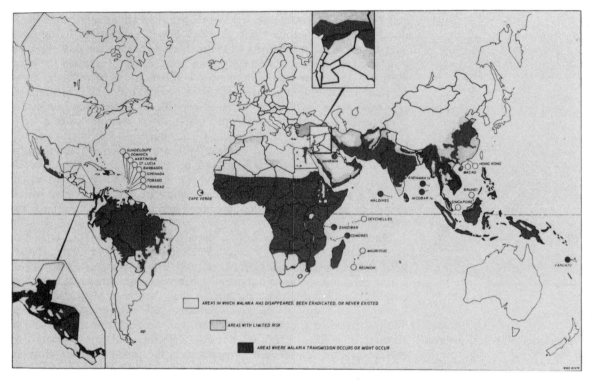

52.3 Status of malaria, 1979. (*Reproduced from Health Information for International Travel, Supplement, Morbidity and Mortality Weekly Report, Vol. 30, 1981, U.S. Government Printing Office.*)

Factors influencing intensity

Clinical manifestations muted with hyperendemicity

Extent and mortality of malaria

Imported malaria

The intensity of malarial transmission in an endemic area depends upon the density and feeding habits of suitable mosquito vectors and the prevalence of infected humans, who serve as parasite reservoirs. In *hyperendemic* areas (areas where more than half of the population is parasitemic), transmission is usually constant, and disease manifestations are moderated by the development of immunity. Mortality is largely restricted to infants and to nonimmune adults who migrate into the region. When the prevalence of disease is lower, transmission is typically intermittent. In this situation, solid immunity does not develop and the population suffers repeated, often seasonal, epidemics, the impact of which is shared by people of all ages.

At the present time, malaria infects between 200 and 300 million inhabitants of 104 countries throughout Africa, Asia, Latin America, and Oceania (Figure 52.3). One million children, primarily Africans, die of the disease each year. Although endemic malaria disappeared from the United States three decades ago, imported cases continue to be reported, and the recent worldwide resurgence of malaria combined with an increase in international travel has resulted in an increase in their numbers. Approximately 50% of imported cases acquire the disease in Asia, 30% in Africa, and 10% in the Caribbean or Latin America. Forty percent of recent infections have involved American travelers: over half acquired their infection in Africa. Clinical manifestations typically develop within 6 months of arrival of cases in the United States; however, one-third of cases caused by *P. vivax* are delayed beyond that time. Approximately 20% of imported cases and almost all associated fatalities have been caused by the virulent *P. falciparum*. Tragically, most of these cases could have been prevented or successfully treated.

Pathogenesis and Pathology

The fever, anemia, circulatory changes, and immunopathologic phenomena characteristic of malaria are all the result of erythrocytic invasion by the plasmodia.

Fever. Fever, the hallmark of malaria, appears to be initiated by the process of red cell rupture that leads to the liberation of a new generation of merozoites (sporulation). It seems likely that a pyrogenic substance released during this process is responsible for the fever; to date, however, all attempts to detect the presence of a circulating pyrogen have been unsuccessful. Early in malaria, red cells appear to be infected with malarial parasites at several different stages of development, each inducing sporulation at a different time. The resulting fever is irregular and hectic. Eventually one population dominates, sporulation is synchronized, and fever occurs in distinct paroxysms at 48-hr or, in the case of *P. malariae*, 72-hr intervals.

Anemia. Parasitized erythrocytes are phagocytosed by a stimulated reticuloendothelial system or are destroyed at the time of sporulation. At times, the anemia is disproportionate to the degree of parasitism. Depression of marrow function, sequestration of erythrocytes within the enlarging spleen, and accelerated clearance of nonparasitized cells all appear to contribute to the anemia. The mechanisms responsible for the latter are unclear. Intravascular hemolysis, although uncommon, may occur, particularly in falciparum malaria. When hemolysis is massive, hemoglobinuria develops, resulting in the production of dark urine. This process in conjunction with malaria is known as *blackwater fever*.

Circulatory Changes. The high fever results in significant vasodilatation. In falciparum malaria, vasodilatation leads to a decrease in the effective circulating blood volume and hypotension, which may be aggravated by other changes in the small vessels and capillaries. The intense parasitemias this organism is capable of producing and the adhesion of infected red cells to the endothelium of visceral capillaries can impair the microcirculation and precipitate tissue hypoxia, lactic acidosis, and hypoglycemia. Although all deep tissues are involved, the brain is the most intensely affected.

Other Pathogenetic Phenomena. Thrombocytopenia is common in malaria and appears to be related to both splenic pooling and a shortened platelet life span. Both direct parasitic invasion and immune mechanisms may be responsible. There may be an acute transient glomerulonephritis in falciparum malaria and progressive renal disease in chronic *P. malariae* malaria. These phenomena probably result from the host immune response, with deposition of immune complexes in the glomeruli.

Immunity. Once infected, the host quickly mounts an immunologic response that typically limits parasite multiplication and moderates the clinical manifestations of disease. There follows a prolonged recovery period

Marginal notes:

Fever associated with red cell rupture

Synchronization of sporulation

Phagocytosis of parasitized erythrocytes

Destruction of normal erythrocytes

Intravascular hemolysis and blackwater fever

Decreased blood flow to vital organs

Thrombocytopenia and nephritis

marked by recurrent exacerbations in both symptoms and number of erythrocytic parasites. With time, the recrudescences become less severe and less frequent, eventually stopping altogether.

Evidence for antibody-mediated immunity

The exact mechanisms involved in this recovery are uncertain. In simian and probably in human malaria, recovery is known to require the presence of both T and B lymphocytes. It is probable that the T cells act partially through their helper effect on antibody production. Some authorities have suggested that they also play a direct role through lymphokine production by stimulating effector cells to release nonspecific factors capable of inhibiting intraerythrocytic multiplication. The B lymphocytes begin production of stage- and strain-specific antiplasmodial antibodies within the first 2 weeks of parasitemia. With the achievement of high levels of antibodies, the number of circulating parasites decreases. The infrequency with which malaria occurs in young infants has been attributed to the transplacental passage of such antibodies. It is uncertain whether they are directly lethal, act as opsonizing agents, or block merozoite invasion of red cells.

Evidence for antigenic variation of malarial parasites

In simian malaria, the parasite can undergo antigenic variation and thereby escape the suppressive effect of the antibodies. This antigenic variation leads to cycles of recrudescent parasitemia but, ultimately, to production of specific antibodies to the variants, and cure. It seems probable that similar changes occur in humans, leading to the eventual disappearance of erythrocytic parasites. With *P. falciparum* and *P. malariae*, which have no persistent hepatic forms, this results in cure. In the former, the disease typically does not exceed 1 year, but with *P. malariae* the erythrocytic infection can be extremely persistent, lasting in one case up to 53 years. How erythrocytic parasites circulating in numbers too small to be detected on routine blood films escape immunologic destruction remains a puzzle. In a closely related simian malaria, splenectomy results in rapid cure, suggesting that suppressor T cells in the spleen may play a protective role. In infection with *P. vivax* and *P. ovale*, latent hepatic infection may result in the discharge of fresh merozoites into the bloodstream after the disappearance of erythrocytic forms. This phenomenon, known as relapse, is capable of maintaining infection for 3–5 years.

Possible role of suppressor cells in maintenance of erythrocytic parasites

Clinical Manifestations

Incubation period

The incubation period between the bite of mosquito and the onset of disease is approximately 2 weeks; that with *P. malariae* and with strains of *P. vivax* in temperate climates, however, is often more prolonged. Individuals who contract malaria while taking antimalarial suppressants may not experience illness for many months. In the United States, the interval between entry into the country and onset of disease exceeds 1 month in 25% of *P. falciparum* infections and 6 months in a similar proportion of vivax cases.

Malarial paroxysm: cold, hot, and wet stages

The clinical manifestations vary with the species of plasmodia, but typically include chills, fever, splenomegaly, and anemia. The hallmark of disease is the malarial paroxysm. This manifestation begins with a *cold stage*, which persists for 20–60 min. During this time, the patient experiences continuous rigors and feels cold. With the consequent increase in body temperature, the rigors cease and vasodilatation commences, ushering in a *hot stage*. The temperature continues to rise for 3–8 hr, reaching a maximum of 40–41.7°C (104–107°F) before it begins to fall. The *wet stage* consists of a decrease in fever and profuse sweating. It leaves the patient exhausted but otherwise well until the onset of the next paroxysm.

Typical paroxysms when sporulation is synchronized

Typical paroxysms first appear in the second or third week of fever, when parasite sporulation becomes synchronized. In falciparum malaria, synchronization may never take place, and the fever may remain hectic and unpredictable. The first attack is often severe and may persist for weeks in the untreated patient. Eventually the paroxysms become less regular, less frequent, and less severe. Symptoms finally cease with the disappearance of the parasites from the blood.

Cerebral malaria and other severe systemic manifestations with *P. falciparum*

In falciparum malaria, capillary blockage can lead to several serious complications. When the central nervous system is involved (cerebral malaria), the patient may develop delirium, convulsions, paralysis, coma, and rapid death. Acute pulmonary insufficiency frequently accompanies cerebral malaria, killing about 80% of those involved. When splanchnic capillaries are involved, the patient may experience vomiting, abdominal pain, and diarrhea with or without bloody stools. Jaundice and acute renal failure are also common in severe illness. These pernicious syndromes generally appear when the intensity of parasitemia exceeds 100,000 organisms per cubic millimeter of blood. Most deaths occur within 3 days.

Laboratory Diagnosis

Thick and thin blood smears

Malarial parasites can be demonstrated in stained smears of the peripheral blood in virtually all symptomatic patients. Typically, capillary or venous blood is used to prepare both thin and thick smears, which are stained with Wright or Giemsa stain and examined for the presence of erythrocytic parasites. Thick smears, in which erythrocytes are lysed with water before staining, concentrate the parasites and allow detection of very mild parasitemia. Nonetheless, it may be necessary to obtain several specimens before parasites are seen. Artifacts are numerous in thick smears, and correct interpretation requires experience. The morphologic differences among the four species of plasmodia allow their speciation on the stained smear by the skilled observer.

New diagnostic procedures

Serologic tests for malaria are available, but are used primarily for epidemiologic purposes. They are occasionally helpful in speciation and detection of otherwise occult infections. Deoxyribonucleic acid probes and antigen detection procedures have recently been described and may eventually play an important role in the diagnosis of malaria.

Treatment

Need to destroy all forms of the parasite

The adequate treatment of malaria requires the destruction of three parasitic forms: the erythrocytic schizont, the hepatic schizont, and the erythrocytic gametocyte. The first terminates the clinical attack, the second prevents relapse, and the third renders the patient noninfectious to *Anopheles* and thus breaks the cycle of transmission. Unfortunately, no single drug accomplishes all three goals. The present strategy of chemotherapy is shown in Table 52.2.

Chloroquine action and resistance

Termination of Acute Attack. Several agents can destroy asexual erythrocytic parasites. Chloroquine, a 4-aminoquinoline, is that most commonly used. It is rapidly effective against all four species of plasmodia and, in the dosage used, is free of serious side effects. Strains of *P. falciparum* resistant to this agent are present in Latin America, Southeast Asia, and East and Central Africa. They are treated with combinations of quinine, antifolates, and sulfonamides. Chloroquine apparently acts by

Table 52.2 Chemotherapy of Malaria

Stage of Parasite	Clinical Goal	Drug
Erythrocytic schizont	Treat clinical attack	
	All species	Chloroquine
	CRFM	Quinine, antifolates, sulfonamides
	Suppress clinical attack	
	All species	Chloroquine
	CRFM	Antifolates, sulfonamides
Erythrocytic gametocyte	Prevent transmission	
	Relapsing malaria	Chloroquine
	Falciparum malaria	Primaquine
Hepatic schizont	Radical cure	
	Relapsing malaria	Primaquine
	Falciparum malaria	None required

Abbreviations: CRFM = chloroquine-resistant falciparum malaria.

inhibiting the degradation of hemoglobin, thereby limiting the availability of amino acids necessary for growth. It has been suggested that the weak basic nature of chloroquine also acts to raise the pH of the food vacuoles of the parasite, inhibiting their acid proteases and effectiveness.

Need to destroy hepatic schizonts of *P. vivax* and *P. ovale*

Radical Cure. In *P. vivax* and *P. ovale* infections, hepatic schizonts persist and must be destroyed to prevent reseeding of circulating erythrocytes with consequent relapse. Primaquine, an 8-aminoquinoline, is used for this purpose. Unfortunately, it may induce hemolysis in patients with G6PD deficiency. Persons of Asian, African, and Mediterranean ancestry should thus be screened for this abnormality before treatment.

Destruction of Circulating Gametocytes. Chloroquine destroys the gametocytes of *P. vivax, P. ovale,* and *P. malariae,* but not those of *P. falciparum.* Primaquine is, however, effective for this species.

Prevention

Mosquito control

Personal Protection. In endemic areas, mosquito contact can be minimized through the use of house screenings, mosquito netting around beds, and insect repellents. In addition, it is possible to suppress clinical manifestations of infection, should it occur, with a weekly dose of chloroquine. In areas where chloroquine-resistant strains are common, the antifolate pyrimethamine plus a sulfonamide can be taken orally at the same interval. However, as use of this combination is occasionally accompanied by serious side effects, it is recommended only for individuals residing in areas of intense transmission for prolonged periods of time. On leaving an endemic area, it is necessary to eradicate residual hepatic parasites with primaquine before discontinuing suppressive therapy.

Chemoprophylaxis

Attempts at eradication

General. Malaria control measures are directed toward reducing the infected human and mosquito populations to below the critical level necessary for sustained transmission of disease. The techniques employed include those mentioned previously, treatment of febrile patients with effective antimalarial agents, chemical or physical disruption of mosquito breeding areas, and use of residual insecticide sprays. An active international cooperative program aimed at the eradication of malaria resulted in a dramatic decline in the incidence of the disease between 1956 and 1968. Eradication was not achieved, however, as mosquitoes became resistant to some of the chemical agents used, and today malaria still infects 200–300 million inhabitants of Africa, Latin America, and Asia. Tropical Africa alone accounts for 100 million of the afflicted and for most of the 1 million deaths that occur annually as a result of this disease. The long-term hope for progress in these areas now depends upon the development of new technologies. Work on a malaria vaccine is continuing, and it is hoped that effective preparations may become available in this century.

Vaccines. Three advances in the last decade have brought the production of an effective malaria vaccine within reach of medical science for the first time. The establishment of a continuous in vitro culture system provided the large quantities of parasite needed for antigenic analysis. Development of the hybridoma technique allowed the preparation of monoclonal antibodies with which antigens responsible for the induction of protective immunity could be identified. Finally, recombinant DNA procedures enabled scientists to clone and sequence the genes encoding such antigens, permitting the amino acid structure of the antigen to be determined and peptide sequences suitable for vaccine development to be identified.

As immunity to malaria is stage specific, the relative advantages and disadvantages of vaccines prepared against each of the plasmodial stages found in the human host (sporozoite, merozoite, and gametocyte) need to be considered. An effective sporozoite vaccine, by blocking the invasion of hepatocytes by mosquito-introduced sporozoites, would prevent the establishment of the infection within the host and, if widely administered, would interrupt parasite transmission within a community. However, to be effective, a sporozoite vaccine would have to prevent the invasion of all injected sporozoites. Theoretically, if even a single parasite reached and penetrated a liver cell, it would multiply intracellularly and later enter the bloodstream to invade erythrocytes. The patient could develop clinical disease and serve as a reservoir for subsequent transmission to others. A vaccine directed at the erythrocytic or merozoite stage, while preventing neither hepatic nor bloodstream infection, would limit the severity of the parasitemia and thus moderate or abort clinical manifestations of disease. Gametogenesis, and thus parasite transmission, would probably proceed unimpaired. Antibodies formed in response to a gametocyte vaccine might block the union of male and female gametes within the mosquito gut, interrupting parasite transmission. It would, however, neither prevent nor moderate malaria in the immunized patient. The limitations of each vaccine type has led some investigators to advocate the combination of all three in a single polyvalent preparation.

Work on a sporozoite vaccine to *P. falciparum* is the most advanced. Natural immunity to this stage is induced by the circumsporozoite (CS) protein, a substance that covers the parasite surface. A major portion of the CS protein is conserved in all strains, and monoclonal antibodies prepared against it neutralize all sporozoite infectivity. A vaccine containing this conserved region is currently undergoing clinical trials. Early results have not been totally satisfactory, suggesting the inclusion of other peptide sequences may be required.

Growth of malarial parasites in culture

Detecting significant antigens or epitopes

Sporozoite vaccine could help prevent initiation of infection

Erythrocytic stage vaccine could moderate disease

Gametocyte vaccine could prevent transmission

TOXOPLASMOSIS

Toxoplasma

Definition. Like the plasmodia, *Toxoplasma gondii*, the cause of toxoplasmosis, is an obligate intracellular sporozoan. It differs from *Plasmodium* in that both sexual and asexual reproductive cycles occur within the gastrointestinal tract of felines, the definitive host. The disease is transmitted to other host species by the ingestion of oocysts passed in the feces of infected felines.

Toxoplasma can infect most warm-blooded animals, both domestic and wild; they are thus the most cosmopolitan of parasites. Approximately one-half of the human population of the United States has been infected. In the overwhelming majority the infection is chronic, asymptomatic, and self-limiting. Clinical disease presents in three major forms: 1) self-limiting febrile lymphadenopathy; 2) highly lethal infection of immunocompromised patients; and 3) congenital infection of infants.

Life Cycle

Definitive Host. Sexual reproduction of *T. gondii* occurs only in the intestinal tract of felines, most importantly in the domestic cat. Ingested parasites enter the epithelial cells of the ileum by mechanisms that remain poorly defined. Intracellularly, the trophozoites reside within a membrane-bound vacuole and undergo schizogony. With cell rupture, merozoites are released. The merozoites infect adjacent epithelial cells; they then repeat another asexual cycle or eventually differentiate into gametocytes, initiating sexual reproduction. Fusion of the mature male and female gametes leads to the formation of an oval, thick-walled oocyst that is then shed in the feces. In the typical infection, millions of these structures are released daily for 1–3 weeks. The oocysts are immature at the time of shedding and must complete sporulation in the external environment. In this process, two sporocysts, each containing four sporozoites, develop within each oocyst. The time required for sporulation varies from 1 day to 3 weeks, depending upon the ambient temperature and moisture. Once mature, the resistant oocyts may remain viable and infectious for as long as a year.

Intermediate Hosts. After ingestion by a susceptible warm-blooded animal, sporozoites are released from the disrupted oocyst and enter macrophages. Within these cells they are transported through the lymphohematogenous system to all organ systems. Continued intracellular schizogony results in macrophage rupture and release of new parasites, which may invade any adjacent nucleated host cell and continue the asexual cycle. With the development of host immunity, many of the parasites are destroyed. Within the cells of certain organs, particularly the brain, heart, and skeletal muscle, the trophozoites produce a membrane that surrounds and protects them: within this tissue cyst, multiplication continues at a more leisurely pace. Eventually, cysts that measure up to 200 μm in diameter and contain more than a thousand organisms are produced. These cysts may persist intact for the life of the host or rupture, producing parasitologic relapse. If they are ingested by a carnivore, they survive the digestive enzymes and initiate infection in the new host.

Asexual and sexual cycles in felines

Spectrum of disease

Infection in cat ileal cells

Fusion of gametes leads to oocyst formation; shed in feces

Sporulation in external environment

Mature oocysts infect hosts orally

Released sporozoites invade macrophages

Development of cysts

Infection from cysts in meat

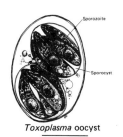

Toxoplasma oocyst

10 μm

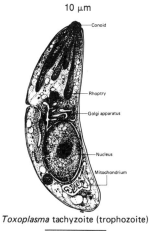

Toxoplasma tachyzoite (trophozoite)

3 μm

Description of Organism

General. *Toxoplasma gondii* was first demonstrated in 1908 in the gondi, an African rodent, by Nicolle and Marceaux. Its name, derived from the Greek *toxo* (arc), is based on the characteristic shape of the organism. All strains of this parasite appear to be closely related antigenically. The major morphologic forms of the parasite are the oocyst, trophozoite, and tissue cyst.

Oocyst. The oocyst is ovoid, measures 10–12 μm in diameter, and possesses a thick wall that makes it resistant to most environmental challenges. It may be destroyed by heat in excess of 66°C and chemicals such as iodine and formalin. In its immature form, the center of the cyst lacks internal structure. With maturation two sporocysts appear, and later four sporozoites may be discerned within each sporocyst. Sporulation does not occur at temperatures below 4°C or above 37°C. This form is responsible for the spread of the parasites from felines to other warm-blooded animals via the fecal-oral route.

Trophozoite. The term *trophozoite* is used in its broadest sense to refer to the asexual proliferative forms responsible for cell invasion. In different stages of the asexual cycle it is referred to by several other terms, including merozoites, and tachyzoite. It is crescent or arc shaped, measures 3×7 μm, and can invade all nucleated cell types. Although trophozoites are obligate intracellular organisms, they may survive extracellularly in a variety of body fluids for periods of hours to days. They cannot, however, survive the digestive activity of the stomach and therefore are not infective on ingestion.

Tissue Cysts. Cysts measure 10–200 μm in diameter. The contained organisms are similar to, but smaller than trophozoites. Tissue cysts are resistant to digestive enzymes, and, like oocysts, are infectious to the animal that ingests them. They survive normal refrigerator temperatures, but are killed by freezing and thawing and by normal cooking temperatures.

Toxoplasma Infections

Prevalence and Distribution

Toxoplasmosis is a cosmopolitan disease that occurs in almost all mammals and many birds. Human infections are found in every region of the globe; in general the incidence is higher in the tropics and lower in cold, arid regions. In the United States, the prevalence of positive serologic test results for the disease increases with age. By adulthood, approximately 50% of Americans can be shown to have circulating antibodies against *T. gondii*.

Transmission

Although it is known that humans may acquire toxoplasmosis in a variety of ways, data on their relative frequency are both meager and conflicting. It is likely that the route of transmission varies from population to population and, perhaps, from age to age within any given area. The most important transmission mechanisms are discussed below.

Significance of feline
infections

Ingestion of Oocysts.   Felinophobes are inclined to the view that the deposition of oocysts in the feces of cats and their subsequent ingestion by
the unsuspecting owner is the most frequent way in which humans acquire
this important infection. Disease epidemics associated with exposure to
infected cats have been reported. Unfortunately, data from studies relating
the frequency of feline exposure to the prevalence of positive serologic
tests are conflicting. Acutely infected cats shed oocysts for only a few
weeks. It has been shown, however, that chronically infected felines can
occasionally reshed oocysts, and prevalence studies have demonstrated
that 1% of domestic cats excrete oocysts at any given time. The large
number of these structures passed during active shedding and their prolonged survival in the external environment greatly enhance their chance

Special hazard to children

of transmission. Particularly at risk are individuals such as children at play,
who may come in close contact with areas likely to be contaminated with
cat feces, and adults responsible for changing kitty litter. It is also possible
that insects can mechanically transfer oocysts to human food.

Cysts killed by normal
cooking

Ingestion of Tissue Cysts.   Tissue cysts have been frequently demonstrated
in meat produced for human consumption. They are most common in
pork (25%) and mutton (10%), less so in beef and chicken (less than 1%).
Although such cysts are killed at normal (well done) cooking temperatures,
an impressive array of epidemiologic information links the handling and/
or ingestion of raw or undercooked meat with serologic and, occasionally,
clinical evidence of disease. Confounding these data is an Indian study
that demonstrated no difference between meat eaters and vegetarians in
the incidence of positive serologic tests.

Congenital.   Approximately 1 of every 500 pregnant women acquires
acute toxoplasmosis, and in one-half of all such cases the infection spreads
to the fetus. The risk of transplacental transmission is independent of the
clinical severity of the disease in the mother, but does correlate with the
stage of gestation at which she is exposed. Fetal involvement occurs in

Transplacental transmission

17% of first trimester and 65% of third trimester infections. Conversely,
the earlier a fetal infection is acquired, the more severe it is likely to be.
Overall, 20% of fetuses experienced severe consequences; a similar proportion develop mild disease. The remainder are asymptomatic.

Miscellaneous.   In addition to causing congenital infection, trophozoites
have been responsible for disease transmission in a number of other situations, including laboratory accidents, transfusions of whole blood and

Laboratory accidents

leukocytes, and organ transplantation. As trophozoites may survive for
several hours in body fluids or exudates of acutely infected humans, it is
possible for infection to occur after contact with such materials.

Blood and organ
transplantation

Immunity and Pathogenesis

In the primary infection, the proliferation of trophozoites results in the
death of involved host cells and the stimulation of a mononuclear inflammatory reaction. In immunodeficient hosts, rapid organism proliferation

Dissemination in
immunosuppressed subjects

continues, producing numerous widespread foci of tissue necrosis. The
consequences are most serious in organs such as the brain, where the
potential for cell regeneration is limited.

In normal hosts, however, acute infection is rapidly controlled with the
development of humoral and cellular immunity. Extracellular parasites are
destroyed, intracellular multiplication is hindered and tissue cysts are

formed. With the exception of the destruction of extracellular parasites, cell-mediated immunity appears to play the principal role in this process. Immunity appears to be lifelong, possibly because of survival of the parasite in the tissue cysts. The cysts, which are found most frequently in the brain, heart, and skeletal muscle, normally produce little or no tissue reaction. The suppression of cell-mediated immunity that accompanies serious illness, or the administration of immunosuppressive agents may lead to the rupture of a cyst and the release of trophozoites. Their subsequent proliferation and the intense antibody reaction to their presence results in an acute exacerbation of the disease.

Clinical Manifestations

In the vast majority of patients, infection with *T. gondii* is completely asymptomatic. Clinical manifestations, when they do appear, vary with the type of host involved. In general, they may be grouped into one of the three syndromes listed below.

Severe manifestations of infection in utero

Congenital Toxoplasmosis. Immune mechanisms are poorly developed in utero. As a result, a large proportion of fetal infections result in clinical illness. If the infection spreads to the central nervous system, the outcome is often catastrophic. Abortion and stillbirth are the most serious consequences. Liveborn children may demonstrate microcephaly, hydrocephaly, cerebral calcifications, convulsions, and psychomotor retardation. Disease of this severity is usually accompanied by evidence of visceral involvement, including fever, hepatitis, pneumonia, and skin rash. Infants infected later in prenatal development demonstrate milder disease. Many appear healthy at birth, but develop epilepsy, retardation, or strabismus months or years later. Probably the most common delayed manifestation of congenital toxoplasmosis is chorioretinitis. This condition, which is thought to result from the reactivation of latent tissue cysts, typically presents during the second or third decade of life as recurrent bouts of eye pain and loss of visual acuity. The lesions are usually bilateral but focal. If the retinal macula is not involved, vision improves as the inflammation subsides. This manifestation accounts for one-quarter of all cases of granulomatous uveitis seen in the United States.

Chorioretinitis

Can mimic infectious mononucleosis

Normal Host. The most common clinical manifestation of toxoplasmosis acquired after birth is asymptomatic localized lymphadenopathy. The cervical nodes are most frequently involved, but nontender enlargement of other regional groups, including the retroperitoneal nodes, also occurs. At times, the adenopathy is accompanied by fever, sore throat, rash, hepatosplenomegaly, and atypical lymphocytosis, thus mimicking the clinical and laboratory manifestations of infectious mononucleosis. Occasionally the normal host will develop severe visceral involvement, which may be manifested as meningoencephalitis, pneumonitis, myocarditis, or hepatitis. Chorioretinitis following postnatally acquired infection, although documented, is highly unusual. Unlike congenitally acquired ocular disease, it occurs during midlife and is generally unilateral.

Immunocompromised Host. In the immunocompromised host, toxoplasmosis is a serious, often fatal disease. If primary infection is acquired while a patient is undergoing immunosuppressive therapy for malignancy or organ transplantation, widespread dissemination of the infection with necrotizing pneumonitis, myocarditis, and encephalitis may occur. More commonly, acute disease in this population results from the activation of chronic, latent infection by immunosuppressive therapy or the acquisition of a concurrent immunosuppressive infection, particularly acquired immunodeficiency syndrome (AIDS). Encephalitis occurs in 50% of such cases and in more than 90% of fatal cases. Toxoplasmic encephalitis is particularly common in AIDS patients, being seen in approximately 10% of those with circulating toxoplasma antibodies. As such, it is a major cause of morbidity and mortality in this patient population.

Reactivation of latent infections with severe manifestations

Severity in AIDS

Laboratory Diagnosis

Demonstration of parasite

The diagnosis may be established by a variety of methods. In acute toxoplasmic lymphadenitis, the histologic appearance of the involved nodes is often pathognomonic. The trophozoite may be demonstrated in tissue with Wright or Giemsa stain. Electron microscopy and indirect fluorescent antibody techniques have also been used successfully on heart transplant or brain tissue obtained by biopsy. Although tissue cysts are selectively stained by periodic acid-Schiff, their presence is not indicative of acute disease. Isolation of the organism can be accomplished by inoculating blood or other body fluids into mice or tissue cultures. Inoculation of other tissues is not usually helpful, as a positive result may only reflect the presence of latent tissue cysts.

Serodiagnosis

Rising titers

Serologic procedures are the primary method of diagnosis. To establish the presence of acute infection, it is usual to demonstrate a fourfold rise in the IgG antibody titer between acute and convalescent serum specimens. As peak titers are often reached within 4–8 weeks, the acute serum must be collected early in the course of illness. Of the many tests developed for the detection of IgG antibodies, the indirect hemagglutination test and the indirect fluorescent antibody test are those most frequently used; they both are sensitive and highly specific. With these tests, titers of 1:1000 or more are usually detected after an acute infection. These levels gradually fall, but may remain high for many years.

Significance of IgM antibody

The detection of IgM antibodies provides a more rapid confirmation of acute infection. As detected by an indirect fluorescent antibody technique, these antibodies arise within the first week of infection, peak in 2–4 weeks, and quickly revert to negative. It also appears that IgM antibodies are produced after reactivation of latent disease. A single high titer (1:80 or more) therefore establishes the presence of acute infection or reactivation. Unfortunately, this test has been difficult to standardize, lacks sensitivity in neonates and immunocompromised (particularly AIDS) hosts and is not widely available. A recently developed enzyme-linked immunosorbent assay for IgM antibody circumvents many of these difficulties, but is neither widely available nor sufficiently sensitive in AIDS patients. Detection of toxoplasma antigen may be a useful adjunctive test in immunocompromised individuals.

Treatment and Prevention

Usually patients do not require therapy unless symptoms are particularly severe and persistent or unless vital organs, such as the eye, are involved. Immunocompromised and pregnant women, however, should be treated if acute infection (or reactivation) is documented (Table 52.3). Routine serial serologic testing of immunocompromised patients and pregnant women would allow early detection of patients and enhance the prospects of a successful outcome. At present, the only proved therapeutic regimen

Combined sulfonamide and pyrimethamine therapy

Table 52.3 Indications for Treatment of Toxoplasmosis[a]

Serologic Criteria	Clinical Criteria
Elevated IgM titers	Potential laboratory acquired infection
Fourfold rise in IgG titers	Pregnant woman
Very high IgG titers (greater than 1:1000)	Neonate
	Immunocompromised patient (including AIDS)
	Severe constitutional symptoms
	Vital organ involvement (including active chorioretinitis)

Abbreviations: Ig = immunoglobulin; AIDS = acquired immunodeficiency syndrome.
[a] Must satisfy one serologic plus one clinical criterion.

available in this country is the combination of sulfonamides and pyrimethamine. Unfortunately, the latter drug is teratogenic and should not be used in the first trimester of pregnancy.

Prevention should be directed primarily at pregnant women and the immunologically compromised host. Hands should be carefully washed after handling uncooked meat. Cysts in meat can be destroyed by proper cooking (56°C for 15 min) or by freezing to −20°C. Cat feces should be avoided, particularly the changing of kitty litter.

CRYPTOSPORIDIOSIS

Cryptosporidia

Definition. Cryptosporidia are small parasites that can infect the intestinal tract of a wide range of mammals including humans. Like other sporozoan parasites, they are obligate intracellular organisms exhibiting alternating cycles of sexual and asexual reproduction. As is true for *Toxoplasma*, both cycles are completed within the gastrointestinal tract of a single host. Long recognized as an important cause of diarrhea in animals, cryptosporidia were not identified as causes of human enteritis until 1976.

Sexual and asexual cycles in a single host

Cause of diarrhea in humans and animals

Life Cycle. Infective oocysts are excreted in the stool of the parasitized animal. Unlike those of *Toxoplasma*, cryptosporidia oocysts are fully mature and immediately infective upon passage in the feces. Following ingestion by another animal, sporozoites are released from the oocyst and attach to the microvilli of the small bowel epithelial cells where they are transformed into trophozoites. These divide asexually by multiple fission (schizogony) to form schizonts containing eight daughter cells known as type 1 merozoites. Upon release from the schizont, each daughter cell attaches itself to another epithelial cell where it repeats the schizogony cycle, producing another generation of type 1 merozoites.

Mature infective oocysts excreted in stool

Sporozoites, trophozoites, and merozoites all attach to epithelial cells

Eventually, schizonts containing four type 2 merozoites are seen. Incapable of continued asexual reproduction, these develop into male (microgamete) and female (macrogamete) sexual forms. Following fertilization, the resulting zygote develops into an oocyst that is shed into the lumen of the bowel. The majority possess a thick protective cell wall that ensures their intact passage in the feces and survival in the external en-

Gametocytes, zygotes, and oocysts

Some oocysts are thin walled and can autoinfect

vironment. Approximately 20% fail to develop the thick protective wall. The cell membrane ruptures, releasing infective sporozoites directly into the intestinal lumen and initiating a new "autoinfective" cycle within the original host. In the normal host, the presence of innate or acquired immunity dampens both the cyclic production of type 1 merozoites and the formation of thin-walled oocysts, halting further parasite multiplication and terminating the acute infection. In the immunocompromised, both presumably continue, explaining why such individuals develop severe, persistent infections in the absence of external reinfection.

Small spherical parasites beneath surface of microvilli

Morphology. Regardless of animal host, all strains of this tiny (2–6 μm) parasite appear morphologically identical and can reasonably be regarded as a single species. They appear as small spherical structures arranged in rows along the microvilli of the epithelial cells. They are readily stained with Giemsa and hematoxylin–eosin. Although they remain external to the cytoplasm of the intestinal epithelial cell, they are covered by a double membrane derived from the reflection, fusion, and attenuation of the microvilli and are thus, by definition, intracellular organisms. Oocysts shed into the intestinal lumen mature to contain four sporozoites; their cell wall provides the unusual property of acid-fastness, allowing them to be visualized with stains generally employed for mycobacteria.

Oocysts are acid-fast

Cryptosporidial Infections

Infection rates highest in young

Epidemiology. Cryptosporidiosis appears to involve most vertebrate groups. In all species, infection rates are highest among the young and immature. Experimental and epidemiologic data suggest that domestic animals constitute an important reservoir of disease in humans. However, outbreaks of human disease in day-care centers, hospitals, and urban family groups indicate that most human infections result from person-to-person transmission. In Western countries, between 1 and 4% of small children presenting to medical centers with gastroenteritis have been shown to harbor cryptosporidia oocysts; in third-world countries the rates have varied from 4 to 11%. In some outbreaks of diarrhea in day-care centers, the majority of attendees were found to have oocysts in their stool.

Animal reservoirs and person–person transmission

Infection rates in adults suffering from gastroenteritis is approximately one-third that reported in children; it has been highest in family members of infected children, medical personnel caring for patients with cryptosporidiosis, male homosexuals, and travelers to foreign countries. Asymptomatic carriage is uncommon. Other enteric pathogens, particularly *Giardia lamblia*, are recovered from a significant minority of infected patients.

Fecal–oral route of infection

Because oocysts are found almost exclusively in stool, the principal transmission route is undoubtedly fecal–oral. The hardy nature of the oocysts makes it likely that there is also indirect transmission via contaminated food, water, and fomites.

Minimal pathology; possible role of toxin

Pathogenesis and Immunity. Although the jejunum is most heavily involved, cryptosporidia have been found throughout the gastrointestinal tract, particularly in immunocompromised subjects. By light microscopy, bowel changes appear minimal, consisting of mild to moderate villous atrophy, crypt enlargement, and a mononuclear infiltrate of the lamina propria. The pathophysiology of the diarrhea is unknown, but its nature and intensity suggest that a choleralike enterotoxin may be involved.

The vital role played by the host's immune status in the pathogenesis of the disease is indicated by both the enhanced susceptibility of the young

Prolonged disease in
immunosuppressed

to infection and the prolonged severe clinical disease seen in immuno-compromised patients. Indirect evidence suggests that resistance to rein-fection is mediated by T lymphocytes, whereas the severity and duration of the primary infection may be influenced by both cellular and humoral mechanisms.

Explosive, self-limiting
diarrhea in immunocompetent
individuals

Clinical Manifestations.   Immunocompetent patients usually note the onset of explosive, profuse, watery diarrhea 1 to 2 weeks after exposure. Typically, the illness persists for 5–11 days and then rapidly abates. Oc-casionally, purging, accompanied by a mild malabsorption and weight loss, continues for up to 1 month. A few patients complain of nausea, anorexia, vomiting, and low-grade fever. Except for its shorter duration, more prom-inent abdominal pain, and relative lack of flatulence, the clinical mani-festations of cryptosporidiosis closely resemble those produced by *G. lam-blia*. Radiographic and endoscopic examinations of the gut are either normal or demonstrate mild, nonspecific abnormalities. Recovery is com-plete, and neither relapse nor reinfection has been reported.

Solid immunity

Cryptosporidiosis has been described in patients with a broad range of immunodeficiencies including childhood malnutrition in third-world countries, AIDS, and congenital hypogammaglobulinemia and in those resulting from cancer chemotherapy and immunosuppressive management of organ transplants. In such patients cryptosporidiosis is usually indolent in onset and manifestations are similar to those seen in normal hosts, but the diarrhea is more severe. Fluid losses of up to 17 L/day have been described. Unless the immunologic defect is reversed, the disease usually persists for the duration of the patient's life. Weight loss is often prom-inent. The prognosis depends upon the nature of the underlying immu-nologic abnormality; half of patients with AIDS die within 6 months. Although other intercurrent infections are usually the direct cause of death, malnutrition and complications of parenteral nutrition contribute.

Severe, prolonged diarrhea in
immunosuppressed including
AIDS patients

Laboratory Diagnosis.   The diagnosis of cryptosporidiosis is established by the recovery and identification of *Cryptosporidium* oocysts in a recently passed or preserved diarrheal stool. Oocyst excretion is most intense dur-ing the first week of illness, tapers during the second week, and generally stops with the cessation of diarrhea. As cryptosporidia oocysts are one of the few acid-fast particles found in feces, a definitive identification can be established with any one of the few acid-fast staining procedures developed for mycobacteria. When direct examinations are negative, concentration procedures are used and the concentrate restained.

Detection of oocysts by acid-
fast stains

Treatment and Prevention.   In the immunocompetent patient, the disease is self-limited and attempts at specific antiparasitic therapy are not war-ranted; rehydration may be required in small children. In the immuno-compromised host, the severity and chronicity of the diarrhea warrants therapeutic intervention. Unfortunately, there is no effective anticryp-tosporidial agent available at this time. The only uniformly successful ap-proach has been the reversal of underlying immunologic abnormalities. When appropriate, withdrawal of cancer chemotherapy agents or immu-nosuppressive drugs may result in a cure.

No specific therapeutic yet in
use

The stools of patients with cryptosporidiosis are infectious. Stool pre-cautions should be instituted at the time the diagnosis is first suspected; for the immunosuppressed patient, this should be whenever diarrhea, re-gardless of presumed etiology, is first noted. This is particularly important in cancer chemotherapy and transplantation units where spread of the

Stool precautions to protect
immunosuppressed

disease from a symptomatic patient to other immunosuppressed patients can have life-threatening consequences.

Additional Reading

Bruce-Chwatt, L.J. 1979. Man against malaria: Conquest or defeat. *R. Soc. Trop. Med. Hyg.* 73:605–617. The world's leading malariologist reviews the successes and failures of the WHO-sponsored Malaria Eradication Program.

Dubey, J.P., Miller, N.L., and Frenkel, J.K. 1970. The *Toxoplasma gondii* oocyst from cat feces. *J. Exp. Med.* 132:636–662. The first demonstration of a sexual form of *T. gondii*, thus establishing its definitive host, method of transmission, and taxonomic status as a coccidian.

Frenkel, J.K., and Ruiz, A. 1981. Endemicity of toxoplasmosis in Costa Rica. Transmission between cats, soil, intermediate hosts and humans. *Am. J. Epidemiol.* 113:254–269. This article is the most comprehensive study on the role of cats in the transmission of toxoplasmosis. It suggests that humans are infected primarily from soil contaminated with cat feces, rather than direct contact.

Godsen, G.N. 1985. Molecular approaches to malaria vaccines. *Sci. Am.* 252:52–59. A highly detailed, clearly written, and beautifully illustrated review of recent efforts to develop malaria vaccines.

Luft, B.J., Brooks, R.G., Conley, F.K. 1984. Toxoplasmic encephalitis in patients with acquired immune deficiency syndrome. *JAMA* 252:913.

Molineaux, L., and Gramiccia, G. 1980. *The Garki Project. Research on the Epidemiology and Control of Malaria in the Sudan Savanna of West Africa.* Geneva: World Health Organization. The most comprehensive study ever undertaken of malaria transmission in holoendemic areas.

Phillips, R.E., and Warrell, D.A., 1986. The pathophysiology of severe falciparum malaria. *Parasitol. Today* 2:271–282. A concise review of the conflicting hypotheses of malaria pathophysiology, including important data recently generated by the authors.

Soave, R., and Armstrong, D. 1986. *Cryptosporidium* and Cryptosporidiosis. *Rev. Infect. Dis.* 8:1012–1023. A recent, readable review of the topic.

53

Rhizopods

James J. Plorde

Rhizopods, or amebas, are the most primitive of the protozoa. They multiply by simple binary fission and move by means of cytoplasmic organelles called *pseudopodia*. These projections of the relatively solid ectoplasm are formed by streaming of the inner, more liquid endoplasm. They move the ameba forward and, incidentally, engulf and internalize food sources found in its path. Most amebas, when faced with a hostile environment, can produce a chitinous, external wall that surrounds and protects them. These forms are referred to as *cysts* and may survive for prolonged periods under conditions that would rapidly destroy the motile trophozoite.

Most amebas free-living

The majority of amebas belong to free-living genera. They are widely distributed in nature, being found in literally all bodies of standing fresh water. Few free-living amebas produce human disease, although two genera, *Naegleria* and *Acanthamoebae*, have been implicated occasionally as causes of meningoencephalitis and keratitis.

Several parasitic amebas; fecal–oral transmission

Several genera of amebas including *Entamoeba, Endolimax*, and *Iodamoeba*, are obligate parasites of the human alimentary tract and are passed as cysts from host to host by the fecal-oral route. Several are devoid of mitochondria, presumably because of the anaerobic conditions under which they exist in the colon. Only one, *Entamoeba histolytica*, regularly produces disease.

Entamoeba histolytica

Description of Organism

Morphology and Physiology. *Entamoeba histolytica* possesses both trophozoite and cyst forms. The trophozoites are microaerophilic, dwell in the lumen or wall of the colon, feed on bacteria and tissue cells, and multiply rapidly in the anaerobic environment of the gut. When diarrhea occurs, the trophozoites are passed unchanged in the liquid stool. Here they can

721

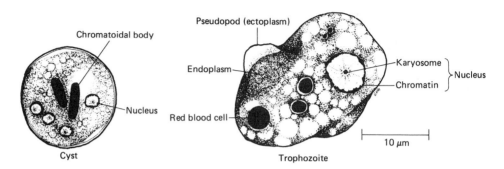

Chromatoidal body

Nucleus

Cyst

Pseudopod (ectoplasm)

Endoplasm

Karyosome

Chromatin

Nucleus

Red blood cell

10 μm

Trophozoite

53.1 *Entamoeba histolytica.*

Trophozoites passed in diarrheal stools; may contain ingested erythrocytes

be recognized by their size (12–20 μm in diameter); directional motility; granular, vacuolated endoplasm; and sharply demarcated, clear ectoplasm with fingerlike pseudopods. Invasive strains tend to be larger and may contain ingested erythrocytes within their cytoplasm (Figure 53.1). Appropriate stains reveal a 3- to 5-μm nucleus with a small central karyosome or nucleolus and fine regular granules evenly distributed around the nuclear membrane (peripheral chromatin). Electron microscopic studies demonstrate microfilaments, an external glycocalyx, and cytoplasmic projections thought to be important for attachment.

Resistant mature quadrinucleate cysts

With normal stool transit time, trophozoites usually encyst before leaving the gut. Initially, a cyst contains a single nucleus, a glycogen vacuole, and one or more large, cigar-shaped ribosomal clusters known as *chromatoid bodies*. With maturation, the cyst becomes quadrinucleate, and the cytoplasmic inclusions are absorbed. In contrast to the fragile trophozoite, mature cysts can survive environmental temperatures up to 55°C, chlorine concentrations normally found in municipal water supplies, and normal levels of gastric acid. *Entamoeba histolytica* can be differentiated from the other amebas of the gut by its size, nuclear detail, and cytoplasmic inclusions (Table 53.1).

Human-to-human infection by ingested cysts

Life Cycle. Humans are the principal hosts and reservoirs of *E. histolytica*. Transmission from person to person occurs when a parasite passed in the stool of one host is ingested by another. Because the trophozoites die rapidly in the external environment, successful passage is achieved only by the cyst. Human hosts may pass up to 45 million cysts daily. Although the average infective dose exceeds 1000 organisms, ingestion of a single cyst has been known to produce infection. After passage through the stomach, the cyst eventually reaches the distal small bowel. Here the cyst wall disintegrates, releasing the quadrinucleate parasite, which divides to form eight small trophozoites that are carried to the colon. Colonization is most intense in areas of fecal stasis such as the cecum and rectosigmoid, but may be found throughout the large bowel.

Cyst releases trophozoites in jejunum

Trophozoites colonize cecum and rectosigmoid

Virulence is strain related; associated with certain zymodeme patterns

Pathogenicity. Normally, *E. histolytica* exists in the gut as a harmless commensal. Occasionally it invades, producing tissue damage; if the damage is sufficiently extensive, clinical disease results. There is a substantial body of data that suggests that virulence is a strain-specific characteristic, and a number of workers feel that pathogenic and nonpathogenic strains can be distinguished by the electrophoretic motility patterns of four tro-

Table 53.1 Some Differential Characteristics of *Entamoeba* Species

Characteristics	E. histolytica	E. hartmanni	E. coli
	Trophozoites		
Cytoplasm	Differentiated[a]	Differentiated	Undifferentiated
Nucleus			
Peripheral chromatin	Fine	Fine	Coarse, irregular
Karyosome	Small, central	Small, central	Large, eccentric
Ingested particles			
Bacteria	No	—	Yes
Red blood cells	Yes	No	No
Size	>12 μm	<12 μm	>12 μm
	Cysts		
Nuclei[b]	1–4	1–4	1–8
Chromatoid bodies	Rods	Rods	Splinters
Size	>10 μg	<10 μm	>10 μm

[a] Sharp differentiation between ectoplasm and endoplasm.
[b] Fine structure similar to that of trophozoites.

phozoitic enzymes. Twenty-two such patterns, or zymodemes, have been identified to date of which nine have been found in strains of *E. histolytica* isolated from patients with clinical disease. Individuals harboring strains with "nonpathogenic" zymodemes seldom mount antibody responses to the organism or demonstrate physical evidence of sustained invasion. In contrast, amebic antibodies are regularly found in individuals harboring amebas with "pathogenic" zymodemes, suggesting that colonization by these strains is followed by tissue invasion. In most cases, however, tissue damage is minimal, and the host is symptom free.

Most infected individuals symptom free

Factors influencing host resistance

Colonic microflora may influence invasiveness

Possible increased virulence with passage

Virulence determinants

The factors that modulate the invasiveness of virulent strains are still poorly understood, but changes in host resistance, the colonic milieu, or the parasite itself may amplify tissue damage and clinical manifestations. Protein malnutrition, high-carbohydrate diets, corticosteroid administration, and pregnancy all appear to render the host more susceptible to invasion. Certain colonic bacteria appear to enhance invasiveness, possibly by providing a more favorable redox potential for survival and multiplication or by facilitating the adherence of the parasite to colonic mucosa. Finally, it is known that the pathogenic strains in the tropics are more invasive than those isolated in more temperate areas, possibly because poor sanitation results in more frequent passage through humans.

Entamoeba histolytica possess a number of mechanisms potentially capable of mediating tissue damage. In an experimental setting, the invasiveness of amebic strains correlates well with their endocytic capacity, ability to produce collagenase and a cytotoxic protein, and, perhaps most importantly, their capacity to lyse host cells that they contact. The latter phenomenon is initiated by specific adherence of the trophozoite to a target cell. Following adherence the ameba releases a pore-forming protein that polymerizes in the target cell membrane, forming large tubular lesions. Cytolysis rapidly follows.

Axenic cultures

Laboratory Growth. Trophozoites are facultative anaerobes that require complex media for growth. Most require the addition of live bacteria for successful isolation. Sterile culture techniques (axenic) have been developed, however, and are essential for the preparation of the purified antigens required for serologic testing and zymodeme typing. The value of culture procedures in the diagnosis of amebiasis remains unestablished.

Amebiasis

Pathology. Amebas contact and lyse colonic epithelial cells, producing small mucosal ulcerations. There is little inflammatory response other than edema and hyperemia, and the mucosa between ulcers appears normal. Trophozoites are present in large numbers at the junction between necrotic and viable tissue. Once the lesion penetrates below the superficial epithelium, it meets the resistance of the colonic musculature and spreads laterally in the submucosa, producing a flasklike lesion with a narrow mucosal neck and a large submucosal body. It eventually compromises the blood supply of the overlying mucosa, resulting in sloughing and a large necrotic ulcer. Extensive ulceration leads to secondary bacterial infection, formation of granulation tissue, and fibrotic thickening of the colon. Occasionally, the granulation tissue is organized into large tumorlike masses known as *amebomas*. The major sites of involvement, in order of frequency, are the cecum, ascending colon, rectum, sigmoid, appendix, and terminal ileum. Amebas may also enter the portal circulation and be carried to the liver or, more rarely, to the lung, brain, or spleen. In these organs, liquefaction necrosis leads to the formation of abscess cavities.

Immunity. Although pathogenic strains of *E. histolytica* elicit both humoral and cellular immune responses in humans, it is still not clear which, and to what degree, they are capable of modulating initial infection or thwarting reinfection. In endemic areas, the prevalence of gastrointestinal colonization increases with age, suggesting that the host is incapable of clearing *E. histolytica* from the gut. However, the relative infrequency with which populations living in these areas suffer repeated bouts of severe amebic colitis or liver abscess indicates that those who experience such infections have protection against recurrent disease.

Patients with invasive disease are known to produce high levels of circulating antibodies. Nevertheless, there is no correlation between the presence or concentration of such antibodies and protective immunity, possibly because pathogenic *E. histolytica* trophozoites have the capacity to aggregate and shed attached antibodies and are resistant to the lytic action of complement. The susceptibility to invasive amebiasis of malnourished populations, pregnant women, steroid-treated individuals, and acquired immunodeficiency syndrome (AIDS) patients indicates that cell-mediated immune mechanisms may be directly involved in the control of tissue invasion, although, as measured by the onset of delayed-type hypersensitivity and T-cell proliferative responses to amebic antigens, they develop slowly, often peaking weeks after recovery from invasive disease. Effector mechanisms appear to include cytotoxic T lymphocytes and lymphokine-activated macrophages, both of which have been shown capable of killing pathogenic amebas in vitro.

The role of immune mechanisms in the pathogenesis of the disease remains speculative. It is possible the presence of immune complexes and neutrophils in amebic abscess cavities contribute to tissue necrosis.

Pathogenic *E. histolytica* strains produce a lectinlike substance that is mitogenic for lymphocytes. It has been suggested that this substance could stimulate viral replication of human immunodeficiency virus (HIV)-infected lymphocytes as does another mitogen, phytohemagglutinin A. As

---

Mucosal ulceration; little inflammatory response

Flasklike lesion of submucosa

Amebomas and metastatic amebic abscesses

Immunity incomplete; does not correlate with antibody response

Trophozoites shed antibody and resist complement lysis

Evidence for significance of cell-mediated immunity

Possible immunopathology

significant numbers of homosexual males carry *E. histolytica*, it is conceivable that this parasite might accelerate the development of AIDS in HIV-infected individuals.

Clinical Manifestations.   Individuals who harbor *E. histolytica* are usually clinically well. In most cases, particularly in the temperate zones, the organism is avirulent, living in the bowel as a normal commensal inhabitant. Spontaneous disappearance of amebas is common among such patients, occuring at the rate of 15% per annum. Serologic data, however, suggest that some asymptomatic carriers possess virulent strains and incur minimal tissue invasion. In this population, the infection may eventually progress to produce overt disease.

Diarrhea, flatulence, and cramping abdominal pain are the most frequent complaints of symptomatic patients. The diarrhea is intermittent, alternating with episodes of normality or constipation over a period of months to years. Typically, the stools consist of one to four loose to watery, foul-smelling passages that contain mucus and blood. Physical findings are limited to abdominal tenderness localized to the hepatic, ascending colonic, and cecal areas. Sigmoidoscopy reveals the typical ulcerations with normal intertwining mucosa.

Fulminating amebic dysentery is less common. It may occur spontaneously in debilitated or pregnant individuals or be precipitated by corticosteroid therapy. Its onset is often abrupt, with high fever, severe abdominal cramps, and profuse, bloody diarrhea and tenesmus. Severe abdominal tenderness and a tender, enlarged liver are common. Sigmoidoscopy reveals extensive rectosigmoid ulceration. Trophozoites are numerous in stools and ulcer aspirates. A number of complications may accompany fulminant disease, including massive hemorrhage and bowel perforation with resulting peritonitis. Amebomas may project into the lumen of the bowel, where they may be mistaken for adenocarcinoma or extend circumferentially around the colon, producing partial obstruction. If tissue destruction is extensive, the colon may be left scarred and irritable despite eradication of the organism, resulting in so-called *postdysenteric colitis*.

Liver abscess presents either acutely or insidiously with fever and tender hepatic enlargement. Most commonly, abscesses occur singly and are localized to the upper outer quadrant of the right lobe of the liver. This localization results in the development of point tenderness overlying the cavity and elevation of the right diaphragm. Liver function is usually well preserved. Isotopic or ultrasound scanning confirms the presence of the lesion. Needle aspiration results in the withdrawal or reddish-brown, odorless fluid free of bacteria and polymorphonuclear leukocytes; trophozoites may be demonstrated in the terminal portion of the aspirate.

Approximately 5% of all patients with symptomatic amebiasis present with a liver abscess. Ironically, fewer than one-half can recall significant diarrheal illness, and *E. histolytica* is demonstrated in the stools of less than one-third. Complications relate to the extension of the abscess into surrounding tissue, producing pneumonia, empyema, or peritonitis. Extension of an abscess from the left lobe of the liver to the pericardium is the single most dangerous complication. It may produce rapid cardiac compression (tamponade) and death or, more commonly, a chronic pericardial disease that may be confused with congestive cardiomyopathy or tuberculous pericarditis.

Epidemiology.   Amebiasis has a worldwide distribution. Infection rates are

Marginal notes:

Relationship usually commensal

Symptoms and signs of intestinal amebiasis

Chronic ulceration with mucus and blood in stool

Fulminating amebic dysentery

Postdysenteric colitis

Hepatic abscess

Complications of hepatic abscess

Worldwide infection; highest rates in warmer climates

higher in warmer climates and may exceed 50% in areas where the level of sanitation is low. Stool surveys in the United States indicate that 1– 5% of the population harbors E. *histolytica*, although the virulence of these strains is uncertain. Invasive disease is both less common and less widely distributed. Reports of amebic liver abscess, for instance, emanate primarily from Mexico, western South America, South Asia, and West and South Africa. For reasons apparently unrelated to exposure, symptomatic illness is much less common in women and children than in men.

Invasive disease rare in United States

In the United States, the incidence of invasive amebiasis decreased sharply over several decades, reaching a nadir of 3500 cases in 1974. Since then, the numbers have steadily increased. Most cases are acquired outside the country. Invasive amebiasis is still seen in institutions for the mentally retarded, Indian reservations, migrant labor camps, and among male homosexuals and victims of AIDS.

Fecal-oral spread

Other modes of transmission

Symptomatic amebiasis is usually sporadic, the result of direct person-to-person fecal-oral spread under conditions of poor personal hygiene. Venereal transmission appears to be particularly common among male homosexuals, presumably the result of oral-anal sexual contact. Food- and water-borne spread occur, occasionally in epidemic form. Such outbreaks, however, are seldom as explosive as those produced by pathogenic intestinal bacteria. An outbreak of intestinal amebiasis due to colonic irrigation at a chiropractic clinic was recently reported.

Epidemics

Laboratory Diagnosis. The diagnosis of intestinal amebiasis depends upon the identification of the organism in stool or sigmoidoscopic aspirates. As trophozoites appear predominantly in liquid stools or aspirates, a portion of such specimens should be fixed immediately to ensure preservation of these fragile organisms for stained preparations. The specimen may then be examined in wet mount for typical motility, concentrated to detect cysts, and stained for definitive identification of E. *histolytica*. Three or more specimens may be required for diagnosis. If trophozoites or cysts are seen, they must be carefully differentiated from those of the commensal parasites, particularly *Entamoeba hartmanni* and *Entamoeba coli* (Table 53.1).

Stool examination for trophozoites and cysts

The diagnosis of extraintestinal amebiasis is more difficult, as the parasite usually cannot be recovered from stool or tissue. Serologic tests are therefore of paramount importance. Typically, results are negative in asymptomatic patients, suggesting that tissue invasion is required for antibody production. Most patients with symptomatic intestinal disease and more than 90% with hepatic abscess have high levels of antiamebic antibodies. Unfortunately, these titers may persist for months to years after an acute infection, making the interpretation of a positive test difficult in endemic areas. At present, the indirect hemagglutination test and the enzyme-linked immunosorbent assay utilizing antigens derived from axenically grown organisms appear to be the most sensitive. Several rapid tests, including latex agglutination and counterimmunoelectrophoresis, are available to smaller laboratories.

Serodiagnosis of extraintestinal amebiasis

Treatment. Treatment is directed toward relief of symptoms, blood and fluid replacement, and eradication of the organism. The drug of choice for eradication is metronidazole. It is effective against all forms of amebiasis, but should be combined with a second agent, such as diloxanide, to improve cure rates in intestinal disease and diminish the chance of recrudescent disease in hepatic amebiasis. Tetracycline, which apparently acts indirectly by altering the bacterial milieu of the gut, may be used as

Primary role of metronidazole and combined therapy

an alternative to diloxanide. Specific contraindications to the use of metronidazole are given in Chapter 54 in the section on Trichomoniasis.

Prevention. As the disease is transmitted by the fecal-oral route, efforts should be directed toward sanitary disposal of human feces and improvement in personal hygienic practices. In the United States, this applies particularly to institutionalized patients and to camps for migrant farm workers. Male homoxexuals should be made aware that certain sexual practices substantially increase their risk of this and other infections.

Naegleria and *Acanthamoeba* Infections

Amebic Meningoencephalitis

Meningoencephalitis due to free-living amebas

Primary amebic meningoencephalitis is caused by free-living amebas belonging to the genus *Naegleria* or *Acanthamoeba*. The disease produced by the former has been better defined; it affects children and young adults, appears to be acquired by swimming in fresh water, and is almost always fatal. *Acanthamoeba* meningoencephalitis is a milder and more chronic illness. *Naegleria* species are found in large numbers in shallow fresh water, particularly during warm weather. *Acanthamoeba* species are found in soil and in fresh and brackish water, and they have been recovered from the oropharynx of asymptomatic humans.

Naegleria infections associated with freshwater swimming

Approximately 140 cases of *Naegleria* meningoencephalitis have been reported, primarily in Great Britain, Czechoslovakia, Australia, and the United States. Serologic studies suggest that inapparent infections are much more common. Most cases in the United States have occurred in the southeastern states. Characteristically, the patients have fallen ill during the summer after swimming or water skiing in small, shallow, freshwater lakes. The Czechoslovakian cases followed swimming in a chlorinated indoor pool, and several have occurred after bathing in hot mineral water. A recent report from Africa suggests the disease may have been acquired by inhaling airborne cysts during the dry, windy season in the sub-Sahara.

Passage to central nervous system across cribriform plate

Histologic evidence suggests that *Naegleria* traverses the nasal mucosa and the cribriform plate to the central nervous system. Here the organism produces a severe hemorrhagic inflammatory reaction that extends perivascularly from the olfactory bulbs to other regions of the brain. The infection is characterized by rapid onset and a brief fatal course.

Purulent bloody cerebrospinal fluid containing *Naegleria* trophozoites

A careful examination of the cerebrospinal fluid often provides a presumptive diagnosis of *Naegleria* infection. The fluid is usually bloody and demonstrates an intense neutrophilic response. The protein level is elevated and the glucose level decreased. No bacteria can be demonstrated on stain or culture. Early examination of a wet mount preparation of unspun spinal fluid will reveal typical trophozoites. Staining with specific fluorescent antibody confirms the identification. To date, only two patients have survived a *Naegleria* infection. Both were diagnosed early, and one was treated with amphotericin B, the other with amphotericin B, miconazole, and rifampin.

Acanthamoeba affects older immunocompromised subjects

The epidemiology of *Acanthamoeba* encephalitis has not been clearly defined. Infections usually involve older, immunocompromised persons, and a history of freshwater swimming is generally absent. The ameba probably reaches the brain by hematogenous dissemination from an unknown primary site, possibly the respiratory tract or skin. Metastatic lesions have been reported. Histologically, *Acanthamoeba* infections produce a diffuse,

Granulomatous lesions

More chronic disease with
spontaneous recovery

necrotizing, granulomatous encephalitis with cysts as well as trophozoites
in the lesions.

The clinical course of *Acanthamoeba* disease is more prolonged than that
of *Naegleria* infection and often ends in spontaneous recovery, although
fatal disease has occurred in immunocompromised hosts. The spinal fluid
usually demonstrates a mononuclear response. *Acanthamoeba* species are
sensitive to a variety of agents, including sulfonamides, clotrimazole, 5-
fluorocytosine, and polymyxin. Studies of clinical efficacy have not been
done.

Other Acanthamoeba *Infections*

Corneal ulcerations

Association with contact lens
use

Treatment usually surgical

Skin lesions, uveitis, and corneal ulcerations have also been reported. The
latter are serious, producing a chronic progressive ulcerative lesion that
may result in blindness. Infection commonly follows mild corneal trauma;
most recently reported cases have been in users of soft contact lenses.
Clinically, severe ocular pain, a paracentral ring infiltrate of the cornea,
and recurrent epithelial breakdown are helpful in distinguishing this entity
from the more common herpes simplex keratitis. The diagnosis can be
confirmed by demonstrating typical wrinkled, double-walled cysts in corneal biopsies or scrapings using wet mounts, stained smears, and/or fluorescent antibody techniques. Culture of corneal tissue and contact lenses
is frequently successful when the laboratory is given time to prepare satisfactory media. Chemotherapy has generally been ineffective. Usually
cure has required corneal transplantation or enucleation of the eye.

Additional Reading

Chesley, A.J., Craig, C.F., Fishbein, M., et al. 1934. Amebiasis outbreak in Chicago. Report of a special committee. *J. Am. Med. Assoc.* 102:369–372. A description of the best known outbreak of amebiasis in the United States. Four-
teen hundred clinical infections and 100 deaths resulted from an inadvertent
connection between the water supply and sewage in two Chicago hotels.

Duma, R.J., Helwig, W.B., and Martinez, A.J. 1978. Meningoencephalitis and
brain abscess due to a free-living amoeba. *Ann. Intern. Med.* 88:468–473. A
useful case report and discussion regarding the taxonomic criteria used to identify free-living amebas producing human disease.

The global problem of amebiasis: Current status, research needs and opportunities
for progress. 1986. *Rev. Infect. Dis.* 8:218–272. This is a series of five papers
covering the current status, epidemiology, pathogenesis, immunology, and diagnosis of amebiasis. It is the most current and comprehensive review of *Entamoeba histolytica* infections.

Martinez-Palomo, A., and Martinez-Baez, M. 1983. Selective primary health care:
Strategies for control of disease in the developing world. X. Amebiasis. *Rev.
Infect. Dis.* 5:1093–1102. This article deals with the difficulties involved in the
early detection and treatment of amebic liver disease.

Moore, M.B., McCulley, J.P., and Luckenbach, M. 1985. *Acanthamoeba* keratitis
associated with soft contact lenses. Am. J. Ophthalmol. 100:396–403. A report
of three patients who developed *Acanthamoeba* keratitis. It discusses the relationship between use of contact lenses and this disease, reviews the literature,
and discusses diagnostic and therapeutic approaches.

Thompson, J.E., Jr., Forlenza, S., and Verma, R. 1985. Amebic liver disease: A
therapeutic approach. *Rev. Infect. Dis.* 7:171. This article deals with the difficulties involved in the early detection and treatment of amebic liver disease.

54

Flagellates

James J. Plorde

Like their amebic cousins, flagellate protozoa are widespread in nature, multiply by binary fission, and move about by means of cytoplasmic organelles of locomotion. Motility, however, is distinctly more vigorous among this group of organisms because of the efficiency of their locomotive apparatus, the flagellum. This organelle arises from an intracellular focus known as a *blepharoplast*, extends to the cell wall as a filamentous *axoneme*, and continues extracellularly as the *free flagellum*. In some species, the blepharoplast is paired with a second cytoplasmic structure known as a *parabasal body*. This structure is believed to be composed of modified mitochondria responsible for the control of flagellar movement. Both structures stain with nucleic acid stains, and they are known collectively as the *kinetoplast*.

In many flagellates the axoneme, before exiting from the cell, lifts a segment of external wall into a longitudinal fold. This *undulating membrane* is thrown into movement as the organism progresses, often imparting to it a characteristic rotary motion.

The long, whiplike free flagella may be single or multiple. The number is distinctive for individual species. When more than one is present, each has its own associated blepharoplast and axoneme.

Although a number of flagellate genera parasitize humans, only four, *Giardia*, *Trichomonas*, *Leishmania*, and *Trypanosoma*, commonly induce disease. The first two comprise noninvasive organisms that inhabit the lumina of the genitourinary or gastrointestinal tract and are spread without benefit of an intermediate host. Disease is of low morbidity and cosmopolitan distribution. *Leishmania* and *Trypanosoma*, on the other hand, are invasive blood and tissue parasites that produce highly morbid, frequently lethal diseases. These *hemoflagellates* require an intermediate insect host for their transmission. As a result, their associated disease states are limited to the semitropical and tropical niches of these intermediate hosts.

Organs and mechanisms of motility

Noninvasive and invasive pathogenic flagellates

Table 54.1 Luminal Flagellates Infecting Humans

Flagellate	Pathogenicity to Humans	Site
Giardia lamblia	+	Intestine
Dientamoeba fragilis	?	Intestine
Chilomastix mesnili	−	Intestine
Enteromonas hominis	−	Intestine
Retortamonas intestinalis	−	Intestine
Trichomonas hominis	−	Intestine
Trichomonas tenax	−	Mouth
Trichomonas vaginalis	+	Vagina

Noninvasive Luminal Flagellates

Luminal flagellates can be found in the mouth, vagina, or intestine of almost all vertebrates, and it is common for an animal host to harbor more than one species. Humans may serve as host and reservoir to eight (Table 54.1), but only two cause disease. Of these, *Giardia lamblia* inhabits the intestinal tract and *Trichomonas vaginalis* inhabits the vagina and genital tract.

These organisms are elongated or oval in shape and typically measure 10–20 μm in length. They often possess a rudimentary cytostome (mouth aperture) and organelles such as sucking discs or axostyles, which assist them to maintain their intraluminal position. They are readily recognized in body fluid or excreta by their rapid motility, and some can be specifically identified in unstained preparations. All can be cultivated on artificial media.

Some luminal flagellates, most notably *T. vaginalis*, possess only a trophozoite stage and are passed from host to host by direct physical contact. Most, including *G. lamblia*, possess both trophozoite and cyst forms. The latter, which is the infective form, is transmitted via the fecal-oral route. Human-to-human infection is thus found in populations where inadequate sanitation or poor personal hygiene favors spread.

Trichomonas vaginalis

Organism. Three members of the genus *Trichomonas* parasitize humans (Table 54.1), but only *T. vaginalis* is an established pathogen. The three species closely resemble one another morphologically, but confusion in identification is rare because of the specificity of their habitats.

Morphology

The *T. vaginalis* trophozoite (Figure 54.1) is oval and typically measures 7 × 15 μm. Organisms up to twice this size are occasionally recovered from asymptomatic patients and from cultures. In stained preparations, a single, elongated nucleus and a small cytostome are observed anteriorly. Five flagella arise nearby. Four immediately exit the cell. The fifth bends back and runs posteriorly along the outer edge of an abbreviated undulating membrane. Lying along the base of this membrane is a cross-striated structure known as the *costa*. A conspicuous microtubule containing a supporting rod or axostyle bisects the trophozoite longitudinally and protrudes through its posterior end. It is thought that the pointed tip of this structure is useful for attachment, and it may be responsible for the tissue

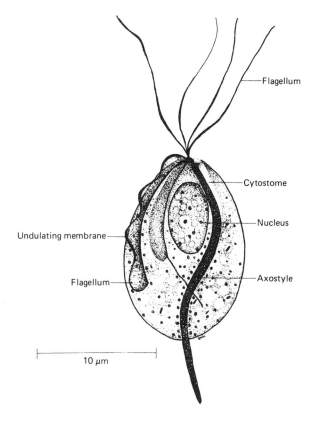

54.1 *Trichomonas vaginalis.*

Flagellum

Cytostome

Nucleus

Undulating membrane

Axostyle

Flagellum

10 μm

Cultivable in vitro

Resistance

Transmission usually sexual

damage produced by the parasite. In unstained wet mounts, *T. vaginalis* is identified by its axostyle and jerky, nondirectional movements.

The organism can be grown on artificial media under anaerobic conditions at pH 5.5–6.0. Soluble nutrients are absorbed across the cell membrane. Particulate material, including bacteria, leukocytes, and occasional erythrocytes, may be ingested through any area of the cell surface. A variety of carbohydrates are fermented by pathways similar to those of anaerobic bacteria. Although it lacks a cyst form, the trophozoite can survive outside of the human host for 1–2 hr on moist surfaces. In urine, semen, and water, it is viable for up to 24 hr, making it one of the most resistant of protozoan trophozoites. Attempts to infect laboratory animals have met with limited success.

Trichomoniasis

Epidemiology. Trichomoniasis is a cosmopolitan disease usually transmitted by sexual intercourse. It is estimated that 3–6 million women in the United States and 180 million worldwide acquire this disease annually, and 25% of sexually active women become infected at some time during their life; 30 to 70% of their male sexual partners are also parasitized, at least transiently. As would be expected, the likelihood of acquiring the disease correlates directly with the number of sexual contacts. Infection is rare in adult virgins, whereas rates as high as 70% are seen among prostitutes, sexual partners of infected patients, and individuals with other venereal diseases. In women, the peak incidence is between 16 and 35 years of age, but there is a relatively high prevalence in the 30 to 50 age group.

Nonvenereal transmission

Occasional neonatal infection

Nonvenereal transmission is uncommon. Transfer of organisms on shared washcloths may explain, in part, the high frequency of infection seen among institutionalized women. Female neonates are occasionally noted to harbor *T. vaginalis*, presumably acquiring it during passage through the birth canal. High levels of maternal estrogen produce a transient decrease in the vaginal pH of the child, rendering it more susceptible to colonization. Within a few weeks, estrogen levels drop, the vagina assumes its premenarchal state, and the parasite is eliminated.

Parasite damages epithelial cells on contact

Pathogenesis and Immunity. Direct contact of *T. vaginalis* with the squamous epithelium of the genitourinary tract results in destruction of the involved epithelial cells and the development of a neutrophilic inflammatory reaction and petechial hemorrhages. The precise pathogenesis of these changes are unknown. The organism is not invasive and extracellular toxins have never been demonstrated. Changes in the microbial, hormonal, and pH environment of the vagina as well as factors inherent to the infecting parasite are thought to modulate the severity of the pathologic changes. Although humoral, secretory, and cellular immune reactions can be demonstrated in most infected women, they are of little diagnostic help and do not appear to produce clinically significant immunity.

Chronic vaginitis

Clinical Manifestations. In women, *T. vaginalis* produces a persistent vaginitis. Although up to half are asymptomatic at the time of diagnosis, most develop clinical manifestations within 6 months. Approximately 75% develop a discharge, which is typically accompanied by vulvar itching or burning (50%), dyspareunia (50%), dysuria (50%), and a disagreeable odor (10%). Although fluctuating in intensity, symptoms usually persist for weeks or months. Commonly, manifestations worsen during menses and pregnancy. Eventually, the discharge subsides, even though the patient may continue to harbor the parasite. In symptomatic patients, physical examination reveals reddened vaginal and endocervical mucosa. In severe cases, petechial hemorrhages and extensive erosions are present. A red, granular, friable endocervix (strawberry cervix) is a characteristic, but uncommon, finding. An abundant discharge is generally seen pooled in the posterior vaginal fornix. Although classically described as thin, yellow, and frothy in character, the discharge more frequently lacks these characteristics.

Vaginitis worsens during pregnancy

Clinical manifestations

Urethritis and prostatitis in men usually asymptomatic

The urethra and prostate are the usual sites of infection in men; the epididymis may be involved on occasion. Infections are usually asymptomatic, possibly because of the efficiency with which the organisms are removed from the urogenital tract by voided urine. Symptomatic men complain of recurrent dysuria and scant, nonpurulent discharge. Acute purulent urethritis has been reported rarely.

Wet mount examination for motile trophozoites

Diagnosis. The diagnosis of trichomoniasis rests on the detection and morphologic identification of the organism in the genital tract. Identification is accomplished most easily by examining a wet mount preparation for the presence of motile organisms. In women, a drop of vaginal discharge is the most appropriate specimen; in men, urethral exudate or urine sediment after prostate massage may be used. Although highly specific when positive, wet mounts are often negative in asymptomatic or mildly symptomatic patients and in women who have douched in the previous 24 hr. Giemsa- and Papanicolaou-stained smears provide little additional

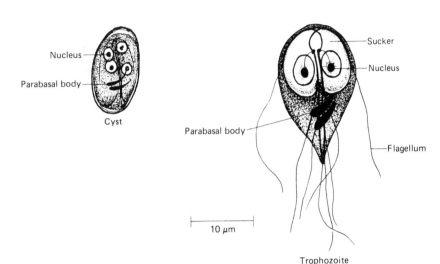

Nucleus

Parabasal body

Cyst

Sucker

Nucleus

Parabasal body

Flagellum

10 μm

Trophozoite

54.2 *Giardia lamblia.*

help. Cultures of urogenital specimens may increase the number of detected cases. Unfortunately, this procedure is not generally available in clinical laboratories and requires several days to complete. Direct detection of parasitic antigen in genital secretions may prove to be an acceptable alternative.

Patients with trichomoniasis should be examined carefully for other venereal disease.

Positive cases should be tested for other sexually transmitted diseases

Treatment. Oral metronidazole (Flagyl) is extremely effective in recommended dosage, curing more than 95% of all infections. Simultaneous treatment of sexual partners may minimize recurrent infections, particularly when single-dose therapy is employed for the index case. Because of metronidazole's disulfiramlike activity, alcohol consumption should be suspended during treatment. Because of its potential teratogenic activity, the drug should never be used during the first trimester of pregnancy. Use in the last two trimesters is unlikely to be hazardous, but should be reserved for patients whose symptoms cannot be adequately controlled with local therapies. High-dose, long-term metronidazole treatment has been shown to be carcinogenic in rodents. No association with human malignancy has been described to date, and in the absence of a suitable alternative drug, metronidazole continues to be used.

Metronidazole; precautions against teratogenic effects

Giardia lamblia

Organism. *Giardia lamblia* was first described by Anton von Leeuwenhoek 300 years ago when he examined his own diarrheal stool with one of the first primitive microscopes. It was not until the past two decades, however, that the cosmopolitan flagellate became widely regarded in the United States as a pathogen. Of the six other flagellated protozoans known to parasitize the alimentary tract of humans, only one, *Dientamoeba fragilis*, has been credibly associated with disease. Definitive confirmation or refutation of its pathogenicity will, it is hoped, not require the passage of another three centuries.

Unlike *T. vaginalis, Giardia* possesses both a trophozoite and a cyst form (Figure 54.2). It is a sting-ray-shaped trophozoite 9–21 μm in length, 5–15 μm in width, and 2–4 μm in thickness. When viewed from the top,

Characteristics of trophozoites

the organism's two nuclei and central parabasal bodies give it the appearance of a face with two bespectacled eyes and a crooked mouth. Four pairs of flagella—anterior, lateral, ventral, and posterior—reinforce this image by suggesting the presence of hair and chin whiskers. These distinctive parasites reside in the duodenum and jejunum, where they thrive in the alkaline environment and absorb nutrients from the intestinal tract. They move about the unstirred mucous layer at the base of the microvilli with a peculiar tumbling or "falling leaf" motility or, with the aid of a large ventral sucker, attach themselves to the brush border of the intestinal epithelium. Unattached organisms may be carried by the fecal stream to the large intestine. In the descending colon, if transit time allows, the flagella are retracted into cytoplasmic sheaths and a smooth, clear cyst wall is secreted. These forms are oval and somewhat smaller than the trophozoites. With maturation, the internal structures divide, producing a quadrinucleate organism harboring two sucking discs, four parabasal bodies, and eight axonemes (Figure 54.2). When fixed and stained, the cytoplasm pulls away from the cyst wall in a characteristic fashion. The mature cysts, which are the infective form of the parasite may survive in cold water for more than 2 months and are resistant to concentrations of chlorine generally used in municipal water systems. They are transmitted from host to host by the fecal-oral route. In the duodenum of a new host, the cytoplasm divides to produce two binucleate trophozoites.

Organisms of the genus *Giardia* are among the most widely distributed of intestinal protozoa; they are found in fish, amphibians, reptiles, birds, and mammals. At first, it was assumed that *Giardia* species found in different animals were host specific, and at least 40 different species were described. It is now known that at least some strains can infect more than a single host species. Unfortunately, there is no general agreement on organism characteristics to be used to define species.

Giardiasis

Epidemiology. Giardiasis has a cosmopolitan distribution; its prevalence is highest in areas with poor sanitation and among populations unable to maintain adequate personal hygiene. In developing countries, infection rates often exceed 10%; in the United States, *G. lamblia* is found in 4% of stools submitted for parasitologic examination, making it this country's most frequently identified intestinal parasite. All ages and economic groups are represented, but young children and young adults are preferentially involved. Children with immunoglobulin deficiencies are more likely to acquire the flagellate, possibly because of a deficiency in intestinal immunoglobulin A. Giardiasis is also common among attendees of day-care centers. Attack rates of over 90% have been seen in the ambulatory non-toilet-trained population (age, 1–2 years) of these institutions, suggesting direct person-to-person transmission of the parasite. The frequency with which secondary cases are seen among family contacts reinforces this probability. Undoubtedly, direct fecal spread is also responsible for the high infection rate among male homosexuals. In several recent studies, the prevalence of giardiasis and/or amebiasis in that population has ranged from 11 to 40% and is correlated closely with the number of oral-anal sexual contacts. Water-borne and, less frequently, food-borne transmission of this organism has also been documented and probably accounts for the frequency with which American travelers to third-world nations acquire infection. Unlike the typical bacterial diarrhea syndrome seen in travelers, the diarrhea begins late in the course of travel and may persist for several weeks. More than 20 water-borne outbreaks of giardiasis have also been reported in the United States. The sources have included untreated pond or stream water, sewage-contaminated municipal water supplies, and chlorinated but inadequately filtered water. In a few of these outbreaks, epidemiologic data have suggested that wild mammals, particularly beavers, served as the reservoir hosts.

Beavers and other mammals possible sources

Pathology, Pathogenesis, and Immunity.   Disease manifestations appear related to intestinal malabsorption, particularly of fat and carbohydrates. Disaccharidase deficiency with lactose intolerance, altered levels of intestinal peptidases and decreased vitamin B_{12} absorption have been demonstrated. The precise pathogenetic mechanisms responsible for these changes remain poorly understood. Mechanical blockade of the intestinal mucosa by large numbers of *Giardia*, damage to the fuzzy coat of the microvilli by the parasite's sucking disc, organism-induced deconjugation of bile salts, altered intestinal motility, accelerated turnover of mucosal epithelium with functional immaturity of transport systems, and mucosal invasion have all been suggested; none correlates well with clinical manifestations. Patients with severe malabsorption have jejunal colonization with enteric bacteria or yeasts, suggesting that these organisms may act synergistically with *Giardia*. Eradication of the associated microorganism, however, has not resulted uniformly in clinical improvement. Jejunal biopsies sometimes reveal a flattening of the microvilli and an inflammatory infiltrate. The demonstration of occasional trophozoites in the submucosa raises the possibility that these changes reflect T-cell-mediated damage. Immunologic reconstitution of experimentally infected nude (T-cell-deficient) mice with lymphoid cells from previously infected animals results in similar mucosal changes. Generally, both malabsorption and the jejunal lesions have been reversed with specific treatment.

Malabsorption syndrome with lactose intolerance

Basis for malabsorption and jejunal pathology remains uncertain

Susceptibility to giardiasis has been related to several factors, including strain virulence, inoculum size, achlorhydria or hypochlorhydria, and immunologic abnormalities. In one experimental study, humans were challenged with varying doses from as few as 10 cysts. They were uniformly parasitized when 100 or more were ingested. Several workers have noted the frequency with which giardiasis occurs in achlorhydric and hypochlorhydric individuals. Although reinfection is common, the frequent occurrence of giardiasis in patients with immunologic diseases, plus the rarity with which it is seen in older adults, suggests that protective immunity, albeit incomplete, does develop in humans. Animal studies suggest that humoral, secretory, and cellular mechanisms are operative.

Predisposing factors

Occurrence in immunocompromised subjects

Clinical Manifestations.   In endemic situations, over two-thirds of infected patients are asymptomatic. In acute outbreaks, this ratio of asymptomatic to symptomatic patients is usually reversed. When they do occur, symptoms begin 1–3 weeks after exposure; they typically include diarrhea, which is sudden in onset and explosive in character. The stool is foul smelling, greasy in appearance, and floats on water. It is devoid of blood or mucus. Upper abdominal cramping is common. Large quantities of intestinal gas produce abdominal distention, sulfuric eructations, and abundant flatus. Nausea, vomiting, and low-grade fever may be present. The acute illness generally resolves in 1–4 weeks; in children, however, it may persist for months, leading to significant malabsorption and weight loss.

Subclinical infections common

Diarrhea, cramping, and flatus

In many adults, the acute phase is often followed by a subacute or chronic phase characterized by intermittent bouts of mushy stools, fla-

Subacute and chronic infections with weight loss

tulence, and "heartburn" and weight loss that persist for weeks or months. At times, patients presenting in this fashion deny having experienced the acute syndrome described previously. In the majority, symptoms and organisms eventually disappear spontaneously. It is not uncommon for lactose intolerance to persist after eradication of the organisms. This condition may be confused with an ongoing infection, and the patient may be subjected to unnecessary treatment.

Laboratory Diagnosis.   The diagnosis is made by finding the cyst in formed stool or the trophozoite in diarrheal stools, duodenal secretions, or jejunal biopsy specimens. In acutely symptomatic patients, the parasite can usually be demonstrated by examining one to three stool specimens, providing appropriate concentration and staining procedures are used. In chronic cases, excretion of the organism is often intermittent, making parasitologic confirmation more difficult. Many of these patients can be diagnosed by examining specimens taken at weekly intervals over 4–5 weeks. Alternatively, duodenal secretions can be collected and examined for trophozoites in trichrome or Giemsa-stained preparations. The organism can be grown in culture, but the methods are not currently adaptable to routine diagnostic work. The value of immunologic tests, including serology and the direct detection of parasite antigen, are under investigation.

Treatment and Prevention.   Three drugs are currently available for the treatment of giardiasis in the United States: quinacrine hydrochloride, metronidazole, and furazolidone. The latter drug is used by pediatricians because of its availability as a liquid suspension, but it has the lowest cure rate. Quinacrine and metronidazole are somewhat more effective (70–95%) and are preferred for patients capable of ingesting tablets. All three agents require 5 to 7 days of therapy. Tinadazole, an oral agent not yet available in the United States, is safe and effective in single-dose treatment. Because of the potential of giardiasis for person-to-person spread, it is important to examine and, if necessary, treat close physical contacts of the infected patient, including playmates at nursery school, household members, and sexual contacts. If possible, treatment should be withheld from pregnant women because of the potential teratogenicity of available drugs.

Hikers should avoid ingestion of untreated surface water, even in remote areas, because of the possibility of contamination by feces of infected animals. Adequate disinfection can be accomplished with halogen tablets yielding concentrations higher than that generally achieved in municipal water systems. The safety of the latter results from additional flocculation and filtration procedures.

Blood and Tissue Flagellates

Of the many genera of hemoflagellates, two are pathogenic to humans: *Leishmania* and *Trypanosoma*. They reside and reproduce within the gut of specific insect hosts. When these vectors feed on a susceptible mammal, the parasite penetrates the feeding site, invades the blood and/or tissue of the new host, and multiplies to produce disease. The life cycle is completed when a second insect ingests the infected mammalian blood or tissue fluid. During the course of their passage through insect and vertebrate hosts, flagellates undergo developmental change. Within the gut of the insect (and in culture media) the organism assumes the promastigote (*Leishmania*) or epimastigote (*Trypanosoma*) form (Figure 54.3). These

---

Marginal notes:

Lactose intolerance may persist

Search for trophozoites and cysts in stool

Duodenal aspirates

Several drugs available

Examination of close contacts

Avoidance of drinking untreated surface water

Leishmania and *Trypanosoma*

Life cycle includes insect host stage

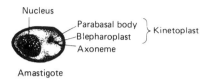

Amastigote

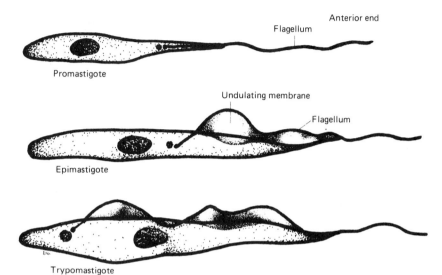

54.3 Stages in the life cycle of the hemoflagellates (Trypanosomidae).

protozoa are motile, fusiform, and have a blunt posterior end and a pointed anterior from which a single flagellum projects. They measure 15–30 μm in length and 1.5–4.0 μm in width. In the promastigote, the kinetoplast is located in the anterior extremity and the flagellum exits from the cell immediately. The kinetoplast of the epimastigote, in contrast, is located centrally, just in front of the vesicular nucleus. The flagellum runs anteriorly in the free edge of an undulating membrane before passing out of the cell. In the mammalian host, hemoflagellates appear as trypomastigotes (*Trypanosoma*) or amastigotes (*Leishmania, Trypanosoma cruzi*). The former circulate in the bloodstream and closely resemble the epimastigote form, except that the kinetoplast is in the posterior end of the parasite. The amastigote stage is found intracellularly. It is round or oval, measures 1.5–5.0 μm in diameter, and contains a clear nucleus with a central karyosome. Although it has a kinetoplast and an axoneme, there is no free flagellum.

The flagellated forms move in a spiral fashion, and all reproduce by longitudinal binary fission. The flagellum itself does not divide; rather, a second one is generated by one of the two daughter cells. The organisms utilize carbohydrate obtained from the body fluids of the host in aerobic respiration.

Promastigote and epimastigote forms in insects

Trypomastigote and amastigote forms in humans

Leishmania

Organism. *Leishmania* species are obligate intracellular parasites of mammals. Several strains can infect humans; they are all morphologically similar, resulting in some confusion over their proper speciation. Definitive identifications of these strains requires isoenzyme analysis, use of mon-

Taxonomy

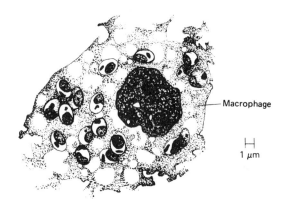

54.4 *Leishmania* within a mononuclear cell.

Macrophage

⊢⊣
1 µm

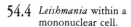

oclonal antibodies, or characterization of kinetoplast DNA. The many strains can be more simply placed in four major groups based on their serologic, biochemical, cultural, nosologic, and behavioral characteristics. For the sake of clarity, these groups will be discussed as individual species in this chapter. Each, however, contains a variety of strains that have been accorded separate species or subspecies status by some authorities.

Organisms can be grown in liquid media

The organisms can be propagated in hamsters and in a variety of commercially available liquid media.

Disease Transmission. It is estimated that over 20 million people worldwide suffer from leishmaniasis and over 400,000 additional individuals acquire the infection annually. *Leishmania tropica* in the Old World and *Leishmania mexicana* in the New World produce a localized cutaneous lesion or ulcer, known popularly as *oriental sore* and *chiclero ulcer. Leishmania braziliensis* is the cause of American mucocutaneous leishmaniasis (espundia), and *L. donovani* is the etiologic agent of kala azar, a disseminated visceral disease.

Disease associations

All four species transmitted by nocturnally feeding sandflies

All four are transmitted by phlebotomine sandflies. These small, delicate, short-lived insects are found in animal burrows and crevices throughout the tropics and subtropics. At night, they feed on a wide range of mammalian hosts. Amastigotes ingested in the course of a meal assume the flagellated promastigote form, multiply within the gut, and eventually migrate to the buccal cavity. When the fly next feeds on a human or animal host, the buccal promastigotes are injected into the skin of the new host. Here, they activate complement by the alternative pathway, are opsonized, taken up by macrophages, lose their flagella and multiply as the rounded amastigote form within the phagolysosome. In stained smears, they take on a distinctive appearance and have been termed *Leishman-Donovan* bodies. Continued multiplication leads to the rupture of the phagocyte and release of the daughter cells. Some may be taken up by a feeding sandfly; most invade neighboring mononuclear cells (Figure 54.4).

Promastigotes injected by fly invade macrophages

Amastigotes released from macrophages can infect feeding sandfly

Continuation of this cycle results in extensive histiocytic proliferation. The course of the disease at this point is determined by the species of parasite and the host's immune response. In the localized cutaneous forms of leishmaniasis, a vigorous cellular immune response results in the development of a positive delayed skin (leishmanin) reaction, lymphocytic infiltration, reduction in the number of parasites, and, eventually, spontaneous disappearance of the primary skin lesion. In infections with *L. braziliensis*, this sequence may be followed weeks to months later by mu-

In localized cutaneous disease, cellular immune responses produce spontaneous cure

Table 54.2 Immune Response to Leishmaniasis

Human Disease	Parasite	Leishmanin Skin Test	Number of Lymphocytes	Number of Parasites	Prognosis	Humoral Antibody Titer
Localized skin ulcer (oriental sore, chiclero ulcer, uta)	L. tropica L. mexicana	Positive	Many	Few	Good	Low
Mucocutaneous lesions (espundia)	L. braziliensis	Positive	Many	Few	Poor	Low
Disseminated cutaneous Ethiopian American	L. tropica[a] L. mexicana[a]	Negative	Few	Many	Poor	High
Disseminated visceral (kala azar)	L. donovani	Negative	Few	Many	Poor	High

[a] Different subspecies from those causing localized skin ulcers

Mucocutaneous metastases in L. braziliensis infections

cocutaneous metastases. These secondary lesions are highly destructive, presumably as a result of the host's hypersensitivity to parasitic antigens.

Some strains of *L. tropica* and *L. mexicana* fail to elicit an effective immune response in certain hosts. Such patients appear to have a selective suppressor T-cell-mediated anergy to leishmanial antigens. Consequently, there is no infiltration of lymphocytes or decrease in the number of parasites. The skin test remains negative, and the skin lesions disseminate and become chronic (diffuse cutaneous leishmaniasis). In infections with *L. donovani*, there is a similar failure of cellular immunity; in this case the organisms are able to disseminate through the bloodstream to the visceral organs, possibly because of a relative resistance of *L. donovani* to the natural microbicidal properties of normal serum. Although dissemination is associated with the development of circulating antibodies, they do not appear to serve a protective function and may, via the production of immune complexes, be responsible for the development of glomerulonephritis. The immune responses in different forms of leishmaniasis are summarized in Table 54.2.

Lack of cellular immune response in disseminated and chronic infections

Localized Cutaneous Leishmaniasis

Epidemiology. The disease is a zoonotic infection of tropical and subtropical rodents. It is particularly common in areas of China, India, Asia Minor, Africa, the Mediterranean littoral, and Central America. In the latter area, *L. mexicana* infects several species of arboreal rodents. Humans become involved when they enter forested areas to harvest chicle for chewing gum and are bitten by infected sandflies. In the eastern hemisphere, the desert gerbil and other burrowing rodents serve as the reservoir hosts of *L. tropica*. Human infection occurs when rural inhabitants come in close contact with the burrows of these animals. In the Mediterranean area, southern Russia, and India, human disease involves urban dwellers, primarily children. In this setting, the domestic dog serves as the reservoir, although sandflies may also transmit *L. tropica* directly from human to human.

Geographic distribution of rodent reservoir and rural transmission to humans

Canine reservoir in urban disease

Clinical Manifestations. Lesions usually appear on the extremities or face (the ear in cases of chiclero ulcer) weeks to months after the bite of the sandfly. They first appear as pruritic papules, often accompanied by regional lymphadenopathy. In a few months the papules ulcerate, producing painless craters with raised erythematous edges, sharp walls, and a granulating base. Satellite lesions may form around the edge of the primary sore and fuse with it. Multiple primary lesions are seen in some patients. Spontaneous healing occurs in 3–12 months, leaving a pitted, depigmented scar. Occasionally the lesions fail to heal, particularly on the ears, leading to progressive destruction of the pinna. A permanent strain-specific immunity follows healing.

Chronic, self-limiting skin ulceration

Strain-specific immunity

Management. In endemic areas, the diagnosis is made on clinical grounds and confirmed by the demonstration of the organism in the advancing edge of the ulcer. Material collected by biopsy, curettage, or aspiration is smeared and/or sectioned, stained, and examined microscopically for the pathognomonic Leishman-Donovan bodies. Material should also be cultured in liquid media. The leishmanin skin test becomes positive early in the course of the disease and remains so for life.

Search for Leishman-Donovan bodies and culture

Pentavalent antimonial agents, amphotericin B, and cycloguanil pamoate have all proved effective chemotherapeutic agents, but are generally reserved for extensive or multiple ulcerations. Secondary bacterial infections are treated with appropriate antibiotics.

Prophylactic measures include the control of the sandfly vector by use of insect repellents and fine mesh screening on dwellings.

Mucocutaneous Leishmaniasis

Epidemiology. *Leishmania braziliensis* causes a natural infection in the large forest rodents of tropical Latin America. Sandflies transmit the infection to humans engaged in opening jungle areas for new settlements.

Rodent reservoir of L. braziliensis

Clinical Manifestations. A primary skin lesion similar to oriental sore develops 1–4 weeks after sandfly exposure. Occasionally it undergoes spontaneous healing. More commonly, it progressively enlarges, often producing large vegetating lesions. After a period of weeks to years, painful, destructive, metastatic lesions of the mouth, nose and, occasionally, perineum appear in 2–50%. Sometimes, decades pass and the primary lesion totally resolves before the metastases manifest themselves. Destruction of the nasal septum produces the characteristic *tapir nose.* Erosion of the hard palate and larynx may render the patient aphonic. In blacks, the lesions are often large, hypertrophic, polypoid masses that deform the lips and cheeks. Fever, anemia, weight loss, and secondary bacterial infections are common.

Primary progressive lesion

Destructive oral and nasal lesions

Management. The diagnosis is made by finding the organisms in the lesions as described for localized cutaneous leishmaniasis. As the propensity to metastasize to mucocutaneous sites is specific to certain species and subspecies, precise identification of the responsible organism as described in the introduction is of clinical import. The leishmanin skin test yields positive results, and most patients have detectable antibodies.

Treatment is accomplished with pentavalent antimonial agents or amphotericin B, as described for kala azar. Advanced lesions are often refractory, and relapse is common. Cured patients are immune to reinfection. Control measures, other than insect repellents and screening of dwellings, are impractical because of the sylvatic nature of the disease.

Diffuse Cutaneous Leishmaniasis

Skin lesions resemble lepromatous leprosy; no cellular immune response

Diffuse cutaneous leishmaniasis is an unusual disease seen primarily in Ethiopia, Brazil, the Dominican Republic, and Venezuela, where it is caused by variants of *L. tropica* and *L. mexicana* that do not stimulate a cellular immune response in the host. Massive dissemination of skin lesions results. The clinical picture bears a striking resemblance to that of lepromatous leprosy. The lesions contain large numbers of organisms, making the diagnosis quite simple. In contrast to all other forms of cutaneous leishmaniasis, the results of the leishmanin skin test are negative. The disease is progressive and very refractory to treatment. Pentamidine and amphotericin B may produce remissions, but cure is rare.

Disseminated Visceral Leishmaniasis (Kala Azar)

Geographic differences in reservoirs and severity

Epidemiology. Kala azar, which is caused by *L. donovani*, occurs in the tropical and subtropical areas of every continent except Australia. Its epidemiologic and clinical patterns vary from area to area. In Africa, rodents serve as the primary reservoir. Human cases occur sporadically, and the disease is often acute and highly lethal. In Eurasia and Latin America, the domestic dog is the most common reservoir. Human disease is endemic, primarily involves children, and runs a subacute to chronic course. In India, the human is the only known reservoir, and transmission is carried out by anthropophilic species of sandflies. The disease recurs in epidemic form at 20-year intervals, when a new cadre of nonimmune children and young adults appears in the community.

Parasites invade macrophages of reticuloendothelial system

Pathogenesis and Pathology. After the host is bitten by an infected sandfly, the parasites disseminate in the bloodstream and are taken up by the macrophages of the spleen, liver, bone marrow, lymph nodes, skin, and small intestine. Histiocytic proliferation in these organs produces enlargement with atrophy or replacement of the normal tissue.

Delayed onset; recurrent fever; chronic disease; diarrhea

Severe systemic manifestations

Clinical Manifestations. Symptoms appear 3–12 months after acquisition of the parasite. Fever, which is usually present, may be abrupt or gradual in onset. It persists for 2–8 weeks and then disappears, only to reappear at irregular intervals during the course of the disease. A double-quotidian pattern (two fever spikes in a single day) is a characteristic, but uncommon, finding. Diarrhea and malabsorption are frequent in Indian cases, resulting in progressive weight loss and weakness. Physical findings include enlarged lymph nodes and liver, massively enlarged spleen, and edema. In light-skinned individuals, a grayish pigmentation of the face and hands is commonly seen, which gives the disease its name (kala azar = black disease). Anemia with resulting pallor and tachycardia are typical in advanced cases. Thrombocytopenia induces petechial formation and mucosal bleeding. The peripheral leukocyte count is usually less than $4000/mm^3$; agranulocytosis with secondary bacterial infections contributes to lethality. Serum immunoglobulin G levels are enormously elevated, but play no protective role. Circulating antigen-antibody complexes are present and

Immune complex glomerulonephritis

are probably responsible for the glomerulonephritis seen so often in this disease.

Search for Leishman-Donovan bodies

Management. The diagnosis is made by demonstrating the presence of the organism in aspirates taken from the bone marrow, liver, spleen, or lymph nodes. In the Indian form of kala azar, *L. donovani* is also found in circulating monocytes. The specimens may be smeared, stained, and examined for the typical Leishman-Donovan bodies (amastigotes in mononuclear phagocytes) or cultured in artificial media and/or experimental animals. Serologic tests are available, but lack sensitivity and specificity. Results of the leishmanin skin test are negative during active disease, but become positive after successful therapy.

High mortality without treatment

The mortality in untreated cases of kala azar is 75–90%. Treatment with pentavalent antimonial drugs lower this rate dramatically. Initial therapy, however, fails in up to 30% of African cases, and 15% of those that do respond eventually relapse. Resistant cases are treated with the more toxic pentamidine or amphotericin B.

Control measures are directed at the *Phlebotomus* vector, with the use of residual insecticides, and at the elimination of mammalian reservoirs by treating human cases and destroying infective dogs.

African Trypanosomiasis (Sleeping Sickness)

Definition. African trypanosomiasis is a highly lethal meningoencephalitis transmitted to humans by bloodsucking flies of the genus *Glossina*. It occurs in two distinct clinical and epidemiologic forms: West African or Gambian sleeping sickness and East African or Rhodesian sleeping sickness. Nagana, a disease of cattle caused by a closely related trypanosome, renders over 10 million square kilometers of Central Africa unsuitable for animal husbandry.

West and East African sleeping sickness

Organism. The trypanosomes that produce these diseases are morphologically and serologically identical. Accordingly, they are considered varieties of a single species, *Trypanosoma brucei*. The three subspecies, known as *T. brucei gambiense*, *T. brucei rhodesiense*, and *T. brucei brucei*, can be distinguished by their biologic and enzymatic characteristics and mitochondrial morphology. All undergo similar development changes in the course of their passage from insect to mammalian host. Upon ingestion by the tsetse fly (*Glossina* sp.) and after a period of multiplication in the midgut, they migrate to the insect's salivary glands and assume the epimastigote form. After a period of weeks they are transformed into metacyclic trypomastigotes, which renders them infectious to mammals. When the fly again takes a blood meal, the parasite is inoculated with the fly's saliva. In the mammal, they continue to multiply extracellularly and eventually invade the bloodstream. During the initial stages of parasitemia, the trypomastigotes elongate to become graceful, slender organisms 30 μm or more in length. For reasons independent of the host's immune response, multiplication eventually slows, and some forms lose their flagella and assume a short, stumpy appearance. Near the end of the episode of parasitemia, both morphologic types may be seen in a single blood specimen. Regardless of their morphology, all trypomastigotes possess a highly immunogenic glycoprotein surface coat. Individual strains of *T. brucei* can change the antigenic character of this coat in a sequential and, at times, predictable fashion. A strain is capable of producing dozens, perhaps hundreds, of these variable antigen types, each of which is encoded in its own structural gene. The genetic repertoire seems to be strain specific. Expression of individual genes appears to be controlled by the sequential duplication and subsequent transfer of each gene (expression-linked copy) to one or more areas of the genome responsible for gene expression.

Three recognized subspecies of *T. brucei*

Development cycle in tsetse fly

Trypomastigote forms in bloodstream of mammalian host

Antigenic variation of glycoprotein coat of trypomastigotes is due to shifting expression of preexisting genes

Epidemiology. The tsetse fly, and consequently sleeping sickness, is confined to the central area of Africa by that continent's two great deserts, the Sahara in the north and the Kalahari in the south. Approximately 50 million people live in this area and 10,000 to 20,000 acquire sleeping sickness annually. Major outbreaks have been reported in several locations within the endemic area over the past two decades. Riverine tsetse flies found in the forest galleries that border the streams of West and Central Africa serve as the vectors of the Gambian disease. Although these flies are not exclusively anthropophilic, humans are thought to be the major reservoir of the parasite. The infection rate in humans is affected by proximity to water, but seldom exceeds 2–3% in nonepidemic situations. Nevertheless, the extreme chronicity of the human disease ensures its continued transmission.

> Humans major reservoir of West African sleeping sickness; chronicity ensures maintenance

Rhodesian sleeping sickness, in contrast, is transmitted by flies indigenous to the great savannas of East Africa that feed on the blood of the small antelope inhabiting these areas. The antelope serves as the major parasite reservoir, although human-to-human and cattle-to-human spread has been documented. Humans typically become infected only when they enter the savanna to hunt or to graze their domestic animals.

> Savanna antelopes are reservoirs of East African trypanosomiasis; humans infected incidentally

Pathology and Pathogenesis. Multiplication of the trypomastigotes at the inoculation site produces a localized inflammatory lesion. After the development of this chancre, organisms spread through lymphatic channels to the bloodstream, inducing a proliferative enlargement of the lymph nodes. The subsequent parasitemia is typically low grade and recurrent. As host antibodies (predominantly IgM) are produced to the surface antigen characteristic of a particular parasitemic wave, they bind to the organism leading to its destruction by lysis and opsonization. The trypomastigotes disappear from the blood, reappearing 3–8 days later as new antigenic variants arise. The recurrences gradually become less regular and frequent, but may persist for weeks to years before finally disappearing. During the course of the parasitemia, trypanosomes localize in the small blood vessels of the heart and central nervous sytem. This localization results in endothelial proliferation and a perivascular infiltration of plasma cells and lymphocytes. In the brain, hemorrhage and a demyelinating panencephalitis may follow.

> Local chancre at site of inoculation and lymphadenitis
>
> Intermittent parasitemia with antigenic shifts
>
> Parasites localize in blood vessels of heart and central nervous system with local vasculitis

The mechanism by which the trypanosomes elicit vasculitis is uncertain. The infection stimulates the production of large quantities of immunoglobulin M (typically 8–16 times the normal limit). In part, this reaction represents specific protective antibodies that are ultimately responsible for the control of the parasitemia. Much, however, consists of nonspecific heterophile antibodies and rheumatoid factor. Antibody-induced destruction of trypanosomes releases nuclear and cytoplasmic antigens with the production of circulating immune complexes. Many authorities believe that these complexes are largely responsible for the anemia and vasculitis seen in this disease.

> High levels of immunoglobulin M
>
> Immune complexes may cause anemia and vasculitis

Clinical Manifestations. The trypanosomal chancre appears 2–3 days after the bite of the tsetse fly as a raised, reddened nodule on one of the exposed surfaces of the body. With the onset of parasitemia 2–3 weeks later, the patient develops recurrent bouts of fever, tender lymphadenopathy, skin rash, headache, and impaired mentation. In the Rhodesian form of disease, myocarditis and central nervous system involvement begin within 3–6 weeks. Heart failure, convulsions, coma, and death follow in 6–9 months. Gambian sleeping sickness progresses more slowly. Bouts of fever often

> Local lesion
>
> Parasitemic manifestations 2–3 weeks later
>
> Central nervous system involvement

persist for years before central nervous system manifestations gradually appear. Spontaneous activity progressively diminishes, attention wavers, and the patient must be prodded to eat or talk. Speech grows indistinct, tremors develop, sphincter control is lost, and seizures with transient bouts of paralysis occur. In the terminal stage, the patient develops a lethal intercurrent infection or lapses into a final coma.

Laboratory Diagnosis.   The diagnosis is made by microscopically examining lymph node aspirates, blood, or cerebrospinal fluid for the presence of trypomastigotes. Often the actively motile organisms can be seen in a simple wet mount preparation; definitive identification requires examination of an appropriately stained smear. If these tests prove negative, they are repeated after concentrating the organisms by centrifugation or filtration. Inoculation of rats or mice can also prove helpful in diagnosing the Rhodesian disease. The patient may also be screened for elevated levels of immunoglobulin M in the blood and spinal fluid or specific trypanosomal antibodies. A card agglutination test, which can be performed on finger-stick blood, can provide serologic confirmation within minutes.

Treatment.   Lumbar puncture must always be performed before initiation of therapy. If the specimen reveals evidence of central nervous system involvement, agents that penetrate the blood-brain barrier must be included. Unfortunately, the most effective agent of this type is a highly toxic arsenical, melarsoprol (Mel B). Although this agent occasionally produces a lethal hemorrhagic encephalopathy, the invariably fatal outcome of untreated central nervous system disease warrants its use. The ornithine decarboxylase inhibitor, DL-α-difluoromethylornithine, appears capable, when used with suramin, of curing central nervous system disease without the serious side effects associated with Mel B. If current field trials prove successful, it will undoubtedly replace the latter agent. If the central nervous system is not yet involved, less toxic agents such as suramin or pentamidine can be used. In such cases, the cure rate is high and recovery complete.

Prevention.   Although a variety of tsetse fly control measures, including the use of insecticides, deforestation, and the introduction of sterile males into the fly population have been attempted, none has proved totally practicable. Similarly, eradication of disease reservoirs by the early detection and treatment of human cases and the destruction of wild game has had limited success. Attempts to develop effective vaccines are currently under way, but are complicated by the antigenic variability of most trypomastigotes. A degree of personal protection can be achieved with insect repellents and protective clothing. Although prophylactic use of pentamidine was once advocated, enthusiasm for this treatment has waned.

American Trypanosomiasis (Chagas' Disease)

Definition.   American trypanosomiasis is a disease produced by *T. cruzi* and transmitted by true bugs of the family Reduviidae. Clinically, the infection presents as an acute febrile illness in children and a chronic heart or gastrointestinal malady in adults.

Organism.   The trypomastigotes of *T. cruzi* closely resemble those of *T. brucei*, and, like them, disseminate from the site of inoculation to circulate in the peripheral blood of their mammalian hosts. Their developmental

---

Margin notes:

Meningoencephalitis, fatal if untreated

Trypomastigotes sought in lymph node aspirates, blood, and cerebrospinal fluid

Animal inoculation

Selection of drugs dependent on whether central nervous system is involved

Transmission of *T. cruzi* by reduviid bugs

cycle, however, differs in several respects. Most significant, *T. cruzi* does not multiply extracellularly. The circulating trypomastigotes must invade tissue cells, lose their flagella, and assume the amastigote form before binary fission can occur. Continued multiplication leads to distention and eventual rupture of the tissue cell. Released parasites revert to trypomastigotes and regain the bloodstream. This new generation of trypomastigotes may invade other host cells, thus continuing the mammalian cycle. Alternatively, they may be ingested by a feeding reduviid and develop into epimastigotes within its midgut. Upon completion of the invertebrate cycle, the parasites migrate to the hindgut and are discharged as infectious trypomastigotes when the reduviid defecates in the process of taking another blood meal. This process can recur at each feeding for as long as 2 years. Infection in the new host is initiated when the trypomastigotes contaminate either the feeding site or the mucous membranes.

Trypanosoma cruzi comprises a number of strains, each with its own distinct geographic distribution, tissue preference, and virulence. They may be distinguished from one another with specific antisera and by differences in their isoenzyme and DNA restriction patterns. All are morphologically identical. In blood specimens, the trypomastigotes can be distinguished from those of *T. brucei* by their characteristic C or U shape, narrow undulating membrane, and large kinetoplast.

Epidemiology. Chagas' disease affects 15 to 20 million people living in South and Central America. Within these areas, it is the leading cause of heart disease, accounting for one-quarter of all deaths in the 25- to 44-year age group. *Trypanosoma cruzi* has been found in both vertebrate and invertebrate hosts in the southwestern United States, and serologic evidence suggests that human infections are not uncommon in this area. To date, however, few have been clinically apparent.

Transmission occurs almost exclusively in rural areas where the reduviid can find harborage in animal burrows and in the cracked walls and thatch of poorly constructed buildings. This large (3-cm), winged insect leaves its hiding place at night to feed on its sleeping hosts. Its predilection to bite near the eyes or lips have earned this pest the nicknames of "kissing bug" and "assassin bug."

In addition to humans, a number of wild and domestic animals, including rats, cats, dogs, opossums, and armadillos, serve as reservoirs. The close association of many of these hosts with human dwellings tends to amplify the incidence of disease in humans and the difficulty involved in its control. Congenital and transfusion-related infections are rapidly increasing problems in endemic areas.

Pathogenesis and Pathology. Multiplication of the parasite at the portal of entry stimulates the accumulation of neutrophils, lymphocytes, and tissue fluid, resulting in the formation of a local chancre or chagoma. The subsequent dissemination of the organism with invasion of tissue cells produces a febrile illness that may persist for 1–3 months and result in widespread organ damage. Any nucleated host cell may be involved, but those of mesenchymal origin, especially the heart, skeletal muscle, smooth muscle, and glial nerve cells, are particularly susceptible. Intracellular multiplication results in formation of a *pseudocyst*, a greatly enlarged and distorted host cell containing masses of amastigotes. With the rupture of the pseudocyst, many of the released organisms disintegrate, eliciting an intense imflammatory reaction with destruction of surrounding tissue. The development of an antibody-dependent, cell-mediated immune response

---

Margin notes (left column):

Mammalian cycle with nondividing extracellular trypomastigotes and dividing intracellular amastigotes

Invertebrate cycle in bug

Bug may remain infectious for up to 2 years

Geographic distribution of Chagas' disease

Nocturnal transmission in rural areas

"Kissing bug"

Other reservoirs and modes of transmission

Local lesion at site of inoculation

Dissemination and invasion of tissue cells

Pseudocysts in host cells

leads to the eventual destruction of the *T. cruzi* parasites and the termination of the acute phase of illness. Parasitic antigens released during this acute phase may bind to the surface of tissue cells rendering them susceptible to destruction by the host's immune response. It has been suggested by some that this results in the production of antibodies that cross-react with host tissue, initiating a sustained autoimmune inflammatory reaction in the absence of systemic manifestation of illness. In the heart, this reaction leads to loss of muscle tissue, interstitial fibrosis, and degenerative changes in the mycocardial conduction system. In the digestive tract, loss of both ganglionic nerve cells and smooth muscle results in dilatation and loss of peristaltic movement, particularly of the esophagus and colon.

Clinical Manifestations. Serologic studies suggest that only one-third of newly infected individuals develop clinical illness. Acute manifestations, when they occur, are seen primarily in children. They begin with the appearance of the nodular, erythematous chagoma 1–3 weeks after the bite of the reduviid. If the eye served as a portal of entry, the patient will present with Romaña's sign: reddened eye, swollen lid, and enlarged preauricular lymph node. The onset of parasitemia is signaled by the development of a sustained fever; enlargement of the liver, spleen, and lymph nodes; and the appearance of peripheral edema or a transient skin rash. Heart involvement results in tachycardia, electrocardiographic changes, and occasionally arrhythmia and enlargement. Newborns may experience acute meningoencephalitis. Clinical manifestations persist for weeks to months. In 5–10% of untreated patients, severe myocardial involvement or meningoencephalitis leads to death.

Chronic disease, the result of end-stage organ damage, is usually seen only in adulthood. Ironically, the majority of patients with late manifestations deny a history of acute illness. The most serious of the late manifestations is heart disease, which may present as arrhythmia, heart block, enlargement with congestive heart failure, and cardiac arrest. In some areas of rural Latin America, as much as 10% of the adult population may show cardiac manifestations. Megaesophagus and megacolon, which are less devastating than the heart disease, are typically seen in more southern latitudes. This geographic variation in clinical manifestations is thought to be attributable to a difference in tissue tropism between individual strains of *T. cruzi*. Megaesophagus leads to difficulty in swallowing and regurgitation, particularly at night. Megacolon produces severe constipation with irregular passage of voluminous stools.

Laboratory Diagnosis. The diagnosis of acute Chagas' disease rests on finding the trypomastigotes from the peripheral blood and their morphologic identification at *T. cruzi*. The methods are similar to those described for diagnosis of African trypanosomiasis. If results are negative, a laboratory-raised reduviid can be fed on the patient, then dissected and examined for the presence of parasites, a procedure known as *xenodiagnosis*. Alternatively, the blood may be cultured in a variety of artificial media or experimental animals. In the diagnosis of chronic disease, recovery of the organisms is the exception rather than the rule, and diagnosis depends upon the clinical, epidemiologic, and serologic findings.

Treatment. The role of treatment in Chagas' disease remains unsettled. Until recently, no effective chemotherapeutic agent was available. At present, nitrofuramox is used to treat acute disease; however, whether

---

Immunity and immunologic damage to heart

Loss of ganglionic and smooth muscle cells in digestive tract

Most infections asymptomatic; acute disease usually in children

Myocardial and central nervous system signs

Chronic cardiac disease in adults

Dilatation of esophagus and colon

Search for trypomastigotes

Xenodiagnosis

Culture usually unrewarding in chronic disease.

this agent is curative or simply suppresses *T. cruzi* is debatable. It appears to have a negligible effect on chronic disease.

Control of reduviid bugs in rural homes

Prevention. The reduviid vector can be controlled by applying residual insecticides to rural buildings at 2- or 3-month intervals. The addition of latex to the insecticide creates a colorless paint that prolongs activity. Fumigants can be used to prevent reinfection. Patching wall cracks, cementing floors, and moving debris and woodpiles away from human dwellings will reduce the number of reduviids within the home. Transfusion-induced disease in endemic areas can be prevented by adding gentian violet to all blood packs before use or by screening potential donors serologically for Chagas' disease. Immunoprophylaxis is not available at present.

Additional Reading

Adler, S. 1959. Darwin's illness. *Nature* (London) 184:1102–1103. The author describes Charles Darwin's 40-year illness and offers convincing arguments that it represented Chagas' disease acquired during Darwin's round-the-world expedition on H.M.S. *Beagle.*

Barker, D.C. 1987. DNA diagnosis of human leishmaniasis. *Parasitol. Today* 3:177–184. This article describes the techniques available for the characterization of leishmanial DNA and their utility in the separation of these organisms.

Jordan, A.M. 1979. Trypanosomiasis control and land use in Africa. *Outlook Agric.* 10:2123. This article discusses the impact of animal trypanosomiasis on the utilization of land in tropical Africa.

Marsden, P.D. 1984. Selective primary health care: Strategies for control of disease in the developing world. XIV. Leishmaniasis. *Rev. Infect. Dis.* 6:736–744. An excellent concise review of the agent, clinical disease, epidemiology, and control.

Marsden, P.D. 1984. Selective primary health care: Strategies for control of disease in the developing world. XVI. Chagas' disease. *Rev. Infect. Dis.* 6:855–865. Another excellent review of the etiology, disease, epidemiology, and disease control methods.

Moore, G.T., Cross, W.M., McGuire, C.D., et al. 1969. Epidemic giardiasis at a ski resort. *N. Engl. J. Med.* 281:402–407. This and the report of Walzer et al. are two of the early studies to document the pathogenicity of *Giardia lamblia* and its transmission via water supplies.

Pearson, R.D., Wheeler, D.A., Harrison, L.H. et al. 1983. The immunology of Leishmaniasis. *Rev. Infect. Dis.* 5:907–927.

Phillips, S.C., Mildvan, D., Williams, D.C., et al. 1981. Sexual transmission of enteric protozoa and helminths in a venereal-disease clinic population. *N. Engl. J. Med.* 305:603–606. These authors establish that homosexual men have a higher prevalence with *Entamoeba histolytica* and *Giardia lamblia* and that the association between these infections and oral–anal sex is significant.

Rein, M.F., and Muller, M. 1984. *Trichomonas vaginalis.* In *Sexually Transmitted Diseases.* Holmes, K.K., Mardh, P.A., Sparling, P.H., Wiesner, P.J., Eds. New York: McGraw-Hill Book Co., Chap 50, pp. 525–536. Most recent comprehensive review of this parasite and associated disease.

Stevens, D.P. 1985. Selective primary health care: Strategies for control of disease in the developing world. XIX. Giardiasis. *Rev. Infect. Dis.* 7:530–535. A brief summary of the worldwide problem with giardiasis with discussion of the relative roles of chemotherapy, sanitation, and immunization in the control of this disease.

Teixeira, A.R.L. 1979. Chagas' disease: Trends in immunological research and prospects for immunoprophylaxis. *Bull. WHO* 57:697–710. The current state of knowledge regarding the immunopathogenesis of chronic Chagas' disease is lucidly recapitulated.

Walzer, P.D., Wolfe, M.S., and Schultz, M.G. 1971. Giardiasis in travelers. *J. Infect. Dis.* 124:235–237.

55

Intestinal Nematodes

James J. Plorde

James J. Plorde

The intestinal nematodes have cylindric, fusiform bodies covered with a tough acellular cuticle. Sandwiched between this integument and the body cavity are layers of muscle, longitudinal nerve trunks, and an excretory system. A tubular alimentary tract consisting of a mouth, esophagus, midgut, and anus runs from the anterior to the posterior extremity. Highly developed reproductive organs fill the remainder of the body cavity. The sexes are separate; the male worm is generally smaller than his mate. The female, which is extremely prolific, can produce thousands of offspring, generally in the form of eggs. Typically, the eggs must incubate or embryonate outside of the human host before they become infectious to another person; during this time, the embryo repeatedly segments, eventually developing into an adolescent form known as a *larva*. In some species of nematodes, offspring develop to the larval stage in the uterus of the worm. The duration and site of embryonation differ with each worm species and determine how it will be transmitted to the new host. In many cases, eggs of nematodes that dwell within the human gastrointestinal tract are carried to the environment in the feces and embryonate on the soil for a period of weeks before becoming infectious. The egg may then be ingested with contaminated food. In some species, the egg hatches outside of the host, releasing a larva capable of penetrating the skin of a person who comes in direct physical contact with it. Obviously, intestinal nematodes are principally found in areas where human feces are deposited indiscriminately or used for fertilizer.

There are six intestinal nematodes that commonly infect humans: *Enterobius vermicularis* (the pinworm), *Trichuris trichuria* (the whipworm), *Ascaris lumbricoides* (the large roundworm), *Necator americanus* and *Ancylostoma duodenale* (the hookworms), and *Strongyloides stercoralis* (Table 55.1). Together they infect more than one-quarter of the human race, producing embarrassment, discomfort, malnutrition, anemia, and occasionally death. Other closely related nematodes of animals that may oc-

Significance of duration and site of embryonation

Members of group

Nematode

749

Table 55.1   Intestinal Nematodes

Human Parasite	Animal Parasite	Human Disease
Enterobius vermicularis (pinworm)		Enterobiasis
Trichuris trichuria (whipworm)		Trichuriasis
	Capillaria philippinensis	Intestinal capillariasis
Ascaris lumbricoides (large roundworm)		Ascariasis
	Ascaris suum	Ascariasis
	Anisakis sp.	Anisakiasis
	Toxocara canis	Toxocariasis (visceral larva migrans)
	Toxocara cati	
Necator americanus (hookworm)		Hookworm disease
Ancylostoma duodenale (hookworm)		
	Ancylostoma braziliense	Cutaneous larva migrans
Strongyloides stercoralis		Strongyloidiasis

casionally infect humans are also listed in Table 55.1, but will not be discussed here.

The adults of each of the six nematodes listed previously can survive for months or years within the lumen of the gut. The severity of illness produced by each depends upon the level of adaptation to the host it has achieved. Some species have a simple life cycle that can be completed without serious consequences to the host. Less well-adapted parasites, on the other hand, have more complex cycles, often requiring tissue invasion and/or production of enormous numbers of offspring to ensure their continued survival and dissemination. Within a given species, disease severity is related directly to the number of adult worms harbored by the host. The greater the worm load or worm burden, the more serious the consequences. As nematodes do not multiply within the human, small worm loads may remain asymptomatic and undetected throughout the life span of the parasite. Repeated infections, however, will progressively increase the worm burden and, at some point, induce symptomatic disease. Although humans can mount an immune response that will eventually lead to the expulsion of worms, it is slow to develop and incomplete. It is therefore the frequency and intensity of reinfection, more than the host's immune response, that determine the worm burden.

Long survival in gut lumen

Relationship of parasitic adaptation to disease

Importance of worm load and repeated infection

Immune response slow and incomplete

Life Cycles

The life cycles of the intestinal nematodes are summarized in Table 55.2. *Enterobius vermicularis* (pinworm), the best adapted of the intestinal nematodes, has the simplest life cycle. It feeds, grows, and copulates within the gut of its host before transiting the anus to deposit its eggs on the perineal skin. The eggs embryonate within hours and are subsequently transported to the same, or a new, host via fingers or dust. Following their inhalation or ingestion, the eggs are swallowed and hatch in the bowel lumen, completing the cycle. The only significant difference between this

Enterobius vermicularis is the best adapted intestinal nematode

Table 55.2 Life Cycles of Intestinal Nematodes

Parasite	Route of Infection	Migration in Body	Diagnostic Form	Site of Embryonation	Infective Form	Free-Living Cycle
Enterobius vermicularis	Mouth	Intestinal	Egg	Perineum	Egg	No
Trichuris trichuria	Mouth	Intestinal	Egg	Soil	Egg	No
Ascaris lumbricoides	Mouth	Pulmonary	Egg	Soil	Egg	No
Necator americanus[a]	Skin	Pulmonary	Egg	Soil	Filariform larvae	No
Stronglyoides stercoralis	Skin	Pulmonary	Rhabditiform larvae	Soil; intestine[b]	Filariform larvae	Yes

Reproduced with permission from Plorde, J.J. in Isselbacher et al. *Harrison's Principles of Internal Medicine,* 9th ed. 1980. McGraw-Hill, Inc. Table 206–3, p. 891.

[a] Also *Ancylostoma duodenale.*

[b] Intestine only in cases of autoinfection.

and the life cycle of *Trichuris trichuria* (whipworm) is that the eggs of the latter are passed in the stool and must incubate on soil before becoming infectious. This relatively minor difference has profound epidemiologic ramifications, because *Trichuris* can be passed only in populations that practice indiscriminate defecation and live in climates suitable for the maturation of eggs in the soil.

Other nematodes have increasingly complex life cycles

Ascaris lumbricoides is transmitted in a manner similar to *T. trichuria.* However, after hatching from the egg in the gut lumen, ascarid larvae penetrate the bowel wall and migrate through the host's liver and lung before returning, older and more sedentary, to the protective environment of the gut lumen. This maladaptive sojourn of juvenile worms through the host tissue is also seen in the life cycles of the hookworms and *Strongyloides stercoralis.* In contrast to *Ascaris,* however, the eggs of the latter two nematodes hatch shortly before or after they are passed in the stool of the original host, resulting in the seeding of the external environment with larval forms capable of penetrating human skin. Transmission is effected when a new host comes into physical contact with the contaminated soil. The adaptation of *S. stercoralis* is the least satisfactory of the intestinal nematodes and, in an evolutionary sense, appears to have occurred quite recently. In addition to the hookwormlike cycle described above, it has the twin capacities to complete its life cycle entirely within the body of the host or to survive in the external environment as a free-living soil organism.

Strongyloides stercoralis is least well adapted

Parasites and Diseases

Enterobiasis

Common name is pinworm

Organism. The adult female is a 10-mm-long, cream-colored worm with a sharply pointed tail, characteristics that have given rise to the common name *pinworm.* Running longitudinally down both sides of the body are small ridges that widen anteriorly to finlike alae. The seldom seen male is smaller (3 mm) and possesses a ventrally curved tail and copulatory spicule. The clear, thin-shelled, ovoid eggs are flattened on one side and measure 25 × 50 μm (Figure 55.1).

Adults inhabit cecum

Life Cycle. The adult worms lie attached to the mucosa of the cecum.

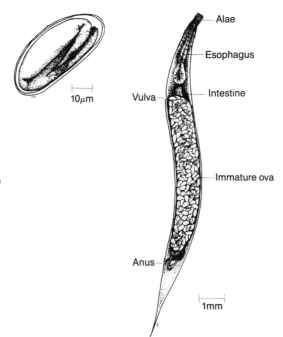

55.1 Female pinworm (*Enterobius vermicularis*) and embryonated egg.

Female transits anus at night to deposit eggs on perineum

Eggs infectious to host and others shortly after deposition

Ingested eggs hatch and larvae mature to adults in intestine

As her period of gravidity draws to a close, the female migrates down the colon, slips unobserved through the anal canal in the dark of the night, and deposits 20,000 sticky eggs on the host's perianal skin, bedclothes, and linens. The eggs are near maturity at the time of deposition and become infectious shortly thereafter. Handling of bedclothes or scratching of the perianal area to relieve the associated itching results in adhesion of the eggs to the fingers and subsequent transfer to the oral cavity during eating or other finger–mouth maneuvers. Alternatively, the eggs may be shaken into the air (for example, during making of the bed), inhaled, and swallowed. The eggs subsequently hatch in the upper intestine and the larvae migrate to the cecum, maturing to adults and mating in the process. The entire adult-to-adult cycle is completed in 2 weeks.

Epidemiology. The pinworm is the oldest and most widespread of the helminths. Eggs have been found in a 10,000-year-old coprolith, making this nematode the oldest demonstrated infectious agent of humans. It has been estimated to infect at least 200 million people worldwide, 30–40 million in the United States alone. In that country and in western Europe, it is the single most common cause of human helminthiasis. Infection is more common among the young and poor, but may be found in any age or economic class. The incidence in white individuals is significantly higher than that in blacks.

Infects 30–40 million in United States

Resistant infective eggs

The eggs are relatively resistant to desiccation and may remain viable in linens, bedclothes, or house dust for several days. Once infection is introduced into a household, other family members are rapidly infected.

Pathogenesis and Immunity. The adult worms produce no significant intestinal pathology and do not appear to induce protective immunity.

Clinical Manifestations. *Enterobius vermicularis* seldom produces serious

Nocturnal pruritis ani

disease. The most frequent symptom is pruritis ani (anal itching). This symptom is most severe at night and has been attributed to the migration of the gravid female. It may lead to irritability and other minor complaints. In severe infections, the intense itching may lead to scratching, excoriation, and secondary bacterial infection. In female patients, the worm may enter the genital tract, producing vaginitis, granulomatous endometritis, or even salpingitis. It has also been suggested that migrating worms might carry enteric bacteria into the urinary bladder in young women, inducing an acute bacterial infection of the urinary tract. Although this worm is frequently found in the lumen of the resected appendix, it is doubtful that it plays a causal role in appendicitis. Perhaps the most serious effect of this common infection is the psychic trauma suffered by the economically advantaged when they discover that they, too, are subject to intestinal worm infection.

Occasional infection of female genitourinary tract

Laboratory Diagnosis. Eosinophilia is usually absent. The diagnosis is suggested by the clinical manifestations and confirmed by the recovery of the characteristic eggs from the anal mucosa. Identification is accomplished by applying the sticky side of cellophane tape to the mucocutaneous junction, then transferring the tape to a glass slide and examining the slide under the low-power lens of a microscope. Occasionally, the adult female will be seen by a parent of an infected child or recovered with the cellophane tape procedure.

Anal cellophane tape test for ova

Treatment and Prevention. Several highly satisfactory agents, including pyrantel pamoate and mebendazole, are available for treatment. Many authorities believe that all members of a family or other cohabiting group should be treated simultaneously. In severe infections, retreatment after 2 weeks is recommended. Although cure rates are high, reinfection is extremely common. It need not be treated in the absence of symptoms.

All family members may need treatment

Reinfection common

Trichuriasis

Organism. The adult whipworm is 30–50 mm in length. The anterior two-thirds is thin and threadlike, whereas the posterior end is bulbous, giving the worm the appearance of a tiny whip. The tail of the male is coiled, that of the female straight. The female produces 3000–10,000 oval eggs each day. They are of the same size as pinworm eggs, but have a distinctive thick brown shell with translucent knobs on both ends (Figure 55.2).

Whipworm

Life Cycle. *Trichuris trichuria* has a life cycle that differs from that of the pinworm only in its external phase. The adults live attached to the colonic mucosa by their thin anterior end. While retaining her position in the cecum, the gravid female releases her eggs into the lumen of the gut. These pass out of the body with the feces and, in poorly sanitated areas of the world are deposited on soil. The eggs are immature at the time of passage and must incubate for at least 10 days (longer if soil conditions, temperature, and moisture are suboptimal) before they become fully embryonated and infectious. Once mature, they are picked up on the hands of children at play or of agricultural workers and passed to the mouth. In areas where human feces are used as fertilizer, raw fruits and vegetables may be contaminated and later ingested. Following ingestion, the eggs hatch in the duodenum, and the released larvae mature for approximately

Adults inhabit cecum

Eggs must mature in soil

No direct person-to-person transmission

Larvae from ingested eggs mature to adults in intestines

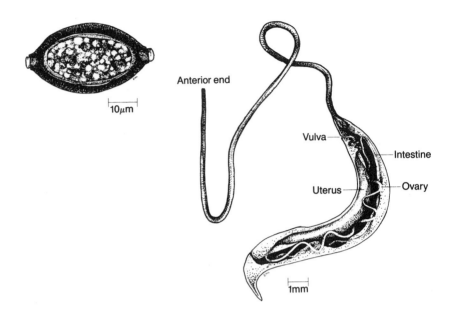

55.2 Female whipworm (*Trichuris trichura*) and unembryonated egg.

1 month in the small bowel before migrating to their adult habitat in the cecum.

Epidemiology. Although it is less widespread than the pinworm, the whipworm is a cosmopolitan parasite, infecting approximately 1 billion people throughout the world. It is concentrated in areas where indiscriminate defecation and a warm, humid environment produce extensive seeding of soil with infectious eggs. In tropical climates, infection rates may be as high as 80%. Although the incidence is much lower in temperate climates trichuriasis affects 2 million individuals throughout the rural areas of the southeastern United States. Here it occurs primarily in family and institutional clusters, presumably maintained by the poor sanitary habits of toddlers and the mentally retarded. Although the intensity of infection is generally low, adult worms may live 4–8 years.

Pathogenesis and Immunity. Attachment of adult worms to the colonic mucosa and their subsequent feeding activities produce localized ulceration and hemorrhage (0.005 ml blood per worm per day). The ulcers provide enteric bacteria with a portal of entry to the bloodstream and, occasionally, a sustained bacteremia results. A decrease in the prevalence of trichuriasis in the postadolescent period and the demonstration of acquired immunity in experimental animal infections suggest that immunity may develop in naturally acquired human infections.

Clinical Manifestations. Light infections are asymptomatic. With moderate worm loads, damage to the intestinal mucosa may induce nausea, abdominal pain, and diarrhea. Occasionally, a child may harbor 800 worms or more. In these situations, the entire colonic mucosa is parasitized, with significant mucosal damage, blood loss, and anemia. The shear force of the fecal stream on the bodies of the worms may produce prolapse of the colonic or rectal mucosa through the anus, particularly when the host is straining at defecation or childbirth. The sudden appearance of a prolapsed

Margin notes (left column):

Associated with defecation on soil and warm, humid climate

Longevity of worms

Local colonic ulceration provides potential entry point for bacteria

Colonic damage with severe infection

Colonic or rectal prolapse

rectum teeming with hundreds of wriggling whipworms has been known to produce nausea and lightheadedness in uninitiated obstetricians.

Laboratory Diagnosis. In light infections, stool concentration methods may be required to recover the eggs. Such procedures are almost never necessary in symptomatic infections, as they inevitably produce more than 10,000 eggs per gram of feces, a density readily detected by examining 1–2 mg of emulsified stool with the low-power lens of a microscope. A moderate eosinophilia is common in such infections.

Stool examination for eggs

Treatment. Infections should not be treated unless they are symptomatic. Mebendazole is the drug of choice. Although the cure rate is only 60–70%, more than 90% of the adult worms are usually expelled, rendering the patient asymptomatic. Prevention requires the improvement of sanitary facilities.

Ascariasis

Organism. *Ascaris lumbricoides*, a short-lived worm (6–18 months), is the largest and most common of the intestinal helminths. Measuring 150–350 mm in length, it dwarfs its fellow gut roundworms and brings an unexpected richness to our mental image of a parasite. Its firm, creamy cuticle and more pointed extremities differentiate it from the common earthworm, which it otherwise resembles in both size and external morphology. The male is slightly smaller than the female and possesses a curved tail with copulatory spicules. His mate passes 200,000 eggs daily, whether she is fertilized or not. Eggs are elliptic in shape; measure 35 × 55 μm; and have a rough, mammilated, albuminous coat over their chitinous shells. They are highly resistant to environmental conditions and may remain viable for up to 6 years in mild climates (Figure 55.3).

Earthworm-sized roundworm

Prolonged viability of eggs

Adults inhabit small intestine

Life Cycle. The adult ascarids live high in the small intestine, where they actively maintain themselves by dint of muscular activity. The eggs are deposited into the intestinal lumen and passed in the feces. Like those of *Trichuris*, the eggs must embryonate in soil, usually for a minimum of 3 weeks, before becoming infectious. The similarity to *Trichuris* ends, however, with the ingestion of the eggs by the host. After hatching, the larvae penetrate the intestinal mucosa and invade the portal venules. They are carried to the liver, where they are still small enough to squeeze through that organ's capillaries and exit in the hepatic vein. They are then carried to the right side of the heart and subsequently pumped out to the lung. In the course of this migration, the larvae increase in size. By the time they reach the pulmonary capillaries, they are too large to pass through to the left side of the heart. Finding their route blocked, they rupture into the alveolar spaces, are coughed up, and subsequently swallowed. After regaining access to the upper intestine, they complete their maturation and mate.

Eggs must mature in soil; infection by ingestion

Larvae from ingested eggs enter bloodstream, pass through alveoli and via respiratory tract and esophagus to intestines

Epidemiology. More than 1 billion of the world's population, including 4 million Americans, are infected. Together they have been estimated to pass more than 25,000 tons of *Ascaris* eggs into the environment annually. Like trichuriasis, with which it is coextensive, ascariasis is a disease of warm climates and poor sanitation. It is maintained by small children who defecate indiscriminately in the immediate vicinity of the home and pick up infectious eggs on their hands during play. Geophagia is common and

Epidemiology similar to that of *Trichuris*

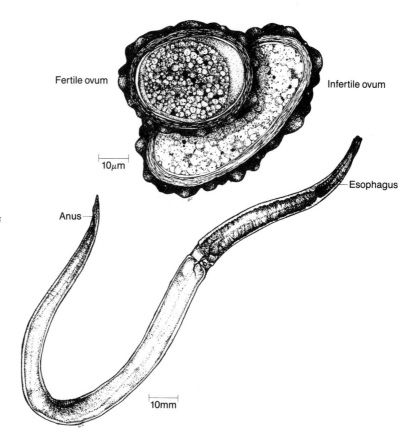

Fertile ovum

Infertile ovum

10μm

Esophagus

Anus

10mm

55.3 Female *Ascaris lumbricoides* worm and fertile and infertile eggs.

may result in massive worm loads. The parasite may also be acquired through ingestion of egg-contaminated food by the host; in dry, windy climates, eggs may become airborne and be inhaled and swallowed. In tropical areas, the entire population may be involved. Isolated infected family clusters are more common in temperate climes.

Pathogenesis and Immunity.   There is convincing evidence that ascariasis induces a protective immune response in the host. Moreover, the severity of pulmonary damage induced by the migration of larvae through the lung appears to be related in part to an immediate hypersensitivity reaction to larval antigens.

Clinical Manifestations.   Clinical manifestations may result from either the migration of the larvae through the lung or the presence of the adults in the intestinal lumen. Pulmonary involvement is usually seen in communities where transmission is seasonal; the severity of symptoms is related to the degree of hypersensitivity induced by previous infections and the intensity of the current exposure. Fever, cough, wheezing, and shortness of breath are common. Laboratory studies reveal eosinophilia, oxygen desaturation, and migratory pulmonary infiltrates. Death from respiratory failure has been noted occasionally.

Hypersensitive pulmonary reactions to larval migration

If the worm load is small, infections with adult worms may be completely asymptomatic. They come to clinical attention when the parasite is vomited up or passed in the stool. This situation is most likely during

Asymptomatic infections with small worm loads

episodes of fever, which appear to stimulate the worms to increase motility. Most physicians who have worked in underdeveloped countries have had the disconcerting experience of observing an ascarid crawl out of a patient's mouth, nose, or ear during an otherwise uneventful evaluation of fever. Occasionally an adult worm will migrate to the appendix, bile duct, or pancreatic duct, causing obstruction and inflammation of the organ. Heavier worm loads may produce abdominal pain and malabsorption of fat, protein, carbohydrate, and vitamins. In marginally nourished children, growth may be retarded. Occasionally a bolus of worms may form and produce intestinal obstruction, particularly in children. Worm loads of 50 are not uncommon, and as many as 2000 worms have been recovered from a single child. In the United States, where worm loads tend to be modest, obstruction occurs in 2 per 1000 infected children per year. The mortality in these cases is 3%.

Laboratory Diagnosis. The diagnosis is generally made by finding the characteristic eggs in the feces. The extreme productivity of the female ascarid generally makes this task an easy one, except when the atypical-appearing unfertilized eggs predominate. The pulmonary phase of ascariasis is diagnosed by the finding of larvae and eosinophils in the sputum.

Treatment and Prevention. Pyrantel pamoate and mebendazole are both highly effective; the latter is preferred if *T. trichuria* is also present. Communitywide control of ascariasis can be achieved with mass therapy administered at 6-month intervals. Ultimately, control requires adequate sanitation facilities.

Hookworm Infections

Organism. Two species, *N. americanus* and *A. duodenale*, infect humans. Adults of both species are pinkish-white and measure about 10 mm in length (Figure 55.4). The head is often curved in a direction opposite that of the body, giving these worms the hooked appearance from which their common name is derived. The males have a unique fan-shaped copulatory bursa, rather than the curved, pointed tail common to the other intestinal nematodes. The two species can be readily differentiated by the morphology of their oral cavity. *Ancylostoma duodenale*, the Old World hookworm, possesses four sharp toothlike structures, whereas *N. americanus*, the New World hookworm, has dorsal and ventral cutting plates. With the aid of these structures, the hookworms attach to the mucosa of the small bowel and suck blood. The fertilized female releases 10,000–20,000 eggs daily. They measure 40×60 μm, possess a thin shell, and are usually in the two- to four-cell stage when passed in the feces (Figure 55.4).

Life Cycle. For all practical purposes, the life cycles of the two hookworms, *N. americanus* and *A. duodenale*, are identical. The eggs are passed in the feces at the 4- to 8-cell stage of development and, on reaching soil, hatch within 48 hr, releasing *rhabditiform larvae*. These move actively through the surface layers of soil, feeding upon bacteria and debris. After doubling in size, they molt to become infective *filariform larvae*, which may survive in moist conditions without feeding, for up to 6 weeks. On contact with human skin, they penetrate the epidermis, reach the lymphohematogenous system, and are passively transported to the right side of the heart and onward to the lungs. Here they rupture into alveolar

Malabsorption and occasional obstruction with heavy worm loads

Stool examination for eggs

N. americanus and *A. duodenale* infect humans

Eggs mature and release rhabditiform larvae in soil

Infective larvae penetrate skin; then follow same path as *Ascaris* larvae to gut

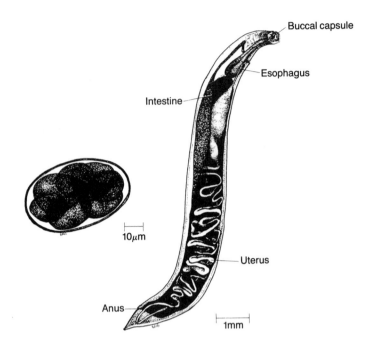

55.4 Female hookworm (*Necator americanus*) and egg.

Buccal capsule

Esophagus

Intestine

Uterus

Anus

10μm

1mm

spaces and, like juvenile ascarids, are coughed up, swallowed, and pass into the small intestine, where they mature to adulthood.

Epidemiology. Hookworm infection is found worldwide between the latitudes of 45° N and 30° S. Transmission requires deposition of egg-containing feces on shady, well-drained soil, development of larvae under conditions of abundant rainfall and high temperatures (23–33°C), and direct contact of unprotected human skin with resulting filariform larvae. Infections become particularly intense in closed, densely populated communities, such as tea and coffee plantations. *Necator americanus* is found in the tropical areas of Asia, Africa, and America, as well as the southern United States, where it was introduced with the African slave trade. *Ancylostoma duodenale* is seen in the Mediterranean basin, the Middle East, northern India, China, and Japan. It has been estimated that together these two worms extract over 7 million L of blood each day from 700 million individuals scattered around the globe, including 700,000 in the United States.

Pathogenesis and Immunity. Each adult *A. duodenale* extracts 0.2 ml of blood daily and *N. americanus* 0.03 ml of blood. Additional blood loss may be related to the tendency of the worms to migrate within the intestine, leaving bleeding points at old sites of attachment. As the adults may survive 2–14 years, the accumulated blood loss may be enormous. The infection elicits both a humoral antibody response and immediate hypersensitivity reaction in the host, but evidence that these moderate the infection is lacking. The peripheral and gut eosinophilia characteristic of this disease may play a role in the destruction of worms and/or modulation of the immediate hypersensitivity reaction.

Clinical Manifestations. In the overwhelming majority of infected patients, the worm burden is small and the infection asymptomatic. Clinical

Larvae hatch under hot moist conditions and traverse unprotected skin

Geographic distribution

Migrate in intestines feeding on blood; bleeding from old attachment sites

Peripheral and gut eosinophilia

Most infections asymptomatic

manifestations, when they do occur, may be related to the original penetration of the skin by the filariform larva, the migration of the larva through the lung, and/or the presence of the adult worm in the gut. Skin penetration may produce a pruritic erythematous rash and swelling, popularly known as *ground itch*. This manifestation is more common in infection with *N. americanus*, generally occurs between the toes, and may persist for several days. It is probably the result of prior sensitization to larval antigens.

Pulmonary manifestations may mimic those seen in ascariasis, but are generally less frequent and less severe. In the gut, the adult worm may produce epigastric pain and abnormal peristalsis. The major manifestations, however—anemia and hypoalbuminemia—are the result of chronic blood loss. The severity of the anemia depends upon the worm burden and intake of dietary iron. If iron intake exceeds iron loss resulting from hookworm infection, a normal hematocrit will be maintained. Commonly, however, dietary iron is ingested in a form that is poorly absorbed. As a result, severe anemia may develop over a period of months or years. In children, this condition may often precipitate heart failure or kwashiorkor. Mental, sexual, and physical development may be retarded.

Laboratory Diagnosis. The diagnosis is made by examining direct or concentrated stool for the distinctive eggs. As they are nearly identical in the two species, precise identification of the causative worm is generally not attempted. Quantitative egg counts can permit accurate estimation of worm load. If the stool is allowed to stand too long before it is examined, the eggs may hatch, releasing rhabditiform larvae. These larvae closely resemble those of *S. stercoralis* and must be differentiated from them.

Treatment and Prevention. The anemia must be corrected. When it is mild or moderate, iron replacement is adequate. More severe anemia may require blood transfusions. The two most widely used antihelminthic agents, pyrantel pamoate and mebendazole, are both highly effective. Prevention requires improved sanitation.

Strongyloidiasis

Organism. *Strongyloides stercoralis* may measure only 2 mm in length, making it the smallest of the intestinal nematodes. The male, which is seldom seen, is probably eliminated from the gut soon after copulation; some authorities believe that the female can conceive parthenogenetically. Be that as it may, the gravid female penetrates the mucosa of the duodenum, where she deposits her eggs. In severe infections, the biliary and pancreatic ducts, the entire small bowel, and the colon may be involved. The eggs hatch quickly, releasing rhabditiform larvae that reenter the bowel lumen and are subsequently passed into the stool. These larvae, which measure about 16×200 µm, can be distinguished from the similar larval stage of the hookworms by their short buccal cavity and large genital primordium (Figures 55.5 and 55.6).

Life Cycle. Three different life cycles have been described for this nematode. The first, or *direct* cycle, is similar to that observed with the hookworms. After rhabditiform larvae are passed in the stool, they molt on soil to become filariform larvae. Filariform larvae can penetrate human skin. After transport to the lung in the vascular system they are coughed up and swallowed and mature to adults in the small bowel. In the second,

Margin notes

Pruritis at site of skin penetration

Pulmonary manifestations

Iron deficiency anemia caused by blood loss from intestinal worms

Detection of eggs in stool

Eggs deposited beneath duodenal mucosa; rhabditiform larvae reenter bowel

Three possible developmental cycles:
1. Resembles hookworm cycle except that larvae passed in stool.
2. Internal and external autoinfection produces increasing worm load.
3. Free-living adults develop and propagate in soil, producing infective larvae

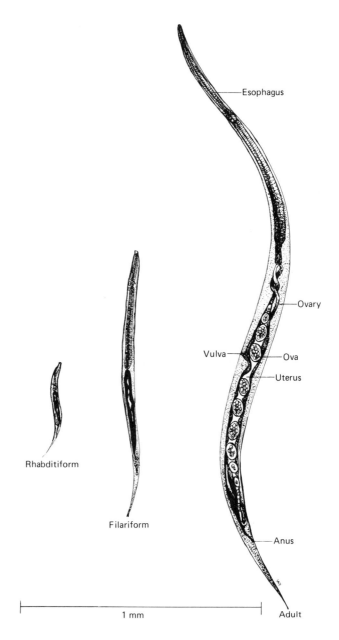

55.5 *Strongyloides stercoralis* worm and rhabditiform and filariform larvae.

or *autoinfective* cycle, the rhabditiform larva's passage through the colon to the outside world is delayed by constipation or other factors, allowing it to transform into an infective filariform larva while still within the body of its host. This larva may then invade the internal mucosa (internal autoinfection) or perianal skin (external autoinfection) without an intervening soil phase. Thus, *S. stercoralis*, unlike any of the other intestinal nematodes, has the capacity to multiply within the body of the host. The worm burden may increase dramatically, and the infection persist indefinitely without the need for reinfection from the environment, often with dire consequence to the host. In the third, or *free-living* cycle, the rhabditiform larvae, after passage in the stool and deposition on the soil, develop into free-living adult males and females. These adults may propagate

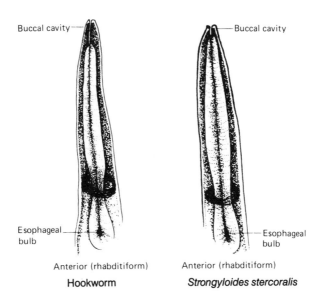

Buccal cavity — Buccal cavity

Esophageal bulb — Esophageal bulb

Anterior (rhabditiform)   Anterior (rhabditiform)

Hookworm   *Strongyloides stercoralis*

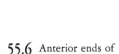

55.6 Anterior ends of hookworm and *Strongyloides stercoralis* rhabditiform larvae.

through several generations of free-living worms before infective filariform larvae are again produced. This cycle creates a soil reservoir that may persist even without continued deposition of feces.

Epidemiology. The distribution of *S. stercoralis* parallels that of the hookworms, although it is less prevalent in all but tropical areas. It infects 400,000 individuals throughout the rural areas of Puerto Rico and the southeastern sections of the continental United States. Although, like hookworm infection, it is generally acquired by direct contact of skin with soil-dwelling larvae, infection may also follow ingestion of filariform-contaminated food. Transformation of the rhabditiform larvae to the filariform stage within the gut can result in seeding of the perianal area with infectious organisms. These larvae may be passed to another person through direct physical contact or autoinfect the original host. In debilitated and immunosuppressed patients, transformation to the filariform stage occurs within the gut itself, producing marked autoinfection or hyperinfection.

Pathogenesis and Immunity. Invasion of the intestinal epithelium may accelerate epithelial cell turnover, alter intestinal motility, and induce acute and chronic inflammatory lesions, ulcerations, and abscess formation, all of which may play a role in the malabsorptive syndrome that frequently characterizes clinical disease. Drug- or malnutrition-related immunosuppression appears to accelerate the metamorphosis of rhabditiform to filariform larvae within the bowel lumen, enhancing the frequency and intensity of autoinfection. There is little evidence that protective immunity develops in the infected host.

Clinical Manifestations. Patients with strongyloidiasis do not generally give a history of ground itch. They do, however, manifest the pulmonary disease seen in both ascariasis and, less often, in hookwork infection. The intestinal infection itself is usually asymptomatic. With heavy worm loads, however, the patient may complain of epigastric pain and tenderness, often aggravated by intake of food. In fact, peptic-ulcer–like pain associated with peripheral eosinophilia strongly suggests the diagnosis of strongy-

Geographic distribution and penetration of skin like that of hookworm

Autoinfection and infection by ingestion of filariform larvae also occurs

Damage to intestinal mucosa may cause malabsorptive syndrome

Immunosuppression enhances risk of autoinfection by accelerating larval development

Pulmonary and intestinal manifestations

loidiasis. With widespread involvement of the intestinal mucosa, vomiting, diarrhea, paralytic ileus, and malabsorption may be seen.

External autoinfection gives lesions of buttocks and back

External autoinfection produces transient, raised, red, serpiginous lesions over the buttocks and lower back that reflect larval invasion of the perianal area. If the patient is not treated, these lesions may recur at irregular intervals over a period of decades; they are particularly common after recovery from a febrile illness. Over 25% of British and American servicemen imprisoned in Southeast Asia during World War II continued to demonstrate such lesions prior to diagnosis and treatment some 40 years after exposure.

Hyperinfection in immunosuppressed host

Massive hyperinfection may occur in immunosuppressed patients, producing severe enterocolitis and widespread dissemination of the larvae to extraintestinal organs, including the heart, lungs, and central nervous system. The larvae may carry enteric bacteria with them, producing Gram-negative bacteremia and occasionally Gram-negative meningitis. Unrecognized and untreated, it usually results in death.

Rhabditiform larvae in stool or duodenal aspirates

Laboratory Diagnosis. The diagnosis is usually made by finding the rhabditiform larvae in the stool. Preferably, only fresh specimens should be examined to avoid the confusion induced by the hatching of hookworm eggs with the release of their look-alike larvae. The number of larvae passed in the stool varies from day to day, often requiring the examination of several specimens before the diagnosis of strongyloidiasis can be made. When absent from the stool, larvae may sometimes be found in duodenal aspirates or jejunal biopsy specimens. If the pulmonary system is involved, the sputum should be examined for the presence of larvae. Serologic tests of adequate sensitivity and specificity have been recently developed, but are not generally available.

Treatment essential

Treatment and Prevention. All infected patients should be treated to prevent the buildup of the worm burden by autoinfection and the serious consequences of hyperinfection. The drug of choice is thiabendazole. In hyperinfection syndromes, therapy must be extended for a week. The cure rate is significantly less than 100%, and stools should be checked after therapy to see if retreatment is indicated. Patients who have resided in an endemic area at some time in their lives should be examined for the presence of this parasite both before and during steroid treatment or im-

Special precautions with hyperinfected patients

munosuppressive therapy. Medical personnel caring for patients with hyperinfection syndromes should wear gowns and gloves, as stool, saliva, vomitus, and body fluids may contain infectious filariform larvae.

Additional Reading

Blumenthal, D.S. 1977. Intestinal nematodes in the United States. *N. Engl. J. Med.* 297:1437–1439.

Davis, A. 1985. Intestinal helminths. In *Epidemiology and the Community Control of Disease in Warm Climate Countries.* 2nd ed. Robinson, D., Ed. Edinburgh: Churchill Livingstone, Chap. 24.

Irga-Siegman, Y., Kapila, R., Sen, P., et al. 1981. Syndrome of hyperinfection with *Strongyloides stercoralis. Rev. Infect. Dis.* 3:397–407.

Pelletier, L.L., Jr. 1984. Chronic strongyloidiasis in World War II Far East ex-prisoners of war. *Am. J. Trop. Med. Hyg.* 33:55–61.

Stevens, D.P. 1978. Quantitative techniques. *Clin. Gastroenterol.* 7:231–238. The relationship of worm burden to severity of disease and need for therapy is discussed.

Wagner, E.D., and Eby, W.C. 1983. Pinworm prevalence in California elementary school children and diagnostic methods. *Am. J. Trop. Med. Hyg.* 32:998–1001.

56

Tissue Nematodes

James J. Plorde

The nematodes discussed in this chapter induce disease through their presence in the tissues and lymphohematogenous system of the human body. They are a heterogenous group. Three of them, *Toxocara canis*, *Trichinella spiralis*, and *Ancylostoma braziliense*, are natural parasites of domestic and wild carnivores. Although capable of infecting humans, they cannot complete their life cycle in this host. Humans therefore serve only as injured bystanders, rather than major participants, in the life cycle of these parasites (Table 56.1).

The remaining four major nematodes, *Wuchereria bancrofti, Brugia malayi, Loa loa,* and *Onchocerca volvulus*, are members of a single superfamily (Filarioidea), and all utilize humans as their natural definitive host (Table 56.1). The thin, threadlike adults live for years in the subcutaneous tissues and lymphatic vessels, where they discharge their liveborn offspring or *microfilariae*. These progeny circulate in the blood or migrate in the subcutaneous tissues until they are ingested by a specific bloodsucking insect. Within this vector, they transform into filariform larvae capable of infecting another human when the invertebrate host again takes a blood meal.

The nematodes considered, the diseases caused, and the usual routes of infection in humans are listed in Table 56.1.

Toxocariasis

Organism

Cycle in canines resembles ascariasis in humans

Toxocara canis is a large, intestinal ascarid of canines, including dogs, foxes, and wolves. Each female worm discharges approximately 200,000 thick-shelled eggs daily into the fecal stream. After reaching the soil, these eggs embryonate for a minimum of 2–3 weeks. Thereafter, the eggs are infectious to both canines and humans and, in moist soil, may remain so for

Table 56.1   General Characteristics of Tissue Nematodes

Parasite	Disease	Usual Source of Human Infection
Toxocara canis	Toxocariasis (visceral larva migrans)	Ingestion of ova from canine stools
Trichinella spiralis	Trichinosis	Ingestion of improperly cooked pork
Ancylostoma braziliense	Cutaneous larva migrans	Soil contaminated with dog or cat feces
Major filarial worms		
Wuchereria bancrofti, Brugia malayi	Lymphatic filariasis (elephantiasis)	Mosquito
Onchocerca volvulus	Onchocerciasis (river blindness)	*Simulium* flies
Loa loa (eye worm)	Loiasis (Calabar swellings)	Deer flies

months to years. When ingested by a young dog, the larvae exit from the eggshell, penetrate the intestinal mucosa, and migrate through the liver and the right side of the heart to the lung. Here, like the offspring of *Ascaris lumbricoides*, they burst into the alveolar air spaces and are coughed up and swallowed; thereafter, they mature in the small bowel. In fully grown dogs, most of the migrating larvae pass through the pulmonary capillaries and reach the systemic circulation. These larvae eventually filter out and encyst in the tissues. Hormonal changes and/or diminished immunity in the pregnant bitch stimulate the larvae to migrate; some penetrate the placenta to infect the unborn pups. Approximately 4 weeks after parturition, both the puppies and the lactating mother begin to pass large numbers of eggs in their stools.

> Transplacentally infected puppies and infected lactating bitches excrete numerous ova

When humans ingest infectious eggs, the liberated larvae are small enough to pass through the pulmonary capillaries and reach the systemic circulation. Rarely does the organism break into the alveoli and reach the intestine to complete its maturation to adulthood. Larvae in the systemic circulation continue to grow. When their size exceeds the diameter of the vessel through which they are passing, they penetrate its wall and enter the tissue.

> Transmission to humans by ingestion of ova; larvae invade tissues

Epidemiology

Toxocara canis is a cosmopolitan parasite. The infection rate in the 50 million dogs inhabiting the United States is very high; over 80% of puppies and 20% of older animals are involved. As "man's best friend" deposits more than 3500 tons of feces daily in the streets, yards, and parks of America, there is a real health risk to our sons and daughters. In areas where studies have been done, between 10 and 30% of soil samples taken from public parks have contained viable *Toxocara* eggs. Moreover, serologic surveys of humans indicate that approximately 4–20% of the population has ingested these eggs at some time. The incidence of infection appears to be higher in the southeastern sections of the country; presumably the warm, humid climate prolongs survival of the eggs, thereby in-

> Extent of contamination of soil with ova

creasing exposure. The presence of puppies in the home increases the risk of infection. Clinical manifestations occur predominantly among children 1–6 years of age; many have a history of geophagia, suggesting that disease transmission results from direct ingestion of eggs in the soil. Most infections are subclinical, but the incidence of overt disease, although difficult to assess, is certainly underreported. Serious ocular infection by larvae is frequently seen by ophthalmologists.

Children are most often infected

Infection much commoner than disease, but disease underreported

Clinical Manifestations

Invasion of any tissues by larvae

Larvae that reach the systemic circulation may invade any tissue of the body, where they can induce necrosis, bleeding, and the formation of eosinophilic granulomas. The liver, lungs, heart, skeletal muscle, brain, and eye are involved most frequently. The severity of clinical manifestations is related to the number and location of these lesions and the degree to which the host has become sensitized to larval antigens. In a subsequently criticized study in the early 1950s, investigators fed 200 embryonated eggs to each of two severely retarded young children. During the subsequent 14 months of observation, the children remained well, but demonstrated a persistent eosinophilic leukocytosis. Children with more intense infection may have fever and an enlarged, tender liver. Those who are seriously ill may develop a skin rash, an enlarged spleen, asthma, recurrent pulmonary infiltrates, behavioral changes, focal neurologic defects, and convulsions. Illness often persists for weeks to months. Death may result from respiratory failure, cardiac arrhythmia, or brain damage. In older children and adults, systemic manifestations are uncommon. Eye invasion by larvae is more common. Typically, unilateral strabismus (squint) or decreased visual acuity causes the patient to consult an ophthalmologist. Examination reveals granulomatous endophthalmitis, which is usually a reaction to a larva that is already dead; it is sometimes mistaken for malignant retinoblastoma, and an unnecessary enucleation is performed.

Disease results from mechanical effects and hypersensitivity

Disseminated disease can occur

Ocular manifestations and granulomatous endophthalmitis

Laboratory Diagnosis

Liver biopsy

Eosinophilia

Serodiagnosis

Stool examination is not helpful, as the parasite seldom reaches adulthood in humans. Definitive diagnosis requires demonstration of the larva in a liver biopsy specimen or at autopsy. A presumptive diagnosis may be made based on the clinical picture, on eosinophilic leukocytosis, and on elevated antibody titers to blood group antigens, particularly the group A antigen. Recently, an enzyme-linked immunosorbent assay (ELISA) utilizing larval antigens was developed, providing clinicians for the first time with a reasonably sensitive and specific serologic test. Unfortunately, many patients with related ocular infections remain seronegative.

Treatment and Prevention

Role of corticosteroids

Corticosteroid treatment may be lifesaving if the patient has serious pulmonary, myocardial, or central nervous system involvement. The efficacy of specific antihelminthic therapy is still uncertain. Prevention requires control of indiscriminate defecation by dogs and repeated worming of household pets. Worming must begin when the animal is 3 weeks of age and be repeated every 3 months during the first year of life and twice a year thereafter.

Need for worming of dogs

Trichinosis

Organism

Intestinal parasite of many flesh-eating mammals

The adult *T. spiralis* lives in the duodenal and jejunal mucosa of flesh-eating animals, throughout the world, particularly swine, rodents, bears, canines, felines, and marine mammals. Although thought to be members of a single species, arctic, temperate, and tropical strains of *Trichinella* demonstrate biologic differences. In all cases the tiny (1.5-mm) male copulates with his outsized (3.5-mm) mate and, apparently spent by the effort, dies. Within a week, the inseminated female begins to discharge offspring. Unlike those of most nematodes, these progeny undergo intrauterine embryonation and are released as second stage larvae. The birthing continues for the next 4–16 weeks, resulting in the generation of some 1500 larvae, each measuring 6 × 100 μm. From their submucosal position, they find their way into the vascular system and pass from the right side of the heart through the pulmonary capillary bed to the systemic circulation, where they are distributed throughout the body. Larvae penetrating tissue other than skeletal muscle disintegrate and die. Those finding their way to striated muscle continue to grow, molt, and gradually encapsulate over a period of several weeks. Calcification of the cyst wall begins 6–18 months later, but the contained larvae may remain viable for 5–10 years. The muscles invaded most frequently include the extraocular muscles of the eye, the tongue, the deltoid, pectoral, and intercostal muscles, the diaphragm, and the gastrocnemius. If a second animal feeds on the infected flesh of the original host, the encysted larvae are freed by gastric digestion, penetrate the columnar epithelium of the intestine, and mature just above the lamina propria.

Larvae reach striated muscle and encapsulate

Eating infected flesh spreads the disease

Epidemiology

Swine infected by eating rats, or meat in garbage

Trichinosis is widespread in carnivores. Among domestic animals, swine are most frequently involved. They acquire the infection by eating rats or garbage containing cyst-laden scraps of uncooked meat. Human infection, in turn, results largely from the consumption of improperly prepared pork products. In the United States, most outbreaks have been traced to ready-to-eat pork sausage prepared in the home or in small, unlicensed butcheries. Disease incidence is highest in Americans of Polish, German, and Italian descent, presumably because of their custom of producing and eating such sausage during holidays. Recent outbreaks have been reported among Indochinese refugees, apparently related to undercooking of fresh pork. Outbreaks have also followed feasts of wild pig in California and Hawaii. At present, approximately 10% of human cases, particularly those in Alaska and other western states, have been attributed to consumption of bear meat. One outbreak among Alaskan Eskimos followed the ingestion of *Trichinella*-infected walrus. Each year, a few cases are acquired from ground beef intentionally but illegally adulterated with pork.

Human infection from undercooked pork

Infection from bear and walrus meat

Human infections are found worldwide, with the exception of Asia and Australia. In the United States, the prevalence of cysts found in the diaphragms of patients at autopsy has declined from 16.1 to 4.2% over a period of 30 years. This decline has been attributed to decreased consumption of pork and pork products; federal guidelines for the commercial preparation of such foodstuffs; the widespread practice of freezing pork, which kills all but arctic strains of *Trichinella*; and legislation requiring the thorough cooking of any meat scraps to be used as hog feed. Nevertheless, it is estimated that more than 1.5 million Americans carry live

Human infections still widespread; most are subclinical

Trichinella in their musculature and that 150,000–300,000 acquire new infection annually. Fortunately, the overwhelming majority are asymptomatic, and only about 100 clinically recognized cases are reported annually to federal officials. In other areas of the world, infection is more commonly acquired from sylvatic sources, including wild boar, bush pigs, and warthogs.

Pathogenesis, Pathology, and Immunity

Larvae in striated muscle, heart, and central nervous system

Acute inflammatory reaction

Eosinophil mediated destruction of larvae

The pathologic lesions of trichinosis are related almost exclusively to the presence of larvae in the striated muscle, heart, and central nervous system. Invaded muscle cells enlarge, lose their cross-striations, and undergo a basophilic degeneration. Surrounding the involved area is an intense inflammatory reaction consisting of neutrophils, lymphocytes, and eosinophils. With the development of specific IgG and IgM antibodies, eosinophil-mediated destruction of circulating larvae begins, production of new larvae is slowed, and the expulsion of adult worms is hastened. A vasculitis demonstrated in some patients has been attributed to deposition of circulating immune complexes in the walls of the vessels.

Clinical Manifestations

Initial diarrhea

Symptoms depend on extent of larval invasion of muscle

More severe complications

One or two days after the host has ingested tainted meat, the newly matured adults penetrate the intestinal mucosa, producing nausea, abdominal pain, and diarrhea. In mild infections, these symptoms may be overlooked, except in a careful retrospective analysis; in more serious infections, they may persist for several days and render the patient prostrate. Larval invasion of striated muscle begins approximately 1 week later and initiates the longer (6 weeks) and more characteristic phase of the disease. Patients in whom 10 or fewer larvae are deposited per gram of tissue are usually asymptomatic; those with 100 or more generally develop significant disease; and those with 1000–5000 have a very stormy course that occasionally ends in death. Fever, muscle pain, muscle tenderness, and weakness are the most prominent manifestations. Patients may also display eyelid swelling, a maculopapular skin rash, and small hemorrhages beneath the conjunctiva of the eye and the nails of the digits. Hemoptysis and pulmonary consolidation are common in severe infections. If there is myocardial involvement, electrocardiographic abnormalities, tachycardia, or congestive heart failure may be seen. Central nervous system invasion is marked by encephalitis, meningitis, and polyneuritis. Delirium, psychosis, paresis, and coma can follow.

Laboratory Diagnosis

Eosinophilia

Serodiagnosis

The most consistent abnormality is an eosinophilic leukocytosis that appears during the second week of illness and persists for the remainder of the clinical course. Eosinophils typically range from 15 to 50% of the white cell count and in some patients may induce extensive damage to the cardiac endothelium. In severe or terminal cases, the eosinophilia may disappear altogether.

There are a number of valuable serologic tests, including complement fixation, indirect fluorescent antibody, and bentonite flocculation. Significant antibody titers are generally absent before the third week of illness, but may then persist for years. Recently, an ELISA capable of detecting specific antibody formation during the first week of illness was developed.

Muscle biopsy

Biopsy of the deltoid or gastrocnemius muscle during the third week will usually reveal encysted larvae.

Treatment

Use of corticosteroids

Patients with severe edema, pulmonary manifestations, myocardial involvement, or central nervous system disease are treated with corticosteroids. The value of specific antihelminthic therapy remains controversial. The mortality of symptomatic patients is 1%, rising to 10% if the central nervous system is involved. Mebendozole halts the production of new larvae, but in severe infection, the destruction of tissue larvae may provoke a hazardous hypersensitivity response in the host. This may be moderated with corticosteroids.

Prevention

Pork should be cooked to an internal temperature of at least 76.6°C, frozen at −15°C for 3 weeks, or thoroughly smoked before it is ingested. *Trichinella* in the flesh of arctic animals may survive freezing for a year or more. All strains may survive apparently adequate cooking in microwave ovens due to the variability in the internal temperatures achieved.

Cutaneous Larva Migrans

Caused usually by larvae of dog and cat hookworms

Filariform larvae penetrate and migrate in human skin

Cutaneous larva migrans, or creeping eruption, is an infection of the skin caused by the larvae of a number of animal and human parasites, most commonly the dog and cat hookworm *Ancylostoma braziliense*. Eggs discharged in the feces of infected animals and deposited on warm, moist, sandy soil develop filariform larvae capable of penetrating mammalian skin on contact. In the United States, parasite transmission is particularly common in the beach areas of the southern Atlantic and Gulf states.

Local and pulmonary manifestations

Although larvae do not develop further within humans, they may migrate within the skin for a period of weeks to months. Clinically, the patient notes a pruritic, raised, red, irregularly linear lesion 10 to 20 cm long. Skin excoriation from scratching enhances the likelihood of secondary bacterial infection. Half of infected patients develop Loeffler's syndrome of transient, migratory pulmonary infiltrations associated with peripheral eosinophilia. The syndrome most probably reflects pulmonary migration of larvae. Larvae are rarely found in either sputum or skin biopsies, and the diagnosis must be established on clinical grounds.

Larvae do not develop to adult forms in humans

The disease responds well to oral or topical thiabendazole. Antihistamines and antibiotics may be helpful in controlling pruritis and secondary bacterial infection, respectively.

Lymphatic Filariasis

Definition

Lymphatic filariasis encompasses a group of diseases produced by certain members of the superfamily Filarioidea that inhabit the lymphatic system of humans. Their presence induces an acute inflammatory reaction, chronic lymphatic blockade, and, in some cases, grotesque swellings of the extremities and genitalia known as *elephantiasis*.

Table 56.2 Differentiation of Microfilariae

Parasite	Location	Sheath	Size (μm)	Nuclei of Tail	Periodicity
Wuchereria bancrofti	Blood	Yes	360	None	Usually nocturnal
Brugia malayi	Blood	Yes	220	Two	Nocturnal
Loa loa	Blood	Yes	275	Continuous	Diurnal
Onchocerca volvulus	Skin	No	300	None	None

Organisms

Adult worms in lymphatic vessels

The two agents most commonly responsible for lymphatic filariasis are *Wuchereria bancrofti* and *Brugia malayi*. Both are threadlike worms that lie coiled in the lymphatic vessels, male and female together, for the duration of their decade-long life span. The female *W. bancrofti* measures 100 mm in length, the male, 40 mm. *B. malayi* adults are approximately half these sizes. The gravid females produce large numbers of embryonated eggs. At oviposition, the embryos uncoil to their full length (200–300 μm) to become microfilariae. The shell of the egg elongates to accommodate the embryo and is retained as a thin, flexible sheath. Although the offspring of the two species resemble each other, they may be differentiated on the basis of length, staining characteristics, and internal structure (Table 56.2). The microfilariae eventually reach the blood. In most *W. bancrofti* and *B. malayi* infections, they accumulate in the pulmonary vessels during the day. At night, in response to changes in oxygen tension, they spill out into the peripheral circulation, where they are found in greatest numbers between 9 PM and 2 AM. A Polynesian strain of *W. bancrofti* displays a different periodicity, the peak concentration of organisms occurring in the early evening. Periodicity has an important epidemiologic consequence, as it determines the species of mosquito to serve as vector and intermediate host. Within the thoracic muscles of the mosquito, microfilariae are transformed first into rhabditiform and then into filariform larvae. These larvae actively penetrate the feeding site when the mosquito takes its next meal. Within the new host, the parasite migrates to the lymphatic vessels, undergoes a series of molts, and reaches adulthood in 6–12 months.

Microfilariae develop from ova

Periodicity of microfilariae in peripheral blood

Mosquito is essential vector and intermediate host

Epidemiology

Geographic distribution

Lymphatic filariasis currently infects about 250 million individuals in Africa, Latin America, the Pacific Islands, and Asia; more than three-quarters of these cases are concentrated in the latter continent. *Wuchereria bancrofti*, transmitted primarily by mosquitoes of the genus *Anopheles* or *Culex*, is the more cosmopolitan of the two species; it is found in patchy distribution throughout the poorly sanitated, densely crowded urban areas of all three continents. A small endemic focus once existed near Charleston, South Carolina, but died out in the 1920s. Moreover, some 15,000 *W. bancrofti* infections were acquired by American servicemen during World War II. The same infection has recently been found in approximately 7% of Haitian refugees to the United States.

Brugia malayi, transmitted by mosquitoes of the genus *Mansonia*, is confined to the rural coastal areas of Asia and the South Pacific. Strains with an unusual periodicity have been found in animals. Humans are the

Humans are the only vertebrate hosts

only known vertebrate host for this parasite and for *W. bancrofti*. In the eastern Indonesian archipelago, a closely related species, *Brugia timori*, is transmitted by night-feeding anopheline mosquitoes.

Pathology and Pathogenesis

Pathologic changes, which are confined primarily to the lymphatic system, can be divided into acute and chronic lesions. In acute disease, the presence of molting adolescent worms and dead or dying adults stimulates infiltration by lymphocytes, plasma cells, and eosinophils, hyperplastic changes in the lymphatic endothelium, and thrombus formation (that is, acute lymphangitis). These developments are followed by granuloma formation, fibrosis, and permanent lymphatic obstruction. Repeated infections eventually result in massive lymphatic blockade. The skin and subcutaneous tissues become edematous, thickened, and fibrotic. Dilated vessels may rupture, spilling lymph into the tissues or body cavities. Bacterial cellulitis often supervenes and contributes to tissue damage.

Acute lymphongitis, fibrosis, and lymphatic obstruction

Lymphatic blockade with repeated infections

Clinical Manifestations

Mild infections often go unnoticed. With a larger worm load, the patient experiences onset of fever, lymphadenitis, and lymphangitis 8–12 months after exposure. The fever is typically low grade; in more serious cases, however, temperatures as high as 40°C, chills, muscle pains, and other systemic manifestations may be seen. Classically, the lymphadenitis is first noted in the femoral area as an enlarged, red, tender lump. The inflammation spreads centrifugally down the lymphatic channels of the leg. The vessels become enlarged and tender, the overlying skin red and edematous. In Bancroftian filariasis, the lymphatic vessels of the testicle, epidididymis, and spermatic cord are frequently involved, producing a painful orchitis, epididymitis, and funiculitis; inflamed retroperitoneal vessels may simulate acute abdomen. Epitrochlear, axillary, and other lymphatic vessels are involved less frequently. The acute manifestations last a few days and resolve spontaneously, only to recur periodically over a period of weeks to months. With repeated infection, permanent lymphatic obstruction develops in the involved areas. Edema, ascites, pleural effusion, hydrocele, and joint effusion result. The lymphadenopathy persists and the palpably swollen lymphatic channels may rupture, producing an abscess or draining sinus. Rupture of intraabdominal vessels may give rise to chylous ascites or urine. In patients heavily and repeatedly infected over a period of decades, elephantiasis may develop. Such patients may continue to experience acute inflammatory episodes.

In India, Pakistan, Sri Lanka, Indonesia, and Southeast Asia an aberrant form of filariasis is seen. This form, termed *tropical eosinophilia*, is characterized by an intense eosinophilia, elevated levels of IgE, high titers of filarial antibodies, the absence of microfilariae from the circulating blood, and a chronic clinical course marked by massive enlargement of the lymph nodes and spleen (children) or chronic cough, nocturnal bronchospasm, and pulmonary infiltrates (adults). Microfilariae have been found in the tissues of such patients, and the clinical manifestations may be terminated with specific antifilarial treatment. It is believed that this syndrome is precipitated by the removal of circulating microfilariae by an IgG-dependent, cell-mediated immune reaction. Microfilariae are trapped in various tissue sites where they incite an eosinophilic inflammatory response, granuloma formation, and fibrosis.

Lymphadenitis and lymphangitis

Relapses of acute manifestations

Effects of repeated infection

Elephantiasis

Tropical eosinophilia syndrome

Laboratory Diagnosis

Eosinophilia

Eosinophilia is usually present during the acute inflammatory episodes, but definitive diagnosis requires the demonstration of microfilariae in the blood or lymphatic, acitic, or pleural fluid. They are sought in Giemsa- or Wright-stained thick and thin smears. The major distinguishing features of these and other microfilariae are listed in Table 56.2. As the appearance of the microfilariae is usually periodic, specimen collection must be properly timed. If this procedure proves difficult, the patient may be challenged with the antifilarial agent diethylcarbamazine. This drug stimulates the migration of the microfilariae from the pulmonary to the systemic circulation and enhances the possibility of their recovery. If the parasitemia is scant, the specimen may be concentrated before it is examined. Once found, the microfilariae must be differentiated from those produced by other species of filariae. A number of serologic tests have been employed for the diagnosis of microfilaremic disease, but until recently they have lacked adequate sensitivity and specificity. Circulating filarial antigens can be found in most microfilaremic patients and also in some seropositive amicrofilaremic individuals. Antigen detection may, thus, prove to be a specific indicator of active disease. Tropical eosinophilia is diagnosed as described previously.

Timing of search for microfilariae in the blood

Treatment

Diethylcarbamazine eliminates the microfilariae from the blood and kills or injures the adult worms, resulting in long-term suppression of the infection or parasitologic cure. Frequently, the dying microfilariae stimulate an allergic reaction in the host. This response is occasionally severe, requiring the use of antihistamines and corticosteroids. The role of ivermectin, a promising new antihelminthic agent, in the treatment of lymphatic filariasis has not yet been established. The tissue changes of elephantiasis are irreversible, but the enlargement of the extremities may be ameliorated with pressure bandages or plastic surgery. Control programs combine mosquito control with mass treatment of the entire population.

Killing of microfilariae may stimulate allergic response

Onchocerciasis

Definition

Onchocerciasis or *river blindness*, produced by the skin filaria *O. volvulus*, is characterized by subcutaneous nodules, thickened pruritic skin, and blindness.

Organism

Adults in subcutaneous tissue, skin, and eye

The 20- to 50-mm adults lie in coiled masses within fibrous subcutaneous nodules. The female gives birth to more than 2000 microfilariae each day of her 15-year life span. These progeny lose their sheaths soon after leaving the uterus, exit from the fibrous capsule, and migrate for up to 2 years in the subcutaneous tissues, skin, and eye. Ultimately they die or are ingested by black flies of the genus *Simulium*, which breed along the banks of turbulent, fast-moving streams. After transformation into filariform larvae, they are transmitted to another human host. There they molt repeatedly over 6–12 months before reaching adulthood and becoming encapsulated.

Transmitted by *Simulium* fly

Epidemiology

Important cause of blindness in affected areas

Onchocerciasis infects approximately 50 million persons, rendering 5% of them blind. Most of the afflicted live in tropical Africa, but foci of infection are also located in Yemen and Latin America. It has been suggested that the disease was introduced into South America by West Africans enslaved and transported to the New World for the purpose of mining gold in the mountain streams of Venezuela and Columbia. The Central American foci date from Napoleon III's use of Sudanese troops to support his invasion of Mexico in 1862. The disease still persists on the high slopes of the Sierra, where coffee plantations lie along the rapidly flowing streams that serve as breeding places for *Simulium* species.

Clinical Manifestations

Subcutaneous nodules

The subcutaneous nodules that harbor the adult worms can be located anywhere on the body, generally over bony prominences. In Mexico and Guatemala, where the fly vector typically bites the upper part of the body, they are concentrated on the head; in South America and Africa, they are found primarily on the trunk and legs. Although nodules may number in the hundreds, most infected individuals have less than 10. They are firm, freely movable, and measure 1–3 cm in diameter. Unless the nodule is located over a joint, pain and tenderness are unusual. Of greater consequence to the patient are the side effects of the presence of microfilariae in the tissues. An immediate hypersensitivity reaction to antigens released by dead or dying parasites results in acute and chronic inflammatory reaction. In the skin, this reaction is manifested as a papular or erysipelaslike rash with severe itching. In time, the skin thickens and lichenifies. As subepidermal elastic tissue is lost, wrinkles and large skin folds or *hanging groins* are formed. In parts of Africa, fibrosing, obstructive lymphadenitis may result in elephantiasis. Invasion of the eye, however, causes the most devastating lesions. Punctate keratitis, iritis, and chorioretinitis can lead to a decrease in visual acuity and, in time, total blindness. In Central America, eye lesions may be seen in up to 30% of infected patients. In certain communities in West Africa, 85% of the population has ocular lesions and one-half of the adult male population is blind.

Hypersensitivity reactions to microfilariae

Lesions become chronic

Laboratory Diagnosis

Microfilariae seen in skin or eye samples

The diagnosis is made by demonstrating the microfilariae in a thin skin sample taken from an involved area. When the eye is involved, the organism may sometimes be seen in the anterior chamber with the help of a slit lamp.

Treatment and Prevention

Treatment-induced hypersensitivity reactions

Traditionally, diethylcarbamazine has been used to kill the microfilariae. Treatment was begun with very small doses to prevent rapid parasite destruction and the attendant allergic consequences. This consideration is particularly important when the eye is involved, as a treatment-induced inflammatory reaction can damage it further. Unfortunately, diethylcarbamazine does not destroy the adult worms, which must be removed by surgical excision or killed with a second, more toxic agent, suramin. Recently, the new microfilaremic agent, ivermectin, has been demonstrated to be more effective than diethylcarbamazine. More importantly, it does not appear to induce the severe allergic manifestations seen with the latter agent. No satisfactory methods of control have yet been developed. Application of insecticides to the vector's breeding waters must be sustained for decades to disrupt transmission permanently, as the parasite is so long-lived within humans. With the introduction of ivermectin, mass treatment or chemoprophylaxis may now be possible.

Loiasis

Loiasis is a filarial disease of West Africa produced by the eye worm, *L. loa*. The long-lived adults migrate continuously through the subcutaneous tissues of humans at a maximum rate of about 1 cm/hr. During migration, they produce localized areas of allergic inflammation termed *Calabar swellings*. These egg-sized lesions persist for 2–3 days and may be accompanied by fever, itching, urticaria, and pain. At times, the adult worms may cross the eye subconjunctivally, producing intense tearing, pain, and alarm.

The female produces sheathed microfilariae, which are found in the bloodstream during daytime hours. Deer flies of the genus *Chrysops* serve as vectors.

The diagnosis is made by recovering the adult worm from the eye or by isolating the characteristic microfilariae from the blood or Calabar swellings. Eosinophilia is constant. Diethylcarbamazine destroys both adults and microfilariae, but must be administered cautiously to avoid marked allergic reactions. The role of ivermectin remains to be defined.

Adults migrate through subcutaneous tissues

Calabar swellings and subconjunctival migration

Demonstration of adult in eye or microfilaria in blood

Additional Reading

Barrett-Connor, E., Davis, C.F., Hamburger, R.N., and Kagan, I. 1976. An epidemic of trichinosis after ingestion of wild pig in Hawaii. *J. Infect. Dis.* 133:473–477.

Edeson, J.F.B. 1972. Filariasis. *Br. Med. Bull.* 28:60–65. A brief, succinct review of a complicated subject.

Margolis, H.S., Middaugh, J.P., and Burgess, R.D. 1979. Arctic trichinosis: Two Alaskan outbreaks from walrus meat. *J. Infect. Dis.* 139:102–105. A report of two unusual outbreaks of trichinosis.

Taylor, H.R. 1985. Review of the immunologic aspects of Onchocerciasis: An introduction. *Rev. Infect. Dis.* 7:787–788. This article introduces an issue of this journal devoted to a review of onchocerciasis.

Worley, G., Green, J.A., Frothingham, T.E., et al. 1984. *Toxocara canis* infection. Clinical and epidemiological associations with seropositivity in kindergarten children. *J. Infect. Dis.* 149:591–597.

57

Cestodes

James J. Plorde

Cestodes are long, ribbonlike helminths that have gained the common appellation of *tapeworm* from their superficial resemblance to sewing tape. Their appearance, number, and exaggerated reputation for inducing weight loss have made them the best known of the intestinal worms. Although improvements in sanitation have dramatically reduced their prevalence in the United States, they continue to inhabit the bowels of many of its citizens. In some parts of the world, indigenous populations take purgatives monthly to rid themselves of this, the largest and most repulsive of the intestinal parasites.

Cestodes

Morphology

Absence of gut

Scolex, neck, and segmented body

Attachment mechanisms

Each proglottid a hermaphroditic unit

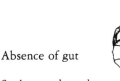

Cestode

Like all helminths, tapeworms lack vascular and respiratory systems. In addition, they are devoid of both gut and body cavity. Food is absorbed across a complex cuticle, and the internal organs are embedded in a solid parenchyma. The adult is divided into three distinct parts: the "head" or *scolex*; a generative *neck*; and a long, segmented body, the *strobila*. The scolex typically measures less than 2 mm in diameter and is equipped with four muscular sucking discs used to attach the worm to the intestinal mucosa of its host. (In one genus, *Diphyllobothrium*, the discs are replaced by two grooves, or *bothria*.) As a further aid in attachment, the scolex of some species possesses a retractable protuberance, or *rostellum*, armed with a crown of chitinous hooks. Immediately posterior to the scolex is the neck from which individual segments, or *proglottids*, are generated one at a time to form the chainlike body. Each proglottid is a self-contained hermaphroditic reproductive unit joined to the remainder of the colony by a common cuticle, nerve trunks, and excretory canals. Its male and female gonads mature and effect fertilization as the segment is pushed further and further from the neck by the formation of new proglottids. When the segment reaches gravidity, it releases its eggs by rupturing, disintegrating, or passing them through its uterine pore. The eggs of the genus *Taenia* possess a solid shell and contain a fully developed, six-hooked (hexacanth) embryo. The eggs of *Diphyllobothrium latum*, in contrast, are immature at the time of deposition and possess a covered aperture, or *operculum*, through which the embryo exits once fully developed.

Life Cycle

With the exception of that of *Hymenolepis nana*, further development of all cestodes requires the passage of the larvae through one or more intermediate hosts. Eggs of the genus *Taenia* pass in the stool of their definitive host, reach the soil, and are ingested by the specific intermediate. They hatch within its gut, and the released embryos penetrate the intestinal mucosa, find their way through the lymphohematogenous system to the tissues, and encyst therein. From the germinal lining of this cyst, immature scolices or *protoscolices* are formed. A cyst with a single such structure is known as a *cysticercus* (or, in the case of *H. nana*, a cysticercoid); a cyst with multiple protoscolices is known as a *coenurus*. In some species of tapeworm, daughter cysts, each containing many protoscolices, are formed within the mother or *hydatid* cyst. The cycle for all is completed when the definitive host ingests the cyst-ridden flesh of the intermediate host. After digestion of the surrounding meat in the stomach, the cyst is freed, and the protoscolex everts to become a scolex. Following attachment to the mucosa, a new strobila is generated.

Diphyllobothrium latum, whose eggs are immature upon release, requires two intermediates to complete its larval development. The egg must reach fresh water before the operculum opens and a ciliated, free-swimming larva, or *coracidium*, is released. The coracidium is then ingested by the first intermediate host, a copepod, in which it is transformed into a larva (*procercoid*). When the copepod is, in turn, ingested by a freshwater fish, the larva penetrates the musculature of the fish to form an elongated and infectious larva, the *plerocercoid*. Life cycles and characteristics of important intestinal and tissue tapeworms infecting humans are summarized in Table 57.1.

Clinical Disease

The clinical consequences of tapeworm infection in humans depend on whether the patient serves as the primary or the intermediate host. In the former case, the adult worm is confined to the lumen of the gut, and the consequences of the infection are typically minor. Taeniasis saginata and diphyllobothriasis are prime examples. In contrast, when the patient serves as the intermediate host (for example, for *Echinococcus granulosus*), larval development produces tissue invasion and frequently serious disease. The capacity of *H. nana* and *Taenia solium* to utilize humans as both primary and intermediate hosts is unique.

Beef Tapeworm Infection

Organism

Taenia saginata, the beef tapeworm, inhabits the human jejunum, where it may live for up to 25 years and grow to a maximum length of 10 m. Its 1-mm scolex lacks hooklets, but possesses the four sucking discs typical

Margin notes

Release of eggs

Eggs of *Taenia* ingested by intermediate host

Infectious cysts of *Taenia* form in tissues of intermediate

Definitive host ingests cysts in flesh of intermediate hosts to yield adult intestinal worms

D. latum requires two intermediates, a copepod and a freshwater fish, to complete cycle

Clinical effects depend on whether humans are definitive hosts or intermediate hosts

T. saginata inhabits human jejunum

Table 57.1 Intestinal and Tissue Tapeworms

Stage	*Diphyllobothrium latum*	*Taenia saginata*	*Taenia solium*	*Hymenolepis nana*	*Echinococcus granulosus*	*Echinococcus multilocularis*
Adult						
Definitive host	Humans, cats, dogs	Humans	Humans	Humans, rodents	Dogs, wolves	Foxes
Location	*Gut lumen*[a]	*Gut lumen*	*Gut lumen*	*Gut lumen*	Gut lumen	Gut lumen
Length (m)	3–10	4–6	2–4	0.02–0.04	0.005	0.005
Attachment device	Grooves	Discs	Discs, hooklets	Discs, hooklets	Discs, hooklets	Discs, hooklets
Mature segment	Broad	Elongated	Elongated	Broad	Elongated	Elongated
Egg						
Maturation status	Nonembryonated	Embryonated	Embryonated	Embryonated	Embryonated	Embryonated
Distinguishing characteristics	Operculate	Radial striations	Radial striations	Polar filaments	Radial striations	Radial striations
Larval development in humans	No	No	Yes	Yes	Yes	Yes
Larva						
Intermediate host	Copepods, fishes	Cattle	Swine, humans	Humans, rodents	Herbivores, humans	Field mice, humans
Location	Tissue	Tissue	*Tissue*	*Gut mucosa*	*Tissue*	*Tissue*
Form	Procercoid (copepod) Plerocercoid (fish)	Cysticercus	Cysticercus	Cysticercoid	Hydatid cyst	Hydatid cyst

[a] Sites of human infection appear in italics.

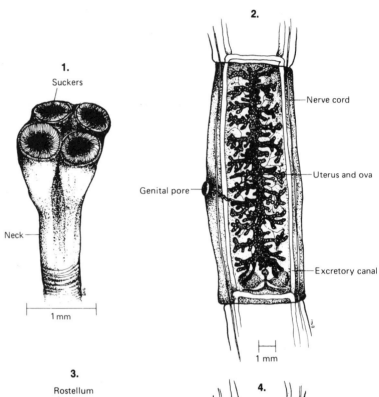

1.
Suckers

Neck

A

1 mm

2.

Nerve cord

Genital pore

Uterus and ova

Excretory canal

1 mm

57.1. (A) *Taenia saginata*;
(B) *Taenia solium*.
(1 and 3) Scolices; (2 and 4)
gravid proglottids; (5) ova
(indistinguishable between
species).

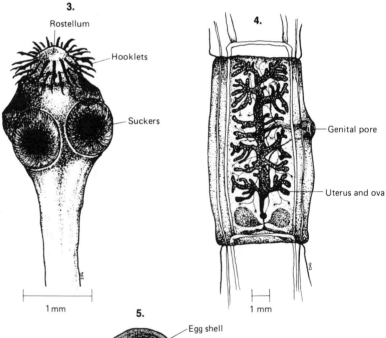

3.
Rostellum

Hooklets

Suckers

B

1 mm

4.

Genital pore

Uterus and ova

1 mm

5.

Egg shell

Hooklet

Hexacanth larvum

10 μm

of most cestodes (Figure 57.1-1). The creamy white strobila consists of 1000–2000 individual proglottids. The terminal segments are longer (20 mm) than they are wide (5 mm) and contain a large uterus with 15–20 lateral branches; these characteristics are useful in differentiating them from those of the closely related pork tapeworm, *T. solium*. When fully gravid, strings of terminal proglottids break free from the remainder of the strobila. These muscular segments may crawl unassisted through the anal canal or be passed intact with the stool. Proglottids reaching the soil eventually disintegrate, releasing their distinctive eggs. These eggs are 30–40 μm in diameter, spherical, and possess a thick, radially striated shell (Figure 57.1-5). In appropriate environments, the hexacanth embryo may survive for months. If ingested by cattle or certain other herbivores, the embryo is released, penetrates the intestinal wall, and is carried by the vascular system to the striated muscles of the tongue, diaphragm, and hindquarters. Here it is transformed into a white, ovoid (5 × 10 mm) cysticercus (*Cysticercus bovis*). When present in large numbers, cysticerci impart a spotted or "measley" appearance to the flesh. Humans are infected when they ingest inadequately cooked meat containing these larval forms.

Gravid proglottids passed in stool

Eggs ingested by herbivore intermediates

Cysticerci in bovine striated muscle

Humans infected by eating inadequately cooked infected meat

Epidemiology

Indigenously acquired disease rare in United States

In the United States, sanitary disposal of human feces and federal inspection of meat have nearly interrupted transmission of *T. saginata*. At present, less than 1% of examined carcasses are infected. Nevertheless, bovine cysticercosis is still a significant problem in the southwestern area of the country where cattle become infected in feedlots or while pastured on land irrigated with sewage or worked by laborers without access to sanitary facilities. Shipment of infected carcuses can result in human infection in other areas of the United States. In countries where sanitary facilities are less comprehensive and undercooked or raw beef is eaten, *T. saginata* is highly prevalent. Examples include Kenya, Ethiopia, the Middle East, Yugoslavia, and parts of the Soviet Union and South America.

Clinical Manifestations

Clinical symptoms usually mild

Most infected patients are asymptomatic and become aware of the infection only through the spontaneous passage of proglottids. The proglottids may be observed on the surface of the stool or appear in the underclothing or bed sheets of the alarmed host. Passage may occur very irregularly and can be precipitated by excessive alcohol consumption. Some patients report epigastric discomfort, nausea, irritability (particularly after passage of segments), diarrhea, and weight loss. Occasionally the proglottids may obstruct the appendix, biliary duct, or pancreatic duct.

Laboratory Diagnosis

Adhesive cellophane tape technique and stool examination for eggs and proglottids

The diagnosis is made by finding eggs or proglottids in the stool. Eggs may also be distributed on the perianal area secondary to rupture of proglottids during anal passage. The adhesive cellophane tape technique described for pinworm can be used to recover them from this area. With this procedure, 85–95% of infections are detected, in contrast to only 50–75% by stool examination. As the eggs of *T. solium* and *T. saginata* are morphologically identical, it is necessary to examine a proglottid to identify the species correctly.

Treatment

The drug of choice is niclosamide, which acts directly on the worm. It is a highly effective single-dose oral preparation. Two other effective agents, praziquantel and mebendazole, have not yet been approved for treatment of taeniasis.

Prevention

Sewage disposal, meat inspection, and adequate cooking

Ultimately, control is best effected through the sanitary disposal of human feces. Meat inspection is helpful, as the cysticerci are readily visible. In areas where the infection is common, thorough cooking is the most practical method of control. Internal temperatures of 56°C or more for 5 min or longer will destroy the cystecerci. Salting or freezing for 1 week at −15°C or less is also effective.

Pork Tapeworm Infection

Organism

Like the beef tapeworm, which it closely resembles, *T. solium* inhabits the human jejunum, where it may survive for decades. It can be distinguished from its close relative only by careful scrutiny of the scolex and proglottids; *T. solium* possesses a rostellum armed with a double row of hooklets (Figure 57.1-3). The strobila is generally smaller than that of *T. saginata*, seldom exceeding 5 m in length or containing more than 1000 proglottids. Gravid segments measure 6 × 12 mm and thus appear less elongated than those of the bovine parasite (Figure 57.1-4). Typically, the uterus has only 8–12 lateral branches. Although the eggs appear morphologically identical to those of *T. saginata*, they are infective only to swine and, perhaps reflecting a genetic proximity we would prefer to overlook, humans. Both pigs and people become intermediate hosts when they ingest food contaminated with viable eggs. Some authorities have suggested that humans may be autoinfected when gravid proglottids are carried backward into the stomach during the act of vomiting, initiating the release of the contained eggs. It seems more likely to this author that autoinfection results from the transport of the eggs from the perianal area to the mouth on contaminated fingers.

T. solium strobila shorter than in *T. saginata*

Eggs infective to swine and to humans

Regardless of the route, an egg reaching the stomach of an appropriate intermediate host hatches, releasing the hexacanth embryo. The embryo penetrates the intestinal wall and may be carried by the lymphohematogenous system to any of the tissues of the body. Here it develops into a 1-cm, white, opalescent cysticercus over 3–4 months. The cysticercus may remain viable for up to 5 years, eventually infecting humans when they ingest undercooked and "measley" flesh. The scolex everts, attaches itself to the mucosa, and develops into a new adult worm, thereby completing the cycle.

Tissue cysticerci in humans and swine

Epidemiology

T. solium rarely found in United States

Although infected swine are still occasionally found in the United States, human disease is rarely acquired in this country. It is, however, widely distributed throughout much of the world and is particularly common in eastern Europe, Asia, Africa, and Latin America.

Clinical Manifestations

Major clinical manifestations caused by reaction to cysticerci

The signs and symptoms of infection with the adult worm are similar to those of taeniasis saginata. Clinical manifestations are totally different when humans serve as intermediate hosts. Cysticerci develop in the subcutaneous tissues, muscles, heart, lungs, liver, brain, and eye. As long as the number is small and the cysticerci are viable, tissue reaction is moderate and the patient asymptomatic. The death of the larva, however,

Eosinophilia

stimulates a marked inflammatory reaction, fever, muscle pains, and eosinophilia. Patients with lesions of the central nervous system may present with meningoencephalitis, epilepsy, and other neurologic or psychiatric manifestations.

Laboratory Diagnosis

Presence of adult worm diagnosed from proglottids

Infection with the adult worm is diagnosed as described for *T. saginata*. Cysticercosis is suspected when an individual who has been in an endemic area presents with neurologic manifestations or subcutaneous nodules. Roentgenograms of the soft tissues often reveal calcified cysticerci. Similarly, multiple small brain masses may be detected by computed tomography, radioisotope scanning, or ultrasonography. The diagnosis is con-

Biopsy for cysticerci

firmed by demonstrating the larva in a biopsy sample of a subcutaneous nodule or specific antibodies in the circulating blood. Enzyme-linked immunosorbent assays detect antibodies in 80–95% of infected patients, but may yield false-positive results in a number of other helminthic infections.

Treatment and Prevention

Infection with the adult worm is approached in the manner described for *T. saginata*. At present, no approved medical therapy is available for cysticercosis, although clinical trials suggest that praziquantel is effective. Concomitant corticosteroid administration may minimize the inflamma-

Surgery occasionally needed for cysticercosis

tory response to dying cysticerci. Surgery may be required in some cases of cerebral and ocular cysticercosis.

Fish Tapeworm Infection

Organism

The adult *D. latum* attaches to the ileal mucosa with the aid of two sucking grooves (bothria) located in an elongated fusiform scolex (Figure 57.2A). In life span and overall length, it resembles the *Taenia* species discussed

D. latum has broad proglottids

previously. The 3000–4000 proglottids, however, are uniformly wider than they are long, accounting for this cestode's species designation as well as one of its common names, the broad tapeworm. The gravid segments contain a centrally positioned, rosette-shaped uterus unique among the tapeworms of humans. Unlike those of the *Taenia* species, ova are released through the uterine pore. Over 1 million oval (55 × 75 μm) operculate eggs are released daily into the stool (Figure 57.2B).

Eggs release coracidia in water

On reaching fresh water they hatch, releasing ciliated, free-swimming larvae or coracidia. If ingested within a few days by small freshwater crus-

Crustacean and fish intermediates; humans infected by ingesting inadequately cooked fish

taceans of the genus *Cyclops* or *Diaptomus*, they develop into procercoid larvae. When the crustacean is ingested by a freshwater or anadromous marine fish, the larvae migrate into the musculature of the fish and develop into infectious plerocercoid larvae. Humans are infected when they eat improperly prepared freshwater fish containing such forms.

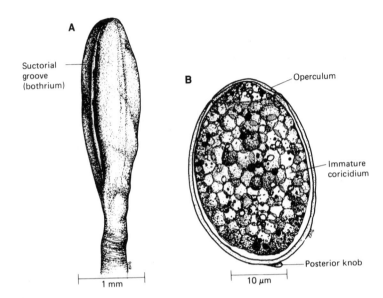

57.2 *Diphyllobothrium latum.*
(A) Scolex. (B) Ovum.

Epidemiology

Worldwide distribution

Fish tapeworms are found wherever raw, pickled, or undercooked fresh-water fish from fecally contaminated lakes and streams is eaten by humans. Human infections have been described in the Baltic and Scandinavian countries, Russia, Switzerland, Italy, Japan, and Chile. The worm, brought to North America by Scandinavian immigrants, is now found in Alaska, Canada, the midwestern states, and Florida. It was shown recently that infectious plerocercoid larvae may develop in anadromous salmon, and human cases have been traced to the ingestion of fish freshly taken from Alaskan waters. The increasing popularity of raw fish dishes such as Japanese sushi and sashimi may lead to increased prevalence of this disease in the United States. Among Ontario Indians, infection is acquired by eating fresh salted fish. Even when fish is appropriately cooked, individuals may become infected by sampling the flesh during the process of preparation.

Worm found in Alaska, Midwest, and Florida

Clinical Manifestations

Occasional intestinal obstruction

Vitamin B_{12} deficiency

Most infected patients are asymptomatic. On occasion, however, they have complained of epigastric pain, abdominal cramping, vomiting, and weight loss. Moreover, the presence of several adult worms within the gut has been known to precipitate intestinal or biliary obstruction. Forty percent of fish tapeworm carriers demonstrate low serum levels of vitamin B_{12}, apparently as a result of the competition between the host and the worm for ingested vitamin. Studies have shown that a worm located high in the jejunum may take up 80–100% of vitamin B_{12} given by mouth. Approximately 0.1–2% of patients develop macrocytic anemia. They tend to be elderly, to have impaired production of intrinsic factor, and to have worms located high in the jejunum. In many, folate absorption is also diminished. Lysolecithin, a tapeworm product, may also contribute to the anemia. Neurologic manifestations of vitamin B_{12} deficiency occur, sometimes in the absence of anemia. They include numbness, paresthesia, loss of vibration sense, and, rarely, optic atrophy with central scotoma.

Laboratory Diagnosis

Demonstration of eggs in stool

The diagnosis is established by finding the typical eggs in the stool. As *D. latum* produces large numbers of ova, identification is usually accomplished without the need for concentration techniques.

Treatment and Prevention

Fish rendered noninfectious at −10°C for 48 hr

Treatment is carried out as described for *T. saginata* infections. When anemia or neurologic manifestations are present, parenteral administration of vitamin B_{12} is also indicated. Personal protection can be accomplished by thorough cooking of all salmon and freshwater fish. Devotees of raw fish may choose to freeze their favorite dish at −10°C for 48 hr before serving. Ultimately, control of diphyllobothriasis is accomplished only by prohibiting the discharge of untreated sewage into lakes and streams.

Hydatid Disease

Definition

Hydatid disease or echinococciasis is a tissue infection of humans caused by larvae of *Echinococcus granulosus* and *Echinococcus multilocularis*. The former, the more common infection, is that discussed herein.

Organism

Adult in canines

The adult *E. granulosus* inhabits the small bowel of dogs, wolves, and other canines, where it survives for a scant 12 months. The scolex, like that of the genus *Taenia*, possesses four sucking discs and a double row of hooklets. The entire strobila, however, measures only 5 mm in length and contains but three proglottids; one immature, one mature, and one gravid.

Wide range of herbivores and humans serve as intermediates

The latter segment splits either before or after passage in the stool, releasing eggs that appear identical to those of *T. saginata* and *T. solium*. A number of mammals may serve as intermediates, including sheep, goats, camels, deer, caribou, moose, and, most important, humans. When one

Larvae from ingested eggs penetrate to portal or systemic circulation

of these hosts ingests eggs, they hatch, and the embryos penetrate the intestinal mucosa and are carried by the portal blood to the liver. Here, many are filtered out in the hepatic sinusoids. The rest traverse the liver and are carried to the lung, where most lodge. A few pass through the pulmonary capillaries, enter the systemic circulation, and are carried to the brain, heart, bones, and other tissues. Many of the larvae are phagocytosed and destroyed. The survivors form a cyst wall composed of an

Cysts and daughter cysts develop in tissues

external laminated cuticle and an internal germinal membrane. The cyst fills with fluid and slowly expands, reaching a diameter of 1 cm over 5–6 months. Secondary or daughter cysts form within the original hydatid. Within each of these daughter cysts, new protoscolices are produced from the germinal lining. Some break free, dropping to the bottom of the cyst to form *hydatid sand*. When hydatid-containing tissues of the intermediate

Cycle completed with ingestion of cysts by canine

host are ingested by a canine, thousands of scolices are released in the intestine to develop into adult worms.

Epidemiology

Pastoral infections maintained by dogs feeding on viscera of herbivores

There are two major epidemiologic forms of echinococciasis, pastoral and sylvatic. The more common pastoral form has its highest incidence in Australia, New Zealand, South and East Africa, the Middle East, Central

Europe, and South America, where domestic herbivores such as sheep, cattle, and camels are raised in close contact with dogs. Although approximately 200 human cases are reported each year in the United States, most were acquired elsewhere. Indigenous cases do occur, however, particularly among Basque sheep farmers in California, southwestern Indians and some Utah shepherds. Animal husbandry practices that permit dogs to feed on the raw viscera of slaughtered sheep allow the cycle of transmission to continue. Shepherds become infected while handling or fondling their dogs. Eggs retained in the fur of these animals are picked up on the hands and later ingested.

Sylvatic echinococciasis is found principally in Alaska and western Canada, where wolves act as the definitive host and moose or caribou as the intermediate. In two counties in California, a second cycle involving deer and coyotes has been described. When hunters kill these wild deer and feed their offal to accompanying dogs, a pastoral cycle may be established.

Hand-to-mouth infection of humans

Sylvatic cycle in Alaska and western Canada

Clinical Manifestations

The enlarging hydatid cysts produce tissue damage by mechanical means. The clinical presentation depends on their number, site, and rate of growth. Typically, there is a latent period of 5–20 years between acquisition of infection and subsequent diagnosis. Intervals as long as 75 years have been reported occasionally.

In sylvatic infections, two-thirds of the cysts are found in the lung, the remainder in the liver. Most patients are asymptomatic when the lesion is discovered on routine chest X-ray or physical examination. Occasionally, the patient may present with hemoptysis, pain in the right upper quadrant of the abdomen, or a tender hepatic mass. Significant morbidity is uncommon, and death extremely rare. In the pastoral form of disease, 60% of the cysts are found in the liver, 25% in the lung. One-fifth of all patients show involvement of multiple sites. The hydatid cysts, which grow more rapidly (0.25–1 cm/year) than the sylvatic lesions, may reach enormous size. Twenty percent eventually rupture, inducing fever, pruritis, urticaria, and, at times, anaphylactic shock and death. Release of thousands of scolices may lead to dissemination of the infection. Rupture of pulmonary lesions also induces cough, chest pain, and hemoptysis. Liver cysts may break through the diaphragm or rupture into the bile duct or peritoneal cavity. The majority, however, present as a tender, palpable hepatic mass. Intrabiliary extrusion of calcified cysts may mimic the signs of acute cholecystitis; complete obstruction results in jaundice. Bone cysts produce pathologic fractures, whereas lesions in the central nervous system are often manifest as blindness or epilepsy. Cardiac lesions have been associated with conduction disturbances, ventricular rupture, and embolic metastases. A recent study has suggested that circulating antigen–antibody complexes may be deposited in the kidney, initiating membranous glomerulonephritis.

Disease caused by mechanical effects of cysts after many years

Pulmonary cysts predominate in sylvatic disease, hepatic in pastoral

Cysts may attain large size

Rupture leads to hypersensitivity manifestations and dissemination

Severe effects of cerebral cysts

Laboratory Diagnosis

On chest X-ray, pulmonary lesions present as slightly irregular, round masses of uniform density devoid of calcification. In contrast, more than one-half of hepatic lesions display a smooth, calcific rim. Computer tomography or ultrasonic scanning may reveal either a simple fluid-filled cyst or daughter cysts with hydatid sand. Because of the potential for an anaphylactoid reaction and dissemination of infection, diagnostic aspira-

Radiologic and tomographic appearance

Aspiration of cysts
contraindicated

Serologic diagnosis

tion is contraindicated. In patients with ruptured pulmonary cysts, however, scolices may be demonstrated in the sputum. In most cases, confirmation of the diagnosis requires serologic testing. Unfortunately, current procedures are not totally satisfactory. Indirect hemagglutination and latex agglutination tests are positive in 90% of patients with hepatic lesions and 60% of those with pulmonary hydatid cysts. When using hydatid cyst fluid or soluble scolex antigen, the presence of an "arc 5" in the immunoelectrophoresis test appears to be more specific. An adaption of this test to an enzyme-linked immunoelectrodiffusion technique appears to provide a rapid, sensitive diagnostic test. Other serologic tests are in the process of evaluation.

Treatment

Surgical extirpation

The only definitive therapy available at this time is surgical extirpation. Patients with pulmonary hydatid cysts of the sylvatic type and small calcified hepatic lesions require surgery only if they become symptomatic or the cysts increase dramatically in size over time. All other lesions should be excised or drained and irrigated with hypertonic saline, silver nitrate, or cetrimide to kill the protoscolices and prevent metastatic infection. Medical therapy using high-dose albendazole and praziquantel are experimental, but may be considered when surgery is contraindicated.

Prevention

Infected dogs should be wormed, and infected carcasses and offal burned or buried. Hands should be carefully washed after contact with potentially infected dogs.

Additional Reading

Craig, P.S., Zeyhle, E., and Romig, T. 1986. Hydatid disease: Research and control in Turkana. II. The role of immunological techniques for the diagnosis of hydatid disease. *Trans. Roy. Soc. Trop. Med. Hyg.* 80:183–192. One of a series of papers examining a population of Kenyans that suffers the highest incidence of echinococciasis in the world.

Jones, T.C. 1978. Cestodes. *Clin. Gastroenterol.* 7:105–128. An extensive review.

Loo, L., and Braude, A. 1982. Cerebral cysticercosis in San Diego. A report of 23 cases and a review of the literature. *Medicine.* 61:341–359.

Ruttenber, A.J., Weniger, B.G., Sorvillo, F., Murray, R.A., and Ford, S.L. 1984. Diphyllobothriasis associated with salmon consumption in Pacific Coast states. *Am. J. Trop. Med. Hyg.* 33:455–459.

Wilson, J.F., Diddams, A.C., and Rausch, R.L. 1968. Cystic hydatid disease in Alaska: A review of 101 autochthonous cases of *Echinococcus granulosus* infection. *Am. Rev. Respir. Dis.* 98:1–15. The unique characteristics of sylvatic *Echinococcus granulosus* infections in Alaska are discussed.

58

Trematodes

James J. Plorde

Of the myriad relationships that have developed between helminth and human over the millennia of our mutual existence, none has proved more destructive to our health and productivity than that forged with the indomitable flukes. Typically, the adults live for decades within human tissues and vascular systems, where they resist immunologic attack and produce progressive damage to vital organs. Morphologically, trematodes are bilaterally symmetric, vary in length from a few millimeters to several centimeters and possess two deep suckers from which they derive their name ("body with holes"). One surrounds the oral cavity; the other is located on the ventral surface of the worm. These organs are used for both attachment and locomotion; movement is effected in a characteristic "inchworm" fashion. The digestive tract begins at the oral sucker and continues as a muscular pharynx and esophagus before bifurcating to form bilateral ceca that end blindly near the posterior extremity of the worm. Undigested food is vomited out through the oral cavity. The excretory system consists of a number of hollow, ciliated "flame cells" that excrete waste products into interconnecting ducts terminating in a posterior excretory pore.

The reproductive systems vary and serve as a means for dividing the trematodes into two major categories: the hermaphrodites and the schistosomes. The adult hermaphrodite contains both male and female gonads and produces operculate eggs. The schistosomes have separate sexes, and the fertilized female deposits only nonoperculated offspring. The two groups have similar life cycles. The major differential features are summarized in Table 58.1. Eggs are excreted from the human host and, if they reach fresh water, hatch to release ciliated larvae called *miracidia*. These larvae find and penetrate a snail host specific for the trematode species. In this intermediate host, they are transformed by a process of asexual reproduction into thousands of tail-bearing larvae or *cercariae*, which are released from the snail over a period of weeks and swim about vigorously

Morphology

Inchworm locomotion

Reproductive systems

Eggs hatch in fresh water to release miracidia which infect snails

Snail releases cercariae in water

789

Table 58.1 General Characteristics of Trematodes

Characteristic	Trematode Type	
	Blood	Tissue/Intestinal
Genus	*Schistosoma*	*Paragonimus, Clonorchis, Opisthorchis, Fasciola*
Morphology		
Adult	Oral and ventral suckers	Oral and ventral suckers
	Blind gastrointestinal tract	Blind gastrointestinal tract
	Slender, wormlike	Flat, leaflike
Egg	Nonoperculate	Operculate
Biology		
Sexes	Separate	Hermaphroditic
Intermediates	One	Two
Life span	Long	Long

Schistosoma cercariae infect humans through skin.

Paragonimus and *Clonorchis* have second intermediate host

in search of their next host. In the case of schistosomal cercariae, this host is the human. When they come in contact with the skin surface, they attach, discard their tails, and invade, thereby completing their life cycle. The cercariae of the hermaphroditic flukes encyst in or upon an aquatic plant or animal, where they undergo a second transformation to become infective *metacercariae*. Their cycle is completed when the second intermediate host is ingested by a human. Of the many trematodes that infect humans, only five will be discussed: the blood flukes, all of which are members of the genus *Schistosoma (S. mansoni, S. haematobium,* and *S. japonicum),* and the lung (*Paragonimus* spp.) and liver (*Clonorchis sinensis*) flukes, which are hermaphroditic (Figure 58.1). Basic details of other hermaphroditic tissue and intestinal flukes are listed in Table 58.2.

Paragonimiasis (Lung Fluke Infection)

Organism

Several *Paragonimus* species may infect humans. *Paragonimus westermani,* which is widely distributed in East Asia, is the species most fequently involved. The short, plump (10 × 5 mm), reddish-brown adults are characteristically found encapsulated in the pulmonary parenchyma of their definitive host. Here they deposit operculate, golden-brown eggs, which are distinguished from similar structures by their size (50 × 90 μm) and prominent periopercular shoulder. When the capsule erodes into a bronchiole, the eggs are coughed up and spat out or swallowed and passed in the stool. If they reach fresh water, they embryonate several weeks before the ciliated miracidia emerge through the open opercula. After invasion of an appropriate snail host, 3–5 months pass before cercariae are released. These larval forms invade the gills, musculature, and viscera of certain crayfish or freshwater crabs, in which, over 6–8 weeks, they transform into metacercariae. When the flesh of these second intermediate hosts is ingested by humans, the metacercariae encyst in the duodenum and burrow through the gut wall into the peritoneal cavity. The majority continue their migration through the diaphragm and reach maturity in the lungs 5–6 weeks later. Some organisms, however, are retained in the intestinal wall and mesentery or wander to other foci such as the liver, pancreas, kidney, skeletal muscle, or subcutaneous tissue. Young worms migrating

Adults encapsulate in lung

Capsule erodes into bronchiole, eggs coughed up; cycle continues if eggs reach water with susceptible snail

Crayfish and freshwater crabs second intermediate hosts

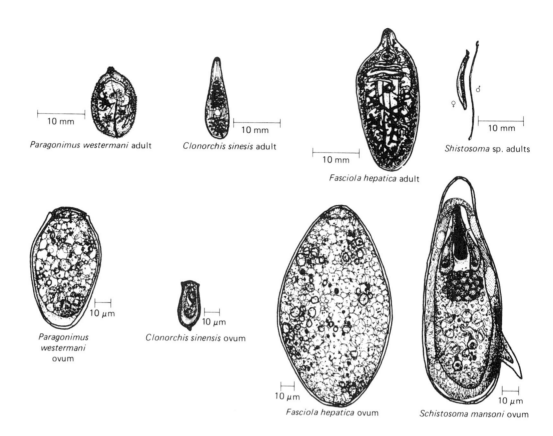

10 mm

Paragonimus westermani adult

10 mm

Clonorchis sinesis adult

10 mm

Fasciola hepatica adult

10 mm

Shistosoma sp. adults

Paragonimus westermani ovum

10 μm

Clonorchis sinensis ovum

10 μm

Fasciola hepatica ovum

10 μm

Schistosoma mansoni ovum

10 μm

58.1 Adult flukes and eggs.

through the neck and jugular foramen may encyst in the brain, the most common ectopic site.

Nonhuman definitive hosts

In addition to humans, other carnivores, including the rat, cat, dog, and pig, may serve as definitive hosts. Immature ectopic adults in the striated muscles of the pig may infect humans after ingestion of undercooked pork.

Epidemiology

Although most of the 3 million human infections are concentrated in Far Eastern nations such as Korea, Japan, China, Taiwan, the Philippines, and Indonesia, paragonimiasis has recently been described in India, Africa, and Latin America. *Paragonimus kellicotti,* a parasite of mink, is widely distributed in eastern Canada and the United States, but rarely produces human infection. Aproximately 1% of recent Indochinese immigrants to this country are infected with *P. westermani.* Infection of the snail host, which is typically found in small mountain streams located away from human habitation, is probably maintained by animal hosts other than humans. Human disease occurs when food shortages or local customs expose individuals to infected crabs. When these crustaceans are prepared for cooking, juice containing metacercariae may be left behind on the working surface and contaminate other foods subsequently prepared in the same area. Fresh crab juice, which is used for the treatment of infertility in the Cameroons and of measles in Korea, may also transmit the disease. In the

Infected snails often found in mountain streams

Humans infected by ingesting infected crustaceans

Table 58.2   Intestinal and Tissue Trematodes

	Paragonimus	Clonorchis	Opisthorchis	Fasciola	Fasciolopsis	Heterophyes/ Metagonimus
			Distribution			
Geographic	Asia, Africa, Central America	Japan, China, Taiwan, Vietnam	Asia, Eastern Europe	Worldwide	East and Southeast Asia	Asia, USSR, Mediterranean
Infected population (in millions)	3	20	4	—	10	—
			Adult Worms			
Reservoir hosts	Domestic and wild animals	Cats, dogs	Domestic and wild animals	Sheep and other herbivores	Pigs	Fish-eating mammals
Location in body	Lungs, CNS	Biliary tract	Biliary tract	Biliary tract	Small intestine	Small intestine
Length (mm)	7–12	10–25	10	20–30	20–75	1–2
Life span (years)	4–6	20–30	20–30	10–15	0.5	1
			Eggs			
Characteristics	Operculated	Operculated	Operculated	Operculated	Operculated	Operculated
Size (μm)	80–100	26–30	26–30	130–150	130–150	26–30
Location[a]	Sputum, stool	Bile, stool	Bile, stool	Bile, stool	Stool	Stool
			Larvae			
First intermediate	Snail	Snail	Snail	Snail	Snail	Snail
Second intermediate	Freshwater crab and crayfish	Freshwater fish	Freshwater fish	Watercress and other aquatic plants	Water chestnut and other aquatic plants	Freshwater fish

Abbreviation: CNS = central nervous system.
[a] Diagnostic specimens.

Orient, crabs are frequently eaten after they have been lightly salted, pickled, or immersed briefly in wine (drunken crab), practices that are seldom lethal to the metacercariae. Children living in endemic areas may be infected while handling or ingesting crabs during the course of play.

Clinical Manifestations

Formation of lung cysts

Secondary infection of ruptured cysts

Chronic pulmonary abscess

Other infected sites

The presence of the adult worm in the lung elicits an eosinophilic inflammatory reaction and, eventually, the formation of a 1- to 2-cm fibrous capsule that surrounds and encloses the parasite. With the onset of oviposition, the capsule swells and erodes into a bronchiole, resulting in expectoration of the brownish eggs, blood, and an inflammatory exudate. Secondary bacterial infection of the evacuated cysts is common, producing a clinical picture of chronic bronchitis or bronchiectasis. When cysts rupture into the pleural cavity, chest pain and effusion can result. In severe infection, the patient may develop chronic pneumonia or a nonresolving lung abscess, a clinical picture closely resembling that of pulmonary tuberculosis. The confusion is compounded by the frequent coexistence of the two diseases. Adult flukes in the intestine and mesentery produce pain, bloody diarrhea, and, on occasion, palpable abdominal masses. In approximately 1% of Oriental cases, parasites lodge in the brain and produce a variety of neurologic manifestations, including epilepsy, paralysis, homonymous hemianopsia, optic atrophy, and papilledema.

Laboratory Diagnosis

Search for eggs in sputum, pleural fluid, and feces

Eggs are usually absent from the sputum during the first 3 months of overt infection; however, repeated examinations will eventually demonstate them in more than three-quarters of infected patients. When a pleural effusion is present, it should be checked for eggs. Stool examination is frequently helpful, particularly in children who swallow their expectorated sputum. Approximately 50% of patients with brain lesions will demonstrate calcification on X-ray films of the skull. The cerebrospinal fluid in such cases shows elevated protein levels and eosinophilic leukocytosis. A diagnosis in these cases, however, often depends on the detection of circulating antibodies. Their presence usually correlates well with acute disease and disappears with successful therapy.

Serodiagnosis

Treatment and Prevention

The disease responds well to bithionol or praziquantel therapy. Control requires adequate cooking of shellfish before ingestion.

Clonorchiasis (Liver Fluke Infection)

Organism

Flukes of the genera *Fasciola, Opisthorchis,* and *Clonorchis* may all infect the human biliary tract and, at times, produce manifestations of ductal obstruction. *Clonorchis sinensis,* the Chinese liver fluke, is the most important and is discussed herein. Essential details of other hermaphroditic tissue and intestinal trematodes are listed in Table 58.2. The small, slender (5 × 15 mm) adult survives up to 50 years in the biliary tract of its host by feasting on the rich mucosal secretions. A cone-shaped anterior pole, a large oral sucker, and a pair of deeply lobular testes arranged one behind the other in the posterior third of the worm serve to distinguish it from other hepatic parasites. Approximately 2000 tiny (15 × 30 μm) ovoid eggs are discharged daily and find their way down the bile duct and into the fecal stream. The exquisite urn-shaped shells have a discernible shoulder at their opercular rim and a tiny knob on the broader posterior pole. On reaching fresh water, they are ingested by their intermediate snail host, transformed into cercariae, and released to penetrate the tissues of freshwater fish, in which they encyst to form metacercariae. If the latter host is ingested by a fish-eating mammal, the larvae are released in the duodenum, ascend the common bile duct, migrate to the bile capillaries, and mature to adulthood over 30 days.

Adults in biliary tract

Eggs in feces

Snails first intermediate host, fish second

Metacercariae from ingested fish migrate to biliary system

In addition to humans, rats, cats, dogs, and pigs may serve as definitive hosts.

Epidemiology

Geography

Mechanism of transmission to humans

Clonorchiasis is endemic in the Far East, particularly in Korea, Japan, Taiwan, the Red River Valley of Vietnam, the Southern Chinese province of Kwantung, and Hong Kong. In previous years, parasite transmission was perpetuated by the practice of fertilizing commercial fish ponds with human feces. Recent improvements in the disposal of human waste have diminished acquisition of the disease in most countries. However, the extremely long life span of these worms is reflected in a much slower decrease in the overall infection rate. In some villages in southern China,

High attack rate

Ingestion of uncooked fish

the entire adult population is infected. A recent survey of stool specimens from immigrants from Hong Kong to Canada showed an infection rate of more than 15% overall and 23% in adults between 30 and 50 years of age. The disease is acquired by eating raw, frozen, dried, salted, or pickled fish. Commercial shipment of such products outside of the endemic area may result in the acquisition of worms far from their original source.

Clinical Manifestations

Light infection usually asymptomatic

Severe hepatic and biliary manifestations from heavy worm loads

Migration of the larvae from the duodenum to the bile duct may produce fever, chills, mild jaundice, eosinophilia, and liver enlargement. The adult worm induces epithelial hyperplasia, adenoma formation, and inflammation and fibrosis around the smaller bile ducts. In light infection, clinical disease seldom results. However, numerous reinfections may produce worm loads of 500–1000, resulting in the formation of bile stones and sometimes bile duct carcinoma in patients with severe, long-standing infections. Calculus formation is often accompanied by asymptomatic biliary carriage of *Salmonella typhi*. Dead worms may obstruct the common bile duct and induce secondary bacterial cholangitis, which may be accompanied by bacteremia, endotoxin shock, and hypoglycemia. Occasionally, adult worms are found in the pancreatic ducts, where they can produce ductal obstruction and acute pancreatitis.

Laboratory Diagnosis

Search for eggs in feces and duodenal aspirates

Eosinophilia common in acute disease

Definitive diagnosis requires the recovery and identification of the distinctive egg from the stool or duodenal aspirates. In mild infections, repeated examinations may be required. As most patients are asymptomatic, any individual with clinical manifestations of disease in whom *Clonorchis* eggs are found must be evaluated for the presence of other causes of illness. In acute symptomatic clonorchiasis, there is usually leukocytosis, eosinophilia, elevation of alkaline phosphatase levels, and abnormal radioisotopic and ultrasonographic liver scans. Cholangiograms may reveal dilatation of the intrahepatic ducts and small filling defects compatible with the presence of adult worms.

Treatment and Prevention

Praziquantel has proven to be an effective therapeutic agent. Prevention requires thorough cooking of freshwater fish and sanitary disposal of human feces.

Schistosomiasis (Blood Fluke Infection)

Organism

Inhabit portal vascular system

The schistosomes are a group of closely related flukes that inhabit the portal vascular system of a number of animals. Of the five species known to infect humans, three—*Schistosoma mansoni, Schistosoma haematobium,* and *Schistosoma japonicum*—are of primary importance, infecting over 200 million individuals worldwide. The remaining two are found only in limited areas of Africa (*Schistosoma intercalatum*) and Southeast Asia (*Schistosoma mekongi*) and will not be discussed in detail.

The adults of these species can be distinguished from the hermaphroditic trematodes by the anterior location of their ventral sucker, by their

Sexually differentiated

cylindric bodies, and by their reproductive systems (that is, separate sexes). They are differentiated from one another only with difficulty. The 1- to 2-cm male possesses a deep ventral groove, or *gynecophoral canal*, in which he carries the longer, more slender female in life-long copulatory embrace. After mating in the portal vein, the conjoined couple utilize their suckers to ascend the mesenteric vessels against the flow of blood. Guided by unknown stimuli, *S. japonicum* enters the superior mesenteric vein, eventually reaching the venous radicals of the small intestine and ascending colon; *S. mansoni* and *S. haematobium* are directed to the inferior mesenteric system. The destination of the former is the descending colon and rectum; the latter, however, passes through the hemorrhoidal plexus to the systemic venous system, ultimately coming to rest in the veins of the bladder and other pelvic organs. On reaching the submucosal venules, the worms initiate oviposition. Each pair deposits 300 (*S. mansoni*) to 3000 (*S. japonicum*) eggs daily for the remainder of its 4- to 35-year life span. Enzymes secreted by the enclosed miracidium diffuse through the shell and digest the surrounding tissue. Ova lying immediately adjacent to the mucosal surface rupture into the lumen of the bowel (*S. mansoni, S. japonicum*) or bladder (*S. haematobium*) and are passed to the outside in the excreta. Here, with appropriate techniques, they may be readily observed and differentiated. The eggs of *S. mansoni* are oval, possess a sharp lateral spine, and measure 60×140 μm. Those of *S. haematobium* differ primarily in the terminal location of their spine. The eggs of *S. japonicum*, in contrast, are more nearly circular, measuring 70×90 μm. A minute lateral spine can be visualized only with care.

When the eggs are deposited in fresh water, the miracidia hatch quickly. Upon finding a snail host appropriate for their species, they invade and are transformed over 1–2 months into thousands of forked-tailed cercariae. When released from the snail, these infectious larvae swim about vigorously for a few days. Cercariae coming in contact with human skin during this time attach, discard their tails, and penetrate. The resulting *schistosomula* enter small venules and find their way through the right side of the heart to the lung. After a delay of several days, the parasites enter the systemic circulation and are distributed to the gut. Those surviving passage through the intestinal capillary bed return to the portal vein, where they mature to sexually active adults over 1–3 months.

S. mansoni reaches colon and rectum and S. haematobium reaches veins of bladder and pelvic organs

Eggs deposited submucosally, rupture to lumina, and pass outside

Miracidia invade snail

Cercariae from snail become schistosomula, traverse human skin and vascular system to portal vein

Epidemiology

Most important of helminthic infections

The widespread distribution and extensive morbidity of schistosomiasis makes it the single most important helminthic infection in the world today. Currently, more than 200 million individuals in 74 countries are infected. The continued presence of the parasite depends upon the disposal of infected human excrement into fresh water, the availability of appropriate snail hosts, and the exposure of humans to water infected with cercariae. The construction of modern sanitation and water purification facilities would break this cycle of transmission, but exceeds the economic resources of most endemic nations. Paradoxically, several massive land irrigation projects launched over the past two decades for the express purpose of speeding economic development have resulted in the dispersion of infected humans and snails to previously uninvolved areas.

Spread to areas served by new irrigation projects

Geographic distribution

Schistosoma mansoni, the most widespread of the blood flukes, is the only one present in the Western Hemisphere. Originally introduced by African slaves, it is now found in Venezuela, Brazil, Surinam, Puerto Rico, the Dominican Republic, St. Lucia, and several other Caribbean islands.

Dependence on snail host

As a suitable snail host is lacking, transmission does not occur within the continental United States; however, nearly half a million individuals residing there have acquired schistosomiasis elsewhere. Puerto Rican, Yemenite, and Southeast Asian populations are those predominantly involved. In the Eastern Hemisphere, the prevalence of *S. mansoni* infection is highest in the Nile Delta and the tropical section of Africa. Isolated foci are also found in East and South Africa, Yemen, Saudi Arabia, and Israel.

Schistosoma haematobium is largely confined to Africa and the Middle East, where its distribution overlaps that of *S. mansoni*. *Schistosoma japonicum* affects the agricultural populations of several Far Eastern countries, including Japan, China, the Philippines, and the Celebes. The closely related *S. mekongi* is found in the Mekong and Mun River valleys of Vietnam, Thailand, Cambodia, and Laos.

Age-related susceptibility

Within endemic areas, there are wide variations in both infection rates and worm loads. In general, both peak in the second decade of life and then decrease with advancing age. This finding has been explained in part by changes in the intensity of water exposure and in part by the slow development of immunity. Most infected patients carry fewer than 10 pairs of worms in the vascular system and, accordingly, lack clinical manifestation of disease. Individuals who develop much heavier loads as a result of repeated infections may experience serious morbidity or mortality.

Pathogenesis and Clinical Manifestations

There are three major clinicopathologic stages in schistosomiasis: The first stage is initiated by the penetration and migration of the schistosomula. The second or intermediate stage begins with oviposition and is associated with a complex of clinical manifestations. The third or chronic stage is characterized by granuloma formation and scarring around retained eggs.

Local and systemic hypersensitivity reactions

Early Stage. Within a few hours of penetrating the skin, a large proportion of the schistosomula die. Immediate and delayed hypersensitivity to parasitic antigens results in an intensely pruritic papular skin rash. As the viable schistosomula begin their migration to the liver, the rash disappears and the patient experiences fever, headache, and abdominal pain for 1–2 weeks.

Serum sickness-like illness

Intermediate Stage. One to two months after primary exposure, patients with severe *S. mansoni* or *S. japonicum* infections experience the onset of an acute febrile illness that bears a striking resemblance to serum sickness. It has been suggested that the onset of oviposition leads to a state of relative antigen excess and the formation of soluble immune complexes. Indeed, high levels of such complexes have been demonstrated in the peripheral blood and correlate well with the severity of illness. In addition to the fever and chills, patients experience cough, urticaria, arthralgia, lymphadenopathy, splenomegaly, abdominal pain, and diarrhea. Sigmoidoscopic examination reveals an inflamed colonic mucosa and petechial hemorrhages; occasionally, patients with *S. japonicum* infection will develop clinical manifestations of encephalitis. Typically, leukocytosis, marked peripheral eosinophilia, and elevated levels of IgM, IgG, and IgE immunoglobulins are present. This symptom complex is commonly

Katayama syndrome

termed the *Katayama syndrome;* it may persist for 3 months or more and occasionally results in death.

Chronic Schistosomiasis.   Approximately one-half of all deposited eggs reach the lumen of the bowel or bladder and are shed from the body. Those retained induce inflammation and scarring, initiating the final and most morbid phase of schistosomiasis. Soluble antigens excreted by the eggs stimulate the formation of T-cell-mediated eosinophilic granulomas. Early in the infection, the inflammatory response is vigorous, producing lesions more than 100-fold larger than the inciting egg itself. Obstruction of blood flow is common. With time, the host's inflammatory response moderates, leading to a significant decrease in granuloma size. Fibroblasts stimulated by factors released by both retained eggs and the granulomas lay down scar tissue, rendering the earlier, granuloma-induced vascular obstruction permanent. As would be expected, the severity of tissue damage is directly related to the total number of eggs retained.

In *S. haematobium* infection, the bladder mucosa becomes thickened, papillated, and ulcerated. Hematuria and dysuria result; repeated hemorrhages produce anemia. In severe infections the muscular layers of the bladder are involved, with loss of bladder capacity and contractibility. Vesicoureteral reflux, ureteral obstruction, and hydronephrosis may follow. Progressive obstruction leads to renal failure and uremia. Calcification of the bladder wall is occasionally seen, and approximately 10% of patients harbor urinary tract calculi. Secondary bacterial infections are common. Chronic *Salmonella* bacteruria with recurrent bouts of bacteremia have been reported from Egypt. In the same country, bladder carcinoma is frequently seen as a late complication of disease.

In *S. mansoni* and *S. japonicum* infections, the bowel mucosa is congested, thickened, and ulcerated. Polyposis has been reported from Egypt, but not elsewhere. Patients experience abdominal pain, diarrhea, and blood in the stool. Eggs deposited in the larger intestinal veins may be carried by the portal blood flow back to the liver, where they lodge in the presinusoidal capillaries. The resulting inflammatory reaction leads to the development of periportal fibrosis and hepatic enlargement. The frequency and severity with which the liver is involved are gentically determined and associated with the HLA type of the patient. In most cases, liver function is well preserved. Infected individuals who subsequently acquire hepatitis B virus develop chronic active hepatitis more frequently than those free of schistosomes. The presinusoidal obstruction to blood flow can result in the serious manifestations of portal obstruction. Eggs carried around the liver in the portosystemic collateral vessels may lodge in the small pulmonary arterioles, where they may produce interstitial scarring, pulmonary hypertension, and right ventricular failure. Occasionally, eggs may be deposited in the central nervous system, where they may cause epilepsy or paraplegia.

Some differences between the clinical presentation of schistosomiasis mansoni and that of schistosomiasis japonicum have been noted. Manifestations of the latter disease typically occur earlier in the course of the infection and tend to be more severe. When involvement of the central nervous system develops, it is more likely to occur in the brain than the spinal cord. On the other hand, immune complex nephropathy and recurrent *Salmonella* bacteremia are more likely to be seen in hepatosplenic *S. mansoni* infections. The latter phenomenon is apparently related to the ability of *Salmonella* to parasitize the gut and integument of the adult fluke, providing a persistent bacterial focus within the portal system of the infected patient. This focus cannot be eradicated without treatment of the schistosomal infection.

Inflammatory and fibrotic reactions to retained eggs cause chronic disease

Bladder lesions with *S. haematobium*

Chronic urinary carriage of *Salmonella*

Bowel, liver, and pulmonary damage in *S. mansoni* and *S. japonicum* infections

Recurrent *Salmonella* bacteremia in *S. mansoni* infection

Immunity

Major manifestations from effects of cell-mediated immunity

The major clinicopathologic manifestations of schistosomiasis result from the host's cell-mediated immune response to the presence of retained eggs. With time, the intensity of this reaction is muted; granulomas formed in the later stages of infection are smaller and less damaging than those formed early. The mechanisms responsible for this modulation are not fully understood. Present evidence suggests that both suppressor T-cell activity and antibody blockade are involved. The correlation in humans between HLA types A1 and B5 and the development of hepatosplenomegaly suggests that the extent of the immunoregulation is influenced, at least in part, by the genetic background of the host.

Antigenic disguise by adult parasite

As evidenced by their prolonged survival, the adult worms are remarkably well tolerated by their hosts. In part, this tolerance may be attributable to the ability of the developing parasites to disguise themselves by absorbing host molecules, including immunoglobulins, blood group glycolipids, and histocompatibility complex antigens. Antibodies formed against the immature worms before they have acquired host antigens, however, are effective in protecting the host from reinfection. Schistosomula that pentrate the skin after the primary infection are coated with specific antibody, bound to eosinophils, and destroyed. Although protection is not complete, the 60–80% kill rate is highly effective in controlling the intensity of parasitism. This condition, in which adult worms from a primary infection can survive in a host resistant to reinfection, has been termed *concomitant immunity*. It may be experimentally reproduced by exposing subjects to irradiated cercariae incapable of reaching full maturity.

Concomitant immunity

Laboratory Diagnosis

Search for *S. haemotobium* eggs in urine

Definitive diagnosis requires the recovery of the charcteristic eggs in urine, stool, or biopsy specimens. In *S. haematobium* infections, eggs are most numerous in urine samples obtained at midday. When examination of the sediment yields negative results, eggs may sometimes be recovered by filtering the urine through a membrane filter. Cystoscopy with biopsy of the bladder mucosa may be required for the diagnosis of mild infection. Eggs of *S. mansoni* and *S. japonicum* are passed in the stool. Concentration technqiues such as formalin-ether or gravity sedimentation are necesssary when the ova are scanty. Results of rectal biopsy may be positive when those of repeated stool examinations are negative.

***S. mansoni* and *S. japonicum* eggs in stool; rectal biopsy**

Determination of egg viability

Because dead eggs may persist in tissue for a long time after the death of the adult worms, active infection is confirmed only if the eggs are shown to be viable. This confirmation may be obtained by observing the eggs microscopically for movement of flame cell cilia or by hatching them in water. Quantitation of egg output is useful in estimating the severity of infection and in the following response to treatment.

Currently available serologic tests possess sensitivities exceeding 90%, but cannot reliably distinguish active from inactive disease. It is probable that this shortcoming will be alleviated by tests using defined antigens from different life stages of the schistosomes.

Treatment

Treatment of hypersensitivity reactions

No specific therapy is available for the treatment of schistosomal dermatitis or the Katayama syndrome. Antihistamines and corticosteroids may be helpful in ameliorating their more severe manifestations. In the late stage of schistosomiasis, therapy is directed at interrupting egg de-

Anthelmintic drugs

position by killing or sterilizing the adult worms. As the severity of clinical and pathologic manifestations is related to the intensity of infection, therapy is usually reserved for patients with moderate or severe active infections.

Several anthelmintic agents may be used. Praziquantel, which is active against all three species of schistosomes, is the agent of choice for *S. japonicum*. In addition to praziquantel, metrifonate may be used for *S. haematobium* and oxamniquine for *S. mansoni*.

Control and Prevention

Sanitary disposal of feces

Molluscicides

Vaccines

It has proved both difficult and expensive to control this deadly disease. Programs aimed at interrupting transmission of the parasite by the provision of pure water supplies and the sanitary disposal of human feces are often beyond the economic reach of the nations most seriously affected. Similarly, measures to deny snails access to newly irrigated lands are expensive. Chemical molluscicides have been shown effective in limited trials, but have been less successful when used over large areas for prolonged periods. Mass therapy of the infected human population has, until recently, been severely limited by the toxicity of effective agents. It is possible that the agents developed most recently will prove more suitable for this purpose. At present, programs that have incorporated all of these control measures have been the most successful.

Currently, there is intense interest in developing a vaccine suitable for human use. A vaccine made from irradiated *Schistosoma bovis* cercariae, developed for cattle, appears to confer a significant degree of protection against infection. Similar vaccines are not available for human populations until questions concerning safety and suitability for widespread field use are satisfactorily resolved. Monoclonal antibodies have been successfully used to identify a number of schistosomula and adult antigens thought to be capable of inducing protective immunity. A number of such defined antigen vaccines are undergoing study.

Additional Reading

Johnson, R.J., Jong, E.C., Dunning, S.B., Carberry, W.L., et al. 1985. Paragonamiasis, Diagnosis and the use of praziquantel in treatment. *Rev. Infect. Dis.* 7:200–206. Discusses the clinical presentation, diagnosis and treatment of paragonamiasis presenting in Southeast Asian immigrants to the United States.

Nash, T.E., Cheever, A.W., Ottensen, E.A., and Cook, J.A. 1982. Schistoma infection in humans: Perspectives and recent findings. *Ann. Intern. Med.* 97:740–754.

Rim, H.J. 1986. The current pathology and chemotherapy of Clonorchiasis. *Korean J. Parasitol.* 24: (suppl monograph series 3)1–141. The most comprehensive recent review of this disease.

Seah, S.K. 1978. Digenetic trematodes. *Clin. Gastroenterol.* 7:87–104. A number of trematode infections are discussed.

Strickland, G.T. 1982. Schistosomiasis: Eradication or control? *Rev. Infect. Dis.* 4:951–954.

Lichtenberg, F. Von 1985. Conference on contended issues of immunity to schistosomiasis. *Am. J. Trop. Med. Hyg.* 34:78–85. Introduction to conference dealing with the evidence for protective immunity, mechanisms of immunologic killing, and future prospects for vaccines against the schistosomes.

Warren, K.S. 1982. Selective primary health care: Strategies for control of disease in the developing world. I. Schistosomiasis. *Rev. Infect. Dis.* 4:715–726. This article and the Strickland article discuss lucidly the limitations of current control strategies and offer alternative approaches, including directed mass therapy.

59

Skin and Wound Infections

John C. Sherris and
Kenneth J. Ryan

Skin Infections

Microbial infections of the skin can result from invasion from an external source by certain bacteria, viruses, fungi, or parasites or from such organisms reaching the skin through the bloodstream as part of a systemic disease. Blood-borne involvement may be evidenced by rashes in many viral and bacterial infections, such as measles, varicella, meningococcal septicemia, and secondary syphilis, or may yield more chronic skin lesions in granulomatous diseases, such as blastomycosis, tuberculosis, and syphilis. Skin lesions remote from sites of infection can be produced by some bacterial toxins, such as the erythrogenic toxin of *Streptococcus pyogenes* (group A streptococcus), exfoliatin, or the toxic shock toxin of some strains of *Staphylococcus aureus*. They can also result from immunologic responses to microbial antigens that have reached the skin. Thus, there are manifold skin manifestations of infections; however, this chapter will be restricted to the discussion of *direct* infections that may occur in the Western Hemisphere.

The skin is an organ system with multiple functions, including protection of the tissues from external microbial invasion. Its keratinized stratified epithelium prevents direct microbial invasion under normal conditions of surface temperature and humidity, and its normal flora, pH, and chemical defenses tend to inhibit colonization by many pathogens (Chapters 9 and 10). However, the skin is subject to repeated minor traumas that are often unnoticed, but that destroy its integrity and allow organisms to gain access to its deeper layers from the external environment. The surface is also penetrated by ducts of pilosebaceous units and sweat glands, and microbial invasion can occur along these routes, particularly if the ducts are obstructed.

Infections in Hair Follicles, Sebaceous Glands, and Sweat Glands

Folliculitis. Folliculitis is a minor infection of the hair follicles and is usually caused by *S. aureus*. As it is often associated with areas of friction and of sweat gland activity, it is seen most frequently on the neck, face, axillae, and buttocks. Blockage of ducts with inspissated sebum, as in acne vulgaris, predisposes to this condition. Folliculitis can also be caused by *Pseudomonas aeruginosa,* and this form of the disease has become more common in recent years with the popularity of hot tubs and whirlpool baths. Unless these facilities are thoroughly cleansed and adequately chlorinated, they can grow large numbers of pseudomonads at their normal operating temperatures, causing extensive folliculitis on areas of the body that have been immersed. The lesions subside rapidly when the insult is discontinued. Occasionally folliculitis may be caused by infection with *Condida albicans.* Such cases are particularly common in immunocompromised hosts.

Acne vulgaris also involves inflammation of hair follicles and associated sebaceous glands. The comedo of acne results from multiplication of *Propionibacterium acnes,* the predominant anaerobe of the normal skin, behind and within inspissated sebum. Organic acids produced by this organism are believed to stimulate an inflammatory response and thus contribute to the disease process. The primary cause of the disease, however, is hormonal influences on sebum secretion that occur at puberty, and the disease usually resolves in early adult life.

Furuncles. The furuncle is a small staphylococcal abscess that develops in the region of a hair follicle. Furuncles may be solitary or multiple and may constitute a troublesome recurrent disease. Spread of infection to the dermis and subcutaneous tissues can result in a more extensive multiloculated abscess, the carbuncle. These lesions and their treatment are considered in Chapter 15.

Treatment. Folliculitis and individual furuncles are normally treated locally by measures designed to establish drainage without the use of antibiotics. Chronic furunculosis may require attempts to eliminate nasal carriage of *S. aureus,* which is sometimes the source of the infection. Antimicrobics are not usually required unless surrounding cellulitis develops. Severe acne can often be treated effectively with topical drying agents. Prolonged administration of low oral doses of tetracycline is often effective, although the reason for the therapeutic response is uncertain.

Infections through Minor or Inapparent Skin Lesions

Minor or inapparent skin lesions serve as the route of infection in many localized skin infections and in some systemic diseases, such as syphilis and leptospirosis.

Infection of Keratinized Layers. The only organisms that can utilize the keratin on cells, hairs, and nails are the dermatophyte fungi. The dermatophytes are particularly well adapted to these sites, cannot grow at 37°C, and fail to invade deeper layers. The clinical manifestations of these infections result from the inflammatory and delayed hypersensitivity responses of the host, and the desquamation induced by these processes is a major factor in the ultimate control of the infection by removing infected skin. In candidiasis, control involves cell-mediated immune mechanisms,

Staphylococcal and *Pseudomonas* infections of hair follicles

Propionibacterium acnes contributes to inflammation of acne

Staphylococcal furuncles are small skin abscesses

Hypersensitivity and inflammatory response to dermatophytes
Cell-mediated immune defects in chronic candidiasis

and chronic *Candida* skin and nail infections are often associated with defects in cellular immunity. The clinical manifestations of these diseases are described in Chapters 46 and 47.

Infection of Other Skin Layers.   Pyoderma, also termed *impetigo,* is a common, sometimes epidemic skin lesion. This disease is caused by *S. pyogenes* and occasionally, by streptococci of other groups although the lesion frequently becomes secondarily infected with *S. aureus.* The initial lesion is often a small vesicle that develops at the site of invasion and ruptures with superficial spread characterized by skin erosion and a serous exudate, which dries to produce a honey-colored crust. The exudate and crust contain numerous infecting streptococci.

Epidemic impetigo is most common in childhood and under conditions of heat, humidity, poor hygiene, and overcrowding. The infection may be spread by fomites such as shared clothing and towels. It is often caused by nephritogenic strains of *S. pyogenes,* particularly in the tropics, and acute glomerulonephritis may result. Rheumatic fever is not associated with streptococcal lesions of the skin. Treatment is usually with penicillin or erythromycin and topical antimicrobics or skin antiseptics to limit spread.

Bullous impetigo is a distinct disease caused by strains of *S. aureus* (usually phage type 71) that produce exfoliatin. It is most common in small children, but may occur at any age. The infection is characterized by large serum-filled bullae (blisters) within the skin layers at the site of infection Minor infections are treated topically; bullous impetigo in infants, however, is a serious disease that usually requires systemic antimicrobic treatment. Epidemic spread may occur under conditions similar to those described for streptococcal impetigo.

Erysipelas is a rapidly spreading infection of the deeper layers of the dermis that is almost always caused by *S. pyogenes.* It is associated with edema of the skin, marked erythema, pain, and systemic manifestations of infection, including fever and lymphadenopathy. As the infection is intradermal, *S. pyogenes* cannot usually be isolated from the skin surfaces. The disease can progress to septicemia or local necrosis of skin. It is serious and requires immediate treatment with penicillin or another β-lactam antibiotic with high activity against streptococci. Erythromycin is an alternative agent; however, erythromycin-resistant strains of *S. pyogenes* have become common in areas in which the antimicrobic has been widely used.

Cellulitis is not a skin infection per se, but can develop by extension from skin or wound infections. It usually presents as an acute inflammation of subcutaneous connective tissue with swelling and pain and often with marked constitutional signs and symptoms. It can be caused by many pathogenic bacteria, but *S. aureus* and *S. pyogenes* are most common. Enteric Gram-negative rods, clostridia, and other anaerobes may also cause cellulitis as a complication of wound infections, particularly in the immunocompromised host and the uncontrolled diabetic.

A relatively uncommon but important form of cellulitis that also involves the dermis is caused by *Haemophilus influenzae* type b. The infection develops most often in children. It is manifested by a warm, painful, bluish swelling that advances rapidly and is associated with fever, bacteremia, and considerable toxicity. Sepsis or meningitis may develop subsequently. Infections caused by ampicillin-sensitive strains respond rapidly to that antimicrobic, but resistant strains are becoming more common. Chloramphenicol or a third-generation cephalosporin is effective in almost all cases.

Skin Ulcers and Granulomatous Lesions

Many acute and subacute skin infections are characterized by ulceration or a granulomatous response. Some are sexually transmitted and are discussed in Chapter 70. Others derive from systemic infection and are not direct infections of skin. A few examples of direct infections, which pose special diagnostic problems are considered herein.

Herpetic paronychia can mimic staphylococcal infections

Herpes simplex virus can invade through the skin to produce a local vesicular lesion followed by ulceration. The lesion may then recur in the infected area. Primary herpetic lesions of the finger can mimic staphylococcal paronychia very closely, as well as produce lymphangitis and local and lymph node enlargement with pain and fever. The lesions are sterile on bacterial culture.

Skin diphtheria

Skin diphtheria, which remains common in some tropical areas, also occurred endemically among the transient population of the West Coast of the United States during the 1970s and early 1980s. The organism gains access through a wound or insect bite and causes chronic erosion and ulceration of the skin, sometimes with evidence of the systemic effects of diphtheria toxin.

Swimmer's granuloma

Mycobacterium marinum produces a self-limiting granuloma, usually of the forearms and knees. The organism usually enters through superficial abrasions from rocks or swimming pool walls. Infections with *Mycobacterium ulcerans* are more serious and produce progressive ulceration, but are limited to tropical areas and do not occur in the United States or Europe.

Necrotic ulcerations in immunocompromised host

Bacterial synergistic gangrene

Several rare forms of necrotic spreading skin ulceration tend to develop in immunosuppressed hosts, in diabetics, and as complications of abdominal surgery. These lesions include bacterial synergistic gangrene, apparently caused by a peptostreptococcus and *S. aureus*, streptococcal gangrene associated with *S. pyogenes* infection, and infection with a variety of opportunistic fungi. Variants of these conditions produce extensive and spreading necrotic cellulitis. Although unsuccessful at times, the major form of treatment is to excise the infected tissues widely and supplement such surgery with massive chemotherapy.

Fungal and parasitic ulcerations

Several primary fungal diseases are associated with cutaneous ulceration or cellulitis, including mycetoma and chromoblastomycosis, which involve the feet, and sporotrichosis, in which ulceration often develops from infected subcutaneous lymph nodes and vessels. Likewise, some parasites directly infect and ulcerate the skin, as in cutaneous leishmaniasis and cutaneous amebiasis. These latter two diseases are not contracted in the United States.

Wound Infections

Wounds subject to infection can be surgical, traumatic, or physiologic. The latter include the endometrial surface, after separation of the placenta, and the umbilical stump. Traumatic wounds comprise such diverse damage as deep cuts, compound fractures, frostbite necrosis, and thermal burns.

Sources of infection

Sources of infection include 1) the patient's own normal flora; 2) infectious material from carriers or other infected individuals that may reach the wound (for example, on fomites, on the hands of attendants, or through the air); and 3) pathogenic organisms from the inanimate environment that can contaminate the wound through soil, clothing, and other foreign material. Examples of such infections include contamination of a penetrating stab wound to the abdomen by colonic flora, contamination of a clean surgical wound in the operating room with *S. aureus* spread by dust from the clothing of a perineal carrier, and introduction of spores of *Clostridium tetani* into the tissues on a splinter.

Classification of Wounds

Surgical and traumatic wounds can be classified according to the extent of potential contamination. This criterion corresponds to the risk of infection and carries important implications regarding surgical treatment and chemoprophylaxis.

Clean, clean contaminated, and dirty wounds

Clean wounds are surgical wounds made under aseptic conditions that do not traverse infected tissues or extend into sites with a normal flora. Clean contaminated wounds are operative wounds that extend into sites with a normal flora (except the colon) without known contamination. Contaminated wounds include fresh surgical and traumatic wounds with a major risk of contamination, such as incisions entering nonpurulent infected tissues. Dirty and infected wounds include old, infected traumatic wounds, wounds substantially contaminated with foreign material, and wounds contaminated with spillage from perforated viscera.

Infection rates in clean surgical wounds without chemotherapy should be less than 1%, whereas untreated dirty wounds have a high probability of infection. Similar considerations apply to the chance of infection developing in a placental site or on the umbilicus. A normal delivery without retained products will rarely be followed by endometrial infection. A prolonged delivery after rupture of the membranes with retained placental fragments poses an increased risk of infection. In some rural cultures in Africa, soil is applied to the umbilical stump, and neonatal tetanus is common, whereas it is almost unknown in the Western world.

Factors Contributing to Infection Probability

Various factors, in addition to those indicated previously, contribute to the probability of a wound becoming infected.

Contaminating dose of organisms

The contaminating dose of microorganisms and their virulence can be critical and, all other things being equal, the chance of infection developing increases progressively with the contaminating dose.

Vascular integrity in wound

The physical and physiologic condition of the wound also influences the probability of infection. Areas of necrosis, vascular strangulation from excessively tight sutures, hematomas, excessive edema, poor blood supply, and poor oxygenation all compromise normal defense mechanisms and substantially reduce the dose of organisms needed to initiate infection. Thus, removal of necrotic tissue and the surgeon's skill, gentleness, and attention to detail are major factors in preventing the development of infection.

Nutritional and immunologic status and inflammatory response

The general health, nutritional status, and ability of the patient to mount an inflammatory response are also major determinants of whether a wound infection develops. Infection rates are higher in the elderly, the obese, uncontrolled diabetics, and those on immunosuppressive or corticosteroid therapy. Nutritional deficiencies enhance the risk of infection, and new approaches to avoid protein-calorie malnutrition in patients with severe burns, for example, have led to substantial reductions in serious clinical infections.

Critical period of contamination of surgical wounds

There is strong evidence that the critical period determining whether contamination of surgical wounds proceeds to infection lies within the first 3 hr after contamination. It is for this reason that prophylactic chemotherapy of some surgical wounds and procedures can be restricted to the immediate perioperative period. There is general agreement that extending such prophylaxis beyond 24 hr increases the chance of complications without reducing the risk of infection.

Etiologic Agents

Some major causes of skin and wound infections are shown in Table 59.1. *Staphylococcus aureus* remains the single most common source of infection of clean surgical wounds; however, the number of infections caused by opportunistic Gram-negative organisms is now increasing. This finding reflects the extension of surgical intervention to more patients whose defenses are compromised or who would have been unacceptable surgical risks before the introduction of new technical and therapeutic procedures. Infections with *S. pyogenes* are now uncommon; however, because of their tendency to spread and cause septicemia, wound or puerperal infections by this organism can be devastating if not treated rapidly.

Anaerobic Gram-negative wound infections have been reported increasingly in the last two decades or so as a result of the higher incidence of such infections in immunocompromised patients and better laboratory recognition. Most infecting organisms derive from normal floral sites and the majority are *Bacteroides* often in combination with anaerobic Gram-positive cocci and facultative aerobic bacteria. They tend to be associated with necrosis, which may spread subcutaneously, and with thrombophlebitis, which may lead to bacteremia with the possible development of metastatic hepatic, pulmonary, or cerebral abscesses. Most postpartum uterine infections are now caused by Gram-negative anaerobes or anaerobic Gram-positive cocci; they can range from self-limiting infections associated with little or no constitutional symptoms to severe infections of the uterus with pelvic thrombophlebitis. Human bite wounds are particularly subject to anaerobic infections. In contrast, infected bites of domestic animals (dogs, cats) are almost always due to *Pasteurella multocida*.

Burns and areas of necrosis resulting from vascular stasis or insufficiency are subject to infection with the same organisms that predominate in postsurgical wound infections; *P. aeruginosa* causes particlarly serious infections in burns, however, with loss of skin grafts and a high risk of septicemia and death. If the fluid electrolyte and nutritional deficiencies of a burned patient can be controlled, the greatest hazard to life is infection.

Tetanus remains a threat to the unimmunized or inadequately immunized individual, particularly from heavy contamination of puncture wounds or introduction of foreign bodies such as splinters, soil, or clothing into the subcutaneous tissues. The pathogenesis, treatment, and prevention of the disease are discussed in Chapter 18. It is worth repeating that a low oxidation-reduction potential in the tissue as a result of necrosis or the presence of foreign material is essential for the multiplication of *C. tetani,* that the organism never spreads beyond the site of the local lesion, and that adequate circulating antibody from tetanus toxoid immunization will prevent the development of the disease.

Gas gangrene (clostridial myositis) is also discussed in some detail in Chapter 18. It can develop within a few hours of traumatic injury and lead to rapid death. *Clostridium perfringens* is the most common contributor to the infection, and its α-toxin is the major cause of the spreading tissue damage and muscle death. Other aerobic and anaerobic bacteria are invariably present and sometimes play an important etiologic role. The dis-

---

Predominance of post surgical staphylococcal infections; increasing proportion of opportunistic Gram-negative infections

S. pyogenes infection rare but serious

Bacteroides and anaerobic Gram-positive coccal infections

Burn infections and *P. aeruginosa*

Clostridial infections: tetanus and gas gangrene

Table 59.1   Major Causes of Primary Skin and Wound Infections

Syndrome	Bacteria	Fungi	Viruses
Skin			
Pyoderma (streptococcal impetigo)	*Streptococcus pyogenes*		
Bullous impetigo	*Staphylococcus aureus*		
Folliculitis	*Pseudomonas aeruginosa*	*Candida albicans*	
	Staphylococcus aureus		
Acne	*Propionibacterium acnes*[a]		
Furuncles and carbuncles	*Staphylococcus aureus*		
Erysipelas	*Streptococcus pyogenes*		
Cellulitis	*Streptococcus pyogenes*		
	Staphylococcus aureus		
	Haemophilus influenzae		
	Miscellaneous bacteria		
Intertrigo[b]	*Staphylococcus aureus*	*Candida albicans*	
	Enterobacteriaceae		
Chronic ulcers[c]	*Treponema pallidum*	*Sporothrix*	Herpes virus
	Haemophilus ducreyi		
	Corynebacterium diphtheriae		
	Nocardia species		
	Mycobacterium (*marinum* and *ulcerans*)		
Wounds			
Surgical (clean)	*Staphylococcus aureus*		
	Enterobacteriaceae		
	Streptococcus pyogenes		
Surgical (dirty)[d]	*Staphylococcus aureus*		
	Enterobacteriaceae		
	Gram-negative anaerobes		
	Peptostreptococci		
Traumatic	*Clostridium* (*tetani*, *perfringens*, and *septicum*)		
	Pseudomonas aeruginosa		
	Organisms listed under surgical wounds[e]		
Postpartum endometrial	Gram-negative anaerobes		
	Peptostreptococci		
	Streptococcus pyogenes		
	Clostridium perfringens		
Neonatal umbilical	*Staphylococcus aureus*		
	Clostridium tetani		
Burns	*Pseudomonas aeruginosa*	*Candida albicans*	
	Staphylococcus aureus		
	Enterobacteriaceae		
Animal bites	*Pasteurella multocida*		

[a] *P. acnes* is contributary but primary etiology is noninfectious.
[b] Infection in moist skin folds (eg, groin).
[c] Usually begin as nodules or pustules.
[d] Etiology determined by the origin of the contaminating flora (eg, abdominal versus gynecological).
[e] Infection with indigenous flora depends on nature and site of trauma.

ease is always associated with muscle trauma and necrosis, which provide the conditions for anaerobic multiplication. Compound fractures, gunshot wounds, and similar extensive injuries that allow entry of clostridial spores set the stage for the disease. Prevention involves surgically debriding all necrotic or potentially necrotic tissue as soon as possible, leaving the wound unsutured, and administering high-dose chemoprophylaxis, in which penicillin is the agent of choice.

Prevention and Treatment

Immunization and prevention of wound and burn infections

Epidemiologic approaches to the prevention of wound infection and the appropriate uses of chemoprophylaxis are considered in Chapters 13 and 72. Recently, however, there has been increasing interest in the possibilities of immunization against the types of organisms that may infect a particular patient, for example, one who has suffered a burn recently or is to undergo certain types of major surgery. Some degree of protection from *P. aeruginosa* infection has been achieved with both active and passive immunization, and the degree of toxicity and risk of septicemia are reduced. It has been shown that immunization with the common antigen of *Escherichia coli,* an antigen it shares with many other Gram-negative organisms, provides a broad range of increased immunity to Gram- negative (including *P. aeruginosa*) infections in experimental animals. However, the clinical application of these findings to burns and severe trauma remains to be established.

Severe wound infections are almost always treated with a combination of surgical and chemotherapeutic approaches. Necrotic tissue and contaminated foreign bodies, such as sutures, must be removed, pockets of pus opened, and drainage established. This approach permits access of the appropriate antibiotics to viable tissues in which they can act.

Additional Reading

Simor, A.E., Roberts, F.J., and Smith J.A. Cumitech No 23. Smith, J.A. (Ed). Infections of the skin and subcutaneous tissues. Washington D.C. American Society for Microbiology. An excellent, clearly illustrated, and well-referenced review.

60

Bone and Joint Infections

C. George Ray

Infections of bones and joints may exist separately or together. Both are most common in infancy and childhood. They are usually caused by blood-borne (hematogenous) spread to the infected site, but can also result from local trauma with secondary infection. Sometimes there may be local spread from a contiguous soft tissue infection, often associated with the presence of a foreign body at the site of the primary wound.

The local effect of such infections can be devastating if they are in-adequately treated, because inflammation and resultant tissue necrosis may produce irreparable damage. The presence of pus under pressure can com-promise normal blood flow and even cause destruction of blood vessels with avascular necrosis of tissue. When this condition develops a *sequestrum* can result, in which a part of the cartilage or bone becomes totally sep-arated from its blood supply and cannot be incorporated into the healing process. In some patients, sequestrum formation can lead to a smoldering chronic infection with draining sinuses and loss of functional integrity. Normal growth of the affected site can be severely impaired in the infant or child, particularly when the epiphysis is involved.

Sequestrum formation

Chronic infection with draining sinuses

Growth impairment in children

Bacteremia and metastatic spread

In the acute phase of infection, bacteremia may also cause sepsis and metastatic infections in sites such as the lungs and heart. The result may be fatal.

Osteomyelitis

Clinical signs of acute hematogenous osteomyelitis

The onset of acute hematogenous osteomyelitis is usually abrupt, but can sometimes be quite insidious. It is classically characterized by localized pain, fever, and tenderness to palpation over the affected site. More than one bone or joint may be involved as a result of blood spread to multiple sites. With progression, the classic signs of heat, redness, and swelling may develop. Laboratory findings often include leukocytosis and elevated acute-phase reactants, such as the sedimentation rate. Osteomyelitis caused by a contiguous focus of infection is usually associated with the

Spread from local infections

Table 60.1   Common Causes of Acute Osteomyelitis

Situation	Usual Causative Organism
Age group	
Neonates (<1 mo)	*Staphylococcus aureus*; group B streptococci; Gram-negative rods (eg, *Escherichia coli, Klebsiella, Proteus, Pseudomonas*)
Older infants, children, adults	*Staphylococcus aureus*
Special problems	
Chronic hemolytic disorders (eg, sickle cell disease)	*Staphylococcus aureus; Streptococcus pneumoniae; Salmonella* species
Infection after trauma or surgery	*Staphylococcus aureus; Streptococcus pyogenes*; Gram-negative aerobic or anaerobic bacteria
Infection after puncture wound of foot	*Pseudomonas aeruginosa; Staphylococcus aureus*

presence of local findings of soft tissue infection, such as skin abscesses and infected wounds.

Extension to joint

When osteomyelitis occurs in close proximity to a joint, septic arthritis may develop by direct spread through the epiphysis (usually in infants) or by lateral extension through the periosteum into the joint capsule. Such extension is particularly common in hip and elbow infections.

Etiologic Agents

Age-related etiologies

The most common causes of acute osteomyelitis and those associated with special circumstances are shown in Table 60.1. It is clear that age plays a significant role in influencing the relative frequency of the various infective agents, particularly in early infancy; however, most infections are caused by *Staphylococcus aureus*.

Staphylococcal osteomyelitis

Chronic granulomatous osteomyelitis

Low-grade smoldering infections may also occur with the organisms listed in Table 60.1; however chronic granulomatous processes also require consideration, including tuberculosis, coccidioidomycosis, histoplasmosis, and blastomycosis. These latter infections usually result from systemic dissemination, and the lesions develop slowly over a period of months. Occasionally bone tumors or cysts and leukemia must also be considered in the differential diagnosis.

General Diagnostic Approaches

Blood cultures, direct aspirates, and bone scans

The primary goals of diagnosis are to establish the existence of infection and to determine its cause. The following procedures are generally employed:

1. Blood cultures, because many infections are associated with bacteremia.
2. Radionuclide scanning or magnetic resonance imaging to demonstrate evidence of localized infection.
3. Direct staining, culture and histology of needle aspirates, or biopsy of periosteum or bone.

Table 60.2   Common Causes of Septic Arthritis

Age Group	Usual Causative Organism
Neonate (<1 mo)	*Staphylococcus aureus;* group B streptococci; Gram-negative rods (eg, *Escherichia coli, Klebsiella, Proteus, Pseudomonas*)
1 mo–4 yr	*Haemophilus influenzae* type b; *Staphylococcus aureus; Streptococcus pyogenes; Streptococcus pneumoniae; Neisseria meningitidis*
4–16 yr	*Staphylococcus aureus*
16–40 yr	*Neisseria gonorrhoeae; Staphylococcus aureus*
>40 yr	*Staphylococcus aureus*

X-rays may be normal in early stages of infection

4. X-rays of affected sites, which often appear normal in the early stages of infection. The first changes seen are swelling of surrounding soft tissues, followed by periosteal elevation. Demineralization of bone and calcification of the periosteum and surrounding soft tissues may not become apparent for 2 weeks or more after the onset of symptoms.

General Principles of Management

Bactericidal antimicrobics

In acute infections, early intervention is important. Management includes vigorous use of bactericidal antimicrobics, which must often be continued for several weeks to ensure a bacteriologic cure and prevent progression to chronic osteomyelitis. Surgical drainage is also essential if there is significant pressure from the localized, purulent process.

Surgery and prolonged therapy for chronic osteomyelitis

In chronic osteomyelitis, sequestrum formation is frequent and sinuses may develop that drain the bone abscess to the surface. The infection is persistent, and treatment becomes extremely difficult. Such patients often require long-term antibiotic treatment (months to years) combined with surgical procedures to drain the abscesses and remove necrotic, infected tissues in an attempt to control infection while preserving the integrity of the affected bone.

Septic Arthritis

Clinical signs of arthritis

The usual clinical features of septic arthritis include onset of pain, which is often abrupt and accompanied by fever. Single or multiple joints may be involved. Tenderness and swelling of the affected joints and frequently other signs of local inflammation are present. Attempts to move the joints, either actively or passively, result in severe pain. In infants, the symptoms may be somewhat nonspecific; local swelling or excessive irritability with unwillingness to move the affected extremity (pseudoparalysis) may be the only clues to the diagnosis.

Common Etiologic Agents

Age-related etiologies

The major causes of septic arthritis are listed in Table 60.2. Although *S. aureus* infection can occur at any age, there are some significant age-specific relationships to other bacterial causes. There is a high frequency of group B streptococcal infections in neonates, whereas in children between 1 month and 4 years of age, *Haemophilus influenzae* type b accounts for up

Table 60.3 Findings in Synovial Fluid in Various Forms of Arthritis

Laboratory Test	Normal	Septic Bacterial Arthritis	Trauma, Degenerative Joint Disease	Rheumatoid Arthritis, Gout
Clarity and color	Clear	Opaque, yellow to green	Clear, yellow	Translucent, yellow; or opalescent
Viscosity	High	Variable	High	Low
White blood cells/mm³	<200	25,000–100,000	200–2000	2000–20,000
Polymorphonuclear cells (%)	<25	>75	25–50	≥50
Glucose level (relative to simultaneous blood glucose level)	Nearly equal	<25%	Nearly equal	50–80%

to 75% of all cases. *Neisseria gonorrhoeae* is implicated in most cases of septic arthritis in young adults.

Tuberculous, spirochetal, and fungal arthritis

Subacute or chronic infective arthritis should prompt consideration of tuberculosis, Lyme disease, syphilis, and deep mycosis such as coccidioidomycosis or *Candida* infection. Arthritis attributable to *Candida* infection is particularly likely in immunocompromised patients.

Self-limiting viral or *Mycoplasma*-associated arthritis

Viruses and *Mycoplasma* can also cause acute arthritis in single or multiple joints. Such illnesses have been associated with rubella, hepatitis B, mumps, parvovirus B19, varicella, Epstein-Barr virus, Coxsackie virus, and adenovirus infections, as well as with *Mycoplasma pneumoniae* and *Mycoplasma hominis.* These arthritides are usually self-limiting and rarely require specific therapy. Some bacterial infections of sites other than joints

Reactive arthritis

may be associated with noninfectious (reactive) arthritis, possibly resulting from deposition of circulating immune complexes and complement in synovial tissues, leading to inflammation. This has occurred with intestinal infections caused by *Yersinia enterocolitica, Campylobacter jejuni,* and some *Salmonella* species and also as a delayed sequela after successful treatment of sepsis due to *Neisseria meningitidis* or *H. influenzae.*

Noninfectious causes of arthritis must also be considered in the differential diagnosis. They can closely mimic septic arthritis. Examples include inflammatory collagen vascular disease such as rheumatoid arthritis, gout, traumatic arthritis, and degenerative arthritis.

General Diagnostic Approaches

Blood culture

In acute cases, blood cultures are often useful because bacteremia may be present. The definitive diagnosis is established by examination of synovial fluid removed from the joint by needle aspiration (arthrocentesis). As other noninfectious causes must be considered, it is important to analyze the chemical and cellular characteristics of the fluid in addition to performing a Gram stain and culture. Table 60.3 summarizes the major findings in synovial fluid in normal and various disease states. Septic bacterial arthritis is usually associated with grossly purulent fluid containing more than 25,000 white blood cells per cubic millimeter, predominantly polymorphonuclear cells. The glucose level in the synovial fluid is usually less than 25% of that in the blood.

Needle aspiration

Characteristics of synovial fluid

In viral, tuberculous, and fungal arthritis, as well as in partially treated bacterial arthritis, cell counts are usually lower, and mononuclear cells may constitute a greater proportion of the inflammatory cells. Occasionally, biopsy of the synovial membrane may be required to resolve the diagnosis. Histologic examination and culture of the tissue are particularly helpful in distinguishing granulomatous from rheumatoid disease.

In most cases of acute septic arthritis, the blood culture and/or synovial fluid culture will yield the specific etiologic agent. One major exception is *N. gonorrhoeae,* which can be difficult to isolate from these sources. When this organism is suspected, it is often wise to include cultures of other sites of potential infection or colonization, such as the urethra, cervix, rectum, and pharynx, as well as skin lesions.

Gonococci may be difficult to isolate from joint fluid

General Principles of Management

Prompt, vigorous, systemic antimicrobial therapy is required as soon as diagnostic tests suggest a bacterial cause. This treatment usually must be continued for 3–6 weeks, depending upon the etiologic agent and the clinical response to therapy.

Drainage of pus under pressure is also an important aspect of management. In cases of hip joint involvement, open surgical drainage is often necessary because collateral blood supply to the hip joint is relatively limited, and pus under pressure can lead to irreversible avascular necrosis of the tissues with permanent crippling. It is also difficult to evaluate the amount of pus that may be present because of the extensive overlying muscle. Other joints can usually be managed by simple aspiration of pus whenever it reaccumulates significantly during the acute phase of infection.

61

Eye, Ear, and Sinus Infections

C. George Ray

Eye Infections

Ocular infections can be divided into those that primarily involve the external structures—eyelids, conjunctiva, sclera, and cornea—and those that involve internal sites.

The major defense mechanisms of the eye are the tears and the conjunctiva, as well as the mechanical cleansing that occurs with blinking of the eyelids. The tears contain secretory immunoglobulin A antibodies and lysozyme, and the conjunctiva possesses numerous lymphocytes, plasma cells, neutrophils, and mast cells, which can respond quickly to infection by inflammation and production of antibody and interferon. The internal eye is protected from external invasion primarily by the physical barrier imposed by the sclera and cornea. If these are breached (for example, by a penetrating injury or ulceration), infection becomes a possibility. In addition, infection may reach the internal eye via the blood-borne route to the retinal arteries and produce chorioretinitis and/or uveitis. Such infections are a particularly common problem in immunocompromised patients.

Other causes of inflammation of the external or internal eye can involve autoimmune or allergic mechanisms, which may be provoked by infectious agents or diseases such as rheumatoid arthritis.

Common Clinical Features

Blepharitis is an acute or chronic inflammatory disease of the eyelid margin. It can take the form of a localized inflammation in the external margin (hordeolum or sty) or a granulomatous reaction to infection and plugging of a sebaceous gland of the eyelid (chalazion).

Dacryocystitis is an inflammation of the lacrimal sac. It usually results from partial or complete obstruction within the sac or nasolacrimal duct,

Defenses of the eye

Sites of infections and definitions

where bacteria may be trapped and initiate either an acute or a chronic infection.

Conjunctivitis is a term used to describe inflammation of the conjunctiva; it may extend to involve the eyelids, the cornea (keratitis), or the sclera (episcleritis). Extensive disease involving the conjunctiva and cornea is often called *keratoconjunctivitis.* Progressive keratitis can lead to ulceration, scarring, and blindness.

Ophthalmia neonatorum is an acute, sometimes severe, conjunctivitis or keratoconjunctivitis of newborn infants.

Endophthalmitis is rare, but often leads to blindness even when treated aggressively. The term refers to infection of the aqueous or vitreous humor, usually by bacteria or fungi.

Uveitis consists of inflammation of the uveal tract—iris, ciliary body, and choroid. Although most inflammations of the iris and ciliary body (iridocyclitis) are not of infectious origin, some agents have been implicated. The acute disease may be associated with severe eye pain, redness, and photophobia; other cases may progress quite silently, with decreased visual acuity as the only symptom in the late stages. The most common infective involvement of the uveal tract is chorioretinitis, in which inflammatory infiltrates are seen in the retina; this infection can lead to destruction of the choroid and inflammation of the optic nerve (optic neuritis) and may extend into the vitreous humor to cause endophthalmitis. If the disease is not treated adequately, the end result can be blindness.

Common Etiologic Agents

The major infectious causes of various inflammatory diseases of the eye are listed in Table 61.1. *Staphylococcus aureus* is the principal offender in bacterial infections of the eyelid and cornea. *Haemophilus influenzae* and *Streptococcus pneumoniae* are common causes of acute bacterial conjunctivitis. In young infants, *Neisseria gonorrhoeae* and *Chlamydia trachomatis* are significant causes of external eye disease, contracted from the mother's birth canal, that must be diagnosed and treated promptly. Chronic conjunctivitis or keratoconjunctivitis at any age must also prompt consideration of *C. trachomatis* infection. Herpes simplex is also a major cause of chronic conjunctivitis, especially in infections of the external structures, and specific therapy is available. Epidemic conjunctivitis or keratoconjunctivitis is most commonly associated with a variety of adenovirus serotypes. Outbreaks have been associated with inadequately chlorinated swimming pools, contaminated equipment or eyedrops in physicians' offices, and communal sharing of towels, which facilitates direct transmission. Chorioretinitis is frequently a manifestation of systemic disease (for example, histoplasmosis, tuberculosis); it is particularly common in immunocompromised patients, who are liable to develop disseminated *Candida,* cytomegalovirus, or *Toxoplasma gondii* infections. Endophthalmitis may also result from blood-borne dissemination or by contiguous spread as a result of injury (for example, corneal ulcerations). In the latter situation, iatrogenic infection by agents such as *Pseudomonas* species can be induced by contaminated eye drops, etc.

Infection of the soft tissues surrounding the eye (periorbital or orbital cellulitis) is potentially severe and can spread to involve the functions of the eye itself. Major causes are *S. aureus, H. influenzae,* and *Streptococcus pyogenes.*

Blepharitis and keratitis

Acute conjunctivitis

Chronic conjunctivitis

Epidemic adenovirus conjunctivitis

Chorioretinitis

Endophthalmitis

Periorbital cellulitis

Table 61.1 Major Infectious Causes of Eye Disease

Disease	Bacteria and *Chlamydia*	Viruses	Fungi	Parasites
Blepharitis	*Staphylococcus aureus*			
Dacryocystitis	*Streptococcus pneumoniae;* *Staphylococcus aureus*			
Conjunctivitis; keratitis; keratoconjunctivitis	*Streptococcus pneumoniae;* *Haemophilus influenzae;* *Haemophilus aegyptius;* *Streptococcus pyogenes;* *Staphylococcus aureus;* *Chlamydia trachomatis;* *Neisseria gonorrhoeae;* *Neisseria meningitidis*	Adenoviruses; herpes simplex; measles; varicella–zoster	*Fusarium* species *Aspergillus* species	*Acanthamoeba* (keratitis)
Ophthalmia neonatorum	*Neisseria gonorrhoeae;* *Chlamydia trachomatis*	Herpes simplex		
Endophthalmitis	*Staphylococcus aureus;* *Pseudomonas aeruginosa;* other Gram-negative organisms		*Candida* species *Aspergillus* species	
Iridocyclitis	*Treponema pallidum*	Herpes simplex; varicella–zoster		
Chorioretinitis	*Mycobacterium tuberculosis*	Cytomegalovirus; herpes simplex	*Histoplasma capsulatum; Coccidioides immitis; Candida* species	*Toxoplasma gondii; Toxocara canis*

General Diagnostic Approaches

In external bacterial infections of the eye, etiologic diagnoses can usually be established by Gram stain and culture of surface material or, in the case of viral infections, by tissue culture. Conjunctival scrapings for *C. trachomatis* can be prepared for immunofluorescent or cytologic examination and for appropriate culture. Infections of internal sites pose a more difficult problem. Some, such as acute endophthalmitis, may require removal of infected aqueous humor for microbiologic studies. Infections involving the uveal tract may require indirect methods of diagnosis, such as serologic tests for toxoplasmosis and deep mycoses, blood cultures to demonstrate evidence of disseminated disease (for example, *Candida* sepsis), and efforts to demonstrate infection in other sites (for example, chest radiography and sputum culture to diagnose tuberculosis). Careful ophthalmologic examination using slit lamps and retinoscopy often helps to suggest specific etiologic agents based on the morphology of the lesions observed.

General Principles of Management

Topical agents for superficial bacterial and herpes simplex infections

Various topical antimicrobial agents have been used effectively in external eye infections of presumed or proved bacterial origin. In addition, topical antiviral treatment is available for herpes simplex infections, but has not been proved efficacious for other viral diseases of the eye.

Severe infections, whether external or internal, require specialized treatment that nearly always includes ophthalmologic consultation because they may threaten vision. Systemic infection associated with eye disease (for example, fungemia, tuberculosis) must be treated vigorously with appropriate antimicrobial agents.

Ear Infections

Most infections of the ear involve the external otic canal (otitis externa) or the middle ear cavity (otitis media), which contains the ossicles and is enclosed by bony structures and the tympanic membrane.

Otitis externa

Factors of importance in the pathogenesis of otitis externa include local trauma, furunculosis, foreign bodies, or excessive moisture, which can lead to maceration of the external ear epithelium (swimmer's ear). Occasionally, external otitis occurs as an extension of infection from the middle ear, with purulent drainage through a perforated tympanic membrane.

Pathogenesis of otitis media and predisposing factors

The eustachian tube, which vents the middle ear to the nasopharynx, appears to play a major role in predisposing patients to otitis media. The tube performs three functions: ventilation, protection, and clearance via mucociliary transport. Viral upper respiratory infections or allergic conditions can cause inflammation and edema in the eustachian tube or at its orifice. These developments disturb its functions, of which ventilation may be the most important. As ventilation is lost, oxygen is absorbed from the air in the middle ear cavity, producing negative pressure. This pressure in turn allows entry of potentially pathogenic bacteria from the nasopharynx into the middle ear, and failure to clear these normally can result in colonization and infection. Other factors that can lead to compromise of eustachian tube function include anatomic abnormalities, such as tissue hyperptrophy or scarring around the orifice, muscular dysfunction associated with cleft palate, and lack of stiffness of the tube wall. The latter is common in infancy and early childhood and improves with age. It may explain in part why otitis media occurs most often in infants 6–18 months old, then decreases in frequency as patency of the eustachian tube becomes established.

Common Clinical Features

Otitis externa is characterized by inflammation of the ear canal, with purulent ear drainage. It can be quite painful, and cellulitis can extend into adjacent soft tissues. A common form is associated with swimming in water that may be contaminated with aerobic, Gram-negative organisms such as *Pseudomonas* species. "Malignant" otitis externa is a considerably more severe form of external ear canal infection that can progress to invasion of cartilage and adjacent bone, sometimes leading to cranial nerve palsy and death. It is seen most frequently in elderly patients with diabetes mellitus and in immunocompromised hosts of any age. *Pseudomonas aeruginosa* is the most common causative pathogen.

P. aeruginosa in swimming pool and malignant otitis externa

Acute bacterial otitis media

Otitis media is arbitrarily classified as acute, chronic, or serous (secretory). *Acute otitis media,* nearly always caused by bacteria, is often a complication of acute viral upper respiratory illness. Fever, irritability, and acute pain are common, and otoscopic examination will reveal bulging of the tympanic membrane and poor mobility and obscuration of normal anatomic landmarks by fluid and inflammatory cells under pressure. In some cases, the tympanic membrane will also be acutely inflamed, with blisters (bullae) on its external surface (myringitis). If treated inadequately, the infection can progress to involve adjacent structures such as the mastoid air cells (mastoiditis) or lead to perforation with spontaneous drainage

Myringitis

Table 61.2 Common Causes of Ear Infection

Otitis externa	*Pseudomonas aeruginosa* is common; occasionally *Proteus* species, *Escherichia coli*, and *Staphylococcus aureus*; bacteria found in otitis media may also be recovered if the process is secondary to middle ear infection with perforation and drainage through the tympanic membrane; fungi, such as *Aspergillus* species, are occasionally implicated
Acute otitis media	
<3 mo old	*Streptococcus pneumoniae*, group B streptococci, *Haemophilus influenzae*, *Staphylococcus aureus*, *Pseudomonas aeruginosa*, and Gram-negative enteric bacteria
>3 mo old	*Streptococcus pneumoniae* and *Haemophilus influenzae* are most common; others include *Streptococcus pyogenes*, *Branhamella catarrhalis*, and *Staphylococcus aureus*
Chronic otitis media	Mixed flora in 40% of cases cultured. Common organisms include *Pseudomonas aeruginosa*, *Haemophilus influenzae*, *Staphylococcus aureus*, *Proteus* species, *Klebsiella pneumoniae*, *Branhamella catarrhalis*, and Gram-positive as well as Gram-negative anaerobic bacteria
Serous otitis media	Same as chronic otitis media; however, many more of these effusions are sterile, with relatively few acute inflammatory cells

Perforation of tympanic membrane

through the tympanic membrane. Potential acute, suppurative sequelae include extension into the central nervous system and sepsis.

Chronic otitis media is usually a result of acute infection that has not resolved adequately, either because of inadequate treatment in the acute phase or because of host factors that perpetuate the inflammatory process (for example, continued eustachian tube dysfunction, caused by allergic or anatomic factors, or immunodeficiency). Sequelae include progressive destruction of middle ear structures and a significant risk of permanent hearing loss.

Risk of hearing loss

Serous otitis media may represent either a form of chronic otitis media or allergy-related inflammation. It tends to be chronic, causing hearing deficits, and is associated with thick, usually nonpurulent secretions in the middle ear.

Common Etiologic Agents

The usual causes of ear infections are listed in Table 61.2 *Streptococcus pneumoniae* is the single most common cause of acute otitis media after the first 3 months of life, accounting for 35–40% of all cases. *Haemophilus influenzae* is also common, particularly in patients less than 5 years of age. Viruses and *Mycoplasma* are rare primary causes of acute or chronic otitis media; however, they predispose patients to superinfection by the bacterial agents.

General Diagnostic Approaches

The diagnosis is established on the basis of clinical examination. Tympanometry can be performed in suspected cases of otitis media to detect the presence of fluid in the middle ear and to assess tympanic membrane function. The specific etiology of otitis externa can be determined by culture of the affected ear canal; one must keep in mind, however, that surface contamination and normal skin flora may lead to mixed cultures, which can be confusing. In otitis media, the most precise diagnostic method is careful aspiration with a sterile needle through the tympanic membrane after decontamination of the external canal. Gram stain and

External ear cultures often confusing

Gram stain and culture of aspirates in special cases of otitis media
Respiratory tract cultures unhelpful

culture of such aspirates is highly reliable; however, this procedure is generally reserved for cases in which etiologic possibilities are extremely varied, as in young infants, or when clinical response to the usual antimicrobial therapy has been inadequate. Respiratory tract cultures, such as those from the nasopharynx, cannot be relied upon to provide an etiologic diagnosis.

General Principles of Management

Topical treatment of otitis externa

Except in severe cases, otitis externa can usually be managed by gentle cleansing with topical solutions. The Gram-negative bacteria most commonly involved are often susceptible to an acidic environment, and otic solutions buffered to a low pH (3.0 or less), as with 0.25% acetic acid, will often be effective. Various preparations are available, many of which also contain antimicrobics.

Antimicrobic therapy for otitis media

Acute otitis media requires prompt antimicrobial therapy and careful follow-up to ensure that the disease has resolved. The choice of antimicrobic is usually empirical, designed specifically to cover the most likely bacterial pathogens because direct aspiration for diagnostic purposes is usually unnecessary. In the usual case these pathogens would be *S. pneumoniae* and *H. influenzae*.

If there is extreme pressure with severe pain, drainage of middle ear exudates by careful incision of the tympanic membrane may be necessary.

In patients with chronic or serous otitis media, management can be more complex, and it is often advisable to seek otolaryngologic consultation to determine further diagnostic procedures as well as to plan medical and possible surgical measures.

Sinus Infections

The paranasal sinuses (ethmoid, frontal, and maxillary) all communicate with the nasal cavity. In health, these sinuses are air-filled cavities lined with ciliated epithelium and are normally sterile. They are poorly developed in early life and, in contrast to otitis media, sinus infections are a rare problem in infancy.

Factors predisposing to sinusitis

The pathogenesis of sinus infection can involve several factors, most of which act by producing obstruction or edema of the sinus opening, which impedes normal drainage. Consequently, bacterial infection and inflammation of the mucosal lining tissues develop. Predisposing factors may be 1) local, such as upper respiratory infections producing edema of antral tissues, mucosal polyps, deviation of the nasal septum, enlarged adenoids, or a tumor or foreign body in the nasal cavity or 2) systemic, such as allergy, cystic fibrosis, or immunodeficiency. Occasionally, maxillary sinusitis can result from extension of a maxillary dental infection.

Common Clinical Features

Signs and symptoms vary according to which sinuses are affected and whether the illness is acute or chronic. Fever is sometimes present; cough, nasal discharge, fetid breath, pain over the affected sinus, headache, and tenderness to percussion over the frontal or maxillary sinuses are all features that may appear in different combinations and suggest the diagnosis.

Complications

Complications of sinusitis can include extension of infection to nearby

Table 61.3   Common Causes of Sinus Infection

Acute sinusitis	*Streptococcus pneumoniae* and *Haemophilus influenzae* are most common; also *Streptococcus pyogenes, Staphylococcus aureus*, and *Branhamella catarrhalis*
Chronic sinusitis	Same as for acute sinusitis; also Gram-negative enteric bacteria and anaerobic Gram-negative and Gram-positive bacteria; mixed aerobic and anaerobic infections are relatively common; *Mucor* species may be found in compromised patients (eg, those with diabetes mellitus)

soft tissues, such as the orbit, and occasionally spread, either directly or via vascular pathways, into the central nervous system.

Common Etiologic Agents

Table 61.3 summarizes the usual etiologies of sinus infections. Respiratory viruses are also occasional direct causes, but are most important as predisposing factors to bacterial superinfection of inflamed sinuses and their antral openings. Together, *S. pneumoniae* and *H. influenzae* account for more than 60% of cases of acute sinusitis. Mucormycosis (zygomycosis), an unusual fungal infection, is a specific sinus infection that may be seen in compromised hosts, such as those with severe diabetes mellitus. It has a particular tendency to spread progressively to adjacent tissues and to the central nervous system and is very difficult to treat.

General Diagnostic Approaches

Gram stain and cultures of sinus aspirates

Radiographic studies of the sinuses will confirm the diagnosis. If it becomes necessary to determine the specific infectious agent, fluid should be obtained directly from the affected sinus by needle puncture of the sinus wall or by catheterization of the sinus antrum after careful decontamination of the entry site. Gram smears and cultures are then made. Cultures of drainage from the antral orifices or nasal secretions are unreliable because of contaminating aerobic and anaerobic normal flora.

Cultures of sinus drainage unreliable

General Principles of Management

In uncomplicated acute sinusitis, prompt antimicrobial therapy is initiated. The choice of antimicrobics is usually empirical, based on the most likely bacterial causes and their usual susceptibility. For example, amoxicillin is effective against nearly all strains of *S. pneumoniae* and most strains of *H. influenzae*. Additional therapy consists of topical vasoconstricting agents, which may reduce edema of the antral orifices and facilitate drainage.

Severe, complicated acute infections and chronic sinusitis often require otolaryngologic consultation. In such cases, it is often necessary to obtain cultures directly from the sinuses to select specific antimicrobial therapy, consider the need for surgical procedures to adequately remove the pus and inflammatory tissues, and correct any anatomic obstruction that may exist.

62

Dental and Periodontal Infections

Murray R. Robinovitch

Dental caries, chronic marginal periodontal disease, and the sequelae of these two diseases constitute the majority of oral and dental infections. In both, the source of the causative bacteria is the microbial plaque that forms on the teeth. Thus, although dental caries and chronic marginal periodontal disease are distinctly different, the prevention and/or halting of the progression of these diseases relies upon the elimination of dental plaque from the tooth surfaces. In addition to causing caries and chronic marginal periodontitis, the bacteria of dental plaque play a role in acute necrotizing ulcerative gingivitis (Vincent's infection), another important oral infection.

Dental plaque

Dental plaque is a soft, adherent dental deposit that forms as a result of bacterial colonization of the tooth surface. It is rather insoluble, as well as adherent, and thus resists removal by water spray or mouth rinsing. Only more vigorous means such as tooth brushing and flossing between the teeth will remove it. It consists almost entirely of bacterial cells (1.7×10^{11} cells/g wet weight).

Caries production by plaque bacteria

Dental caries is the progressive destruction of the mineralized tissues of the tooth, primarily caused by the production of organic acids resulting from the glycolytic metabolic activity of plaque bacteria. The basic characteristic of the carious lesion is that it progresses inward from the tooth surface, be that the enamel-coated crown or the cementum of the exposed root surface, involving the dentin and finally the pulp of the tooth. From here, infection can extend out into the periodontal tissues at the root apex or apices.

Chronic periodontal infection

Chronic marginal periodontal disease encompasses two separate disease entities: gingivitis and periodontitis. These diseases are believed to be related in that gingivitis is thought to be an early stage leading ultimately to periodontitis. The term *gingivitis* is used when the inflammatory condition is limited to the marginal gingiva and bone resorption around the necks of teeth has not yet appeared. *Periodontitis* is used to connote the

823

stage of chronic marginal periodontal disease in which there is progressive loss of tooth support. Periodontitis can also lead to periodontal abscess when the chronic inflammatory state around the necks of the teeth becomes acute at a specific location.

Chronic marginal periodontitis is responsible for most tooth loss in people more than 35–40 years of age. The adjectives *chronic* and *marginal* indicate that the disease progresses slowly and results in the progressive destruction of the supporting tissues of the tooth (periodontal ligament and alveolar bone) from the margins of the gingiva toward the apices of the roots of the teeth.

Acute periodontitis

There is also an acute form of periodontitis that affects young children (prepubertal periodontitis), a form with an age of onset of around puberty that affects adolescents and results in more rapid loss of tooth support (juvenile periodontitis), and an adult form of the disease that progresses quite rapidly (rapidly progressive periodontitis). These diseases are thought to be caused by plaque organisms different from those responsible for chronic marginal periodontitis and/or an altered host resistance to the disease.

Dental Plaque

The formation of dental plaque is the result of a very specific colonization of tooth surfaces by oral bacteria. The mineralized tooth surface is always coated with a thin organic film called the *dental cuticle* or *pellicle.* This coating results from adsorption and binding of specific salivary macromolecules, mainly proteins and glycoproteins, to the tooth surface. As this cuticle or pellicle can form in a matter of minutes after the tooth surface is exposed to the oral fluid, bacteria never interact directly with the mineralized tooth surface. Instead, bacterial adherence to the tooth, which begins the colonization of the tooth surface, is mediated by this organic film.

Attachment of bacteria to dental pellicle

Plaque comprises many species of bacteria, including anaerobes

A number of oral bacteria among the complex indigenous oral flora adhere readily to the cuticle-coated tooth. Primary among them are Gram-positive cocci, such as *Streptococcus sanguis,* and short Gram-positive rods, which are the initial colonizers. After 2–4 days, fusiform and filamentous organisms appear. Anaerobic vibrios, spirochetes, and Gram-negative, motile, anaerobic organisms appear at about 6–10 days. Thus, as the dental plaque increases in thickness, Gram-negative anaerobic organisms appear and multiply. The extent and complexity of involved bacteria is shown in Figure 62.1. Dental plaque would coat the tooth surfaces uniformly but for its physical removal during chewing and other oral activities. Characteristically, plaque remains in the non–self-cleansing areas of the teeth such as pits and fissures, along the margins of the gingiva, and between the teeth. In addition to this supragingival plaque, the sulcus around the tooth and periodontal pockets, which are pathologic extensions of the sulcus. This nonadherent zone contains subgingival plaque. Subgingival plaque differs from supragingival plaque in that the former has an adherent zone next to the tooth surface and a nonadherent zone between that and the epithelial cells lining the sulcus, containing large numbers of Gram-negative, free-swimming, anaerobic microorganisms. Supragingival plaque lacks the nonadherent zone.

Plaque accumulates in non–self-cleansing areas of teeth and gingiva

Supragingival and subgingival plaque

As the causative organisms of both dental caries and chronic marginal periodontal disease are believed to be in the dental plaque, a prime method for maintaining oral health is regular home care practices for plaque removal. Dental plaque cannot be effectively dispersed by chemical or en-

Removal of plaque by oral hygiene

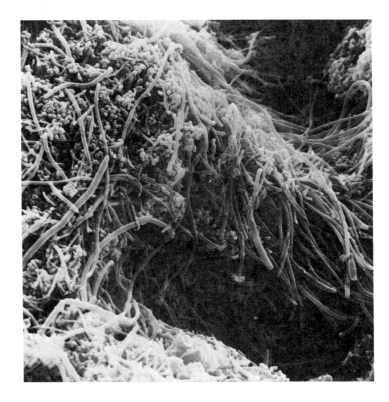

62.1 Scanning electronmicrograph of supragingival plaque.(*Kindly provided by Dr. W. Fischlsweiger and Dr. Dale Birdsell.*)

zymatic means, and the use of antibiotics for prophylactic inhibition of plaque formation cannot be clinically justified, although patients undergoing long-term antibiotic treatment for other medical reasons demonstrate a lower incidence of caries and periodontal disease. Antiseptic substances that bind to tooth surfaces and inhibit plaque formation, such as the *bis*-biguanides, chlorhexidine and alexidine, have been shown to be effective in reducing plaque, caries and gingival inflammation. Recently, the U.S. Food and Drug Administration approved a commercial preparation containing 0.12% chlorhexidine for use in controlling dental plaque and associated disease. This prescription drug along with tooth brushing and flossing constitute the available means for routine elimination of the causative organisms of caries and periodontal disease.

Antiseptics in control of plaque and gingivitis

Dental Caries

Greatest cause of tooth loss in child and young adult

Dental caries is the single greatest cause of tooth loss in the child and young adult. Its onset can be very soon after the eruption of the teeth. The first carious lesions usually develop in pits or fissures on the chewing surfaces of the deciduous molars and result from the metabolic activity of the dental plaque that forms in these sites. Later in childhood, the incidence of carious lesions on smooth surfaces increases; these lesions are usually found between the teeth. The factors involved in the formation of a carious lesion are 1) a susceptible host or tooth; 2) the proper microflora on the tooth; and 3) a substrate from which the plaque bacteria can produce the organic acids that result in tooth demineralization.

Factors in caries development

The newly erupted tooth is most susceptible to the carious process. It gains protection against this disease during the first year or so by a process of posteruptive maturation believed to be attributable to improvement in the quality of surface mineral on the tooth.

Protective effects of saliva

Saliva provides protection against caries, and patients with dry mouth (xerostomia) suffer from high caries attack rates unless suitable measures are taken. In addition to the mechanical flushing and diluting action of saliva and its buffering capacity, the salivary glands also secrete several antibacterial products. Thus, saliva is known to contain lysozyme, a thiocyanate-dependent sialoperoxidase, and immunoglobulins, principally those of the secretory immunoglobulin A class. The individual importance of these antibacterial factors in unknown, but they clearly play some role in determining the ecology of the oral microflora.

Protective effect of fluoride

Proper levels of fluoride, either systemically or topically administered, result in dramatic decreases in the incidence of caries (50–60% reduction by water fluoridation, 35–40% reduction by topical application). In the case of systemic fluoridation, the protective effect is thought to result from the incorporation of fluoride ions in place of hydroxyl ions of the hydroxyapatite during tooth formation, producing a more perfect and acid-resistant mineral phase of tooth structure. Topical application of fluoride is believed to achieve the same result on the surface of the tooth by initial dissolution of some of the hydroxyapatite, followed by recrystallization of apatite that incorporates fluoride ions into its lattice structure. Another important mode of action, namely, the promotion of remineralization of incipient carious lesions by fluoride ions present in the oral fluid, has recently been proposed as an important anticaries mechanism of fluoride. In any event, fluoridation represents the most effective means known to rendering the tooth more resistant to the carious process.

Role of microflora

The microbial basis of dental caries is well established, and Koch's postulates have been fulfilled for a number of microorganisms that cause the disease. This confirmation was achieved by using gnotobiotic (sterile) animals whose oral cavities could be colonized with a single organism. At times during the past half-century, a single microorganism was considered responsible for all caries; *Lactobacillus acidophilus* was regarded in this manner in the 1920s, and *Streptococcus mutans* enjoyed this reputation beginning in the 1960s. Currently, it is safe to say that any oral microorganism with a mechanism for colonizing the tooth surface or preexisting plaque and the ability to produce acid (acidogenic) and survive its action (aciduric) can be cariogenic. Organisms isolated from human carious lesions and shown to be cariogenic in gnotobiotic animals include some strains of *S. mutans, Streptococcus salivarius, Streptococcus sanguis, L. acidophilus, Lactobacillus casei, Actinomyces viscosus,* and *Actinomyces naeslundii,* but not all strains of these species are cariogenic in humans. Studies in human subjects indicate that *S. mutans* is a major etiologic agent for smooth surface caries and possibly for pit, fissure, and root surface caries as well. *Lactobacillus* species may represent secondary invaders of the established caries lesion, but *S. mutans* is thought to be the main initiator of this disease.

Several species may be cariogenic, but *S. mutans* is most important

Demineralization by acid production from carbohydrate breakdown

Cariogenic organisms must be provided with an appropriate substrate for glycolysis to cause tooth demineralization, and dietary monosaccharides and disaccharides such as glucose, fructose, sucrose, lactose, and maltose are readily utilized by most oral bacteria. These carbohydrates permeate the dental plaque, are absorbed by the bacteria, and are metabolized so rapidly that organic acid products accumulate and cause the pH of the plaque to drop to levels sufficient to demineralize the tooth structure. Production of acid and the decreased pH are maintained until the substrate supply is exhausted. Obviously, high-sugar-content foods that

Significance of degree and duration of acid production

adhere and have long oral clearance times are more cariogenic than less retentive foodstuffs such as sugar-containing liquids. Once the substrate is exhausted, the plaque pH returns slowly to its resting level. Frequency of application of substrate is extremely important, as the plaque pH may never reach a normal resting level.

Importance of extracellular polyglycans from sucrose; adherence and carbohydrate storage

Dietary sucrose is also used in the synthesis of extracellular polyglycans such as dextrans and levans by some microorganisms that possess glucose transferase or fructose transferase enzymes on their cell surfaces. Synthesis of polyglycans is considered an additional virulence factor for two reasons: 1) The polyglycan-producing microorganisms are usually aggregated in its presence, which is believed to aid in the colonization of the tooth surface. *Streptococcus mutans* is a major cariogenic microorganism that acts in this way. 2) Extracellular polyglycan production may increase cariogenicity by serving as an extracellular storage form of substrate. Certain microorganisms synthesize extracellular polyglycan when sucrose is available, but then break it down into monosaccharide units to be used for glycolysis when dietary carbohydrate is exhausted. Thus, these microorganisms can prolong acidogenesis beyond the oral clearance time of the substrate.

Prolongation of acidogenesis from intracellular glycogen stores

Some oral bacteria also use dietary monosaccharides and disaccharides internally to form glycogen, which is stored intracellularly and used for glycolysis after the dietary substrate has been exhausted; thus, the period of acidogenesis is again prolonged and the cariogenicity of the microorganism increased. It is therefore clear that the ability to synthesize extracellular or intracellular storage polysaccharides, to colonize tooth surfaces, and to produce and survive in acid contributes to the microorganism's cariogenicity.

Complicating pulp and periapical infections

The most common complications of dental caries are extension of the infection into the pulp chamber of the tooth (pulpitis), necrosis of the pulp, and extension of the infection through the root canals into the periapical area of the periodontal ligament. Periapical involvement may take the form of an acute inflammation (periapical abscess), a chronic nonsuppurating inflammation (periapical granuloma), or a chronic suppurating lesion that may drain into the mouth or onto the face via a sinus tract. A cyst may form within the chronic nonsuppurating lesion as a result of inflammatory stimulation of the epithelial rests normally found in the periodontal ligament. If the infectious agent is sufficiently virulent or host resistance is low, the infection may spread into the alveolar bone (osteomyelitis) or the fascial planes of the head and neck (cellulitis) or ascend along the venous channels to cause septic thrombophlebitis. As most carious lesions represent a mixed infection by the time cavities have developed, it is not surprising that most oral infections resulting from the extension of carious lesions are mixed and frequently caused by anaerobic organisms.

More severe complications

Chronic Marginal Periodontal Disease

Role of subgingival plaque

Both chronic marginal gingivitis and periodontitis are now believed to be caused by certain bacteria in the dental plaque lying next to the gingival tissues. Thus, subgingival plaque found within the gingival crevice or the sulcus around the necks of the teeth is thought to house the etiologic agent(s). The characteristic histopathologic picture of gingivitis is of a marked inflammatory infiltrate of polymorphonuclear leukocytes, lymphocytes, and plasma cells in the connective tissue that lies immediately adjacent to the epithelium lining the gingival crevice and attached to the tooth. Collagen is lost from the inflamed connective tissue. There does

Tissue destruction by bacterial products

Probable role of immunological mediators of tissue damage

Bacterial source of the disease is outside the affected tissues

Development of periodontitis and bone resorption

Periodontal abscess may result

Organisms involved in chronic periodontitis

Acute juvenile periodontitis and phagocyte defects

not seem to be any direct invasion of the gingival tissues by intact bacteria, at least in the early stages of the disease.

It has been proposed that tissue destruction is mediated by bacterial substances that pass through the epithelial barrier and cause either direct or indirect injury. Bacterial products that could cause direct injury to the tissues include toxins, such as endotoxin and leukocidins, and enzymes, such as hyaluronidase and collagenase. Several mechanisms for indirect injury of the periodontal tissues have been proposed. These hypotheses include initiation of an unresolvable inflammatory response with excessive release of the lysosomal contents of polymorphonuclear leukocytes; activation of complement, which further magnifies the inflammatory response; and development of a host of humoral and cell-mediated immune responses, which can also magnify the inflammatory response as well as lead to tissue destruction through lymphokine release. Many oral bacteria have been found to contain potent polyclonal B-lymphocyte activators, leading some investigators to propose that periodontal pathogens release these substances in lesions. Polyclonal B-lymphocyte activation could promote an exaggeration of the inflammatory response and further tissue injury through enhanced antibody and lymphokine production. Regardless of the mechanisms of tissue destruction, the true source of the disease, namely, the causative bacteria, remains outside the gingival tissues and is therefore not susceptible to the body's defense mechanisms. For this reason, the disease continues to progress unless the dental plaque is removed and the involved tooth is kept plaque-free. If these measures are taken, chronic marginal gingivitis can resolve completely and the tissues return to normal.

As the disease progresses, a point may be reached at which the alveolar bone around the necks of the teeth is resorbed; the condition is then no longer termed gingivitis, but *periodontitis*. With resorption of the bone the attachment of the periodontal ligament is lost and the gingival sulcus deepens into a periodontal pocket. If unchecked, bone resorption progresses to loosening of the tooth, which may ultimately fall out. Occasionally, the neck of a periodontal pocket becomes constricted, the bacteria proliferate, causing an acute inflammatory response in the occluded pocket, and a periodontal abscess results. This acute exacerbation requires drainage in the same way as abscesses elsewhere for the patient to obtain relief from the symptoms.

Chronic marginal gingivitis will develop within 2 weeks in those who fail to practice effective tooth cleansing. It is not known whether particular species of plaque bacteria are responsible for gingival inflammation, but among those suspected of pathogenicity in the case of chronic marginal periodontitis are anaerobic Gram-negative rods (*Bacteroides gingivalis, Bacteroides melaninogenicus* subspecies *intermedius, Wolinella recta, Fusobacterium nucleatum*), *Eikenella corrodens,* and some large spirochetes. Many of these organisms produce periodontal disease in monoinfected animals.

There is some evidence that the causative agents in rapidly progressing periodontal disease may differ from those associated with chronic marginal disease. In the condition known as juvenile periodontitis, a small anaerobic Gram-negative rod (*Actinobacillus actinomycetemcomitans*) and several species of another genus (*Capnocytophaga*) have been indicted based on studies of the flora of disease sites. In addition, it has been found that a significant proportion of patients with this condition demonstate high serum antibody titers to *A. actinomycetemcomitans.* Of interest, also, is the fact that many of these patients have neutrophil chemotactic or phagocytotic defects.

Acute Necrotizing Ulcerative Gingivitis

Acute necrotizing ulcerative gingivitis is also known as *Vincent's infection* or *trench mouth*. This disease is distinctly different from chronic marginal periodontal disease. It has an acute onset, frequently associated with periods of stress and poor oral hygiene. There is rapid ulceration of the interdental areas of the gingiva, resulting in destruction of the interdental papillae. The inflammatory condition can quickly lead to pathologic bone resorption. Unlike chronic marginal periodontal disease, acute necrotizing ulcerative gingivitis is painful. As the oral epithelium is destroyed, the causative bacteria come into direct contact with the underlying tissues and may invade them. Spirochetes and fusiform bacteria have been implicated; thus, the term *fusospirochetal disease* has been used to describe this infection, which can also be manifested as ulceration in other areas of the pharynx or oral cavity. The disease may be treated with systemic antibiotics for immediate relief of symptoms, but resolution is dependent on thorough professional cleaning of the teeth and institution of good home care. Further details of fusospirochetal disease are provided in Chapter 26.

Acute onset with painful ulcerative lesions

Fusospirochetal etiology

Dental Plaque and Oral Flora in the Compromised Patient

As it can be the source of transient bacteremia, dental plaque must be viewed as a hazard in the compromised patient. The best example is the patient with heart valve damage as a result of a congenital anomaly, rheumatic fever, or a heart prosthesis. If transient bacteremia develops, the blood-borne bacteria may form vegetative growths in the heart and cause bacterial endocarditis (Chapter 68). Such patients should always be placed on a course of prophylactic antibiotic therapy before any dental procedure is performed, including routine dental prophylaxis.

It has also been established that dental plaque organisms and other oral bacteria may give rise to serious systemic infections in patients whose host defense mechanisms are compromised. Patients who have undergone extensive radiation treatment of the jaw area, for example, are prone to develop osteomyelitis. Furthermore, one of the most frequent sources of fatal infections in leukemic patients is the oral cavity. Therefore, for these patients scrupulous home care and professional dental treatment are required.

Endocarditis from oral flora

Other severe opportunistic infections in the immunocompromised

Additional Reading

Genco, R.J., and Mergenhagen, S.E., Eds. 1982. *Host-Parasite Interactions in Periodontal Diseases.* Washington, D.C.: American Society for Microbiology.

Newbrun, E. 1989. *Cariology.* 3rd ed. Chicago: Quintessence Publishing Co.

Newman, M.G., and Nisengard, R., Eds. 1988. *Oral Microbiology and Immunology.* Philadelphia: W.B. Saunders Co.

These are authoritative reviews of caries and periodontal disease and new advances in understanding these conditions.

63

Upper Respiratory Tract Infections and Stomatitis

C. George Ray

Most upper respiratory infections caused by viruses

Upper respiratory infections usually involve the nasal cavity and pharynx, and most (more than 80%) are caused by viruses. Like middle and lower respiratory illnesses, the diseases of the upper respiratory tract are named according to the anatomic sites primarily involved. *Rhinitis* (or coryza) implies inflammation of the nasal mucosa, *pharyngitis* denotes pharyngeal infection, and *tonsillitis* indicates an inflammatory involvement of the tonsils. Because of the close proximity of these structures to one another, infections may simultaneously involve two or more sites (for example, rhinopharyngitis or tonsillopharyngitis). All such infections are grouped under the general term *upper respiratory infections. Stomatitis* is a term used to describe infections primarily localized to the mucous membranes of the oral cavity. These infections can sometimes also involve the tongue (glossitis) or the gingival and periodontal tissues (gingivostomatitis or acute necrotizing ulcerative gingivitis (Chapter 62)).

Other infections considered herein are peritonsillar abscess (quinsy), or retrotonsillar abscess, and retropharyngeal abscess. These infections are the result of direct invasion from mucosal sites and localization in deeper tissues to produce inflammation and abscess formation.

Common Clinical Features

The common cold

Rhinitis is the most common manifestation of the common cold. It is characterized by variable fever, inflammatory edema of the nasal mucosa, and an increase in mucous secretions. The net result is varying degrees of nasal obstruction; the nasal discharge may be clear and watery at the onset of illness, becoming thick and sometimes purulent as the infection progresses over several days.

Inflammatory exudate

Pharyngitis and tonsillitis are associated with pharyngeal pain (sore throat) and the clinical appearance of erythema and swelling of the affected tissues. There may be exudates, consisting of inflammatory cells overlying

831

the mucous membrane, and petechial hemorrhages; the latter may be seen in viral infections, but tend to be more prominent in bacterial infections. Viral infections, particularly herpes simplex, may also lead to the formation of vesicles in the mucosa, which quickly rupture to leave ulcers. Pharyngeal candidiasis can also erode the mucosa under the plaques of "thrush." On rare occasions, the local inflammation may be sufficiently severe to produce *pseudomembranes,* which consist of necrotic tissue, inflammatory cells, and bacteria. This finding is particularly common in pharyngeal diphtheria, but may be mimicked by fusospirochetal infection (Vincent's angina) and sometimes by infectious mononucleosis. In acute tonsillitis or pharyngitis of any etiology, regional spread of the infecting agents with inflammation and tender swelling of the anterior cervical lymph nodes is also common.

Stomatitis is inflammation of the oral cavity. Multiple ulcerative lesions of the oral mucosa, seen most frequently with severe primary herpes simplex infections, may extend to the tongue, lips, and face. In extreme cases, the pain may be so severe that the patient requires relief with topical anesthetics during the usual 9- to 12-day period of acute symptoms. *Candida* species can also invade oral surfaces to produce plaques identical to those of pharyngeal thrush. This infection is particularly common in young infants.

Aphthous stomatitis is a recurrent disease of the oral mucosa characterized by single or multiple painful ulcers with irregular margins, usually 2–10 mm in diameter. Healing usually occurs in a few days. The term commonly used to describe this condition is *canker sore.* The cause is unknown. It can easily be confused with recurrent herpes simplex lesions and, like herpes, tends to recur in relation to stress, menses, local trauma, and other nonspecific stimuli.

A severe, gangrenous stomatitis that progresses beyond the mucous membranes to involve soft tissues, skin, and sometimes bone can complicate a variety of acute illnesses in patients who are severely debilitated and whose oral hygiene is poor. This infection, called *noma* or *cancrum oris,* is rarely seen in the United States. Typical cases occur among children with severe protein–calorie malnutrition or other immune compromise. Measles will sometimes precipitate noma. Etiologic agents thought to be involved include *Fusobacterium* and *Bacteroides* species, as well as *Pseudomonas aeruginosa.*

Milder forms of stomatitis are seen in a variety of other common viral infections. Examples include Koplik's spots in measles, buccal or palatal ulcers in chickenpox, and similar phenomena in some enteroviral infections such as hand-foot-and-mouth disease.

Peritonsillar abscesses are usually a complication of tonsillitis. They are manifested by local pain, and examination of the pharynx reveals tonsillar asymmetry with one tonsil usually displaced medially by the abscess. This infection is most common in children more than 5 years of age and in young adults. If not properly treated, the abscess may spread to adjacent structures. It can involve the jugular venous system, erode into branches of the carotid artery to cause acute hemorrhage, or rupture into the pharynx to produce severe aspiration pneumonia.

Retropharyngeal abscesses occur most frequently in infants and children less than 5 years of age. They can result from pharyngitis or from accidental perforation of the pharyngeal wall by a foreign body. The infection is characterized by pain, inability or unwillingness to swallow, and, if the pharyngeal wall is displaced anteriorly near the palate, a change in phonation (nasal speech). The neck may be held in an extended position to

Vesicles and ulcerated lesions

Pharyngeal pseudomembranes

Lymphadenitis

Herpetic and *Candida* stomatitis

Aphthous stomatitis (canker sores)

Noma

Tonsillar asymmetry

Complications

Bulging of anterior
pharyngeal wall

relieve pain and maintain an open upper airway. Examination of the pharynx will usually reveal anterior bulging of the pharyngeal wall; if this finding is not apparent, lateral X-rays of the neck may demonstrate a widening of the space between the cervical spine and the posterior pharyngeal wall. The complications of retropharyngeal abscesses are basically the same as those described for peritonsillar abscesses; in addition, the suppurative process can extend posteriorly to the cervical spine to produce osteomyelitis or inferiorly to cause acute mediastinitis.

Oral and pharyngeal lesions
in immunocompromised hosts

May be portal of entry for
systemic infection

In the immunocompromised patient, all of the various forms of stomatitis and pharyngitis described previously can be accentuated. Leukemia, agranulocytosis, chronic ulcerative colitis, congenital or acquired immunodeficiency (eg, acquired immunodeficiency syndrome), and treatment with cytotoxic or immunosuppressive drugs are commonly associated with such lesions. The marked damage to mucosal tissues that sometimes occurs can provide a portal of entry into deeper structures and then to the systemic circulation, creating a risk of bacterial or fungal sepsis. Conversely, oral lesions may also result from dissemination of infection from other remote sites. Examples include disseminated histoplasmosis and sepsis caused by *Pseudomonas* species.

Common Etiologic Agents

Predominance of viral
infections

S. pyogenes and C. diphtheriae
infections
Gonococcal pharyngitis

Table 63.1 lists the more common causes of upper respiratory infections and stomatitis. Viral infections predominate. The most frequent bacterial cause to be considered is *Streptococcus pyogenes*. *Corynebacterium diphtheriae*, although very rare in the United States, is a major pathogen that continues to cause infection in many other countries and must not be overlooked, particularly if clinical and epidemiologic findings suggest this possibility. *Neisseria gonorrhoeae*, isolated from adults with symptomatic pharyngitis in whom no other etiologic agent can be demonstrated, must now be considered a pharyngeal pathogen that is usually transmitted by oral-genital contact. Other bacteria occasionally implicated in acute pharyngitis and tonsillitis include *Corynebacterium pyogenes*, *Corynebacterium ulcerans*, *Francisella tularensis*, and β-hemolytic streptococci other than those of Lancefield group A; these are rare causes that are not specifically sought except in very unusual situations.

In patients with purulent rhinitis, sinusitis should also be considered in the differential diagnosis (Chapter 61). Unilateral and foul-smelling purulent discharge suggests the presence of a foreign body in the nose.

General Diagnostic Approaches

Viral infections

Although viruses cause the vast majority of upper respiratory infections, they are generally not amenable to specific therapy, and laboratory tests for viral infections are usually reserved for investigating outbreaks or in cases in which the illness seems unusually severe or atypical.

Laboratory diagnosis of S.
pyogenes infections

The primary diagnostic approach in pharyngitis and tonsillitis is to determine whether there is a bacterial cause requiring specific treatment. The only reliable method is to collect a throat swab for culture, taking care to thoroughly swab the tonsillar fauces as well as the posterior pharynx, and to include any purulent material from inflamed areas. Cultures are usually made only to detect the presence or absence of *S. pyogenes*.

For the laboratory diagnosis of diphtheria or pharyngeal gonorrhea, the clinical suspicion should be indicated to the laboratory so that specific cultures for *C. diphtheriae* or *N. gonorrhoeae* may be made.

Table 63.1   Major Infectious Causes of Upper Respiratory Disease

Disease	Viruses	Bacteria and Fungi
Rhinitis	Rhinoviruses; adenoviruses; coronaviruses; parainfluenza viruses; influenza viruses; respiratory syncytial virus; some Coxsackie A viruses	Rare
Pharyngitis or tonsillitis	Adenoviruses; parainfluenza viruses; influenza viruses; rhinoviruses; Coxsackie A or B virus; herpes simplex virus; Epstein-Barr virus	*Streptococcus pyogenes; Corynebacterium diphtheriae; Neisseria gonorrhoeae*
Stomatitis	Herpes simplex virus; some Coxsackie A viruses	*Candida* species; *Fusobacterium* species and spirochetes
Peritonsillar or retropharyngeal abscess	None	*Streptococcus pyogenes* (most common); oral anaerobes such as *Fusobacterium* species; *Staphylococcus aureus* (rare); *Haemophilus influenzae* (usually in infants)

Evidence for pathogenic role of opportunists

Candida species, fusospirochetal bacteria, *Pseudomonas* species, and other Gram-negative organisms are often found in pharyngeal or oral specimens from healthy individuals as well as in certain infections. Their probable pathogenic significance in association with disease in these sites, largely based on the appearance of the lesions and the presence of the organisms in large numbers, can be supported by histologic demonstration of tissue invasion by the organisms. It is important to remember that other

Pathogens that may be present in normal flora but do not cause pharyngitis

bacterial pathogens such as *Streptococcus pneumoniae, Staphylococcus aureus, Haemophilus influenzae,* and even *Neisseria meningitidis* may be present in the pharynx. These organisms are *not* primary etiologic agents in rhinitis, pharyngitis, and tonsillitis, and their presence in the throat does *not* implicate them as causes of the illnesses; they should instead be regarded as colonizers.

The laboratory diagnosis of causes of peritonsillar and retropharyngeal abscesses is based on Gram staining and culture of purulent material obtained directly from the lesion, including anaerobic cultures.

General Principles of Management

Viral infections of the upper respiratory tract can only be treated symptomatically. If *S. pyogenes* is the cause, penicillin therapy is required; if the patient is allergic to penicillin, an alternative is chosen (eg, erythromycin or a cephalosporin). Therapeutic levels of the antibiotic should be maintained for at least 10 days. Such treatment prevents suppurative or toxi-

Ten days of therapeutic levels of penicillin needed for *S. pyogenes* infections

genic complications (for example, pharyngeal abscess, cervical adenitis, and scarlet fever) and the development of acute rheumatic fever. The latter, a serious complication, may occur in 1–3% of patients in certain population groups if they are not adequately treated. In addition, treatment of acute streptococcal infections can aid in reducing spread of the organisms to other persons. When the duration of therapy is less than 10 days, the risk of relapse and failure to eradicate the organisms is significantly increased.

Corynebacterium diphtheriae infections involve more complex management, which includes antitoxin as well as antimicrobic treatment (detailed in Chapter 17). Infections caused by *N. gonorrhoeae* are treated with appropriate antimicrobics (Chapter 19).

The management of stomatitis includes maintenance of adequate oral hygiene. If invasive *Candida* infection is present, topical and/or systemic antifungal therapy is sometimes necessary. Vincent's angina and other fusospirochetal infections are usually treated with systemic penicillin therapy as well as with appropriate dental and periodontal care. There is no specific, widely accepted treatment for aphthous stomatitis. Peritonsillar and retropharyngeal abscesses are treated aggressively with antimicrobics and often require surgical drainage, taking care to prevent accidental aspiration of the abscess contents into the lower respiratory tract.

64

Middle and Lower Respiratory Tract Infections

C. George Ray and
Kenneth J. Ryan

Middle Respiratory Tract Infection

For the purpose of this discussion, the middle respiratory tract will be considered to comprise the epiglottis, surrounding aryepiglottic tissues, larynx, trachea, and bronchi. Inflammatory disease involving these sites may be localized (for example, laryngitis) or more widespread (for example, laryngotracheobronchitis). The majority of severe infections occur in infancy and childhood. Disease expression varies somewhat with age, partly because the diameters of the airways enlarge with maturation and because immunity to common infectious agents increases with age. For example, an adult with a viral infection of the larynx (laryngitis) who was exposed to the same virus in childhood will have a relatively better immune response; in addition, the larger diameter of the larynx in the adult permits greater air flow in the presence of inflammation. An infant or child with the same infection in the same site can develop a much more severe illness, known as *croup,* which can lead to significant obstruction of air flow.

Most severe middle tract infections occur in infancy and childhood

Common Clinical Features

Epiglottitis: risk of acute airway obstruction

Epiglottitis is often characterized by the abrupt onset of throat and neck pain, fever, and inspiratory stridor (difficulty in moving adequate amounts of air through the larynx). Because of the inflammation and edema in the epiglottis and other soft tissues above the vocal cords (supraglottic area), phonation becomes difficult (muffled phonation or aphonia), and the associated pain leads to difficulty in swallowing. If this disease is not treated promptly, death may result from acute airway obstruction.

Laryngitis and croup

Laryngitis or its more severe form, croup, may have an abrupt onset (spasmodic croup) or develop more slowly over hours or a few days as a result of spread of infection from the upper respiratory tract. The illness is characterized by variable fever, inspiratory stridor, hoarse phonation,

837

and a harsh, barking cough. In contrast to epiglottitis, the inflammation is localized to the subglottic, laryngeal structures, including the vocal cords. It sometimes extends to the trachea (laryngotracheitis) and bronchi (laryngotracheobronchitis), where it is associated with a deeper, more severe cough that may provoke chest pain and variable degrees of sputum production. When vocal cord inflammation is severe, transient aphonia may result.

Bronchitis

Bronchitis or tracheobronchitis may be a primary manifestation of infection or a result of spread from upper respiratory tissues. It is characterized by cough, variable fever, and sputum production, which is often clear at the onset but may become purulent as the illness persists. Auscultation of the chest with the stethoscope often reveals coarse bubbling rhonchi, which are a result of inflammation and increased fluid production in the larger airways.

Association of chronic bronchitis with smoking, air pollution, and other diseases

Chronic bronchitis is a result of long-standing damage to the bronchial epithelium. A common cause is cigarette smoking, but a variety of environmental pollutants, chronic infections (for example, tuberculosis), and defects that hinder normal clearance of tracheobronchial secretions and bacteria (for example, cystic fibrosis) can be responsible. Because of the lack of functional integrity of their large airways, such patients are susceptible to chronic infection with members of the oropharyngeal flora and to recurrent, acute flare-ups of symptoms when they become colonized and infected by viruses and bacteria, particularly nontypable *Haemophilus influenzae* and *Streptococcus pneumoniae*. A vicious cycle of recurrent infection may evolve, leading to further damage and increasing susceptibility to pneumonia.

Nontypable *H. influenzae* and *S. pneumoniae* in exacerbations of chronic bronchitis

Common Etiologic Agents

Most subglottic middle airway infections are viral

With the exception of epiglottitis, acute diseases of the middle airway are usually caused by viral agents (Table 64.1). When acute airway obstruction is present, noninfectious possibilities must also be considered, such as aspirated foreign bodies and acute laryngospasm or bronchospasm caused by anaphylaxis.

General Diagnostic Approaches

When a viral etiology is sought, the usual method of obtaining a specific diagnosis is by inoculation of cell culture with material from the nasopharynx and throat. Acute and convalescent sera can also be collected to determine antibody responses to the common respiratory viruses and *Mycoplasma pneumoniae*. In bacterial infections, the following approaches are valuable.

High incidence of bacteremia in *H. influenzae* epiglottitis

Local culture collection contraindicated in acute epiglottitis

Epiglottitis.   *Haemophilus influenzae* type b, the most common cause of epiglottitis, produces an associated bacteremia in 85% of cases or more. Attempts to obtain local cultures from the epiglottis or throat are contraindicated because they may provoke acute reflex airway obstruction in patients who have not undergone intubation to ensure proper ventilation; furthermore, the yield is lower than that of blood culture. In addition, other bacterial agents that cause epiglottitis less frequently can often be isolated from the blood. The exception is *Corynebacterium diphtheriae* infection, in which local cultures of the nasopharynx or pharynx are required.

Laryngotracheitis and Laryngotracheobronchitis.   Although most cases of

Table 64.1   Major Causes of Acute Middle Respiratory Tract Disease

Syndrome	Viruses	Bacteria	Percentage Caused by Viruses
Epiglottitis	Rare	*Haemophilus influenzae* type b most common; also *Streptococcus pyogenes, Streptococcus pneumoniae, Corynebacterium diphtheriae, Neisseria meningitidis*	10
Laryngitis and croup	Parainfluenza virus, influenza virus, adenoviruses; occasionally respiratory syncytial virus, rhinoviruses, coronaviruses, echoviruses	Rare	90
Laryngotracheitis and laryngotracheobronchitis	Same as for laryngitis and croup	*Haemophilus influenzae* type b; *Staphylococcus aureus*	90
Bronchitis	Parainfluenza virus; influenza virus; respiratory syncytial virus; adenoviruses; measles	*Bordetella pertussis; Bordetella parapertussis; Haemophilus influenzae; Mycoplasma pneumoniae; Chlamydia pneumoniae*	80

laryngotracheitis and laryngotracheobronchitis have a viral etiology, a severe purulent process is seen occasionally. Gram staining and culture of sputum or, better yet, of purulent secretions obtained by direct laryngoscopy help to establish the causative agent. Blood cultures are again useful in such cases when a bacterial etiology is suspected.

Acute Bronchitis.   A major bacteriologic consideration in acute bronchitis, especially in infants and preschool children, is *Bordetella pertussis*. Deep nasopharyngeal cultures plated on the appropriate media constitute the best specimens. Gram staining and examination of nasopharyngeal smears by direct fluorescent antibody methods are also useful adjuncts to establishing the diagnosis. When purulent sputum is produced, Gram staining and culture may be useful in suggesting other bacterial causes (Table 64.1). An exception is *M. pneumoniae* infection, which is most readily diagnosed by serologic testing of acute and convalescent sera.

Nasopharyngeal specimens for diagnosis of pertussis

Sputum examination for other bacteria

Serodiagnosis of Mycoplasma infection

General Principles of Management

Maintenance of airway

The primary initial concern is ensuring an adequate airway. It is particularly crucial in epiglottitis, but can become a major issue in laryngitis or laryngotracheobronchitis as well. Thus, some patients will require placement of a rigid tube that provides communication between the tracheobronchial tree and the outside air (a nasotracheal tube or a surgically placed tracheostomy). Other adjunctive measures, such as highly humidified air and oxygen, may also provide relief in acute diseases involving the structures in and around the larynx. In proved or suspected bacterial infections,

Chemotherapy for bacterial infections

specific antimicrobic therapy is required; other treatment, such as antitoxin administration in diphtheria, may also be necessary.

Lower Respiratory Tract Infection

Lower respiratory tract infection develops with invasion and disease of the lung, including the alveolar spaces and their supporting structure, the interstitium, and the terminal bronchioles. Infection may occur by extension of a middle respiratory tract infection, aspiration of pathogens past the upper airway defenses, or, less commonly, by hematogenous spread from a distant site such as an abscess or an infected heart valve. When infection develops through the respiratory tract, there is usually some compromise of the upper airway mechanisms for filtering or clearing inhaled infectious agents. The most common are those that impair the epiglottic and cough reflexes; such as drugs, anesthesia, stroke, and alcohol abuse. Toxic inhalations and cigarette smoking may also interfere with the normal mucociliary action of the tracheobronchial tree. In healthy persons, the most common antecedent to lower respiratory infection is infection of the middle respiratory structures (usually viral), allowing an otherwise innocuous aspiration of oropharyngeal flora to reach the lower tract and progress to disease rather than undergo rapid clearance. Some small infectious particles can accomplish airborne passage through the middle airway and bypass mucociliary defenses; if they can survive or multiply in alveolar macrophages, they may produce a primary infection. Examples include arthroconidia of *Coccidioides immitis* and cells of *Mycobacterium tuberculosis.*

Infection can be by inhalation, aspiration, extension from middle tract, or blood-borne

Infection through air passages associated with compromised local defenses

Clinical Features

Acute pneumonia is an infection of the lung parenchyma that develops over hours to days and, if untreated, runs a natural course lasting days to weeks. The onset may be gradual, with malaise and slowly increasing fever, or sudden, as with the bed-shaking chill associated with the onset of pneumococcal pneumonia. The only early symptom referable to the lung may be cough, which is caused by bronchial irritation. In adults the cough becomes productive of sputum, which is purulent material generated in the alveoli and small air passages. In some cases the sputum may be blood streaked, rusty in color, or foul smelling. Labored or difficult breathing (dyspnea), rapid respiratory rate, and sometimes cyanosis are signs of increasing loss of alveolar air-exchange surface through spread of exudate. Chest pain from involvement of the pleura is common. Physical signs on auscultation reflect the filling and eventual consolidation of alveoli by fluid and inflammatory cells. Consolidation of an entire area adjacent to the chest wall results in dullness to percussion over the site.

Origin and characteristics of sputum

Clinical signs of acute pneumonia

The radiologic pattern of inflammatory changes in the lung is very useful in the diagnosis of pneumonia and for clinical differentiation into likely etiologic categories. The most common pattern is patchy infiltrates related to multiple foci centering on small bronchi (bronchopneumonia), which may progress to a more uniform consolidation of one or more lobes (lobar pneumonia). A more delicate, diffuse, or "interstitial" pattern, which is also common, is particularly associated with viral pneumonia.

Radiologic changes

Chronic pneumonia has a slow insidious onset that develops over weeks to months and may last for weeks or even years. The initial symptoms are the same as those of acute pneumonia (fever, chills, and malaise), but they develop more slowly. Cough can develop early or late in the illness. As

Symptoms and signs of chronic pneumonia

the disease progresses, appetite and weight loss, insomnia, and night sweats are common. Cough and sputum production may be the first indication of a vague constitutional illness referable to the lung. Bloody sputum (hemoptysis), dyspnea, and chest pain appear as the disease progresses. The physical findings and radiologic features can be similar to those of acute pneumonia, except that the diffuse interstitial infiltrates of viral pneumonia are uncommon. There may be parenchymal destruction and the formation of abscesses or cavities communicating with the bronchial tree. The clinical features of chronic pneumonia may be due to a number of infectious agents or noninfectious causes such as neoplasms, vasculitis, allergic conditions, infarction, radiation or toxic injury, and diseases of unknown etiology (for example, sarcoidosis).

Pleural effusion is the transudation of fluid into the pleural space in response to an inflammatory process in adjacent lung parenchyma. It may result from a wide variety of causes, both infectious and noninfectious. *Empyema* is a purulent infection of the pleural space that develops when the infectious agent gains access by contiguous spread from an infected lung through a bronchopleural fistula or, less often, by extension of an abdominal infection through the diaphragm. Symptoms are usually insidious and related to the primary infection until enough exudate is formed to produce symptoms referable to the chest wall or to compromise the function of the lung. The physical and radiologic findings are characteristic, with dullness to percussion and localized opacities on X-ray that can be demonstrated by appropriate manipulation of the patient. In contrast to noninfectious effusions, empyema is frequently loculated.

Lung abscess is usually a complication of acute or chronic pneumonia caused by organisms that can cause localized destruction of lung parenchyma. It may occur as part of a chronic process or as an extension of an acute, destructive pneumonia, often after aspiration of oral or gastric contents. The symptoms of lung abscess, which are usually not specific, resemble those of chronic pneumonia or an acute pneumonia that has failed to resolve. Persistent fever, cough, and the production of foul-smelling sputum are typical. Lung abscess can be diagnosed and localized with certainty only radiologically; it appears as a localized area of inflammation with single or multiple excavations or as a cavity with an air–fluid level. Multiple abscesses may develop as a result of blood-borne infection.

Common Etiologic Agents

The infectious agents that cause lower respiratory infection most frequently are listed in Table 64.2. The etiology of acute pneumonia is strongly dependent on age. More than 80% of pneumonias in infants and children are caused by viruses, whereas less than 10–20% of pneumonias in adults are viral. The reasons are probably the same as those indicated previously for middle respiratory tract infections. Influenza and other viruses, however, may provide the initial predisposition toward bacterial infection. Viruses are extremely rare as a cause of chronic as opposed to acute lower respiratory tract infections, although some symptoms of the acute infection, such as cough, may persist for weeks until the bronchial damage has healed. Influenza virus is noteworthy as a cause of acute life-threatening pneumonia, even in previously healthy young adults. Pneumonia caused by bacteria such as enteric Gram-negative rods, *Pseudomonas,* and *Legionella* is primarily limited to patients with serious debilitating underlying disease or as a complication of hospitalization and its procedures (nosocomial infection). *Klebsiella pneumoniae* has been known to produce

---

Abscesses and cavities may develop

Noninfectious causes of chronic pneumonia

Infectious or noninfectious pleural effusions

Empyema is a purulent infection of pleural space

Lung abscess frequently follows aspiration pneumonia

Blood-borne infection may give multiple abscesses

Most pneumonias are viral in infants and children

Viral infections predispose to acute bacterial pneumonia

Gram-negative pneumonias in debilitated hosts

Table 64.2 Major Causes of Lower Respiratory Tract Infection

Syndrome	Viruses	Common Bacteria	Fungi	Other Agents
Acute pneumonia	Influenza[a] Parainfluenza Adenovirus Respiratory syncytial (infants)[a]	*Streptococcus pneumoniae* *Staphylococcus aureus* *Haemophilus influenzae* Enterobacteriaceae *Legionella* Mixed anaerobes (aspiration) *Pseudomonas aeruginosa*[b]	*Candida albicans*[b] *Aspergillus* species	*Mycoplasma pneumoniae* *Pneumocystis carinii*[b] *Chlamydia trachomatis* (infants) *Chlamydia pneumoniae*
Chronic pneumonia	Rare	*Mycobacterium tuberculosis,* Other Mycobacteria; *Nocardia*	*Coccidioides immitis*[c] *Blastomyces dermatitidis*[c] *Histoplasma capsulatum*[c] *Cryptococcus neoformans*	*Paragonimus westermani*[c]
Lung abscess	None	Mixed anaerobes *Actinomyces* *Nocardia* *Staphylococcus aureus*[d] Enterobacteriaceae[d] *Pseudomonas aeruginosa*[b,d]	*Aspergillus* species	*Entamoeba histolytica*
Empyema	None	Mixed anaerobes *Staphylococcus aureus*[d] *Streptococcus pneumoniae*[d] Enterobacteriaceae *Pseudomonas aeruginosa*[b,d]	Rare	

[a] Occurrence limited to seasonal epidemics.
[b] Primarily infects the immunologically compromised host.
[c] Geographically limited.
[d] Infection develops during or after acute pneumonia.

Pneumococcus is commonest cause of acute bacterial pneumonia

community-acquired pneumonia under conditions similar to those for *S. pneumoniae* infection. At any age, the pneumococcus is the most common bacterial cause of acute pneumonia, and Gram-negative infections other than *Haemophilus* are rare in children unless they have cystic fibrosis. Acute and subacute pneumonia can be due to *Chlamydia*. *Chlamydia trachomatis* is almost exclusively limited to infants less than 7 months of age, but recent data indicate that *Chlamydia pneumoniae* strain TWAR commonly infects young adults and may produce both bronchitis and pneumonia.

Causes of lung abscess

Lung abscess and empyema follow infections with the more destructive organisms or massive aspiration of mixed anaerobic flora from the oropharynx. Several clinical clues can suggest some of the etiologic agents, given a typical clinical syndrome. For example, *Nocardia* and mycobacteria, which are strict aerobes, tend to produce upper lobe infiltrates, whereas

Anaerobic abscesses from aspiration pneumonia

aspiration pneumonia caused by anaerobes tends to develop in the most dependent parts of the lung. Textbooks on infectious disease should be consulted for further details regarding these features.

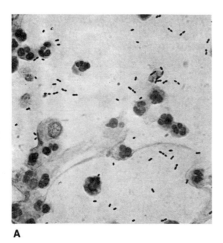
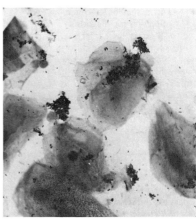

64.1 Comparison of findings in sputum and saliva. True sputum (A) should show an abundance of inflammatory cells and no squamous epithelial cells. In acute bacterial pneumonia, large numbers of a single organism are usually present. This Gram smear shows large numbers of polymorphonuclear leukocytes and *Streptococcus pneumoniae.* Saliva (B) typically contains squamous epithelial cells and a mixed bacterial population.

A   B

Diagnosis

The degree of difficulty in establishing an etiologic diagnosis for a lower respiratory tract infection depends on the number of organisms produced in respiratory secretions, whether the causative species is normally found in the oropharyngeal flora, and how easily it is grown. In the presence of typical clinical findings, the isolation of influenza virus from the throat or of *M. tuberculosis* from sputum is sufficient for diagnosis of influenza or tuberculosis, because these organisms are not normally found in such sites. The same cannot be said for *S. pneumoniae* and most bacterial pathogens, as they may be found in the throat in a significant number of healthy persons (Chapter 9).

Sputum collection and evaluation: problems of contamination

The examination of expectorated sputum has been the primary means of diagnosing the causes of bacterial pneumonia, but this approach has several advantages and disadvantages. The advantages are ease of collection and absence of risk to the patient. The primary disadvantage is the confusion that results from contamination of the sputum with oropharyngeal flora in the process of expectoration and excessive contamination with saliva. Efforts to remove saliva from sputum by washing or to accomplish interpretive differentiation of infective from normal flora by quantitative culture (as with urine specimens) (Chapter 66) have been unsuccessful. The quality of a sputum sample can be enhanced by collection early in the morning (just after the patient arises), careful instruction of the patient, and occasionally by the use of saline aerosols (induced sputum) under the supervision of an inhalation therapy specialist. The worst results can be expected when the physician's only involvement is writing an order, which is then passed down the ward chain of command to an orderly, who directs the patient to put his "sputum" in a cup placed at the bedside.

Microscopic characteristics of sputum and saliva

Microscopic examination before culture of direct Gram smears of specimens alleged to be sputum has proved useful. Polymorphonuclear leukocytes and large numbers of a single morphologic type of organism are typical findings in sputum from patient with bacterial pneumonia. Squamous epithelial cells from the oropharynx and a mixed bacterial population are characteristic of saliva (Figure 64.1). Unfortunately, most specimens are a mixture of both, which makes interpretation more difficult. Studies have shown that more than 10–25 squamous epithelial cells per low-power ($\times$10) microscopic field are evidence of excessive salivary contamination,

64.2 Techniques of specimen collection for diagnosis of lower respiratory tract infection. (A) Expectorated sputum must pass through the area above the larynx, which contains the normal oropharyngeal flora. The "sputum" may then be a mixture of both true sputum and other secretions. (B) Invasive collection techniques bypass the oropharyngeal flora to collect the purulent material directly. Some infections, such as empyema or lung abscess, may only be reached by direct aspiration or surgical procedures. Transtracheal aspiration collects material from below the larynx via a catheter inserted through the cricothyroid membrane.

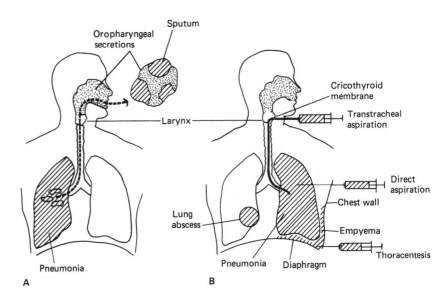

Salivary specimens should not be cultured

Transtracheal aspiration, direct transpleural aspiration, and open biopsy: risks and benefits

Use of bronchoalveolar lavage in *P. carinii* infection

Value of blood culture in acute pneumonia

Anaerobic infections cannot be diagnosed from sputum

and such specimens should not be cultured because the results may be misleading. Thus, the direct Gram smear is crucial to the use of expectorated sputum for diagnosis of acute bacterial pneumonia. The smear may be useful in the absence of cultural results, but cultures are useless without a Gram smear to assess specimen quality.

Another approach is to attempt a more direct collection from the lung using methods that bypass the oropharyngeal flora. This approach may be used in patients who are not producing sputum or in cases where analysis of expectorated sputum has been inconclusive. The major techniques are shown in Figure 64.2. In transtracheal aspiration, a puncture is made in the cricothyroid membrane and a catheter advanced deep into the tracheobronchial tree to aspirate sputum directly. This method is useful in diagnosis of both pneumonia and lung abscess. Any aspiration method that involves initial passage through the upper airway (including bronchoscopy) is less reliable than transtracheal aspiration, because the collection instruments may become contaminated with oropharyngeal secretions. Aspirates from tracheostomies are also of limited value, because these sites become colonized with Gram-negative bacteria within hours of their implantation. Direct aspiration through the chest wall can be used for diagnosis of pneumonia or empyema if the involved area can be well localized and is at the lung periphery. In some cases an open lung biopsy is the only way to obtain diagnostic material. Recently, the technique of bronchoalveolar lavage has been shown to demonstrate organisms, such as *Pneumocystis carinii*, that were previously only seen in open lung biopsies. Bacteremia may occur in acute pneumonia, particularly in its early stages, and a positive blood culture will serve to confirm a diagnosis based on clinical findings or those of expectorated sputum culture.

Once an appropriate specimen is obtained, diagnosis is usually readily made by culture using the methods described in Chapter 14 and in the sections on the individual etiologic agents. Only specimens collected by one of the invasive techniques should be used for anaerobic culture, because expectorated sputum is invariably contaminated with oropharyngeal

Serodiagnosis in *Mycoplasma* infection

anaerobes and results are meaningless. With some agents (*S. pneumoniae, H. influenzae*), detection of circulating antigen in the blood or urine by counterimmunoelectrophoresis, latex agglutination, or coagglutination may establish the diagnosis. In the case of *Mycoplasma pneumoniae* infection, serodiagnosis is usually the only practical procedure and is frequently helpful during the course of the disease (see Chapter 24). It is probable that serodiagnostic procedures will also be used as the primary method for diagnosis of *Chlamydia pneumoniae*.

Management

The general principles of management of lower respiratory tract infections are similar to those of middle tract infections. Drainage or surgical measures are needed more often as adjuncts to antimicrobial therapy in cases of chronic pneumonia, lung abscess, and empyema. When bacterial infection is considered, empirical therapy is usually given until the results of cultures and antimicrobial susceptibility tests are available. Treatment may vary from penicillin alone for a previously healthy individual in whom the most reasonable nonviral possibility is *S. pneumoniae,* to multiple drugs for a debilitated or immunocompromised patient, in whom the possibilities are much broader.

65

Enteric Infections and Food Poisoning

Kenneth J. Ryan

Acute infections of the gastrointestinal tract are among the most frequent of all illnesses, exceeded only by respiratory tract infections such as the common cold. Diarrhea is the most common manifestation of these infections; however, because it is usually self-limiting within hours or days, most of those afflicted do not seek medical care. Nonetheless, in the United States gastrointestinal infection remains one of the three most common syndromes seen by physicians who practice general medicine. Worldwide, diarrheal disease remains one of the most important causes of morbidity and mortality among infants and children. It has been estimated that in Asia, Africa, and Latin America, depending on socioeconomic and nutritional factors, a child's chance of dying of a diarrheal illness before the age of 7 years can be as high as 50%. In developed countries mortality is very much lower, but still significant. This chapter will summarize the known etiologies and epidemiologic circumstances of these infections, as well as diagnostic methods and some aspects of management. Chapters on the individual etiologic agents should be consulted for details.

High mortality from diarrheal diseases in developing countries

Clinical Features

The most prominent clinical features of gastrointestinal infections are fever, vomiting, abdominal pain, and diarrhea. Their presence varies with different diseases and different stages of infection. The occurrence of diarrhea is a central feature, and its presence and nature form the basis for classification of gastrointestinal infections into three major syndromes: watery diarrhea, dysentery, and enteric fever.

Watery Diarrhea

The most common form of gastrointestinal infection is the rapid development of frequent intestinal evacuations of a more or less fluid character known as diarrhea (*dia-* + the Greek *rhein,* to flow through, as a stream).

847

Nausea, vomiting, fever, and abdominal pain may also be present, but the dominant feature is intestinal fluid loss. Diarrhea is produced by pathogenic mechanisms that attack the proximal small intestine, the portion of the bowel in which more than 90% of physiologic net fluid absorption occurs. The purest form of watery diarrhea is that produced by enterotoxin-secreting bacteria such as *Vibrio cholerae* and enterotoxigenic *Escherichia coli*, which cause fluid loss without fever. Other common pathogens that damage the epithelium, such as rotaviruses, also cause fluid loss, but are more likely to cause fever and vomiting as well. Most cases of watery diarrhea run an acute but brief (1–3 days) self-limiting course. Exceptions are those caused by *V. cholerae*, which usually produces a more severe illness, and those caused by *Giardia lamblia*, which produces a watery diarrhea that may last for weeks.

Loss of fluid from proximal small intestine

Dysentery

Dysentery begins with the rapid onset of frequent intestinal evacuations, but the stools are of smaller volume than in watery diarrhea and contain blood and pus. If watery diarrhea is the "runs," dysentery is the "squirts." Fever, abdominal pain, cramps, and tenesmus are frequent complaints. Vomiting occurs less often. In dysentery the focus of pathology is the colon. Organisms causing dysentery can produce inflammatory and/or destructive changes in the colonic mucosa either by direct invasion or by production of cytotoxins. This damage produces the pus and blood seen in the stools, but does not result in substantial fluid loss because the absorptive and secretory capacity of the colon is much less than that of the small bowel. Dysenteric infections generally last longer than the common watery diarrheas, but most cases still resolve spontaneously in 2–7 days.

Colonic infection with inflammation

Pus and blood in stools

Enteric Fever

Enteric fever is a systemic infection, the origin and focus of which are the gastrointestinal tract. The most prominent features are fever and abdominal pain, which develop gradually over a few days in contrast to the abrupt onset of the other syndromes. Diarrhea is usually present, but may be mild and not appear until later in the course of the illness. The classic enteric fever is typhoid fever, which is produced by *Salmonella typhi* and described in detail in Chapter 20. The pathogenesis of enteric fever is more complex than that of watery diarrhea or dysentery. It generally involves penetration of the mucosa of the distal small bowel with subsequent spread outside the bowel to the biliary tract, liver, mesentery, or reticuloendothelial organs. Bacteremia is common, occasionally causing metastatic infection in other organs. Typhoid fever is the only infection for which these events have been well studied. Although it is usually self-limiting, enteric fever carries a significant risk of serious disease and even death. The duration of illness is not well established except for typhoid fever, which lasts 3–4 weeks when untreated.

Serious systemic disease with lymphoid and reticuloendothelial invasion

Etiology

In the past 20 years, great advances have been made in our understanding of gastrointestinal infections. Before the late 1960s, fewer than 20% of the infectious syndromes described previously could be linked to a specific etiologic agent by any diagnostic method. The organisms listed in Table

65.1 now account for 60–80% of cases, although diagnostic methods for all of them are not yet available in many laboratories. The primary clinical syndrome caused by each agent is also listed in Table 65.1 but should not be regarded as absolute because symptoms and signs vary significantly from patient to patient and even at different times in the course of the same illness. For example, *Shigella* infections frequently go through a brief watery diarrhea stage before localizing in the colon, and *Campylobacter* enteritis usually begins with fever, malaise, and abdominal pain, followed by dysentery. In any single case the clinical findings may suggest a range of etiologic agents, but are not sufficiently specific to be diagnostic of any single organism.

The epidemiologic setting of the infection is of great importance in assessing the relative probability of each of the agents listed in Table 65.1. When combined with clinical findings, the differential diagnosis can usually be limited to two or three organisms. The major epidemiologic settings are 1) endemic infection; 2) epidemic infection; 3) traveler's diarrhea; 4) food poisoning; and 5) hospital-associated diarrhea.

Importance of epidemiologic setting in preliminary diagnosis

Endemic Infections

By definition, endemic diarrheas are those that occur sporadically in the usual living circumstances of the patient (from the Greek *endemos,* dwelling in a place). Some organisms are endemic worldwide, whereas others are geographically limited. There are also seasonal variations and age-related attack rates within the endemic foci. In developed countries the most common causes of endemic gastrointestinal infections are rotaviruses, parvo/picornaviruses, *Campylobacter, Salmonella,* and *Shigella.* All are more common in infants and children because they are more prone to fecal—oral spread and because development of immunity is related to age. Rotaviruses account for 40–60% of diarrheal infections occurring during the cooler months in infants and children less than 2 years of age, but are uncommon in older persons.

Higher frequency in infants and children

The geographically limited agents (Table 65.1) are common only in the endemic areas listed. These distributions are not fixed, making it necessary to keep abreast of geographic changes in the distribution of established agents as well as the recognition of new ones. For example, cholera has long been limited to warm-climate river deltas in Asia, Africa, and the Middle East, but recently an endemic focus of *V. cholerae* in the United States was discovered off the Gulf Coast of Louisiana and Texas.

Geographic limitations of some agents

Epidemic Infections

Under certain epidemiologic conditions some of the organisms responsible for endemic infections can spread beyond the family unit to cause epidemics involving regional, national, and even international populations. The intestinal diseases most frequently associated with epidemics are typhoid fever, cholera, and shigellosis. For all three, epidemics are related to the failure of basic public health sanitary measures. For example, *S. typhi* and *V. cholerae* may be spread for some distance through the community water supply, a route blocked by modern sewage and water treatment practices. When these procedures are not employed or are interrupted by equipment failure or natural disasters (floods, earthquakes), these diseases can and do recur in epidemic form. Epidemics of shigellosis may be water-borne under the same conditions, but *Shigella* dysentery is more typically a disease "of wars and armies, and of crowds and move-

Spread of typhoid, cholera, and shigellosis where hygiene is poor or after major disasters

Table 65.1 Features of Infectious Gastrointestinal Syndromes

| Organism | Common Distribution | Clinical Syndrome | Pathogenic Mechanism | Stool Microscopy | Laboratory Diagnosis[a] | | | | |
| | | | | | Culture | | Toxin in Stools | Serology | |
					Stool[b]	Blood		Antibody Detection	Antigen Detection
1. *Salmonella serotypes*	Worldwide	Dysentery	Mucosal invasion	PMNs	+	–	–	–	–
2. *Salmonella typhi*	Tropical, developing countries	Enteric fever	Penetration, spread	Monocytes	+	+	–	+	–
3. *Shigella* sp.	Worldwide	Dysentery	Mucosal invasion, cytotoxin	PMNs, RBCs	+	–	–	–	–
4. *Shigella dysenteriae* (Shiga)	Tropical, developing countries	Dysentery	Mucosal invasion, cytotoxin	PMNs, RBCs	+	+	–	–	–
5. *Campylobacter fetus*	Worldwide	Dysentery	Unknown	PMNs, RBCs	+	–	–	–	–
6. *Escherichia coli* (EIEC)	Worldwide	Dysentery	Mucosal invasion	PMNs, RBCs	+[c]	–	–	–	–
7. *Escherichia coli* (ETEC)	Worldwide[d]	Watery diarrhea	Enterotoxin(s)	–	+[c]	–	–	–	–
8. *Escherichia coli* (EHEC)	Worldwide	Watery diarrhea	Cytotoxin	RBCs	+[c]	–	–	–	–
9. *Escherichia coli* (EPEC)	Worldwide[d]	Watery diarrhea	Adherence	–	+[c]	–	–	–	–

	Distribution	Clinical presentation	Mechanism	Diagnostic method				
10. *Vibrio cholerae*	Asia, Africa, Middle East, Louisiana	Watery diarrhea	Enterotoxin	–	+	–	–	–
11. *Vibrio parahemolyticus*	Seacoast	Watery diarrhea	Unknown	–	+	–	–	–
12. *Yersinia enterocolitica*	Worldwide	Enteric fever[e]	Penetration, spread	–	+	+	–	–
13. *Clostridium difficile*	Worldwide	Dysentery	Cytotoxin, enterotoxin	–	+	–	+	–
14. *Clostridium perfringens*	Worldwide	Watery diarrhea	Enterotoxin	–	+	+	–	–
15. *Bacillus cereus*	Worldwide	Watery diarrhea	Enterotoxin	–	+	–	–	–
16. Rotavirus	Worldwide	Watery diarrhea	Mucosal destruction	Electron microscopy[f]	–	–	–	+
17. Parvo/picornavirus	Worldwide	Watery diarrhea	Mucosal destruction	Electron microscopy[f]	–	–	–	–
18. *Giardia lamblia*	Worldwide	Watery diarrhea	Mucosal irritation	Flagellates, cysts	–	–	–	–
19. *Entamoeba histolytica*	Worldwide[d]	Dysentery	Mucosal invasion	Amebas, PMNs	–	–	+	–

Abbreviations: RBCs = *red blood cells;* PMNs = *polymorphonuclear leukocytes;* EIEC = *enteroinvasive* E. coli; ETEC = enterotoxigenic E. coli; EHEC = enterohemorrhagic E. coli; EPEC = enteropathogenic E. coli.

[a] Positive sign indicates procedure is useful and usually available in clinical laboratories.

[b] Which cultures are done routinely depends on the laboratory and/or physician's request.

[c] Organism may be isolated in culture, but demonstration of pathogenic potential (toxin production etc) is limited to specialized laboratories.

[d] Organism is more common in developing countries.

[e] Infection may also manifest watery diarrhea or dysentery.

[f] Appropriate methods may be available in only a limited number of laboratories.

ment."* The very low infecting dose of *Shigella* can make spread through direct contact reach epidemic proportions when crowding and poor sanitary facilities are combined.

Although such epidemics are usually associated with the 19th century, it is clear that the potential remains. In the late 1970s large epidemics of both typhoid fever and shigellosis spread through Central and South America. In 1973 more than 200 cases of typhoid fever in Florida were associated with a defective chlorinator in the local water system.

Traveler's Diarrhea

Travelers from developed to less developed countries all too frequently experience a diarrheal illness in the first week that is usually brief but can be serious. The common names applied to this syndrome, such as "Delhi belly" and "Montezuma's revenge," reflect geographic associations and the cumulative frustration of those forced to spend part of their vacation next to the toilet rather than the swimming pool.

The most extensive studies of traveler's diarrhea has involved travelers from the United States to Latin American countries, particularly Mexico. In nearly one-half of these cases the diarrhea is caused by enterotoxigenic strains of *E. coli* acquired during travel. *Shigella* infections account for another 10–20%, and the remaining cases are attributable to various pathogens or unknown causes. Ingestion of uncooked or incompletely cooked foods is the most likely source of infection, but most epidemiologic studies have not shown specific food associations. An exception is the strong relationship between toxigenic *E. coli* diarrhea and the consumption of salads containing raw vegetables. "Don't drink the water" still seems like sound advice for travelers to countries where hygiene remains poor, but the adage is not well supported by studies relating infection to water or ice consumption.

Predominant role of enterotoxigenic E. coli

Food Poisoning

Many gastrointestinal infections involve food as a vehicle of transmission. The term *food poisoning,* however, is usually reserved for instances in which a single meal can be incriminated as the source. This situation typically arises when multiple cases of the same gastrointestinal syndrome develop at the same time among persons whose only common experience is a meal shared at a social event or restaurant. The probable etiologic agent can usually be assessed from knowledge of the incubation period, the food vehicle, and the clinical findings.

The most common causes of food poisoning are shown in Table 65.2. Some are not infections but intoxications, caused by ingestion of a toxin produced by bacteria in the food before it was eaten. Intoxications generally have shorter incubation periods than infections and may involve extraintestinal symptoms (for example, botulism). Infectious food poisoning does not differ from endemic diarrheal infections caused by the same species. The length of the incubation period and the severity of the symptoms are generally related to the number of organisms in the infecting dose.

The epidemiologic circumstances of food poisoning vary with the eti-

Single-source outbreaks

Diseases from ingestion of preformed toxin

Infectious diseases

---

* Christie, A.B. 1974. *Infectious Disease, Epidemiology and Clinical Practice.* 2nd ed. New York: Churchill Livingstone, p. 137.

Table 65.2 Clinical and Epidemiologic Features of Food Poisoning

Etiology	Percentage of Reported Outbreaks[a]	Typical Incubation Period	Primary Clinical Findings	Characteristic Foods
Intoxication[b]				
Bacillus cereus (vomiting toxin)	1–2	1–6 hr	Vomiting	Rice
Clostridium botulinum	5–15	12–72 hr	Neuromuscular paralysis	Improperly preserved vegetables, meat, fish
Staphylococcus aureus	15–25	2–4 hr	Vomiting	Meats, custards, salads
Chemical[c]	20–25	0.1–48 hr	Variable	Variable
Infections[d]				
Bacillus cereus (diarrheal toxin)	1–2	6–24 hr	Watery diarrhea	Meat, poultry, vegetables
Clostridium perfringens	5–15	9–15 hr	Watery diarrhea	Meat, poultry
Salmonella	10–30	6–48 hr	Dysentery	Poultry, eggs, meat
Shigella	2–5	12–48 hr	Dysentery	Variable
Vibrio parahemolyticus	1–2	10–24 hr	Watery diarrhea	Shellfish
Trichinella spiralis	5–10	3–30 days	Fever, myalgia	Meat, especially pork
Hepatitis A	1–3	10–45 days	Hepatitis	Shellfish

[a] Based on documented outbreaks reported to the Centers for Disease Control, Atlanta (variable from year to year).
[b] Disease caused by toxin in food at time of ingestion.
[c] Includes heavy metals, monosodium glutamate, mushrooms, and various toxins of nonmicrobial origin.
[d] Disease caused by infection after ingestion.

Association with deficiencies in food preparation and storage temperature

ologic agent, but virtually always involve a breach in the recommended procedures for handling food. The organisms may be present as contaminants in raw food before cooking or introduced by a carrier or contaminated utensil involved in preparation. Causes of bacterial food poisoning include failure to kill the organisms by adequate cooking, almost always followed by a period of warming (incubation) long enough for the organisms to multiply to infectious numbers or, in the case of toxigenic disease, to produce sufficient toxin to cause disease. In 80–90% of investigated outbreaks of bacterial food poisoning, the most important contributing factor is the use of improper storage temperatures for the food. This factor may obtain in home-cooked meals as well as those prepared in restaurants, in schools, or at large social events such as church picnics. An example of typical circumstances for a *Salmonella* outbreak is provided in Chapter 20.

Frequency of reported outbreaks

The relative frequency of each etiologic agent and the foods most frequently involved are also shown in Table 65.2. This information is based on outbreaks investigated by public health agencies but, because of differences in reporting rules and practices, may not reflect the actual incidence of each. Large outbreaks, restaurant-associated outbreaks, and outbreaks involving serious illness with hospitalization or death are all more likely to be reported to health authorities than are mild diarrheas after a dinner party. In recent years, of the 400–500 outbreaks (10,000–15,000 cases) reported each year in the United States, fewer than 200 are "solved." Food poisoning characterized by a short incubation period (for example, *Staphylococcus aureus*) is more likely to be recognized because it can easily be associated witl. a specific meal and because the food itself may still be available for examination. There are also large geographic differences in reporting. For example, in 1979, New York City, in which 50% of the state population resides, reported 98% of New York State's food-borne outbreaks, and Connecticut reported more outbreaks than all of the southeastern states combined.

Approaches to determing the cause of microbial food poisoning

Sampling problems aside, the food poisoning syndromes listed in Table 65.2 are well recognized, with *Salmonella, Clostridium perfringens,* and *S. aureus* accounting for more than 70% of those for which a microbial etiology can be found. For bacterial infections such as *Salmonella* and *Shigella,* which are not normal members of the stool flora, establishing the diagnosis by isolating the causative organism is relatively easy. If the circumstances indicate *C. perfringens* or *S. aureus* food poisoning, investigation will involve cultures of vomitus, stool from several cases, and the suspect food. In some cases, toxin detection will be required to establish the etiology and source. Such investigations are best coordinated by public health authorities, who can also address the legal and community implications of the outbreak. For example, one investigation of *Salmonella* food poisoning led to the discovery that the owner of a restaurant was keeping and slaughtering chickens at the restaurant. Although this practice may have provided very fresh chicken, it guaranteed *Salmonella* contamination of the entire kitchen.

Hospital-Associated Diarrhea

The hospital environment should not allow spread of the usual causes of endemic intestinal infection. When such infection occurs, it can usually be traced to an employee who continues working while ill or to contaminated food prepared outside the hospital that is "smuggled" in by the patient's friends. Two special causes of hospital-associated diarrhea are caused by *E. coli* in infants and *C. difficile* in patients treated with antimicrobial agents. The relative role of enterotoxigenic and enteropathogenic strains of *E. coli* in nursery outbreaks of diarrhea is discussed in Chapter 20. The disease is highly infectious among newborns. Fortunately, such outbreaks have become rare. *Clostridium difficile* accounts for more than 90% of cases of a syndrome that ranges from mild diarrhea to fulminant pseudomembranous colitis during or after treatment with antibiotics. The disease is mediated by a cytotoxin and/or an enterotoxin produced in vivo by *C. difficile.* The responsible toxigenic *C. difficile* may be resident in the patient's intestinal flora before administration of antimicrobics or be acquired in the hospital. Rotaviruses can also cause hospital outbreaks in infants.

Roles of pathogenic *E. coli* strains, *C. difficile,* and rotaviruses

Laboratory Diagnosis

Laboratory diagnostic procedures, summarized in Table 65.1, include microscopic examination, culture, toxin detection, and serologic procedures. The relative value of each is different for the various etiologies. The diagnostic approach therefore requires that the physician assess the clinical and epidemiologic features of the case, decide which organisms are potential causes, and provide this assessment to the laboratory so that appropriate procedures will be used.

Microscopic Examination

Stool cytology

Microscopic examination is of limited value in the assessment of bacterial infections. The presence of polymorphonuclear leukocytes or blood in the stool correlates with organisms that produce disease by invasion, particularly colonic invasion. The leukocytes may be seen in unstained or methylene-blue-stained wet mount preparations; the absence of fecal leukocytes, however, does not exclude invasive diarrhea. The observation and morphologic characterization of amebas and flagellates on wet or stained preparations are the primary means by which amebic (*Entamoeba histolytica*) and flagellate (*G. lamblia*) infections are diagnosed. Direct electron microscopy can be used to diagnose viral diarrhea, as the rotaviruses and parvo/picornaviruses have a characteristic morphology but cannot be grown in cell culture.

Direct detection of intestinal parasites

Electron microscopic detection of rotaviruses and parvo/picornaviruses

Culture

Blood cultures: positive in early stages of enteric fever

Isolation of the etiologic agent is the primary means by which bacterial enteric infection is diagnosed. In enteric fever the organism is typically present in the blood in the early stages of disease. Blood cultures are, however, usually negative in watery diarrhea and dysenteric infections, and stool culture must be relied upon for diagnosis. Fortunately, several good selective media have been developed for both direct plating and enrichment culture, which allow isolation of the infecting organism in the presence of a predominant normal flora. Selective media are then used for the various enteric pathogens (see Chapter 14). Media routinely employed may vary between clinical laboratories, but should include those appropriate for *Salmonella, Shigella,* and *Campylobacter fetus.* Three or four primary plates and one or two enrichment broths are required. After incubation the enrichment broths are subcultured to new sets of selective plates, and suspect colonies on all plates are screened with multiple biochemical tests. Diarrhea caused by *E. coli* is a special problem, because none of the methods that define the enterotoxigenic, invasive, or other pathogenic mechanisms is practical for clinical laboratories.

Stool culture on selective media

Toxin Assay

Cytopathic effect on cell culture of *C. difficile* toxin

The B cytotoxin of *C. difficile* can be detected by its cytopathic effect in a cell culture system. In most clinical cases, enough toxin is present for direct detection in a stool specimen. This assay is currently available only in reference laboratories. A method that detects the *C. difficile* A toxin by latex agglutination has been developed, but its application to clinical illness is still controversial. *Escherichia coli* enterotoxin can be assayed from cultures in specialized laboratories, but not directly from stool specimens. A DNA probe for the toxin gene developed by recombinant DNA techniques can be applied directly to colonies to detect enterotoxigenicity.

Colony DNA hybridization probe

Serologic Diagnosis

At present, antibody detection is useful in the diagnosis of amebic dysentery caused by *E. histolytica* and of typhoid fever. Both are considered ancillary to the primary diagnostic tests, which involve specific detection of the organism by microscopic and cultural methods. Reagents are commercially available for the detection of rotavirus antigen in stool by enzyme-lined immunosorbent assay or radioimmunoassay. These methods have a sensitivity roughly comparable to that of electron microscopy. Serologic methods have been described for many other causes of gastrointestinal infection, but are not generally used because of lack of sensitivity, specificity, or availability of reagents.

Other Causes of Intestinal Infection

Despite recent advances in defining the etiologies of enteric infections, there are surely more to be discovered. Organisms not listed in Table 65.1, such as *Aeromonas, Citrobacter, Plesiomonas,* and other, have occasionally been associated with intestinal infections, but the evidence for their enteropathogenicity is not yet strong enough to interpret their isolation from individual cases. At our present state of knowledge it is not useful to attempt isolation of these organisms unless strong epidemiologic evidence, such as food-borne outbreak, supports interpretation of the results.

Treatment

Maintenance of fluid and electrolyte balance

In most gastrointestinal infections the primary goal of treatment is relief of symptoms, with particular attention to maintaining fluid and electrolyte balance. The effect of common antidiarrheal medications such as bismuth compounds (Pepto-bismol) or antispasmotics (Lomotil) is variable depending on the etiology. In general, they may be helpful for the watery diarrhea caused by enterotoxins, but not for dysentery caused by mucosal invasion, and antispasmotics may be harmful or dangerous in the latter instance. Antimicrobial agents are usually not indicated for self-limited watery diarrhea, but are required for more severe dysenteric infections. Some enteric infections, such as typhoid fever, are always treated with antimicrobics. More information on therapy is given in the individual chapters, but texts on infectious diseases should be consulted for specific recommendations.

Factors influencing decisions on antimicrobic therapy

66

Urinary Tract Infections

James J. Plorde

A physycyen, truely, can lyttel descerne Ony maner sekeness wythout syght of uryne.

Hawes, S. 1509. *The Pastime of Pleasure* (The Oxford English Dictionary)

The examination of urine has been used to assist medical practitioners in the diagnosis and management of human illness for centuries. So great an emphasis did medieval physicians place on the color, sediment, smell, and even taste of this effluent that a urine-filled flask became the symbol of their profession. This fluid, which so faithfully reflects the maladies of the urinary tract, is produced by the kidney, collected by the renal pelvis, and transported through the ureters to the bladder for storage. Here it remains until the discomfort of bladder distention stimulates its evacuation via the urethra. Bacterial colonization of the urine within this tract (*bacteriuria*) is common and can, at times, result in microbial invasion of the tissues responsible for the manufacture, transport, and storage of urine. Infection of the upper urinary tract, consisting of the kidney and its pelvis, is known as *pyelonephritis*. Infection of the lower tract may involve the bladder (*cystitis*), urethra (*urethritis*), or prostate (*prostatitis*), the genital organ that surrounds and communicates with the first segment of the male urethra. Because all portions of the urinary tract are joined by a fluid medium, infection at any site may spread to involve other areas of the system.

It has been estimated that approximately 10% of humans are afflicted with a urinary tract infection at some time during their lives. The exact prevalance is age and sex dependent. Approximately 1% of male infants acquire infection but, unexpectedly, few show evidence of congenital urinary tract abnormalities. Thereafter, infection in the male is uncommon until the sixth decade of life, when enlargement of the prostate interferes with emptying of the bladder. In contrast, the prevalence of bacteriuria in schoolage girls is 1–2% and as many as 5% eventually are involved at some time during their childhood years. Although most recover unev-

Definitions

Prevalence of bacteriuria

857

entually, this population group is at substantially increased risk of recurrent urinary tract infection during adult life. Accordingly, the prevalence of bacteriuria in the female population increases gradually with time, reaching 5% in women of childbearing age and 10–20% in postmenopausal women. These infections may be symptomatic or asymptomatic, acute or chronic, singular or recurrent. At times they can produce permanent damage to the kidney.

Pathogenesis

Host Factors

Ascending infections in women of childbearing age

Contribution of adherence and anatomic factors to colonization and infection

Infections are seen most frequently in women of childbearing age. They are caused by gut flora, which reach the bladder via the urethra, after colonization of the vagina, external periurethral area, and distal urethra. The circumstances that lead to this colonization are not fully understood, but it is known that certain strains of *Escherichia coli* adhere more readily to vaginal and urinary epithelial cells and possess other properties that distinguish them from nonuropathogenic *E. coli*. In addition, epithelial cells from the introitus of infection-prone women support bacterial adherence to a greater extent than cells from controls. Thus, both host and bacterial properties are of importance in pathogenesis. Bacteria can reach the bladder more easily in the female host than in the male because the urethra is shorter, lies in close proximity to the moist perirectal area, and is subjected to the massaging effect of sexual intercourse. Once in the bladder, organisms that cause cystitis can multiply in the contained urine.

Catheter-associated infections

Bacteria can also be carried easily to the bladder in both men and women by passage of a catheter or other instrument, such as a cystoscope. This mode of transmission constitutes the most common single cause of hospital-acquired bacteriuria in either sex. A single transient catheterization of the bladder induces bacteriuria in approximately 1% of ambulatory and 10% of bed-ridden patients. An indwelling catheter, by providing a fluid-filled conduit for the migration of organisms from the external environment to the bladder, is more frequently associated with urinary tract infection. Even with meticulous attention to aseptic technique, most patients harboring a catheter for more than 2 weeks develop infection.

The factors that determine whether the bacteriuria persists after the removal of the initiating event include the number and type of bacteria introduced and the adequacy of the host's response to these organisms. In the overwhelming majority of cases, the number of bacteria is small and the host's defense mechanisms prove adequate. The urine itself is inhibitory to anaerobes and other fastidious organisms that are part of the normal flora of the urethral mucosa, and these bacteria seldom cause persistent infections. Even organisms known for their ability to multiply in urine may be inhibited when exposed to the very high osmolality and concentration of urea and hydrogen ions that characterize the urine of many normal individuals. It is likely that the moderation of these urinary parameters during pregnancy accounts, at least in part, for the increased incidence of bacteriuria in this population. The antibacterial properties of the bladder mucosa and the few neutrophils that reach the surface contribute to the clearance of introduced organisms. Perhaps the most important of the host defenses, however, is the act of voiding. The constant flushing of contaminated urine from the body and its dilution with newly formed, uncontaminated urine eliminates bacteria or maintains their num-

Inhibitory properties of concentrated urine

Flushing effects of micturation

Causes and effects of interference with urine flow

bers at low levels. Any interference with this clearing mechanism results in bacterial multiplication and a greatly increased probability of developing or sustaining an infection. The interference may be by mechanical obstruction to urine flow (stone, stricture, or hypertrophied prostate), neurogenic impairment of bladder control (spinal cord injury, multiple sclerosis), or functional impairment, such as the vesicoureteral reflux seen in many children with urinary tract infections. The latter appears to result from the effect of the inflammatory reaction, which interferes with the integrity of the vesicoureteral junction and allows regurgitation of urine from the bladder into the ureters. Such reflux, not only returns a pool of infected urine to the bladder after voiding is completed, but also can carry bacteria to the renal pelvis and thus initiate infection in a previously uninvolved kidney. A similar functional abnormality has been described in pregnant women. The hormonal changes in pregnancy lead to a decrease in bladder tone, diminished ureteral peristalsis, and dilatation of the renal pelvis and ureters. All enhance the likelihood of reflux and explain, at least in part, the frequency with which pregnant women with bacteriuria develop upper urinary tract disease. Congenital or acquired anatomic derangements of the vesicoureteral junction produce similar results.

Infections in pregnancy

Blood-borne infections

Occasionally, urinary tract infection occurs when bacteria seed the renal parenchyma directly from the blood. It is possible to infect the kidneys of experimental animals by intravenous injection of a variety of bacterial species other than Gram-negative bacilli. Hematogenous pyelonephritis in humans is uncommon, however, except during periods of sustained *Staphylococcus aureus* bacteremia.

Microbial Factors

Fecal origin of infecting organisms

Determinants of uropathogenicity of *E. coli*

Human feces contain a rich diversity of bacterial species. Surprisingly, only a few regularly produce urinary tract infection. In fact, *Escherichia coli* accounts for more than 90% of acute infections in patients with structurally normal urinary tracts. The factors responsible for this extraordinary monopoly are incompletely understood, but the relative resistance of *E. coli* to the inhibitory effects of vaginal fluid, its possession of pili that aid its attachment to the epithelial cells of the urinary tract, and its motility appear to contribute to its effectiveness as a uropathogen. Some or all of these features, however, are found in other, less successful, enteric species. It has been shown that the relationship of *E. coli* to acute symptomatic urinary tract infection is limited to relatively few of the O/H/K serotypes of this organism found in the stool. These uropathogenic *E. coli* all possess the P pilus (see Chapter 20), α-hemolysin, and/or aerobactin, which are chromosomally mediated virulence properties.

Infections associated with few serotypes and P pilus

Chronic and recurrent infections

Patients with urinary tract abnormalities that interfere with the free flow of urine are particularly apt to experience chronic or recurrent infection. This exposes them to multiple courses of antimicrobial therapy, which eventually leads to the replacement of antibiotic-susceptible strains of *E. coli* with more resistant pathogens. Hospitalized patients are particularly susceptible to cross-infection with nosocomial strains of *Proteus, Providencia, Pseudomonas, Klebsiella, Enterobacter, Serratia,* coagulase-negative staphylococci, and enterococci, many of which are passed directly from catheterized patient to catheterized patient on the hands of medical personnel. Once established in the urinary tract, *Proteus* strains appear to be particularly virulent. Experimental evidence suggests that *Proteus mirabilis* possesses pili that facilitate its adherence to the mucosa of the renal pelvis. In addition, urease production by all species of *Proteus* leads to

Nosocomial infections with opportunists

Effects of urease activity of *Proteus*

hydrolysis of urea, formation of ammonium hydroxide, and alkalinization of the urine. The elevated pH in the urine is directly toxic to renal cells and stimulates the formation of magnesium and ammonium phosphate struvite urinary calculi (stones), which can contribute to the chronicity of the infection by producing ureteral obstruction and sheltering the bacteria from the patient's defensive mechanisms and the physician's antimicrobial agents. Species of *Klebsiella,* because of their more limited urease production or through production of an extracellular polysaccharide slime layer, are also associated with the presence of urinary calculi.

Stone formation

Staphylococcus saprophyticus, a coagulase-negative, novobiocin-resistant, urease-positive staphylococcus, is now recognized as the cause of as much as 20% of symptomatic urinary tract infections in young, sexually active women. *Staphylococcus aureus* infections usually result from the bacteremic seeding of the urinary tract, as described previously.

S. saprophyticus infections

Yeasts, particularly species of *Candida,* may be isolated from catheterized patients receiving antibacterial therapy and from diabetics, but they seldom produce symptomatic disease. *Chlamydia trachomatis,* in contrast, can produce the acute urethral syndrome described subsequently.

Candida infections

Chlamydia infections

Common Clinical Features

The clinical manifestations of urinary tract infection are variable. Approximately one-half of infections do not produce recognizable illness and are discovered incidentally during a general medical examination. Infections in infants produce symptoms of a nonspecific nature, including fever, vomiting, and failure to thrive. Manifestations in older children and adults, when present, often suggest the diagnosis and sometimes the localization of the infection within the urinary tract.

Urethritis

Infections confined to the urethra are characterized by painful urination (dysuria) and discharge of mucoid or purulent material from the urethral orifice. They are most commonly produced by sexually transmitted agents. This syndrome is discussed more fully in Chapter 70.

Dysuria and discharge

Cystitis

The symptoms of cystitis—dysuria, frequent voiding (frequency), and an imperative "call to toilet" (urgency)—are similar to those of urethritis. This symptom complex is, in fact, produced by irritation of the mucosal surface of the urethra as well as the bladder. Unlike urethritis associated with sexually transmitted agents, cystitis is produced by the multiplication of enteric organisms in the bladder urine. It is clinically distinguished from urethritis by a more acute onset, more severe symptoms, the presence of bacteriuria, and, in approximately half, hematuria. The urine is often cloudy and malodorous and occasionally frankly bloody; unlike patients with urethritis, those with cystitis often experience pain and tenderness in the suprapubic area. Fever and systemic manifestations of illness are usually absent unless the infection spreads to involve the kidney. Approximately one-third of women presenting with dysuria and frequency lack cultural evidence of either bacteriuria or sexually transmitted disease. Use of more sensitive culturing techniques in such patients has defined an acute urethral syndrome associated with the presence in the urethra of small numbers

Urgency, frequency, and dysuria

Causative bacteria multiply in urine

Suprapubic tenderness and turbid urine

Acute urethral syndrome

of enteric bacteria (usually *E. coli*) or agents of sexually transmitted infections, such as *C. trachomatis*.

Pyelonephritis

Fever, flank pain, and systemic signs

The typical presentation of upper urinary infection consists of flank pain and fever that exceeds 38.3°C. These findings may be preceded or accompanied by manifestations of cystitis. Rigors, vomiting, diarrhea, and tachycardia are present in the more severely ill. Physical examination reveals tenderness over the costovertebral areas of the back and, occasionally, evidence of septic shock. In the absence of obstruction, the clinical manifestations usually abate within a few days, leaving the kidneys functionally intact. It has been estimated, however, that 20–50% of pregnant women with acute pyelonephritis give birth to premature infants, one of the most serious consequences of urinary tract infection. In the presence of obstruction, a neurogenic bladder, or vesicoureteral reflux, clinical manifestations are more persistent, occasionally leading to necrosis of the renal papillae and progressive impairment of kidney function with chronic bacteriuria. If a renal calculus or necrotic renal papilla impacts in the ureter, severe flank pain with radiation to the groin occurs.

Association with premature delivery

Chronic pyelonephritis

Prostatitis

Symptoms and signs

Infection of the prostate is typically manifested as pain in the lower back, perirectal area, and testicles. In acute infection, the pain may be severe and accompanied by high fever, chills, and the signs and symptoms of cystitis. Inflammatory swelling can lead to obstruction of the neighboring urethra and urinary retention. On rectal palpation, the prostate is boggy and exquisitely tender. Response to antibiotic therapy is good, but occasionally abscess formation, epididymitis, and seminal vesiculitis or chronic infection develop. Typically, acute prostatitis develops in young adults; however, it can also follow placement of an indwelling catheter in an older man. Patients with chronic prostatitis seldom give a history of an acute episode. Many are totally without symptoms; others experience low-grade pain and dysuria. Periodic spread of prostatic organisms to the urine in the bladder produces recurrent bouts of cystitis. In fact, chronic prostatitis is probably the major cause of recurrent bacteriuria in men.

Acute prostatitis in young men

Chronic prostatitis

General Diagnostic Approaches

Specimen Collection

Contamination of voided urine

The diagnosis of urinary tract infection is based on examination of the normally sterile urine for evidence of bacteria or an accompanying inflammatory reaction. Critical to this examination is the use of appropriate techniques for specimen collection. Urine is most easily obtained by spontaneous micturation. Unfortunately, voided urine is invariably contaminated with urethral flora and, in the case of the female, vaginal secretions, which can confound the results of laboratory testing. Although the contaminants can never be completely eliminated, their quantity may be diminished by carefully cleansing the periurethrum before voiding and allowing the initial part of the stream to flush the urethra before collecting a specimen for examination. This clean-voided midstream urine collection procedure is preferred to catheterization for routine purposes because it avoids the risk of introducing organisms into the bladder. When the lab-

Clean-voided urine collection

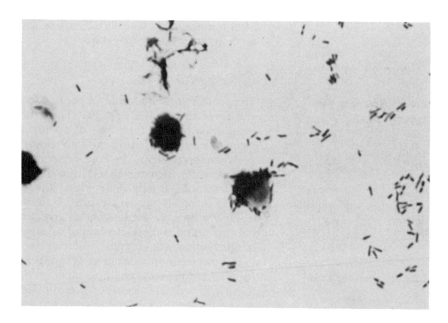

66.1 Gram stain of an uncentrifuged clean voided urine specimen from a patient with an acute *E. coli* urinary tract infection. Some degenerating polymorphonuclear leukocytes and numerous Gram-negative rods are present.

oratory examination of such a specimen produces equivocal results or the patient cannot comply with the requirements of the clean-voided technique, catheterization may be needed. Alternatively, urine may be aspirated from the bladder with a needle and syringe. In this procedure, the patient refrains from voiding until the bladder is distended. The suprapubic skin is then disinfected and a small needle passed through the skin into the bladder. The procedure has proved to be safe and well tolerated.

Suprapubic aspiration

Microscopic Examination

Pyuria

Approximately 90% of patients with acute symptomatic urinary tract infection have pyuria (that is, more than 10 white cells/mm^3 of urine). This finding is also common, however, in a number of noninfectious diseases. More specific is the presence of white cell casts, which occur almost exclusively, although not uniformly, in patients with acute pyelonephritis. The most sensitive and specific microscopic procedure is a Gram-stained smear of uncentrifuged urine (Figure 66.1). The presence of at least one organism per oil-immersion field is almost always indicative of bacterial infection. The absence of white cells and bacteria in several fields makes the diagnosis unlikely, but does not rule it out, especially in young women with acute, symptomatic infection who may be infected with smaller numbers of organisms.

Direct Gram staining

Chemical Screening Tests

Detection of leukocyte esterase and nitrite

A number of nonmicroscopic urinary screening tests have been commercially marketed within the past several years. The most successful detects leukocyte esterase from inflammatory cells and nitrite produced from urinary nitrates by bacterial nitrate reductase. Although technically simpler, the sensitivity and specificity of these products are similar to that of microscopic examination. Like microscopic examination, they do not reliably detect bacteriuria below the level of 10^5 organisms/ml.

Urine Culture

Significance of bacterial counts with clean-voided, catheterized, and suprapubic specimens

Urine specimens collected even by the clean-void midstream procedure contain small numbers of bacterial contaminants. This finding can be distinguished from true bacteriuria only with quantitative cultures, which allow colony counts. Contaminated specimens usually yield less than 1000 colonies of mixed bacterial flora per milliliter of urine. In urinary tract infections, in contrast, more than 100,000 colonies of a single bacterial species are generally seen. Occasionally colony counts fall between these two values. If the patient is asymptomatic, the culture should be repeated. In symptomatic patients, counts in this range are considered significant if a single bacterial species, especially a typical uropathogen, is isolated. Intermediate counts on urine specimens collected by catheterization or suprapubic aspiration are always considered significant because contamination is minimal in such specimens. Colony counts must be performed

Prevention of growth in urine after collection

on freshly collected or specimens refrigerated to prevent bacterial growth from occurring before processing.

Miscellaneous Studies

Blood cultures

If acute pyelonephritis or prostatitis is suspected, blood cultures should be obtained to exclude bacteremia. Infected children, men, and those who experience a relapse of urinary tract infection should be investigated with intravenous pyelography to allow detection and correction of any factor causing predisposition to infection.

General Principles of Management

The principal goal in the treatment of urinary tract infection is eradication of the offending organism from the urine and tissues. In simple isolated instances of cystitis in a young woman, the diagnosis may be confirmed by a simple Gram smear of urine and treatment for an assumed *E. coli*

Short course treatment of uncomplicated cystitis

infection given empirically. Many antimicrobics are successful in controlling such infections, and knowledge of the susceptibility of community-acquired *E. coli* in a particular area serves as the best guide. In many cases, single-dose or 3-day therapy has been shown to be as effective as a course covering longer periods. Sulfonamides and trimethoprim alone or in combination and nitrofurantoin are the agents most commonly used.

Need to establish microbial diagnosis in other cases

For cystitis in children, pregnant women, men, diabetics, those who have been symptomatic for more than 1 week, and in those with acute pyelonephritis, it is imperative to establish the presence of bacteriuria with one or, in asymptomatic bacteriuria, two quantitative urine cultures. Therapy must be prolonged. Except in cases of clinical emergency, it should be delayed until the diagnosis is established. As bacteriuria may persist despite the spontaneous abatement of symptoms, the success of

Test of cure in more complex cases

treatment in patients with upper tract disease should be checked with follow-up urine cultures. The first should be obtained 48–72 hr after initiation of therapy. If the offending microorganism is still present at that time, the chemotherapeutic agent should be withdrawn and a substitute selected on the basis of susceptibility tests. If bacterial clearance has been achieved, the therapeutic course should be completed and repeat cultures obtained 2 weeks after termination of therapy. Sterile cultures at this time suggest eradication of the bacteriuria. A recurrence is classified as either

Investigation and treatment of recurrences

relapse or *reinfection*. Relapses are infections produced by the organism responsible for the initial infection that generally occur within 2 weeks of discontinuing therapy. They usually indicate an upper urinary tract infection or, in a male case, prostatitis, and require the initiation of a urologic evaluation. If an abnormality causing predisposition to urinary tract infection is discovered, it should be corrected whenever possible. If none is found, prolonged antibiotic therapy should be administered in hopes of eradicating the residual focus of infection.

Reinfections (recurrences caused by a new species or serotype) are usually indicative of a bladder infection. They respond readily to standard courses of treatment. Some patients, usually women of childbearing age, suffer repeated bladder reinfections. Those with several symptomatic episodes annually may be helped with long-term, low-dose chemoprophylaxis. In women whose recurrences are related to sexual activity, administration of the chemoprophylactic agent may be limited to immediately after intercourse.

Patients experiencing an episode of severe acute pyelonephritis should usually be hospitalized and treated, at least initially, with appropriate parenteral antibiotics. This treatment is particularly important if Gram-negative bacteremia is suspected. Milder cases can be managed with oral medications in an outpatient setting. Asymptomatic bacteriuria developing in a patient with an indwelling catheter often remits spontaneously after the removal of the catheter. It need not be treated unless the patient is at high risk of sepsis because of an underlying problem. Symptomatic infections in catheterized patients require treatment.

Prophylaxis in patients prone to reinfection

Treatment of pyelonephritis and catheter-associated infections

Additional Reading

Farrar, W.E. Jr. 1983. Infections of the urinary tract. *Med. Clin. North Am.* 67:187. An up-to-date review of the topic and of the management of urinary tract infections in office practice.

Gleckman, R.A. 1987. Treatment of urinary tract infections in adults. *Antimicrob. Agents Chemother.* 31:1–5. This is a review of studies dealing with the appropriate treatment duration of different categories of urinary tract infections.

Latham, R.H., et al. 1985. Laboratory diagnosis of urinary tract infection in ambulatory women. *JAMA* 254:3333–3336.

Lipsky, B.A., and Plorde, J.J. 1985. Laboratory diagnosis of urinary tract infections in men. *Clin. Microbiol. Newsletter* 7:121–124.

Pezzlo, M. 1988. Detection of urinary tract infections by rapid methods. *Clin. Microbiol. Rev.* 1:268–280. This is a comprehensive review of recently introduced screening tests for urinary tract infections.

67

Central Nervous System Infections

C. George Ray

Anatomy and
pathophysiology

The cerebrum, cerebellum, brain stem, spinal cord, and their covering membranes (meninges) constitute the central nervous system (CNS). Because of the unique anatomic and physiologic features of the CNS, infections in this site can represent unique challenges to the microbiologist and clinician.

The CNS is encased in a rigid, bony vault, and it is highly vulnerable to the effects of inflammation and edema: its critical life-regulatory functions and the metabolic requirements to sustain these functions can also be easily disrupted by infection, with resultant local acidosis, hypoxia, and destruction of nerve cells. Thus, the effects of increased pressure, biochemical abnormalities, and tissue necrosis can be profound and sometimes irreversible.

One specialized defense mechanism of the CNS is the *blood-brain barrier*, which serves to minimize passage of infectious agents and potentially toxic metabolites into the cerebrospinal fluid (CSF) and tissues, as well as to regulate the rate of transport of plasma proteins, glucose, and electrolytes. When CNS infection develops, however, this barrier also poses difficulties in control; some antimicrobial agents and host immune factors, such as immunoglobulins and complement, do not pass as readily from the blood to the site of infection as they do to other tissues.

Within the brain are the ventricles, which are cavities in which CSF is actively produced, primarily by specialized structures called the *choroid plexuses*. The CSF fills the lateral ventricles in each half of the brain, circulates into a central third ventricle, and then passes through the cerebral aqueduct to emerge through foramina at the brain stem. From cisterns at the base of the brain, the CSF circulates in the subarachnoid space over the entire CNS, including the spinal cord, to supply nutrients and serve as a hydraulic cushion for these tissues. It is reabsorbed primarily by the major venous system in the meninges. Obstruction of the normal flow of CSF in either the internal (ventricular) or external (subarachnoid) systems

865

can result in increased intracranial pressure, because production of CSF by the choroid plexuses will continue within the ventricles. Such impairment of flow or normal reabsorption can occur during certain infections as a result of inflammation or subsequent fibrosis, leading to dilatation of the ventricles, compression of brain tissue, and a condition known as *hydrocephalus*.

Routes of Infection

Blood-borne spread

Most CNS infections appear to result from blood-borne spread; for example, bacteremia or viremia resulting from infection of tissue at a site remote from the CNS may result in penetration of the blood-brain barrier. Examples of infectious agents that commonly infect the CNS by this route are *Haemophilus influenzae, Neisseria meningitidis, Streptococcus pneumoniae, Mycobacterium tuberculosis*, and viruses such as enteroviruses and mumps. The initial source of infection leading to bloodstream invasion may be occult (for example, infection of reticuloendothelial tissues) or overt (for example, pneumonia, pharyngitis, skin abscess or cellulitis, or bacterial endocarditis).

Direct spread from infected focus

Occasionally, the route of infection is from a focus close to or contiguous with the CNS. These possible sources include otitis media, mastoiditis, sinusitis, or pyogenic infections of the skin or bone. Infection may extend directly into the CNS, indirectly via venous pathways, or in the sheaths of cranial and spinal nerves.

Traumatic, surgical, or congenital lesions

In some cases, a contiguous or distant infectious focus may not be necessary to produce CNS infection. If an anatomic defect exists in the structures encasing the CNS, infectious agents may readily gain access to the vulnerable site and establish themselves. Such defects may be traumatically or surgically induced or result from congenital malformations. For example, fractures of the base of the skull may produce an opening between the CNS and the sinuses, nasal passages (defects in the cribriform plate), mastoid, or middle ear. All of these sites are contiguous with the upper respiratory tract, which enables a potentially pathogenic member of the respiratory flora to gain ready access to the CNS. Neurosurgical procedures also create transient communications between the external environment and the CNS that can be readily contaminated. This risk can be compounded when foreign bodies, such as shunts or external drainage tubes, must be left in place for the treatment of hydrocephalus. These foreign bodies, when colonized, can serve as chronic foci of infection. Congenital defects, such as meningomyeloceles or sinus tracts through the cranium or spine, may also be sources. The latter may be overlooked; the orifice of the sinus may be a small cleft on the skin surface, or occasionally it may open internally into the intestinal tract. Recurrent purulent meningitis or unusual pathogens in an otherwise healthy host should prompt a careful search for such defects.

Implanted foreign bodies

Intraneural pathways

Perhaps the least common route of CNS infection is via intraneural pathways. Agents capable of direct intraneural spread to the CNS include rabies virus (presumably along peripheral sensory nerves), herpes simplex virus (often, but not exclusively, via the trigeminal nerve root or sacral nerves), and perhaps some togaviruses.

Abscesses

Abscesses of the CNS deserve special mention. Although relatively uncommon compared with other CNS infections, they represent a special microbiologic and clinical problem. Such abscesses may be within the tissues of the CNS (for example, brain abscess, see Figure 67.1) or localized in the subdural or epidural spaces. They sometimes develop as a

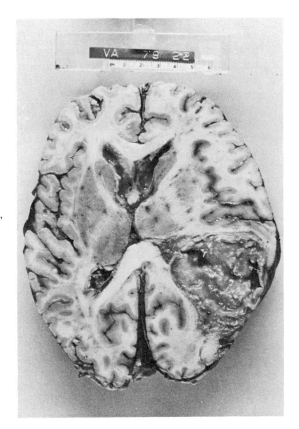

67.1 Coronal section of a brain, demonstrating a poorly encapsulated abscess.

complication of pyogenic meningitis. More commonly, abscesses of the CNS result from embolization of bacteria or fungi from a distant focus, such as endocarditis or pyogenic lung abscess; extension from a contiguous focus of infection (for example, sinusitis or mastoiditis); or a complication of surgery or nonsurgical trauma.

Common Clinical Features

Several terms commonly applied to CNS infections need to be understood. *Purulent meningitis* refers to infections of the meninges associated with a marked, acute inflammatory exudate and is usually caused by a bacterial infection. Such infections frequently involve the underlying CNS

Acute onset

tissue to a variable degree, and it is now appreciated that often the ventricular system is also involved (ventriculitis). Most cases of purulent meningitis are acute in onset and progression and are characterized by fever,

Serious prognosis if untreated

stiff neck, irritability, and varying degrees of neurologic dysfunction that, if untreated, usually progress to a fatal outcome. Large numbers of polymorphonuclear leukocytes are present in the CSF of established cases.

Chronic meningitis has a more insidious onset, with progression of signs and symptoms over a period of weeks. This is usually caused by myco-

Granulomatous infection

bacteria and fungi that produce granulomatous inflammatory changes, but occasionally protozoal agents are responsible (see Table 67.3). The cellular response in the CSF reflects the chronic inflammatory nature of the disease.

Aseptic meningitis is a term used to describe a syndrome of meningeal inflammation associated mostly with an increase (pleocytosis) of lymphocytes and other mononuclear cells in the CSF and absence of readily cultivable bacteria or fungi. It is associated most commonly with viral infections and is often self-limiting. The syndrome can also occur in syphilis and some other spirochetal diseases, as a response to the presence of drugs or radioopaque substances in the CSF, or from tumors or bleeding involving the meninges or subarachnoid space. The primary site of inflammation is in the meninges without clinical evidence of involvement of the neural tissue. Such patients may have fever, headache, a stiff neck or back, nausea, and vomiting.

Aseptic meningitis is most commonly of viral etiology

Other causes

Encephalitis also implies a primary viral etiology; however, acute or chronic demyelinating diseases with or without inflammation are included. This latter group includes the *postinfectious* or *allergic* encephalomyelitis syndromes, in which the etiology and pathogenesis are not always clearly defined. Clinically, this term is reserved for patients who may or may not show signs and CSF findings compatible with aseptic meningitis, but who also show objective evidence of CNS dysfunction (for example, seizures, paralysis, disordered mentation, and the like). Many clinicians use the term *meningoencephalitis* to describe patients with both meningeal and encephalitic manifestations.

Viral and post-infectious etiology

Meningoencephalitis

Poliomyelitis refers to the selective destruction of anterior motor horn cells in the spinal cord and/or brain stem, which leads to weakness or paralysis of muscle groups and occasionally respiratory insufficiency. It is usually associated with aseptic meningitis, sometimes with encephalitis. The polioviruses are the major causes of this syndrome, although Coxsackie viruses (primarily type A7) and other enteroviruses, such as enterovirus 71, have been implicated. The hallmark of poliomyelitis is asymmetric flaccid paralysis.

Viral destruction of anterior horn cells

Paralysis

Two other nervous system syndromes presumably associated with infection deserve brief mention. Acute polyneuritis, an inflammatory disease of the peripheral nervous system, is characterized by symmetric flaccid paralysis of muscles. In most cases, no specific etiology is found; some, however, have been associated with *Corynebacterium diphtheriae* toxin and infections by cytomegalovirus or Epstein-Barr virus. Reye's syndrome (encephalopathy with fatty infiltration of the viscera) is an acute, noninflammatory process, usually observed in childhood, in which cerebral edema, hepatic dysfunction, and hyperammonemia develop within 2–12 days after onset of a systemic viral infection. Although the influenza A and B and varicella–zoster viruses have been most frequently implicated in this syndrome, the precise pathogenesis is not yet known. Concomitant salicylate therapy is believed to be a contributory factor.

Acute polyneuritis

Reye's syndrome

Common Etiologic Agents

The causes of CNS infections are numerous, as illustrated in Tables 67.1, 67.2, and 67.3. Acute purulent meningitis is usually caused by one of three organisms: *Haemophilus influenzae* type b, *Neisseria meningitidis,* or *Streptococcus pneumoniae.* The major exception is neonatal infection, in which *Escherichia coli* or group B streptococci are most frequently implicated. However, many other bacteria can occasionally cause the disease if they gain access to the meninges.

Acute purulent meningitis

Of the viral causes of acute CNS disease, the categories most commonly encountered are the enteroviruses, mumps, herpes simplex, Epstein-Barr virus, and arthropod-borne viruses. In the United States, enteroviruses account for the greatest proportion of infections. Viral CNS infections can be manifested clinically as aseptic meningitis, encephalitis, or, with

Acute viral disease

Table 67.1   Common Causes of Purulent Central Nervous
System Infections

Age Group	Agent
Newborns (<1 mo old)	Group B streptococci and *Escherichia coli* (most common); *Listeria monocytogenes; Klebsiella* species; other enteric Gram-negative bacteria
Infants and children	*Haemophilus influenzae* type b; *Neisseria meningitidis; Streptococcus pneumoniae*
Adults	*Streptococcus pneumoniae; Neisseria meningitidis*
Special circumstances	
Meningitis or intracranial abscesses associated with trauma, neurosurgery, or intracranial foreign bodies	*Staphylococcus aureus; Staphylococcus epidermidis; Streptococcus pneumoniae;* anaerobic Gram-negative and Gram-positive bacteria; *Pseudomonas* species
Intracranial abscesses not associated with trauma or surgery	Microaerophilic or anaerobic streptococci, anaerobic Gram-negative bacteria (often mixed aerobic and anaerobic flora of upper respiratory tract origin)

poliovirus and some other enterovirus infections, poliomyelitis. The age of the patient and the season of occurrence help somewhat in predicting some of the agents that may be involved, as illustrated in Table 67.2; other epidemiologic, ecologic, and clinical factors associated with these infections are discussed in the individual chapters on specific virus groups.

Slow viral infections   Slow viral infections of the CNS, such as subacute sclerosing panencephalitis (due to measles or sometimes congenital rubella), acquired immunodeficiency syndrome encephalopathy (associated with human immunodeficiency virus), progressive multifocal leukoencephalopathy (due to certain papovaviruses), and Creutzfeldt–Jacob disease ("unconventional" viruses), are discussed in Chapters 33, 41, 42, and 43, respectively.

Chronic meningitis   Other important causes of CNS infections (Table 67.3) that must not be overlooked include *Mycobacterium tuberculosis* and the deep mycoses (especially *Cryptococcus neoformans* and *Coccidioides immitis*). These chronic infections can be insidious in onset and can mimic other processes in the clinical findings and CSF examination, thus delaying consideration of the proper diagnosis.

Noninfectious diseases mimicking infections   Finally, there are noninfectious causes of CNS disease to be considered in the differential diagnosis. These include 1) metabolic disturbances, such as hypoglycemia, diabetic coma, and hepatic failure; 2) toxic conditions, such as those caused by bacterial toxins (diphtheria, tetanus, botulism), insect toxins (tick paralysis), poisons (lead), and drug abuse; 3) mass lesions, such as acute trauma, hematoma, and tumor; 4) vascular lesions, such as intracranial embolus, aneurysm, and subarachnoid hemorrhage; and 5) acute psychiatric episodes.

General Diagnostic Approaches

Lumbar puncture   Except in unusual circumstances, in which severe increases in intracranial pressure make the procedure dangerous, a lumbar puncture is the first step in the workup of a patient with suspected CNS infection. The CSF

Table 67.2 Primary Acute Viral Infections of the Central
Nervous System

Agent	Major Age Group Affected	Seasonal Predominance
Enteroviruses (Coxsackie A, Coxsackie B, echoviruses, polioviruses)	Infants, children	Summer-fall
Mumps	Children	Winter-spring
Herpes simplex		
Type 1	Adults	None
Type 2	Neonates, young adults	None
Arboviruses		
Western equine encephalitis	Infants, children	Summer-fall
St. Louis encephalitis	Adults over 40 yr old	Summer-fall
California encephalitis	School-aged children	Summer-fall
Eastern equine encephalitis	Infants, children	Summer-fall
Rabies	All ages	Summer-fall
Measles	Infants, children	Spring
Varicella–zoster	Infants, children	Spring
Lymphocytic choriomeningitis	Adults	None
Epstein-Barr virus	Children, young adults	None
Other (myxoviruses, paramyxoviruses, cytomegaloviruses, adenoviruses, etc)	Infants, children	Variable

Table 67.3 Other Causes of Central Nervous System Infections

Disease	Agent
Chronic granulomatous infection	*Mycobacterium tuberculosis*[a]
	Coccidioides immitis
	Cryptococcus neoformans
	Histoplasma capsulatum
Parasitic infection	
Protozoa	*Toxoplasma gondii*[b]
	Trypanosoma
	Naegleria (ameba) species
Nematodes	*Toxocara* species
	Trichinella spiralis
	Angiostrongylus cantonensis
Cestodes	*Taenia solium* (cysticercosis)
Other	*Leptospira* species
	Treponema pallidum
	Borrelia burgdorferi

[a] Tuberculous meningitis can appear as acute or chronically progressive disease.
[b] Toxoplasmosis of the central nervous system is usually seen in congenital infections or immunocompromised hosts.

Table 67.4 Findings of Cerebrospinal Fluid Analysis: Normal versus Infection

Clinical Situation	Leukocytes/ mm³	%Poly- morpho- nuclears	Glucose (% of blood)	Protein (mg/dl)
Children and Adults				
Normal	0–5	0	≥60	≤30
Viral infection	2–2000 (80)[a]	≤50	≥60	30–80
Pyogenic bacterial infection	5–5000 (800)	≥60	≤45[b]	>60
Tuberculosis and mycoses	5–2000 (100)	≤50	≤45	>60
Neonates				
Normal (term)	0–32 (8)	≤60	≥60	20–170 (90)
Normal (preterm)	0–29 (9)	≤60	≥60	65–150 (115)

[a] Numbers in parentheses represent mean values.
[b] Usually very low.

Cells, protein, and glucose in CSF

pressure is determined at the time of the procedure, and CSF is removed for analysis of cells, protein, and glucose. Ideally, the glucose content of the peripheral blood is determined simultaneously for comparison with that in the CSF. Table 67.4 presents guidelines for interpretation of results of CSF analysis; these guidelines represent generalizations, however, and must not be considered as absolute findings in all cases. For example, although a patient with bacterial, mycobacterial, or fungal meningitis will usually have a glucose level in the CSF of less than 40 mg/dl, or less than half the blood glucose level (hypoglycorrhachia), this finding may not be present in the early stages of infection. Although uncommon, viral infections of the CNS occasionally produce low glucose values in the CSF; in addition, the early stages of viral infection may be associated with a preponderance of polymorphonuclear leukocytes. It is clearly important to recognize that viral CNS infections can exist with a negligible CSF cell count. This sometimes also occurs in the early stages of bacterial meningitis.

Interpretation of findings

Realizing the limitations, it is possible to make some general interpretations that are helpful in the diagnosis. Viral CNS infections are usually associated with a preponderance of lymphocytes, a normal glucose value, and a normal or moderately elevated protein level in the CSF. In contrast, acute bacterial meningitis usually causes a CSF pleocytosis consisting primarily of polymorphonuclear cells, a low glucose value, and a high protein level. Mycobacterial and fungal infections are more commonly associated with lymphocytosis (and sometimes moderate eosinophilia) in the CSF; like the acute bacterial infections, however, they tend to lower glucose and increase protein levels markedly.

Normal values for CSF are also shown in Table 67.4. No polymorphonuclear cells should appear in normal CSF, but as many as five lymphocytes/mm³ may be found in health. Neonatal CSF is considerably more difficult to interpret, as cell counts are often elevated in the absence of infection; glucose values, however, should be within the normal range.

Direct staining and culture

The other major procedures that must be performed on all CSF samples in which any infection is suspected include bacterial cultures and Gram

Tests for free antigens

Other laboratory tests

staining. If the CSF is grossly purulent and the patient untreated, a Gram stain of the uncentrifuged CSF or of its centrifuged sediment will frequently show the infecting organism and indicate the specific diagnosis. According to the clinical indications and results of CSF cytology and chemistry, other microbiologic tests may be used, including viral cultures, special stains and cultures for fungi and mycobacteria, and immunologic methods to detect fungal or bacterial antigens (for example, latex agglutination for *Cryptococcus* or selected bacteria).

Tests on specimens other than CSF are selected on the basis of the clinical diagnostic possibilities. If acute bacterial meningitis is suspected, blood cultures should be used to ensure the diagnosis. Viral cultures of the pharynx, stool, or rectal swabs may provide indirect evidence of CNS infection. Herpes simplex encephalitis poses a unique situation: to establish the diagnosis, a biopsy specimen of the brain is sometimes required to demonstrate viral antigen by immunofluorescence and/or growth of virus. Other studies may include acute and convalescent sera for viral serology and serologic tests to detect antibodies to certain fungi, such as *Coccidioides immitis*.

Intracranial abscesses can often be detected with radiologic techniques, such as brain scanning. A definitive etiologic diagnosis is established by careful aerobic and anaerobic culture of the contents of the abscess.

General Principles of Management

Chemotherapy

In bacterial, mycobacterial, and fungal infections of the CNS, prompt and aggressive antimicrobial therapy is required. The duration of treatment varies from as little as 10 days for uncomplicated bacterial meningitis to 12 months or longer for tuberculous meningitis and several years for some cases of fungal meningitis.

Correction of metabolic defects and of raised intracranial pressure

In addition to antimicrobial therapy, correction of associated metabolic defects (acidosis, hypoxia, saline depletion, inappropriate antidiuretic hormone secretion) is necessary. Increased intracranial pressure as a result of vasogenic edema or hydrocephalus must be monitored and controlled accordingly; osmotic agents such as intravenous mannitol are often used to control acute cerebral edema, and neurosurgical shunting procedures may be needed to treat progressive hydrocephalus. Abscesses often require drainage.

Abscess drainage

Treatment of viral infections

Except for those with herpes simplex encephalitis, which may respond to early treatment with antiviral agents, patients with viral infections of the CNS receive supportive care only. This therapy includes specific attention to the metabolic and ventilatory problems that may develop in severe cases.

68

Intravascular Infections, Bacteremia, and Endotoxemia

C. George Ray and
Kenneth J. Ryan

In many cases the presence of circulating microorganisms in the blood is either a part of the natural history of the infectious disease or a reflection of serious, uncontrolled infection. Depending on the class of agent involved, this process is described as *viremia, bacteremia, fungemia*, or *parasitemia*. Viremia is usually a very early, even prodromal, event accompanied by fever, malaise, and other constitutional symptoms, such as muscle aches. With the exception of a few specific infections, the detection of viremia does not play a role in the diagnosis or management of viral infections. The presence of bacteremia defines some of the most serious and life-threatening situations in medical practice, and it has a marked impact on the management and outcome of bacterial infections. This chapter will focus on the causes and implications of bacteremia and, to a lesser extent, fungemia. Diseases in which parasitemia is a feature are covered in Chapters 51–54.

Association of bacteremia with sepsis

The terms *sepsis* and *septicemia* are used somewhat loosely, but generally refer to the clinical symptom complexes associated with bacteremia. They include fever, chills, hypotension, shock, and evidence of spread to multiple body systems. The clinical findings may develop acutely, as in Gram-negative septic shock, or slowly, as in most forms of infective endocarditis.

Bacteremia from intravenous contaminated devices

Transient bacteremia

Bacteremia or fungemia may also result from microbial growth on the inner or outer surfaces of intravenous devices. Clinical manifestations may be minor initially, but may later become severe. Because the bloodstream is sterile in health, bacteremia is considered potentially serious regardless of the symptoms present; however, transient bacteremia may occur when there is manipulation or trauma to a body site that has a normal flora. After such events, species indigenous to the site may appear briefly in the blood, but are soon cleared. Such transient bacteremias usually have no immediate clinical significance, but they are important in the pathogenesis of infective endocarditis.

873

Intravascular Infection

Intracardiac infections (endocarditis) and those primarily involving veins (thrombophlebitis) or arteries (endarteritis) are usually caused by bacterial agents, although fungi, rickettsiae, chlamydiae, and even viruses have been occasionally implicated. This discussion will focus primarily on the bacterial causes, because they are the most numerous and important. Infections of the cardiovascular system are usually extremely serious and, if not promptly and adequately treated, can be fatal. They commonly produce a constant shedding of organisms into the bloodstream that is often characterized by continuous, low-grade bacteremia (1–20 organisms/ml of blood) in untreated patients.

Infective Endocarditis

Sites of endocardial infection

The term *infective endocarditis* is preferable to the commonly used term *bacterial endocarditis*, simply because not all infections of the endocardial surface of the heart are caused by bacteria. Most infections occur on natural or prosthetic cardiac valves, but can also develop on septal defects, shunts (for example, patent ductus arteriosus), or the mural endocardium. Infections involving coarctation of the aorta are also classified as infective endocarditis because the clinical manifestations and complications are similar.

The pathogenesis of infective endocarditis involves several factors that, if concurrent, result in infection:

Cardiac abnormalities and hemodynamic effects

1. The endothelium is altered to facilitate colonization by bacteria and deposition of platelets and fibrin. Most infections involve the mitral or aortic valves, which are particularly vulnerable when abnormalities such as valvular insufficiency, stenosis, intracardiac shunts (for example, ventricular septal defect), or direct trauma (for example, catheters) exist. The turbulence of intracardiac blood flow that results from such abnormalities can lead to further damage to endothelial surfaces and facilitates platelet and fibrin deposition. These factors produce a potential nidus for colonization and infection.

Bacteremia with normal flora as infection source

2. Transient bacteremia is common, but usually of no clinical importance. Often seen for a few minutes after a variety of dental procedures, it has also been shown to develop after normal childbirth and manipulations such as bronchoscopy, sigmoidoscopy, cytoscopy, and some surgical procedures. Even simple activities such as tooth brushing or chewing candy can cause such bacteremia. The organisms responsible for transient bacteremia are usually common surface flora of low pathogenicity, such as viridans streptococci. Other, more virulent strains may also be involved, however; for example, intravenous drug abuse may lead to transient bacteremia with *Staphylococcus aureus* or a variety of Gram-negative aerobic and anaerobic bacteria. Whether the organisms causing bacteremia (or fungemia) are of high virulence or not, they can colonize and multiply in the heart if local endothelial changes are suitable.

Adherence and development of vegetation

3. Bacteremic organisms adhere to the damaged surface, followed by complement activation, inflammation, fibrin, and platelet deposition and further endothelial damage at the site of colonization. The resulting entrapment of organisms in the thrombotic "mesh" of platelets, fibrin, and inflammatory cells leads to a mature vegetation, which protects

<table>
<tr><td>Embolization</td><td>the organisms from host humoral and phagocytic immune defenses, and to some extent from antimicrobial agents. As a result, the infection can be exceedingly difficult to treat. The vegetation can also create greater hemodynamic alterations in terms of obstruction to flow and increased turbulence. Parts of vegetations may break off and be deposited in smaller blood vessels (embolization) with resultant obstruction and secondary sites of infection. Emboli may be transported to the brain or coronary arteries, for example, with disastrous results.</td></tr>
</table>

Embolization

the organisms from host humoral and phagocytic immune defenses, and to some extent from antimicrobial agents. As a result, the infection can be exceedingly difficult to treat. The vegetation can also create greater hemodynamic alterations in terms of obstruction to flow and increased turbulence. Parts of vegetations may break off and be deposited in smaller blood vessels (embolization) with resultant obstruction and secondary sites of infection. Emboli may be transported to the brain or coronary arteries, for example, with disastrous results.

Circulating immune complexes

Another phenomenon shown to contribute to infective endocarditis syndrome is the development of circulating immune complexes of microbial antigen and antibody. These complexes can activate complement and contribute to many of the peripheral vascular manifestations of the disease, including nephritis, arthritis, and cutaneous vascular lesions.

Host immune and hyperimmune responses

Frequently, there is a widespread stimulus to host cellular and humoral immunity, particularly if the infection continues for more than a couple of weeks. This condition is characterized by hyperglobulinemia, splenomegaly, and the occasional appearance of macrophages in the peripheral blood. Some patients will develop circulating rheumatoid factor (IgM anti-IgG antibody), which may play a deleterious role by blocking IgG opsonic activity and causing microvascular damage. Antinuclear antibodies, which also appear occasionally, may contribute to the pathogenesis of the fever, arthralgia, and myalgia that is often seen.

In summary, infective endocarditis involves an initial complex of endothelial damage or abnormality, which facilitates colonization by organisms that may be circulating through the heart. This colonization, in turn, leads to the propagation of a vegetation, with its attendant local and systemic inflammatory, embolic, and immunologic complications.

Acute, subacute, and chronic infective endocarditis

Common Clinical Features.   Infective endocarditis has often been classified by the progression of the untreated disease. The acute course is generally fulminant with high fever and toxicity, and death may occur in a few days or weeks. Subacute endocarditis progresses to death over 6 weeks to 3 months, and chronic cases continue for longer than 3 months. These latter two forms of the disease are characterized by low-grade fever, night sweats, weight loss, and vague constitutional complaints. The clinical course is substantially related to the virulence of the infecting organism; *S. aureus*, for example, usually produces acute disease, whereas infections by the otherwise avirulent viridans streptococci are more likely to be subacute or chronic. Before the advent of antimicrobial therapy, death was considered inevitable in all cases. Physical findings often include a new or changing heart murmur, splenomegaly, various skin lesions (petechiae, splinter hemorrhages, Osler's nodes, Janeway's lesions), and retinal lesions.

Cardiac, embolic, and immunologically mediated complications

Complications include the risk of congestive heart failure as a result of hemodynamic alterations, rupture of the chordae tendinae of the valves, or perforation of a valve. Abscesses of the myocardium or valve ring can also develop. Other complications relate to the immunologic and embolic phenomena that can occur. The kidney is commonly affected, and hematuria is a typical finding. Renal failure, presumably from immune complex glomerulonephritis, is possible. Left-sided endocarditis can readily lead to coronary artery embolization and "mycotic" aneurysms; the latter will be discussed later in this chapter. In addition, more distant emboli to the central nervous system can lead to cerebral infarction and infection. Right-sided endocarditis often causes embolization and infarction or infection in the lung.

Table 68.1 Common Etiologic Agents in Infective Endocarditis

Agent	Approximate Percentage of Cases
Viridans streptococci (several species)	30–40
Group D streptococci (enterococci)	5–18
Other streptococci	15–25
Staphylococcus aureus	10–27
Staphylococcus epidermidis	1–3
Enterobacteriaceae and *Pseudomonas*	2–13
Fungi (*Candida* sp., *Aspergillus* sp., etc)	2–4

Streptococci most common cause

Culture-negative endocarditis

Predisposing factors to unusual etiologies

Common Etiologic Agents. Table 68.1 summarizes the most common causes of infective endocarditis. α-hemolytic streptococci and enterococci are involved in most cases. In the so-called culture-negative group, infective endocarditis is diagnosed on clinical grounds, but cultures do not confirm the etiologic agent. This group of patients is difficult to treat, and the overall prognosis is considered poorer than when a specific etiology has been determined. Negative cultures may result from 1) prior antibiotic treatment; 2) fungal endocarditis with entrapment of these relatively large organisms in capillary beds; 3) fastidious, nutritionally deficient, or cell-wall-deficient organisms that are difficult to isolate; 4) infection caused by obligate intracellular parasites, such as chlamydiae (*Chlamydia psittaci*), rickettsiae (*Coxiella burnetii*), or viruses; 5) immunologic factors (for example, antibody acting on circulating organisms); or 6) subacute endocarditis involving the right side of the heart, in which the organisms are filtered out in the pulmonary capillaries.

Some special circumstances alter the relative etiologic possibilities, for example, intravenous drug addiction, prosthetic valves, and immunocompromise. The major associations in these cases are summarized in Table 68.2.

General Diagnostic Approaches. The diagnosis of infective endocarditis is usually suspected on clinical grounds; however, the most important di-

Table 68.2 Etiologic Agents More Commonly Observed in Special Circumstances

Situation	Agent
Intravenous drug abuse	*Staphylococcus aureus*; group D streptococci; Enterobacteriaceae and *Pseudomonas*; fungi
Prosthetic valve infection	*Staphylococcus epidermidis*; *Staphylococcus aureus*; Enterobacteriaceae and *Pseudomonas*; diphtheroids; *Candida* and *Aspergillus* sp.
Immunocompromise, chronic illness	Any of the above organisms

Blood cultures

agnostic test for confirmation is the blood culture. In untreated cases, the organisms are generally present continuously in low numbers (1–20/ml) in the blood. If an adequate volume of blood is obtained, the first culture will be positive in over 95% of culturally confirmed cases. Most authorities recommend three cultures over 24 hr to ensure detection, and an additional three if the first set is negative. Multiple cultures yielding the same organism support the probability of an intravascular or intracardiac infection. In acute endocarditis, the urgency of early treatment may require collection of only two or three cultures within a few minutes so that antimicrobial therapy can begin.

Other specific cardiologic procedures can delineate the nature of the lesion, size of vegetations, and progression of disease.

Need for bactericidal antimicrobics

Use of antimicrobic combinations

Parenteral therapy; blood level may need monitoring

General Principles of Management.   Because of the nature of the lesions and their pathogenesis, response to therapy may be slow and cure is sometimes difficult. Therefore, specific antimicrobial therapy must be aggressive, using agents that are bactericidal (rather than bacteriostatic) and can be given in amounts that will achieve high continuous blood levels without causing toxicity to the patient. Treatment may involve a single antimicrobial if the organism is highly susceptible in vitro, or antimicrobial combinations if synergistic effects are possible (for example, a penicillin and an aminoglycoside for enterococcal endocarditis). Parenteral therapy is begun to produce adequate blood levels, and the patient may need to be monitored frequently to ensure antimicrobial activity in the serum sufficient to kill the organisms without causing unnecessary toxicity. Therapy is usually prolonged, lasting longer than 4 weeks in most cases. In some cases, surgery may be required to excise the diseased valve and replace it with a valvular prosthesis. The decision for surgery is sometimes difficult, requiring consultation with both a cardiologist and a surgeon.

Candidates for antimicrobial prophylaxis

Prophylaxis with dental work

Prophylaxis can sometimes prevent the development of endocarditis in persons with known congenital or acquired cardiac lesions that predispose to bacterial endocarditis. When they undergo procedures known to cause transient bacteremia (for example, dental manipulations or surgical procedures involving the upper respiratory, gastrointestinal, or genitourinary tracts), administration of high doses of antimicrobics is begun just before the procedure and continued for 6–12 hr thereafter. An example of prophylaxis is the case of a patient with rheumatic valvular disease who is planning to undergo dental work. The organism most likely to produce transient bacteremia would be a penicillin-sensitive member of the oral flora, especially viridans streptococci. Thus, an intramuscular dose of penicillin within 30 min before the procedure, followed by a high dose of intramuscular or oral penicillin 6 hr later, would be expected to afford protection. Several regimens similar to this approach are recommended, depending upon the patient, the nature of the procedure, and the organisms that might be expected to be involved.

Mycotic Aneurysm

The term *mycotic aneurysm* is somewhat misleading, as it suggests infection by fungi. Originally used by William Osler to describe the mushroom-shaped arterial aneurysm that can develop in patients with infective endocarditis, the term now applies to infection with any organism that causes inflammatory damage and weakening of an arterial wall with subsequent aneurysmal dilatation. This sequence can progress to rupture, with a fatal outcome.

Pathogenesis of intraarterial infection

Arterial infection can result from direct extension of an intracardiac infection or from septic microemboli from a cardiac focus, with seeding of vasa vasorum within the arterial wall. These infections frequently complicate infective endocarditis. Other pathogenetic factors include 1) seeding of a previously damaged arterial intima by bacteria from a distant infection (the intima may have been altered by atherosclerotic plaques, vascular thrombi, congenital malformations, or trauma; 2) trauma to the arterial wall with direct contamination; and 3) spread from a contiguous focus of infection directly into the artery.

The clinical features vary according to the site of involvement. Common findings may include pain at the site of primary arterial supply (for example, back or abdominal pain in abdominal aortic infections) and fever. In many cases, a pulsatile mass may be palpated.

Etiologic agents similar to those of infective endocarditis

The etiologic agents are similar to those listed in Tables 68.1 and 68.2 for infective endocarditis, and diagnostic measures (for example, blood culture) are also the same. *Salmonella* species and *S. aureus* are particularly common offenders in this disease. Management requires vigorous, prolonged antimicrobial therapy. Surgical excision and vascular grafting are often necessary.

Suppurative Thrombophlebitis

Categories

Suppurative (or septic) thrombophlebitis is an inflammation of a vein wall frequently associated with thrombosis and bacteremia. There are four basic forms: superficial, pelvic, intracranial venous sinus, and portal vein infection (pylephlebitis). With the steadily increasing use of intravenous catheters, the incidence of superficial thrombophlebitis has risen and represents a major complication in hospitalized patients.

Pathogenesis

The pathogenesis of suppurative thrombophlebitis appears to first involve thrombus formation, which may result from trauma to the vein, extrinsic inflammation, hypercoagulable states, stasis of blood flow, or combinations of these factors. The thrombotic site is then seeded with organisms, and a focus of infection is established. In superficial thrombophlebitis, an intravenous cannula or catheter may cause local venous wall trauma, as well as serve as a foreign body nidus for thrombus formation. Infection will evolve if bacteria are introduced by intravenous fluid, local wound contamination, or bacteremic seeding from a remote infected site.

Intravenous catheter associated thrombophlebitis

Deep thrombophlebitis from extension of neighboring infection

Thrombophlebitis of pelvic, portal, or intracranial venous systems most often occurs as a result of direct extension of an infectious process from adjacent structures, or from venous and lymphatic pathways near sites of infection. For example, infections of intracranial venous sinuses usually result from orbital or sinus infections (causing cavernous sinus thrombophlebitis) or from infections of the mastoid and middle ear (causing lateral and sagittal sinus thrombophlebitis). Pelvic thrombophlebitis is a potential result of intrauterine infection (endometritis), particularly after pelvic surgery or 2–3 weeks after childbirth. Pelvic or intraabdominal infections may also spread to the portal venous system to produce pylephlebitis.

Signs and symptoms depend on site involved

Common Clinical Features. Clinical manifestations vary according to the site of involvement. Common features often include fever and inflammation over the infected vein. Signs of septicemia may also be present. Pelvic or portal vein thrombophlebitis is usually associated with high fever, chills, nausea, vomiting, and abdominal pain. Jaundice may develop in portal vein infections.

Table 68.3 Common Etiologic Agents in Suppurative Thrombophlebitis

Site	Agent
Superficial veins (saphenous, femoral, antecubital, etc)	*Staphylococcus aureus*; Gram-negative aerobic bacilli
Pelvic veins, portal veins	*Bacteroides* sp.; microaerophilic or anaerobic streptococci; *Escherichia coli*; β-hemolytic streptococci (group A or B)
Intracranial venous sinuses (cavernous, sagittal, lateral)	*Haemophilus influenzae, Streptococcus pneumoniae*; β-hemolytic streptococcus (group A); anaerobic or microaerophilic streptococci; *Staphylococcus aureus*

Intracranial thrombophlebitis varies in its presentation. Headache, facial or orbital edema, and neurologic deficits are variably present: for example, cavernous sinus thrombophlebitis often causes palsies of the third, fourth, fifth, and sixth cranial nerves. A major clue to the diagnosis is the presence of recent or current infection in adjacent structures (for example, mastoids, sinuses).

Extension of infection, septic embolization, and bacteremia may occur

Complications of thrombophlebitis include extension of suppurative infection into adjacent structures, further propagation of thrombi, bacteremia with sepsis, and septic embolization. Embolization, particularly from pelvic or leg veins, is to the lungs, and pulmonary embolism with infarction may be the primary manifestation of the remote infection.

Common Etiologic Agents. The major infectious causes of suppurative thrombophlebitis are outlined in Table 68.3. In superficial thrombophlebitis, which often follows intravenous therapy, organisms that are common nosocomial offenders predominate (*S. aureus*, Gram-negative aerobes). Deeper infections are more frequently caused by organisms that reside on adjacent mucous membranes (for example, *Bacteroides* species in intestinal and vaginal sites) or commonly infect adjacent sites (for example, *Haemophilus influenzae* and *Streptococcus pneumoniae* in acute otitis media and sinusitis).

General Diagnostic Approaches. The diagnosis is often suspected on clinical grounds and from associated events known to create predisposition to such infections (for example, surgery, presence of indwelling venous cannulas). Direct cultures of the infected site or blood cultures will usually yield the infecting organism, because bacteremia is often present. Cultures of purulent material from adjacent infected sites may also suggest the etiologic agent.

Direct culture and blood culture

Radiologic procedures, including scanning methods, may be necessary to localize the process and support the diagnosis. In some cases, surgical exploration is required, both for definitive treatment and obtaining specimens for cultures.

Selection of chemotherapy

General Principles of Management. Antimicrobial agents are an important aspect of treatment, with the choice of antimicrobics based upon culture results. In the absence of microbiologic data, therapy is chosen to cover the most likely possibilities listed in Table 68.3. Other important aspects of management include prompt removal of possible offending sources, such as intravenous catheters, vigorous treatment of adjacent infections, and sometimes surgical excision and drainage. Severe cases may also benefit from systemic anticoagulant therapy to prevent further propagation of thrombi and embolization.

Many cases are preventable. Unnecessary, long-term intravenous cannulation should be avoided. Whenever possible, it is better to use short needles such as "scalp vein" cannulas than venous catheters or plastic cannulas. Careful asepsis is essential with all intravenous procedures to prevent contamination of intravenous fluids, tubing, and the site of venous entry.

Removal of source of infection

Intravenous Catheter Bacteremia

Source of endocarditis and metastatic infection

A variant of intravascular infection develops when a medical device such as an intravenous catheter or any of several types of monitoring devices placed in the bloodstream becomes colonized with microorganisms. The event itself does not have immediate clinical significance but, unlike transient bacteremia from manipulation of normal floral sites, the bacteremia is continuous. This persistence greatly increases the chances of secondary complications such as infective endocarditis and metastatic infection, depending on any underlying disease and the virulence of the organism involved.

The organisms involved are usually those found in the skin flora, such as *Staphylococcus epidermidis* or *S. aureus*. In debilitated patients already on antimicrobial therapy, *Candida* species may be involved. Occasionally the sources of contamination are the intravenous solutions themselves rather than the skin. In these cases, members of the Enterobacteriaceae, *Pseudomonas*, or other Gram-negative rods are more likely.

Discrepancies between degree of bacteremia and clinical manifestations

The clinical findings in catheter bacteremia are usually mild despite the large numbers of organisms in the bloodstream (Figure 68.1). Signs of inflammation may or may not be present, in addition to low-grade fever. Management is by removal of the contaminated catheter. Antimicrobial therapy often will not eradicate the organisms in the presence of a foreign body (the catheter).

Bacteremia from Extravascular Infection

Although bacteremia is a more constant feature of intravascular infection, most cases of clinically significant bacteremia are the result of extravascular infection. In these cases, the organisms drained by the lymphatics or otherwise escaping from the infected focus reach the capillary and venous circulation through the lymphatic vessels. Depending on the magnitude of the infection and the degree of local control, these organisms may be filtered in the reticuloendothelial system or circulate more widely, producing bacteremia or fungemia. The process is dependent on the timing and interaction of multiple events and is thus much less predictable than the bacteremia of intravascular infection. If the infection is extensive and uncontrolled, such as an overwhelming staphylococcal pneumonia, there may be hundreds or even thousands of organisms per milliliter of blood, a poor prognostic sign. An intraabdominal abscess may only seed a few organisms intermittently until it is discovered and drained. Most infections that produce bacteremia fall between these extremes, with bloodstream invasion more common in the acute phases and intermittent at other times.

Bacteremia more variable than with intravascular infection

68.1 Patterns of bacteremia.
The magnitude and timing of bacteremia for six typical patients (**A–F**) are depicted. These findings have implications for blood culture sampling plans. Cases such as **A** and **B** will only be detected by cultures taken early in their course. Cases such as **C** and particularly **D** are more variable and more likely to be detected by cultures spaced over the time period shown. Continuous bacteremia (**E** and **F**) should be detected by any sampling plan. It could be confused with transient bacteremia on single blood cultures, as both are caused by organisms of low virulence (viridans streptococci, *Staphylococcus epidermidis*); in cases such as **E** and **F**, however, bacteremia is sustained, whereas cases of transient bacteremia will yield multiple positive results only if they are collected at or near the same time.

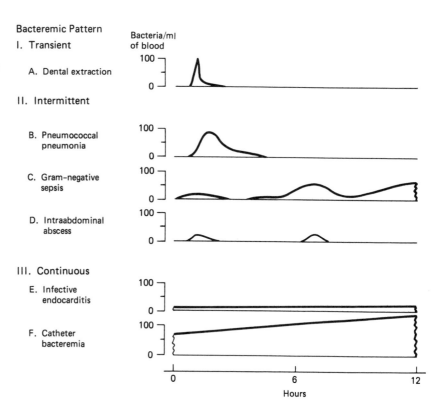

Bacteremic Pattern

I. Transient

   A. Dental extraction

II. Intermittent

   B. Pneumococcal pneumonia

   C. Gram-negative sepsis

   D. Intraabdominal abscess

III. Continuous

   E. Infective endocarditis

   F. Catheter bacteremia

Bacteria/ml of blood

Hours

Association with severe infections such as meningitis

The causative organisms and the frequencies with which they usually produce bacteremia (or fungemia) are listed in Table 68.4. There is considerable overlap, and the probability of bacteremia is dependent on the site as well as the organism. Any organism producing meningitis is likely to produce bacteremia at the same time. Infections with *H. influenzae* type b are usually bacteremic whether the site is the meninges, epiglottis, or periorbital tissues. Meningitis caused by *S. pneumoniae* can be expected to be bacteremic, but only 20–30% of pneumococcal pneumonias yield positive blood cultures.

Bacteremia from respiratory, urinary, wound, and other primary sites of infection

The most common sources of bacteremia are urinary tract infections, respiratory tract infections, and infections of skin or soft tissues, such as wound infections or cellulitis. The frequency with which any organism causes bacteremia is related to both its propensity to invade the bloodstream (Table 68.4) and how often it produces infections. For example, cases of *Escherichia coli* bacteremia are common, attributable in part to the fact that *E. coli* is the most frequent cause of urinary tract infection, a disease with a high prevalence but low incidence of associated bacteremia.

Gram-Negative Septic Shock

Gram-negative shock may develop in patients with bacteremic infections caused by Gram-negative rods such as the Enterobacteriaceae, *Pseudomonas aeruginosa*, and Gram-negative cocci, such as *Neisseria meningitidis*. Once fully developed, the shock and organ failure may be irreversible and are responsible for the high mortality (25–60%) associated with Gram-negative sepsis.

Association with bacteremic Gram-negative infections

Table 68.4 Frequency of Detection of Bloodstream Invasion by Bacteria and Some Fungi During Significant Infections at Extravascular Sites

Large (>90%) Proportion of Cases	
Haemophilus influenzae type b	*Brucella[a]*
Neisseria meningitidis	*Salmonella typhi*
Streptococcus pneumoniae (meningitis)	*Listeria*
Variable (10–90%) Depending on Stage and Severity of Infection	
β-hemolytic streptococci	Enterobacteriaceae
Streptococcus pneumoniae	*Pseudomonas*
Staphylococcus aureus	*Bacteroides*
Neisseria gonorrhoeae	*Clostridium* (myositis and endometritis)
Leptospira[a]	Anaerobic cocci
Borrelia[a]	*Candida*
Acinetobacter	*Cryptococcus neoformans[a]*
Shigella dysenteriae	
Small (<10%) Proportion of Cases	
Shigella (except *S. dysenteriae*)	*Pasteurella multocida*
Salmonella enteritidis	*Haemophilus,* noncapsulated
Campylobacter jejuni[a]	
Isolation Too Rare to Justify Attempt	
Vibrio (intestinal infections)	*Clostridium tetani*
Corynebacterium diphtheriae	*Clostridium botulinum*
Bordetella pertussis	*Clostridium difficile*
Mycobacterium[b]	*Legionella[c]*

[a] Isolation and/or demonstration requires special methods or prolonged incubation.

[b] *Mycobacterium avium-intracellulare* infections in acquired immunodeficiency syndrome patients often yield positives.

[c] Infrequent isolation may be due to inadequate cultural methods.

Pathophysiology

The initial events in Gram-negative shock appear to be vasodilatation with resultant decreased peripheral resistance and increased cardiac output. The patient is flushed and febrile. Capillary leakage and reduced blood volume follow, leading to a whole series of events identical to those seen in shock resulting from blood loss. These manifestations include vasoconstriction, reflex capillary dilatation, and local anoxic damage. Once this stage is reached, the patient may develop hypotension and hypothermia, and acidosis, hypoglycemia, and coagulation defects ensue with failure of highly perfused organs such as the lungs, kidneys, heart, brain, and liver.

Direct effects of endotoxin

The mechanisms involved in Gram-negative septic shock have been studied extensively in experimental animals. Most of the features seen in humans can be produced with the lipopolysaccharide endotoxin of the Gram-negative cell wall, although there is some variation between animal species and with different endotoxin preparations. The central events associated with the effect of endotoxin are 1) release of vasoactive substances

such as histamine, serotonin, noradrenaline, and plasma kinins, which may
cause arterial hypotension directly and trigger coagulation abnormalities;
2) disturbances in temperature regulation, which may be direct central
nervous system effects or, in the case of the early febrile response, mediated by interleukin 1 and tumor necrosis factor released from macrophages; 3) plasma complement depletion; and 4) direct metabolic effects
in which endotoxin disturbs the mechanisms for controlling glucose metabolism. Oxidative phosphorylation by liver mitochondria is also impaired, and the action of corticosteroid hormones may be affected.

Immune mechanisms may also be involved, as there are similarities
between some features of endotoxin shock and allergic reactions. If so,
previous sensitization by enterobacterial antigens in the gastrointestinal
flora would be required. The acute events could then be triggered by the
endotoxin released during the bacteremic phase of an infection. It is of
interest in this regard that sterile (gnotobiotic) animals are resistant to the
effects of endotoxin.

Although the clinical and physiologic features described previously are
typical of Gram-negative bacteremia with endotoxemia, they are not invariably present and are not reliable for distinguishing these cases from
other overwhelming causes of bacteremia without endotoxic effects. The
sudden appearance of one or more of these features, however, should
alert the physician to the possibility of Gram-negative septic shock, because management requires more than antimicrobial therapy. Other primary therapeutic measures include maintenance of adequate tissue per-
fusion through careful fluid and electrolyte management and the use of
vasoactive amines.

Blood Culture

The primary means for establishing a diagnosis of sepsis is by blood culture. The microbiologic principles involved are the same as with any culture. A sample of the patient's blood is obtained by aseptic venipuncture
and cultured in an enriched broth or, after special processing, on plates.
Growth is detected, and the organisms are isolated, identified, and tested
for antimicrobial susceptibility. Because of the importance of blood cultures in the diagnosis and therapy of most bacterial and fungal infections,
considerable attention must be paid to details of sampling if the prospects
of obtaining a positive culture are to be maximized. In recent years older
dogma has been replaced by a more scientific approach based on clinical
studies of blood culture procedures. The approach to blood culture must
be tailored to the individual patient, as no single procedure is best for all.
The important features are as follows.

Venipuncture. Before venipuncture, the skin over the vein must be carefully disinfected to reduce the probability of contamination of the blood
sample with skin bacteria. Although it is not possible to "sterilize" the
skin, quantitative counts can be markedly reduced with a combination of
70% alcohol and an antiseptic containing iodine. Mechanical cleansing is
as important as use of the antiseptic. Blood may be drawn with a needle
and syringe or into a sterile blood collection tube containing an anticoagulant free of antimicrobial properties. Sodium polyanethol sulfonate is
currently preferred, as other anticoagulants such as citrate and ethylene-
diaminetetraacetic acid have antibacterial activity. Blood should not be
drawn through indwelling venous or arterial catheters unless it cannot be
obtained by venipuncture.

Number of organisms in
blood often <1/ml

Volume. The number of organisms present in blood is often low (less than 1 organism/ml) and cannot be predicted in advance. Thus, small samples yield fewer positive cultures than larger ones. For example, as the volume sampled increases from 2 to 20 ml, the diagnostic yield increases by 30–50%. Samples of at least 10 ml should be collected from adult patients. The same principles apply with infants and young children, but the sample size must be reduced to take account of the smaller total blood volume of a child. Although it should be possible to obtain at least 1 ml, smaller volumes should still be cultured because bacteremia at levels of more than 1000 bacteria/ml is found in some infants.

Number. If the volume is adequate, it is rarely necessary to collect more than two or three blood cultures to achieve a positive result. In intravascular infections (for example, infective endocarditis), a single blood culture will be positive in more than 95% of cases. Studies of sequential blood cultures from bacteremic patients without endocarditis have yielded 80–90% positive results on the first culture, more than 90–95% with two cultures, and 99% in at least one of a series of three cultures.

Timing. The best timing schedule for a series of two or three blood cultures is dependent on the bacteremic pattern of the underlying infection and the clinical urgency of initiating antimicrobial therapy. Figure 68.1 illustrates some typical bacteremic patterns that can be related to the probability of obtaining positive blood cultures. Transient bacteremia is usually not detected, because organisms are cleared before the appearance of any clinical findings suggesting sepsis. The continuous bacteremia of infective endocarditis is usually readily detected, and timing is not critical. Intermittent bacteremia presents the greatest problem, because fever spikes generally occur after, rather than during, the bacteremia. Little is known about the periodicity of bloodstream invasion, except that the bacteremia is more likely to be present and sustained in the early acute stages of infection. Closely spaced samples are less likely to isolate the organism than those spaced an hour or more apart. In urgent situations, when antimicrobial therapy must be initiated, two or three samples should be collected at brief intervals and therapy begun as soon as possible. It is generally not useful to collect blood cultures while the patient is receiving antimicrobics unless none were collected before therapy or there is a change in the clinical course suggesting superinfection. The laboratory should be advised when such cultures are submitted, because it is sometimes possible to inactivate an antimicrobic, for example, with β-lactamases.

Timing of intermittent
bacteremia not predictable

Interference of antimicrobic
therapy with blood culture
results

Automated and direct plating
procedures

Laboratory processing. The basic blood culture procedure of incubating blood in an enriched broth is quite simple, but considerable effort must be expended to ensure detection of the broadest range of organisms in the least possible time. Daily examination of cultures for a week or more and a routine schedule of stains and/or subcultures of apparently negative cultures are required to detect organisms such as *H. influenzae* or *N. meningitidis* which usually do not produce visual changes in the broth. An automated blood culture system that measures radioactively labeled carbon dioxide released into the atmosphere from labeled carbon sources in the broth may be used in place of the conventional visual and cultural examinations. Direct plating of blood onto blood or chocolate agar is accomplished in a system that concentrates the specimen by centrifugation following lysis of the erythrocytes. This is particularly useful for bacterial quantification and rapid identification. Modifications of blood culture procedures have been shown to improve recovery of certain classes of mi-

Special cultural conditions for yeasts and anaerobes

croorganisms. Isolation of fungi is favored by ensuring maximum aerobic conditions in direct plating systems and broth bottles. Conversely, anaerobes are recovered best when a highly reduced environment is provided for plates and broths. Some bacteria, such as *Leptospira*, will not be isolated by routine blood culture procedures. The laboratory must be notified in advance so special media can be employed.

Problems in distinguishing infection with organisms from normal floral contamination

Interpretation. As the blood is normally sterile, the interpretation of blood cultures growing a pathogenic organism is seldom a problem. The major decision is the differentiation of agents causing transient bacteremia and skin contaminants from those opportunists associated with an intravascular or extravascular infection. Transient bacteremia is of short duration (Figure 68.1), is associated with manipulation of or trauma to a site possessing a normal flora, and involves species indigenous to that site. Despite skin disinfection, 2–4% of venipunctures result in contamination of the culture with small numbers of cutaneous flora such as *S. epidermidis*, corynebacteria (diphtheroids), and propionibacteria. The presence of these organisms in blood cultures can be considered a result of skin contamination unless quantitative procedures indicate large numbers (more than 5 organisms/ml) or repeated cultures are positive for the same organism. These findings should suggest diseases such as infective endocarditis or catheter bacteremia.

69

Infections of the Fetus and Newborn

C. George Ray

The usual 10-month period from conception through birth and the first 4 weeks of extrauterine life is one of unusual susceptibility to infection, but also a time at which special defenses acquired from the mother are operating.

Intrauterine protection of fetus

1. During normal development, the fetus is in a protected intrauterine environment, with fetal membranes serving as a physical barrier to external infection and the placenta contributing, with maternal immunity, to protection against many blood-borne infections. Transplacental transmission of specific immunoglobulins, particularly of the immunoglobulin G class (IgM does not normally cross the placental barrier), continues to provide some immunologic protection to the infant for weeks to months after birth, while lymphokines from the mother can provide transient cell-mediated immune support. If the infant is breast-fed, specific immunoglobulins (predominantly of the IgA class) in maternal colostrum afford some protection against pathogens that involve or invade through the infant's gastrointestinal tract.

Passive immunity from mother

Immaturity of fetal immune system and suppression of maternal cell-mediated immunity

2. On the other hand, the fetal immune system is immature, and there is relative suppression of maternal cell-mediated immunity as pregnancy progresses. These immune deficiencies serve an important biologic purpose, as they protect fetus and mother from activation of specific immunologic recognition and response mechanisms to differences in their histocompatibility locus antigens. If these processes did not occur normally, the fetus could be immunologically rejected by the mother or the fetal immune mechanisms activated to respond against maternal antigens in a form of "graft versus host" disease.

3. Specific and nonspecific immune responses begin to develop in early fetal life, perhaps as early as 8 weeks of gestation; however, a nearly normal immunocompetent state is usually not achieved until the infant

887

Specific deficiencies of neonate

is more than 2 years of age. Deficiencies commonly seen in the early period include poor antibody response to T-independent polysaccharide antigens, decreased phagocytic capability and variability in intracellular killing of certain infectious agents, lower levels of complement components, and decreased opsonic capacity.

Teratogenic effects of infection

4. Cell growth and organ differentiation are at their highest rates in the fetal–neonatal period, making the host especially susceptible to permanent damage when an infectious process intervenes.

Factors influencing risk of infection

The actual risk of infection and the types of pathogens encountered are influenced by a variety of interacting factors, including the state of maternal health and susceptibility to specific agents, adequacy of fetal and neonatal nutrition, integrity of fetal membranes, and degree of maturity at birth. This chapter will outline the major types of infection of concern to those caring for the fetus and neonate and the general approaches to their diagnosis. Specific biologic characteristics and aspects of prevention and treatment for each of the agents have been addressed in previous chapters.

Definitions

Times and sources of infection

A number of terms are commonly used to describe the infections that can affect the fetus and newborn. *Prenatal infections* include those acquired by the mother and/or fetus at any time before birth. When fetal infection develops, it is usually either blood-borne to the placenta, with subsequent spread to the fetus (transplacental), or by the ascending route from the vagina through torn or ruptured fetal membranes. *Natal infections* are those acquired during delivery. They are often caused by agents in the maternal genital tract, but occasionally by organisms introduced from exogenous sources through attendants, fetal monitors, or other instruments. *Postnatal infections*, which constitute the remainder of the group, include all infections acquired after delivery throughout the newborn (or neonatal) period, defined as the first 4 weeks of life.

Another commonly used term is *congenital infection*, which describes infection occurring at any time before or at birth (prenatal or natal). Consequently, the infection is usually still active in the newborn period and sometimes persists for months or years.

Perinatal infection is often used to include a period extending from 20–28 weeks of gestation to 7–28 days after birth. The term will not be used in this chapter.

Chorioamnionitis is an inflammatory response to infectious agents involving the chorionic and amnionic fetal membranes. It usually results from entry of pathogens from the vagina through tears or ruptures in the membranes, and it places the fetus at risk of direct exposure just before or at delivery. The risk of chorioamnionitis increases rapidly when membranes have been ruptured for longer than 12 hr before birth. When infection is by the bloodborne maternal route, there may be evidence of infection of the placenta, termed *placentitis*. Endometritis may be observed occasionally if the infection is an extension from a maternal pelvic focus along venous or lymphatic pathways.

Sepsis is a term employed to indicate a severe systemic bacterial infection associated with bacteremia.

Table 69.1   Modes of Infection and Major Agents

Mode	Agents		
	Bacteria	Viruses	Other
Prenatal Transplacental	*Listeria monocytogenes; Mycobacterium tuberculosis* (rare); *Treponema pallidum*	Rubella; cytomegalovirus; enteroviruses; Epstein-Barr virus; human immunodeficiency virus; parvovirus B19	*Toxoplasma gondii; Plasmodium* sp.
Ascending	Group B streptococci; *Escherichia coli; Listeria monocytogenes*	Cytomegalovirus; herpes simplex	*Chlamydia trachomatis; Mycoplasma hominis; Ureaplasma urealyticum*
Natal	Group B streptococci; *Escherichia coli; Listeria monocytogenes; Neisseria gonorrhoeae*	Herpes simplex; cytomegalovirus; enteroviruses; hepatitis B; varicella–zoster; human immunodeficiency virus	*Chlamydia trachomatis*
Postnatal	*Escherichia coli*; group B streptococci; *Listeria monocytogenes*; miscellaneous Gram-negative bacteria; *Staphylococcus aureus; Staphylococcus epidermidis; Clostridium tetani*	Cytomegalovirus; herpes simplex; enteroviruses; varicella–zoster; respiratory syncytial virus; influenza viruses	

Common Etiologic Agents

Table 69.1 lists the major pathogens affecting the fetus and newborn, according to the usual modes of acquisition. Some, such as *Mycobacterium tuberculosis* and *Plasmodium* species, are exceedingly rare, but require consideration in certain clinical and epidemiologic circumstances. It should also be noted that some pathogens that commonly affect older infants and children are quite rarely observed in newborns. This phenomenon is partially attributable to the protective effect of maternally derived immunity to organisms such as *Haemophilus influenzae* type b, *Streptococcus pneumoniae, Neisseria meningitidis*, and mumps and measles viruses, but also reflects less opportunity for exposure to some agents early in life. Some organisms, such as *Staphylococcus aureus*, very rarely cause prenatal or natal infections, but commonly colonize in the postnatal period and most often cause disease after the first week of life.

If one views the fetus as existing normally in a protected, "germ-free" intrauterine environment before emerging into a milieu of potential pathogens, it is easy to see how the newborn can be colonized with the first organisms encountered, some of which can cause disease. The initial external pathogenic flora often acquired can include organisms frequently present in the maternal genital tract, such as group B streptococci and *Escherichia coli, Neisseria gonorrhoeae, Listeria monocytogenes, Chlamydia trachomatis*, and herpes simplex virus, all of which are important causes of natal infection.

Postnatal infections may be late manifestations resulting from prenatal or natal colonization by pathogens such as those mentioned previously, but additional organisms may be acquired after birth. Particular risks in-

Rarity of some childhood infections in infancy

Postnatal S. aureus infections

Sources of colonization with pathogens

Factors determining common neonatal infections

clude contamination of the nursery environment by a variety of Gram-negative bacteria, staphylococci, and some common viruses (Table 69.1) and attendants who are infected with or carrying such organisms. The risks are increased if the infant is born prematurely or otherwise physically compromised, and they are amplified by prolonged hospitalization and invasive procedures such as respiratory intubation, mechanical ventilation, and intravenous treatment, as well as by blood or blood product transfusions.

Risks of prematurity, prolonged hospitalization, and invasive procedures

Effect of Prenatal Infection on Pregnancy and Intrauterine Development

All of the agents indicated in Table 69.1 as causing prenatal infections have the potential of creating an adverse pregnancy outcome, either as a result of compromising the health of the mother or by directly affecting the fetus. The effect can be untimely termination of pregnancy resulting in abortion, stillbirth, or prematurity, as well as developmental defects and fetal malnutrition.

Common Clinical Features, Diagnosis, and Management

Acute Bacterial Sepsis

When a physician first encounters a sick newborn, the primary concern is whether the illness represents sepsis and/or meningitis caused by bacteria. This determination is important, because treatment is both feasible and extremely urgent. Clinical disease apparent at birth or developing within the first 3 days of life (early onset) has usually been acquired prenatally. Mortality can exceed 70%, even with prompt treatment. Later onset of symptoms is commonly associated with natal or postnatal acquisition of pathogens; however, these infections can also be exceedingly severe. If meningitis develops, the overall mortality, even with treatment, ranges from 25 to 40%, and permanent neurologic damage may occur in 30–50% of survivors. The two pathogens most commonly associated with neonatal sepsis and meningitis are group B streptococci and *E. coli*.

Severity of neonatal infections

Group B streptococci and E. coli sepsis and meningitis

Diagnostic clues

The diagnosis of neonatal infections is based first on clinical suspicion. There is sometimes a history of recent maternal febrile illness immediately before or at birth. Other suggestive features include fetal distress, prolonged rupture of membranes, foul-smelling amnionic fluid, and premature delivery. The first signs and symptoms of illness in the infant may be subtle and extremely variable, including respiratory distress, apneic episodes, cyanosis, irritability, unexplained jaundice, tachycardia, poor feeding, abdominal distention, and fever. Initial laboratory findings often include either leukocytosis, with an increased proportion of immature neutrophils, or leukopenia. The development of seizures, hypotension, or disseminated intravascular coagulation indicates a particularly grave prognosis.

Cultures of blood and cerebrospinal fluid

Initial therapy

Diagnostic tests for suspected infections must be initiated as quickly as possible, followed by empirical antimicrobial therapy while waiting for culture results. The major tests include examination and culture of cerebrospinal fluid and a blood culture. The antimicrobics initially chosen are those known to be effective against the pathogens most commonly encountered. They often include penicillin or ampicillin for the streptococci (also useful for *L. monocytogenes*) and an aminoglycoside such as gentamicin for *E. coli*.

Other Bacterial and Chlamydial Infections

Chlamydial and gonococcal conjunctivitis

Although *N. gonorrhoeae* and *C. trachomatis* are common natally acquired infections, they are usually not associated with sepsis. Both can produce a severe conjunctivitis in the newborn that requires prompt diagnosis and treatment. Gonococcal ophthalmia is usually apparent in the first 5 days after birth, whereas the onset of chlamydial conjunctivitis is frequently delayed until after the first week of life.

Chlamydial infant pneumonia syndrome

Another significant illness associated with natally acquired *C. trachomatis* infection is infant pneumonia syndrome. The onset of respiratory symptoms is often delayed, with most cases occurring between 2 weeks and 6 months of age. This illness is also considered in Chapter 29.

Postnatal infections by *S. aureus*

Localized infections, such as cutaneous or subcutaneous abscesses, show a particular association with postnatally acquired *S. aureus* and occasionally with various Gram-negative bacteria. If the newborn is affected by a staphylococcal strain that produces exfoliative toxin, the local lesion may be relatively trivial in contrast to the more widespread effect of circulating toxin on the skin, which is termed the *staphylococcal scalded-skin syndrome*. Prompt treatment with an antistaphylococcal antimicrobial agent results in resolution of the disease within 2 weeks, usually with complete healing.

Scalded skin syndrome

Syphilis

Congenital syphilis

Prenatal infection by *Treponema pallidum* (congenital syphilis) is unusual in the United States, but if left untreated, the organism can produce long-term damage, often without apparent signs or symptoms in the newborn period. To minimize these risks, serologic screening is recommended for all pregnant women when first seen in early gestation and at delivery. An alternative to testing the mother at delivery is to screen sera from newborn infants. In addition, serologic testing is recommended whenever clinical or epidemiologic circumstances suggest the possibility of exposure at any time during pregnancy. Prompt treatment of infected mothers during pregnancy, preferably with penicillin, will markedly reduce the risk of fetal infection. Similar treatment is also effective for the infected infant. Congenital syphilis is described also in Chapter 70.

TORCH Complex

Toxoplasmosis, rubella, cytomegalovirus, herpes simplex, and other infections

Common clinical manifestations

Delayed manifestations

When bacterial, spirochetal, and chlamydial infections have been reasonably excluded from consideration, other possibilities can best be remembered by the convenient acronym TORCH (*t*oxoplasmosis, *o*ther, *r*ubella, *c*ytomegalovirus, *h*erpes simplex). This term comprises major infections that can be particularly severe if acquired prenatally. There is often significant overlap of clinical manifestations associated with the various agents in the TORCH complex. Common features may include low birth weight, rash, jaundice, and hepatosplenomegaly. On the other hand, many infants with TORCH infections can go undiagnosed, because the clinical signs may be inapparent at birth, only to appear weeks, months, or even years later. For example, congenital cytomegalovirus infection may be manifested only as mild mental retardation and/or hearing loss that may not become apparent until after the first year of life. Toxoplasmosis also presents a dilemma. It is estimated that as many as 1 in 200 pregnancies in the United States is complicated by primary infection with *Toxoplasma gondii*, which is usually subclinical. Of these cases, approximately 45% result in fetal infection, but only 8–11% of the infected offspring demonstrate clinical symptoms in the newborn period. The remainder are at risk, however, and can ultimately develop neurologic deterioration and/ or chorioretinitis, which may not be recognized until 5 or more years later. These observations only partially illustrate the importance of TORCH complex infections and our relative impotence in controlling many of them.

Of the array of miscellaneous agents grouped in the "other" category, three viruses deserve specific mention. If the mother has active infection with hepatitis B virus during pregnancy, the risk of natal or postnatal transmission to the infant is high (range, 20–80%, depending on the status of virus activity). Although it is unlikely that clinical disease will be apparent in the newborn period, it is important to undertake specific measures to prevent infection in the infant when the mother is infected. They include immediate administration of hepatitis B immune globulin after birth as well as immunization of the infant with hepatitis B vaccine. The chance of maternal transmission of the human immunodeficiency virus, either transplacentally or natally, has not yet been precisely established, but is estimated to be between 30 and 50%. No means of prevention other than avoidance of pregnancy is currently known. Primary varicella is infrequent in pregnancy. If the mother develops varicella less than 5 days before or 2 days after delivery, however, the risk of severe neonatal varicella is significant, with a mortality of approximately 20%. It is recommended that the infant be given varicella–zoster immune globulin (or zoster immune globulin) immediately in an attempt to prevent or modify subsequent disease. Maternal zoster infections are not associated with a significant risk to the offspring, presumably because of adequate transplacental transmission of specific antibody.

The approach to a suspected TORCH complex infection requires some thought in selection of appropriate tests. The appendix summarizes the major clinical and historic features of specific agents and the diagnostic procedures that can be used. The following general comments should also be kept in mind:

1. Clinical and epidemiologic data are used as much as possible in ascertaining likely specific agents.

2. Probabilities must be weighed; for example, congenital cytomegalovirus infection is by far the most frequent TORCH complex agent encountered in the United States (more than 90% of all proved cases).

3. Potentially treatable infections must be considered first. If toxoplasmosis or herpes simplex is suggested by the historic and clinical findings, it may be controlled by prompt and aggressive therapy. Other infections, which are potentially preventable by early specific immunoglobulin therapy of the infant, include maternal varicella and hepatitis B infections. The remaining agents involved in the TORCH array are not amenable to specific therapy at present. Their importance lies more in long-term prognosis, planning of continuing care, and epidemiologic management.

4. Serologic testing, when indicated, should be done on both infant and maternal sera collected at the same time to facilitate interpretation of specific antibody titer levels in the infant. This approach is based upon the following principles: passive transplacental transmission of IgG antibodies occurs, but these maternal antibodies normally wane and disappear in the infant over 3–6 months. If the infant is actively infected, it usually produces its own specific antibodies to the agent, which then

Sources, risks, and prevention of hepatitis B infection

Human immunodeficiency virus transmission

Neonatal varicella from infected mother

Focus on treatable conditions

Value of comparisons of maternal and infant antibody titers

persist for much longer periods. Thus, a specific antibody titer in the infant's serum during the first month of life equal to or less than that of the mother may merely reflect passive transfer, and does not support a diagnosis of active infection. On the other hand, if the infant's titer is significantly higher than the mother's (fourfold or greater) or rises progressively in serial samples obtained in later months, active infection by the agent in question is suggested.

Determination of infant IgM antibodies

In active congenital and neonatal infections, the infant's early responses often include IgM antibodies. As maternal IgM antibodies rarely cross the placental barrier, specific IgM antibody determinations early in life may be useful for the diagnosis of congenital toxoplasma, rubella, and cytomegalovirus infections. However, both false-positive and false-negative results have been noted. The presence of rheumatoid factor has been a major cause of false-positive results. Tests that show promise of high specificity include solid-phase IgM assays with antihuman IgM as a "capture" antibody and enzyme-linked antibody markers.

Lack of value of nonspecific tests

Nonspecific tests, such as quantitation of total IgM or IgA or detection of rheumatoid factor, have limited or no usefulness. Negative results do not rule out infection, and positive results must be regarded cautiously. Other tests, such as lymphocyte stimulation with specific antigens, show some promise, but are not yet available in enough centers to recommend them routinely.

Conclusion

Fetal and neonatal infections remain a highly significant and often frustrating challenge. They can be severe, and permanent sequelae are common. At the onset of infection, clinical signs and symptoms are often exceedingly subtle; thus, the physician must be quickly alerted to the infectious possibilities, particularly when specific treatment is available.

Of all of these infections, the most preventable is rubella, and assurance of immunity before conception is a mandatory goal. Better control of the remainder may become possible in the future with newer bacterial and viral vaccines, better early diagnostic methods, and improved treatment methods.

Appendix

TORCH Complex: Salient Features and Diagnostic Tests

Toxoplasmosis

Suggestive clinical findings. Chorioretinitis (found in more than 90% of symptomatic neonatal cases); lymphadenopathy.

Maternal history. Usually negative; occasional cervical lymphadenopathy during pregnancy.

Tests of choice. Specific maternal and infant antibody titers; follow-up titers may be helpful.

Other Infections

The list of causes includes enteroviruses, hepatitis B, human immunodeficiency virus, varicella–zoster, Epstein-Barr virus, arthropod-borne viruses, malaria, and tuberculosis. As the agents in this category most commonly encountered are the enteroviruses, the features summarized here pertain primarily to them.

Suggestive clinical findings. Sepsislike syndromes; meningitis; myocarditis (findings are variable).

Maternal history. Fever common at or near parturition.

Tests of Choice. Viral cultures of throat, rectum, and cerebrospinal fluid.

Rubella

Suggestive clinical findings. Congenital malformations, often multiple. In severe cases, "celery stalking" of metaphyses of long bones may be seen in early radiographs (see also cytomegalovirus).

Maternal history. Rubellalike illness or epidemiologic history of exposure in early pregnancy is common. If available, maternal serologic and immunization history can aid in supporting or refuting this diagnostic possibility.

Tests of choice. Maternal and infant antibody titers, including IgM-specific antibody testing in the infant. Serial determinations over 6 months may be of additional help. Culture is not a readily available routine test in most hospitals; special arrangements must be made.

Cytomegalovirus

Suggestive clinical findings. None very specific in differentiating infection from most others in the group. Statistically, cytomegalovirus is the most common congenital infection encountered. In florid cases, early radiographs of the long bones may resemble those of congenital rubella (celery stalking).

Maternal history. Usually none; occasionally, an account of a mononucleosislike syndrome may be elicited.

Tests of choice. Urine culture is the most sensitive test. If results are negative, this diagnosis is highly unlikely; if positive, the diagnosis is supported (especially if cultures are done in the first 3 weeks of life). With advancing age of the infant, however, positive cultures may require careful interpretation before an unequivocal diagnosis is made.

Herpes Simplex

Suggestive clinical findings. Cutaneous vesicles and/or ocular or mucous membrane ulcerations; however, these lesions may not become apparent until other signs of illness have developed.

Maternal history. Up to 70% have no history of genital lesions or symptoms. Others may have a history of recent primary symptomatic infection. It is also important to ascertain whether genital lesions were known to exist in recent sexual partners.

Tests of choice. Culture of lesions; immunofluorescent and cytologic studies may be available for rapid diagnosis. If no lesions are present, throat culture is also a valuable source. Brain biopsy and urine and cerebrospinal cultures may also be necessary in some cases. Maternal cultures, if positive, may give indirect support regarding etiology.

70

Sexually Transmitted Diseases

Lawrence Corey

Sexually transmitted infections are now major public health problems in all population groups and social strata. Over the last three decades some of the most important worldwide pandemics have been due to sexually transmitted disease (STDs). These include infections due to *Neisseria gonorrhoeae*, sexually acquired chlamydia trachomatis, genital herpes simplex virus, genital papillomavirus, and the most recent and most worrisome, human immunodeficiency virus (HIV). Table 70.1 lists the major sexually transmitted pathogens and the disease syndromes associated with them. The most important are discussed in this chapter.

Gonorrhea

Spectrum of disease

Gonorrhea is an acute pyogenic infection of columnar and transitional epithelium caused by *N. gonorrhoeae*. The urethra, endocervix, anal canal, pharynx, and conjunctivae can be infected directly. Spread of the organism along contiguous mucosal surfaces results in endometritis, salpingitis, peritonitis, and bartholinitis in the female host and epididymitis in the male. Systemic complications of bacteremic spread (gonococcemia) include inflammation of tendon sheaths (tenosynovitis), arthritis, dermatitis, myopericarditis, hepatitis, endocarditis, and meningitis. The microbiology of this organism is discussed in Chapter 19.

Prevalence

The prevalence and clinical manifestations of gonorrhea differ according to the patient population surveyed. In private practice, *N. gonorrhoeae* has been isolated in from 0.5 to 2% of women; however, a much higher prevalence (approaching 20%) has been found in women reporting to venereal disease clinics who are under 30 years of age, unmarried, and of low socioeconomic status. The risk of transmission of gonorrhea from an

Table 70.1 Sexually Transmitted Agents and Diseases Caused

Agent	Disease or Syndrome
Bacterial	
Neisseria gonorrhoea	Urethritis; cervicitis; proctitis; pharyngitis; conjunctivitis; endometritis; pelvic inflammatory disease; perihepatitis; bartholinitis; disseminated gonococcal infection
Chlamydia trachomatis	Nongonococcal urethritis; epididymitis; cervicitis; salpingitis; inclusion conjunctivitis; infant pneumonia; trachoma; lymphogranuloma venereum
Ureaplasma urealyticum	Nongonococcal urethritis
Treponema pallidum	Syphilis
Haemophilus ducreyi	Chancroid
Calymmatobacterium granulomatis	Granuloma inguinale
Viral	
HIV	AIDS; AIDS-related complex (ARC); perinatal and congenital AIDS; aseptic meningitis; subacute neurological syndromes; persistent generalized adenopathy; asymptomatic infection
Herpes simplex virus	Primary and recurrent genital herpes; aseptic meningitis; neonatal herpes
Papillomavirus	Condylomata accuminata; laryngeal papilloma of newborn; association with cervical carcinoma
Cytomegalovirus	Heterophil-negative infectious mononucleosis; congenital birth defects
Hepatitis B virus	Hepatitis B, acute and chronic infections
Molluscum contagiosum virus	Genital molluscum contagiosum
Protozoan	
Trichomonas vaginalis	Trichomonal vaginitis
Fungal	
Candida albicans	Vulvovaginitis; penile candidiasis
Ectoparasitic	
Phthirus pubis	Pubic louse infestation
Sarcoptes scabiei	Scabies

Abbreviations: HIV = human immunodeficiency virus; AIDS = acquired immunodeficiency syndrome; ARC = AIDS-related complex.

infected woman to a man during one sexual exposure is estimated to be about 30%, whereas the risk of transmission from an infected man to a woman is higher (approximately 70%).

Clinical Manifestations

May be symptomatic or asymptomatic

Urethritis and urethral discharge in men

Gonococcal infection of the genital tract may be symptomatic or asymptomatic in men or women. Persons with symptomatic disease generally have sexual contacts with ignored or absent symptoms. The most common manifestation of gonococcal infection in men is urethritis with purulent discharge, dysuria, frequency, and meatal erythema. The usual incubation period is 2–7 days after exposure. In the absence of treatment, symptoms

Cervicitis in women

Spread to upper genital tract

Salpingitis and PID

Association of PID with
intrauterine devices
Risk of infertility and ectopic
pregnancy after salpingitis

Disseminated gonococcal
infection; bacteremia; skin
manifestations; arthritis

persist for an average of 8 weeks, and unilateral epididymitis will develop in 5–10% of cases.

In women, gonorrhea is manifested by discharge and pain associated with infection of the cervix. Characteristically, the endocervix is dusky red and friable with mucopurulent yellow exudate emanating from the endocervical os. Urethral infection causes urinary frequency and dysuria. Upward spread of the gonococcus to the endometrium causes endometritis associated with abnormal menstrual bleeding and midline abdominal pain. Further extension into the fallopian tubes results in pelvic inflammatory disease (PID) or acute salpingitis. The symptoms of gonococcal PID include bilateral lower abdominal pain, tenderness localized to the fallopian tubes and ovaries, fever, chills, and leukocytosis. The onset is generally during or shortly after menses, and the risk is increased in women using an intrauterine contraceptive device. The inflammatory response to gonococcal infection of the upper genital tract can result in scarring or dysfunction of the fallopian tubes and a decrease in fertility. The average risk of infertility is 13% after one episode of salpingitis, 35% after two episodes, and 75% after three or more episodes. In addition, salpingitis appears to increase the risk of subsequent ectopic pregnancies. Occasionally, spread of gonococci into the upper abdomen may lead to gonococcal perihepatitis with abdominal pain bilaterally or in the right upper quadrant, tenderness, and a hepatic friction rub. This diagnosis is often confused with acute cholecystitis.

Spread beyond the pelvic area can produce disseminated gonococcal infection (DGI), which may proceed through two phases. The first is an early bacteremic phase characterized by fever, asymmetric tenosynovitis, and petechial, papular, or hemorrhagic skin lesions on the distal extremities. Without treatment, the systemic manifestations of bacteremia may subside only to be followed by infection at another site, most often an isolated joint. Septic arthritis may develop without a prior history to suggest bacteremia. The infection occasionally leads to endocarditis or meningitis. In contrast to strains causing urethritis, those causing disseminated gonococcal infection are usually resistant to killing by serum, often produce asymptomatic infections, have more fastidious growth requirements, and are usually sensitive to penicillin. In areas where penicillinase-producing *N. gonorrhoeae* are common, they may cause DGI.

Diagnosis

A presumptive diagnosis of gonococcal infection may be made when Gram staining of the infected material reveals typical Gram-negative intracellular diplococci. In experienced hands, the sensitivity of the Gram stain exceeds 95% for urethral exudates from men and 60% for endocervical exudates from women. Cultures of exposed sites, such as the pharynx, urethra, cervix, and anal canal, should be obtained from all patients in whom the disease is suspected, except for men with smear-positive urethritis.

Value of Gram smear of
urethral exudate in men

Treatment

Currently, recommended treatment of gonorrhea has undergone change because of the emergence of penicillin-resistant *N. gonorrhoeae* and the frequent association between *N. gonorrhoeae* and *C. trachomatis* infection. In areas where penicillinase-producing gonococci are rare and concurrent chlamydial infection is not expected, high single-dose oral therapy

Role of penicillins

with ampicillin or amoxicillin is used with probenecid to block renal excretion and raise and prolong blood levels. Third-generation cephalosporins such as ceftriaxone are effective. High-dose intramuscular injection of procaine penicillin G with probenecid can also be used. A course of oral tetracycline is effective for tetracycline-susceptible strains and will treat simultaneous chlamydial infection; however, antimicrobics curative with single high doses are usually preferable because of difficulty in ensuring patient compliance and the increasing emergence of tetracycline-resistant strains. It should be remembered the treatment plan must also include the sexual partner. The emergence of β-lactamase-producing gonococci (Chapter 19) has made it important to follow treatment with cultural tests for cure. At present, spectinomycin is a drug of choice for penicillinase-producing strains or when their presence is likely because of epidemiologic associations (disease contracted in Southeast Asia) or of treatment failure with penicillin G. Some of the newer third-generation cephalosporins, such as ceftriaxone and cefotaxime, are being used increasingly for the treatment of gonococcal infections because of effectiveness against strains resistant to penicillin and/or spectinomycin.

The Centers of Disease Control periodically reviews treatment recommendations for all sexually transmitted disease and details of these recommendations are published periodically in the *Morbidity and Mortality Weekly Report*. They are also available through local health departments.

Syphilis

Syphilis is a chronic systemic infection caused by *Treponema pallidum*, which is usually sexually transmitted. The primary lesion is an ulcer with regional lymphadenopathy. Secondary syphilis is a bacteremic stage associated with generalized mucocutaneous lesions. This stage is followed by a latent period of subclinical infection that lasts for many years and eventually leads to tertiary syphilis in 30–50% of untreated cases. Tertiary syphilis may present as aortitis, central nervous system disease, or destructive mucocutaneous, musculoskeletal, and parenchymal lesions. *Treponema pallidum* and the pathogenesis of the different syphilitic stages are discussed in Chapter 26.

Epidemiology

Nearly all cases of noncongenital syphilis are acquired by sexual contact with infectious lesions. Fomite spread is extremely rare, and transmission by blood transfusion has essentially been eliminated. Most cases of syphilis occur in individuals 18–24 years of age. In the United States, the incidence is highest in nonwhite urban residents and among homosexual or bisexual men. About one-third of sexual contacts of those with infected primary or secondary lesions will develop the disease. New cases of syphilis must be reported to health departments to permit identification and treatment of contacts.

Primary Syphilis

Syphilis must always be considered in the differential diagnosis of a genital ulcer. The median incubation period from contact until the appearance of the primary syphilitic chancre is about 21 days; the period is proportional to the size of the infecting inoculum. The chancre (Figure 70.1A) develops at the site of infection. Typically, it begins as an indurated,

Margin notes:

Single-dose therapy preferable

Agents for β-lactamase-producing strains

Frequency in homosexual and bisexual men

Incubation period about 21 days

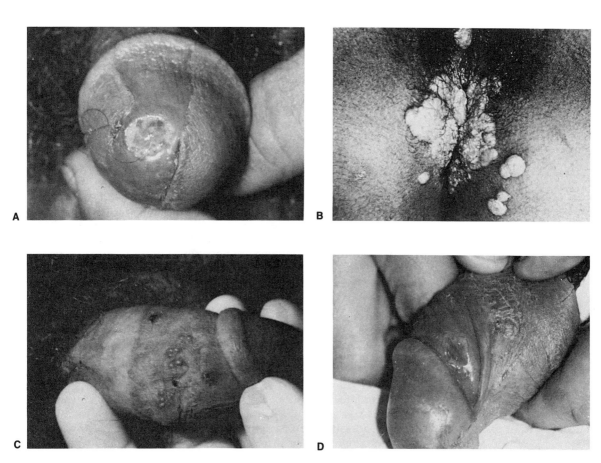

70.1 Some manifestations of sexually transmitted diseases. (A) Syphilitic chancre, showing rolled borders and indurated margin. Lesion is nontender when touched. (B) Condylomata lata in secondary syphilis. (C) Multiple grouped vesicles of genital herpes. (D) Chancroid infection. Lesion is tender and ulcerated. Patient also had a large, fluctant inguinal lymph node.

painless papule, usually of the penis, external genitalia, anal area, or lips, that becomes ulcerated. Bilateral, firm, nonsuppurative, painless enlargement of the inguinal lymph nodes usually develops within 1 week of the primary lesion and may persist for months. Primary lesions teeming with *T. pallidum* can be found by dark-field or direct fluorescent antibody microscopy. They heal spontaneously after 4–6 weeks.

Primary chancre; many spirochetes present

Secondary Syphilis

Secondary syphilis may develop 2–10 weeks after the primary lesion has healed. It is characterized by a symmetric mucocutaneous maculopapular rash and generalized nontender lymph node enlargement with manifestations of systemic infection. Skin lesions are distributed on the trunk and extremities, often including the palms, soles, and face, and can mimic a variety of infectious and noninfectious skin eruptions. About one-third of cases develop painless mucosal warty erosions called *condylomata lata* (Figure 70.1B). These erosions usually develop in warm, moist sites such as the genitals and perineum. They are often elevated and pale or

Rashes and systemic manifestations

Condylomata lata

pink and must be differentiated from infectious genital warts (condylomata accuminata). The nontreponemal (cardiolipin antigen) and treponemal (eg, FTA) tests are invariably positive in secondary syphilis. Large numbers of *T. pallidum* are present in all lesions, and dark-field or direct fluorescent antibody examination of exudate from secondary lesions readily establishes the diagnosis. In one-third of untreated cases, host immune responses appear to resolve the infection. In the remainder the illness enters a dormant or latent state.

Many spirochetes present in lesions; serologic tests positive

Latent Syphilis

Serologic tests positive in absence of clinical signs

Latent syphilis is characterized by positive results of serologic tests in the absence of clinical signs or symptoms or of abnormal findings in cerebrospinal fluid. It is divided into two stages. Early latent syphilis, which occurs within 2 years of infection, is potentially transmissible because relapses associated with spirochetemia are possible. Late latent syphilis, which occurs more than 2 years after infection, is associated with immunity to relapse and resistance to reinfection: About one-third of cases do not progress beyond this stage.

Tertiary Syphilis

About one-third of patients with untreated syphilis will develop clinically evident tertiary manifestations (that is, cardiovascular syphilis, neurosyphilis, or gumma formation). Tertiary syphilis may appear as early as 5 years after infection, but characteristically occurs after 15–20 years. Neurosyphilis may be manifested as meningovascular syphilis, general paresis, or tabes dorsalis. Meningovascular syphilis involves diffuse gummatous and obliterative vascular changes of the meninges associated with increased cells and protein in the cerebrospinal fluid and focal neurologic changes. In general paresis, there is extensive cortical degeneration of the brain, and, unlike other tertiary syphilitic diseases, large numbers of *T. pallidum* are found in the affected areas. Some changes develop in the cerebrospinal fluid, but the major disease manifestations are personality changes ranging from decreased memory to hallucinations or frank psychosis. Delusions of grandeur are characteristic but not diagnostic, as they have been known to occur in healthy politicians, professors, or senior house staff. Tabes dorsalis involves demyelination of the posterior columns and dorsal roots and damage to dorsal root ganglia. The latter produces ataxia; wide-based gait; foot slap; and loss of the sensations of position, pain, and temperature. Not all patients with central nervous system involvement have symptomatic disease. The diagnosis of asymptomatic neurosyphilis is made in those who have a reactive serum treponemal antibody test (for example, FTA-ABS) with increased cells and protein and a reactive cardiolipin (eg, VDRL) test in the cerebrospinal fluid.

Can develop many years after infection

Meningovascular syphilis

General paresis

Tabes dorsalis

Asymptomatic neurosyphilis

The most characteristic lesion of late cardiovascular syphilis is the development of an aneurysm of the ascending and transverse segments of the aortic arch as a result of gummatous changes in the middle coat of the aorta and loss of elasticity. This aneurysm can lead to aortic valve incompetence, pressure necrosis of structures adjacent to the aorta, or rupture of the aorta.

Cardiovascular syphilis

Aortic aneurysm

The isolated gumma is a granulomatous reaction to *T. pallidum* infection. It occurs most often in skin, bones, or joints, but may involve any organ. Clinical manifestations of gumma are similar to those of other mass-producing lesions in the tissues, such as tumors. The diagnosis of a gumma involves serologic evidence of the disease and characteristic histologic

Gummata

Table 70.2 Frequency of Positive Serologic Tests in
Untreated Syphilis

Stage of Syphilis	Frequency (%)		
	VDRL[a]	FTA[b]-ABS	MHA[c]-TP
Primary	70	80	80
Secondary	100	100	100
Latent or late	70	98	98

[a] Nontreponemal antigen test.
[b] Fluorescence treponemal antibody test.
[c] Treponemal microhemagglutination test.

features. Because of its protean sites of attack, syphilis, like tuberculosis, is a great mimic of other diseases.

Congenital Syphilis

The fetus is susceptible to syphilis only after the fourth month of gestation, and adequate treatment of an infected mother before that time will prevent fetal damage. Thereafter, treatment of the mother involves treatment of an already infected fetus. Because active syphilitic infection is devastating to the infant, routine serologic testing is performed in early pregnancy and should be repeated in the last trimester in women at high risk of acquiring syphilis. Untreated maternal infection may result in fetal loss or congenital syphilis, which is analogous to secondary syphilis in the adult, with involvement of the eyes, meninges, bones, and skin. Anemia, jaundice, and thrombocytopenia may also occur, and the disease in the infant must be differentiated from other congenital infections such as toxoplasmosis, rubella, and cytomegalovirus.

Importance of routine serologic testing of pregnant women
Fetal death or possible severe compromise

Diagnosis

All primary and secondary lesions should be evaluated by dark-field examination by an expert or by direct fluorescent antibody staining. The surface of a lesion is gently abraded and squeezed to express a drop of serous transudate, which is then examined directly for characteristic motile treponemes by dark-field microscopy or for the presence of *T. pallidum* by direct fluorescent antibody staining of a smear. A positive test is diagnostic of syphilis.

The basis of treponemal and nontreponemal serologic tests for *T. pallidum* infection is discussed in Chapter 26. Table 70.2 illustrates the frequency of positive test results in untreated syphilis by stage of disease for the VDRL, FTA, and microhemagglutination tests. Treponemal tests are highly specific, but remain positive after cure. Nontreponemal tests such as the VDRL or RPR are less specific, but the titers reflect the activity of disease and can be used as a test of cure. The VDRL titers should decrease at least fourfold after successful treatment of primary, secondary, or early latent syphilis, and 75% of primary and 40% of secondary cases revert to completely negative within 3–12 months. Failure of titers to decrease suggests inadequate therapy. An initial decrease followed by an increase during the first year suggests reinfection or relapse. The VDRL type test results are falsely negative in 25% of patients with early primary

Direct dark-field examination and direct fluorescent antibody staining

Serodiagnosis

Specificity of treponemal antigen tests

Nontreponemal test titers decline with cure

False-negative and false-positive nontreponemal test results

syphilis and 25–30% of those with late or late latent syphilis. Many acute conditions that cause cell damage result in transient false-positive VDRL results. Chronic (more than 6 months) false-positive results are associated with drug addiction, autoimmune diseases, and aging.

Treatment

Penicillin is agent of choice

Treponema pallidum is killed by low concentrations of penicillin G; long exposure to the drug is required in established disease, however, probably because of the long generation time of the organism and its inaccesssibility in some lesions. There is no evidence of resistance of *T. pallidum* to penicillin, which remains the antimicrobic of choice. Erythromycin, tetracyclines, chloramphenicol, and cephalosporins are alternative antibiotics in penicillin-hypersensitive patients.

Jarisch-Herxheimer reaction

Fever, chills, myalgia, headache, tachycardia, leukocytosis, and vasodilatation, known as the *Jarisch-Herxheimer reaction*, may develop 2–24 hr after penicillin treatment of syphilis is begun. This reaction occurs in about one-half of patients with primary syphilis, 90% of those with secondary syphilis, and 25% of those with latent disease. In secondary syphilis, erythema and edema of the mucocutaneous lesions may occur. The pathogenesis of the reaction is not completely understood, but appears to result from an immune response to release of antigen by large numbers of lysed spirochetes.

Prevention

At present, no vaccine against syphilis is available. Prevention and control depends upon detection and treatment of infectious cases. Because about one-third of those exposed to syphilis will develop disease, prophylactic therapy of all sexual contacts with penicillin G is recommended.

Genital Herpes Simplex

Genital herpes simplex virus (HSV) infection has emerged as a disease of increasing public health importance. It differs from other sexually transmitted diseases in the chronicity of the infection and the frequency of recurrences. The biology of this organism is described in Chapter 37. Genital HSV infections can be caused by viral types 1 or 2. The symptoms and signs of acute infection are similar for both HSV-1 and HSV-2.

Epidemiology

High prevalence

As genital herpes is not a reportable disease in the United States, the annual incidence is unknown; however, approximately half a million new cases have been estimated to occur yearly. It is the most common cause of genital ulceration in industrialized nations. Antibody prevalence data indicate that the incidence of genital herpes depends on the past sexual activity of the population studied. In some, such as prostitutes, HSV-2 antibody is detected in up to 80% of individuals. It is estimated that in middle-class American populations, the prevalence of antibody to HSV-2 is approximately 15–30%. Genital herpes infection is contracted by direct spread. It may be transmitted by asymptomatic shedding of virus from the cervix, urethra, semen, or from seemingly trivial small unnoticed lesions on the penile or vulvar skin.

Primary Herpes Infection

The mean incubation period from sexual contact to onset of lesions is 5 days. Lesions begin as small erythematous papules that soon form vesicles and then pustules. Within 3–5 days the vesiculopustular lesions break to

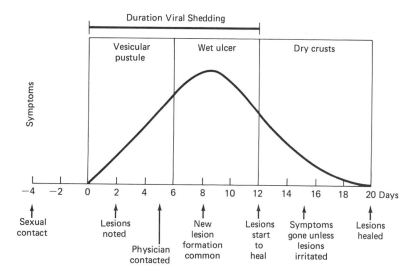

70.2 Typical course of first episode of herpetic infection.

Painful ulcerating vesicles

Multiple primary lesions

Inguinal adenopathy

Systemic manifestations

Other complications

form painful coalesced ulcers that subsequently dry; some form crusts and heal without scarring (Figure 70.2). With primary disease the genital lesions are usually multiple (mean, 20), bilateral, and extensive (Figure 70.1C). The urethra and cervix are also infected frequently, with discrete or coalesced ulcers on the exocervix. Bilateral tenderness of the inguinal lymph nodes and slight enlargement are usually present, are most apparent during the second week of the disease, and may persist as long as 1–2 months after infection. Lymph nodes do not become suppurative as in *Haemophilus ducreyi* infection. About one-third of patients show systemic symptoms such as fever, malaise, and myalgia, and 10% develop aseptic meningitis with neck ridigity and severe headache. Other complications include herpetic pharyngitis and autoinoculation of virus to other body sites, including fingers, lips, buttocks, and thighs. Bacterial superinfection is very uncommon. First episodes of disease usually abate after 20–30 days of illness.

Recurrent Infection

In contrast to primary infection, recurrent genital herpes is a disease of shorter duration, usually localized in the genital region, without systemic symptoms. One of the characteristic symptoms is prodromal paresthesia in the perineum, genitalia, or buttocks 12–24 hr before the appearance of lesions. Recurrent genital herpes usually presents with grouped vesicular lesions in the external genital region. Local symptoms such as pain and itching are mild and last for 4–5 days. The mean duration of viral shedding is 4 days, and lesions usually last for 10–14 days.

Grouped vesicular lesions on genitalia; no systemic manifestations

At least 80% of patients with primary genital HSV-2 infection develop recurrent episodes of genital herpes within 12 months. Genital HSV-1 infection appears to recur less frequently. In cases that recur, the median number of recurrences is four or five per year. They are not evenly spaced, and some patients experience a succession of monthly attacks followed by a period of quiescence. Most recurrences result from reactivation of virus from S_3–S_4 dorsal root ganglia. Rarely, recurrent infections may be due to reinfections with different strains of HSV-2.

Neonatal Herpes Infection

Acquisition from birth canal

High mortality of untreated systemic disease

The major complication of genital herpes is transmission of infection to the infant. Most herpes in the newborn is due to acquisition of disease at birth by contact with HSV-infected genital secretions. In the United States about 0.5–1% of women excrete HSV from the genital tract at the onset of labor and about 6% of infants born through infected birth canals will develop neonatal herpes. Infants appear uniquely susceptible to HSV dissemination into the central nervous system or visceral organs. Untreated, the mortality of neonatal herpes approaches 65%, and neurologic sequelae are high in those who survive. Antiviral therapy has reduced the mortality to about 10%. Women with either symptomatic or asymptomatic genital HSV infections should be followed to determine if active HSV infection or lesions are present at the time of labor. If lesions are present, cesarean delivery is indicated to avoid contact of the infant with the virus.

Diagnosis

Viral culture

Tzanck test

Although some genital HSV infections can be diagnosed clinically, the etiologic diagnosis of any genital ulceration should be determined; confirmation is best made by viral culture of the fluid from a fresh lesion. A smear prepared from the base of the lesions and treated with either Giemsa or Papanicolaou stain may show intranuclear inclusions or multinucleated giant cells typical of herpes (Tzanck test). This test is less sensitive than viral culture.

Treatment and Prevention

The antiviral agent acyclovir has been used to shorten the course of primary and recurrent episodes, but it does not affect the latent state of the virus in the dorsal nerve root ganglia. Patients with genital herpes should not have sexual activity until lesions are completely healed.

Chancroid

Painful nonindurated ulcer

Inguinal bubo may develop

Antimicrobic therapy

Chancroid, a disease caused by *H. ducreyi*, is characterized by painful genital ulcerations and suppurative inguinal adenopathy. It is common in tropical areas, although outbreaks have occurred in Canada and the United States. The classic chancroid ulcer is a superficial, exudative, ragged ulcer measuring 1–2 cm (Figure 70.1D). It is painful and tender, but nonindurated. Involvement of the inguinal lymph nodes appears rapidly and may develop into an abscess within a node (bubo), which can rupture. The differential diagnosis includes genital herpes and syphilis; some distinguishing features are listed in Table 70.3. Genital HSV lesions may be difficult to differentiate from chancroid, although inguinal adenopathy in genital herpes is usually discrete and nonsuppurative. Microbiologic diagnosis of chancroid by culture on a special selective medium should be attempted in all cases. Successful therapy has been achieved with sulfonamides, sulfonamide–trimethoprim, erythromycin, or a third-generation cephalosporin.

Lymphogranuloma Venereum

Caused by *C. trachomatis* L$_1$, L$_2$, or L$_3$ serovars

Lymphogranuloma venereum (LGV) is a sexually transmitted infection caused by *C. trachomatis* strains of the L$_1$, L$_2$, or L$_3$ serovars. The clinical course is characterized by transient genital lesions followed by multilocular

Table 70.3   Causes of Genital Ulcerations

Disease	Type of Lesion	Type of Inguinal Adenopathy[a]
Genital herpes	Multiple grouped lesions; vesicles to coalesced ulcers	Tender on palpation
Chancroid	Tender, shallow, painful, ulcerated lesion	Suppurative
Syphilis	Nontender, indurated	Rubbery consistency
Lymphogranuloma venereum	Painless, small ulceration, usually healed at time of presentation	Suppurative
Granuloma inguinale	Chronic indolent, papular lesions	"Pseudobubo" caused by induration of subcutaneous tissue in inguinal area

[a] Involvement of inguinal lymph nodes.

suppurative involvement of the inguinal lymph nodes. The primary genital lesion is usually a painless ulcer or papule, which heals in a few days and may go unnoticed. The most common presenting complaint is inguinal adenopathy. Nodes are initially discrete, but as the disease progresses they become matted and suppurative (bubos). The skin over the node may become thin and multiple draining fistulas develop. Systemic symptoms such as fever, chills, headaches, arthralgia, and myalgia are common. Late complications include urethral or rectal strictures and perirectal abscesses and fistulas. In homosexual men, LGV strains can cause a hemorrhagic ulcerative proctitis. The most satisfactory method for diagnosis is isolation of an LGV strain of *C. trachomatis* from aspirated bubos. In 80–90% of patients, the LGV complement fixation test is positive (titer of more than 1:64) shortly after the appearance of the bubo. The treatment of choice for acute LGV is tetracycline. Lymph nodes should also be aspirated to prevent rupture.

Granuloma Inguinale

Granuloma inguinale is a very uncommon disease characterized by chronic, persistent genital papules or ulcers. It is caused by *Calymmatobacterium granulomatis*, a Gram-negative bacillus morphologically and antigenically similar to *Klebsiella*. The genital ulcerations persist for months and may extend into the inguinal region. The diagnosis of granuloma inguinale is usually made by examination of impression smears from biopsy specimens of the lesion. Wright- or Giemsa-stained smears demonstrate clusters of encapsulated coccobacilli in the cytoplasm of mononuclear cells. These aggregates, called *Donovan bodies*, are considered diagnostic. *Calymmatobacterium granulomatis* has been isolated in culture using specialized media containing egg yolk. Tetracycline is the treatment of choice.

Acquired Immunodeficiency Syndrome

Acquired immunodeficiency syndrome has become a devastating and unanticipated epidemic disease, the full consequence of which will become clear with the passing years. Its disastrous course is a result of the fact

HIV attacks T4 lymphocytes and macrophages (see Chapter 73)

that the HIV virus attacks the very cells, T4 helper-inducer lymphocytes and macrophages, that are involved in the control of most viral diseases. Because of the importance of this problem it is being handled in a special chapter (Chapter 73). The basic virology of HIV is considered in Chapter 41 along with other retroviruses.

Genital Warts

Many genome types

Genital wart virus infections are caused by the human papilloma virus (HPV). There are over 50 genome types of HPV, of which types 6, 11, 16, 18, and 32 are the predominant cause of genital warts. Within the past decade, HPV infections are believed to have increased 10-fold in industrialized nations, and in most cases are sexually transmitted. Of particular concern is the epidemiologic and molecular evidence linking certain HPV types to the development of cervical carcinoma. This association is reviewed in Chapter 42.

Some types associated with carcinoma of the cervix

Two major clinical forms of genital warts exist. One manifests as easily recognized warty lesions on genital skin termed *condylomata accuminata*. The other has been recognized only recently as flat and often unrecognized condylomata of genital mucosal and/or skin surfaces. They can be detected by applying a dilute acetic acid solution to the musocal or skin surface and examining the area under 10–40× magnification. In women, HPV types 16, 18, and 31 are usually associated with these flat or subclinical warts and are the viral types commonly associated with cervical dysplasias, carcinoma in situ, or invasive cervical cancer.

Warty condylomata accuminata

Flat lesions due to the HPV types associated with cervical dysplasia

Perinatal transmission of HPV infection to infants may also occur occasionally and be manifested by the development of laryngeal papillomas in the infant. These lesions are usually due to HPV types 6 and 11.

Treatment is primarily ablative

Current treatment of HPV is undergoing modification, but at present is mainly designed to destroy or remove the affected epithelium. Recurrences are common due to survival of virus in the basal layers of the epithelium. Systemic and local interferon therapy has shown some promise as a treatment.

Other Specific Diseases

Several specific skin diseases may be acquired by sexual contact, including scabies and pubic louse infestation. Details should be sought in textbooks of dermatology or venereology.

Clinical Syndromes of Multiple Etiology

Nongonococcal urethritis, cervicitis, epididymitis, vaginitis, and PID may have multiple etiologies. The range of known infecting organisms is shown in Table 70.1, and the clinical manifestations are discussed below.

Nongonococcal Urethritis

The terms *nongonococcal urethritis* (NGU) and *postgonococcal urethritis* are used to describe cases not attributable to infection by *N. gonorrhoeae*. Patients present with dysuria and/or urethral discharge. In men, urethritis is established when purulent exudate is produced by milking the urethra from the base of the penis to the meatus. In the absence of expressible discharge, the presence of polymorphonuclear leukocytes in a urine sediment or on a urethral swab suggests urethritis.

C. trachomatis

U. urealyticum and HSV

The major cause of NGU is *C. trachomatis*, which accounts for 30–50% of cases. *Ureaplasma urealyticum* appears to be responsible for an additional 30% of cases. Herpes simplex virus has been implicated as the etiologic agent in about 2% of cases. About one-fourth of all cases have no established etiology; response to tetracycline therapy in some of these cases, however, indicates that an infectious etiology is likely.

NGU is now much more common than gonorrhea

The age distribution of patients with NGU is similar to that of patients with gonococcal urethritis, but the ratio of NGU to gonorrhea is highest for individuals of high socioeconomic status. In most Western industrialized nations, NGU is now three times as common in men as gonococcal urethritis, possibly because treatment of sexual contacts of patients with NGU is not generally emphasized. This finding may also explain why cervical infection with *C. trachomatis* has been found to be several times more common than gonococcal infection in most population studies.

Clinical manifestations similar to gonorrhea, but usually less urethral discharge

Clinical signs and symptoms of NGU are similar to those of *N. gonorrhoeae* infection. Patients present with urethral discharge, dysuria, and meatal swelling. There tends to be less urethral discharge with NGU than with gonococcal urethritis, but the diseases cannot be differentiated clinically in the individual patient. Gram stain of urethral exudate in the untreated patient with NGU demonstrates the presence of neutrophils, but not the Gram-negative intracellular gonococci seen in gonorrhea. Where available, specific cultural diagnosis of *C. trachomatis*, *U. urealyticum*, or HSV can be attempted. In practice, most patients in whom smear and cultured results are negative for gonococci are treated empirically without a specific etiologic diagnosis.

Therapy

Chlamydial postgonococcal urethritis

Tetracycline is usually effective, but approximately one-third of patients with nonchlamydial NGU fail to respond or have recurrences after treatment. Some are caused by tetracycline-resistant strains of *U. urealyticum*, but others may be related to HSV or unknown pathogens. Alternative drugs include erythromycin or a combination of spectinomycin and a sulfonamide. Postgonococcal urethritis appears in men 2–3 weeks after curative penicillin treatment of gonorrhea. It is usually due to *C. trachomatis* infection that was acquired simultaneously with gonorrhea, but which has a much longer incubation period. Penicillin therapy cures only the *N. gonorrhoeae* component of this mixed infection.

Epididymitis

Gonococcal and chlamydial infection in young men

Enterobacterial and S. epidermidis infection commoner in older men

Unilateral swelling of the epididymis is a common clinical illness seen in sexually active men. It is usually quite painful, with fever and acute unilateral swelling of the testicle that is sometimes confused with testicular torsion. In the preantibiotic era, approximately 10–15% of untreated gonococcal infections resulted in epididymitis. In developed countries, the two most common causes of epididymitis are *N. gonorrhoeae* and *C. trachomatis*. In men over 35 years of age and in homosexual men, *Enterobacteriaceae* and *S. epidermidis* may also cause the disease, probably from reflux of infected urine into the epididymis. This condition is often associated with obstruction by the prostate gland. Treatment depends on demonstration of the etiologic agent in urethral specimens or epididymal aspirates.

Cervicitis

Gonococcal, chlamydial, and HSV infections most common

The microbial etiology of cervical infections is varied; *N. gonorrhoeae* and *C. trachomatis* cause endocervicitis, and HSV can infect the stratified squamous epithelium of the ectocervix. The major clinical manifestation of cervicitis is a mucopurulent vaginal discharge. The cervix is friable and inflamed, and polymorphonuclear leukocytes are present in the exudate. Viral, chlamydial, and gonococcal cultures are needed to demonstrate the etiologic agent. Occasionally, other pathogens such as cytomegalovirus and *Trichomonas vaginalis* are associated with symptomatic cervicitis. Therapy depends on the etiologic agent involved.

Vaginitis and Vaginal Discharge

Symptomatic vaginal discharge may accompany salpingitis, endometritis, cervicitis, or a simple vaginitis. Evaluation includes pelvic examination, cervical cultures for *N. gonorrhoeae* and *Chlamydia trachomatis*, and microscopic examination of the discharge. Measurement of the pH of the discharge may also be helpful. Pelvic examination is valuable in determining whether uterine, adnexal, or cervical tenderness is present and whether the source of the discharge is the cervix or the vagina.

Candida vaginitis

The clinical and laboratory findings vary with the etiologic agent. *Candida albicans* generally produces a vulvovaginitis associated with pruritis and erythema of the vulvar area and a discharge with the consistency of cottage cheese. Microscopic demonstration of yeast and pseudomycelia in a potassium hydroxide preparation of the exudate confirms the diagnosis. *Candida* vaginitis can be treated with local nystatin or with miconazole.

Trichomonas infection

Trichomonas vaginalis typically produces a foamy, purulent vaginal discharge. The pH is variable (usually greater than 5.0), and numerous polymorphonuclear cells and motile trichomonads will be seen on a wet mount examination. Metronidazole is effective therapy for *T. vaginalis* vaginitis. Sexual partners should also be treated.

Bacterial vaginosis associated with anaerobic overgrowth

Bacterial vaginosis (BV), previously termed *nonspecific vaginitis*, is the commonest form of vaginitis in women. BV is associated with overgrowth of the vaginal anaerobic flora, a high concentration of a small Gram-negative rod (*Gardnerella vaginalis*) in the vagina, and a number of other organisms. At one time *G. vaginalis* was believed to be the cause of the disease, but it is now clear that it is probably of multiple etiology and more a result of disturbance in anaerobic flora than of any specific organism.

Clue cells in bacterial vaginosis

The vaginal discharge of BV is yellowish, homogenous, and adherent to the vaginal wall. The pH is greater than 5.0. Addition of KOH to the vaginal secretions produces a fishy smell as a result of volatilization of amines. The Gram stain shows a shift from the usual lactobacillary flora to one of many Gram-negative coccobacilli. Clue cells, which are vaginal epithelial cells heavily coated with *G. vaginalis*, may also be seen.

Metronidazole treatment

Metronidazole is the most effective agent in treatment, although ampicillin will also be successful in 70% of cases. Relapses are common. It is uncertain whether treatment of sexual partners has any effect on the remission rate.

Pelvic Inflammatory Disease

Multiple etiologies; *N. gonorrhoeae* predominant

Clinical manifestations of PID vary, but generally include lower abdominal pain elicited by movement of the cervix or palpation of the adnexal or endometrial areas. In most clinical studies, about one-half of all cases of PID are caused by *N. gonorrhoeae*. Nongonococcal PID has a complex and sometimes polymicrobial etiology, including *C. trachomatis*, *Bacteroides*, anaerobic streptococci, and *Mycoplasma hominis* alone or in various combinations. In general, nongonococcal PID is milder than that associated

Higher incidence with use of intrauterine devices

with *N. gonorrhoeae* infection. The incidence of PID is 5–10 times higher in women with intrauterine devices than in those not using this form of contraception. The diagnosis is established most reliably by culture of peritoneal aspirates from the vaginal cul-de-sac.

Additional Reading

Holmes, K.K., Mardh, P.A., Sparling, F., et al, eds. 1989. *Sexually Transmitted Diseases*. New York: McGraw-Hill. 2nd ed. This treatise on sexually transmitted diseases is the definitive textbook on the subject.

Sexually Transmitted Disease Treatment Guidelines. 1989. *Morbid. Mortal. Weekly Rep. Suppl.* 38(S-8). Details of recommended therapy are provided.

71

Infections in the Immunocompromised Patient

Lawrence Corey

Immunocompromised patients are those with some disorder or deficit in host defense mechanisms that predisposes them to increased frequency and morbidity or infections. Many such infections are caused by organisms that are members of the normal flora in health; they gain the ability to infect because of disruptions or disorders of the skin or mucosal barriers, neutropenia (shortage of neutrophils), impairment of phagocyte chemotaxis or intraphagocytic killing, and defects in antibody production or cell-mediated immunity. An immunocompromised state may result from trauma, the use of cytotoxic or immunosuppressive therapeutic agents, or genetic abnormalities, or it may be acquired as, for example, in acquired immunodeficiency syndrome (Chapter 73).

In evaluating nontraumatic defects in host defenses, it is useful to categorize them as 1) defects in nonspecific immune responses (for example, the phagocytic response); 2) defects in the complement system; 3) defects in antibody-mediated immunity; and 4) defects in cell-mediated immunity. Each of these tends to be associated with infections caused by specific groups of organisms (Table 71.1 and appendix). For example, neutropenia and disorders of phagocytosis are often associated with infections by Gram-positive cocci, Enterobacteriaceae and *Pseudomonas*, and sometimes fungi. In contrast, patients with defects in cell-mediated immunity tend to have severe viral, parasitic, and fungal infections or disease caused by bacteria that can multiply intracellularly (for example, mycobacteria). Those with defects in antibody production, such as agammaglobulinemia, are prone to infection with encapsulated organisms such as *Streptococcus pneumoniae* and *Haemophilus influenzae*.

In many immunosuppressed patients, several specific deficits in host defense mechanisms may be present concurrently. For example, cytotoxic drugs and glucocorticoids may impair phagocytosis, cell-mediated immunity, and humoral immunity and cause ulcerations of mucosal barriers, particularly of the oropharynx and gastrointestinal tract. Such patients are

Different types of immunocompromise are associated with different infecting organisms

Combined immune defects often are present

Table 71.1   Infections in the Compromised Host

Type of Compromise	Examples	Pathogens
↓ Leukocyte number or functions	Myelocytic leukemias Chronic granulomatous disease Granulocytopenia Acidosis Burns	Extracellular bacteria[a] Opportunistic fungi
↓ Humoral immune response	Lymphocytic leukemias Multiple myeloma Nephrosis Antimetabolites Hypogammaglobulinemia Children with AIDS	Encapsulated and other extracellular bacteria[a] Enteroviruses *Pneumocystis* *Giardia*[b]
↓ Complement deficits	Genetic deficiencies	Extracellular bacteria[a] *Neisseria*[c]
↓ Cellular immune response	Hodgkin's disease Steroids Uremia Antimetabolites Malnutrition AIDS	Intracellular bacteria[d] *Nocardia* *Candida* and fungi of systemic mycoses Most viruses *Pneumocystis* Protozoa[e] *Strongyloides*
↓ Reticuloendothelial system function	Splenectomy Chronic hemolysis	*Pneumococci* *Salmonella* *Listeria*

Abbreviations: AIDS = acquired immunodeficiency syndrome.
[a] Bacteria that are unable to multiply in phagocytes.
[b] Associated with IgA deficiency.
[c] Associated with C5, C6, C7, and C8 deficiencies.
[d] Bacteria capable of multiplying in unactivated macrophage.
[e] Includes *Toxoplasma* and *Cryptosporidium*.

susceptible to the range of organisms associated with each of the individual deficits.

Defects in Epithelial Barriers

Defects in mucosal barriers allow access to the tissue by organisms that normally colonize the skin, gastrointestinal tract, or upper airway. Burns, extensive trauma, or decubitus ulcers remove the epithelial defense of the skin; however, less obvious factors, such as inhalation of toxic materials and immunosuppressive therapy, may cause the damage to mucosal surfaces that predisposes to attachment and replication of potentially pathogenic organisms and can cause loss of host clearing mechanisms (for example, ciliary function). Defects in intestinal mucosal barriers are often associated with infections caused by Gram-negative aerobic and anaerobic enteric bacteria from the gut flora. Staphylococcal, streptococcal, or pneumococcal infections of the lung are particularly likely when the respiratory epithelium is damaged, whereas *Pseudomonas aeruginosa* infections are a common feature of severe burns. Bacteremia is a common complication of severe infections of these types.

Table 71.2   Disorders of Phagocytosis and Intracellular Phagocytic Killing

Chemotactic Defects	*Ingestion*
Complement component deficiency	Actin-myosin dysfunction
Immunoglobulin deficiency	Drugs (colchicine, tetracycline, cyclophosphamide)
Intrinsic defects	Hyperosmolar states
"Lazy leukocytes"	Acute infections
Burns	*Degranulation*
Hyperimmunoglobulin syndrome (Job's syndrome)	Chédiak-Higashi syndrome
Collagen vascular disease	
Opsonization	*Killing*
Immunoglobulin deficiency	Lysosomal enzyme deficiency
Complement component deficiency	Chronic granulomatous disease
Interference by immune complexes (system lupus erythematosus)	Glucose-6-phosphate dehydrogenase deficiency
Inhibition by drugs	Drugs (phenylbutazone, chloramphenicol)
Sickle cell anemia	Glutathione reductase deficiency

Defects in Numbers or Functions of Phagocytes

When the natural barriers of the skin and mucosal surfaces are breached, the next major line of defense is the circulating phagocyte. To defend against infection, there must be an adequate number of these cells, which must be able to move to the site of infection and ingest and kill invading organisms. Numerous defects in these processes have been described.

Neutropenia

Causes and significance of neutropenia

Although normal neutrophil granulocyte counts vary greatly according to the age, sex, and race of the patient, the usual value is 2500–7500 cells/ mm³ of blood in adults. Neutropenia may result from inherited or acquired diseases, use of cytotoxic drugs, or adverse reactions to therapeutic agents such as chloramphenicol. If the neutrophil count decreases to less than 500 cells/mm³, especially less than 100 cells/mm³, the incidence of in-

Neutropenia associated infections

fections increases markedly. Severe neutropenia is accompanied most frequently by bacterial infections caused by the pyogenic Gram-positive cocci, Enterobacteriaceae, *P. aeruginosa*, and *H. influenzae*. Fungal infections with *Candida, Aspergillus*, or the Phycomycetes are also common.

Defects in Chemotaxis and Leukocytic Function

Inadequate function or failure of chemotaxis

Occasionally, defects in phagocytic defenses are caused by inadequate leukocyte chemotaxis or function (Table 71.2). Deficiencies of complement or immunoglobulins can decrease chemoattractants at the site of an infection, and certain metabolic diseases such as diabetes and uremia can alter the microenvironment of leukocytes to reduce their mobility and responsiveness to tactic stimuli. This phenomenon has also been shown to occur in immune complex diseases such as lupus erythematosus. In each case, removal of the leukocyte to a normal environment restores its mobility and ability to respond chemotactically.

Several genetic diseases produce specific defects in granulocyte bactericidal mechanisms that result in an immunocompromised host. Because they frequently diminish life span, these illnesses are usually seen in children. That most studied is chronic granulomatous disease, an X-linked disease of childhood associated with frequent pyogenic infections, usually caused by *Staphylococcus aureus*. The basic deficit is an inability to generate superoxide in phagocytes. In another disease, the Chédiak-Higashi syndrome, neutrophil lysosomes fail to fuse with the phagosome and the cells fail to destroy ingested organisms. These children also suffer recurrent infections with pyogenic organisms.

> **Chronic granulomatous disease due to lack of superoxide production**
>
> **Chédiak-Higashi disease; failure lysosome–phagosome fusion**

The spectrum of infections in patients with phagocytic dysfunction is wide and includes repeated bouts of cellulitis, pharyngitis, perirectal and other abscesses, pneumonia, osteomyelitis, and bacteremia. Many pyogenic organisms other than staphylococci can be involved. Antimicrobic treatment given either therapeutically or prophylactically has helped greatly in the care of these patients, but they still suffer repeated bouts of infection that may ultimately prove fatal. Techniques have been developed to allow rapid collection and transfusion of functioning leukocytes in sufficient numbers to benefit some patients. Recent evidence suggests that recombinant gamma interferon may also be of benefit for patients with chronic granulomatous disease.

> **Sites and causes of infection with phagocyte dysfunction**

Defects in Humoral and Cell-Mediated Immunity

Antibody Deficiency

Several congenital and acquired disorders can lead to inadequate synthesis of immunoglobulins as a result of deficiency or dysfunction of B lymphocytes. The most common and least serious is immunoglobulin A deficiency, which is associated with increased risk of gastrointestinal tract infection, especially with the parasite *Giardia lamblia*. Individuals with severe defects in IgG and IgM production (hypogammaglobulinemia or agammaglobulinemia) are prone to recurrent infections with encapsulated organisms such as *S. pneumoniae* or *H. influenzae*, which require opsonization for adequate phagocytosis (Chapter 10). Sinusitis, otitis media, bacterial pneumonia, and bacteremia are the most common types of infection. Selective deficiency in immunoglobulin production may also occur in multiple myeloma and certain types of chronic lymphocytic leukemia that involve monoclonal proliferation of one immunoglobulin-producing cell line and relative deficiencies of cells producing other antibodies. These patients are also prone to infections by systemically invasive organisms.

> **IgA deficiency and giardiasis**
>
> **IgG and IgM deficiency and susceptibility to encapsulated organisms**
>
> **Antibody deficiency in multiple myeloma and lymphocytic leukemia**

Repeated injections of immunoglobulins (immune serum globulin) may decrease the incidence and morbidity of infections in patients with agammaglobulinemia. In those capable of some immune responses, the use of pneumococcal vaccine may provide a degree of protection against overwhelming infection with this organism.

> **Treatment with immune serum globulin**
>
> **Use of pneumococcal vaccine**

Complement Deficiency

Defects of the complement system also predispose the patient to many infections. Individuals with deficiencies in C3 are prone to infections with encapsulated organisms that require opsonization and to a range of in-

> **Opsonization defects with C3 deficiency**

fections similar to those seen in patients with hypogammaglobulinemia. Those with deficiencies in later components are prone to develop recurrent bacteremia caused by *Neisseria meningitidis* or *Neisseria gonorrhoeae* if they are infected with these species. Patients with defects in the early complement components, C1, C2, or C4, have less of a problem than those with later complement deficiencies, because they retain the ability to utilize the alternative complement pathway to activate C3 and hence C5–C9.

Systemic Neisseria infections in C5–8 deficiencies

Most serious defects involve both classic and alternative pathways

Disorders in Cell-Mediated Immunity

Cell-mediated immunity is the part of the immune system that involves previously sensitized thymus-derived lymphocytes and is independent of circulating antibody. Both congenital and acquired abnormalities of the cell-mediated immune system are possible. Congenital abnormalities, which are uncommon, include thymic dysplasia syndrome, ataxia telangiectasia, and severe combined immunodeficiency (both T- and B-cell deficiency). A much more common defect develops in patients on treatment with immunosuppressive or cytotoxic agents that damage both macrophage precursors and T lymphocytes. Cytotoxic chemotherapy for cancer with cyclophosphamide and other antimetabolites has these effects and also inhibits humoral immune responses. Glucocorticoids can have multiple effects, causing neutropenia, lymphopenia, and monocytopenia through suppression of cell production, inhibition of mobilization of neutrophils to the site of inflammation, and interference with cell-mediated immune responses by altering the responsiveness of monocytes and macrophages to lymphokines. In addition, glucocorticoids impair the function of cells lining the mucosal surfaces, thus increasing the chance of microbial invasion by this route. Combinations of glucocorticosteroids and immunosuppressive drugs are essential in the treatment of certain diseases, but are particularly likely to interfere with the ability of a patient to combat new or established infections.

Rare congenital abnormalities

Effects of immunosuppressive or cytotoxic drugs on T cells and macrophages

Multiple effects of glucocorticoids

A detailed analysis of the infections associated with the different causes of cell-mediated and combined immune deficits is beyond the scope of this chapter. In general, defects in cell-mediated immunity are associated with increased susceptibility to infection with some opportunistic pathogens, particularly facultative or obligate intracellular pathogens (appendix). Because of the wide range of potential infecting organisms, the sites of infection associated with defects in cell-mediated immunity are varied. They include superficial skin infections, lung infections, pharyngitis, otitis, sinusitis, bacteremia, and abscesses. Infections with multiple organisms are common. Clinical recognition and treatment of these infections is often difficult, because they may be relatively silent. Laboratory diagnosis can also be difficult, because many of the organisms listed in the appendix require special culture media and grow slowly; others cannot be grown at all. It must be remembered that colonization of a peripheral site by an opportunistic organism does not necessarily mean that it is the cause of invasive disease. Thus, isolation of *Candida albicans* from the urine or the pharynx does not indicate that it is the cause of a concurrent renal abscess pneumonitis. Diagnostic procedures such as biopsy of involved organs are often needed to identify the causative agent.

Increased susceptibility to intracellular pathogens

Difficulties in clinical and laboratory diagnosis of infections

Attempts to enhance cell-mediated immune responses specifically or nonspecifically with agents that have shown some activity in animals generally have had little if any effect in reducing the frequency and severity of opportunistic infections in humans. Transfer factor has been used with

Attempts to enhance deficient cell-mediated immunity

limited success. It is a substance of low molecular weight secreted by circulating lymphocytes that can passively transfer delayed hypersensitivity to nonreactive individuals. Clinical trials with recombinant interferon gamma and interleukin 2 are currently under way.

Treatment of Infections in Immunocompromised Patients

Successful treatment of infections in the compromised host depends on recognition of the deficit, early diagnosis, and prompt intervention. This requires recognition of the organisms most likely to be involved in the infection and is urgent in the case of classes of bacteria with short generation times. The index of suspicion must be very high, because the signs and symptoms of infection that are seen in immunocompetent individuals may be lacking. For example, in neutropenia the clinical signs of infection and even of abscess formation may not be apparent when the patient is first seen because of lack of reaction to the disease. It is thus usually necessary to initiate microbic treatment before results of culture and antibiotic susceptibility tests are available. Broad-spectrum antimicrobic coverage is used initially and replaced with narrower-spectrum agents, when the etiologic agent and its susceptibility are known, to reduce the risk of superinfection. In general, bactericidal antimicrobics are needed to control infections when host defenses are inadequate, and with severe infections a combination of synergistic agents may be necessary to provide increased bactericidal action.

Patients with neutropenia have high rates of infection, and mortality may be as high as 20–30% if bacteremia develops. Therefore, short-term prophylactic antibiotic treatment has been advocated for these cases and can be effective in preventing infection until the neutrophil count improves. Selection of resistant organisms and "breakthrough" bacteremia as a result of overwhelming infection are major risks in these susceptible patients, and the physician must be alert to the possibility of superinfection with other pathogens during treatment.

Need for early diagnosis and treatment

Use of bactericidal agents

Antimicrobic prophylaxis in neutropenia

Problems of resistance and superinfection during prophylaxis

Additional Reading

Rubin, R.H., and Young, L.S., Eds. 1988. *Clinical Approach to Infection in the Compromised Host.* 2nd ed. New York: Plenum Press. Highly recommended for further reading and as a source of references.

Appendix 71.1 Agents Commonly Infecting Immunocompromised Patients

Agent	Decreased Phagocytosis	Complement Deficiencies	Hypo- or Agamma-globulinemia	Defects in Cell-Mediated Immunity
Bacteria				
Staphylococcus aureus and β-hemolytic streptococci	+ + +	+ +	+ +	
Streptococcus pneumoniae	+ + +	+	+ + +	
Enterobacteriaceae	+ + +	+	+	
Pseudomonas aeruginosa	+ + +	+ +	+	
Haemophilus influenzae	+	+	+ + +	
Salmonella species	+	+		+ + +
Listeria monocytogenes				+ + +
Mycobacterium species				+ + +
Legionella				+ + +
Nocardia asteroides				+ + +
Neisseria species		+ +	+	
Fungi				
Candida species Systemic	+ +			
Chronic mucocutaneous				+ + +
Aspergillus species	+ + +			
Phycomyces species	+ + +			
Cryptococcus neoformans				+ + +
Coccidioides immitis				+ + +
Histoplasma capsulatum				+ + +
Viruses				
Herpes simplex			+	+ + +
Varicella–zoster			+ +	+ + +
Cytomegalovirus				+ + +
Epstein-Barr				+ + +
Papovaviruses				+ +
Enteroviruses			+ + +	
Hepatitis B				+ + +
Influenza			+	+
Adenoviruses			+	+ + +
Parasites				
Pneumocystis carinii[a]			+ +	+ + +
Giardia lamblia			+ +	+
Toxoplasma gondii				+ + +
Stronglyoides sterocoralis				+ + +
Cryptosporidium				+ + +

Note: Number of pluses indicates relative susceptibility to the organisms listed according to the immune deficits.
[a] *Pneumocystic carinii* may be a fungus.

72

Nosocomial Infections and Hospital Infection Control

Kenneth J. Ryan

Nosocomial is a medical term for hospital associated. Nosocomial infections are those that arise during hospitalization as a complication of another illness. The purpose of hospital infection control is prevention of nosocomial infections by application of epidemiologic concepts and methods.

The shining example of the fundamental importance of epidemiology in detection and control of nosocomial infections is the work of Ignaz Semmelweis, between 1847 and 1849, which preceded the microbiologic discoveries of Pasteur and Koch. His recognition, definition, and solution of the problem of childbed (puerperal) fever will be outlined as much as an example of still-valid epidemiology as for its historic importance.

Semmelweis and control of childbed fever

Semmelweis was assistant obstetrician at the Vienna General Hospital, where more than 7000 infants were delivered each year. Childbed fever (puerperal endometritis), which we now know was caused primarily by *Streptococcus pyogenes* (group A), was a major problem accounting for 600–800 maternal deaths per year. By careful review of hospital statistics, Semmelweis clearly showed that the death rate in one of the two divisions of the hospital was 10 times that in the other. Division I, which had the high mortality, was the teaching unit in which all deliveries were by obstetricians and students. In Division II, all deliveries were by midwives. No similar epidemic existed elsewhere in the city of Vienna. Mortality was very low in mothers delivering at home.

Semmelweis postulated that the key difference between Divisions I and II was participation of the physicians and students in autopsies. One or more cadavers were dissected daily, some from cases of childbed fever and other infections. Hand washing was perfunctory, which Semmelweis believed to allow the transmission of "invisible cadaver particles" by direct contact between the mother and the physician's hands during examinations and delivery. In 1847, as a countermeasure, he required hand washing with a chlorine solution until the hands were slippery and the odor of the cadaver was gone. The results were dramatic. The full effect of the chlorine

Demonstration of critical importance of hand washing in infection control

Table 72.1 Childbed Fever at the Vienna General Hospital

Year	Division I (Teaching Unit)			Division II (Midwife Unit)		
	Births	Maternal Deaths	Per- centage	Births	Maternal Deaths	Per- centage
1846[a]	4010	459	11.4	3754	105	2.7
1848[b]	3556	45	1.3	3219	43	1.3

[a] No hand washing.
[b] First full year of chlorine hand washing.

hand washing can be seen by comparing mortality in the two divisions for 1846 and 1848 (Table 72.1). The mortality in Division I was reduced to that of Division II, and both were below 2%.

Unfortunately, because of his personality and failure to publish his work until 1860, Semmelweis' contribution was not generally appreciated in his lifetime. As his frustration mounted over lack of acceptance of his ideas, he became abusive and irrational, eventually alienating even his early supporters. Some believe that he also suffered from presenile dementia (Alzheimer's disease). He died in an insane asylum in 1865, unaware that his concept of spread via direct contact would later be recognized as the most important mechanism of nosocomial infection and that hand washing would remain the most important means of infection control in hospitals.

Nosocomial Infections

Definitions of nosocomial infections

Infections associated with any hospitalization may be divided into two categories, community acquired and nosocomial. The Centers for Disease Control (CDC) in Atlanta defines community infections as those present or incubating at the time of hospital admission. All others are considered nosocomial, including those that appear within 14 days of hospital discharge. For example, a case of chickenpox erupting on the fifth hospital day would be classified as community acquired (incubating), but the same infection would be nosocomial if the patient had been in the hospital beyond the limits of the known incubation period (20 days). A staphylococcal skin infection appearing 12 days after discharge would be called nosocomial despite the distinct possibility that it was acquired at home. The purpose is to identify all infections that are truly a complication of hospitalization, at the risk of including a few others that were acquired

Special infection hazards to hospitalized patients

elsewhere. It is important to recognize the peculiar infection hazards posed by the hospital: it is there that the most seriously infected and most susceptible patients are housed and often cared for by the same staff. Antimicrobic therapy, by reducing competing flora, may create a predisposition to hospital-acquired infection often with resistant organisms.

Sources

Endogenous infections

The infectious agents responsible for nosocomial infections arise from various sources. Many are endogenous, originating from the patient's own normal flora. The factors involved in the pathogenesis of such infections are essentially the same in or out of the hospital. They include any debilitating disease plus the additional risks imposed by treatments that breach the normal defense barriers. Surgery, urinary or intravenous catheters, and invasive diagnostic procedures all may provide normal flora

Exogenous infections

with access routes to usually sterile sites. The risk of infection is generally related to the extent of the trauma and the severity of the underlying illness. Minimizing or controlling both is the primary preventive measure. Of particular concern in infection control are nosocomial infections in which the source of organisms is the hospital rather than the patient. These sources include hospital personnel, the environment, and medical equipment.

Hospital cross-infection routes

Dangers of infected medical attendants

Infection from carriers

Hospital Personnel.   Physicians, nurses, students, therapists, and any others who come in contact with the patient may transmit infection. Transmission of an organism causing infection in one patient to another patient is called *cross-infection.* The vehicle of transmission is most often the inadequately washed hands of a medical attendant. Another source is the infected medical attendant. Many hospital outbreaks have been traced to hospital personnel, particularly physicians, who continue to care for patients despite an overt infection. Transmission is usually by direct contact, although airborne transmission is also possible. A third source is the person who is not ill but is carrying a virulent strain. *Staphylococcus aureus* and group A streptococcal infections are those in which carriers are most frequently involved. Nasal carriage is most important, but sites such as the perineum and anus have also been involved in outbreaks. An occult carrier is less often the source of nosocomial infection than a physician covering up a boil or a nurse minimizing "the flu." The carrier is difficult to detect unless the epidemic strain has distinctive characteristics or the epidemiologic circumstances indicate a single person.

Environmental contamination least important source

Environmental Sources.   The hospital air, walls, floors, linens, and the like are not sterile and thus could serve as a source of organisms causing nosocomial infections, but importance of this route of infection has generally been exaggerated. With the exception of the immediately vicinity of an infected individual or a carrier, transmission through the air or on fomites is much less important than that caused by personnel or equipment. Exceptions are instances in which organisms are numerous and patients particularly susceptible or when a particular site is unusually vulnerable (valvular heart surgery).

Infection from equipment that crosses epithelial or other defenses

Medical Devices.   Much of the success of modern medicine is related to medical devices that support or monitor basic body functions. By their very nature, devices such as catheters and respirators carry a risk of nosocomial infection, because they bypass normal defense barriers, providing microorganisms access to normally sterile fluids and tissues. Most of the recognized causes are bacterial or fungal. The risk of infection is related to the degree of debilitation of the patient and various factors concerning the design and management of the device.

Any device that crosses the skin or a mucosal barrier will allow flora in the patient or environment to gain access to deeper sites around the outside surface. Possible access inside the device (for example, in the lumen) adds another and sometimes greater risk. In some devices, such as urinary catheters, contamination is avoidable; in others, such as respirators, complete sterility is either impossible or impractical to achieve.

Bacterial growth in moist environment

The risk of contamination leading to infection is increased if the organisms can multiply within the system. This process requires moisture, because no bacteria or fungi will grow in a totally dry system. The nutrient content and temperature of the available fluid largely determine which organism will survive and multiply. In general, Gram-positive bacteria such as staphylococci require near-physiologic fluid, whereas many of the Gram-negative rods are much less demanding. Once organisms such as *Pseudomonas, Acinetobacter*, and members of the Enterobacteriaceae gain access, they can frequently multiply in an environment containing water and little else.

Even with proper growth conditions, many hours are required before contaminating organisms become numerous. Detailed studies of catheters and similar devices show the risk of infection begins to increase after 24–48 hr and is cumulative even if the device is changed or disinfected at intervals. It is thus important to discontinue transcutaneous procedures as soon as medically indicated.

Need to remove transcutaneous and urethral devices as soon as possible

The medical devices most frequently associated with nosocomial infections are listed below. The infectious risk of others can be estimated from the principles discussed previously. New devices are constantly being introduced into medical care, occasionally without adequate consideration of their potential to cause nosocomial infection.

Urinary Catheters. The infectious risk of a single urinary catheterization has been estimated at 1–5%. Indwelling catheters carry a risk that may be as high as 10% for each day the catheter is in place. The major preventive measure is maintenance of a completely closed system through the use of valves and aspiration ports designed to prevent bacterial access to the inside of the catheter or collecting bag. The urine itself serves as an excellent culture medium once contamination occurs.

Closed urinary drainage systems

Vascular Catheters. Needles and plastic catheters placed in veins (or, less often, in arteries) for fluid administration, monitoring vital functions, or diagnostic procedures are a leading cause of nosocomial bacteremia. These sites should always be suspected as a source of organisms whenever blood cultures are positive with no apparent primary site for the bacteremia. Contamination may originate from the skin flora with growth in the catheter tip or somewhere in the lines, valves, bags, or bottles of intravenous solutions proximal to the insertion site. The latter circumstance usually involves Gram-negative rods, whereas infections originating from the catheter tip are predominantly staphylococcal. Preventive measures include aseptic insertion technique and appropriate care of the lines, including changes at regular intervals.

Sources of intravenous contamination from medical devices

Respirators. Machines that assist or control respiration by pumping air directly into the trachea have a great potential for infection if the aerosol they deliver becomes contaminated. Bacterial growth is significant only in the parts of the system that contain water; in systems using nebulizers, bacteria can be suspended in water droplets small enough to reach the alveoli. This combination of circumstances has been documented as a cause of lung infection when large numbers of Gram-negative rods contaminate the respirator aerosol. These organisms include *Pseudomonas*, Enterobacteriaceae, and a wide variety of environmental bacteria such as *Acinetobacter, Flavobacter*, and *Alcaligenes*. The primary control measure is periodic disinfection of the tubing, reservoirs, and nebulizer jets. Studies of contamination indicate that equipment should be changed every 24–48 hr.

Nebulizer contamination

Hemodialysis. Bacterial infections of shunts and cannulas, a possible complication of chronic hemodialysis, are generally similar in origin to other infections arising from catheterization. Contamination of the dialysis fluid or artificial kidney is now an uncommon problem, but remains possible

Table 72.2 Nosocomial Infection Rates, Frequencies, and Most Common Pathogens

Infection	Infections/10,000 Hospital Discharges[a,b]	Percentage of All Nosocomial Infections[b]	Most Common Pathogens
Primary bacteremia[a]	7–30	3–7	*Staphylococcus aureus; Escherichia coli; Klebsiella*
Surgical wound	52–98	18–27	*Staphylococcus aureus; Escherichia coli*
Lower respiratory tract	35–72	14–18	*Klebsiella; Staphylococcus aureus; Pseudomonas aeruginosa*
Urinary tract	112–151	34–46	*Escherichia coli;* group D streptococci; *Pseudomonas aeruginosa*
Cutaneous	15–33	4–8	*Staphylococcus aureus*
All others	23–70	8–16	*Staphylococcus aureus; Escherichia coli*

[a] Data from 1979 National Nosocomial Infection Study, published by Centers for Disease Control in March 1982.

[b] Ranges reflect differences among community, community-teaching, federal, municipal, and university hospitals.

[c] No documented site of origin.

Risk of hepatitis B and HIV cross-infection

because the fluid contains bacterial nutrients and is maintained at body temperature. A far greater problem in hemodialysis units is the risk of transmission of hepatitis B or human immunodeficiency virus (HIV) infections as a result of the many procedural manipulations involving blood. Control requires meticulous attention to procedures that prevent direct contact with blood, such as the use of gloves and gowns. Identification of hepatitis B and HIV carriers so that they can be treated separately is very important. Most units have established serologic surveillance procedures to detect both carriers and evidence of transmission among patients and staff.

Etiologic Agents and Infection Rates

The rates and relative frequencies of the most common forms of nosocomial infection are shown in Table 72.2, together with the most common etiologic agents for each. These data are taken from the 1979 National Nosocomial Infections Study, a voluntary surveillance program directed by the CDC. Using the CDC definition of nosocomial infection, the rates in U.S. hospitals range between 0.8 and 8.9%. Most have nosocomial infection rates of 3–5%. If extrapolated to the more than 40 million persons hospitalized in the United States each year, this percentage translates to well over 1 million cases annually.

Differences in infection rates between hospitals

The ranges shown in Table 72.2 reflect differences among community, community–teaching, federal, municipal, and university hospitals. In general, the rates are lowest in community hospitals and highest in municipal and university hospitals. This finding probably reflects differences in the types of patients treated in these institutions. For example, municipal hospitals usually have a higher proportion of elderly and debilitated patients and university hospitals a higher proportion of immunosuppressed patients. Both groups are more susceptible to infection and tend to have prolonged hospital stays. Table 72.2 also shows that urinary tract infections are the most common nosocomial infections, constituting one-third to one-half of all cases. Most of these infections are associated with the use of urinary catheters.

Urinary tract infections most common

The most common pathogens isolated are *Escherichia coli* and *S. aureus*, which together account for 25–30% of nosocomial infections. Other members of the Enterobacteriaceae, group D streptococci, *Pseudomonas aeruginosa*, and *Candida* species are also common causes. In general, the organisms most resistant to antimicrobics, such as *Klebsiella, Serratia*, and *Pseudomonas*, are much more common as causes of hospital-acquired than of community-acquired infections. For example, although Table 72.2 shows *E. coli* to be the most common cause of urinary infection in the hospital, its proportion (32%), is much smaller than its share of community-acquired urinary infections, which exceeds 90%. Other organisms such as the group A streptococcus are currently uncommon, but occasionally cause outbreaks of serious infections, including puerperal fever.

Antimicrobic resistant organisms more common in hospitals

Viruses tend to be underestimated in, or excluded from, surveys of nosocomial infections, because most hospitals still lack adequate viral diagnostic laboratories. Respiratory viruses such as influenza virus and respiratory syncytial virus have been shown to spread in hospitals by droplet inhalation or direct contact. Some of the highly infectious viruses, such as varicella (chickenpox, herpes zoster) and rubella (German measles), have caused outbreaks among susceptible patients and medical staff.

Viral infections

Hepatitis B and, very occasionally, HIV viruses can be responsible for hospital-associated infections in which transmission is from patient to medical staff, rather than the reverse. The primary mechanism for transmission of both viruses in the health care setting is by blood or blood products. This may occur by contact of patient's blood with a mucosal surface or through accidents involving breaks in the skin, such as needle sticks. Transmission is much more likely with hepatitis B virus than with HIV. Prospective studies of needle stick and other events resulting in substantial contamination with HIV-positive blood have documented seroconversions, but the risk appears to be well below 0.1%. Exposure to other body fluids of acquired immunodeficiency syndrome (AIDS) patients is of theoretical concern, but has not been shown to lead to transmission of the virus in the health care setting.

Infection Control

Infection control is the sum of all the means used to prevent nosocomial infections. Historically such methods have been developed as an integral part of the study of infectious diseases, often serving as key elements in the proof of infectious etiology. Semmelweis' hand washing is the first example. Later in the 19th century, Joseph Lister achieved a dramatic reduction in surgical wound infections by infusion of a phenolic antiseptic into wounds. This local destruction of organisms was known as *antisepsis* and sometimes included liberal applications of disinfectants, including sprays to the environment. As it became recognized that contamination of wounds was not inevitable, the emphasis gradually shifted to preventing contact between microorganisms and susceptible sites, a concept called

Change from antisepsis to asepsis

asepsis. Asepsis, which utilizes the methods of sterilization and disinfection discussed in Chapter 11, is the central concept of infection control. The measures taken to achieve asepsis vary, depending on whether the circumstances and environment are most similar to the operating room, hospital ward, or outpatient clinic.

Asepsis

Surgical aseptic procedures, rituals, and attitudes

Operating Room.   The surgical suite and operating room represent the most controlled and rigid application of aseptic principles. The procedure begins with the use of an antiseptic scrub of the skin over the operative site and the hands and forearms of all who will have contact with the patient. The use of sterile drapes, gowns, and instruments serves to prevent spread through direct contact, and caps and face masks reduce airborne spread from personnel to the wound. As all students learn the first time they scrub, even the manner of dressing and moving in the operating room are rigidly specified, and those involved assume a strict aseptic attitude as well as their masks and gowns. In some hospitals the air entering the operating room is filter sterilized, but this practice is expensive and its value unproved. The level of bacteria in the air is generally more related to the number of persons and amount of movement in the operating room than to incoming air. The net effect of these procedures is to draw a sterile curtain around the operative site, thus minimizing contact with microorganisms. Surgical asepsis is also employed in other areas where invasive special procedures such as cardiac catheterization are performed.

Hospital Ward.   Although theoretically desirable, strict aseptic procedures as used in the operating room are impractical in the ward setting. Asepsis is practiced by the use of sterile needles, medications, dressings, and other items that could serve as transmission vehicles if contaminated. A "no touch" technique for examining wounds and changing dressings eliminates direct contact with any nonsterile item. Invasive procedures such as catheter insertion and lumbar punctures are done under aseptic precautions similar to those used in the operating room. In all circumstances hand washing between patient contacts is the single most important aseptic precaution.

Critical importance of hand washing

Outpatient Clinic.   The general aseptic practices used on the hospital ward are also appropriate to the outpatient situation as preventive measures. The potential for cross-infection in the clinic or waiting room is obvious, but has been little studied regarding preventive measures. Patients who may be infected should be segregated whenever possible using techniques similar to those of hospital ward isolation. The examining room may be used in a manner analogous to the private rooms on a hospital ward. This approach is difficult because of patient turnover, but should be attempted for infections that would require strict or respiratory isolation in the hospital.

Isolation Procedures

Patients with infections pose special problems, because they may transmit their infections to other patients either directly or by contact with a staff member. This additional risk is managed by the techniques of isolation, which separate the infected patient from others on the ward. The appropriate isolation techniques vary with the communicability of the infectious

Table 72.3 Category-Specific Isolation Techniques Used in Hospitals to Prevent Spread of Infection

Isolation Category	Route of Transmission Blockage	Isolation Techniques	Typical Situation
Strict	All, or on clothing or fomites	Private rooms;[a] gowns; gloves; masks; all articles[b]	Congenital rubella; chicken pox; plague (pneumonic); generalized staphylococcal infections
Respiratory	Respiratory route	Private rooms;[a] masks; contaminated articles[b]	Measles; pertussis; tuberculosis
Enteric	Contact spread from stools	Private room;[a] gowns;[c] gloves;[d] contaminated articles[b]	*Salmonella; Shigella*, hepatitis
Contact	Contact spread from lesions: infected wounds	Private room (desirable);[d] gowns;[d] gloves;[e] masks;[e]	Infected burns;[f] draining wounds[f]
Blood and body fluid	Contact spread from blood or body fluids	Private room;[f] gloves	Hepatitis or human immunodeficiency virus infections
Protective	Staff to patient	Private room;[a] masks	Agranulocytosis; extensive burns; immunosuppression

[a] Door must be closed.
[b] Articles contaminated with pus or potentially infected secretions must be wrapped or otherwise handled for future sterilization or disinfection.
[c] For those touching patient.
[d] Contact with infectious material.
[e] Wound or burn infections with *Staphylococcus aureus* or group A streptococci that cannot be easily contained by dressings require strict isolation.
[f] Poor hygiene or child.

agent and the route(s) of transmission. These criteria have been formalized into specific isolation categories recommended by the CDC for use in hospitals. The isolation categories most commonly used are listed in Table 72.3 with the general techniques required for each.

Recognition of the risk posed to health care workers by the AIDS epidemic has caused a reexamination of these category-specific isolation procedures, because there have been a number of documented transmissions of HIV to hospital personnel from patients not known to carry the virus at the time they were initially seen. Thus, limiting protective measures to known AIDS or known HIV-positive persons is no longer considered safe. This problem has been addressed by the concept of *universal precautions* in which the use of protective measures, such as gowns, gloves, and goggles, is determined solely by the probability of contact with blood

Table 72.4 Universal Precautions Used to Protect Medical and Laboratory Personnel[a,b]

Risk Level[b]	Route of Transmission	Isolation Techniques	Typical Situation
Low	None[c]	None[c]	General patient care; contact with intact skin
Moderate	Contact spread from body fluids	Gloves; gowns[d]	Blood drawing; dressing changes
High	Contact splash and aerosol spread from body fluids	Gloves; gowns; eye/face protection	Suctioning; bronchoscopy; emergency procedures; surgery

[a] When infection is present, appropriate category specific measures are added.
[b] The primary determinant is the potential risk for contact with the patient's body fluids, particularly, blood.
[c] Except hand washing (appropriate for all care).
[d] If clothes could become soiled.

or body fluids without regard to the patient's diagnosis. These are illustrated in Table 72.4. The category-specific measures are still appropriate for other infections when they include procedures not already implemented under *universal precautions*. It is the physician's responsibility to recognize the presence of infection and to institute the appropriate isolation restrictions.

Organization

Modern hospitals are required by regulatory agencies to have formal infection control programs. Although the exact arrangements vary among hospitals, all have an Infection Control Committee and some kind of epidemiology service.

The Infection Control Committee. The Infection Control Committee is composed of representatives of various medical and surgical services, as well as of pathology, hospital administration, nursing, housekeeping, food services, central supply, and other hospital departments. The chairman is usually a microbiologist, infectious disease specialist, pathologist, or some other person with a special interest in and knowledge of infection control. The committee is a policy-making and review body. The institution's infection control procedures and information on the status of nosocomial infections in the hospital are periodically reviewed by the committee. When epidemiologic circumstances warrant it, the committee may have to take drastic action such as closing a hospital unit or suspending a physician's privileges.

The Epidemiology Service. The epidemiology service is the working arm of the Infection Control Committee. Its functions are performed by one or more epidemiologists who usually have a nursing background. This work requires familiarity with clinical microbiology, epidemiology, infectious disease, hospital procedures, and immense tact. The main activities are as follows.

1. *Patient surveillance.* It is necessary to collect ongoing information about the frequency and nature of nosocomial infections in the hospital to detect deviations from the institutional or national norm. Such reviews are conducted by the epidemiologist and reported to the Infection Control Committee.

2. *Environmental surveillance.* Routine sampling of the microbial flora of the hospital (air, floors, and the like) is of no value, but programs to sample some of the medical devices known to be nosocomial hazards can be useful. The epidemiology service usually oversees such programs, although the sampling itself may be done by others.

3. *Outbreak investigation.* On-the-spot investigation of true or potential outbreaks allows early implementation of preventive measures. This activity is probably the single most important function of the epidemiology service. Suspicion of an increased number of infections may be communicated to the epidemiologist by a physician, nurse, or microbiologist or be indicated by surveillance data. An investigation must then be conducted to verify the facts and establish basic epidemiologic associations. The primary concern is cross-infection, in which a virulent organism is being transmitted from patient to patient. Solution of the problem may require additional microbiologic investigations, such as bacteriophage typing of *S. aureus.* Other circumstances may indicate the failure of ward personnel to follow an established procedure, such as aseptic care of closed-drainage urinary catheters.

4. *Education.* The epidemiology service should take the initiative in education of the hospital staff regarding infection control. This information may be imparted informally as rounds are made on hospital wards or in the course of surveillance or outbreak investigation. Formal in-service teaching sessions on subjects such as urinary catheter care, isolation procedures, and the like are also important. All hospital personnel, from housekeeping to medical staff, must be involved in continual review of infection control procedures, because the most common problem is behavioral. It cannot be stressed sufficiently that the most important procedure for preventing cross-infection is adequate hand washing between contacts with patients.

Summary

The prevention of nosocomial infections is contingent on basic and applied knowledge drawn from all parts of this book. Applied with common sense, these principles can both prevent disease and reduce the costs of medical care.

Additional Reading

Garner, J.S., and Simmons, B.P. 1983. Guideline for isolation precautions in hospitals. *Infect. Control* 4:245–325.

Centers for Disease Control. 1989. Guidelines for prevention of transmission of human immunodeficiency virus and hepatitis B virus to health-care and public safety workers. MMWR 38:S6:1–37.

The traditional category specific isolation approach and the more recent *"universal precautions"* approach are outlined in these two publications.

73

Acquired Immunodeficiency Syndrome

Lawrence Corey
and John C. Sherris

There must now be few literate people in the world who are unaware of the acquired immunodeficiency syndrome (AIDS) pandemic and of its basic features. It is caused by the human immunodeficiency viruses HIV-1 and HIV-2. These viruses disable the immune system and thus predispose to a wide range of opportunistic infections and some tumors. The viruses can also cause damage to brain cells, and the dementia that ensues is one of the most serious effects of the disease. The nature of the causative retroviruses (Chapter 41), their impact on the immune system (Chapters 8 and 41), and many of the opportunistic infections that afflict AIDS patients have been considered elsewhere in the book. The purpose of this chapter is to give a broader overview of AIDS and associated syndromes and to consider the epidemiology, diagnosis, and treatment of HIV infection and the possibilities for control in the future.

Historical Background

AIDS first recognized in 1981

The AIDS syndrome was first recognized in the United States in 1981, when it became apparent that an unusual number of rare skin cancers (Kaposi's sarcoma) and opportunistic infections were occurring among male homosexuals. These patients were found to have a marked reduction in T4 lymphocytes carrying the CD4 marker and were subject to a wide range of opportunistic infections normally controlled by an intact immune system. The disease was found to progress relentlessly to a fatal outcome and was first identified in male homosexuals, hemophiliacs who were receiving blood-derived coagulation factors, and intravenous (IV) drug abusers.

Associated with reduction in T4 lymphocytes

Recognition of groups at particular risk

First isolation of the human immunodeficiency virus (HIV-1)

In 1982 the virus now known as HIV-1 was isolated in France by Montagnier and his colleagues and, in 1983, was shown by Gallo and his coworkers to be responsible unequivocally for the disease and its immunological manifestations. Within an amazingly short time thereafter, the

Characterization of the virus

mode of replication of the virus, its genome, and most of the products that it encodes were characterized. It was recognized to be a virus of extraordinary complexity and variability that would be unusually difficult to control because of its affinity for the master cell of the immune system.

Determination of modes of transmission

Growth of the virus in cell culture and isolation of its products allowed development of effective test procedures for detecting HIV infection. These almost eliminated the risk of transmission by blood transfusion and allowed assessment of the modes of transmission of the disease and the extent of infection nationally and worldwide. It became apparent that heterosexual transmission could occur and that the infection could be transmitted from mother to infant either by intrauterine spread or during the birth process. It was also found that the disease had its greatest prevalence in parts of Africa where the spread was predominantly heterosexual.

Heterosexual spread in Africa

Isolation of HIV-2, a second virus of AIDS

Retrospective serological studies with material saved from patients with immune deficiencies indicate that the disease was already occurring in Africa in the 1950s and in the United States in the 1970s. In 1985, a related but distinct virus, HIV-2, was also found to be endemic in parts of West Africa and to also cause AIDS. To date, this virus has been relatively restricted geographically although infections with it have occurred in western Europe. In the last several years, simian immunodeficiency viruses have been discovered that cause a disease in monkeys analogous to AIDS. These agents are genomically more closely related to HIV-2 than to HIV-1 and provide some insight into the biologic heritage of their human counterparts.

Clinical Manifestations

Infection with HIV results in a wide spectrum of disease varying from silent infection to the presence of multiple opportunistic infections and cerebral damage. The initial infection with HIV is usually asymptomatic, although in some cases a mononucleosislike illness develops 1–6 weeks after infection and lasts for about 2–6 weeks. This is manifested by fever, malaise, lymphadenopathy, hepatosplenomegaly, arthralgias, and rash. Sometimes there is also a mild aseptic meningitis. Whether or not these early manifestations of infection occur, the virus persists and integrates into the genome of some host cells, and the individual is thus infected for life.

Initial infection is often asymptomatic, but may be mononucleosislike

Latent period of years before major symptomatic disease

The initial infection is followed by an asymptomatic period that, in most cases, continued for years before the disease becomes clinically apparent. During this time virus can be isolated from blood, semen, and the cervix. Between 15 and 35% of infected individuals will develop significant disease within 6 years of infection, and the number continues to increase thereafter. It is expected that nearly all HIV-infected individuals will eventually develop some clinical aspects of this infection.

General lymphadenopathy syndrome, AIDS-related complex, and AIDS

Disease can be manifested as

1. Persistent generalized lymphadenopathy syndrome (PGL) characterized by multiple enlarged lymph nodes.

2. AIDS-related complex (ARC), which is a constellation of signs and symptoms consisting of fever, fatigue, diarrhea, weight loss, night sweats, and immunologic abnormalities.

3. The fully developed AIDS syndrome, which involves the occurrence of opportunistic infections, a neoplasm, or central nervous system damage in a person with HIV infection.

Table 73.1 Summary of CDC Classification System for HIV Infection

Group I	Acute infection
Group II	Asymptomatic infection[a]
Group III	Persistent generalized lymphadenopathy[a]
Group IV	Other diseases
Subgroup A	Constitutional disease
Subgroup B	Neurologic disease
Subgroup C	Secondary infectious diseases
Category C-1	Specified secondary infectious diseases listed in CDC surveillance definition for AIDS[b]
Category C-2	Other specified secondary infectious diseases
Subgroup D	Secondary cancers[b]
Subgroup E	Other conditions

[a] Patients in groups II and III may be subclassified on the basis of laboratory evaluation.

[b] Includes those patients whose clinical presentation fulfills the definition of AIDS used by CDC for national reporting.

One commonly used clinical classification for HIV infections is that developed by the Centers for Disease Control (CDC) (Table 73.1).

As the disease progresses, the number of T4 cells declines; there is an increasing immune deficiency; and opportunistic infections become more frequent, severe, and difficult to treat. One of the best markers of the severity of AIDS is the number or proportion of T4 cells. Those with overt AIDS almost always have less than 400 T4 cells/μL of blood (normal = 800–1200 cells/μL). The mechanisms by which HIV causes T-cell destruction and immunologic abnormalities are considered in Chapter 41.

Patients with fully developed AIDS experience a wide spectrum of infections depending on the severity of their immune defect, and the opportunistic organisms in their normal flora or with which they come in contact (Table 73.2). Some clinical manifestations of AIDS may thus vary by locale. For example, disseminated histoplasmosis is a common complication in the Midwest of the United States, and disseminated toxoplasmosis in France. These infections are uncommon in areas where the diseases are not endemic. The diversity and anatomic sites of infection vary between patients, and any one patient may have several infections. The most common infection is pneumocystosis, and approximately 50% of patients develop *Pneumocystis carinii* pneumonia. In the past, about a quarter of all AIDS patients developed Kaposi's sarcoma, but the number of cases has been falling in the United States despite increasing numbers of cases of AIDS. The reasons for this change are unknown. Mycobacteria of the avium–intracellulare complex are very common sources of infection, and AIDS patients are highly susceptible to tuberculosis. Oral thrush and esophagitis due to *Candida albicans* and meningitis due to *Cryptococcus* are commonly encountered fungal infections. Persistent progressive mucocutaneous herpes simplex and varicella–zoster infections are common. Disseminated cytomegalovirus infection is often seen and presents as fever and with visceral (e.g., adrenal) organ involvement. Cytomegalovirus chorioretinitis may result in serious visual impairment, or deafness may occur.

As the duration of survival of AIDS patients has extended, an increasing number are developing neurological manifestations of the disease and lymphoid neoplasms, especially non-Hodgkins lymphomas. The HIV is a neurotropic virus and is isolated from the cerebrospinal fluid of 50–70% of

Severity of disease increases with declining T4 lymphocyte numbers

Fully developed AIDS is associated with severe opportunistic infections

50% develop *P. carinii* pneumonia

Mycobacterial, fungal, and viral infections

Neurologic and lymphomatous complications of later stages

Table 73.2 Common Opportunistic Infections in AIDS Patients

Protozoan infections
  Pneumocystosis

  Toxoplasmosis

  Isosporosis belli

  Cryptosporidiosis

Fungal infections
  Cryptococcosis

  Candidiasis

  Histoplasmosis (disseminated)

Mycobacterial infections
  Disseminated tuberculosis (especially extrapulmonary)

  Mycobacterium avium–intracellulare complex infections

Viral infections
  Persistent mucocutaneous herpes simplex

  Disseminated and pulmonary cytomegalovirus infection

  Disseminated varicella–zoster

  Progressive multifocal leukoencephalopathy

patients with CDC class III or IV infection. Central nervous system involvement may be asymptomatic, but many patients develop a subacute neurologic illness that produces clinical symptoms varying from mild cognitive dysfunction to severe dementia. In children, a lymphocytic interstitial lung disease often occurs, possibly due to direct HIV infection of the lung. The disease spectrum in Africa is similar in many regards to that seen in the Western world, but many more patients present with severe intractable wasting and diarrhea called *slim disease*. Tuberculosis is also more commonly encountered in AIDS patients in Africa, reflecting the higher incidence of the disease in the population in general.

> Fully developed AIDS has a fatal course at present

The 2-year mortality of AIDS, once the disease has been fully established was initially 75%, with nearly all cases eventually dying of opportunistic infections or neoplasms. Recent advances in therapy have slowed progression of the disease, but have not thus far prevented its relentless progress.

Epidemiology of HIV Infection

Transmission

> Transmission often from exchange of blood or body fluids during sexual contact

The HIV virus is transmitted between humans by exchange of blood or body fluids; occasional transmission has occurred with transplanted organs. The virus has been demonstrated in particularly high titers in semen and cervical secretions, and the majority of cases have resulted from sexual contact. Infection is facilitated by breaks in epithelial surfaces, which provide direct access to the underlying tissues or bloodstream. The relative fragility of the rectal mucosa probably contributed to the predominance of the disease among male homosexuals in western countries. Until serological tests for the infection became available, about 2% of cases were acquired through blood transfusion, and about 50% of hemophiliacs

> Some infections in the past resulted from blood transfusions or injected blood products

treated with coagulation factors derived from pooled blood sources became infected. Testing of donors and the use of recombinant or specially treated coagulation factors have now minimized or eliminated these sources of infection. Transmission of infection by blood is now largely associated with sharing of unsterilized needles and syringes by IV drug abusers, and this has been an increasing source of the disease. In some areas of the United States, as many as 50% of IV drug abusers have been infected. Infants can acquire the disease transplacentally or perinatally from mothers who have been infected by their sexual partners or by IV drug abuse. Between a quarter and a half of infants born to infected mothers will develop AIDS within 2 years, and it appears at present that they will all die.

Blood transmission through shared needles and syringes by drug abusers

Transmission of infection to health care workers after accidental sticks with potentially contaminated needles is very rare (considerably less than 1% of occurrences), presumably because the amounts of infectious virus in the blood of infected cases is small and larger volumes or repeated exposures are needed for a significant chance of infection. Nevertheless, occasional cases have occurred both from clinical and laboratory exposure, and the universal precautions described in Chapter 72 should be applied to minimize the already small risk.

Risk of transmission from accidental needle sticks is very low

Transmission does not occur through day-to-day nonsexual contact with infected individuals or through insect vectors. This is because of the fragility of the virus and the need for direct mucosal or blood contact. It is of interest that the virus has been detected in saliva, tears, urine, and breast milk. With the possible exception of breast milk, these sources have not been shown to be infectious.

No transmission by day-to-day nonsexual contact or by insects

Occurrence

In the United States the highest prevalence rates of HIV infections are in homosexual and bisexual males, IV drug abusers, prostitutes, and sexual partners of HIV-infected persons. In some areas of the United States, 40–60% of homosexual males attending sexually transmitted disease clinics were found to be infected. Rates in prostitutes vary from 0 to 40%, depending partly on the degree of associated drug abuse. Prevalence rates in the heterosexual population in general are currently less that 1%, but have been increasing.

Infection in United States is commonest in male homosexuals, bisexuals, drug abusers, prostitutes, and sex partners of infected individuals

In contrast to the situation in the Western world, heterosexual transmission is the primary route of transmission in Africa where there is an approximately equal distribution of infection and disease between the sexes. This may be due to a high frequency in affected areas of ulcerative genital lesions due to other sexually transmitted diseases that facilitate passage of virus into the tissues during heterosexual intercourse.

Most infections in Africa are transmitted heterosexually

Genital ulcerative lesions from other infections may facilitate spread

Acquired immunodeficiency syndrome has been reported in over 140 countries at the time of this writing, and it has been estimated that as many as 10 million people are infected with HIV worldwide. In the United States, over 85,000 cases had been reported by mid-1989, and it is believed that well over a million people are infected. It is predicted that over 250,000 cases of AIDS will develop by 1991, almost all having already been infected and in the latent phase of the disease. In the United States, the major foci of the disease are in areas with high male homosexual populations and in areas of poverty and drug abuse.

Present extent of the problem

The epidemiology of HIV infection is changing in the United States as the pandemic evolves and as the modes of transmission become more generally understood. The homosexual communities that were first af-

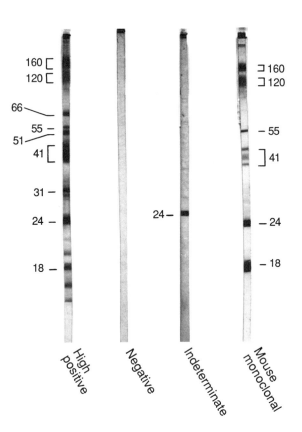

73.1 Western blot detection of HIV-1 antibodies. Note that the "High Positive" serum exhibits antibodies to the HIV-1 envelope glycoproteins of 160, 120 and 41 kilodaltons (kD), to the gag (core) proteins of 24 and 18 kD, and to other HIV proteins (55 and 51 kD). The "Indeterminate" serum exhibits antibody to only the gag (core) 24 kD protein. The mouse monoclonal blot is a positive control and contains antibodies to key HIV antigens. A positive sample should exhibit antibodies to both envelope and gag proteins, or to both envelope proteins (41 and 120/160 kD).

flicted have modified their behavior and adopted prophylactic procedures that are tending to prevent new infections. On the other hand, the number and proportion of heterosexually transmitted, drug abuse-related, and neonatal cases is increasing, particularly among the poor and disadvantaged racial minorities. On a worldwide scale, the disease continues to spread rapidly in Africa and South America. In some areas of Africa, up to one-tenth of the population is infected. The impact on the future development of these countries will be severe and the health care systems throughout the world will be hard pressed to meet the challenge of AIDS in the 1990s.

Increasing proportion of infections in heterosexuals, drug abusers, and newborns in the United States

Laboratory Diagnosis of HIV Infection

Diagnosis is most commonly made by demonstrating antibody to the virus or its components. Initial screening tests are made using whole viral lysates as the target antigens in enzyme-linked immunosorbent assay tests (see Chapter 14). These have a high level of sensitivity, but occasional false positives occur, and specificity thus varies according to the frequency of disease in the population tested. Tests made with HIV-1 do not detect antibody to HIV-2. Because false positives occur, positive ELISA tests are confirmed by a Western blot analysis to detect antibodies to specific viral proteins. In this procedure, viral proteins are separated by electrophoresis, transferred to nitrocellulose paper, incubated with antisera, and antibody bound to the individual proteins is detected by enzyme-labeled anti-human globulin sera (see Figure 73.1). Sera from infected patients have antibodies that react with the envelope glycoproteins, or core pro-

ELISA screening tests use viral lysates as antigens

Specificity of positive screening tests confirmed by Western blots

teins, or both. Envelope and the core p24 antigen have been expressed in *Escherichia coli* from recombinant plasmids and have also been used in Western blot studies.

Antibodies may not be detectable for several weeks after infection

The combination of ELISA and Western blots gives a high degree of specificity to test results, but antibody is not detectable by these procedures in the first 2–4 weeks after infection, a period during which the individual can be infectious to others. During and after this time virus may be grown in mixed lymphocytic cell culture (see Chapter 41), but may not be detected for up to a month. Thus, the process is complex and expensive and has little direct clinical utility. More usefully, viral core antigen (the p24 antigen) can often be detected by sensitive immunologic tests in the early stages of the disease, and exploitation of the polymerase chain reaction, which amplifies part of the genome of the virus, should allow its detection by hybridization techniques in the early stages of the disease before serological tests become positive.

Viral core antigen may be detected before serodiagnostic tests become positive

Recent evidence indicates that occasional individuals may remain seronegative for up to 20 months after infection even though HIV or virally encoded DNA can be detected in blood lymphocytes. This indicates the limitations of any single diagnostic test for this disease.

Therapy of AIDS

Zidovudine slows or controls progression but does not cure

At present, zidovudine (see Chapter 13) is the only agent specifically preventing HIV replication that has been shown to be clinically valuable. It has significant toxicity for bone marrow cells, and its use is frequently complicated by anemia, which often requires transfusion. It is a drug that controls the spread of progression of the disease, but is ineffective against integrated virus and is, thus, not curative. The virus has been demonstrated to develop resistance in some cases during the course of therapy. Several other antiretroviral drugs are under development. These include reverse transcriptase inhibitors such as dideoxyinosine or agents that block binding of the virus to the T4 lymphocyte (recombinant soluble CD4 receptor). Treatment directed toward controlling or preventing opportunistic infections is an important part of AIDS therapy. It is complicated by the severe immune deficiency that develops in the disease and is often suppressive rather than curative. Chemoprophylaxis is now being increasingly used.

Other antiretroviral agents under development

Treatment of opportunistic infections is complicated by the immunosuppression

One serious and often lethal complication that has been particularly difficult to control is *P. carinii* infection. Sulfonamide–trimethoprin therapy has proven unusually toxic in AIDS patients, and systemic pentamidine treatment has not been effective in the long term. Recently, pentamidine aerosols given prophylactically have reduced the frequency of pneumocystosis and helped prolong the periods of freedom from this serious opportunistic disease.

Prophylactic pentamidine aerosols can prevent or delay pneumocystosis

Prevention of AIDS

Social changes and the spread of AIDS

The spread of AIDS has been facilitated by changing sexual mores, increased drug abuse, and, in some parts of the world, by disruption of family and tribal units as a consequence of industrialization and urbanization. These factors, obviously, are not subject to early change. Immediate prevention has to be based on education about the means of transmission and easy access to condoms and safe needles for those large numbers of people who continue to place themselves at risk. The epidemiological and laboratory methods used to control foci of other major epidemic diseases pose particular problems in AIDS control at present.

Immediate prevention is dependent on education

Possibilities for
vaccines, chemoprophylaxis,
and chemotherapy

Quite apart from questions of potential discrimination against infected individuals and the calamitous effects of false positive serological test results on the individual, the sheer magnitude and cost of case finding and contact tracing at present limit this approach.

There is much research under way to develop vaccines against the virus, but the marked mutability of HIV greatly complicates this approach, although conserved epitopes of the surface glycopeptides provide possible targets. The passage of virus between fused cells and in syncytia protects it from antibody neutralization in established disease. The most affected cells are those that contribute to cell-mediated immunity. Nevertheless, the possibility that immunization with a vaccine may block the earliest process of infection is being explored.

Another approach involves chemoprophylaxis beginning during the clinically silent phase of the disease using agents that specifically block reverse transcriptase or the products or processes used for viral assembly. Agents with these properties can be expected to be developed and may well control, but probably not cure the disease. Such an approach will require widespread testing for infection and provision of the financial resources needed for this and for the drugs involved.

Need for financial resources
to control the disease

Further Reading

Institute of Medicine, National Academy of Sciences. 1989. *Confronting AIDS. Update 1988*. Washington D.C.: National Academy Press. A recent publication giving an overview of the current state of AIDS and of new developments in research.

Kulstad, R., Ed. 1986. *AIDS. Papers from Science 1982–1985*. Washington D.C.: The American Association for the Advancement of Science, pp. 1–617. A compendium of the early articles on AIDS including the classic papers describing the association between HIV and the syndrome.

Turner, C.F., Miller, H.G., and Moses L.E., Eds. 1989. *AIDS. Sexual Behavior and Intravenous Drug Use*. Washington D.C.: National Academy Press, pp. 1–568. An excellent compendium on current problems in controlling HIV infection.

Advancing Fronts in Medical Microbiology

Predicting future developments in a scientific discipline is risky, but some current areas of intense interest will certainly be in the forefront of medical microbiology in the next few years.

Approaches to Taxonomy, Identification, and Genome Detection

Direct analysis of the microbial genome is becoming increasingly important in taxonomy, identification, and diagnosis. Comparisons of ribosomal RNAs, which are highly conserved in nature, are providing evolutionary information that allows a firmer basis for the allocation of bacteria to families and genera. DNA:DNA homology techniques bring these approaches to the species level, and using probes for essential parts of the genome can result in specific identification of organisms or detection of genes encoding key virulence factors such as toxins. The processes by which these analyses can be accomplished are simplified with the use of nonradioactive detection systems and are thus becoming a part of the armamentarium of the clinical diagnostic laboratory. Whole-cell DNA restriction patterns and two-dimensional gel separation of whole-cell proteins are also proving of value in identification and can be analyzed by computer pattern recognition. They may be expected to be developed increasingly as identification tools that can be effective down to the subspecies level.

Specific microbial nucleic acid sequences can often be detected directly in clinical material or in cultures when present in sufficient quantity. An immensely powerful new tool, the polymerase chain reaction, now allows amplification of otherwise undetectable DNA sequences (or DNA copies of RNA) in clinical material to the point at which they can be recognized by specific probes. This approach is being applied particularly to detecting latent viral nucleic acid present in minute quantities in host cells, and is

937

rapidly extending knowledge of human immunodeficiency virus infection and of latent herpesvirus infections. It will certainly help in clarifying whether latent viruses are involved in some chronic neurological and other diseases of unknown etiology.

Plasmid Epidemiology and Fingerprinting

Comparisons of electrophoretic patterns of plasmid DNA and of its restriction endonuclease digests is an established epidemiological procedure for staphylococci and enteric Gram-negative rods and is certain to be extended to the full range of bacteria that may be encountered in hospital and community epidemics. The procedure is also proving of value in helping determine whether isolates of a bacterial species from the same patient at different times are identical. This will be helpful, for example, in determining the significance of blood culture isolates of coagulase-negative staphylococci.

Detection of Virulence Determinants and Immunizing Antigens

In recent years there has been rapid progress in characterizing determinants of virulence of some pathogenic organisms at the molecular level and in identifying the antigens that elicit effective immune responses against them. This area of investigation can be expected to accelerate and provide substantial benefits in therapy, diagnosis, and improved vaccines. Advances have exploited techniques to separate the multiple antigens of an organism and detect antibodies in polyclonal antisera that react with them. Specific monoclonal antibodies can then be made for detection and isolation of the relevant antigens, and the genes that encode them can be cloned in a nonpathogenic organism by recombinant DNA techniques so that their products can be produced and studied in a safe and defined environment. Even though virulence is frequently polygenic, these approaches may allow the detection of key virulence determinants in organisms such as mycobacteria, treponemas, and eukaryotic parasites and open the way to development of effective vaccines.

Vaccine Development

Prevention of important infections by vaccines is developing along three main lines. Specific immunizing antigens and epitopes detected by procedures such as those described above are being isolated and in some cases synthesized. Their use reduces the breadth of the antigenic stimulus while increasing its specificity. Small peptides, however, although eliciting highly specific responses, may fail to produce the levels of response obtained with whole organisms and may thus require the immunostimulating effect of adjuvants such as aluminum hydroxide to make them effective immunizing agents. Immunization with T-independent polysaccharide antigens such as capsular material from *Haemophilus influenzae* and *Neisseria meningitidus* has been relatively ineffective in early childhood when most infections occur. Conjugation with a protein such as diphtheria toxoid has greatly reduced this problem because it allows recognition by T cells and enhanced antibody production by B cells. Combinations of protein and polysaccharide immunizing agents exploiting this approach can be expected to be used increasingly in the future.

Because of continued antigenic stimulus, live vaccines offer considerable advantages in producing prolonged immunity and in stimulating sIgA-mediated immunity at the site of a potential infection. Pragmatic approaches to selecting attenuated vaccine strains are being replaced by procedures in which specific determinants of virulence are deliberately altered by procedures such as insertional mutagenesis, or genetic determinants of immunizing antigens are added to the genome of an avirulent strain that has the capacity to colonize potential sites of infection. It has also been shown that genes for more than one immunizing antigen can be added to the genetic makeup of the vaccinia virus, can be expressed, and can elicit both T- and B-cell immune responses. The practical application of this approach would exploit the vast experience of the use of vaccinia virus in humans. Thus, we may anticipate a continued extension of the use of vaccines to protect against a range of diseases that have not so far been amenable to this approach or which required crude vaccines that were often associated with an appreciable incidence of adverse effects.

Genetic Determinants of Susceptibility to Infection

Differences in individual or racial immunity to particular infections, or in the ability of different individuals to respond to vaccines are coming under increased study. Some differences are due to genetic variations in Class II MHC encoded host cell antigens that can influence their ability to associate with particular microbial antigenic epitopes or to present them in the needed configuration for T-cell recognition. As the range of these genetic associations and their mechanisms becomes increasingly understood, the possibilities of targeting prophylactic measures to particular individuals or of altering antigenic epitopes to allow a more general response become of increasing interest. It would also be very helpful clinically to be able to identify those at particular risk of serious infection.

Antimicrobics and New Approaches to Therapy

Advances in therapy of infections are occurring on several fronts. There seems to be no slowing in the development of new β-lactam antimicrobics that resist the increasing range of bacterial β-lactamases. The success of the quinolones also indicates that completely new classes of antibacterials may be synthesized or discovered in the future. More effective and less toxic antiparasitics can be expected to be developed because of the enormous worldwide burden of ill health from parasitic diseases and because of the development of resistance of earlier agents, particularly by the malarial parasite. Similar developments will certainly occur with antiviral agents. We can also anticipate introduction of some dramatically different approaches to treatment. The therapeutic use of free receptors that are the specific points of viral attachment to cells may be applicable to the prevention or treatment of some viral diseases; for example, the CD4 receptor for the human immunodeficiency virus has shown promise in experimental systems for preventing or slowing the progress of this otherwise unrelenting infection. Similarly, human monoclonal antibodies may inhibit attachment of organisms or toxins to target cells and thus meet the promise of serotherapy by avoiding the adverse immunological responses to sera from animal sources and the difficulties in obtaining large amounts of hyperimmune human sera. Another promising approach under exploration is the use of recombinant cytokines such as interleukin 2 and the interferons to stimulate the immune response during the course of an infection or to inhibit viral replication. There is particular interest in approaches to activating and expanding the pool of natural killer cells because of their ability to recognize and destroy host cells expressing foreign or abnormal antigens on their surface. The main thrust of this work has been directed at tumor cells, but virally infected cells may also be targets and subject to attack in the early stages of an infection before an immunological response is mounted, or later so that liberated virus is neutralized by specific antibody. Thus, we may expect an increasing emphasis on stimulating host defense mechanism as an adjunct to chemotherapy of a variety of infectious diseases.

Rapid and Simple Diagnostic Procedures

Nucleic acid probes and rapid antigen detection techniques using monoclonal antibodies on particulate carriers or with enzyme-linked detection procedures have been developed for the diagnosis of many infections. Some are available in kit form and can give results within minutes. There are some problems with sensitivity when the tests are applied directly to clinical material because of the small numbers of organisms that may be present; however, when combined with short periods of enrichment culture, they appear very promising when applied to the diagnosis of an infection for which there are a limited number of likely etiologic agents. These approaches may not only speed diagnostic results but also reduce the costs of the more traditional labor-intensive procedures; they can be of particular value in developing countries where simple and inexpensive methods are urgently needed for diagnosis of the more serious endemic and epidemic infection. At the other end of the spectrum, laboratory diagnosis is being increasingly automated in developed countries, and the advantages in speed, reproducibility, and precision can be expected to be of substantial help in the care of the infected patient in the future.

In short, the outlook for improvements in understanding, diagnosis, and control of infectious diseases is very bright, and the field of medical microbiology is likely to continue to be one of great activity and promise in the future.

Appendix: Additional Pathogenic Organisms

Summary of Some Additional Pathogenic or Potentially Pathogenic Organisms Not Considered in the Body of the Text

Organism	Disease	Comment
Bacteria		
Bartonella bacilliformis	Verruga peruvana (skin) Oroya fever (systemic)	Small Gram-negative bacillus transmitted by Sandlfy vector. Limited to Andes mountain regions. Organism invades erythrocytes producing hemolytic anemia in Oroya fever.
Streptobacillus moniliformis	Rat-bite fever	Highly pleomorphic Gram-negative bacillus of oropharynx of rodents. Produces high fever, rash, and septic or pneumonic complications. Most infections follow rodent bites.
Spirillum minor	Rat-bite fever	Gram-negative spiral organism with polar flagella. Habitat and epidemiology similar to *Streptobacillus moniliformis*. Disease manifests as fever, rash, and local lesion with lymphadenitis.
Viruses		
Rift Valley fever virus	Rift Valley fever	Febrile illness sometimes complicated by hemorrhage, encephalitis, and blindness. Occurs as mosquito-borne epizootics in sub-Sahara Africa and Egypt. Produces disease in sheep, cattle, and humans.
Fungi		
Pseudoallescheria (Petriellidum) boydii	Pseudoallescheriasis	A free-living ascomycete that may produce infectious features similar to those of *Aspergillus* infection especially in the immunocompromised.
Prototheca wickerhamii	Chronic skin papilloma-like lesions, wound infections and bursitis	Alga-like unicellular fungus.

Protozoa

CILIATES

Balantidium coli	Balantidiasis	Large colonic protozoan of swine, found primarily in tropics. Human infection may produce a diarrheal illness resembling amebiasis.

FLAGELLATES

Dientamoeba fragilis	Diamentamoebiasis	A noninvasive intestinal amebo-flagellate related to *Trichomonas*. Uncommonly, infection produces acute or recurrent diarrhea.

SPOROZOA

Isospora belli	Isosporiasis	Coccidian parasite resembling *Cryptosporidium* seen in areas of low sanitation and in patients with AIDS. Watery diarrhea is seen in acute infections, malabsorption and weight loss in chronic disease.
Sarcocystis spp	Sarcocytosis	Coccidian parasite that produces intestinal infection in carnivores (definite hosts) and large tissue cysts in herbivores. Human infections of animal origin are seen in Latin America and Asia. They may be intestinal producing diarrhea, or muscular producing painful swellings.
Babesia spp	Babesiosis	Tick-transmitted intraerythrocytic parasites of animals resembling the falciparum malaria agent. In N. America, human infections found primarily in off-shore islands of New England. Usually characterized by prolonged fever and mild to moderate hemolytic anemia.

Helminths

NEMATODES

Anasakis spp	Anasakiasis	Intestinal ascarids of sea mammals. Larval stages are found in flesh of several marine fish. Humans are infected by eating uncooked fish. Parasite may be vomited or burrow into mucosa producing abdominal pain.
Capillaria philippinensis	Capillariasis	Intestinal nematodes of birds related to *Trichuris*. Inhabitants of Philipines and Thailand become infected when they ingest raw fresh water crustaceans and fish which serve as intermediate hosts. Invasion of intestinal mucosa produces severe diarrhea and malabsorption.
Trichostrongylus spp	Trichostrongyliasis	Worldwide parasite of herbivores. Humans are infected by ingesting leafy plants contaminated with larvae. Most infections are asymptomatic. Abdominal pain and diarrhea may occur.

Angiostrongylus cantonesis	Eosinophilic meningitis	Nematode parasite of mammals of the Far East and tropical areas of the Pacific. Human ingestion of raw snails or fresh water crustaceans serving as intermediate hosts results in larval invasion of the CNS and meningitis.
Dracuncula mediensis	Dracunculiasis	The "guinea worm" is the largest nematode of humans. Humans in south Asia, Middle East, and Africa are infected by drinking water containing infected fresh water fleas. Adult worm migrates to subcutaneous tissues of the legs and penetrates skin to discharge its eggs.

Cestodes

Taenia multiceps	Coenurosis	A dog tapeworm. Larval invasion of human subcutaneous tissues, eyes, and CNS occurs following ingestion of eggs from feces of an infected dog.

Trematodes

Fasciolopsis buski	Fasciolopsiasis	The largest intestinal trematode of humans inhabits duodenum and jejunum of humans and swine in the Far East and Southeast Asia. Human infection follows ingestion of fresh water plants containing infective metacercariae. Heavy infections may produce diarrhea, malabsorption and edema.
Heterophyes heterophyes	Heterophyiasis	One of several minute intestinal flukes found in the Far East, Middle East, Brazil, USSR, and Hawaii. Humans are infected by ingesting second intermediate hosts such as fresh water fish, shrimp and reptiles. Heavy infections may produce diarrhea.
Fasciola hepatica	Fascioliasis	Worldwide liver fluke of sheep and other herbivores. Human infection acquired by ingesting watercress and other water plants containing infective metacerceria. Following migration to liver, clinical manifestations resemble clonorchiasis.
Opisthorchis spp	Opisthorchiasis	Liver fluke found in eastern Europe, USSR, and Far East. Fresh water fish serve as second intermediate host. Human infection follows ingestion of raw or undercooked fish. Clinical disease resembles clonorchiasis.

Historical Appendix

Some Major Figures Contributing to Knowledge of Medical Microbiology

1670–1800

Antony Van Leeuwenhoek

At the beginning of this period, he developed single-lensed microscopes which allowed him to see and describe microorganisms in numerous environmental and biological samples.

Edward Jenner

In 1798 reported on the efficacy of cowpox vaccination against smallpox.

1800–1860

Ignaz Semmelweiss and Oliver Wendell Holmes.

Described the epidemiology, contagiousness, and measures for prevention of puerperal fever.

Florence Nightingale

Showed that post-traumatic infection and epidemic diseases in hospital could be reduced by cleanliness and disinfection. Established the basis of modern hospital hygiene.

1860–1900

Louis Pasteur

Between 1857–1880 demonstrated that fermentation was a microbial process, and that there was no spontaneous generation of microbes. He developed pasteurization to control contamination of wines, vinegar, and beer. He demonstrated the microbial cause of many diseases of plants,

1860–1900
(Continued)

insects, and mammals, and developed attenuated vaccines for anthrax and rabies.

Joseph Lister

Developed the techniques of antiseptic surgery for preventing surgical wound infections.

Robert Koch

Isolated the causative agents of anthrax, tuberculosis, and cholera and conclusively demonstrated their etiologies. Developed various staining procedures and the use of solid media for pure culture techniques.

Patrick Manson

First showed that a parasite of humans (Filaria) had a developmental phase in an insect (mosquito).

Elie Metchnikoff

Discovered the role of phagocytic cells in immunity.

Hans Christian Gram

Developed the staining procedure that carries his name.

Emil von Behring

Discovered the neutralization of diphtheria toxin by antitoxin.

Dmitri Ivanowksi

Described a filterable non-bacterial agent (virus) as the cause of tobacco mosaic disease.

Paul Ehrlich

Postulated the side chain reaction theory of antibody production and action.

Ronald Ross

Conclusively demonstrated the role of the anopheline mosquito in the transmission of malaria.

Jules Bordet

Described the lysis of some Gram-negative bacteria by antibody and complement.

1900–1925

August von Wasserman

Developed the first serologic test for syphilis.

1900–1925
(Continued)

Walter Reed

Reported studies in 1902 which established that yellow fever virus, the first recognized human virus, could be transmitted by mosquito bites.

Paul Ehrlich

Defined the principles of chemotherapy and developed salvarsan as the first effective chemotherapeutic for syphilis.

Peyton Rous

Discovered a virally transmitted sarcoma of chickens.

Frederick Twort and Felix d'Herelle

Independently discovered bacterial viruses (bacteriophages).

Alexander Fleming

Discovered lysozyme.

1925–1945

Fred Griffith

Described the phenomenon of pneumococcal transformation.

Alexander Fleming

Reported his discovery of penicillin, and its antibacterial characteristics, in 1929.

Max Theiler

Developed the mouse model as a susceptible mammalian host for the isolation, propagation, and study of arboviruses.

Ernest Goodpasture

Showed that some viruses could be grown in the laboratory in the developing chick embryo.

Gerhard Domagk

Discovered the first of the sulfonamide antimicrobics.

Max Delbrück

Began a series of studies on bacteriophages that ultimately helped elucidate the fundamental relationships of DNA, RNA, and protein in living systems.

Ernst Chain, Howard Florey and their colleagues

Produced and purified penicillin to the point of clinical trials in the early 1940s.

1925–1945
(Continued)

Oswald Avery, Colin MacLeod, and Maclyn McCarty

Showed that pneumococcal transformation was determined by DNA from the donor strain.

Salvador Luria and Max Delbrück

Showed that bacterial mutations occurred spontaneously and were not directed by the environment.

1945–1965

Joshua Lederberg and Edward Tatum

Demonstrated genetic exchange in bacteria by conjugation.

John Enders, Frederick Robbins, and Thomas Weller

Grew the poliomyelitis virus in cell culture opening the way to vaccine production.

Norton Zinder and Joshua Lederberg

Discovered genetic exchange mediated by bacteriophage in *Salmonella* (transduction).

James Watson, Francis Crick, and Maurice Wilkins

Described the double helical structure of DNA in 1953.

Jonas Salk

Developed the inactivated poliomyelitis vaccine in 1955.

Albert Sabin

Developed the live attenuated poliomyelitis vaccine.

Alick Isaacs

Discovered interferon.

Jacques Monod and Francis Jacob

Reported their studies on enzyme regulation leading to recognition of promoters, regulatory proteins, and the role of mRNA.

Tomoichiro Akiba, Kunitaro Ochiai, Susumu Mitsuhashi, Tsutomu Wantanabe, and others

Discovered that multiple drug resistance was encoded on transmissible plasmids (R factors).

Carlton Gajdusek

Described the epidemiology of the first recognized slow virus disease (Kuru), and the unique characteristics of the etiologic agent.

1965–1985

Baruch Blumberg

Reported the discovery of "Australia antigen" in 1967, and later confirmed its association with hepatitis B virus.

Howard Temin and David Baltimore

Independently described reverse transcriptase in RNA tumor viruses.

Herbert Boyer, Stanley Cohen and others

Developed techniques for in vitro splicing of DNA.

Cesar Milstein and George Köhler

Developed the procedures for production of monoclonal antibodies.

Luc Montagnier and Robert Gallo

Independently isolated the virus causing AIDS and defined its activity on human immunocytes.

Glossary

The glossary is intended as an adjunct to the index for rapid reference. It includes words and phrases that have not been defined in the text or that have been defined but are used frequently in later chapters.

The list of prefixes and suffixes at the beginning of each alphabetical section includes word elements used in combined form. The meaning of many words can be derived from the prefixes and suffixes listed and therefore have not been included in the glossary.

A

Prefixes
A-, An- Without
Anthropo- Relationship to humans
Arthro- Pertaining to joints
Auto- Self, or arising from within
Auxo- Pertaining to growth

Suffix
algia Pain

Acanthosis Hyperplasia and thickening of prickle cell layer of skin

Accessory sinuses Blind-ended cavities in bone draining into nasal cavity

Achlorhydria Absence of hydrochloric acid in stomach

Acidosis Increased acidity of body fluid

Aciduric Resistant to effects of acid

Acid fast Describes an organism that resists acid decolorization after straining

Addison's disease Result of primary deficiency of production of adrenal hormones

Adenocarcinoma Malignant tumor derived from glandular epithelium

Adhesin Surface component of a microbe that binds to a cell receptor

Adrenal Important endocrine glands situated above the kidneys

Adnexa (uterine) Fallopian tubes and ovaries

Aerobactin A hydroxamate siderophore produced by many bacteria

Agammaglobulinemia Absence of immunoglobulins in the blood

Agglutinate Clumping

Agranulocytosis Failure of white blood cell production in bone marrow

Allele Alternate forms of a gene at the same chromosomal locus

Alloantigen An antigen that exists in alternate allelic forms

Allosteric Property of a protein that leads to a change in conformation and function associated with attachment of a smaller effector molecule

Alveoli (lung) Microscopic air sacs in lung

Ameboma A local inflammatory mass caused by an amebal infection

Amniotic fluid Fluid in amniotic sac surrounding the fetus

Anaerobe   Microorganism that multiplies only in the absence of oxygen

Analog   Structurally or functionally similar substance or property

Anamnestic   Enhanced immunological memory response on reexposure to antigen

Anaphylaxis   Immediate and severe antibody-mediated hypersensitivity reaction

Anneal   Subject to controlled heating and cooling to achieve a particular property

Anergic   Absence of ability to respond to antigen

Aneurysm   Localized abnormal dilatation of blood vessel

Anicteric   Absence of clinical jaundice

Anorexia   Loss of appetite

Anoxia   Lack of adequate oxygenation of blood or tissues

Anterior horn cell   Motor neuron in the anterior gray matter of the spinal cord

Antibiogram   Pattern of in vitro susceptibilities to different antibiotics

Antibody   An immunoglobulin molecule that interacts with the antigen that elicited its production

Antigen   A substance that elicits a specific immunological response or reacts with antibody in vitro. *See* Immunogen and Hapten

Antiserum   Serum containing specific antibodies

Antitussive   Substance that helps control coughing

Antitoxin   An antibody that neutralizes an exotoxin

Aplastic anemia   Failure of red cell production in bone marrow

Aphonia   Loss of speech

Apnea   Temporary absence of breathing

Aqueduct of Sylvius   Canal connecting the third and fourth ventricles of the brain

Arachidonic acid   Precursor of prostaglandins

Arachnoid   The middle of three membranes that cover the brain and spinal cord (meninges)

Arrythmia   Irregularity of heartbeat

Arteriole   Smallest artery leading to capillary

Arthralgia   Pain in a joint

Aryepiglottis   Related to the epiglottis and the arytenoid cartilage

Ascites   Fluid in a peritoneal cavity

Asepsis   Exclusion of pathogenic organisms

Ascus   A sac. In mycology, a specialized structure containing spores termed ascospores

Asphyxia   Suffocation

Astrocyte   Connective tissue cell of the central nervous system

Ataxia   Disturbance of muscular coordination

Ataxia telangiectasia   Hereditary disorder causing ataxia and permanent dilatation of some blood vessels

Atelectasis   Collapse of part of lung

Atherosclerosis   Hardening of the arteries

Atrophy   Wasting

Attenuated   Reduced in virulence, e.g., organisms in a live vaccine

Autochthonous flora   Organism with intimate and permanent association with an epithelial surface

Autoimmunity   An immune response against the body's own tissues

Autolysis   Lysis of a cell by its own enzymes

Autonomic   Relates to involuntary nervous system controlling cardiac, vascular, intestinal, and other functions

Auxotroph   Bacterial mutant that has lost the ability to synthesize an essential nutrient or metabolite

Axenic   Refers to pure cultures of a microorganism without presence of a contaminating or symbiotic organism

Axon   The extension of a neuron that conducts nerve impulses

Avascular   Absence of blood vessels or blood supply

B

Prefixes

Bio-   Pertaining to life

Blepharo-   Pertaining to the eyelid

Brady-   Slowing

Broncho-   Pertaining to the bronchial tree

Suffix

-blast   Precursor cell

Bacteremia   Bacteria in the blood

Bacteriocins   Proteins produced by one bacterium that kill another of the same or other species

Bacteriophage   Bacterial virus

Bacteriostasis   Inhibition of bacterial growth without killing

Bacteruria   Bacteria in the urine

Bartholin's glands   Lubricating glands on either side of the vaginal opening

Basophil   Polymorphonuclear leucocyte with basophilic granules

Basophilic   Stains with a basic dye

Biliary   Pertaining to the bile and bile ducts

Bilirubin   A bile pigment

Biotype   Subtype within a species characterized by physiologic properties

Bleb   *See* Bulla

Blepharoplast   Basal body of a cilium or flagellum

Blepharal   Pertaining to the eyelids

Blood-brain barrier Functional barrier preventing passage of large molecules to the brain parenchyma

Bolus Rounded mass that may obstruct (e.g., fecal bolus) or a concentrated mass (e.g., an antibiotic) given rapidly and intravenously

Bothria Paired sucking grooves in the head of the fish tapeworm (Diphyllobothrium)

Bradycardia Unusually slow heartbeat

Bronchial tree Bronchi and bronchioles that conduct gases to and from the lung alveoli

Bronchiectasis Pathologic dilatation of terminal bronchi

Bronchiole Smallest subdivision of bronchial tree

Bubo Swollen, inflamed, infected lymph node

Buccal Pertaining to the cheek

Bulla Blister or vesicle containing semi-purulent fluid

Bursa Sac filled with fluid, e.g., protecting a joint or tendon

C

Prefixes

Cardio- Pertaining to the heart

Chole- Pertaining to bile

Cysto- Pertaining to the bladder

Cyto- Pertaining to the cell

Suffix

-cidal Killing

Calculus Pathological stone, e.g., renal or gallbladder calculus

Calmodulin A protein present in eukaryotic cells that activates some essential enzymes when it has bound calcium

Carbuncle A necrotic staphylococcal infection of skin and subcutaneous tissue which has spread from infected furuncles

Carcinoma Malignant growth of epithelial cells

Cardiolipin A phospholipid occurring naturally in mitochondrial membranes against which antibodies are formed in syphilitic infection

Cardiomyopathy Disease of heart muscle

Capillary The smallest blood vessel connecting the arterial and venous systems

Capsid The outer protein coat of a virus that protects its nucleic acid

Capsomeres Subunits of viral capsids

Caseous Cheesy in consistency

Catalase Enzyme that catalyses the reduction of toxic hydrogen peroxide to oxygen and water

Cell-mediated immunity Immune reactions in which T lymphocytes play the pivotal role

Cellulitis Inflammation of subcutaneous tissue

Cementum Layer of modified bone on tooth root

Cerebrospinal fluid Fluid that fills spaces within and surrounding the central nervous system

Cervical Pertaining to the neck or uterine cervix

Cervix The constricted portion of an organ. Usually refers to the lower part of the uterus

Chancre Cutaneous lesion that develops at the site of an infection. Most often used to describe the primary syphilitic lesion

Chemoprophylaxis Use of antimicrobics to prevent infection

Chemotaxis Attraction of a motile cell

Chelator Compound that binds metallic ions

Chitin Polysaccharide forming exoskeletons of some insects or cell walls of some fungi

Cholangitis Inflammation of the bile ducts

Cholestasis Interruption of the flow of bile

Cholecystitis Inflammation of the gallbladder

Cholinergic nerves Nerve fibers that release acetylcholine as a mediator at their effector terminals

Chordae tendinae Small tendons that connect papillary muscles of the heart to the cusps of the atrio-ventricular valves

Chorea Rapid purposeless involuntary movements

Chorioallantoic membrane The outer membrane surrounding an avian embryo within the egg shell

Chorionic membrane The outer extraembryonic membrane from which the placenta originates

Chorioretinitis Inflammation of choroid and retina of the eye

Choroid plexus Vascular invagination into the cerebral ventricles. Produces the cerebrospinal fluid

Chromatin Complex of DNA and histones making up the chromosomes of eukaryotic cells

Chronic Granulomatous Disease Genetic disorder causing absence of H_2O_2 production and myeloperoxidase activity of phagocytes. Results in repeated infections with catalase positive bacteria

CIE *See* Counterimmunoelectrophoresis

Cilia Surface structures of some eukaryotic cells that beat rhythmically to move mucus over surfaces or confer motility on some single-celled organisms

Cirrhosis Fibrosis and nodular regeneration of the liver with loss of function

Cistron The smallest functional genetic unit. A gene

Clone Identical progeny of a single cell, gene, or genes

CMI *See* Cell-mediated immunity

Co-agglutination Agglutination involving two organisms, one of which acts as an inert particle coated with specific antibody to the other

Coarctation Stricture or narrowing (e.g., of the aorta)

Co-cultivation Process that can be used for unmasking latent virus by growing susceptible cells with those from affected tissue

Codon The three nucleotides encoding an amino acid or a chain termination signal

Collagen Fibers of connective tissue

Coloboma A defect of the eye

Colostrum Initial secretion of the breast after delivery (contains antibodies and lymphocytes)

Comedo Blocked sebaceous duct with retention of sebum (blackhead)

Commensal Organism of the normal flora that has a symbiotic relationship with the host

Complement A system of serum proteins that act in sequence to mediate inflammatory and some immune responses

Condyloma acuminatum A wart-like infectious benign growth that occurs on the genitalia and in the anal canal

Conidia Asexual fungal reproductive spore-like bodies

Conidiophore Fungal structure that bears conidia

Copepod Minute fresh water fleas that serve as intermediate hosts for some parasites

Coprolith Stony, hard stool

Cornea Clear, anterior portion of the eyeball

Coracidium The ciliated free swimming embryo of certain tapeworms

Cortex The outer layer of an organ

Corticosteroid Steroid hormone from adrenal gland; some are anti-inflammatory

Coryza Catarrhal rhinitis, e.g., from the common cold

Counterimmunoelectrophoresis A technique for increasing the sensitivity and speed of the immunodiffusion procedure by the application of an electrophoretic field (*see* Immunodiffusion)

Crepitation A crackling or rattling sound

Cribriform plate Area of bone above nasal cavity through which pass the olfactory nerves

Croup Manifestations of laryngeal obstruction from inflammation or other causes

Curare A plant extract that produces generalized paralysis by acting at neuro-muscular junctions

Cuticle Skin or surface layer

CSF *See* Cerebrospinal fluid

Cyanosis Blue color of skin caused by lack of oxygen

Cysticercus Larval form of tapeworm enclosed in a cyst

Cystic fibrosis Congenital disease of secreting glands affecting pancreas, respiratory tract, and sweat glands. Associated with viscid respiratory mucus and chronic respiratory infections

Cystoscope Instrument for examining inside the urinary bladder

Cytokine Hormone-like intercellular messenger molecule, eg, lymphokine and interleukin

Cytology The study of cells rather than of tissues and organs

Cytoplasm Cellular contents excluding the nucleus

Cytosol Liquid portion of cytoplasm

Cytosome The body of a cell apart from its nucleus

Cytostome The mouth opening of certain ciliated protozoa

D

Prefixes

Dermo- Pertaining to the skin

Dys- Difficult or painful

Dalton Atomic mass unit that gives the same number as atomic weight

Decubitus ulcer Pressure sore (bed sore)

Debridement Removing foreign matter and dead tissue

Dendritic Branched

Demyelination Loss of nerve sheaths

Dermatophyte Fungus that causes skin infections

Dermis Skin connective tissue immediately below the epidermis

Desquamation Loss of skin epithelial cells

Dextran A polymer of D-glucose

Dimorphism Occurring in two morphologic forms under different conditions

Diploid Possessing two sets of chromosomes

Diverticulum Blind-ended extrusion from a hollow organ

Ductus arteriosus Fetal blood vessel connecting the pulmonary artery to the descending aorta

Dysentery Pain and frequent defecation resulting from inflammation of the colon or other intestines, with blood and pus in the stool

Dyspareunia Difficult or painful intercourse

Dysphagia Difficulty in swallowing

Dysplasia Histological evidence of possible premalignant changes in cells

Dyspnea Shortness of breath

Dysuria Difficult or painful urination

E

Prefixes

Ecto-   Outside or outer
Endo-   Within
Entero-   Pertaining to intestines
Epi-   Upon or additional to
Erythro-   Red

Suffixes

-ectomy   Surgical removal of
-emia   Of the blood

Ecchymosis   Bruise

Ecthyma   Eroded, scabbed lesion of the skin

Ectopic pregnancy   Fetal development outside the uterus (usually in the Fallopian tubes)

Ectoplasm   Clear layer of cytoplasm near the cell membrane of amebas

Edema   Excessive fluid in tissues

Elastosis   Disorder of fibro-elastic proteins

Electrophoresis   Procedure for separating charged particles by differences in their migration in an electric field

ELISA   *See* Enzyme-linked immunosorbent assay

Embolism   Sudden blockage of an artery

Emphysema (pulmonary)   Irreversible enlargement of alveolar sacs of lung

Empyema   Pus in a body cavity (e.g., pleural cavity)

Encephalitis   Inflammation of brain tissue

Endarteritis   Inflammation of the inner coat of an artery or arteriole

Endemic   A disease which is continuously present at sub-epidemic levels in a particular region, locality, or group

Endogenous   Originating within an organism

Endometrium   Interior epithelial lining of the uterus

Endonuclease   Enzyme of a class that hydrolyzes internal bonds of DNA or RNA. Involved in synthesis and breakdown of nucleic acids

Endophthalmitis   Inflammation of interior tissues of the eye

Endoplasm   Central portion of cytoplasm of cell

Endoplasmic reticulum   Ramifying membranes within the cytoplasm of eukaryotic cells

Endospore   Bacterial spore

Endotoxin   Lipid A toxic moiety of bacterial cell wall lipopolysaccharide

Enteric   Pertaining to the intestinal tract

Enteric fever   Typhoid or similar systemic *Salmonella* or *Yersinia* infection

Enterobactin   A phenolate siderophore produced by *E. coli* and some other enteric species of bacteria

Enterochelin   Synonym for Enterobactin

Enucleation (ocular)   Removal of an eye intact

Enzootic   Disease present at low levels at all times in an animal community

Enzyme-linked Immunosorbent Assay   A method for detecting antigen-antibody reactions by labeling one of the reagents with detectable enzyme

Eosinophil   Polymorphonuclear leucocyte with eosinophilic granules

Epicardium   Outer lining of the heart

Epidemic   A disease which rapidly affects many people in a circumscribed period of time

Epididymis   Tubular structure attached to the testes in which spermatozoa mature

Epigastrium   Upper central region of the abdomen overlying the stomach

Epiglottis   Movable structure overlying and protecting the larynx

Epiphysis   Growing end of bone

Episome   Plasmid or viral DNA that can replicate extrachromosomally or can integrate into chromosome

Epitope   Structural part of an antigen that determines specificity of an antigen–antibody reaction (also called antigenic determinant)

Epitrochlear node   Lymph node above inner side of elbow

Erythema   Red color caused by dilatation of blood vessels

Erythrocyte   Red blood cell

Erythema nodosum   Red raised skin nodules usually on the legs. Usually a manifestation of a hypersensitivity reaction

Eschar   Necrotic scab-like area of skin

Etiology   Cause of a disease

Eukaryote   Organism comprising one or more cells containing true nuclei

Eustachian tube   Tube connecting the middle ear and the nasopharynx

Exanthem   Disease in which skin rashes are major manifestations

Exocrine glands   Glands excreting their products to skin, intestinal, respiratory, or genito-urinary tracts

Exotoxin   Toxic protein liberated from a bacterial cell

F

Facultative   When describing bacteria without a qualification means ability to grow aerobically or anaerobically

Fallopian tubes   Tubes extending from ovaries to uterus

Fascia   Sheets of specialized connective tissue

Fauces   Area between the mouth and the pharynx. Bounded by the tonsils, soft palate, and base of tongue

Febrile   Having a raised temperature

Felinophobe   Cat hater

Fibrin   Insoluble protein of blood clots

Fibrinogen   Precursor of fibrin

Fibroblast   Specialized cell producing collagen and elastic connective tissue

Fibrosis   Formation of collagenous connective tissue

Fimbriae   Very fine fibrils on the surface of a bacterium analagous to the larger pili. Often referred to as pili

Fistula   An abnormal passage from a hollow organ (e.g., intestine)

Flaccid   Loose; absence of muscle tone

Flagellum   Organelle of motion of bacteria and some eukaryotic cells

Fluke   Flat parasitic worm (trematode)

Fluorochrome   A fluorescent dye

Follicle   A small sac or cavity

Folliculitis   Usually describes localized inflammation of hair follicles without the purulence of furuncles

Fomites   Inanimate objects transmitting infectious agents

Foramina   Outlets to cavities

Fulminant   Rapid and severe development (e.g., of an infection)

Fungemia   Fungi in the bloodstream

Funiculitis   Inflammation of a cord-like structure, usually the spermatic cord

Furuncle   Purulent infection of a hair follice; a boil

Fusiform   Tapering at both ends

G

Prefixes

Gastro-   pertaining to the stomach

Gingivo-   pertaining to the gums

Suffix

-genic   arising from, origin

Ganglion   Group of nerve cells outside the spinal cord

Gangrene   Death of tissue

Gametocyte   Male or female sexual cell of the malarial parasite found in the blood of humans and transmissible to mosquitoes

Genital primordium   First recognizable embryonic genital structure. Assists in distinguishing hookworm from *Strongyloides* larvae

Genome   The total gene complement of an organism

Genotype   The genetic constitution of an organism

Geophagia   Eating soil

Giemsa stain   A combination of basic and acidic dyes used to stain blood smears and to demonstrate some protozoa

Gingival crevice   Area between the tooth and the gums

Glaucoma   Excessive pressure in eyeball that can lead to blindness

Glia   Supporting cells of the central nervous system (neuroglia)

Glomerulus   Microscopic organ of specialized capillaries in the kidney that filters waste products from the blood

Glottis   The sound-producing area of the larynx

Glucans   Polymers of glucose

Gnotobiotic animals   Animals reared under aseptic conditions which may either be sterile ("germ free") or in which defined microflora are introduced

Gonads   Ovaries or testes

Granulocyte   Polymorphonuclear leucocyte of the neutrophil, basophil, or eosinophil series

Granuloma   Chronic inflammatory lesion infiltrated with macrophages and lymphocytes and accompanied by fibroblast activity

Gravid   Pregnant

Guillain-Barré syndrome   Febrile polyneuritis with muscle weakness; may lead to paralysis

Gumma   Tertiary syphilitic granulomatous lesion, usually without demonstrable spirochetes

H

Prefixes

Hemo-, Hema-   Pertaining to blood

Hepato-   Pertaining to the liver

Hetero-   Of different origin

Hyper-   Greater than, above normal

Hypo-   Less than, below normal

Halophilic   Preferring or requiring a high salt content (e.g., for growth)

Haploid   Half the number of chromosomes of eukaryotic tissue cells (*see* Meiosis) or number of chromosomes in asexual organisms

Hapten   A small molecule that can react with a specific antibody but does not elicit antibody production unless attached to a larger molecule

Helminth   A parasitic worm

Hemagglutination   Agglutination of erythrocytes

Hematocrit   Volume of erythrocytes in blood as a percentage of the total volume of blood (adult normal = 45%)

Hematoma   Extravasation of blood into the tissues causing a swelling

Hematogenous   Derived from blood. Spread by the bloodstream

Hematopietic system   Precursor cells that produce blood cells

Hematoxylin-eosin stain   Commonly used histological stain. Hematoxylin stains nuclei blue. Eosin is a red counter stain

Hematuria   Blood in the urine

Hemianopsia   Loss of vision in half the visual field

Hemoglobulinemia   Free hemoglobin in the blood

Hemolysin   A substance or enzyme causing lysis of erythrocytes

Hemolysis   Liberation of hemoglobin from red cells

Hemolytic-uremic syndrome   A syndrome that includes hemolytic anemia, thrombocytopenia, and evidence of renal disease

Hemoptysis   Coughing up of blood

Hemothorax   Blood in the pleural cavity of the chest

Hepatocellular   Pertaining to liver cells (hepatocytes)

Hepatocytes   Liver cells

Hepatoma   Malignant tumor of liver cells

Heterologous   Derived from a different clone, strain, species or tissue

Heterophil antibody   Antibody reacting with an antigen other than that which elicited its production

Heteroploid   Eukaryotic cell with abnormal number of chromosomes

Heterotroph   An organism that requires organic carbon for nutrition

Heterozygous   Possessing different alleles at a particular genetic locus in a diploid cell

Hexacanth   A tapeworm embryo containing six pairs of hooklets

Hexamer   In virology, a capsomer comprising six subunits

Hilar lymph nodes   Nodes at the root of the lung

Histiocyte   Tissue macrophage

Histocompatibility   Antigens on tissue cells that are recognized by the host as self or foreign

HIV-1 or -2   Abbreviation for human immunodeficiency viruses, the cause of AIDS

Hodgkin's disease   A malignant lymphoma initially affecting groups of lymph nodes

Homeostasis   Tendency to stability of conditions within a complex biologic system

Homonymous hemianopsia   Blindness affecting the same half of the visual field in each eye

Homozygous   Possessing the same alleles at a particular genetic locus in a diploid cell

Humoral   Usually relates to antibody immunity as opposed to cellular immunity

Hyaline   Clear and transparent

Hyaluronic acid   Acid mucopolysaccharide comprising the ground substance of connective tissue. Also found in synovial fluids

Hybridization   Process in which denatured, single stranded nucleic acids from different sources are annealed. Homologous sequences form double strands that can be detected and quantified

Hybridoma   A clone derived from fused cells of different origin, e.g., from an antibody producing lymphocyte and a tumor cell

Hydrocele   Fluid accumulation within the scrotum

Hydrocephalus   Pathological accumulation of cerebrospinal fluid in the ventricles of brain

Hydronephrosis   Accumulation of urine in the renal pelvis due to obstruction of urinary flow. Associated with atrophy of the renal parenchyma

Hyperalimentation   Intravenous administration of nutrients for treatment of actual or potential malnutrition

Hyperammonemia   Excessive amounts of ammonia in the blood

Hyperbaric oxygen   Oxygen under increased pressure relative to the atmosphere

Hyperemia   Increased blood flow to a tissue

Hypernatremia   Increased serum sodium

Hyperplasia   Increase in the number of cells in a tissue

Hypersensitivity   Exaggerated and harmful immune response to a normally innocuous antigenic stimulus

Hypertension   Increased blood pressure

Hypertonic   Of higher osmotic pressure than fluid on the other side of a semi-permeable membrane (e.g., cell membrane)

Hypertrophy   Enlargement of an organ due to increase in size of its cells. Note distinction from hyperplasia.

Hypha   A fungal filament

Hypochlorhydria   Reduced hydrochloric acid in the stomach

Hypoglycemia   Blood sugar below normal levels

Hypotension   Low blood pressure

Hypothalamus   Portion of the brain that forms the floor and part of the lateral wall of the third ventricle

Hypothermia   Serious reduction in body temperature

Hypoxia   Decreased oxygen supply to the tissues

I

Prefixes

Inter-   Between

Intra-   Within

Suffix

-itis   inflammation

Icosahedron   A solid geometric shape having 12 vertices. Serves as the structural basis for many viruses

Icteric   Pertaining to jaundice

Idiopathic   Of unknown origin

Ig   Abbreviation for immunoglobulin antibodies. Classes include IgG, IgM, IgA, IgD, IgE, and sIgA

Ileitis   Inflammation of the lower ileum

Ileum   Portion of the small intestine between the jejunum and the cecum

Inclusion body   A morphologically distinct intracellular mass of viruses or virus components

Infarct   Interference with the blood supply producing local death of tissue

Intrapartum   Occurring during the process of childbirth

Isotonic   Of the same osmotic pressure as a solution on the other side of a semi-permeable membrane

In vitro   Occurring in the test tube

In vivo   Occurring in the living animal

Immunocompromise   Deficiency in some components of the body's immune mechanisms

Immunocyte   Cell of the lymphoid series that responds to an antigenic stimulus by producing antibodies or initiating cell mediated immune processes

Immunodiffusion   A procedure involving diffusion of antigen and antibody towards each other in a gel. A visible precipitate develops where optimal concentrations interact

Immunofluorescence   A serologic procedure using antibody labeled with a fluorescent dye which allows visible detection of sites of reaction with antigen

Immunogen   An antigen that induces an immune response

Immunoglobulins   Large class of glycoproteins that constitute the antibodies produced in response to antigenic stimuli.

Impetigo   Superficial purulent skin infection; pyoderma

Isoantigen   Normal substance present in one individual that may elicit an antibody response in another

Interferon   Class of cytokine proteins. When produced by virally infected cells they inhibit viral replication in these and adjacent cells

Interstitial   Spaces between the cells of a tissue

Intertriginous   Pertaining to area between folds of the skin

Intima   Inner lining of a blood vessel

Intrathecal   Within the membranes of the spinal cord

Introitus   An opening

Interleukin   Class of cytokine produced by macrophages or T cells that mediate immune responses

Integument   Skin

J

Janeway's lesions   Painless macular lesions of palms and soles seen in acute bacterial endocarditis

Jejunum   Portion of small intestine between duodenum and ileum

K

Kaposi's sarcoma   Multiple malignant vascular tumors. Occur most commonly as a complication of AIDS

Karyosome   Area of chromatin concentration in a cell nucleus

Karotype   Size, structure, and organization of chromosomes within a cell

Keratin   Major protein of the skin, hair, and nails

Keratitis   Inflammation of the cornea of the eye

Kilobase   Unit to describe the lengths of a nucleotide sequence. One kilobase = 1000 nucleotides

Kinetoplast   Structure at the base of a protozoal flagellum

Kupffer cells   Fixed phagocytic cells of the liver sinusoids. Part of the reticulo-endothelial system

Kwashiorkor   Condition caused by severe protein malnutrition in children

Prefixes

Lympho-   Pertaining to the lymphatic system

Leuco-   White; relating to a leukocyte

Lipo-   Relating to fats or lipids

Suffix

-lytic   Pertaining to lysis

Labia   Structures of the external female genitalia

Lactoferrin   Iron-binding protein present in milk, other secretions, and granules of neutrophil leukocytes

Lamina propria   Connective tissue supporting the epithelial cells of a mucous membrane

Latex beads   Used to adsorb soluble antigens. The treated beads agglutinate with specific antibody

Leukocyte   White blood cells including granulocytes, lymphocytes, and monocytes

Leukemia   Malignant tumor of white blood cells

Leukocytosis   Increased blood leukocyte count

Leukopenia   Abnormally low leukocyte count

Leukotrienes   Products of arachidonic acid that mediate inflammatory and allergic reactions

Ligand   One component of a complex involving the binding of molecules or structures

Lobar   Related to a lobe of the lung

Lophotrichous   Describing several flagella at one or both ends of a bacillus

Lumen   Cavity within a tubular organ

Lupus erythematosus (systemic)   Autoimmune inflammatory disease of skin, joints, and other tissues

Lymph   Tissue fluid derived from the blood stream and passing to the lymphatics

Lymphangitis   Inflammation of lymphatic vessels

Lymphadenitis   Enlarged, inflamed lymph nodes

Lymphocytosis   Increased blood lymphocyte count

Lymphokine   Cytokine produced by lymphocytes

Lymphoma   Tumor of lymphatic tissues

Lymphoreticular   Relating to the reticulo-endothelial system

Lysis   Dissolution of cells

Lysozyme   Enzyme that breaks down peptidoglycan

Lysosome   Granules of cells that contain hydrolytic digestive enzymes

M

Prefixes

Macro-   Large

Mega-   Large

Micro-   Small

Myo-   Pertaining to muscle

Suffixes

-metry   measure

-megaly   Enlargement. Usually of an organ

Macrocytic anemia   Anemia characterized by large erythrocytes

Macrophage   Tissue phagocyte derived from blood mononuclear cells

Macule   A flat lesion of skin rash

Masseter   Major muscle controlling movement of the lower jaw

Mast cell   Connective tissue cell analogous to the blood basophil. Granules contain heparin, histamine, and other vasoactive mediators

Mastitis   Inflammation of the breast

Mastoid   Process of temporal bone behind the ear that contains air cells

Matrix   Extracellular substance of tissues

Meatus   Orifice

Meckel's diverticulum   Congenital diverticulum of the lower part of the ileum

Mediastinum   Mid-portion of the chest including heart, bronchial bifurcation, and esophagus

Medulla   The inner portion of an organ within the cortex

Medulla oblongata   Portion of central nervous system between the brain and spinal cord

Megacolon   Dilatation of the colon

Meiosis   Cellular divsison process yielding haploid gametes

Meninges   The membranes covering the brain and the spinal cord

Meningomyelocele   Malformation of vertebral column with protrusion of meninges

Mentation   Mental activity; thinking

Merozoite   A stage in the life cycle of a sporozoan parasite resulting from asexual division; a daughter cell

Mesenchymal   Derived from the embryonic mesoderm layer

Mesentery   Fold of peritoneum surrounding the intestinal tract and attaching it to the posterior abdominal wall

Mesophile   A microbe that grows best at temperatures of approximately those of the body

Mesosome   A complex invagination of the bacterial cell membrane

Metastases   Satellite tumors or infections spread through lymphatics or the blood stream from a primary site

Microaerophilic   Can grow only in less than the atmospheric concentration of oxygen, or anaerobically.

Microcephaly   Small head with failure of development of the brain

Microphthalmia   Failure to develop normal sized eyes

Mitochondria   Complex cytoplasmic organelles of eukaryotic cells involved in oxidative phosphorylation

Mitogen   Substance that increases the normal frequency of mutations

Mitral valve   Valve between the left atrium and ventricle of the heart

Monoclonal   Derived from a single cell

Monocyte   Large mononuclear phagocyte of the blood. Precursor of the macrophage

Monolayer   A single layer of cultured eukaryotic cells on a glass or plastic surface

Monotrichous   Possessing a single flagellum

Morphology   The shape, size, and form of an organism or cell

Mordant   Substance that enhances the effect of a stain

Mutagen Substance that increases the mutation rate of cells or organisms

Mucolytic Substance that dissolves mucus

Multiple sclerosis Chronic disorder involving disseminated focal damage to nerve cells

Myalgia Pain in the muscles

Mycelium A mass of fungal hyphae

Mycetoma A localized granuloma or lesion caused by a fungus

Mycosis A fungal infection

Myelin Component of the myelin sheath around the axon of a neuron which increases the conduction velocity of the nerve impulse

Myelitis Inflammation of the spinal cord

Myeloma Malignant tumor derived from bone marrow cells

Myocardium Heart muscle

Myringitis Inflammation of the tympanic membrane of the ear

N

Prefixes

Neo- New

Nephrito- Pertaining to the kidney

Neuro- Pertaining to the central nervous system or nerves

Nares Interior of the nostrils

Nasal turbinates Three scroll-like bony projections from the lateral wall of the nasal cavity (nasal conchae)

Nasolacrimal duct Duct draining the conjunctiva into the nasal cavity

Necrosis Death of tissue

Neoplasm Tumor

Nephritogenic Producing inflammation of the kidneys

Neurone Nerve and its nerve cell

Neuromotor synapses Connections between nerve endings and muscle

Neutrophils Major class of polymorphonuclear phagocytic leukocytes

Neutropenia Reduced number of circulating neutrophil leukocytes

NGU Abbreviation for "nongonococcal urethritis"

Nidus Focus of infection, a cluster

Noma A gangrenous condition spreading from the oral cavity to the skin; seen in undernourished children

Nosocomial Acquired within a hospital

Nucleocapsid The nucleic acid-protein complex found inside an enveloped virus

Nucleoid The double stranded circular DNA genome of a bacterium

Nucleolus Round body within a eukaryotic nucleus that is the site of synthesis of ribosomal RNA

O

Prefixes

Oligo- Small, few

Onco- Pertaining to tumors

Osteo- Pertaining to bone

Oro- Pertaining to the mouth

Oto- Pertaining to the ear

Suffix

-oscópy Use of an instrument to see within a viscus or vessel

Occult Hidden, inapparent

Olfactory Pertaining to the sense of smell

Olfactory bulb Terminal enlarged portion of the olfactory tract from which the olfactory nerves emerge

Oligodendroglia Specialized connective tissue of the central nervous system

Oncogene Gene whose activation is associated with malignant change and progression

Ontogeny Origin and course of development of an individual organism

Operculum A lid or cover

Operon Operator gene and the adjacent structural gene(s) that it controls

Ophthalmia Severe inflammation of the eye

Opisthotonos Severe spasm of back muscles leading to hyperextension of the spine

Opportunist A microorganism that only causes disease when the body's defenses are compromised or bypassed

Opsonin Antibody or complement component that facilitates phagocytosis when bound to a microorganism

Orbit Skull cavity that contains the eyeball

Orchitis Inflammation of a testis

Organelles Membrane-bound cytoplasmic structures of eukaryotic cells, e.g., mitochondria

Organogenesis Formation of the organs of the body

Osler's nodes Skin papules, usually of hands and feet, seen in bacterial endocarditis

Ossicles Small bones (e.g., of hearing)

Osteomyelitis Inflammation of bone marrow and adjacent bone

Oviparous Producing eggs from which the embryo is released outside the body

Oxidase Oxidation-reduction enzyme that catalyses transfer of electrons to molecular oxygen with formation of water

P

Prefixes

Pan- All, throughout
Para- Beside, abnormal
Peri- Around, covering
Pleo- More
Pleuro- Relating to the pleura
Poly- Many, repeated
Pro- Before, a precursor
Pseudo- False
Pyo- Producing pus

Suffixes

-pathy denoting disease
-penia decreased numbers
-phobia fear of, repulsion
-phylia affection for

Pandemic Worldwide severe epidemic
Panencephalitis Inflammation of all tissues of the brain
Papilla Small nipple-like swelling
Papilledema Edema of the optic nerve and adjacent retina
Papilloma Warty tumor of the epithelium
Papule Small, firm elevated nodule on the skin
Parasite An organism that lives on and at the expense of another organism
Parasitism Describes the relationship between parasite and host
Parenchymal Substance of body organs in contrast to their covering
Parenteral Administration by injection rather than by mouth
Paresis Paralysis
Paresthesias Disorders of sensation; tingling
Paronychia Infection of nail fold
Parotid glands Salivary glands beneath the cheek
Parturition The process of giving birth
Pathogenic Cause of disease
Pathognomonic Diagnostic, distinctive
Pentamer A polymer of viral capsid having five structural units
Peptidoglycan High molecular weight cross-linked polymer forming the rigid structure of the bacterial cell wall
Peptone Protein hydrolysed product used as a source of aminoacids in bacterial culture media
Periapical Beside the root of a tooth
Pericardium Membranous lining around the heart
Perineum Area between vulva or scrotum and the anus
Periodontal Area around the tooth including supporting tissues

Periosteum Membrane around the bone
Perioplasm Area between the outer and cell membranes of a Gram-negative bacterium. Contains the peptidoglycan layer
Peristalsis Normal contractile waves of a hollow organ
Peristome The mouth and surrounding areas of certain ciliated protozoa
Peritrichous Presence of multiple flagella around a bacterial cell
Permease A protein of the bacterial cell membrane transport system
Petechiae Small hemorrhages in the skin
Peyer's patches Lymphoid follicles in the ileum
Phage Common abbreviation for bacteriophage
Phagocyte A cell that ingests foreign material
Phagolysosome The digestive vacuole formed by fusion of the cell lysosomes with the phagocytic vacuole
Phenotype The properties expressed by the complete genome under particular conditions
Pheromone Hormone-like substance that elicits a favorable or attraction response in an individual of the same species
Phonation Speech
Photophobia Intolerance of light
Phylogeny Pertaining to the evolution of a species
PID Abbreviation for pelvic inflammatory disease
Pilo-sebaceous Unit of hair follicle and sebaceous gland
Pilus Fibrillar structure on the surface of a bacterial cell
Pinocytosis Uptake of fluids into a cell by a mechanism analogous to phagocytosis
Plaque A patch or flat area. An area of lysis in fixed host cells by an infecting virus
Plasma Non-cellular component of whole blood
Plasmid Extrachromosomal circular double stranded DNA molecule
Plasmin Derived from plasminogen—dissolves fibrin
Platelet Small anucleate cell involved in filling small holes in blood vessels and in clotting mechanisms
Pleocytosis Increased number of cells in a particular area
Pleomorphism Variation in shape and size
Pleura Membrane covering the lungs and thoracic cavity enclosing the pleural space
Pleurisy Inflammation of the pleura
Pleurodynia Pain caused by inflammation or irritation of the pleura
Pneumonitis Inflammation of the lung
Pneumothorax Air in the pleural cavity

Polyarthralgia Pain in several joints

Polycistronic Encoding two or more proteins, e.g., polycistronic mRNA

Polyclonal activation Simultaneous activation of different antibody producing clones of lymphocytes

Polymerase chain reaction Continuous enzyme-mediated amplification of a nucleotide sequence that allows its detection and analysis

Polymorphonuclear Two or more lobes to the nucleus

Polymyositis Inflammation of many muscles

Polyneuritis Inflammation of many nerves

Polyp A sessile benign or malignant tumor of a mucous membrane (usually of colon)

Polyposis Presence of many polyps

Porin Protein of outer membrane pores of Gram-negative bacteria

Portal venous system Veins carrying blood from the intestinal tract to the liver

Premenarchal Prepubertal years in the female (before onset of menses)

Prepuce Foreskin

Proctoscopy Use of an instrument to examine interior of rectum

Prodromal Initial symptoms before the characteristic manifestations of disease develop

Proglottid One of the segments of the body of a tapeworm

Prokaryote Organism lacking a true nucleus. Possesses a single chromosome

Prophage Complete bacterial virus genome integrated in the chromosome

Prophylaxis Measures or treatments designed to prevent disease

Prostaglandins Derivatives of arachidonic acid that mediate a variety of biologic reactions including inflammation

Prostate gland Gland surrounding the male urethra which produces part of the seminal fluid

Prosthesis Artificial replacement of a missing part of the body

Proteinuria Protein in the urine indicating a renal abnormality

Prothrombin Precursor of thrombin; thrombin activates the terminal blood clotting mechanism

Protomer Protein subunit of a viral capsomere

Protoplasm The viscid colloidal solution that makes up living matter

Protoplast A Gram-positive bacterium that has lost its cell wall

Prototroph Bacterial strains with complete synthetic pathways from which auxotrophs may be derived

Protozoan A unicellular member of the animal kingdom

Proventriculus An enlargement of the alimentary tract of an invertebrate that precedes the stomach

Provirus Complete viral genome integrated into a eukaryotic genome

Pruritis Itching

Pseudopod A pseudopodium. Moving extrusion of the cytoplasm of an amoeboid cell that brings about movement or ingestion of food particles

Psychophile A microorganism that grows best or exclusively at low temperatures

Puerperal Following childbirth

Purpura Multiple hemorrhages in the skin, mucous membrane, or other organs

Pustule Pus in an infected hair follicle or sweat gland producing a visible inflammatory swelling

Pyelonephritis Infection of the pelvis and tissues of the kidney

Pylephlebitis Inflammation in the portal venous system

Pyogenic Producing pus and pustular lesions

Pyuria Pus in the urine

R

Prefix

Rhino- Pertaining to the nose

Radioimmunoassay A method for detecting antigen-antibody reactions that utilizes a radioisotope as a readily detectable label

Rales Crackling respiratory sounds heard with the stethoscope

Receptor Component of the cell surface to which another substance or organism attaches specifically

Redox potential Oxidation-reduction potential

Reduviid A large winged "cone-nosed" insect

Renal Pertaining to the kidney

Repressor A regulatory protein that binds to an operator sequence and inhibits expression of the adjacent gene

Reservoir of infection Natural habitat or source of an infecting organism

Reticuloendothelial system System of phagocytic monocytes, particularly those in the spleen, bone marrow, and lymph nodes

Retinoblastoma Malignant tumor of the retina

Retrovirus RNA virus, the genome of which is transcribed into DNA by its reverse transcriptase

Reverse transcriptase RNA-directed DNA polymerase

Rhinorrhea Continuous discharge of watery mucus from the nose

RIA *See* Radioimmunoassay

Rhonchi Coarse snoring or rattling respiratory sounds heard with a stethoscope

Romana's sign Unilateral opthalmia, edema of the eyelids, and enlarged draining lymph nodes

Rostellum Portion of tapeworm head that contains hooklets or other attachment organs

S

Prefixes

Sub- Below

Supra- Above

Spleno- Relating to the spleen

Suffix

-scopy Denotes use of an instrument for visual examination of a hollow viscus, e.g., bronchoscopy

Salpingitis Inflammation of the fallopian tubes

Saprophyte Organism living on dead organic material in the environment

Sarcoidosis Disease of unknown etiology characterized by granulomatous lesions of many tissues and organs

Sarcolemma Membrane surrounding muscle fibers

Schizogany Asexual reproduction in sporozoa producing merozoites by multiple nuclear fusion followed by cytoplasmic segregation

Schizont The multinucleated stage of a sporozoan undergoing schizogany

Sclera White part of the eyeball

Scolex The attachment organ or head of a tapeworm

Scotoma A blind spot in the visual field

Sebaceous Relating to sebum and sebum production

Sebum Waxy secretion of sebaceous glands

Seminal vesicles Sacs in which semen is stored prior to ejaculation

Septicemia Evidence of systemic disease associated with presence of organisms in the blood (see bacteremia)

Sepsis A term often used synonymously with septicemia, but applied particularly to infants and children with severe life-threatening infections

Sequelae Results occurring subsequent to an infection or other disease

Sequestrum Necrotic bony fragment

Seroconversion Development of antibodies in response to an infection

Serodiagnosis Diagnosis of an infection by serologic procedures

Serotype Subtype of species detectable with specific antisera

Serpiginous Moving irregularly from one place to another, snake-like

Serum Liquid part of blood separable after clotting

Shunt Deviation of blood or other body fluids, e.g., from artery to vein

Sickle cell anemia Hereditary anemia associated with crescent-shaped erythrocytes resulting from an abnormal hemoglobin

Siderophore Compound that binds iron

Sigmoid colon Lower portion of the colon between descending colon and rectum

Sinus 1. A tract leading from an infected area or hollow viscus to the surface
2. A wide venous blood channel
3. Accessory nasal sinuses which are blind sacs draining to the nasopharynx

Sinusoid A wide thin-walled venous passage. Smaller than a sinus

Slime layer Term sometimes used for polysaccharide surface components of bacteria that do not constitute a morphologic capsule

Spasticity Excessive tone of muscles leading to awkward movement

Spheroplast A circular, osmotically unstable, Gram-negative rod that has lost its peptidoglycan layer

Sphincter Circular muscle controlling a natural orifice

Splanchnic Pertaining to the viscera

Sporogony Sexual reproduction process in sporozoan parasites leading to formation of oocysts and sporozoites

Sporozoite Motile, elongated, infective stage of sporogony

Sprue A chronic form of intestinal malabsorption

Squamous epithelium Composed of layers of flattened cells

Stasis Stagnation or cessation of flow of body fluids

Stenosis Reduction in diameter of a blood vessel or tubular organ

Steroids Derivatives of cholestrol including hormones, some of which have anti-inflammatory effects

Sterol Lipid-soluble steroid with long aliphatic side chains. Present in eukaryotic cell membranes as cholesterol or ergosterol

Stevens Johnson syndrome A serious allergic reaction, characterized by multiple blister-like lesions of skin and mucous membrane

Stomatitis Inflammation of the mouth

Strabismus Squint

Stratum corneum Outer keratinized part of the skin

Stridor Harsh respiratory sound due to partial respiratory obstruction

Strobila Chain of segments making up the body of a tapeworm

Subarachnoid Cerebro-spinal fluid containing area between the middle (arachnoid) and inner (pia mater) layers of the meninges

Subdural Between the outer (dura mater) and middle (arachnoid) layers of the meninges

Submandibular Below the jaw

Subphrenic Below the diaphragm

Sulcus Groove

Suppurative Producing pus

Surfactant A substance that acts on a surface to reduce surface tension, e.g., a detergent

Sylvatic Pertaining to the woods. Commonly applied to nonurban plague whether occurring in wooded or prairie land

Symbiont An organism living on or in close association with another

Synapse A connection between neurons for nerve impulse transmission

Syncytium A multinucleate mass of fused cells

Syndrome Group of clinical manifestations characterizing a particular disease or condition

Synergistic Enhanced rather than additive effect of two agents or processes acting together

Synovium Lining membrane of a joint, tendon, or bursa

T

Prefixes

Tachy- Increased rate, swift

Thermo- Pertaining to heat

Thrombo- Pertaining to thrombosis

Tracheo- Pertaining to the trachea

Trans- Across

Tachypnea Abnormally rapid rate of breathing

Tamponade (cardiac) Increased fluid or constriction around the heart leading to interference in cardiac function

T cells Thymus derived immunocytes: helper, suppressor, and cytotoxic T cells

Tenesmus Ineffective and painful straining at stool or urination

Tenosynovitis Inflammation of a tendon sheath

Teratogenic Causing abnormalities of fetal development

Thalassemia Hereditary hemolytic anemia resulting from abnormal hemoglobin synthesis

Thermophile Bacteria with an optimal growth temperature of over 50°C

Thrombocyte See platelet

Thrombophlebitis Inflammation of a vein with thrombosis; may release infected emboli

Thrombus A blood clot developing in vivo

Thymus A lymphoid organ located in the anterior upper portion of the mediastinum. The site of maturation of T cells

Titer Highest dilution of an active substance (e.g., antibody in serum) that still causes a discernable reaction (e.g., an agglutination reaction)

Tracheostomy Surgically produced artificial air passage to the trachea

Transcriptase DNA-directed RNA polymerase

Transferrin Serum protein that binds and transports iron

Transovarial Passage of infectious agents to progeny by way of the egg. Usually occurs in ticks and mites

Transposon A DNA segment carrying one of more recognizable genes that can move between plasmid and between plasmid and chromosome in both directions

Trimester Usually means a three-month period of pregnancy

Trismus Spasm of the masseter muscle; lockjaw

Trophozoite The motile feeding stage of a protozoan parasite

Tropism Having an affinity for a particular organ, or moving towards or away from a particular stimulus

Tumorigenesis The property of causing tumors

Turgor pressure Osmotic pressure of the cellular contents

Tympanic membrane Eardrum

U

Suffix

-uria Pertaining to urine

Ureter Tube carrying urine from the kidney to bladder

Urethra Tube carrying urine from the bladder to the exterior

Uremia Toxic accumulation of nitrogenous metabolites due to renal insufficiency

Urticaria Local edema and itching of the skin

Ultrasonograph Picture of deep organs of the body derived from reflection of ultrasonic waves

Uropathic Causing disease of the urinary tract

Uvea Inner vascular coat of the eyeball, including the iris

Uvula Small extension hanging from the back of the soft palate

V

Prefix

Vaso- pertaining to blood vessels

Vacuolate Forming small holes of vacules

Vacuole Microscopic hole or cavity

Vagotomy Surgical cutting of the vagus nerve

Vasa vasorum Small blood vessels in walls of veins and arteries

Vasculitis Inflammation of blood vessels

Vector An aminate transmitter of disease, e.g., an insect

Venipuncture Insertion of a hypodermic needle into a vein—usually to draw blood

Ventricle Fluid cavity, e.g, chamber of the heart

Vesicle Small fluid filled cavity, e.g, a blister-like lesion of the skin

Viscera Interior organs of the body, e.g., the intestinal tract

Vesicoureteral junction Junction of ureter with the urinary bladder

Vestibular function Function of the vestibular branch of the eighth cranial nerve concerned with the body's equilibrium

Viremia Presence of a virus in the blood stream

Virion A complete virus particle

Viropexis Viral entry into the cell by phagocytosis

Viruria Viruses in the urine

Vitreous humor The clear viscous fluid in the posterior chamber of the eye

Viviparous Developing young within the body as opposed to oviparous

W

Weil-Felix test Test for agglutinating antibodies to certain strains of *Proteus* that develop in the course of some rickettsial infections

Western blot Test for antibodies to specific proteins separated by gel electrophoresis

Whitlow Abscess of the terminal pulp of the finger. Also paronychia

Wright's stain Stain for blood cells that has similar properties to Giemsa stain

X

Xenodiagnosis Recovery of a parasite by allowing an arthropod to feed on the patient and seeking the parasite in the arthropod

Xerostomia Dry mouth from dysfunction of the salivary glands

Z

Zoonosis A disease transmissable to humans from an animal host or reservoir

Zygote The cell that results from fusion of male and female gametes

Index

The page ranges given for citations of organisms, which are covered in detail, include considerations of habitat, morphology, antigenic structure, cultural characteristics, virulence determinants, pathogenesis of disease, antimicrobic susceptibility, and life cycles when appropriate. Only unusual properties, those of special interest, or those discussed elsewhere in the text, are included as subcitations.

A similar approach has been adopted for specific diseases, in which the major citation includes clinical manifestations, immunology, epidemiology, laboratory diagnosis, prevention, and treatment, when these are covered in the text. Pages cited for individual antimicrobics include consideration of structure, mode of action, spectrum, and resistance mechanisms when appropriate. As with the citations for organisms, subcitations for diseases and antimicrobics relate to unusual characteristics or those considered elsewhere in the text.

The marginal headings in the cited pages should be used to find the specific information needed.